GLOBAL SURGERY AND ANESTHESIA MANUAL

Providing Care in Resource-Limited Settings

GLOBAL SURGERY AND ANESTHESIA MANUAL

Providing Care in Resource-Limited Settings

Edited by

John G. Meara

Craig D. McClain, David P. Mooney, Selwyn O. Rogers, Jr

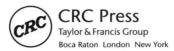

CRC Press
Taylor & Francis Group
Boca Raton London New York

CRC Press is an imprint of the
Taylor & Francis Group, an **informa** business

CRC Press
Taylor & Francis Group
6000 Broken Sound Parkway NW, Suite 300
Boca Raton, FL 33487-2742

Printed on acid-free paper
Version Date: 20140818

International Standard Book Number-13: 978-1-4822-4730-5 (Paperback)

Library of Congress Cataloging-in-Publication Data

Global surgery and anesthesia manual : providing care in resource-limited settings / editor, John G. Meara.
   p. ; cm.
   Includes bibliographical references and index.
   ISBN 978-1-4822-4730-5 (paperback : alk. paper)
   I. Meara, John G., editor.
   [DNLM: 1. General Surgery. 2. Postoperative Complications--prevention & control. 3. Anesthesia. 4. International Cooperation. 5. Poverty Areas. 6. World Health. WO 140]

RD81
617.9'6--dc23
        2014028483

**Visit the Taylor & Francis Web site at
http://www.taylorandfrancis.com**

**and the CRC Press Web site at
http://www.crcpress.com**

Contents

Section I   Introduction

Section II   Anesthesia

Section III   Non-Trauma

Section IV   Trauma

Foreword

Paul E. Farmer

In the spring of 2008, writing in *World Journal of Surgery*, Jim Yong Kim and I—both internists with long experience in the delivery of health care in settings of poverty—referred to surgery as "the neglected stepchild of global health."[1] We argued that this was the case because the dominant means of financing surgical care excluded those in greatest need of such services. If anything, the term "neglected" was a euphemism, because all pathologies afflicting the world's poorest were, by definition, neglected:

> The truth is even more unpleasant: within poor countries, surgical services are concentrated almost wholly in cities and reserved largely for those who can pay for them. In Haiti, for example, a community-based survey conducted in the 1980s suggested that rates of caesarean delivery in a large area of southern Haiti were close to zero; maternal mortality was pegged at 1,400 per 100,000 live births. Yet among the affluent of that same country, rates of caesarean delivery do not vary much from those registered in the United States. Careful scrutiny of local inequalities of risk and access to care reveals that in poor countries, even minor surgical pathologies are often transformed through time and inattention into lethal conditions. Congenital abnormalities such as cleft palate remain life-long afflictions rather than pediatric surgical disease. In addition to surgical abdomens, severe trauma (from road accidents more often than from intentional violence) and other potentially fatal pathologies remain a massive burden of untreated disease that weighs on the lives, and productivity, of the world's bottom billion.[1]

The assessment seemed to have struck a chord among our surgical colleagues, in part because there had been, even by 2008, significant advances in non-surgical care for people living both with serious illness *and* in extreme poverty. But these advances were very recent ones, as we knew from our work with Partners In Health, an organization we co-founded in the late 1980s, and as academic physicians working and teaching in places like Haiti, Peru, Rwanda, and Lesotho.

What a difference a decade makes. Just look at the past one: by the year 2003, the world's leading infectious killer of young adults was acquired immunodeficiency syndrome (AIDS), which along with an airborne illness fanned by epidemic human immunodeficiency virus (HIV), had led (along with several other pathogens and pathogenic forces, including divestment from public health systems) to a massive reversal of public-health gains in many of the world's poorest countries, especially in Africa. A mere decade ago, it's easy to imagine that predictions of imminent improvement might have been greeted with weary skepticism by those living with (and dying from) AIDS and in dire poverty. But by the year 2008, when Kim and I wrote, significant investments in *health care delivery* were beginning to drop mortality due to AIDS in many of these same settings, including the rural areas in which most Africans lived. By the time this important and long-overdue volume, *Global Surgery and Anesthesia Manual*, goes to press, the return on investments such as those made possible by new programs (the two largest being the U.S. President's Emergency Plan for AIDS Relief and the Global Fund to Fight AIDS, Tuberculosis, and Malaria, but these often spurred, in turn, increased national resources for programs to prevent and treat these pathogens) is even more evident. Case-fatality rates attributable to these three pathogens have plummeted and epidemics have shrunk, as would be expected when both prevention and care are increased. In one striking example, we recently reported that over the past decade Rwanda has witnessed the sharpest decrease in mortality ever recorded in human history.[2] By 2013, only 10 years into "the delivery decade," both prevention and care have been strengthened; life expectancy has resumed its upward trend in many of the most affected regions; and new HIV infections have at last started to decline.[3] With regards to AIDS, the prevention-versus-care debate has at last been improved to one about how best to integrate prevention and care. This improvement in the terms of debate may be one of the chief returns on the investments of the past decade.

If we are at the end of the delivery decade, was our 2008 diagnosis about surgery overly pessimistic? Alas, no. The term "neglected stepchild" was, if anything, euphemistic. While long-standing inattention to deaths due to epidemic disease has diminished somewhat, the same successes cannot yet be heralded for global surgical disease. To mix metaphors a bit, it was hard to call for a renaissance, because prior efforts to make access to safe surgical care a priority for the poor were, beyond a few short-term exceptions, too often linked to war or to natural disasters, mostly still-born.

But there is hope on the horizon. In the past several years, interest in "global surgery" has experienced something of a growth spurt, which has also led to a greater, if imperfect, understanding of the burden of surgical disease as well as increasing knowledge of who has access to surgical care that is both safe and indicated. Much of that knowledge is summarized in *Global Surgery and Anesthesia Manual*, which allows me to repeat, with some chagrin, that surgery (along with effective therapy for malignancies, which often includes surgical care and effective anesthesia, and with major mental illness) remains a neglected stepchild even if things have started to look up. New information about the know-do gap reminds us our previous assessment was euphemistic in part because it is not only the bottom billion or so who miss out.

One assessment cited here suggests that two billion people do not have access to safe surgical care, but this figure counts those with access to an operating theater with a functional pulse oximeter—surely a paltry measure of access to safe surgical care. Those lucky enough to live out long and fruitful lives and never need such services are just that—fortunate. But because the majority of the world's families will not know such good fortune—to never need any sort of surgical care—we are a long way from any safety net that covers even two billion souls. And adding proper pain control to the list of requisite items shrinks that number, that fortunate few, still more.

The *Global Surgery and Anesthesia Manual* describes scores of procedures required to avert suffering, debility, or premature death, and many of them require much more than trained surgical personnel and rudimentary monitoring capacity. Some require only short-term anesthesia, but not all are pain-free after even the most expert surgical care, as defined in this important manual. Work in a hospital with even modest patient flow—for example, 25,000 ambulatory visits per year—reveals the *routine* need for procedures ranging from laparotomy for small-bowel obstruction to open-fracture repair; biliary, urologic, and oncologic breast procedures; and a great deal of burn debridement and plastic reconstruction. This volume also reminds us that patients in low- and middle-income countries (LMICs) will require complex hepatobiliary, thoracic, and neurosurgical procedures. Furthermore, in settings in which gastroenterologists are few and far between, it is the surgical services that perform endoscopy. In other words, global surgery cannot be only about caesarean delivery and the drainage of abscesses, even if these procedures are necessary parts of even the most modest efforts to promote primary care, especially in rural areas or wherever referrals are difficult. Nor can global surgery flourish as an academic field as long as its primary activities are restricted by its practitioners' narrow enthusiasms or training rather than the burden of surgical disease in populations thus far shut out of modern medical care. Global surgery, long restricted to short-term visiting surgical efforts and largely funded independently, must become a legitimate, and legitimated, academic endeavor.

Perhaps the biggest challenge, felt by all those who work in settings of privation, is traumatic injury, a leading cause of death among young adults in much of the world. Often, this is not a question of geography so much as one of socioeconomic status: In many of the world's cities, poverty still traps many in need of surgical services. They're effectively marooned on an island or in a desert. This is why one of the headings of the first chapter in an early and important textbook of what today would be called global surgery, first published in 1987, is titled "Referral is mostly a myth."[4] It is also the reason that the south side of Chicago, the third-largest city in the United States, can be termed a "trauma desert" in which the absence of any Level II Trauma Center means longer transport times, and higher mortality, for injured patients, many of them from gun-shot wounds.[5]

If "trauma deserts" can exist in some of the poorer corners of the largest cities in high-income countries (HICs), it's easy to imagine them as a vast Sahara, stretching, oasis-free, across the poorest reaches of the world. In launching the first academic medical center outside of Haiti's capital city, which in 2010 was close to the epicenter of an earthquake that revealed that entire nation to be a trauma desert, it quickly became clear that elective procedures would command little attention from an overworked surgical staff.

So why is there no, say, "Global Fund for Surgery"? Why isn't surgical care better addressed in national health plans? Let me raise and dismiss a couple of commonly cited reasons, and explore a couple more.

One pernicious explanation given in explaining surgery's status as a neglected stepchild is that surgical care is not a ranking priority in settings of poverty. Reasons for surgery's neglect in the new arena of global health are many, but lack of global burden of surgical disease has never been among them. Initial analysis suggested the global burden of diseases requiring surgical intervention comprised over 11% of the overall global disease burden[6]; updates show that 11.2% of the world's disability-adjusted life years (DALYs) are due to injuries alone.[7] These numbers will continue to rise as premature deaths from vaccine-preventable illness and epidemic disease drop. As noted, injuries are the leading cause of deaths among children and young adults in much of the developing world; and maternal mortality will remain high in settings in which surgical delivery and modern contraceptive methods are not readily available to women living in poverty.

Others claim that too much attention is paid to infectious diseases. This is absurd: As any historian of surgical care would note, it was antisepsis and antibiotics that helped make possible the revolution in surgical care. These components of adequate medical care are not, and were never, in competition with each other; in most HICs, the majority of nosocomial infections occur in surgical patients.[8] The same holds true for modern oncology. It is true, however, that since the earliest days of modern public health, attention—and therefore resources, always scant—focused primarily on "communicable" disease. This attention was undoubtedly justifiable and has led, over the past half-century, to positive results: the eradication of smallpox, the near eradication of polio, and a drop in deaths due to vaccine-preventable illnesses. But such efforts were narrowly defined (or "vertical"), long-overdue, and grossly underfunded. There is little evidence that such efforts crowded out attention to surgical care; there was no "lion's share" for any of the diseases of poverty, regardless of etiology. For years, as noted, many in public health argued that AIDS *treatment* was unlikely to prove feasible or cost-effective. This was true for all of the chronic infectious diseases of poverty—a long list (some of it leading to surgical disease, also neglected). The delivery decade began only recently and when novel funding streams from organizations (such as the Global Fund) and programs (such as PEPFAR) freed providers serving the destitute sick from the pernicious prevention-rather-than-care logic of international health at the close of the twentieth century. As understanding of pathogenesis and burden of disease evolves, the lines between "communicable" and "non-communicable" continue to blur. But all diseases of poverty remain, at this writing, neglected. Fighting our own socialization for scarcity remains a ranking challenge within global health.

A more credible explanation for inattention to surgical disease among the poor is that it requires substantial investment in infrastructure. The provision of high-quality surgical care requires not only surgeons, anesthesiologists, nurses, operating rooms, and assured supply chains, but also adequate lighting, clean water, increased nursing staff and appropriate postoperative follow-up. Emergency medical services and referral need to be more than a myth. This high "activation energy" requirement has long served as a deterrent; many have claimed that such care is simply not possible in settings of poverty and privation, places where electricity and a safe water supply are as rare as pulse oximeters. Our own experience in Haiti interrogates that claim. It is true that significant investment in systems able to provide complex surgical care in the places in which we work is still vanishingly rare. But in the spring of 2013, the University Hospital of Mirebalais opened its doors to patients—including patients in need of surgery—in the country's rural Central Plateau. This public-sector facility, built by Partners In Health, has opened close to 300 beds, six state-of-the-art operating theaters, and an emergency department. As required for teaching hospitals (and, as an aspirational aside, Level I trauma centers), it also has a surgical residency program, the first established outside of the capital city. The facility will soon open an intensive care unit, and thus be capable of serving as a tertiary referral center for the most complex cases. It is powered largely by solar energy and treats its own wastewater on site. The vast majority of employees are Haitian; the hospital is the largest employer in the region and one study has concluded that each dollar invested in its construction has returned almost two to the local economy.[9] It has also helped to reverse the brain drain: The chief of surgery is a senior Haitian surgeon who for decades worked in the United States because such facilities were not available in his home country. A similar story describes both the Chief of Medicine and the Chief of Nursing.

Another credible contributor to the relative neglect is confusion about such claims—from those about burden of disease to those about extravagant attention to infectious diseases and the general unfeasibility of surgical care in such settings—among the academic leaders of surgery and anesthesia. Such confusion arises in part because such infrastructure is absent in settings of poverty and thus so are the leaders. In our 2008 commentary, Jim Yong Kim and I—despite our rather grim assessment—also offered a prescription: "We need our surgical colleagues to speak fluently about rebuilding infrastructure, training personnel, and delivering high-quality care to the very poorest ... To bring a greater number of surgeons into the campaign for public health unrestricted by ability to pay will involve enlarging the horizons of both the surgical and public health professions."

In the intervening 6 years, those horizons have expanded faster and more broadly than we thought possible. For example, a consortium of US academic institutions—including those represented by many of those who wrote and edited this volume—initiated a 7-year-long effort to address Rwanda's dearth of surgical professionals.[10] This represents, surely, the largest movement of surgical faculty from regions in which they abound to one from which they have been absent. An academic field of global surgery—under the leadership of surgeons like John Meara and now with a comprehensive manual in the form of this textbook—can continue to bring us closer to the goal of global health equity. As Meara and I noted in a recent commentary, the time has come to merge the fields of academic surgery and

global health equity.[11] Meara and his colleagues have, in effect, launched a new field. The Program in Global Surgery and Social Change at Harvard Medical School, the Center for Surgery and Public Health at Brigham and Women's Hospital, and the Fellowship in Global Surgery at Boston Children's Hospital are examples of innovative models that seek to train a new generation of surgeons skilled not only with management of surgical disease but also with management of resources. This textbook offers another groundbreaking step forward in making that vision a reality. It is, as far as I know, the first of its kind: a thorough, expert compilation of best practices across the spectrum of global surgical services (including anesthesia). I recommend this timely volume to all those who are interested in delivering high-quality surgical care to communities across the globe. A hospital like the University Hospital of Mirebalais should not be a novelty in a world full of trauma deserts. Clean facilities with appropriate equipment and staff capable of providing high-quality medical and surgical services should be available to all, regardless of ability to pay. That is the goal of global health equity.

REFERENCES

1. Farmer PE, Kim JY. Surgery and global health: a view from beyond the OR. *World Journal of Surgery*. 2008;32:533–6.
2. Farmer PE, Nutt CT, Wagner CM, et al. Reduced premature mortality in Rwanda: lessons from success. *BMJ*. 2013;346:f64.
3. Farmer PE. Chronic infectious disease and the future of health care delivery. *New England Journal of Medicine*. 2013;369:2424–36.
4. King MH et al. *Primary Surgery: Non-Trauma*, vol. 1. Oxford: Oxford University Press, 1987.
5. Crandall M, Sharp D, Unger E, et al. Trauma deserts: distance from a trauma center, transportation times, and mortality from gunshot wounds in Chicago. *American Journal of Public Health*. 2013;103(6):1103–9.
6. Debas HT, Gosselin R, McCord C, Thind A. Surgery. In: *Disease Control Priorities in Developing Countries*. 2nd ed. Washington, DC: World Bank, 2006.
7. Murray CJL, Vos T, Lozano R, et al. Disability-adjusted life years (DALYs) for 291 diseases and injuries in 21 regions, 1990–2010: a systematic analysis for the Global Burden of Disease Study 2010. *Lancet*. 2012;380(9859):2197–223.
8. Lewis SS, Moehring RW, Anderson DJ, et al. Increasing rates of methicillin-resistant *Staphylococcus aureus* in academic hospitals: a result of active surveillance? *Infection Control and Hospital Epidemiology*. 2013;34:105–106.
9. Pantal MA, Faure PA, Jerome JG, et al. The economic impact of the Mirebalais National Teaching Hospital on the Haitian economy. Working paper, 7 Nov 2013. http://parthealth.3cdn.net/3392f391b7abb45ec7_qjm6bawoj.pdf
10. Binagwaho A, Kyamanywa P, Farmer PE, et al. Human resources for health program in Rwanda—a new partnership. *New England Journal of Medicine*. 2013;369:2054–2059.
11. Farmer PE, Meara JG. Commentary: the agenda for academic excellence in "global" surgery. *Surgery*. 2013;153(3):321–2.

Preface

John G. Meara
Craig D. McClain
Selwyn O. Rogers, Jr.
David P. Mooney

As global surgery is becoming recognized as a necessary public health intervention, access to safe surgery and anesthesia is being redefined as a universal human right. Surgery is an essential, cost-effective measure that will strengthen health systems and improve patient outcomes. There is a high global burden of surgical disease, and it impacts nearly every face of health care, including maternal and child health, non-communicable diseases, infectious diseases, and trauma. As we consider the distribution and determinants of surgical disease, we are reminded of the need for academic partnerships and long-term collaborative relationships between visiting and local surgical teams.

This clinical guide offers practical knowledge for providing surgical services in low- and middle-income countries (LMICs) for teams of care providers, both local and visiting.

The organization is simple: We divided the book into introductory topics, anesthesia and perioperative care, and trauma surgery. Our work is written by a group of culturally and academically diverse clinicians with the goal of being accessible to all providers and settings; it is not only for fully trained surgeons and anesthesia providers. Each chapter is enriched by at least one commentary from a surgeon or anesthesiologist in an LMIC who shares their first-hand perspective of the realities and complexities of providing surgical care in LMICs. It is our hope that this manual will empower you as providers to deliver evidence-based care, and inspire you to continue to work to eliminate health disparities with the ultimate goal of providing access to safe, affordable, high-quality surgery and anesthesia for all.

Authors

Olusegun I. Alatise, MD, FWACS
Senior Lecturer/Consultant Surgeon
Department of Surgery
Obafemi Awolowo University
Ile-Ife, Osun State, Nigeria

Emmanuel A. Ameh, MBBS, FWACS, FACS
Professor of Pediatric Surgery
Ahmadu Bello University and Ahmadu Bello University
  Teaching Hospital
Zaria, Nigeria

Paul T. Appleton, MD
Clinical Instructor in Orthopaedic Surgery
Harvard Medical School
Beth Israel Deaconess Medical Center
Boston, Massachusetts, USA

Marcel Tunkumgnen Bayor, B.Pharm (Hons), MSc, PhD
Senior Lecturer
Kwame Nkrumah University of Science and Technology
  (KNUST)
Department of Pharmaceutics
Faculty of Pharmacy and Pharmaceutical Sciences College of
  Health Sciences, KNUST
Kumasi, Ghana

Regan Bergmark, MD
Resident Surgeon
Department of Otolaryngology-Head and Neck Surgery
Massachusetts Eye and Ear Infirmary and Harvard Medical
  School
Clinical Fellow in Otology and Laryngology
Harvard Medical School
Boston, Massachusetts, USA

Robert M. Boucher, MD, MPH, FACS
Chief of Staff
Wilmington VA Medical Center
Wilmington, Delaware, USA
Consultant in Otolaryngology—Head and Neck Surgery
Visiting Otolaryngologist
Partners in Health/Zanmi Lasante
Clinique Bon Sauveur, Cange and Hôpital Universitaire de
  Mirebalais
Mirebalais, Haiti
Lecturer in Otology and Laryngology
Harvard Medical School
Boston, Massachusetts, USA

Susan Miller Briggs, MD, MPH, FACS
Associate Professor of Surgery
Harvard Medical School
Affiliate Faculty
Department of Global Health and Social Medicine, Harvard
  Medical School
Director, International Trauma and Disaster Institute
Massachusetts General Hospital
Department of Surgery
Boston, Massachusetts, USA

Jill Buckley, MD
Associate Professor
Urologic Trauma and Reconstructive Surgery
Department of Urology
University of California, San Diego
La Jolla, California, USA

Matthew C. Bujak, MD, PT, FRCS(C)
Lecturer
University of Toronto
Department of Ophthalmology and Vision Sciences
Cornea, External Ocular Disease, Refractive Surgery
St. Michael's Hospital
Toronto, Ontario, Canada

Mack Cheney, MD
Kletjian Professor of Global Health
Massachusetts Eye and Ear Infirmary
Professor of Otology and Laryngology
Harvard Medical School
Boston, Massachusetts, USA

Kathryn M. Chu, MD, MPH, FACS
Instructor in Surgery
Harvard Medical School
Courtesy Surgeon
Brigham and Women's Hospital
Affiliate Faculty
Center for Surgery and Public Health
Brigham and Women's Hospital
Boston, Massachusetts, USA
Honorary Assistant Professor in Surgery
University of Rwanda
Consultant Surgeon
University Teaching Hospital
Kigali, Rwanda

Quyen D. Chu, MD, MBA, FACS
Charles Knight Professor of Surgery
Chief of Surgical Oncology
Director of Surface Malignancies
Feist-Weiller Cancer Center
Louisiana State University Health Science Center—Shreveport
Shreveport, Louisiana, USA

Ibrahim M. Daoud, MD, FACS
Associate Clinical Professor of Surgery
University of Connecticut Medical School
Director of Minimally Invasive Surgery and Fellowship
St. Francis Hospital and Medical Center
Hartford, Connecticut, USA

Vladimir Daoud, MD, MS
General Surgery Resident
Tufts Medical Center
Department of Surgery
Tufts University School of Medicine
Boston, Massachusetts, USA

Joseph P. DeAngelis, MD
Director
Sports Medicine Research
Beth Israel Deaconess Medical Center Sports Medicine and
    Shoulder Surgery
Instructor
Harvard Medical School
Boston, Massachusetts, USA

George S. M. Dyer, MD, FACS
Assistant Professor of Orthopaedic Surgery
Program Director
Harvard Combined Orthopaedic Residency
Harvard Medical School
Orthopaedic Upper Extremity Surgeon
Brigham and Women's Hospital
Orthopaedic Advisor
Partners In Health
Boston, Massachusetts, USA

Der Muonir, Edmund, MB ChB, MWACP, MGCP
Specialist Pathologist
Korle-Bu Teaching Hospital
Accra, Ghana
Tamale Teaching Hospital
Tamale, Ghana

J. Kent Ellington, MD, MS
Orthopedic Surgeon
Foot and Ankle Institute – OrthoCarolina
Carolinas Medical Center
Clinical Faculty Orthopaedics
University of North Carolina Charlotte
Department of Biology
Adjunct Professor
Charlotte, North Carolina, USA

Paul E. Farmer, MD, PhD
Kolokotrones University Professor
Harvard University Chair
Department of Global Health and Social Medicine, Harvard
    Medical School
Chief, Division of Global Health Equity
Brigham and Women's Hospital
Co-founder
Partners In Health
Boston, Massachusetts, USA

Ingrid Ganske, MD, MPA
Resident
Harvard Combined Plastic Surgery Residency Program
Massachusetts General Hospital
Boston, Massachusetts, USA

Joel Goldberg, MD, FACS
Associate Surgeon
Division of Colon and Rectal Surgery
Brigham and Women's Hospital
Harvard Medical School
Dana Farber Cancer Institute
Gastrointestinal Cancer Center & Cancer Risk and
    Prevention Clinic
Boston, Massachusetts, USA

Caris Grimes, MBBS
King's Centre for Global Health
King's College London
London, England

Reinou S. Groen, MD, MIH, PhD
Department of Gynecology and Obstetrics
Johns Hopkins Hospital
Baltimore, Maryland, USA

**Mawuli Kotope Gyakobo, BSc, MB, ChB, MSc, PhD,
    FWACP-Fam. Med, Post Doc. Global Health
    & Palliative Medicine**
Fellow
Primary Care/Family Medicine
Consultant
Public Health Physician & Health Policy and
    Planning
Tetteh Quarshie Memorial Hospital
Mampong-Akuapem
Akuapem North District, Ghana
Medical Superintendent
Tetteh Quashie Memorial Hospital
Head of Palliative Medicine Unit
Faculty of Family Medicine
Ghana and West African Colleges of Physicians at Korle-Bu
    Teaching Hospital
Accra, Ghana

Mitchel B. Harris, MD, MS
Professor
Department of Orthopedic Surgery
Harvard Medical School
Chief
Orthopedic Trauma
Brigham and Women's Hospital
Boston, Massachusetts, USA

Ann T. Hau, MD
Staff Anesthesiologist
Department of Anesthesiology
Kapi'olani Medical Center for Women and Children
Honolulu, Hawaii, USA

Joaquim M. Havens, MD
Instructor in Surgery
Harvard Medical School
Division of Trauma
Burns and Surgical Critical Care
Brigham and Women's Hospital
Boston, Massachusetts, USA

**Mykel Hawke, MS, U.S. Army Special Forces
    Captain (*Ret.*)**
Special Ops and Survival Gear Designer
Special Forces Medic, 18d
Medical Service Officer, 70b
NR-EMT-Paramedic, PHTLS, ATLS, ACLS
Combat Anesthesia, Combat Chemical Care
Captain, US Army Special Forces, Retired
US Army Special Forces Command, Reserves
Special Forces Command
Fort Bragg, North Carolina, USA

Kelly C. Hewitt, MD
General Surgery Resident
University of Utah
Salt Lake City, Utah, USA

Robert P. Horne, DDS
Associate Program Director of Oral and Maxillofacial
    Surgery
Section Chief of Facial Trauma
Associate Program Director of Oral and Maxillofacial
    Surgery
Section Chief of Facial Trauma
Christiana Care Hospital System
Wilmington, Delaware, USA

Christopher D. Hughes, MD, MPH
Surgical Resident
University of Connecticut School of Medicine
Department of Surgery
Farmington, Connecticut, USA

Evelyn Jiagge, MD, PhD(c)
Cancer Biology Program
Department of Internal Medicine
University of Michigan Medical School
Ann Arbor, Michigan, USA

T. Peter Kingham, MD, FACS
Assistant Attending
Memorial Sloan-Kettering Cancer Center
New York, New York, USA

Adam L. Kushner, MD, MPH, FACS
Associate
Johns Hopkins Bloomberg School of Public Health
Baltimore, Maryland, USA
Lecturer, Department of Surgery
Columbia University
Founder & Director
Surgeons OverSeas (SOS)
New York, New York, USA

John Y. Kwon, MD
Foot & Ankle/Trauma
Department of Orthopaedic Surgery
Massachusetts General Hospital
Boston, Massachusetts, USA

Abraham Lebenthal, MD
Instructor in Surgery
Harvard Medical School
Brigham and Women's Hospital
Boston, Massachusetts, USA

Christopher S. Lee, MD, FAAP
Assistant Professor of Clinical Anesthesia and Clinical
    Pediatrics
University of Cincinnati
Cincinnati Children's Hospital Medical Center
Cincinnati, Ohio, USA

Felicia Lester, MD, MPH, MS
Assistant Professor
Department of Obstetrics, Gynecology and Reproductive Sciences
University of California San Francisco
San Francisco, California, USA

Guy Lin, MD
Trauma Director
Meir Medical Center
Kfar-Saba, Israel

Allison F. Linden, MD, MPH
General Surgery Resident
Georgetown University Hospital,
Washington, District of Columbia, USA

Marc D. Manganiello, MD
Chief Resident
Urology
Lahey Clinic
Burlington, Massachusetts, USA

Alexi C. Matousek, MD, MPH
Global Health Equity Resident in General Surgery
Brigham and Women's Hospital
Arthur Tracy Cabot Research Fellow
Brigham and Women's Hospital Center for Surgery and Public
    Health
Paul Farmer Global Surgery Research Fellow
Program in Global Surgery and Social Change, Harvard
    Medical School
Boston, Massachusetts, USA

Craig D. McClain, MD, MPH
Senior Associate in Perioperative Anesthesia
Department of Anesthesiology, Perioperative and Pain Medicine
Boston Children's Hospital
Director
Global Pediatric Anesthesiology Fellowship
Assistant Professor of Anaesthesia
Harvard Medical School
Boston, Massachusetts, USA

K. A. Kelly McQueen, MD, MPH
Associate Professor
Department of Anesthesiology
Director
Vanderbilt Anesthesia Global Health & Development
Director
Global Anesthesia Fellowship
Vanderbilt University Medical Center
Nashville, Tennessee, USA

Daniel J. Meara, MS, MD, DMD, FACS
Chair
Department of Oral and Maxillofacial Surgery & Hospital
Dentistry
Program Director
Oral and Maxillofacial Surgery Residency
Director of Research
Oral and Maxillofacial Surgery
Christiana Care Health System
Wilmington, Delaware, USA

Gita N. Mody, MD, MPH
General Surgery Resident
Brigham and Women's Hospital
Center for Surgery and Public Health Arthur Tracy Cabot
    Research Fellow
Brigham and Women's Hospital
Fogarty International Clinical Research Scholar
Boston, Massachusetts, USA

Doreen Nakku
Lecturer
Department of ENT Surgery
Mbarara University of Science and Technology
Mbarara, Uganda

Lisa A. Newman, MD, MPH, FACS
Professor of Surgery
Director
Breast Care Center
University of Michigan
Comprehensive Cancer Center
Ann Arbor, Michigan, USA

Hiep T. Nguyen, MD, FAAP
Pediatric Urology
Cardon Children's Medical Center
Banner Children's Specialists
Mesa, Arizona, USA

Doruk Ozgediz, MD, Msc
Assistant Professor of Surgery
Yale University
New Haven, Connecticut, USA
Advisory Board
Global Partners in Anesthesia and Surgery
Kampala, Uganda

Julian J. Pribaz, MD
Professor of Surgery
Harvard Medical School
Boston, Massachusetts, USA

Raymond R. Price, MD FACS
Director
Graduate Surgical Education
Intermountain Medical Center
Intermountain Healthcare Adjunct
Associate Professor
Department of Surgery, University of Utah
Associate Director
Center for Global Surgery
University of Utah
Salt Lake City, Utah, USA

Joel S. Reynolds, DDS
Chief Resident, Oral and Maxillofacial Surgery
Christiana Care Health System
Wilmington, Delaware, USA

Johanna N. Riesel, MD
Clinical Fellow in Surgery
Massachusetts General Hospital
Department of Surgery
Research Fellow
Program in Global Surgery and Social Change
Harvard Medical School
Boston, Massachusetts, USA

Robert Riviello, MD, MPH
Instructor in Surgery
Harvard Medical School
Director of Global Surgery Programs
Brigham and Women's Hospital Center for Surgery and
    Public Health
Boston, Massachusetts, USA

Selwyn O. Rogers, Jr., MD, MPH, FACS
Chief Medical Officer
University of Texas Medical Branch
Galveston, Texas, USA

Kristen R. Scarpato, MD, MPH
University of Connecticut Urology Department
Storrs, Connecticut, USA

Samuel C. Schecter, MBBS
Clinical Instructor
Division of General Surgery
University of California San Francisco
San Francisco, California, USA

William P. Schecter, MD
Professor of Clinical Surgery Emeritus
University of California, San Francisco at San Francisco
    General Hospital
San Francisco, California, USA

Leal G. Segura, MD
Assistant Professor
Department of Anesthesiology
Mayo Clinic College of Medicine
Rochester, Minnesota, USA

Nadine B. Semer, MD, MPH, FACS
Plastic Surgeon
Los Angeles, California, USA

Navil F. Sethna, MD, FAAP
Associate Professor of Anesthesia
Harvard Medical School
Clinical Director
Mayo Family Pediatric Pain Rehabilitation Center
Boston Children's Hospital
Boston, Massachusetts, USA

Sachita Shah, MD
Assistant Professor, Emergency Medicine
University of Washington School of Medicine
Harborview Medical Center
Seattle, Washington, USA

David S. Shapiro, MD, FACS, FCCM
Director
Surgical Critical Care
Saint Francis Hospital and Medical Center
Hartford
Assistant Professor of Surgery
Site Director
UCONN Surgical Residency
University of Connecticut School of Medicine
Storrs, Connecticut, USA

Andrew K. Simpson, MD, MHS
Spine Surgeon
Texas Back Institute
Dallas, Texas, USA

Stephen R. Sullivan, MD, MPH
Assistant Professor of Surgery (Plastic and Reconstructive) and
    Pediatrics
Co-director
Cleft and Craniofacial Center
Alpert Medical School of Brown University
Rhode Island Hospital and Hasbro Children's Hospital
Providence, Rhode Island, USA

Geoffrey Tabin, MA, MD
John E. and Marva M. Warnock Presidential Endowed Chair
Professor of Ophthalmology and Visual Sciences
Moran Eye Center–University of Utah
Chairman–Himalayan Cataract Project
Salt Lake City, Utah, USA

Amir H. Taghinia, MD, MPH
Assistant Professor of Surgery
Harvard Medical School
Attending Plastic Surgeon
Boston Children's Hospital
Boston, Massachusetts, USA

Simon G. Talbot, MD
Assistant Professor of Surgery
Harvard Medical School
Brigham and Women's Hospital
Boston, Massachusetts, USA

Helena O.B. Taylor, MD, PhD
Assistant Professor of Surgery (Plastic and Reconstructive) and
    Pediatrics,
Co-director
Cleft and Craniofacial Center
Alpert Medical School of Brown University
Rhode Island Hospital and Hasbro Children's Hospital
Providence, Rhode Island, USA

Benjamin J. Thomas, MD
Fellow
International Ophthalmology
John A. Moran Eye Center
University of Utah
Salt Lake City, Utah, USA

Cynthia S. Tung, MD, MPH
Instructor in Anesthesia
Harvard Medical School
Assistant in Perioperative Anesthesia and Pain Medicine
Boston Children's Hospital
Boston, Massachusetts, USA

Gabriela M. Vargas, MD, MS
Clinical instructor
Department of General Surgery
University of Texas Medical Branch
Galveston, Texas, USA

David B. Waisel, MD
Associate Professor of Anesthesia
Harvard Medical School
Senior Associate in Anesthesia
Boston Children's Hospital
Boston, Massachusetts, USA

Jennifer Wall, PA-C, BS, MPAS
Physician Assistant
Brigham and Women's Hospital Burn Center
Boston, Massachusetts, USA
President and Founder of Africa Burn Relief Program
Malawi

Benjamin C. Warf, MD
Associate Professor of Surgery
Director of Neonatal and Congenital Anomalies Neurosurgery
Department of Neurosurgery
Boston Children's Hospital
Affiliate Faculty of Department of Global Health and Social Medicine
Harvard Medical School
Boston, Massachusetts, USA
Senior Medical Director CURE
Hydrocephalus
Director of Research
CURE Children's Hospital of Uganda
Mbale, Uganda

Sierra Washington, MD, MSc
Assistant Professor
Division of Family Planning and Global Health
Department of Obstetrics and Gynecology
Albert Einstein College of Medicine
Bronx, New York, USA

Thomas G. Weiser, MD, MPH
Assistant Professor
Stanford University School of Medicine
Department of Surgery
Section of Trauma and Critical Care
Stanford, California, USA

Mallory Williams, MD, MPH, FACS , FICS, FCCP
Associate Professor of Surgery and Chief
Division of Trauma, Critical Care, and Acute Care Surgery
Department of Surgery
University of Toledo College of Medicine
Trauma Medical Director
Director of the Surgical ICU
University of Toledo Medical Center
Toledo, Ohio, USA

Wendy Williams, JD
Associate Director
Office of Global Surgery and Health
Massachusetts Eye and Ear Infirmary
Boston, Massachusetts, USA

Traci A. Wolbrink, MD, MPH
Associate in Critical Care Medicine
Boston Children's Hospital
Instructor in Anesthesia
Harvard Medical School
Boston, Massachusetts, USA

Nikolaj Wolfson, MD, FRCSC, FACS
Chief of Orthopedics
San Joaquin General Hospital
French Camp, California, USA

Terrance A. Yemen, MD
Director of Pediatric Anesthesia
Associate Professor of Anesthesia and Pediatrics
Department of Anesthesia & Pediatrics
University of Virginia Medical School
Charlottesville, Virginia, USA

Richard N. Yu, MD, PhD
Associate in Urology
Boston Children's Hospital
Instructor in Surgery (Urology)
Harvard Medical School
Boston, Massachusetts, USA

Martin Zammert, MD
Director of Vascular Anesthesia
Department of Anesthesiology, Perioperative and Pain Medicine
Brigham and Women's Hospital
Instructor of Anesthesia
Harvard Medical School
Boston, Massachusetts, USA

Commentators

Nivaldo Alonso, MD, PhD
Associate Professor of Plastic Surgery at University of São Paulo
Director of Craniofacial Service in Hospital das Clinicas da Faculdade de Medicina da Universidade de São Paulo
São Paulo, Brazil

Ankur B. Bamne, MS (Orth)
Clinical Fellow
Department of Knee Surgery and Sports Medicine
Seoul National University Bundang Hospital
Bundang-gu, Gyeonggi-do, Korea

Demberelnyambuu Batsukh, MD
Department of Pediatric Urology
National Center for Maternal and Child Health
Ulaanbaatar, Mongolia

Denise M. Chan, MD
Clinical Instructor
Department of Anesthesiology, Perioperative and Pain Medicine
Stanford University School of Medicine
Stanford, California, USA

Daniel Chimutu, MS II
Orthopedic Clinical Officer
Nkhoma Hospital, Malawi
Lilongwe, Malawi

Jigjidsuren Chinburen
Professor of Clinic
National Medical Science University of Mongolia
Head of HPBSD at National Cancer Center Mongolia
Head of Hepatopancreatic Surgery Department
National Cancer Center
Mongolia Bayan Zurkh District, Ulaanbaatar, Mongolia

Ruth Damuse, MD
Assistant Professor of Basic Immunology, Internal Medicine, Immuno-Hematology
School of Medicine
State University of Haiti Oncology Program Director
Partners in Health:
University Hospital of Mirebalais Centre
Haiti Mirebalais, Haiti

Miliard Derbew, MD, FRCS, FCS - ECSA
Associate Professor of Surgery
Addis Ababa University
School Of Medicine
Addis Ababa, Ethiopia

Rose Dina Premier, DDS
Dental Chief
Mirebalais
Dentist Coordinator
Zanmi Lasante
University Hospital of Mirebalais
Mirebalais, Haiti

Sebastian O. Ekenze, MD
Senior Lecturer
Department of Surgery
University of Nigeria
University of Nigeria Teaching Hospital
Enugu, Nigeria

Ndukauba Eleweke, MBBS, FMCS
Head of Department of Surgery
Consultant General Surgeon and Senior Lecturer
Abia State University Teaching Hospital
Aba/Abia State University
Uturu, Abia State, Nigeria

Tsiiregzen Enkh-Amgalan, MD
HPB Surgeon
International Medical Center, Mongolia
Ulaanbaatar, Mongolia

Ifeoma Ezegwui, MBBS, FMCoph, FWACS
Senior Lecturer and Consultant Department of Ophthalmology
College of Medicine
University of Nigeria Enugu Campus
University of Nigeria Teaching Hospital, Enugu
Enugu, Nigeria

Emmanuel R. Ezeome, MBBS, MA, FWACS, FACS
Professor of Surgery
College of Medicine
University of Nigeria Enugu
Consultant Surgical Oncologist and Bioethicist
Director of Oncology Center
University of Nigeria Teaching Hospital Enugu
Enugu, Nigeria

Charles Furaha, Lt. Col. MD, FC Plast (SA)
Honorary Senior Lecturer
College of Medicine and Health Sciences
University of Rwanda
Plastic Surgeon
Rwanda Military Hospital
King Faisal Hospital
Kigali, Rwanda

Zipporah Gathuya, MbCHb, Mmed (Anaesth) UON
Consultant Paediatric Anaesthesiologist
Gertrudes Children Hospital
Nairobi, Kenya

Ntakiyiruta Georges, MMed, FCSECSA
Senior Lecturer and Academic Head
Department of Surgery School of Medicine
University of Rwanda
Butare, Rwanda

Rodolphe R. Eisenhower Jean-Louis, MD
Hospital Albert Schweitzer
Deschapelles, Haiti

Thaim Buya Kamara, MBChB, FWACS
Consultant Urologist and Head
Department of Surgery
Connaught Hospital
Senior Lecturer and Head
Department of Surgery
College of Medicine and Allied Health Sciences
Freetown, Sierra Leone

Emmanuel Kayibanda, MBCHB, MMED (Dakar University), FCS-ECSA Honorary Associate Professor
College of Medicine and Health Sciences
University of Rwanda
Consultant Surgeon
King Faisal Hospital
Kigali, Rwanda

Clover Ann Lee, MBBCh (Wits), DA (SA), FCA (SA)
Anesthesiologist
University of the Witwatersrand
Johannesburg, South Africa

Ouyang Lizhi, MD
Director
First Department of Breast Cancer
Hunan Provincial Tumor Hospital
Changsha, China

Samuel Abimerech Luboga, MBChB, MMed (Surg), PhD
Associate Professor of Anatomy
Makerere University, Uganda (recently retired)
Privileges at Mulago Hospital and St. Stephen's Hospital (Church of Uganda), Mpererwe
Kampala, Uganda

Thandinkosi E. Madiba, MBChB, MMed, LLM, PhD, FCS (SA), FASCRS
Professor and Head
Department of Surgery
Head
Colorectal Unit
University of KwaZulu-Natal
Durban, South Africa

Tarek Meguid, MD, MPhil, DTM&H, LLB, MSt
Consultant Obstetrician and Gynaecologist
Mnazi Mmoja Hospital, Zanzibar, Tanzania
Associate Professor
School of Health and Medical Sciences, State University of Zanzibar, Tanzania
Zanzibar, Tanzania

Nyengo Mkandawire, BMBS, FRCS, MCh(ORTH), FCS(ECSA)
Professor and Head of Surgery
College of Medicine
University of Malawi
Zomba, Malawi
Adjunct Professor
School of Medicine
Faculty of Health Sciences
Flinders University
Adelaide, South Australia

David Morton, MD, DTM&H
Deputy Medical Director
Nkhoma CCAP Hospital
Nkhoma, Malawi

John Mugamba, MD
Consultant
Ministry of Health, Uganda
Medical Director of CURE Children's Hospital of Uganda
Mbale, Uganda

Wakisa Mulwafu, MBBS(Mlw), FCORL(SA)
ENT Surgeon and Senior Lecturer
College of Medicine
University of Malawi
Lilongwe, Malawi

Francoise Nizeyimana
Resident in Anaesthesia and Critical Care Management
University of Rwanda
Butare, Rwanda

John Nkurikiye, MD, FC Ophth (SA), FEACO
Consultant Ophthalmologist
Rwanda International Institute of Ophthalmology
Dr. Agarwal's Eye Hospital
Kigali, Rwanda

Peter M. Nthumba, MD
Plastic, Reconstructive and Hand Surgeon
Medical Education and Research Director
AIC Kijabe Hospital, Kenya
Kijabe, Kenya
Clinical Assistant Professor
Department of Plastic Surgery
Vanderbilt University Medical Center
Nashville
Department of Plastic Surgery
Chattanooga Unit
University of Tennessee Health Science Center
Knoxville, Tennessee, USA

Ikechukwu A. Nwafor, MBBS, CAS, FWACS
Senior Hospital Consultant Cardiothoracic Surgeon
University of Nigeria Teaching Hospital
Enugu, Nigeria

Wangari Nyaga, MBChB, MMED (Anaesthesia)
Anaesthetist
Overseas Fellow in Anaesthesia and Pain Management
The Children's Hospital at Westmead, Australia
Nairobi, Kenya

Bomi Ogedengbe, BM, BCh, MA (Oxon), FRCOG, FWACS, FICS, FCOGSA (Hons) Professor
Obstetrics and Gynaecology
College of Medicine
University of Lagos
Nigeria Lagos State, Nigeria

Michael O. Ogirima, MB, BS, FMCS(Ortho), FICS, FAOI, FWACS
Reader and Consultant Orthopaedic and Trauma Surgeon
Head of Department and Acting Dean of Faculty of Medicine
President
Nigerian Orthopaedic Association
Department of Orthopaedics and Trauma Surgery
Ahmadu Bello University Teaching Hospital, Zaria
Zaria, Nigeria

E. Oluwabunmi Olapade-Olaopa, MBBS, DUrol, MD, FMedEd, FRCS, FWACS, ACIArb
Professor of Surgery and Honorary Consultant Urologist and Director
Ibadan PIUTA Center
University of Ibadan and University College Hospital
Ibadan, Nigeria

Okechukwu O. Onumaegbu, MD, FWACS
Lecturer and Consultant Burn and Plastic Surgeon
College of Medicine University of Nigeria/ University of Nigeria Teaching Hospital
President
Nigerian Burn Society
Secretary
Pan African Burn Society
Enugu, Nigeria

Sergelen Orgoi, MD, ScD
Head of the Department of Surgery
Health Sciences University of Mongolia
Vice President
Surgical Association of Mongolia
Ulaanbaatar, Mongolia

Jorge Palacios, MD
Director of Postgraduate Plastic Surgery
Universidad Catolica de Guayaquil
Head
Department of Plastic Surgery
Hospital General Luis Vernaza
Guayaquil, Ecuador

Christian Paletta, MD, FACS
Clinical Professor of Surgery
Geisel School of Medicine at Dartmouth
Rwanda Human Resources for Health Program
Plastic Surgeon
Rwanda Military Hospital
King Faisal Hospital and CHUK
Kigali, Rwanda

Okao Patrick, MB, ChB, MMed (Surgery), MIHA
General Surgeon
Partners in Health, Rwanda
Attached to Butaro Cancer Centre of Excellence
Burera, Rwanda

Nakul Raykar, MD
Resident in General Surgery
Harvard Medical School/Beth Israel Deaconess Medical Center
Paul Farmer Global Surgery Research Fellow
Harvard Medical School/Boston Children's Hospital
Boston, Massachusetts, USA

Edgar Rodas, MD, FACS
Founding President of the Cinterandes Foundation
University of Azuay
Former Professor of Surgery
University of Cuenca
Cuenca, Ecuador

Edgar B. Rodas, MD, FACS
University of Cuenca
Cinterandes Foundation, University of Azuay
Cuenca, Ecuador

Nobhojit Roy, MBBS, MS, MPH
Chief of Surgery
BARC Hospital
Visiting Professor of Public Health
Tata Institute of Social Sciences, Mumbai
Mumbai, India

Emile Rwamasirabo, MD, FCS (ECSA)
Honorary Professor
University of Rwanda
Consultant Urological Surgeon
King Faisal Hospital
Kigali, Rwanda

Bin Song, MD, PhD
Resident in Plastic Surgery
Plastic Surgery Hospital
Peking Union Medical College and Chinese Academe of Medical Sciences
Paul Farmer Global Surgery Research Fellow
Harvard Medical School/ Boston Children's Hospital
Boston, Massachusetts, USA
Dongcheng, Beijing, China

Louis-Franck Telemaque, MD, FICS, MSc
Chairman
Department of Surgery at Medicine School (FMP)
General Surgeon
Chief of Service of General Surgery at General University
    Hospital (HUEH), Port-au-Prince, Haiti
Medical Director of General University Hospital (HUEH)
Port-au-Prince, Haiti

L.O.A. Thanni, BSc (Hons), MBChB, FWACS
Professor of Orthopaedics and Traumatology
Olabisi Onabanjo University
Obafemi Awolowo College of Health Sciences
Department of Surgery
Sagamu, Ogun State, Nigeria

Chona Thomas, MS, FRCS, FACS
Senior Consultant Plastic Surgeon
ATLAS Medical Centre (AMC)
Muscat, Oman

Alexandra Torborg, MBChB, DA(SA) and FCA(SA)
Anaesthesiologist
Inkosi Albert Luthuli Central Hospital
Honorary Lecturer
Nelson R. Mandela School of Medicine
University of KwaZuluNatal
Durban, South Africa

Sterman Toussaint, MD
General Surgeon
State University Hospital of Haiti, HUEH
Department of Surgery at FMP/UEH
Surgical Coordinator Zanmi Lasante/PIH, Haiti
Port-au-Prince, Haiti

C.C. Uguru, BDS, FWACS
Senior Lecturer and Consultant
Department of Oral and Maxillofacial Surgery
Faculty of Dentistry
College of Medicine
University of Nigeria Enugu Campus and
University of Nigeria Teaching Hospital
Enugu, Nigeria

Edouard Uwamahoro
Resident in Anaesthesia and Critical Care Management
University of Rwanda
Butare, Rwanda

Koffi Herve Yangni-Angate, MD, FWACS, FICS, FISS
Chairman of Department of Thoracic and Cardio-Vascular
    Surgery University of Bouake, Cote d'Ivoire
Bouake, Cote d'Ivoire

Editors

John G. Meara, MD, DMD, MBA, FACS, FRACS
Editor-in-Chief
Director, Program in Global Surgery and Social Change
Harvard Medical School
Plastic Surgeon-in-Chief
Boston Children's Hospital
Boston, Massachusetts, USA

Craig D. McClain, MD, MPH
Anesthesia Section Editor
Senior Associate in Perioperative Anesthesia
Department of Anesthesiology, Perioperative and Pain
    Medicine
Boston Children's Hospital
Director
Global Pediatric Anesthesiology Fellowship
Assistant Professor of Anaesthesia
Harvard Medical School
Boston, Massachusetts, USA

Selwyn O. Rogers, Jr., MD, MPH, FACS
Non-Trauma Section Editor
Chief Medical Officer
University of Texas Medical Branch
Galveston, Texas, USA

David P. Mooney, MD, MPH, FACS
Trauma Section Editor
Trauma Center Director
Boston Children's Hospital
Assistant Professor of Surgery
Harvard University
Boston, Massachusetts, USA

Project Managers:
Rachel R. Yorlets, MPH
Kiran Jay Agarwal-Harding, MD
Christopher D. Hughes, MD, MPH

Copy Editors/Research Assistants:
Tiffany E. Chao, MD, MPH
Ainhoa Costas Chavarri, MD, MPH
Jacky Fils, MD, MPH
Rowan Gillies, MBBS, FRACS
Sarah L. M. Greenberg, MD, MPH
Lars Hagander, MD, PhD, MPH
Paula Hercule, MD
Marguerite Hoyler, MD
Gino Inverso
Rebecca Maine, MD, MPH
Alexi C. Matousek, MD, MPH
Cecilia T. Ong, MD
Pratik B. Patel, MD
Jordan Pyda, MD
Margarita Ramos, MD
Mike Steer, MD

Section I

Introduction

1

The Global Burden of Surgical Disease

K. A. Kelly McQueen

Introduction

The role of surgery in global health has only recently become a topic of debate within the global public health community. Of course, surgeons have always maintained that surgical interventions have impacted disability and death, especially for traumatic injuries and obstetric emergencies. But the surgical agenda has often been seen as a "luxury" or "too expensive" by the global public health community. The increase in chronic disease has demanded that these assumptions be revisited. Three of the 10 leading causes of death include cardiovascular disease, trauma, and neoplasm,[1] and each of these disease categories often includes surgical intervention[2] at some point in the continuum of the disease process. Therefore, governments, hospitals, policy makers, and donors must now recognize the data supporting the impact and cost-effectiveness of emergency and essential surgery.[3] It is estimated that 2 billion people worldwide have no access to emergency or essential surgery.[4]

Measuring Unmet Surgical Need

The *burden* of disease, or the contribution of a disease or group of diseases to the overall disability and premature death that exists in a population, is a complex estimation reported in disability-adjusted life years (DALYs). One DALY is equal to 1 year of healthy life lost due to death or disability from a disease process. The global burden of disease is a dynamic estimate of global health and is influenced by acute and chronic disease processes as well as by the interventions that impact or avert disease burden. These interventions include vaccines, medicines, and surgery.[5] The dimensions of disease burden include risk factors, causes of disease (International Classification of Diseases), and sequelae.[6]

In 2006, Debas et al. estimated the burden of surgical disease (BoSD) to be 11% of the overall global burden of disease (GBD).[7] The BoSD is equal to the total surgical need in a community, including the *met need* (i.e., the proportion of surgically treatable conditions that are seen and treated), the *unmet need* (i.e., the proportion of surgically treatable conditions that remain unseen and untreated), and the *unmeetable need* (i.e., the proportion of potentially surgically treatable conditions that are so severe that death and/or disability could not be averted even with adequate access to quality surgical care).[8] Despite limited available international data, the initial estimate proposed by Debas

and colleagues was a pivotal beginning for including surgery in the greater global health agenda. Many experts, however, now believe this to be an underestimation and hypothesize that the BoSD may be much greater.[9,10] Surgical interventions are important for a number of diseases that have been defined as surgical conditions.[2] Surgical care provides treatment, cure, and palliation for many conditions, including trauma, complications from childbirth, chronic disease, cancer, congenital anomalies, and cataracts. Important steps are under way to apply global health concepts to the BoSD and to better estimate the actual unmet surgical need in low- and middle-income countries (LMICs).[11,12]

Contributions to the Global Burden of Surgical Disease (Unmet Surgical Need)

Many factors have contributed to a lack of attention to surgical conditions in LMICs. Historically, limited life expectancy and the prevalence of infectious disease demanded that most healthcare expenditures in LMICs be spent on prevention and mitigation of endemic disease. The human immunodeficiency virus (HIV) crisis further impacted this reality, and led to many national expenditures and international contributions being specifically targeted to reduce the incidence of HIV infection, and eventually to treat those infected with antiretrovirals. While HIV/acquired immunodeficiency syndrome (AIDS) remains an important worldwide epidemic, successful treatment of the syndrome has contributed to improving life expectancy in many countries. This combined with the role of globalization, changing regional diet and activity levels, has increased the role of chronic disease, including cardiovascular disease, obesity, diabetes, and cancer. Simultaneously, maternal mortality rates have continued to be unacceptably high even as prenatal treatment improved due to the lack of caesarean sections and surgical intervention for postpartum hemorrhage. As well, trauma and other injuries have been on the rise in most LMICs. The global BoSD has therefore continued to grow, while the resources for this disease group have stagnated or declined.

The global health community has been slow to acknowledge the role of surgical conditions in the global burden of disease. While emergency surgery is acknowledged to be important to global public health, little has been done to implement what is needed to provide emergency surgery. The World Health Organization (WHO) outlines guidelines on surgical procedures that must be available at the district hospital level,[13] but assessments at these facilities reveal that there is no national or international commitment for implementing these guidelines.[14] Only recently has the role of essential surgery been acknowledged as an essential component of the basic right to health.[15] As awareness of the role of chronic disease in the GBD has improved, the surgical solutions for many of these diseases, including breast and cervical cancer, cardiovascular disease, congenital conditions, and ophthalmic pathology, have been disregarded due to the belief that they were not cost-effective or sustainable. Recent studies prove both of these assumptions inaccurate.

National health systems in most LICs have also been reluctant to invest in surgical solutions. While the WHO Guidelines for Surgery at the District Hospital[13] suggests that emergency surgery should be readily available, the reality is that a majority of these facilities have neither obstetricians nor surgeons for emergencies such as caesarean sections, nor anesthesia providers or the equipment required to safely perform an anesthetic. While surgery is often available at the regional or provincial hospital, many of those in need don't reach these facilities in time to treat their surgical disease. Even when surgery is provided at the district hospital level, many patients have poor outcomes due to the absence of providers, equipment, monitors, drugs, and blood products.[16]

What we do know about surgical intervention on a global scale is that the volume is large. Weiser et al. estimated that 234 million surgical procedures are performed annually worldwide, and that a majority of these procedures are performed in high-income countries (HICs).[17] A majority of unmet surgical need occurs in LMICs where human, infrastructural, and financial resources are limited, and many conditions that can be treated surgically are recognized late in the natural course of the disease. The World Health Report from 2006[18] revealed that a majority of the burden of disease is found in Africa, where the fewest health workers are found.

Surgery and Safe Anesthesia in LMICs

Most LMICs have a critical shortage of surgical and anesthesia providers.[18,19] While the WHO tracks numbers of physicians and other healthcare providers per country as a public health indicator,[1] it does not report the number of specialists, such as surgeons and anesthesiologists, in a country. The little that is known about surgical and anesthesia providers is provided by ministries of health (MOH) or national health systems, or in some cases is reported by nongovernmental organizations (NGOs) or individuals working in regions with critical need. Even without solid quantitative information, much can be inferred by overall numbers of reported physicians, hospital beds, life expectancy, and maternal mortality rates reported per capita by the WHO.

The impact of the scarcity of physician and other healthcare providers is nonspecifically revealed by life expectancy at birth and maternal mortality rates. In LMICs in Africa, where health workers are few and the GBD great, the life expectancy range is from 41 years (Sierra Leone) to 65 years (Comoros), with most LMICs reporting life expectancy as mid-40s to mid-50s. In comparison, Canada, the United Kingdom, and the United States report 81, 80, and 78 years, respectively. Of course, life expectancy is impacted by many factors, including those chosen by the WHO as Millennium Development Goals (MDG),[20] which include access to sanitation and clean water, decreasing infectious disease rates including HIV, and decreasing child and maternal mortality. Few indicators reveal the impact of physicians and skilled healthcare providers, including surgical, obstetrical, and anesthesia providers, as clearly as maternal mortality rates. Canada, the United Kingdom, and the United States report death rates during pregnancy and following delivery at 7, 8, and 11 per 100,000 live births. LMICs in Africa report maternal mortality rates between 400 (Comoros) and 2,100 (Sierra Leone) per 100,000 live births.

The Role for Anesthesia

Surgical, obstetric, and anesthesia providers are in short supply in most LMICs. Their numbers have been impacted by brain drain and limited training in recent decades. And while the paucity of surgeons and obstetricians is significant and parallel to the overall shortage of physicians in these countries, there is a growing crisis of limited numbers of anesthesia providers. Many international surgeons and organizations now recognize, much as the Western world did in the 1950s and 60s, that the rate-limiting step in safe surgical outcomes is dependent on safe anesthesia. Anesthesia providers in LMICs, especially those in Africa, are not recognized as the professionals that their surgical counterparts are, and they are not compensated similarly. So even those trained as anesthesiologists and nurse anesthesia providers often leave the profession for more lucrative and respected positions in other medical fields.

Anesthesiologists are a critical component of health systems infrastructure. As perioperative physicians, they provide quality, safe patient care in diverse settings. In LMICs, perhaps even more important than the clinical care they provide, anesthesiologists are responsible for the education and training of physician, nurse, and other anesthesia providers who are essential to the maintenance of an anesthesia system that ensures safe anesthesia outcomes and improved surgical outcomes. The success story of anesthesia safety within HICs with good anesthesia infrastructure and requirements for monitoring are well known.[21] Recent work by the WHO Safe Surgery Saves Lives[22] further substantiates the role of anesthesia and a minimum of basic monitoring (pulse oximetry) in improving safety and decreasing adverse outcomes. Therefore, the role of anesthesia is integral to the BoSD discussion and is critical to meeting the unmet surgical need through the delivery of surgical services.

The role of anesthesia within the BoSD is difficult to appreciate and even more difficult to measure in LMICs where anesthesia providers are critically limited, physiologic monitoring is often absent, outcomes are unknown, and yet surgery continues. It is complicated by limited interest in anesthesia in many countries due to poor reimbursement and lack of professional respect, and by the available infrastructure considerations such as routine medicines, oxygen supplies, pulse oximetry, and other monitoring equipment.[22] History reveals that safe surgery with acceptable outcomes cannot be provided without adequate anesthesia providers and safe anesthesia equipment practices; therefore, to be completely addressed, the BoSD must be considered as a system: infrastructure, surgeons, anesthesiologists, and nurses.

Mortality rates attributable to anesthesia and the lack of monitoring in LMICs are largely unknown. Anesthesia in HICs is incredibly safe[21] due to adequate numbers of physician personnel; supervision of nonphysician personnel; requirements for monitoring; and ample supply of medications, equipment, and blood supplies. Anesthesia monitoring and vigilant personnel are anecdotally reported and witnessed to be absent or rare by international volunteers and others visiting hospitals and clinics in LMICs. But verified mortality rates from these countries are rare. The few published accounts have reported mortality attributed to anesthesia as high as 1 in 133 anesthetics,[23] with other reports of avoidable anesthesia-related death rates as high as 1 in 144 anesthetics[24] and 1 in 504 anesthetics.[25] The United Kingdom–based Confidential Enquiry for Perioperative Death reported mortality from anesthesia as being 1 in 185,000 anesthetics,[26] revealing the true crisis in LMICs. Of even greater concern is that many of the preventable anesthesia deaths occurred in otherwise young, healthy patients, many of whom were undergoing caesarean section.[27]

A New Generation of Surgeons, Obstetricians, and Anesthesiologists

A new generation of physicians is in training in residencies and fellowships. These future anesthesiologists and surgeons have a documented and unprecedented interest in global health. Even the current and future medical students report a high interest in global health, and a desire to use their skills to work outside the United States.

A few academic partnerships have made long-term commitments to LMICs and are partnering to improve the delivery of surgical services, as well as education and training of surgeons and anesthesia providers.[28] Many of these programs in partnership with LMICs believe that education and training must be central to these programs, such that infrastructure will be improved along with the unmet surgical need being met. The future of these partnerships is unclear, but many international surgeons and anesthesiologists are hopeful for the sustainable education, training, and infrastructural improvement that may be possible through these conscientious academic commitments.

Conclusions

Global Public Health is only beginning to recognize the role of anesthesia and surgery within the scope of population health. With chronic disease on the rise, and the role of surgical intervention recognized by the WHO and other organizations especially with regard to the impact of emergency obstetric surgery, trauma, and other abdominal emergency surgical interventions, it is only a matter of time before anesthesiologists and surgeons are critical members of the global health network.

COMMENTARY

Zipporah Gathuya, Kenya

Access to safe anesthesia and pain relief following surgery could be considered a basic human right in the twenty-first century. However, international standards for the safe practice of anesthesia (adopted by the World Federation of Societies of Anaesthesiologists [WFSA] in 1992) are seldom met in LMICs. Perioperative mortality and morbidity rates are high in LMICs when compared to the standards in HICs. However, these rates are relative to the local expectations in LMICs, which reflect the facilities and quality of care that are available.

In rural hospitals in LMICs, most surgical patients, even those with complicated cases, rarely have the benefit of being attended to by a physician anesthetist. Ironically, most surgical patients present very late to hospitals, so they require care from surgeons and anesthetists with expertise in complicated cases but do not receive it as a result of poor infrastructure. Patients sometimes present late because they go to traditional healers before going to the hospital for surgery; common examples include patients with neoplasms, goiters, or Wilms' tumors. There is also a higher burden of complicated cases in LMIC hospitals compared to HIC hospitals because some complications are more common in LMICs; one example is recto-vaginal and vulvo-vaginal fistulae as delivery complications.

2

Ethical Considerations

David B. Waisel
Caris Grimes

Introduction

There are a number of different reasons that surgeons travel from high-income countries (HICs) to operate in low- and middle-income countries (LMICs). These include emergency disaster relief, surgical "missions" that address a specific surgical problem, surgical visits as part of a long-term partnership, or occasionally as individuals. All approaches are valid and needed for specific situations, but unless such trips are carefully constructed, there is a risk of causing harm to local populations and damaging relationships.

For example, imagine a hypothetical situation in which a surgical team flies out on a trip to an LMIC to treat a specific disorder. They do back-to-back operations for a week or two using local resources. There is little or no emphasis on education and training, and they interact little with local doctors. There is no sensitivity to local language or culture. They take plenty of photos of the patients they treat without informed consent for their advertising, fund-raising, and teaching in their home country. They use locally available anesthetics, equipment, and staff, and as a result other areas of work within the hospital inadvertently suffer. Eventually, they fly back to their HIC proud of their achievements on the operating table and exhorting others to do likewise. In the meantime, the hospital has to deal with complications of operations they know nothing about and do not know how to treat. As the anesthetic and equipment supplies have been run down, few operations are performed for the rest of the financial year. Relationships become damaged, and such trips begin to be resented by local healthcare staff.

This chapter is designed to act as a guide to avoid these and other possible unintended consequences of visiting surgical work. The ultimate goal is to build good long-term relationships and make a sustainable, positive impact on local populations through good, ethical, and sustainable practice.

Ethical Basis

The first principle of medical ethics is *primum non nocere,* Latin for "first, do no harm." It is important that individuals and surgical teams do not cause harm, either directly or indirectly, even when intentions are good. This principle of nonmaleficence goes hand in hand with that of beneficence, that medical practice should benefit the patient. In the United Kingdom, the General Medical Council outlines the Duties of a Doctor (Table 2.1), and for surgeons traveling abroad, these duties should be maintained and respected.

TABLE 2.1

Duties of a Doctor[1]

Knowledge, skills, and performance
- Make the care of your patient your first concern.
- Provide a good standard of practice and care.
  - Keep your professional knowledge and skills up to date.
  - Recognize and work within the limits of your competence.

Safety and quality
- Take prompt action if you think that patient safety, dignity, or comfort is being compromised.
- Protect and promote the health of patients and the public.

Communication, partnership, and teamwork
- Treat patients as individuals and respect their dignity.
  - Treat patients politely and considerately.
  - Respect patients' right to confidentiality.
- Work in partnership with patients.
  - Listen to, and respond to, their concerns and preferences.
  - Give patients the information they want or need in a way they can understand.
  - Respect patients' right to reach decisions with you about their treatment and care.
  - Support patients in caring for themselves to improve and maintain their health.
  - Work with colleagues in the ways that best serve patients' interests.

Maintaining trust
- Be honest and open and act with integrity.
- Never discriminate unfairly against patients or colleagues.
- Never abuse your patients' trust in you or the public's trust in the profession.

[1] You are personally accountable for your professional practice and must always be prepared to justify your decisions and actions.

Similarly, as guests with the intention of doing good, volunteers should follow the dictum of "seeking to understand before seeking to be understood." The surgeon or surgical team is there primarily to serve the community. Local practices develop for a reason, and parachuting in with the "right" answers can be alienating and harmful. Read *The Ugly American*[2] for a fuller discussion of the futility of this arrogant approach.

However, ethical absoluteness is not always possible. It is not always practical to bring in "first-world" practices and standards to LMICs, and a pragmatic, sensible approach is needed. Assessing risks and benefits for any given situation is necessary to achieve success in visiting surgical team trips. Willingness, flexibility, and an ability to rigorously think through the issues are required. Flexibility, however, does not mean that anything is permissible. It means that ethical principles are followed, within the constraints of the situation and with respect to local sensitivities.

Essentially, clinicians should adhere to home country standards unless there is a clear reason for not doing so, for which they should be held accountable. For example, if a standard in the home country is to obtain consent before taking photographs of patients, the same standard holds for photos taken on visiting surgical team trips.[3] The canard "teaching people will help future patients" is insufficient to overcome the formalized standard of respect for the patient by obtaining consent. Reasoning that showing the pictures of the patients is permissible because they are getting donated care is unethical and potentially harmful.

Distributive justice should be maintained as much as possible. Distributive justice is the concept of sharing scarce resources based on fairness. Although implementing this principle can be difficult because of different definitions of *fairness,* these problems are mostly irrelevant in global surgical work. It is difficult to think of how one underserved area may be more deserving than another. Some locations are easier to visit, but the principle of distributive justice requires an effort to provide care in less accessible areas.

Adherence to HIC Standards

There are many standards as to how surgery and surgical care should be carried out in HICs. These include who should be performing the operation, timing of the operation, staffing ratios, and equipment standards. How such standards should be enforced within global surgical care delivery, outside of the home country, is critical to the ethical analysis.[4] The core debate surrounding these statements is whether they should be considered an absolute requirement or an aspiration.

For example, a standard may include the requirement for working modern anesthetic machines; dependable oxygen supply; and monitors including capnography, blood pressure, and temperature with similar monitors required in the postoperative period. Anesthesia machines are expected to have a calibrated vaporizer functioning mechanical ventilator. A physician's refusal to operate in the absence of such equipment in an LMIC setting would limit worthwhile visiting surgical team trips.

It is also worth considering what underlies the requirement for machines and monitors and other standards in an LMIC setting. One reason may be to honor a principle that visiting surgical team care should be equivalent to care in more socioeconomically advantaged countries. Underlying this principle may be the one that all people should be treated equally, but adherence to such principles may prevent some people from being treated at all.

Standards endeavor to ensure safe care. Safe care favors patients. But in the absence of an ability to meet such standards, the safety of operating requires a more holistic assessment. The benefit of proceeding with an operation should be considered in light of the risks incurred if the operation does not go ahead. Because many factors play into this decision, sometimes first-world standards can be considered aspirational. This does not mean that they can be ignored, but simply that there needs to be a pragmatic approach as well as an ethically sound one.

Principles in Practice

These are the principles of ethics and guidance as to how they should be applied to surgical trips abroad.

1. Partnership, Partnership, Partnership

The concepts of partnership, solidarity, and accompaniment all describe a common foundation of collaboration that is required for any surgical trip to be successful. Whether they are short-term, one-off trips, such as in disaster relief, or long-term agreements, working together with local healthcare providers or government officials, a sense of team work should be developed which will enhance satisfaction and the quality of care provided. Good relationships are everything, and good operations alone are not enough.

Partnerships and good relationships often have to be built at a wide range of levels. Patients need to feel that the foreign doctors are giving them good treatment and can be trusted. Local healthcare providers should be included and accompanied rather than replaced or ignored. Local leaders should be a real part of the partnership; particularly, if there are any local or regional surgical training programs or surgical initiatives, there is a need to work alongside and in support of these.

2. Communication

Organizations should not assume they know the needs and desires of their hosts. To ensure a successful trip, there should be as much communication as possible with the local healthcare providers to ensure that things go smoothly and that partnership is generated. Often, communication is difficult with remote and rural communities. Therefore, a site visit can be useful for planning future trips. Teams should be sensitive to the possibility of displacing normal care, which may, among other matters, affect local clinicians' incomes.

In some instances, local physicians may need to provide care after the team leaves. Therefore, teams are responsible for training their local colleagues if possible in the operations they are providing, but certainly in the aftercare and possible complications that may ensue. Team members must realize that this may generate extra work for their colleagues locally and may consider compensating them for these services.

Particularly in vertical interventions, efforts should be made to avoid overlap with other groups. Ideally, this could be managed by a central registry providing sufficient information to improve distribution to underserved areas. Practically, it is often a matter of talking to local staff and finding out what else is going on in that area.

In this regard, emergency disaster relief is plagued with overlap. Many of the organizations will shed parochial identity and commit to sharing resources and distributing work for the betterment of all. This process may range from regular meetings of representatives, to generating specialty areas (e.g., a pediatric tent), to developing a healthy and fair market to trade needed equipment. Several organizations, perhaps for geopolitical reasons, may choose to work alone. But those working together should be wary of isolating the intransigent organization. Isolated teams, for example, may refuse to participate in a rotation for staffing triage (or they may insist on their own triage point in which they only take cases that interest them); may refuse to do cases they find uninteresting; or may insist on doing cases when superior expertise is 100 meters away.

Assuming that the central goal in disaster work is a utilitarian approach of providing the best care for the greatest number of people, the goal is to engage any estranged group to become part of the wider team. Shunning the group may limit their usefulness to overall care, but it is often necessary to clarify roles and boundaries between different teams.

3. Sustainability

All surgical trips and partnerships should incorporate a teaching and training program for local healthcare providers as part of their trip. Ideally, such trips should aim to equip the local community so that further visits become unnecessary in the long term; that is, aim for sustainability. This is not just about training on the operating table, but also—and perhaps more crucially— about training on the assessment and diagnosis of disease, pre-operative care, knowing when and when not to operate, and who to transfer. It is imperative that training is also provided for after-care, particularly regarding the management of pain, wounds, and complications. Training should involve more than just the local surgeons and surgical trainees. All healthcare providers seeing patients with surgical problems in rural health clinics as well as in the local hospital need to recognize the patient who needs surgical care. Furthermore, anesthetic staff, scrub and the-ater staff, and nursing staff all need partnership, mentoring, and training. This should be reinforced by the same people going to the same place to build on previous work and previous train-ing time and time again. Sustainability will be achieved through commitment.

However, there are ethical concerns with respect to training nonsurgeons in surgical skills. It may be argued that if in HICs we expect only fully qualified surgeons to operate, why should LMICs be expected to accept a "lower" standard? Although with the advent and empowerment of physician's assistants in many HICs, this does not necessarily hold true. In addition, there are some who argue that if a patient will die without surgery, then better a competent nonphysician surgeon than nobody at all. Certainly, if anyone is going to be trained in operative skills, that training should be accompanied with a plan to allow continued mentoring and supervision, and auditing of complications and outcomes. Finally, surgical trainees accompanying a trip or team should not displace the training of local healthcare providers. The goal of a team or partnership should be to equip local people with the knowledge and skills required, and trainees and trainers need to be particularly sensitive to this.

4. Competence and Limitations

The standard that surgeons should not be operating outside the limits of their competence holds true even when they are in remote areas. Operating in LMICs is not about getting practice for doing things that one would not be allowed to attempt in HICs. Sending trainees to "practice" on susceptible populations is unethical.

However, there are situations where a patient will die if noth-ing is done immediately. In that case, there needs to be a prag-matic assessment of the situation as to whether it is worse to attempt something outside the normal limits of an individual's practice or withhold treatment. There are strong ethical argu-ments on either side. The General Medical Council in the United Kingdom states: "In an emergency, wherever it arises, you must offer assistance, taking account of your own safety, your compe-tence, and the availability of other options for care."[1]

There is a precedent, therefore, for provision of care within certain limits in an emergency situation. A pragmatic approach would be to suggest that surgeons should expect the unexpected, and obtain extra training in areas outside of their normal practice prior to traveling to a remote area to equip them for such situations.

5. Monitoring and Quality

Clinicians have an obligation to monitor and improve the quality of care that they provide, and also the quality of care that their trainees provide. Significant post-operative complications should be documented, and if this is not done by the visiting surgeons, there should be a plan to do this in their absence. This is particu-larly true when local healthcare providers have been trained in a surgical procedure or procedures. A mechanism needs to be put in place to monitor post-operative events and complications, although in rural and remote areas this can be difficult to achieve with patients traveling long distances.

During disaster relief there should be a daily review of poten-tial care concerns and the limited resources should be focused on identifying and rectifying salient problems. This usually involves a fairly rapid plan-do-study-act model that may rely significantly on instinct. When doing such a rapid change model, it is essen-tial to include all types of clinicians because they may recog-nize otherwise unanticipated consequences of proposed changes. Collection of other data should be attempted so that it may be used later in developing recommendations for future trips. Disaster relief groups should have a mechanism for data collec-tion ready for implementation upon initiating disaster relief.

Vertical relief trips should follow a similar, though less intense and more thoughtful, quality improvement practice. Radical process changes are usually less necessary. Long-term commit-ments should have a robust quality improvement system, with plan-do-study-act cycles similar to home institutions.

Organizations have an obligation to ensure that systems are in place to meet ethical obligations to hosts, patients, and vol-unteers.[5] Many of these are logistic and require familiarity with local systems and resources. Perhaps one of the most important obligations of organizations is to ensure that clinicians are prop-erly credentialed and that there is a clear understanding of the type of care a specific clinician can provide. Most organizations that perform vertical and long-term visiting surgical team care perform a hearty vetting; disaster relief groups, often thrown together at the last minute, may be less thorough.

Ideally, surgeons and surgical organizations should participate in a multi-organization registry. There is a distinction between data used solely for internal quality improvement and registry data that may be published. Even information collected ostensi-bly for quality improvement needs to go through an institutional review board process prior to publication.

6. Informed Consent for Procedures

Informed consent is how Western medicine honors the principle of respect for patient autonomy. But how it should be applied in a developing country setting is not so well described. One guideline suggests "team members must tell the truth, respect the patient's autonomy, and deal justly with the patient."[6] This is a very Western view of informed consent, and the question of how it should be applied to patients in LMICs is vital.

On one hand, the goal for informed consent may be based on local culture for theoretical (it is respectful) and practical (it permits the patient to control the extent of communication) reasons. Not honoring local culture may confuse, scare, or cause distrust in the patient. On the other hand, volunteers must consider how local standards differ from home standards, whether it matters, and how it should be handled.

Obtaining consent through an interpreter, particularly a non-medical interpreter, loses nuance. Well-meaning interpreters may circumscribe the discussion out of respect for local cultures. Visiting teams bringing their own translator may improve the transmission of the informed consent. On the other hand, the presence of a foreigner may inhibit interactions.

In disaster relief, the goal is to save lives first, and this should not be at the expense of lengthy, involved written informed consent discussions. In these situations, informed consent should still be obtained, however, even if only verbally or implied. It is always important to remember that informed consent is not a piece of paper or a document; it is the discussion and understanding that results when the healthcare provider communicates with her patients.

If there is uncertainty with how best to obtain informed consent, then discussing the issue with local healthcare providers and partners who usually are from the culture and understand the issues is a good barometer to determine the best way forward. This, like many other issues surgeons encounter, is often made easier by working in partnership and building good local relationships and understanding of local culture.

Finally, just as patients in HICs have every right to refuse information, patients in LMICs have every right to do the same.[7]

7. Informed Consent for Research

Ethical research requires institutional review board approval at the local level. It may also require approval by any nongovernmental organization (NGO) involved, and by the home institution.[8,9] In addition, there is no place for "trying things out" that would otherwise not be done in the home institution. The flexibility that may be applied when obtaining informed consent from individual patients for treatment, particularly in disaster/emergency situations, does not apply to research. The primary distinction is that clinical interventions directly and clearly benefit the patient, while research does not. No claim of beneficence can therefore be made to permit deviation from applicable international research guidelines. In particular, given the desperate conditions, vulnerable patients will feel coerced to participate, regardless of assurances otherwise.

To fulfill ethical requirements, expectations and obligations of the research team members must be clear. It is often best to write these down for clarity and precision. This helps to avoid misunderstanding. In addition, all research projects should be done in partnership with local providers, and in fact some surgical journals are now requiring this for publication.

8. Confidentiality

The principle of confidentiality, which often goes hand-in-hand with informed consent, applies as it would in the home institution or home country. This may particularly apply with the telling of case studies to illustrate points and use of photographs with any patient-identifying characteristics. The patient must have given informed consent to this breach in confidentiality.

9. Patient and Institutional Costs

It is good practice to understand the costs that another surgeon or surgical team incurs from the host institution. These may be direct financial costs, such as the provision of anesthesia and analgesia, or personnel costs such as the removal of healthcare providers from their usual daily work to support the visiting surgical teams. There may also be indirect costs that can be more difficult to quantify. There may also be costs related to follow-up and complications at a later date. Out of respect for the local team and local providers, it is appropriate to attempt to quantify and address these costs. Ideally, teams should come with the anesthesia and analgesia they and the patients require, or be prepared to pay for it.

Patients, although assumed to be the beneficiaries of surgical trips, can also sustain significant individual costs. These are most obvious for elective surgery, where the patient often has to get transportation to the hospital or walk long distances, take time off work, bring family members with them for days, and may be required in some countries to pay for all the equipment and medicines needed during their hospital stay. Before the surgical team embarks on a trip abroad, there should be an attempt to address these issues so as to provide good care with minimal cost to both patient and hosts.

10. Training and Education

As stated above, training should be a mandatory and central part of any surgical trip abroad. The aim of provision of surgical care in trips to LMICs should be to build the local capacity and quality of care such that visiting trips eventually become unnecessary. This will not be achieved without training, education and long-term supervision, mentoring, and partnership. Again, the operative concept is accompaniment.

Training should be holistic and multidisciplinary, and include training of pre- and post-operative management, as well as support the training of theater and nursing staff, wound management, and analgesia. Identification of surgical patients by staff within rural clinics and decision-making around timing of surgery and those that would not benefit from an operation also form part of the training required. There should be plans for long-term mentoring, supervision, and continuing professional development.

11. Local and Cultural Considerations

Cultures differ. What is polite in one culture can be an abomination in another. To avoid offending or being offended, teams must be educated regarding local culture. Ideally, all team members should undergo orientation that should include understanding local customs and practices, as well as enough local language to greet, thank, and say good-bye at minimum.

12. Working with Other Local, Regional and Other NGO Initiatives

Trips are more likely to build successful sustainable partnerships if they incorporate and tailor the trip to work already ongoing in that region. It is worth seeking out other NGOs already working in the area and to ensure that work is not duplicative.

Ethical Aspirations

Those traveling abroad on visiting surgical team trips should aim to benefit patients and communities by good medical practice, creating partnerships, and developing self-sufficiency and sustainability.

Many goals are addressed by a continual or consistently reoccurring presence.[10] A primary goal should be to strengthen the host's healthcare systems.[4,6,11] This can be done at both the administrative and clinical levels. At the clinical levels, a long-term continuous or even intermittent presence of known clinicians working and teaching in the environment, in partnership with their local colleagues, promotes interpersonal respect and greater improvement. It is good for patient care, good for partnership development, and good for development of long-term sustainability, so long as that remains the end goal.

A second goal should be active coalescing of organizations and individual groups. Teamwork may decrease subtle or overt competition, may enable a better distribution of resources, and may enable better achievement of desirable standards.

COMMENTARY

Wangari Nyaga, Kenya

This chapter is written from a surgical point of view. I will add comments that pertain to anesthesiologists and anesthesia providers, because their situation may be unique.

Away from the major hospitals, anesthesia is provided by nonphysician anesthetists in many LMICs, including Kenya and Papua New Guinea. Anesthesia is often considered to be a "secondary" specialty, and it is not viewed with the same respect as surgery. Indeed, many people are surprised when they meet physicians who are trained anesthesiologists. The surgeon is usually a trained physician and often doubles up as the chief of the hospital. Usually, the surgeon runs the show in theater and everyone defers to his opinions. Not surprisingly, many trainee doctors only want to become surgeons. For this reason, it is important that visiting medical teams are viewed as a collaborative team in which ideas, opinions, and advice from both the surgeon and the anesthesiologist are respected and taken into account when making decisions about a difficult case. This can lead to change of perception so that, in the future, the input of the nonphysician anesthetist may be considered in perioperative care. Additionally, more trainee doctors may want to become anesthesiologists, which will ultimately enhance the development of pain medication and critical care.

Apart from providing patient care, the visiting global surgery team also acts as ambassadors for their country and profession. Specialty trainees will often be sent to work with the visiting team as a learning experience. The behavior of the visiting team members can be very influential to the junior doctors and medical students present, and can also attract trainees to a certain specialty. Because of the visiting team's potential impact, the actions of the team should reflect professionalism, mutual respect, cohesiveness, and adaptability.

In addition to equipment and pharmaceuticals, the visiting team should ask the local doctors what else is needed in terms of education. This may mean preparing lectures and educational material that can be presented to a wider audience, such as at the hospital grand rounds. Combined presentations by the anesthesiologist and the surgeon present a more balanced view of perioperative care. It can also be an invaluable learning experience for the visiting team as they learn from their hosts, including rationale for local practices.

As noted earlier in the chapter, partnership is important. The local team plays a vital role in public awareness prior to the visiting doctors' arrivals; otherwise, there would be no patients to be treated. This is especially important for specialized teams.

As there are no set guidelines for visiting teams, it can be difficult for them to prioritize cases. This process should be based on:

- Recommendation by the local surgeon, who is aware of cultural factors.

- Ability of local doctors to care for the patient. Difficult cases should be done earlier so that the patients can be cared for while the visiting team is still present.
- Patient travel. Perhaps patients who come from the remotest and farthest parts should be operated on first, as they may not present again when the team next visits. A disadvantage of this is that the local community may become resentful if their patients are turned away due to time constraints because the ones from farther away were operated on first.

A single visit from the team rarely helps more than a few patients and provides limited training. For this reason, a long-term commitment is most helpful. Repeat visits over time by the same team provides a longer follow-up period for complex cases; additional support in other areas of the hospital (e.g., equipment, consumables, and pharmaceuticals); more opportunities for continuing education; and long-term mentoring for junior trainees. However, this can create unwanted dependence, because many team visits are totally free to patients, but hospital care (at least in Kenya) costs a subsidized fee. For example, if patients know that a surgical team will visit yearly, patients may decide to wait for the next team visit instead of seeking medical care early.

The chapter mentions doing what you normally do in your practice, and I agree with this, although many anesthesiologists may be unfamiliar with practices in LMICs. Many anesthesiologists are unfamiliar with the drugs used in LMICs (e.g., halothane), and this needs to be considered when selecting an individual for a trip. To address this problem, there are now several courses on anesthesia in LMICs; they are offered in Australia, the United Kingdom, and the United States. There is also a concern of unfamiliarity with surgeons who may not have access to endoscopic equipment and are forced to do open operative procedures. To eliminate the problem of unfamiliarity with the local hospital's machines, some visiting teams choose to bring portable anesthesia machines that use sevoflurane. Additionally, this teaches local trainee anesthesiologists to use agents they normally do not use, thus increasing their exposure and knowledge.

In terms of ethics, it is important for visiting teams to be sensitive to the local culture. If the team is purely on a medical visit, it should refrain from sharing any religious or political views, as this can strain the relationship. Visiting teams should also be aware that the process of obtaining consent, including for taking patient photographs, may be unfamiliar. Many of the patients may be illiterate, and verbal consent may be all that is available. This should be recorded in the patients' notes and the team records. A thumbprint is also used in lieu of a signature. Consent may be a cultural issue as well and may be required to be given by a senior, often male, family member.

3

Developing Surgical Capacity: Models of Implementation

Regan Bergmark
Wendy Williams
Johanna N. Riesel
Doreen Nakku
Mack Cheney

The World's Missing Surgeons

Nascent health systems in many low- and middle-income countries (LMICs) are now beginning to grapple more formally with their burden of surgical disease. For several decades, surgery has taken a back seat to the challenges of human immunodeficiency virus (HIV) and malaria. Surgical disease is generally underfunded and has not to date received the energy and attention of the acquired immunodeficiency syndrome (AIDS) epidemic. When the HIV epidemic began, few considered that surgeons would look to the relative success of HIV funding, antiretroviral treatment, and public health programs as a model for noncommunicable disease. Emergency response systems, prompt diagnostic interventions, surgical access, safe anesthesia, postoperative care, and the many support services such as pathology and radiology are all components of effective surgical care. The systematic development of these essential components poses challenges and opportunity for surgical stakeholders.

The question is whether there is an effective way to mobilize resources in high-income countries (HICs) to support safe surgical care in LMICs. Infectious disease specialists, internal medicine physicians, and public health workers have fostered strong international collaborations and have paved the way for new levels of multi-site collaborations. In HIV this has allowed for training of physicians and other clinicians in LMICs, research, development of drug delivery systems, infrastructure development, and community outreach. "Vertical" systems focus on a single disease process, but the infrastructure developed can be used "diagonally" to impact related fields, including noncommunicable and surgical disease. Surgical and procedure- and technology-driven fields are among the last to build a significant "global health" presence. As we build surgical training programs that form on capacity building and are sustainable, we stand to learn from our colleagues who have focused on infectious disease and general public health.

This chapter focuses on models for developing systems of surgical care, with an emphasis on international collaboration and partnership. To date, most surgical models have included visiting surgical team trips, equipment donation, short courses and conferences, exchanges, and more recently robust academic collaborations. These collaborations bring together partners from HICs and LMICs. This chapter outlines the components of a surgical system: clinical care, research, teaching, ancillary services, infrastructure development, and public health. We also provide a description of the parties involved in developing surgical care, including national governments, academic centers, nongovernmental organizations (NGOs), individuals, and international governing bodies such as the World Health Organization (WHO). We briefly discuss funding of surgical systems and also provide specific examples of large-scale partnerships to build surgical capacity.

Direct Clinical Care and Traditional Surgical Missions

Directly caring for surgical patients has been the focus of global surgery for decades. The traditional visiting surgical team model—focused on one or a few surgeons and associated staff addressing a limited range of surgically correctable disease processes—has been a mainstay of providing support to healthcare systems in LMICs. In this model, case volume is emphasized, with the goal of completing a large number of cases in a limited period of time. Typically, the visiting surgical team model focused on a limited range of specific surgical challenges, such as cleft lip and palate, cataract surgery, burn care, and urologic or obstetric care.

Many surgical teams visit the same site(s) repeatedly, and the local surgical team becomes more involved in preoperative assessment and postoperative care. There is often some aspect of teaching, but teaching is usually not the primary goal and there is rarely a formal associated curriculum. Generally, the number and type of surgeries performed are logged, but thorough outcomes measures (as with many international surgical models) are rarely used. Many organizations are well seasoned in building high-volume visiting surgical team trips, such as Operation Smile and Smile Train. Over time their models have evolved to include more teaching and longer-term relationships with local sites or development of centers of excellence, all of which will be discussed below.

Visiting surgical team trips, particularly when run by an academic center, may also have training as a goal, but often it is the HIC resident who is the recipient of surgical training. Trips are seen as an opportunity to manage surgical disease not frequently managed in HICs or to perform a high volume of specific types of cases, such as cleft lip and palate, where more cases may be done in a week than some residents would see over the course of their residency or fellowship.

This model is quite specific to procedural, generally surgical, fields. Potential drawbacks include lack of long-term follow-up, limited pre- and post-operative care for some visiting surgical team trips, minimal teaching, and possible strain on system resources for other types of medical and surgical care during the trip itself. Direct surgical care brings a high level of specialty care but does not address the constant burden of general surgical disease or emergent surgical problems. Typically there are limited data on effectiveness and impact on the healthcare systems.

Surgical Training

Scarcity of surgical care is directly related to a lack of trained surgeons. The human resource needs in LMICs are daunting. Without surgeons it is challenging to train the next generation of surgeons. Training surgeons in the United States and Europe takes over a decade—4–8 years of undergraduate and medical school, and several years of surgical residency and fellowship. Surgery has preserved a guild-like apprenticeship system in HICs, in which apprentices are trained by specialized masters for several years. Apprentices alone, without surgical educators, are insufficient. Task sharing allows nonphysicians to perform traditional physician tasks, including surgery, but someone still must have the skill set to teach operative techniques.

Methods of instruction are similar in LMICs and HICs. Electronic resources including online books and atlases are widely available, and academic learning is often impressive. Conferences and simulation allow for further training. Hands-on experience in the operating room requires mentorship and repetition, and this is more difficult to coordinate in a system with few surgeons. Sabbaticals in HICs or surgeons traveling to areas where there are few surgeons can help support direct surgical training.

The goals of advancing surgical training are met in a variety of ways, including:

1. The creation of formal residency training programs within the country: These are most commonly developed in association with a medical school. Regional accreditation agencies are well established in many regions and are developing in others. Academic institutions in HICs often partner with a LMIC training program to help with a more robust faculty presence and increase teaching and research.

2. Professional societies and the development of regional excellence: Professional societies in each region have led the development of regional standards for training and practice, and often help to provide additional training opportunities. Regional centers can train surgeons who then return to their home to operate and train the next generation of surgeons.

3. Task-shifting surgical training: These surgical training programs are often supported by the local ministry of health, global organizations, or NGOs and focus on teaching critical surgical skills to nonsurgeons, such as general practitioners, nurses, or community health workers. Obstetric care has advanced significantly in some countries with task shifting to allow for safe labor and delivery.

Emphasis on Research

Surgical research in LMICs is in its infancy. There is a need for work in surgical disease pathophysiology and epidemiology, and assessment of surgical safety and surgical outcomes. Many of the above partnerships focused on training also provide support for LMIC research. Doctor Tollefson and Larrabee recommended a research focus on epidemiology, assessing the impact of surgical services with metrics such as the disability-adjusted life year (DALY), determining "benchmarks for quality of care" and assessing cost-effectiveness.[1] Increasing LMIC research capacity is critical. Some academic partnerships have successfully fostered the development of academic surgeons with strong research programs.

Partnerships with Professional Societies: Increasing Training, Surgical Standards, and Research

Medical societies have taken a growing role in the strengthening and standardizing of health systems in their local countries or regions. In addition to offering training opportunities and alternate accreditation programs, professional surgical societies are well placed to provide direct insight into determining the state of surgical capacity and infrastructure constraints. They have often done so in partnership with professional societies in HICs.

The College of Surgeons in East Central and Southern Africa (COSECSA) works with the Royal College of Surgeons in Ireland, the Royal College of Surgeons in Edinburgh, and the Associations of Surgeons of Great Britain and Ireland, among others, to support COSECSA's efforts to provide training programs and increase surgical capacity in its region of activity.[2] COSECSA has developed an accreditation program for surgeons in parallel to country-specific master's degree programs, designating training institutions throughout the region as functional "colleges without walls" and requiring the passing of formal final written and clinical examinations.[3] Working with the University of Toronto (UT), COSECSA provides fundamental support for East African surgeons who have utilized the Ptolemy Project, a program by which East African surgeons may become research affiliates of UT and thereby gain access to its electronic medical library, thereby buoying surgical research capacity.[4]

The Association for Academic Surgery in conjunction with the West African College of Surgeons has held Fundamentals of Surgical Research Courses to balance the continued loss of human and material resources resulting from emigration of medical and scientific personnel.[5] In Rwanda, the Rwanda Surgical Society has served as host for the inaugural Strengthening Rwanda Surgery Meeting, merging and harmonizing the agendas and resources of the foreign NGOs, governmental agencies, and academic medical centers with national counterparts to develop a rational strategy for addressing methods to improve surgical capacity in Rwanda.[6]

Nonphysician Training: Surgical Task Sharing

Shortages of trained health workers particularly impact LMICs. In addition to having fewer medical schools and postgraduate training programs, LMICs must deal with the "brain drain" imposed by emigration of health workers who successfully complete training.[7–10] An internal brain drain also occurs within countries as most physicians and surgeons choose to practice in urban areas and private hospitals, further limiting surgical access for the majority of the population.[11,12] The recent decades of generous international funding for research, training programs, and scholarships in infectious disease have further skewed these numbers, making careers in anesthesia and surgery less attractive for graduating medical students.[11] While all parties agree that developing the surgical and anesthesia infrastructure necessary to address the surgical burden of disease requires the sustainable production of fully trained surgical and anesthesia specialists, most hospitals and health centers currently rely on formal and informal task shifting as an interim solution.[13] Surgical task sharing involves the delegating of certain surgical procedures, such as caesarean sections, hernia repairs, wound care for trauma, and circumcision, to trained but less specialized healthcare workers.

Even without a formalized training program, surgical task sharing is a common practice resulting from understaffing, high patient load, and patients refusing to be referred to urban hospitals due to prohibitive costs.[13] Almost half of all countries in sub-Saharan Africa utilize nonphysician clinicians to perform minor surgical procedures. A survey of surgical rates in Uganda, Mozambique, and Tanzania found that higher surgical rates are likely attributable to greater reliance on mid-level providers as a major source of surgical care. In these countries, nurses, mid-level providers, and general practitioners provide the majority of surgical care, with nearly half of major surgeries performed by nonsurgeons.[14] Studies conducted in Mozambique, Malawi, and Niger show that surgical task shifting may provide access to essential surgical services where otherwise there would be none. Of interest, reviews on caesarean sections performed by nonphysician clinicians and physician specialists in hospitals in Mozambique, Niger, and Malawi show no significant difference in clinical outcomes.[12,15–17]

While task shifting has been shown to be a possible cost-effective, provisional solution to the lack of trained surgeons and anesthesiologists, there are causes for concern. In Uganda, a survey of healthcare managers and health workers showed support for surgical task shifting as a stopgap measure to address the shortage of human resources for health but showed concern with implementing such a policy without appropriate formalized regulations and guidelines, oversight, and support in terms of training, compensation, and resources.[13] While task sharing is already a widespread, informal component of the health system in much of Africa, it does not address existing staff deficits and, without proper supervision, may lead to risks for patients and staff. Absent time allowance for training and recognition of

greater responsibilities, task shifting also threatens to overburden in-country healthcare workers' existing workload.[18]

Case Study: Uganda and Global Partners in Anesthesia and Surgery: Establishment of a Larger Surgical and Anesthesia Residency Program[11]

Uganda is one of the world's poorest countries with a significant surgical workforce shortage and poor infrastructure. The Global Partners in Anesthesia and Surgery and Makerere University (GPAS-MU) collaboration was initiated by defining the reasons for the surgical workforce shortage. There are many reasons for poor access to surgical care. The workforce suffers from attrition to HICs and also from the internal pull away from clinical services to better-compensated and less frustrating positions in research, administration, and public health. Surgical and anesthesia training tends to be longer than for other fields. Compensation is poor in surgery, and there is relatively less funding for residency training (which residents must pay for themselves) than in well-funded fields such as infectious disease, internal medicine, and obstetrics/gynecology. "Poor infrastructure compromises quality of care and leads to demoralization of health care providers," and there is also concern for blood-borne pathogen exposure relative to other fields.[11]

There are two ways to gain surgical training in Uganda. The first is through traditional surgical residency programs in general surgery or a surgical subspecialty at one of the major medical universities: Makerere University College of Health Sciences in Kampala, Uganda; Mbarara University of Science and Technology in Mbarara, southwestern Uganda; or Uganda Martyrs University in Nkozi, Uganda, roughly 50 miles west of Kampala.[13] These surgical training programs include several years of residency training, undertaken after a combined undergraduate/medical school education and 1 year of service as a general medical officer. The second method is to be trained by COSECSA. COSECSA has provided an alternate training route for general medical officers through a 2-year "membership" program or a 5–6 year "fellowship" program, the second of which is similar to standard U.S. or Canadian training.[3] The goal of COSECSA in these programs is to provide increased training opportunities beyond the walls of the standard universities, with matched mentors and examination for entrance into the college at the end of training. COSECSA identifies hospitals where training takes place to allow residents to train away from the understaffed and under-resourced national referral center, for more oversight and supervision.

GPAS is a collaboration borne out of a partnership between Makerere University and Mulago Hospital in Uganda and University of California-San Francisco. This model "shift[s] away from the trainee exchange, equipment donation, and clinical service delivery models. Instead, it focuses on three locally identified objectives to improve surgical and perioperative care capacity in Uganda: workforce expansion, research, collaboration."[19] From 2007 to 2011 this project increased the number of surgical trainees from 20 to 40 and increased the number of anesthesia trainees from 2 to 19. More than 15 peer-reviewed collaborative papers were published, and a surgeon at Mulago was also awarded a research grant resulting in at least one publication.[19,20] They have also have seen an increase in retention of trainees regionally.

The success of this program has been in recruiting, training, and retaining an increasing number of surgeons and anesthesiologists. The partnership used a multipronged approach aimed at undergraduate and graduate education with an emphasis on clinical work and research. They introduced more surgical and anesthesia exposure early in medical school training, including community-based training, which is more hands-on. The GPAS partnership has developed research training including research of surgical treatment of HIV-infected patients.[11] Over the past several years they have developed a "Senior Scholar" position for anesthesia and also for surgery for a graduating resident to continue as a chief resident for 1 year with a focus on teaching the younger residents and mentoring research. In 2012 an orthopedic Senior Scholar position was also awarded.

In spite of these efforts, there is still limited surgical care outside of Kampala. GPAS has used surgical camps in the past—much like in-country visiting surgical team trips—to operate in regions away from the capital for 1 to 2 weeks at a time.[11] This strategy seems to have the same advantages and disadvantages as visiting surgical team trips. Subspecialists have also reached out to more rural regions of Uganda. There were initially efforts to improve the health subdistrict surgical capacity, particularly for obstetric care, but by 2004-2005 only 20 percent of these sites were operational. New partnerships are being established to help develop surgical capacity and training in other parts of the country, including a partnership between Harvard Medical School, Massachusetts Eye and Ear Infirmary, and Massachusetts General Hospital with Mbarara University of Science and Technology-Mbarara Regional Referral Hospital in Mbarara, Uganda.

GPAS states that "Because a purely academic-based model was unable to provide enough funding or dedicated faculty time to support these projects, volunteers were recruited, partnerships were sought, and financial support was obtained through research grants, philanthropic contributions, and local government."[19] GPAS now works with the Association of Anesthetists of Great Britain and Ireland, Mulago Hospital Departments of Anesthesia and Surgery, the Ugandan Ministry of Health, the Mulago Foundation, and many other donors.[21]

Infrastructure Development

Even when surgeons are available to teach, there must be a sufficient volume of cases such that new residents or clinicians can obtain the necessary operative training. That means a sufficient referral or self-referral network, operating room space and equipment, safe anesthesia, and ancillary services such as pathology and radiology to facilitate appropriate diagnosis. A surgical system works only with these components in place.

Equipment donation has also been a strategy for enhancing surgical capacity, but with varying success. Equipment is often shipped or donated with noble intentions; however, no one knows how to use it or repair it: a microscope light burns out and there is no replacement, the CT scanner uses too much power. Basic equipment needs to be available that the users know how to use, take care of, and repair or replace.

Supply line issues are especially important for drug and equipment delivery, particularly for safe anesthesia that is required for safe surgery. Operating rooms need to be available, as well as space for preoperative triage and evaluation and postoperative management. Safe operating rooms also need to include appropriate monitoring equipment and allow postoperative monitoring.

Electronic medical records, whose implementation has been no small feat in HICs like the United States, have also made inroads into LMICs. Tracking, outcomes evaluation, and quality improvement may all potentially be facilitated by electronic records. At minimum, a records system that is of high fidelity and allows patients to be tracked over time is essential, particularly for longer-term problems requiring extensive surgical treatment and monitoring such as oncologic disease.

Ancillary services essential to safe surgery include anesthesia and drug delivery/pharmaceutical access. For cancer surgery, pathology is critical for diagnosis and appropriate treatment. Hospitals with limited pathology often have more extended wait times for curative cancer surgery. Radiologic evaluation is helpful but requires working radiographic equipment, radiation safety knowledge, and expertise with image interpretation. Other ancillary services critical for larger operative cases include a functional and safe blood bank, and an effective laboratory including microbiology.

Telemedicine will play an increasingly important role. Telemedicine allows for consulting on difficult cases remotely, remote teaching, as well as shared conferences such as tumor boards, which allow for collaboration and the sharing of expertise.

More broad-based health systems interventions are beyond the scope of this chapter but involve the creation of hospital and health center networks, referral centers, and emergency response systems. Public health efforts to prevent surgical disease, such as traffic safety, smoking prevention, and cooking safety for burn prevention, are also critical.

Stakeholders

The most critical actors in global surgery are surgeons and parasurgical personnel in LMICs. Academic institutions, academies, and consortia support the field. Academic journals may also collaborate; for example, *The Lancet* recently conducted a commission on global surgery. Local and national government, ministries of health, and international bodies such as the WHO and World Bank may support the development of functional healthcare systems in LMICs.

Funding

The funding of global surgery activity is rapidly evolving. The catalytic philanthropist, government, and NGO funding available for projects in HIV and public health is often not available to programs or research addressing surgical activities. Global surgery shares its roots with more traditional forms of visiting surgical team work and thus is primarily self-funded or supported through individual and corporate donors. Over the last decade, large-scale traditional visiting surgical teams such as Operation

Smile and ReSurge International have added surgical training components including the building of specialized surgical centers in LMICs and on-site physician training programs that are funded through their pre-existing donor network.[22–24] Many of the long-running partnerships between hospitals in the developing world and academic medical centers in HICs began as relationships formed by individual surgeons and only later became associated with institutions.

Academic medical centers have also supported their own faculty members' initiatives through internal funding. At Duke, the Department of Surgery provides five annual global surgery grants for Duke surgical faculty and has supported a variety of programs including neurosurgical capacity-building in Uganda and short-term surgical interventions.[25,26] Some funding and resource sharing results from collaborations among multiple departments, as the University of Virginia's Global Surgery Initiative works with UVA Telemedicine and its Center for Telehealth to support its educational teleconference sessions with the Kigali Health Institute in Rwanda.[27] Even those programs associated with academic institutions derive much of their funding from private sources, utilizing web-based fundraising tools such as direct online donations through websites or crowdsourcing tools and the traditional fund-raising strategies of benefits and galas.[28,29]

As global surgery has been increasingly recognized as an academic field, a few academic fellowships have become available, including the Paul Farmer Global Surgery Clinical and Research Fellowships, the Center for Surgery and Public Health's Arthur Tracy Cabot Fellowship, the AAS/AASF Global Surgery Research Fellowship, and the Operation Smile–based Regan Fellowships, all with a wide range of funding sources. The Paul Farmer Fellowships' funding is balanced among Boston Children's Hospital, Partners in Health, and the Harvard Medical School through its Program in Global Surgery and Social Change.[30] The AAS/AASF Fellowship is funded by the Association for Academic Surgery and the corresponding Foundation through the generosity of its members.[31] The Operation Smile Fellowship is funded by private donors.[32] Corporate funding, specifically funding provided by medical device companies, has been a longtime partner for traditional visiting surgical team trips and remains so as these programs develop more formalized capacity-building elements. The Karl Storz Head and Neck Fellowship at Cape Town University is funded by the Storz Foundation and provides the only opportunity that we know of for fellowship-level head and neck training in sub-Saharan Africa.[33]

At this time, there is limited funding available from the major financiers of global health for surgical capacity-building programs. While the most recent reports from the 2010 Global Burden of Disease Study highlight the growing threat that noncommunicable disease poses on global health, most funding remains directed toward HIV/AIDS, malaria, tuberculosis, or "neglected diseases."[34–36] A handful of smaller foundations, such as Ronald McDonald House Charities, have begun to embrace training initiatives and other surgical capacity-building projects such as IVUmed, a program in association with the University of Utah that has been dedicated to teaching urology in HICs for almost 20 years.[37]

Conclusions

Developing human resource capacity, research, infrastructure, and ancillary services will require sustained effort and investment. Although the magnitude of unmet surgical need is daunting, there are successful models for developing surgical capacity, research, and infrastructure. Training skilled surgeons can be facilitated through twinning programs, academic, and public-private partnerships. Training partnerships are becoming more widespread, but research on effectiveness is sparse. Understanding the unmet needs of communities in LMICs requires increased effort in surgical disease epidemiology. Systems of surgical care require many ancillary services to work together in concert. Surgical outcomes measures need to be more widely tested and implemented to facilitate safe surgical practice. These research needs may be best met if there is significant in-country research capacity. Emphasis should be placed on sharing best practices and evaluation of outcomes. Close evaluation of programs aimed at improving surgical capacity will be critical for ensuring access to safe surgery for all.

Case Study: Human Resources for Health

Human Resources for Health (HRH) is an internationally recognized initiative to strengthen and expand the global health workforce to meet the world's health needs. The WHO has created a department focused on increasing the availability of appropriately trained and accessible health workers to populations around the globe. Recognizing that health delivery cannot be accomplished without infrastructure, financial support, and educated personnel, WHO has taken a systems approach to increasing accessible health care in the post–2015 Millennium Development Goals era.[38] A number of other organizations have also been involved in health systems strengthening, but one notable example is that of the Rwandan Ministry of Health, which has employed the fundamental principles of HRH in a country-wide 7-year plan to upgrade the Rwandan surgical workforce on a national level.

The Rwandan HRH

The Rwandan Human Resources for Health Program HRH was launched in July of 2012 in an effort to generate high-quality sustainable health care for the people of Rwanda by the year 2020. Its vision was born out of collaboration with the Rwandan Government, the Rwandan Ministry of Health, the U.S. Government, and several U.S. institutions as a means to address the need for a larger, more capable and sustainable health workforce in Rwanda.[39]

At the time of this publication, program leadership felt it was too early to report the definitive outcome or impact of the HRH program. However, its very nascency and inherent uniqueness has catapulted Rwanda to the forefront of global health delivery as a potentially reproducible paradigm of successful collaboration in global health systems strengthening.

The Way It Works

Twenty-three U.S. institutions (USI) are partnered with the HRH program to form teaching and mentoring relationships in areas of medicine, nursing and midwifery, dentistry, and health management (see appendix below). Each USI recruits educators in a variety of fields that align with the training needs identified by the Rwandan medical education leadership. USI faculty are specialists who reside in Rwanda, generally for year-long appointments, to help provide high-quality hands-on clinical education. The program is largely predicated on teaching and mentoring. Mentees include the Rwandan post-graduate trainees as well as the faculty from the University of Rwanda College of Medicine and Health Sciences (also known as the "College Faculty"). This partnership takes the form of twinning, a term used to describe the close co-directional mentorship between one U.S. specialist and one Rwandan partner. The USI faculty focuses on a variety of topics ranging from current standards of care to effectual teaching methods. In turn, the USI faculty benefit from the contextual expertise of the College Faculty and trainees in order to modify delivery of care with a focus on local-regional realities in Rwanda. Ideally, these academic collaborations between the USI and Rwandan institutions will forge lasting relationships that will result in long-term impact on local human resources. Through dedicated education, the Rwandan workforce has the ability to expand, thereby addressing the crucial need for a larger, more capable health workforce. This serves to strengthen their residency programs as well as the various departments' abilities to train future specialists via strengthening pedagogy, research skills, administrative skills, and clinical skills.

The USI medical faculty are initially located at the four major referral hospitals in Rwanda (King Faisal Hospital, Centre Hospitalier Universitaire de Kigali [CHUK], Centre Hospitalier Universitaire de Butare [CHUB], and Rwanda Military Hospital). In subsequent years, they will expand to provincial and district hospitals that will be designated as teaching hospitals. The nursing and midwifery faculty are largely at the School of Nursing in addition to the district hospitals where the largest volume of maternal and gynecologic cases is managed. Professional oral health experts are stationed at the new School of Dentistry, working closely with Rwandan faculty to facilitate training. Finally, the health management advisors work mostly with CHUK and the School of Public Health.[40]

In the first year of the program, 91 faculty members from U.S. institutions partnered with 90 Rwandan colleagues across four referral hospitals; seven district hospitals; and eight schools of medicine, nursing and midwifery, and public health.[41]

As the program continues to mature, the goal remains to influence the development of high-quality, sustainable healthcare that will continue once the U.S. partners phase out in 2020.

Funding

The program is nearly entirely funded by the U.S. federal government through the U.S. Agency for International Development (USAID), the U.S. President's Emergency Plan for AIDS Relief (PEPFAR), the Centers for Disease Control and Prevention (CDC), and The Global Fund. The Clinton Health Access Initiative (CHAI) plays a critical unfunded role in providing structural support to the Rwandan Ministry of Health and implementation of the project. Interestingly, this does not represent new funding to Rwanda but rather a reallocation of funds previously committed to Rwanda via third-party consulting agencies, many of them nonprofit organizations. Another novelty of the program is that funds from the U.S. government are granted directly to the Government of Rwanda's Ministry of Health. This arrangement allows funds to be more closely aligned with Rwandan national priorities and health strategy, and results in low overhead fees for the U.S. government.[42] At the end of the 7 years, the Rwandan government hopes to be able to support the program without the assistance of foreign aid by catering to wider catchments of patients as a result of their high-quality care.

Pros and Cons of This Approach

Pros: The Rwandan HRH is unique in that it has created a plan for independence and sustainability. In addition, it ensures that funding is aligned with national goals and health planning. This allows a focus to be placed on high-yield, dedicated education that is designed to continue to pay for itself in the years to come. With the benefit of a 7-year trajectory, the HRH's immediate focus can be on the needs of organizing training programs while maintaining a long-term trajectory of staffing capable and effective health facilities. Its most obvious strength lies in its mission to position Rwandan nationals to be able to address the growing burden of disease with the highest standards of care for the Rwandan people. Doing so by means of sustained relationships between visiting faculty with long-term engagements and Rwandan nationals with a focus on education makes this program a dynamic example of collaboration and systems strengthening.

Cons: This arrangement is not necessarily scalable to other countries with only one nation as the sole provider of financial and educational support. The amount of financial support and resources required to orchestrate such a program in just one country is formidable, yet feasible, as Rwanda is potentially demonstrating. Extending similar programs to additional LMICs may be realistic with dedicated input from other HICs. In other words, the Rwanda HRH program may be able to serve as a model for future collaborations between other LMICs and HICs, but ensuring other sources of twinning faculty and funding may be a challenge. The U.S. government is likely to be able to reproduce such programs in other countries on a continuing basis only if it adopts a similar model of direct funding to ministries of health with good governance in an effort to align with local national goals, decrease funder overhead, and continue zero-sum funding.

APPENDIX: United States Institutions currently partnered with Rwanda HRH Program (10/01/13)

Medicine

- Albert Einstein College of Medicine at Yeshiva University
- Rhode Island Hospital at Brown University
- University Medicine Foundation at Brown University
- University Emergency Medicine Foundation at Brown University

- Columbia University
- Duke University School of Medicine
- Geisel School of Medicine at Dartmouth
- Harvard Medical School
- Brigham and Women's Hospital
- Boston Children's Hospital
- Beth Israel Deaconess Hospital
- University of Texas Medical Branch
- University of Virginia School of Medicine
- Yale School of Medicine

Nursing

- Duke University School of Nursing
- Howard University School of Nursing

- New York University College of Nursing
- University of Illinois at Chicago College of Nursing
- University of Texas Health Science Center at Houston
- University of Maryland School of Nursing

Health Management

- Yale University Global Health Leadership Institute

Oral Health

- Harvard School of Dental Medicine
- University of Maryland at Baltimore

COMMENTARY

Nobhojit Roy, India
Nakul Raykar, USA

The authors have done an excellent job summarizing the key issues in building surgical capacity. Meaningful surgical systems strengthening requires a systematic framework approach for improvements based on local context and provides example opportunity for partnership between HICs and LMICs. Visiting surgical teams, for example, can help boost confidence in local surgical teams that planned and elective procedures can be safely performed in their environment. The more important component of emergency surgery, though, remains a challenge that is not addressed by visiting surgical teams. Instead, coordinated funding and prioritization across the health system is necessary to establish comprehensive surgical care for all citizens, year-round.

Collaborative research, though, may be the most important partnership between HICs and LMICs. The published literature, after all, drives policy change and opinions, and the absence of the LMIC voice should be of significant concern. The LMIC limitations to research capacity include slow Internet access, licensing agreements putting most academic articles behind a paywall, inadequate proficiency with the English language for academic writing and, perhaps most significantly, harried clinical schedules with minimal administrative support. Here, systematic research partnerships between HICs and LMICs focusing on context-appropriate research could provide high value. HICs would contribute high-quality methodology and scientific writing skills, and LMICs would provide large clinical loads and relevant research questions.

Section II

Anesthesia

4

Preparing for a Trip: OR Management

Craig D. McClain

Introduction

Practitioners who are used to working in operating rooms in high-income countries (HICs) may be amazed when they see what can serve as an operating room (OR) in many parts of the less developed world. It is crucial for anesthesia providers to adjust their expectations and focus on how to provide safe and effective care in these challenging environments.[1] Therefore, before leaving their home country, the team must have a realistic understanding of what physical and human resources will be available and plan accordingly. It is imperative for the success of the trip that these unique considerations are planned for before the anesthesiology team leaves their home country. Successful trips have primary plans for the daily running of the OR as well as multiple contingency plans to attempt to optimize the provision of safe care. This chapter will address many questions that anesthesiologists must deal with when organizing a short-term visiting surgical team trip. This chapter will not specifically address the different implications of setting up and managing an OR during a disaster response as that is outside the scope of this discussion.

Setting up a perioperative system is arguably the most important aspect of a short-term trip (Figure 4.1). Without a functioning system in place, safety and efficiency suffers.[2–4] This aspect of care needs to be within the context of a perioperative environment that is already unfamiliar to visiting healthcare providers. There are areas that need to be considered when setting up a system: pre-trip team building, defining team expectations and roles, and assessment of human and physical resources.

Preparation

Familiarity with the other team members prior to arrival at the destination is extremely valuable.[5–7] It is recommended that the members of the team meet (preferably in person but at least via conference call or virtual meeting) at some point prior to the trip. This meeting should provide opportunity for the team members to get to know one another as well as laying down the expectations and roles of each person. Questions and concerns of each team member should be addressed. Leaders within each specialty—surgery, anesthesiology, nursing, etc.—will be identified as well as principles by which the entire team will function on the trip. Consensus on these underlying principles is necessary to ensure both safety and efficiency of care.

One of the guiding principles behind successful short-term visiting surgical team trips is equity among visiting care providers. For example, any team member should have the authority to cancel a case or initiate a thorough discussion of the risks and benefits of proceeding with the case. No team member should be pressured into doing something that is against his or her clinical judgment. The open practice of this principle also serves as a strong positive model for all involved, including less experienced team members and local caregivers. This principle should be defined and agreed upon prior to embarking on the trip.

Other information that needs to be collected before the trip includes the physical makeup of the facilities and identification of local contacts that will aid the team. Questions need to be answered to ensure the safe and efficient delivery of anesthetic care. Information that needs to be obtained includes:

1. Target population. Anesthesiologists will plan and prepare for a pediatric cleft trip much differently than they would for an adult burn trip.

2. Plan for anesthetic delivery. Providers should be clear about the overall plan. Will procedures be done under general anesthesia, regional, or a combination thereof? If general anesthesia will be utilized, will it be via inhaled or intravenous agents? If inhaled agents, is a circle system available or will Mapleson circuits be used? If intravenous agents, are there functional pumps available or the ability to set up drip infusions?

3. Number of simultaneous tables being run. This will influence the size of the team (see below). It is also important to clarify if there will be a local/sedation table, and if the presence of an anesthesiologist at this table is necessary.

4. Anesthesia machines and monitoring equipment. The presence, type, and quality of this equipment at the local site must be assessed prior to the trip and supplemented if necessary. See Figure 4.2.

5. Local availability of controlled drugs. It is crucial to know the medications and IV fluids that are locally available. A reliable local individual must be identified to serve as a liaison for obtaining these things prior to and throughout the trip.

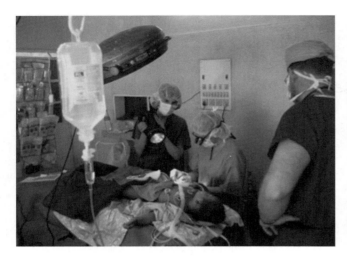

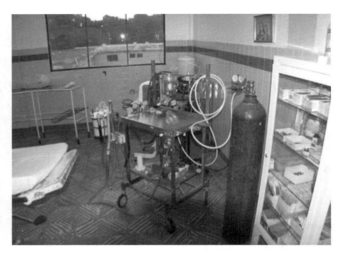

FIGURE 4.1 OR setup typical in LMICs. An OR setup by a team visiting a hospital in Northern India in 2003. Note the lack of reliable electricity and need to improvise lighting with a flashlight. Note also the use of a Mapleson circuit for delivery of inhaled anesthetic agent. In this particular site, there were no anesthesia providers whatsoever. The OR was simply a room in the district hospital with enough space to accommodate two surgical tables. The visiting team had to be completely independent. The team brought all equipment necessary for safe surgery and anesthesia, including instruments, sterilization systems, monitors, vaporizers, and other disposables. Only oxygen and controlled drugs were supplied by the hosts, as they could not provide anything else. Image by Craig D. McClain.

FIGURE 4.2 Anesthesia machine. This depicts a rudimentary anesthesia machine typical of many developing country settings. Image by Craig D. McClain.

6. Local availability of medical-grade oxygen. The team must know whether oxygen will be supplied via cylinders or wall. Wall oxygen is exceedingly rare in developing world settings. If by cylinder, it is useful to bring a wrench and regulator as they may not be available at the site.

7. Local host and liaison. This person will be the contact when issues arise and should be in a political position within the local community to help the visiting team address these issues.

8. Operating and recovery space. Such knowledge will influence case selection and perioperative management.

9. OR access. It needs to be clear if the team will have access to the ORs throughout the day, or if they will be sharing with other surgical teams or local providers.

10. Didactic and teaching opportunities. Close interaction with local providers should be fostered. This interaction can come in many forms, including sharing of clinical responsibilities or bedside exchange of ideas. Often, there will be an opportunity to provide formal, didactic education to local, interested parties. It is useful to try to determine what topics for such lectures would be most useful to local providers before the trip.

The acquisition of such information is helpful for all team members, and can be expanded upon for surgeon preparation. Namely, such preparation should include investigating if there are adequate and appropriate instruments locally, the type of sterilization equipment available, as well as the presence of adequate stock of suture locally. The results of these investigations will determine how much and what type of equipment the surgeons need to bring to perform the procedures safely and effectively.

Surgeons and anesthesia providers must also have a clear understanding of how patients are gathered for evaluation for surgery. Crucial questions involving the patients include:

1. Who are the patients? Most team members engage in these types of trips to help poor people with surgical needs who would be otherwise unable to get such treatment without visiting surgical team intervention. The makeup of the patients needs to be clarified before the trip.

2. How were they gathered? There are a number of methods used to advertise these types of trips to the local population. Some of these methods include posting notices, actively recruiting in rural areas, or simply keeping lists of surgically correctable problems among patients. Knowledge of the method of patient recruitment is important because it will give the provider insight into other issues that surround patient care—potential comorbidities, nutritional issues, transportation concerns, and potential problems with follow-up.

3. Was there any pre-screening prior to the clinic day? Additionally, it must be clear how thorough this medical evaluation was, and the provider level responsible for the evaluation, prior to the team's arrival. Documentation of the evaluation can be requested prior to the trip.

4. Who funds patient travel, food, etc.? This is certainly something that should concern care providers. If a patient is scheduled for several days after the initial screening clinic but lives 10 hours away, will he/she go home and return, or will simply stay and wait? If the patient stays, can he/she, and his/her family, afford lodging and food during the interim?

5. How will follow-up occur? Lack of follow-up is an all too common problem in these environments, and care providers must be proactive in establishing a reasonable system for post-trip care and evaluation. Who will be following up with these patients? How will the visiting surgeons be kept in the loop?

6. What are the contingency plans for complications? In high-income countries (HICs), we are used to having multiple levels of backup in the case of misadventure, such as rapidly accessible diagnostic imaging, specialists available for consultation, and intensive care units. These things are often a luxury or nonexistent in the less developed world. Availability of such services will affect care providers regarding the cases performed and medical conditions they are willing to treat.

Failure to address these issues until arrival in the host country makes the entire process much more complicated and potentially unsafe. Proper preparation will contribute tremendously to the success of the trip, satisfaction of the participants, trust- and relationship-building among the local community, and, most importantly, the safety of the patients.

Human Resources

Trip goals should focus more on quality of care, safety, education, and interaction with local practitioners than on simply performing large numbers of cases. Fortunately, this is rapidly becoming the focus of short-term visiting surgical team trips. An emphasis on sheer case volume can lead to compromises in quality and safety and can sidestep development of the local medical system. Investments in building partnerships with local providers through education, both through formal didactics and informal teaching at the bedside, and shared care responsibilities are invaluable to the long-term sustainability of the local medical system. As an additional but important benefit, effective partnerships with local practitioners can yield future capacity improvement and cost savings for local practitioners and international visiting teams.

The planned number of simultaneous surgical procedures will help determine the size and makeup of the team. Veteran anesthesiologists of these types of visiting surgical team trips recommend that the necessary number of anesthesia providers be the planned number of tables plus one (at least). For example, if the plan is to bring two surgeons and run two operating tables at a time, the number of anesthesia providers should be three. This allows the constant availability of a helpful pair of hands without diverting attention from another patient. The extra person provides another anesthesiologist for induction, airway management, and resuscitation in the event that there is a misadventure. The availability of a "plus one" anesthesia provider also allows a free person to serve other roles:

1. Engage local anesthesia providers and help to integrate the visiting team into the local perioperative structure.
2. Help turn over the OR between cases by replacing anesthesia circuits, cleaning necessary equipment, drawing up fresh drugs, etc., while the anesthesiologists directly delivering the anesthetic can focus on the patient and safely delivering him or her to the recovery area.
3. Address preoperative and PACU issues.
4. Engage in teaching in the perioperative space, especially related to preoperative evaluation and postoperative pain management.

5. Aid in OR management, including addressing workflow issues and changes to the planned schedule.

The surgeons, anesthesiologists, and nurses participating in the care of patients for elective humanitarian trips should be familiar with care for similar patient populations in their everyday practice. For example, it is inappropriate for an anesthesiologist who never cares for small children in her daily practice to go to a low- or middle-income country (LMIC) and care for such patients. Likewise, a surgeon who does not routinely engage in cleft lip repairs domestically should not be performing these procedures on poor kids in the less developed world.

Anesthesia providers should be well versed in delivery of the type of care (e.g., OR anesthesia, regional anesthesia, etc.) they will be providing in the LMIC. Independent practitioners should be board certified or in the process of examination. The Volunteers in Plastic Surgery guidelines echo these sentiments.[4] It is perfectly acceptable (and should be encouraged) for trainees to participate in this type of care, but they should be supervised to the same level that they would be in their home countries. This should not be an environment where trainees practice completely independently. This would not be considered ethical in the United States, United Kingdom, or Canada and should not be acceptable in a less developed country.

Team members should be adaptable and flexible. Practitioners who are extremely rigid and feel unsafe without significant human, facility, and/or equipment backup will not thrive in an LMIC. With the growing general interest in global healthcare delivery, this cannot be stressed enough. Practitioners who do not feel comfortable practicing in such an environment can still get involved by helping cover cases at home for travelling providers or delivering lectures via the Internet to local practitioners at the destination site. Team members should be able to work effectively with other specialties while setting strong positive examples of the team approach to local care providers. Grandstanding and overt displays of ego in the OR are profoundly detrimental to these endeavors and have no place in these settings.

In an LMIC, all care providers will experience stress from a variety of pressures, including but not limited to unfamiliarity, food- and water-borne illness, a level of poverty many are unused to, different living conditions, and the sheer volume of work. The level of stress experienced by teams is often underestimated due to the generally positive experiences people report. It can be quite difficult to be far from home, working in an unfamiliar and stressful environment with unfamiliar equipment, eating unfamiliar food, and dealing with a completely different culture. Team leaders must identify team members whose reaction to such conditions prevents them from performing their role in patient care. It is useful for team leaders to ensure there is adequate decompression time from the direct patient care and opportunities, as a group, to discuss any troubling issues. Leaders should take note of any member who isolates him- or herself and is unwilling to engage in nonmedical group activities such as meals or visits to the homes of the hosts. This can be a sign that the individual is having a difficult time processing the conditions around him or her. Leaders should be prepared to identify these individuals and speak to them privately about their feelings regarding the trip.

Physical Resources

The physical resources of a hospital and operating theater in the developing world may be quite different from those in the more developed world. It is important to have a concept of the limitations that the local operating room and hospital will present prior to leaving one's home country. These limitations will dictate the types of cases that can safely be undertaken, the support available in case of misadventure, the method of anesthesia delivery, the hours that can be worked, and instrument sterilization techniques, among other things. Further, one needs to consider how the presence of a foreign team affects the daily operation of the hospital. Will ORs be closed to allow the visiting team to operate? Will a number of hospital beds be set aside for the team that otherwise would have been utilized? What impact will the team have on the host facility?

Specifically, the team must decide together which cases can safely be done based on this information. If there is no wall oxygen, reliable electricity, or clean running water, the types of cases must be adjusted to reflect these limitations. It would be wise to avoid cases with large amounts of anticipated blood loss, as there is unlikely to a blood bank available. Some hospitals may not have 24-hour staffing for inpatient beds, relying instead on family members to offer basic care after hours. It would be prudent to plan only on cases that could be done as day surgery cases in such a situation. The ability to admit postoperative patients to a staffed floor, or even an intensive care unit, allows a completely different approach to patient care.

OR Management

An individual should be designated daily to be in charge of running the OR. This individual ensures maximum efficiency and safety in the schedule, manages the inevitable daily schedule issues, addresses the preoperative issues on the day of surgery, and deals with the care of the postoperative patients. Rotating the person who serves in this capacity also provides a break from operative care, helping to keep clinicians fresh for cases later in the trip. The anesthesiologist in charge is in an ideal position to deal with common problems such as securing adequate pharmaceutical supplies locally and assuring an adequate oxygen supply. This person can function as the "plus one" anesthesiologist as discussed above. It is common for teams to rotate this responsibility daily among all the anesthesiologists.

The team concept cannot be stressed enough. Self-sufficiency is valuable as well as the ability to multitask. An individual who can do multiple things to help facilitate success is extremely valuable. A mentality of "that's not my job" should be completely unacceptable. Scrub nurses, circulators, anesthesiologists, and surgeons can all facilitate the work of their team members. This may mean that surgeons are taking personal responsibility for their instrument selection and helping with transport, nurses are helping to turn the room over between cases, and anesthesiologists are involved with instrument cleaning and sterilization. A successful trip depends on a strong team dynamic where each member is able to fill multiple roles while being an expert in his or her own specialty.

COMMENTARY

Clover Ann Lee, South Africa

We spend a lot of time during our training and careers referring to "standards" and "norms." It has been my experience that the "textbook" norms, as defined in HICs, are often completely different from those in LMICs, making adequate preparation and communication essential. It is worthwhile to talk to local doctors when you arrive to find out about the local health problems. Let them advise you as to what is considered normal. For example, in a community where malnutrition, malaria, or worms are rife, the majority of children will be anemic by our textbook definitions, but run around happily and are fit for anesthesia. In the same way, children who seem really small for their age and almost fall off standard growth charts may be entirely normal for that region.

When working with the local healthcare providers, there may be barriers in language and education. Language is the most significant challenge for me, and I have found that learning a few basic greetings goes a long way. In terms of education, anesthesia providers may be nurses, who may have only basic medical training; this means that a teaching program designed for someone with advanced medical training is not very helpful. I have been asked to teach nurses how to read an electrocardiogram, and then found that they don't know any basic cardiovascular physiology. We spent the week examining each others' hearts!

Leave your assumptions at home, and don't forget to take spare laryngoscope batteries, antidiarrheals, and plenty of photographs.

5

Pharmacology of Commonly Used Drugs

Leal G. Segura

Introduction

Urban and rural facilities in low- and middle-income countries (LMICs) frequently face shortages of medications and personnel considered essential to anesthetic care in the more developed world. Planning successful anesthetics requires an understanding of these limited resources. Anesthetic plans should also be tailored to this environment, aiming for quick recoveries without the need for frequent postoperative intervention. Clinicians should anticipate shortages and consider bringing their own supplies of essential anesthetic drugs. However, it is important to note that the transport of controlled drugs (e.g., opioids) abroad without proper authorization may be considered illegal. Further, bringing uncommonly used drugs or agents that are not widely available in destination countries limits the ability of visiting clinicians to educate local providers, who will not have access to these medications after the visitor has left. Finally, it is becoming increasingly common for nations to not allow expired drugs through customs, so providers should be aware of this fact as well when planning a visiting surgical team trip.

Inhalational Agents

Inhaled anesthetics are mainstays of anesthetic practice in the more developed world but are often unavailable in LMICs because of cost, inconsistent delivery, and transport issues. Even if supplies of inhaled anesthetics and machines do exist, functional vaporizers to administer them may not, as facilities may lack either the funds or expertise required for their ongoing calibration and maintenance.

In anticipation of anesthesia machines in various states of repair and inconsistent supplies of inhaled anesthetics, those planning anesthetic care in an LMIC should familiarize themselves with the anesthesia machine at the destination facility (if one exists at all), and know which agents and vaporizers (if any) are available. Halothane and ether, which have virtually disappeared from modern anesthetic practice in the more developed world, remain the only available inhaled agents available in many countries.[1-3] Reviewing the pharmacology, hazards, and practical aspects of handling of these agents is essential to unfamiliar providers.

Halothane

Halothane is a volatile halogenated alkane derivative that is rarely used in the more developed world, but it remains the least expensive volatile agent and the most common inhaled anesthetic agent available in many LMICs.

Pharmacodynamics and Pharmacokinetics

Halothane is a relatively soluble anesthetic agent with a sweet, nonpungent odor that makes it suitable for inhalation inductions. Despite its higher solubility, it undergoes greater biotransformation and therefore faster elimination than isoflurane.

The minimal alveolar concentration (MAC) of halothane is 0.75% (1.1% in infants), and it demonstrates a predictable dose-dependent decrease in blood pressure secondary to direct myocardial depression; 2 MAC results in a 50% decrease in cardiac output. Junctional rhythms and bradycardia are common at higher doses, occurring secondary to slowing of sinoatrial node conduction. It also sensitizes the heart to the arrhythmogenic effects of epinephrine, and ventricular arrhythmias are more common than with other volatile agents, particularly in the presence of hypercarbia.

Technical Considerations

Halothane is non-explosive and nonflammable, but it reacts with many metals in the presence of moisture, and rubber and some plastic products will erode when in contact with halothane, in either its vapor or liquid form. Halothane contains thymol as a stabilizer, which can accumulate in vaporizers after use, causing dysfunction of the vaporizer itself or discoloration of the remaining liquid. If discoloration occurs, the liquid should be discarded.

Isoflurane and Sevoflurane

Many facilities in LMICs will have limited, inconsistent, or non-existent supplies of more familiar agents like isoflurane and sevoflurane. Providers planning to use these agents should check availability of functioning agent-specific vaporizers and consider bringing their own supplies of each. Desflurane, which is expensive and requires a specific vaporizer, will almost certainly be unavailable.

Ether

The anesthetic use of diethyl ether, or ether, was first publicly reported in Boston in 1846, but it has disappeared from anesthetic practices in the more developed world, replaced by agents with fewer side effects and fewer safety concerns. However, it continues to be used in some LMICs, as it is cheaply and easily produced.

Pharmacodynamics and Pharmacokinetics

Ether is a highly soluble agent, with a blood/gas solubility coefficient of 12:1, resulting in a slow rise of the alveolar concentration and therefore a slow onset. It acts as a bronchodilator, but also as a respiratory irritant, and inhalation inductions with ether are marked by coughing and significant increases in bronchial secretions, often requiring treatment with glycopyrrolate or atropine. From a cardiovascular standpoint, ether is relatively stable, producing only small variations in heart rate and blood pressure, without the sensitization of cardiac muscle to catecholamines seen with halothane. Ether is also known to cause significant postoperative nausea and vomiting (PONV).[5]

Technical Considerations

Providers encountering ether should be aware of its significant volatility and flammability, particularly when transporting bottles of the agent and especially during cases involving the use of cautery. Low concentrations of ether can burn in the presence of sufficient oxygen or nitrous oxide, and high concentrations become explosive. During storage in open air or in ultraviolet (UV) light, ether can autoxidize and become dangerously explosive; shaking a bottle of autoxidized ether can be enough to trigger explosion.

Nitrous Oxide

Nitrous oxide (N_2O) is an inorganic inhaled anesthetic frequently utilized in the more developed world. It has a low potency and does not produce surgical anesthesia when used alone due to its high MAC (104%), but it is commonly used as a sedative medication by itself or as an adjunct in combination with inhalation or intravenous anesthetics for general anesthesia.

Availability

Despite its relatively low cost, N_2O is rarely available in most LMICs where it is difficult to produce, transport, and store. If N_2O is available, it will be stored in cylinders, as the wall pipeline supplies of N_2O, almost universal in more developed world hospitals, are seldom available and potentially unreliable. In some countries, cylinders containing a mixture of 50% N_2O and oxygen equipped with a demand valve and mouthpiece are used to administer doses of N_2O as needed for sedation during procedures, dressing changes, and childbirth.

Technical Considerations

N_2O is not flammable, but like oxygen, it will support combustion and should be used with caution in the presence of cautery, particularly during surgeries involving the airway.

Anesthetics in LMICs may be performed with older equipment that has not been properly maintained and with limited patient monitoring. Providers in these settings should remember the potentially catastrophic possibility of delivering a hypoxic gas mixture. Oxygen and N_2O are delivered via flowmeters in a series arrangement, with oxygen usually downstream to N_2O. If oxygen is delivered upstream, a leak in the system will cause oxygen to exit the system before N_2O

is added, resulting in the delivery of a higher concentration of N_2O and a hypoxic patient. In addition, some older machines will allow the delivery of a hypoxic air mixture because they will deliver N_2O without the mandatory minimum oxygen flow required by newer machines.

Vaporizers

Modern vaporizers are agent specific, and in some facilities in LMICs, only one vaporizer type may be available. Halothane and isoflurane have virtually the same vapor pressure across a wide range of temperatures, which determines the amount of gas delivered by a vaporizer. Thus, a halothane vaporizer filled with isoflurane allows delivery of the dialed in concentration of isoflurane. Likewise, an isoflurane vaporizer can be filled with halothane. However, it is important to remember that an isoflurane vaporizer has the potential to deliver a 5% concentration of halothane, potentially a dangerously high dose.

A halothane vaporizer could be filled with sevoflurane, which might be more desirable than halothane as an induction agent because of its relative hemodynamic stability and faster onset of action. However, because the vapor pressure of sevoflurane is less than that of halothane, the delivered concentration will be less than that set on the dial of vaporizer and the maximum achievable end-tidal alveolar concentration of sevoflurane will be too low for a rapid inhalation induction or intubation.[4] Occasionally, visiting providers will encounter vaporizers for enflurane, a volatile anesthetic, which is no longer used in the United States. The maximum concentration delivered by an enflurane vaporizer is 7%. Because enflurane and sevoflurane have similar vapor pressures, sevoflurane can be used to fill an enflurane vaporizer, delivering a similar concentration to that on the dial and allowing a speedy induction. Due to significant safety concerns, agents that have dissimilar vapor pressures should not be interchanged in a vaporizer. For example, halothane should not be used in an enflurane vaporizer (see Figure 5.1).

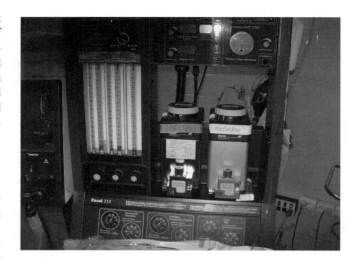

FIGURE 5.1 A photograph of an anesthetic machine from the destination facility for a visiting surgical team trip. Note the enflurane vaporizers relabeled by the anesthetic providers and containing isoflurane and halothane. Practitioners should note that common colors used for medical gases in the United States may be different in other countries. For example, oxygen lines and cylinders are green in the United States but white in many other parts of the world. Image by Robert C. Chantigian.

Analgesics

In the setting of a visiting surgical team trip with limited perioperative resources, agents that produce analgesia without respiratory compromise are ideal. The role of perioperative opioids is limited by their potential for respiratory depression, as resultant hypoxia may remain undetected due to lack of monitors or monitoring personnel, and supplemental oxygen may be scarce or non-existent. Opioids may also increase the risk of PONV and recovery room stays. A multimodal approach to postoperative pain, utilizing non-opioid adjuncts like acetaminophen, nonsteriodal anti-inflammatory drugs (NSAIDs), ketamine, and local anesthetics, will decrease the need for opioids and facilitate earlier postoperative recovery.

Opioids

Short-acting agents like fentanyl used incrementally in low doses (0.5 mcg/kg) may minimize postoperative hypoventilation and desaturation compared to longer duration drugs like hydromorphone, oxymorphone, or even morphine. During general anesthesia, it is useful to maintain spontaneous ventilation, titrating opioid to respiratory rate.

Providers bringing their own supplies of medications may face restrictive transport regulations for opiates. However, facilities in destination countries often have adequate supplies of commonly used medications like fentanyl and morphine. Other less familiar opioid medications may be available. See Table 5.1.

Codeine

Codeine is a weak opioid analgesic, typically available as an elixir combined with acetaminophen. Although it is among the most commonly prescribed opiates in the United States, it has limitations as a therapeutic agent. Codeine is a prodrug that is metabolized to morphine for its therapeutic effect. However, patients exhibit wide pharmacogenetic variation in the metabolism of codeine, resulting in either limited conversion (and inadequate analgesia) or rapid metabolism (and subsequent overdose). An inability to convert codeine to morphine has been described in 7–10% of the Caucasian population.[6] In contrast, over 25% of Ethiopians are defined as ultra-rapid metabolizers.[7] Because of the relatively common presence of rapid metabolizers in the general population, codeine has been discontinued from the

formularies of many U.S. hospitals. However, it is still quite common in less developed settings. Side effects, including nausea, vomiting, and constipation, are common with codeine, particularly higher doses. Intravenous (IV) formulations of codeine are available but not recommended because IV administration has been associated with profound hypotension and seizures.[8,9]

Tramadol

Intravenous and intramuscular formulations of tramadol, not available in the United States, are used in some LMICs. Tramadol is a synthetic analogue of codeine that acts as a weak opioid analgesic. It has noradrenergic and serotonergic properties that contribute to its analgesic effect. Because of these non-opioid receptor effects, it may demonstrate less respiratory depression than other narcotics. An initial adult dose for postoperative pain is 50-100 mg IV; this can be followed every 4-6 hours. Seizures have been reported in patients taking tramadol, and it should be used cautiously in at-risk patients.[10]

Buprenorphine

Buprenorphine is a partial agonist of the mu-receptor, which is more than 20–30 times as potent as morphine, and much longer acting than fentanyl. Like other opioids, Buprenorphine does cause respiratory depression, but this effect plateaus at higher doses, in contrast to pure agonist opioids like fentanyl or morphine.[11]

Buprenorphine can be used as a premedicant (0.3 mg intramuscular [IM]) and postoperative pain control (0.3 mg IV or IM). It can also be used for intraoperative analgesia (2–6 mcg/kg) but should not be used as a sole anesthetic agent.

Meperidine (Pethidine)

Meperidine (Pethidine, Demerol) is a synthetic opioid used for procedural sedation, analgesia, and postoperative shivering. Its peak onset of action is 10–15 minutes, and its duration of action is 2 hours. It undergoes hepatic metabolism to normeperidine, a proconvulsant which is renally excreted. For this reason, it should be used with caution in patients with renal failure, but it has also has been associated with seizures in healthy patients without kidney disease.[12]

TABLE 5.1

Opioid equivalencies

Drug	Potency relative to Morphine	Equianalgesic Doses		IV Doses	
		IV	PO	>6 mo or < 50 kg	> 50 kg
Morphine	1	10 mg	30 mg	0.1 mg/kg q 2–4 hrs	3-5 mg q 2–4 hrs
Fentanyl	80–100	100 mcg	NA	0.5–1.0 mcg.kg q 1–2 hrs	NA
Hydromorphone	5	1.5–2 mg	6–8 mg	0.03 mg/kg q 2–4 hr	0.5–1 mg q 2–4 hr
Codeine	0.1	120 mg	200 mg	Not recommended	
Meperidine(Pethidine)	0.1	75–100 mg	300 mg	0.5–1.0 mg/kg q 2–3 hours	1 mg/kg q 2–4 hr

Created by Leal G. Segura. Adapted from Berde CB, Sethna NF. Analgesics for the Treatment of Pain in Children. Table 3, "Initial guidelines for opioid analgesics." *N Engl J Med* 2002;347:1094–1103.

*Doses should be reduced 25% of per-kilogram recommendations for children < 6 mo.

Opioids should be avoided in children <3 months of age unless continuous monitoring is available.

Non-Opioid Adjuncts (See Table 5.2)

Acetaminophen (Tylenol, United States; Paracetamol, United Kingdom and other countries)

Acetaminophen is an analgesic with a safe therapeutic profile and few contraindications. It produces no respiratory depression and has opioid-sparing properties,[13] either as part of a general anesthetic or regional techniques. Scheduled acetaminophen postoperatively is particularly useful in decreasing the need for supplemental narcotics, particularly when alternated with NSAIDs.

Oral acetaminophen (10–15 mg/kg pediatric; 650–1000 mg for adults), is available in liquid or tablet form and rapidly absorbed. It can be administered preoperatively (with or without additional sedatives like midazolam or ketamine) to decrease opioid requirements during and after surgery.

Rectal acetaminophen can be administered intraoperatively. Peak blood levels are seen 1–2 hours after administration, so it should be given soon after anesthesia is induced in order to achieve maximum benefit.

Intravenous acetaminophen, widely available outside the United States, was first approved for use in the United States in November 2010. Dosing regimens for children are 15 mg/kg every 6 hours or 12.5 mg/kg every 4 hours, with a maximum dose of 75 mg/kg/day (<3.75 mg/day).[14] For adults, doses of 650–1000 mg IV with a maximum dose of 4 mg in 24 hours are recommended.[15]

Nonsteroidal anti-inflammatory drugs

NSAIDs provide effective analgesia by inhibiting the cyclooxygenase enzyme (COX) involved in prostaglandin synthesis. Multiple studies have demonstrated the efficacy of NSAIDs in reducing perioperative pain and opioid consumption, making them useful adjuncts in facilities in LMICs.

Oral ibuprofen is frequently available in LMICs, and easy to administer as a premedication before surgery. Postoperatively, it can be given on a scheduled basis and alternated with Tylenol to minimize narcotic use.

Ketorolac and ibuprofen are the only NSAIDs available for IV injection in the United States, but IV formulations of ketoprofen, diclofenac, and ibuprofen may be encountered in other countries. Ketorolac is nonnarcotic and can be transported to destination countries as multi-dose vials.

One 30 mg IM dose of ketorolac, a nonspecific COX inhibitor, has an analgesic equivalent to 6–12 mg of morphine, without respiratory depression, sedation, or PONV. However, like other nonspecific COX inhibitors, ketorolac may increase risk of surgical and gastrointestinal bleeding. Renal toxicity is possible, particularly in hypovolemic patients receiving long-term doses and those with preexisting renal injury.

Recommended adult doses range from 15–30 mg IV or IM every 6 hours or 0.5 mg/kg IV in children (maximum 30 mg). The lower dose probably offers the same analgesic benefit, but with less risk of side effect.[16] Dosing with ketorolac should be limited to 5 days, as the risk of gastrointestinal and operative site bleeding has been shown to increase with longer therapy.[17]

Ketamine

Ketamine is an N-methyl-d-aspartate (NMDA) antagonist with sedative and analgesic properties. It is the most commonly available anesthetic agent in many LMICs, and it is probably the most frequently used anesthetic drug in the less developed world. It is a versatile drug that can be used as a premedicant; a sole anesthetic agent; a sedative to facilitate regional anesthesia; a sedative for short, painful procedures; or an analgesic supplement during general anesthesia. See Table 5.3. It also provides an opioid sparing effect. See Table 5.3.

Ketamine's utility in LMICs that lack reliable postoperative monitoring or personnel lies in its ability to provide sedation, anesthesia, and analgesia with minimal respiratory compromise. It is particularly useful when supplemental oxygen and mechanical ventilation are unavailable or inconsistent. After administration, the ventilatory response to carbon dioxide and airway muscle tone is preserved. However, when large doses of ketamine are administered rapidly or with concomitant opioids, apnea can occur. Ketamine also increases salivary and tracheobronchial secretions, which can be copious and lead to laryngospasm. Treatment with glycopyrrolate or atropine can prevent accumulation of these secretions, particularly during repeated doses or deeper levels of sedation.

Systemic Effects

Ketamine stimulates the sympathetic nervous system, which leads to relative cardiovascular stability compared to other anesthetic agents like propofol or thiopental. Systemic blood pressure, heart rate, and cardiac output increase after administration, making it a useful agent in hypovolemic patients and those with congenital heart disease. However, providers should use caution when using ketamine in patients who may not tolerate such sympathetic stimulation (i.e., patients with uncontrolled hypertension, severe coronary disease, and severe aortic stenosis). Additionally, ketamine can decrease cardiac output in catecholamine-depleted patients (e.g., long-standing and untreated hypovolemic shock).[18]

Ketamine can also be associated with hallucinations, nightmares, or delirium. The incidence of delirium is higher in adolescents or adults and higher with larger or repeated doses. Administration of a benzodiazepine such as midazolam or diazepam with ketamine can attenuate delirium but may prolong recovery after short procedures.

Routes of Administration

Ketamine can be administered orally, intravenously, intramuscularly, nasally, transmucosally, and rectally, with doses adjusted to the level of sedation required.

Oral or intramuscular ketamine can be administered to facilitate IV access and inhalation inductions in uncooperative patients. Higher doses may provide enough sedation and analgesia for short procedures or painful interventions outside the operating room such as dressing changes. Low-dose ketamine (0.1–0.2 mg/kg) is also a versatile adjunct; it can be used for intraoperative analgesia with or without additional opioids, for postoperative pain relief and as a sedative during regional anesthesia.

Local Anesthetics

Local anesthetics have an important role in anesthesia in the less developed world. See Table 5.4. Field blocks, peripheral nerve blocks, and neuraxial techniques can provide adequate surgical anesthesia alone with or without additional sedation. Local or regional nerve blockade can also provide enough analgesia to make supplemental opioids unnecessary, even in the postoperative setting. There are two classes of local anesthetics, esters and amides.

Mechanism of Action

Local anesthetics act by blocking neuronal voltage-gated sodium channels, interfering with channel activation and subsequent membrane depolarization. The effect of local anesthetics is greatest when nerve fibers are firing rapidly because their affinity for an inactivated or activated channel is much higher than their affinity for channels in the resting state.

Regional Anesthesia Adjuncts

The addition of clonidine (1mcg/kg), an α2-adrenergic receptor agonist, to local anesthetic mixtures can lengthen the duration of nerve blockade and maximize postoperative analgesic benefit. Like clonidine, epinephrine (1:200,000–1:400,000) also activates α2-adrenergic receptors, prolonging block duration and enhancing analgesia. Further, epinephrine causes vasoconstriction, which decreases systemic absorption (and subsequent systemic side effects), and increases neuronal uptake and block duration. This prolongation is more marked with short-acting agents like lidocaine. The duration of longer-acting local anesthetics (bupivacaine, ropivacaine) is largely due to protein binding and remains largely unaffected by vasoconstrictors. Phenylephrine is another vasoconstrictor that can be used as an adjunct for regional anesthesia, but it is less commonly used.

Most LMICs have ample supplies of lidocaine, but providers should bring longer-acting medications if regional anesthetics and field blocks are planned. To minimize bulk, higher concentrations of local anesthetics (bupivacaine 0.25% or 0.5%, ropivacaine 0.5%) can be transported from home in large

TABLE 5.2

Oral and IV dosing of non-opioid analgesics

Drug	PO	IV	Maximum Dose
Acetaminophen	Pediatric: 10–15 mg/kg q 4–6 hours Adult: 650–1000 mg q 4–6 hours	Pediatric: 15 mg/kg Q6 hours or 12.5 mg/kg Q4H Adult: 650-1000 mg Q6 hours	Pediatric: 75 mg/kg/24 hours (3.75 mg/day) Adult: 4 grams/24 hours
Ibuprofen	6 mo–12 yr: 6–10mg/kg q 6–8 hours >12 yr: 200–400 mg q 4–6 hours	Pediatric:10 mg/kg Adult: 400–800 mg Q6 hours	< 60 kg: 40 mg/kg/day PO >60 kg: 2400 mg/day PO 3200 mg/day IV
Diclofenac	1 mg/kg up to 50 mg q 8 hours	1 mg/kg	3 mg/kg up to 150 mg
Ketorolac	0.5 mg/kg q 6–8 hours	Pediatric: 0.5 mg/kg up to 30 mg Adult: 15–30 mg	2 mg/kg/day up to 120 mg/kg/day

Adapted from Berde CB, Sethna NF. Analgesics for the Treatment of Pain in Children. Table 2, "Oral dosage guidelines for commonly used non-opioid analgesics." *N Engl J Med* 2002;347:1094–1103.

TABLE 5.3

Ketamine: Dosing and clinical use

Anesthetic Goal	Dose and Route	Uses	Useful Adjuncts	Comment
Premedication	2–5 mg/kg PO 3–5 mg/kg IM	Facilitates IV placement; may provide enough sedation and analgesia alone for short procedures.	Benzodiazepine adjunct for deeper sedation and prevention of dysphoria (midazolam 0.25–0.5 mg/kg PO or 0.05–0.1 mg/kg IM) Benzodiazepine (midazolam 0.1 mg/kg IM). Antisialagogue for oral secretions (Glycopyrrolate 0.01 mg/kg IM).	IM dosing associated with longer recoveries and nausea and vomiting: if insufficient for procedural conditions, repeat half or full dose effective. Peak onset of IM dose is 5–10 min; duration of action is 15–30 min.
Induction	4–8 mg/kg IM 1–2 mg/kg IV	Intubation with muscle relaxant; surgical conditions for 10–15 min.	Benzodiazepine for deeper sedation Antisialagogue for oral secretions (Glycopyrrolate 0.01 mg/kg).	Hypersalivation and emergence phenomena more common with induction dose.
Analgesic	0.1–0.5 mg/kg IV	Pre- or postoperative analgesia.	Antisialagogue and benzodiazepine after repeated doses.	Apnea may occur when used with opioids. Effective as an analgesic in opioid-tolerant patients.
Procedural Sedation	2–3 mg/kg IM	Short painful procedures (i.e., dressing changes, I&Ds, wound explorations).	Benzodiazepine for prevention of dysphoria (0.1mg/kg up to 2 mg IV midazolam). Antisialagogue for oral secretions.	1-2 mg/kg IV initial dose. Additional incremental doses of 0.5–1 mg/kg can prolong or deepen procedural sedation.

Created by Leal G. Segura. Adapted from Morgan, Jr. GE, Mikhail MS, Murray MJ, eds. *Clinical Anesthesiology*. 4th ed. New York: McGraw-Hill; 2006.

multi-dose vials and then diluted for peripheral nerve or neuraxial blocks.

Muscle Relaxants

Muscle relaxants are neuromuscular blocking agents classified as depolarizing or nondepolarizing based on their mechanism of action. They are most frequently used to facilitate endotracheal intubation or provide muscle relaxation for surgical exposure. In operating rooms in the less developed world, where intra- and postoperative mechanical ventilation may not be possible, muscle relaxants are often avoided. The utility of nondepolarizing muscle relaxants (NDMRs) in LMICs is limited by the accompanying need for specific reversal agents. Without these specific agents, duration of relaxation depends on the gradual redistribution, metabolism, and excretion of NDMRs. Inadequate reversal at the end of an anesthetic can lead to a profoundly weak patient postoperatively who is unable to maintain ventilation.

Succinylcholine (or Suxamethonium Chloride)

Succinylcholine is a depolarizing neuromuscular blocker that provides rapid relaxation (within 30–60 seconds) and short duration (<10 minutes). Most commonly, it is used intravenously to facilitate endotracheal intubation, but it is also used in the emergency treatment of laryngospasm and for rapid-sequence inductions for emergency surgery in nonfasting patients.

The dose of succinylcholine for intubation is 1–1.5 mg/kg IV in adults, 1.5–2 mg/kg IV in older children, and 1.5–3 mg/kg IV in infants. Succinylcholine is also effective when given IM, but larger doses are required. Typical IM doses are 3–4 mg/kg IM in children and 5 mg/kg IM in infants less than 6 months.

Precautions and Contraindications

Some patients are vulnerable to life-threatening hyperkalemia after succinylcholine. Serum potassium increases by 0.5 mEq/L after succinylcholine-induced depolarization, and it should be avoided in patients with preexisting hyperkalemia. In patients with burns, massive trauma, and new onset neurologic disorders (i.e., strokes, paresis, myopathies), succinylcholine can elicit massive hyperkalemia and cardiac arrest due to upregulation of acetylcholine receptors.

The short duration of succinylcholine is due to its rapid metabolism by pseudocholinesterase. One in 50 patients is heterozygous for an atypical pseudocholinesterase gene and will demonstrate a slight prolongation in muscle relaxation (20–30 minutes). Patients who are homozygous for the atypical gene will demonstrate marked prolongation in muscle relaxation (4–8 hours); fortunately, this is rare (1 in 3,000 patients).

Technical Considerations

Despite its classification as an essential medicine by the World Health Organization and its low cost, it remains unavailable to providers in many LMICs.[19] Questionnaire-based surveys

TABLE 5.4

Local anesthetics: Common concentrations, uses, and doses

Drug	Available Concentrations	Routes of Administration	Maximum Dose mg/kg	Block Duration	Potential Complications
Chloroprocaine	1%, 2%, 3%	Epidural, infiltration, peripheral nerve block (PNB).	12	0.5–1	Neuro deficits after unintentional subarachnoid injection; severe back pain post-epidural; decreased analgesia from spinal morphine after epidural administration.
Tetracaine	0.2%, 0.3%, 0.5%, 1%, 2%	Spinal, topical.	3	1.5–6	Neurotoxicity (Cauda Equina Syndrome) after spinal injection.
Lidocaine (Lignocaine)	0.5%, 1%, 1.5%, 2%, 4%, 5%	Epidural, spinal, PNB, topical, IV regional.	4.5 plain 7 with epinephrine	0.75–2	Neurotoxicity (Cauda Equina Syndrome) after spinal injection.
Mepivacaine	1%, 1.5%, 2%, 3%	Epidural, infiltration, PNB.	4.5 plain 7 with epinephrine	1–2	
Ropivacaine	0.2%, 0.5%, 0.75%, 1%	Epidural, spinal, infiltration, PNB.	3	1.5–8	
Bupivacaine	0.25%, 0.5%, 0.75%	Epidural, spinal, infiltration, PNB.	3	1.5–8	
Prilocaine	4%	Topical mixture with lidocaine (EMLA), PNB.	8	0.5–1	Allergy related to PABA. Methemoglobinemia with large doses.
Procaine	1%, 2%, 10%	Spinal infiltration, PNB.	12	0.5–1	
Benzocaine	20%	Topical.	<1sec spray*	0.5–1	Allergy related to PABA. Methemoglobinemia with large doses. Potential overdosing with spray.

Created by Leal G. Segura. Adapted from Morgan, Jr. GE, Mikhail MS, Murray MJ, eds. *Clinical Anesthesiology.* 4th ed. New York: McGraw-Hill; 2006, p. 270, Chapter 14, Table 14-3.

showed succinylcholine was always available to only 64% of providers in Zambia and 54% of providers in Uganda.[1,2]

Succinylcholine in solution will deteriorate with storage at room temperature, but in powder form, it can be stored longer. It undergoes decomposition at higher temperatures, and in hot countries it should be refrigerated if possible. Because facilities in LMICs face shortages of succinylcholine and storage conditions may be unreliable, visiting providers should consider bringing their own supplies.

Nondepolarizing muscle relaxants

NDMRs are even less available to providers in LMICs. In most LMICs, newer and more expensive drugs like rocuronium will be nonexistent, and visiting clinicians may encounter drugs no longer in use at home, such as curare or atracurium. If NDMRs are available, visiting anesthetists will likely need to provide their own supply of reversal agents. Most importantly, providers should consider alternatives to NDMRs, such as deep anesthesia and intubation without paralytics, and should review the pharmacology of less familiar agents.

d-Tubocurarine (Curare)

Curare was the first muscle relaxant used in clinical practice. In the more developed world, it is of historical interest only, but it may be encountered in less developed nations. Providers should be aware of its long duration (similar to pancuronium). Its elimination half-life and duration of action is even longer in the very young and very old and in patients with impaired glomerular filtration. Hypotension is common after administration even in low doses, and is secondary to histamine release and sympathetic ganglion blockade. Decreases in blood pressure can be profound when it is used with halothane, which also acts as a ganglion blocker. Bronchospasm may be seen secondary to histamine release. An intubating dose is 0.3–0.6 mg/kg.[5]

Alcuronium

Alcuronium has never been used in clinical practice in North America, but it may be encountered in other countries. Vagolysis may lead to tachycardia, and hypotension can also occur. It can also be associated with histamine release, and anaphylactoid reactions may be more common than with other muscle relaxants. Initially described as an "intermediate-acting" drug, with initial doses of 0.25 mg/kg IV, alcuronium is actually a relatively long-acting agent, with surgical relaxation lasting 1 hour and complete recovery of neuromuscular transmission after 5 hours without reversal.

Gallamine

Gallamine is another NDMR no longer used in modern anesthetic practices and rarely available in the less developed world. It may produce an increase in heart rate and blood pressure secondary to a vagolysis. Histamine release may occur and anaphylactoid reactions have been reported.

Emergency Medications and Essential Drugs

Anesthesia providers visiting LMICs should bring their own supplies of emergency medications to ensure proper storage. Providers should consider bringing the medications on the suggested list below, which includes commonly used drugs in adult and pediatric resuscitation protocols and perioperative emergencies.

Antiemetics

PONV is a frequent complication even in the developed world, prolonging recovery room stays and delaying discharges. In LMIC perioperative environments, PONV prophylaxis is even more essential. Providers should consider using multi-modal anti-emetic therapy, which has been shown to be more effective than single agents used alone.

Dexamethasone

Dexamethasone is a useful and inexpensive anti-emetic (15–20 mcg/kg up to 8 mg), and its routine use should be considered in the operating room. However, it has multiple uses in the perioperative setting beyond its role as an anti-emetic that make it essential to providers planning surgical interventions abroad. It is effective in treating (and preventing) post-extubation airway edema in adults and children,[22,23] and may be helpful preemptively in severe asthmatics. It is also used as an adjunct in the treatment of anaphylaxis.

Ondansetron

Ondansetron is a 5-HT3 receptor antagonist with a favorable side effect profile routinely used in the prevention of PONV. A typical adult dose is 4 mg IV; pediatric doses range from 50–100 mcg/kg.

Droperidol

Droperidol is a well-studied and effective anti-emetic, which works by blocking dopamine stimulation at the chemoreceptor trigger zone. Although a U.S. Food and Drug Administration (FDA) "black box" warning cautioned that droperidol is associated with QT prolongation and torsades des pointes, the warning itself was based on only 10 reported adverse cardiovascular events in patients receiving 1.25 mg or less of droperidol, and whether droperidol was in fact the cause of these events has been challenged.[24] Other side effects with droperidol are dose-dependent, and low doses (0.625 mg IV in adults; 10–20 mcg/kg IV in children) are effective.

Epinephrine

Epinephrine is a mainstay in advanced cardiac life support (ACLS) and pediatric advanced life support (PALS) protocols and an essential emergency medication used in the treatment of cardiac arrest, anaphylaxis, bronchospasm, hypotension, and, in nebulized form, post-intubation croup.

Epinephrine (1 mg/ml) is available for transport in single-dose 1 ml vials, or 30 ml multi-dose vials. The 1 mg/ml solution can be aerosolized (0.5ml/kg per dose) to treat post-intubation croup, and is as effective as a racemic mixture.

Halothane sensitizes the heart to catecholamines, and supplemental doses of epinephrine can trigger ventricular fibrillation.

Atropine

Atropine (0.4 mg/ml or 1 mg/ml) is a parasympatholytic drug that increases heart rate and improves atrioventricular (AV) nodal conduction. It is used in the treatment of symptomatic bradycardias and second- and third-degree heart blocks. It can also be used to decrease oral secretions and acts as a bronchodilator. Glycopyrrolate, which does not cross the blood-brain barrier, is a preferable agent for those indications because it is less likely to contribute to postoperative delirium and its anticholinergic action is longer.

Calcium Gluconate or Calcium Chloride

Calcium should be available for the treatment of hypocalcemia, hypotension, and during cardiopulmonary resuscitation (CPR) in patients with hypocalcemia, hyperkalemia, and/or hypermagnesemia. It is an inotrope and vasoconstrictor, lasting 10–20 minutes. It is also necessary after massive transfusion when high doses of citrate (in blood products) have been administered. It is also useful after albumin administration as albumin will bind serum calcium.

Calcium can be administered as calcium chloride (10–20 mg/kg/dose) or calcium gluconate (30–60 mg/kg/dose). Caution should be used when infusing calcium through a peripheral IV, as extravasation can cause severe tissue necrosis. Calcium gluconate may have a decreased risk of tissue injury.

Sodium Bicarbonate

Sodium bicarbonate (1 mEq/kg; 4.2% 0.5 mEq/ml; 8.4% 1 mEq/ml) should be available for the treatment of acidosis. It should be noted that sodium bicarbonate can act paradoxically in patients with hypercapnia during CPR, worsening acidosis. It can be administered IV or intraosseously (IO), but not endotracheally, and it can cause tissue injury if it extravasates.

Adenosine

Adenosine is used to terminate supraventricular tachycardias in children and adults by producing sinus bradycardia and temporary AV nodal block within 10–20 seconds.

Adenosine has an extremely short half-life (<10 seconds) because it is metabolized rapidly by erythrocytes and endothelial cells. Therefore, in order for the active drug to reach the heart and achieve clinical effect, it should be administered as a rapid bolus followed by a rapid flush. The PALS dose is 0.1 mg/kg IV with successive doses of 0.2 and 0.4 mg/kg if required. The initial adult dose is 6 mg, followed by 12 mg, if ineffective.

Because of its AV nodal blocking properties, adenosine can produce profound bradycardia, cardiac pauses, and even asystole, which is usually transient. Ventricular arrhythmias and atrial fibrillation can also occur. It can also cause bronchospasm, which is usually mild.

Anti-arrhythmics

Amiodarone is the drug of choice for ventricular tachycardia and fibrillation resistant to defibrillation. The pediatric dose is 5 mg/kg; adults should receive 300 mg initially during ACLS, followed by a repeat dose of 150 mg if necessary. Hypotension is common with IV administration. Amiodarone-associated torsades de pointes has been reported, and the drug should be avoided in patients with prolonged QT intervals.[25,26]

Lidocaine (1–1.5 mg/kg IV, followed by 0.5–0.75 mg/kg every 10 minutes) can be used as an alternative for treatment of ventricular tachyarrhythmias if amiodarone is unavailable.

Magnesium sulfate (2g IV in adults; 25–50 mg/kg in pediatrics) is the drug of choice in polymorphic ventricular tachycardia, or torsades de pointes.

Ephedrine and Phenylephrine

Ephedrine (available in 25 mg or 50 mg, 1 mL ampules) indirectly causes release of norepinephrine, producing increases in heart rate, blood pressure, and cardiac output. It is less potent than epinephrine and therefore useful in the treatment of mild hypotension. A 5–10 mg IV bolus is a typical adult dose, and 0.1 mg/kg is appropriate for infants and children. Intramuscular doses of 25–50 mg can be useful for treatment of anesthesia induced emesis or mild hypotension. In some institutions, ephedrine is considered a controlled substance because it is used in the production of methamphetamine.

Phenylephrine is also used in the treatment of perioperative hypotension, and is particularly useful in the setting of anesthesia-induced peripheral vasodilation (i.e., spinal anesthesia). It is a predominantly α1-agonist, increasing arterial blood pressure through vasoconstriction. A typical adult dose is 50–100 mcg; pediatric doses range from 0.5–1 mcg/kg IV. Continuous infusions (0.25–1 mcg/kg/min) can also be used. Reflex bradycardia can occur, particularly in children.

Naloxone

Naloxone is an opioid antagonist used in the treatment of opioid side effects, including respiratory depression. In the setting of respiratory depression, a reasonable initial dose is 0.25–1 mcg/kg IV repeated every 5 minutes until ventilation improves. However, in the setting of severe respiratory depression and a critically ill patient, low doses may not be effective, and a higher dose (100–400 mcg in an adult) may be required. High doses should be used with caution, however, as hypertension, arrhythmias, and pulmonary edema have been described.[27,28]

In adults, the elimination half-life is 1–1.5 hours. The duration of opioid can outlast the naloxone effect, and respiratory depression can recur. Patients who require the use of naloxone should be monitored for at least 2 hours.

Flumazenil

Flumazenil is a γ-aminobutyric acid (GABA) antagonist that reverses benzodiazepines. For adults, 200 mcg can be administered IV every minute (up to 1 mg) until sedation improves. In children, 10 mcg/kg can be repeated every minute (maximum dose 0.05 mg/kg or 1 mg) until the desired effect is achieved.

Elimination half-life is 1 hour in adults, and even shorter in children. The benzodiazepine effect can outlast the flumazenil, and sedation can recur. As with naloxone, patients receiving flumazenil should be monitored for at least 2 hours.

Albuterol

Albuterol is a selective-ß₂ agonist used in the treatment of acute asthma or bronchospasm. It can be administered as a nebulized solution or a metered-dose inhaler (MDI). Metered-dose inhalers are difficult to administer to small uncooperative children, but they may be more reliable in destination countries, as administration of the nebulized solution to a non-anesthetized patient requires specific equipment and a high-flow oxygen source that are frequently unavailable in LMICs. However, in the operating room, providers can bring adaptors that allow drug delivery through an endotracheal tube. In an awake patient, makeshift spacers can be fashioned from plastic cups by cutting a hole for the MDI in the bottom and placing the open end over the child's mouth and nose.

Glucose

Vials of 50% dextrose should be available for the emergency treatment of symptomatic hypoglycemia (0.5–1 g/kg/dose IV). D50 vials can be diluted in lactated Ringer's or normal saline to supply 1%, 2.5%, 5%, and 10% dextrose infusions as needed for infants and other patients at risk of perioperative hypoglycemia.

Beta-blockers

ß-blockers decrease heart rate, blood pressure, and oxygen consumption, and are indicated in the treatment of myocardial ischemia, hypertrophic cardiomyopathy, and hypertension.

They are used for rate control in supraventricular tachycardia, and also decrease tachycardia and ß-receptor effects in the unlikely setting of thyrotoxicosis and pheochromocytoma.

Esmolol

Esmolol is an extremely short-acting selective ß1-antagonist that decreases heart rate more than blood pressure. It is administered as an IV bolus (0.1–0.5 mg/kg). Side effects, like bradycardia and hypotension, are short-lived as esmolol has an extremely short duration, with an elimination half-life of 9 minutes.

Propanolol

Propanolol is a nonselective ß-receptor blocker that decreases myocardial contractility, heart rate, and arterial blood pressure. It has a much longer elimination half-life (100 min) compared to esmolol. An initial dose depends on sympathetic tone, but a reasonable starting dose is 0.5 mg IV in adults, with incremental additional doses repeated as necessary every 3–5 minutes. In pediatric patients, doses range from 0.01–0.1 mg/kg, but profound bradycardia, hypotension, and AV block can occur. ß2-receptor blockade can cause bronchospasm.

Labetalol

Labetalol acts as both an α-adrenergic receptor and ß-receptor antagonist. It is used as an anti-hypertensive. Like propranolol, it can cause bronchospasm secondary to ß2-receptor blockade. After an initial dose of 0.1–0.25 mg/kg IV, increasing doses can be repeated at 10-minute intervals until blood pressure decreases.

Metoprolol

Metoprolol is a relatively selective B-1 blocking agent with a half-life of around 3.5 hours. Doses of 1–5 mg IV every 5 minutes until rate control is achieved are effective. It is available in IV and oral formulations.

Dantrolene

Dantrolene is the drug of choice in malignant hyperthermia (MH), a rare but potentially catastrophic complication of anesthesia. It is characterized by hypermetabolism, rhabdomyolysis, acidosis, and death if untreated.

The dose of dantrolene is 2.5 mg/kg IV every 5–10 minutes, administered rapidly and through a large bore IV if possible, and repeated until clinical signs of MH are reversed. Preparing dantrolene is labor-intensive and time-consuming. The drug comes in 20 mg vials, each of which needs to be dissolved in 60 ml sterile water.

While dantrolene is the drug of choice in MH, it is unlikely to be available in LMICs. Maintaining a supply of dantrolene is expensive because the drug is costly and has a short shelf life. It needs to be covered in a light-protective bag and requires a supply of sterile water for preparation. Because the mortality of MH is high, providers planning anesthetics in the less developed world should consider bringing dantrolene.

COMMENTARY

Edouard Uwamahoro, Rwanda
Denise M. Chan, USA

In the major referral hospitals in Rwanda, both general and regional anesthesia are administered. We prefer to use regional anesthesia whenever possible, to facilitate faster recovery and minimize postoperative respiratory complications.

For general anesthesia, maintenance in most hospitals is with halothane in 100% oxygen, although some private hospitals have sevoflurane. We see a lot of volume-depleted patients, mostly from trauma or abdominal pathology, and thus our most widely used induction agent is ketamine. Thiopental and propofol are also available, but we use these much less often, even on hemodynamically stable patients, since we have become accustomed to using ketamine. This is especially true with pediatric patients, whom we routinely induce with ketamine. Oftentimes, if a patient is hypotensive and cannot tolerate maintenance with halothane, we use intravenous ketamine boluses instead. Muscle relaxation is with suxamethonium, pancuronium, or vecuronium; cisatricurium is available at one private hospital. We often encounter patients who need a rapid sequence induction but have a contraindication to suxamethonium; without the availability of rocuronium, we must make a clinical decision by weighing risks and benefits.

Opioids are currently limited in Rwanda to fentanyl, morphine, pethidine (meperidine), and tramadol; all of these are given sparingly due to a deficiency of postoperative care. Paracetamol is a mainstay of pain management, but families must purchase it at an outside pharmacy and bring it into the hospital, and thus it is inconsistently administered.

Benzodiazepines such as midazolam and diazepam are available, but we use these primarily for sedation in the intensive care unit. We virtually never premedicate patients before surgery, for a variety of reasons, including cost and lack of preoperative monitoring.

The importance of antiemetics is recognized, but we are limited to dexamethasone and metoclopramide for most patients. Ondanestron must be purchased from a private pharmacy.

Ephedrine is our most commonly used vasopressor, but we also use dopamine and epinephrine infusions as necessary. It would be very helpful to have access to phenylephrine and norepinephrine for hypotensive patients who cannot tolerate an increased heart rate. Other medications such as nitroglycerin, nitroprusside, and most intravenous beta blockers are difficult or impossible to acquire, making the management of unique and complex patients, such as those with pheochromocytoma, extremely challenging.

Spinal anesthesia is preferred for most lower-extremity and urologic procedures, as well as non-emergent Caesarian sections. We use bupivacaine with dextrose and add preservative-free fentanyl or morphine. Continuous epidural analgesia is not possible in our setting, but caudal analgesia is used liberally for infants and young children undergoing almost any procedure at a dermatome level of T_6 or below. Again, because of the paucity of postoperative monitoring, this allows us to minimize opioid use and therefore potential respiratory complications.

As you can see, we are limited in Rwanda to a smaller pool of pharmaceuticals than that which is available in other countries. Even those medications that are usually available can be out of stock for months at a time. Thus we must be flexible and guide our perioperative management according to what is available.

6

Regional Anesthesia

Christopher S. Lee
Navil F. Sethna

Introduction

The practice of medicine in the austere environment requires adaptation to a situation in which there are significant deficiencies in basic infrastructure, equipment, supplies, and human resources. This is all the more true for anesthesia, which typically utilizes a plethora of resources in high-income countries (HICs).

However, regional anesthesia provides advantages that are realized to a greater degree in underdeveloped areas.[1] It can provide excellent operating conditions for the surgeon and limb-specific anesthesia. It can be used as an alternative to general anesthesia in appropriate patients. When used as the sole anesthetic technique, it frequently manifests stable hemodynamics and produces minimal side effects (e.g., sedation, respiratory depression, nausea, and vomiting), allowing for rapid recovery from anesthesia. These advantages must be placed in the context of environments where adequate monitoring is scarce, as is adequate postoperative care. These techniques can provide an awake, pain-free patient at the conclusion of surgery, which is ideal to facilitate a safe postoperative recovery. All these advantages result in far less resource utilization in an austere environment and potentially allow the delivery of safe surgical care to a greater number of individuals. Despite these advantages, there is a real failure rate of these techniques largely depending on the experience of the provider. Therefore, practitioners must be prepared either to supplement the technique with monitored anesthetic care or to convert to general anesthesia.

General Principles

Informed consent: As with any procedure, the anesthesiologist should explain to the patient and/or guardian, when applicable, the details of the technique, including the risks, benefits, and alternatives.[2] The extent of information provided varies and depends on cultural context and details requested by the patient or guardians.

Overcoming language and cultural barriers: Consent should be obtained through an interpreter who is fluent in the patient's native language.

Patient identification and peripheral nerve block (PNB) site marking: Prior to all procedures and sedation, the correct patient and block site should be identified and marked. Another physician or operating nurse involved in the patient's care should confirm the patient's identification and PNB site.[3]

Preoperative evaluation/patient selection: A good preoperative evaluation will determine the appropriate patients for regional techniques.

Designated block area: A dedicated block area can aid in efficiency because all of the necessary drugs, equipment, and staff are in the same area. Moreover, the blocks can be placed preoperatively with adequate setup time and avoidance of operating room (OR) time for these activities.[4,5] The block area should have the following:

- Medications: Sedatives, local anesthetics, and additives for local infiltration and blocks
- Pulse oximetry and preferably other monitors (EKG and noninvasive blood pressure)
- Intravenous supplies
- Ideally, suction and an oxygen source, but this may vary depending on the location
- Resuscitation equipment: airway equipment, including mask, ambu bag, laryngeal mask airway, laryngoscopes, and endotracheal tubes
- Resuscitation drugs, such as 20% intralipid and defibrillator for management of serious cardiovascular and nervous system toxicity due to inadvertent intravascular injection of local anesthetics, but this will be dependent upon resources available

Sedation and Monitoring

When providing sedation for the PNB, the patient should be awake enough to maintain meaningful communication with the provider and make known paresthesias, pain with injection, or symptoms of intravascular injection.

All patients receiving PNB with or without sedation ideally will have standard American Society of Anesthesiologists (ASA) monitoring that includes electrocardiogram (ECG), blood pressure measurement capability, and pulse oximetry. This should be the standard on visiting surgical team trips.

Intravenous (IV) access should be secured prior to performance of all PNBs except for distal field PNBs (e.g., digital nerve block).

Post-block instructions: Inform the patient and the guardians to protect the insensate, impaired part of the body until the effects of the local anesthetic dissipate. Caution the patient about other potential side effects specific to the block (e.g., Horner's syndrome and phrenic nerve block for interscalene block). It could be argued that this communication is even more important in the austere environment because unanticipated adverse effects may increase patient fears and negatively impact the populations' perception of their anesthetic care.

General Contraindications

Infection is an absolute contraindication of nerve blockade when the region of needle placement overlaps the area of local infection or when considering an indwelling catheter in the context of systemic infection.

Coagulopathy, thrombocytopenia, and anticoagulation are relative contraindications for plexus and deeply situated nerve blockade. The risk of hematoma is increased, so patients and family should be informed.

Acute compartment syndrome secondary to swelling, bleeding, or tight cast may lead to acute ischemia, and intense sensory block may mask the pain due to compartment syndrome. Therefore, dilute local anesthetics should be used in patients at risk and patients should be monitored closely for evidence of ischemia.

Patient and/or guardian refusal is an absolute contraindication.

Nerve Localization Techniques

The key to regional anesthesia is guiding the tip of the block needle in close proximity to the target nerve(s) without piercing the nerve to achieve an effective and safe nerve block. There are several methods of confirming the correct placement of the needle tip, including: (1) paresthesia, (2) nerve stimulation, and (3) ultrasound guidance.

Paresthesia technique: Paresthesia presumably occurs when the needle stimulates the nerve by direct contact or indirectly compressing the nerve through pressure on the surrounding tissues. Mechanical or electrical stimulation of the nerve results in sensory nerve depolarization and a shock-like sensation in the distribution of the nerve being stimulated. However, it does not always predict success. Eliciting paresthesia is no longer recommended or considered standard of care because it is associated with discomfort, potential for nerve trauma and post-block persistent neuropathy.[6]

Electrical nerve stimulation technique (Figure 6.1): The principle of nerve stimulation is to use a low electrical current sufficient to stimulate the motor component of a mixed peripheral nerve and elicit painless muscle contraction. Higher current intensity will stimulate the sensory component and cause painful paresthesia. The current required to stimulate a nerve generally varies inversely with the distance between the stimulating needle tip and the target nerve (i.e., the closer the needle tip is to the target nerve, the lower the stimulating current required).

In general, the nerve stimulator black lead (cathode) is the negatively charged stimulating lead. The red lead (anode) is the positively charged returning lead. Useful mnemonics to help remember include: (1) "Black to block." Attach the black lead to the stimulating needle; (2) "Positive to patient." Attach the red lead to the patient.

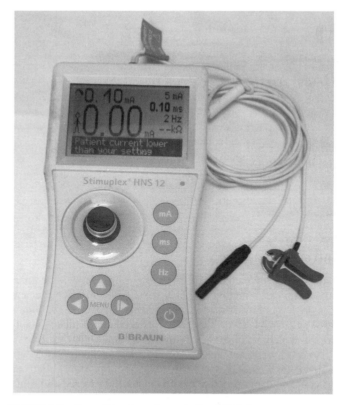

FIGURE 6.1 Nerve Stimulator. Image by Navil F. Sethna.

The electrical current flows from the black to the red via the patient to complete the circuit. The nerve stimulator should have an adjustable current output between 0 and 10 mA and a frequency of 1–2 Hz.

It is preferable to use an insulated needle. These needles concentrate the flow of the current from the needle tip to neural tissue directly without stimulating the surrounding tissue, as is the case with non-insulated needles. Once the needle is through the skin, the nerve stimulator is turned on at 1 mA at 1–2 Hz and 100–200 msec. The needle is advanced until target muscle contraction is visible or the patient reports paresthesia. Once motor response is established, the needle is likely 1–2 cm away. As the needle approaches the nerve, the muscle contraction should get stronger with the same amount of current. The needle is then advanced slowly and the intensity of the current turned down until a minimum current of 0.3–0.8 mA is capable of producing muscle contraction. This minimum current ensures that the needle tip is in close proximity to the target nerve. Signs of intraneural needle tip placement include: (1) muscle contraction with less than 0.3 mA and (2) high-resistance, painful paresthesia, or pain with injection. If it is difficult to inject the first 0.1 mL, stop immediately. In these instances withdraw the needle and reassess. Once the stimulating needle is placed in the desired position, further confirmation of correct needle placement is elicited by cessation of muscle contraction or paresthesia after injection of 0.5–1 mL of local anesthetic. It should be noted that once local anesthetic is injected and the muscle ceases to contract, the ability of the stimulating needle to localize the nerve is lost.

In HICs, the use of this technique has declined in recent years with increased use of ultrasound for localization of the target neural tissue.[6]

Ultrasound-Guided Technique

Ultrasound (US) imaging facilitates nerve localization in several different ways. It enhances visualization of the target nerve and the surrounding structures. It provides real-time assessment of appropriate needle tip position and catheter placement. It visually confirms the spread of the injectate around the target nerve. In addition, it helps identify anomalous anatomy and pathology. Ultrasound provides a clear advantage over peripheral nerve stimulation in patients with distorted anatomy, amputations, contractures, and vascular anomalies. The clinical advantages of ultrasound-guidance are more rapid block onset, smaller volumes of local anesthetic, longer duration of blockade, fewer needle passes, and possible increased success rate. Ultrasound may also potentially improve safety. While it would seem intuitive to consider ultrasound-guidance safer than nerve stimulation, to date, there are no studies to confirm this perception.

For visiting surgical team trips, practitioners who plan to use US-guided PNB techniques should plan on bringing their own, portable US machines, as they are prohibitively expensive in most low- and middle-income countries (LMICs). Practitioners should not count on such technology being available unless they bring it themselves. [7,8] That being said, this technique is becoming more popular and available in LMICs. Further, this presents an opportunity for visiting anesthesiologists to engage local practitioners and offer education on newer techniques that local practitioners would most likely be interested in.

Needle visualization: The path of the needle is directed either out-of-plane or in-plane relative to the ultrasound beam. In the out-of-plane approach, position the probe so that the target neural tissue is in the middle of the probe. The needle is placed in the middle of the probe, parallel to the US beam and at 90 degrees to every plane at the skin; the needle's shaft will appear as a hyperechoic dot, which will be difficult to visualize. Tissue movement and intermittent aspiration/injection of small amounts of solution, such as sterile normal saline solution or 5% dextrose solution, hydrodissecting tissue planes confirm the needle tip location. In the in-plane approach, the probe is positioned so that the target neural tissue is on the edge of the probe furthest from the operator. The needle is placed along the edge of the probe closest to the operator. The needle will appear as a hyperechoic line as it is advanced toward the target. Again, it is recommended to intermittently hydrodissect the tissue planes with sterile saline or 5% dextrose solution to identify the needle tip and avoid puncturing vital tissues.[9] Once the needle tip is immediately adjacent to the target neural tissue, aspirate the needle and inject local anesthetic without resistance. The local anesthetic should surround the nerves in a "doughnut or halo sign" pattern.

Local Anesthetic Dosing

In our practice, we typically use 0.5% ropivacaine for adults. For children, we typically use 0.2% ropivacaine or 0.25% bupivacaine with 1:200,000 epinephrine (unless epinephrine is contraindicated). The volume of local anesthetic is described in Table 6.1.[10] Other choices of local anesthetics that could be used are outlined in Table 6.2.[11] However, keep in mind that the maximum dose for the nerve block is determined by the weight and age of the patient, patient comorbidities, the local anesthetic being used, and other local anesthetic the patient has already received. The toxic dose of local anesthetic is additive within each class of local anesthetic. Therefore, if a patient receives half of the maximum dose of lidocaine via wound infiltration, a practitioner should administer no more than half of the maximum dose of ropivacaine for the block since they are both amide local anesthetics. Children should not receive more than a total of 2.5 mg/kg of bupivacaine or 3 mg/kg of ropivacaine. Moreover, one should avoid the use of denser local anesthetics in pediatric patients due to the risk of local anesthetic toxicity.

Local Anesthetic Toxicity

Accidental intravascular injection, excessive absorption, and overdosing—particularly in newborns, infants, and patients with reduced hepatic function—are the most frequent causes of local anesthetic toxicity. Drug dosing error with amide local anesthetics can lead to cardiovascular collapse and central nervous system toxicity, and death if not treated promptly. With appropriate dosing, the rate of absorption is a major determinant of systemic toxicity and the rate of absorption varies directly with the vascularity of the site of injection. Sites of greatest to least absorption are: intercostal > caudal > epidural > brachial plexus > femoral-sciatic > subcutaneous > intra-articular > spinal.

The central nervous system (CNS) is more susceptible to toxicity than the cardiovascular system. So, the first manifestation of systemic toxicity is CNS excitation. The unbound fraction of the local anesthetic is responsible for the systemic toxicity through

TABLE 6.1

Suggested volume of local anesthetics for peripheral nerve blocks

Block	Adult vol (mL)*	Pediatric vol (mL/kg)*
Brachial plexus	15–20	0.2–0.4
Femoral	15–20	0.3–0.5
Sciatic	20–25	0.3–0.5
Popliteal fossa	15–20	0.3–0.5

From Navil F. Sethna.

* These are suggested volumes of local anesthetic for these particular peripheral nerve blocks. However, the total dose (mg) of local anesthetic should not exceed the safe maximum allowable dose adjusted for body weight and age.

TABLE 6.2

Suggested local anesthetics, maximum recommended doses, duration of action

Local Anesthetic	Class	Max Dose	Duration of Action (shortest to longest)
2-Chloroprocaine	Ester	20 mg/kg	½ hr–1 hr
Procaine	Ester	10 mg/kg	1 hr –1½ hrs
Tetracaine	Ester	1.5 mg/kg	3 hrs–10 hrs
Lidocaine	Amide	7 mg/kg	1 ½ hrs–3½ hrs
Bupivacaine	Amide	2.5 mg/kg	3–10 hrs
Ropivacaine	Amide	3 mg/kg	3–10 hrs
Levobupivacaine	Amide	2.5 mg/kg	3–10 hrs

Adapted from Cote C, Lerman J, Anderson B (eds). *A Practice of Anesthesia for Infants and Children.* Philadelphia: Saunders, 2013: Table 41-2.

binding to the brain neurons. This leads to symptoms such as tinnitus, visual changes, light-headedness, peri-oral numbness, and muscular twitching. If this early prodrome is not treated quickly, these symptoms can progress to extreme anxiety, fear of imminent death, generalized tonic-clonic seizures, loss of consciousness, and respiratory arrest. As the serum level rises, the unbound local anesthetic enters the myocytes in sufficient amount to cause cardiovascular toxicity that can present with arrhythmias or sudden cardiac arrest.

There are several ways to avoid inadvertent intravascular injection of local anesthetics: (1) aspiration for blood prior to injection of local anesthetic, (2) administration of a test dose, (3) fractionated dosing, and (4) monitoring awake/sedated patients for symptoms and signs of systemic toxicity. When administering a test dose, give 0.1 mL/kg of local anesthetic with 1:200,000 epinephrine (maximum 3 mL) and monitor for signs of intravascular injection, including an increase in heart rate greater than 10 beats/minute, blood pressure increase greater than 15 mm Hg, or a lead II T-wave amplitude increase greater than 25%. These changes should occur within 20 seconds of injection and should last approximately 60 seconds. Both the aspiration test and epinephrine test have a false negative response rate. Therefore, the intended total dose of local anesthetics should be administered slowly and fractionated at 3–5 mL every 15–20 seconds while intermittently confirming negative aspiration. Local anesthetic should be administered while monitoring ECG and observing awake/sedated patients for systemic toxicity symptoms and signs.

Sedation with benzodiazepines prior to block performance may mask the early signs of CNS toxicity by increasing the seizure threshold. Another caveat in awake/sedated patients is that the early symptoms of toxicity, such as light-headedness, agitation, and anxiety, could be misinterpreted as fear behavior during an invasive procedure, and the clinician's first inclination may be to deepen sedation, which may lead to further masking of symptoms. Therefore, meaningful communication with awake/sedated patients is essential for early diagnosis of systemic toxicity. In the event systemic toxicity occurs, the management is outlined in Table 6.3.[12]

Upper Extremity Basic Anatomy

The nerve blocks of the upper extremity primarily involve the brachial plexus. The brachial plexus is formed by the five anterior rami of C5–T1 (Figure 6.2).[13] The brachial plexus divides from five roots to three trunks: Superior (C5–6), Middle (C7), and Inferior (C8–T1). Each of the three trunks further divides at the level of the first rib into two divisions, anterior and posterior. The anterior divisions provide innervation to the anterior flexors of the arm, and the posterior divisions provide innervation to the posterior extensors of the arm. As the divisions approach the level of the clavicle, the plexus again reorganizes into three cords (lateral, posterior, and medial), which are oriented around the second part of the axillary artery. The cords then extend beyond the pectoralis minor muscle. They form five terminal branches of the brachial plexus: musculocutaneous (C5–7), median nerve (C6–7), ulnar nerve (C6–T1), axillary nerve (C5–6), and radial nerve (C5–T1). Peripheral nerve blocks can be performed at many junctures along the brachial plexus to provide anesthesia, analgesia, and vasodilatation to the upper extremity. The dermatomal distribution of these nerve roots is illustrated in Figure 6.3.[14]

TABLE 6.3

Treatment of local anesthetic toxicity

1. Discontinue injection of a local anesthetic.
2. Administer oxygen, maintain patent airway & support ventilation if necessary.
3. For CNS excitability & seizures, administer increments and repeat as needed of either iv benzodiazepine (diazepam 0.05–0.1mg/kg; Midazolam 0.05–0.2 mg/kg; smaller doses should be used in neonates and infants) or thiopental 1-2mg/kg.
4. For generalized tonic-clonic seizure succinylcholine (1 mg/kg) may be necessary to terminate the motor component of the seizures and allow effective ventilation.
5. Shock and circulatory arrest should be treated per ACLS and PALS protocols.
6. Intralipid 20% is administered if standard resuscitation effort is unsuccessful. Adult initial dose is 1.5 mL/kg over 1 minute followed by continuous infusion of 0.25 mL/kg/min for 30–60 minutes. Bolus dose may be repeated every 3–5 minutes if asystole persists and infusion may be increased to 0.5 mL/kg/minutes if hypotension persists until hemodynamic stability is achieved; maximum of 8 mL/kg.
7. If available, consider cardiopulmonary bypass should the above measures be unsuccessful.

Neal JM, Weinberg GL, Bernards CM, et al. ASRA practice advisory on local anesthetic systemic toxicity. *Reg Anesth Pain Med.* 2010; 35:152-161, with permission from American Society of Regional Anesthesia and Pain Medicine.

Interscalene Nerve Block

Indications: Surgery of the shoulder or upper arm

Applied anatomy: The block is performed at the level of the C6 transverse process (Chassaignac's tubercle), which is also the level of the cricoid cartilage. At this level, the brachial plexus traverses between anterior and middle scalene muscles. Deposition of local anesthetic occurs around the upper roots (C5, C6) and ensures anesthesia to the shoulder and the upper arm (proximal to the elbow).

Positioning: Supine or sitting with the head up at a 30-degree angle and turned to non-operative side

Landmarks: (1) Upper border of cricoid cartilage (C6 level), (2) Sternal and clavicular heads of sternocleidomastoid muscle (SCM), (3) Clavicle

Needle: 22-gauge, 5 cm short bevel, insulated needle

Nerve stimulation technique: Palpate the lateral border of the SCM at the level of C6 and move your fingers posterior/lateral, letting your fingers fall into the interscalene groove. Having the patient lift his/her head off the bed with the head turned to the contralateral side will accentuate the SCM. Then, have the patient sniff forcefully, which accentuates the interscalene groove. The external jugular vein frequently crosses the SCM at this juncture. If so, initial needle insertion should be posterior to the vein. Place the index and middle fingers of your nondominant

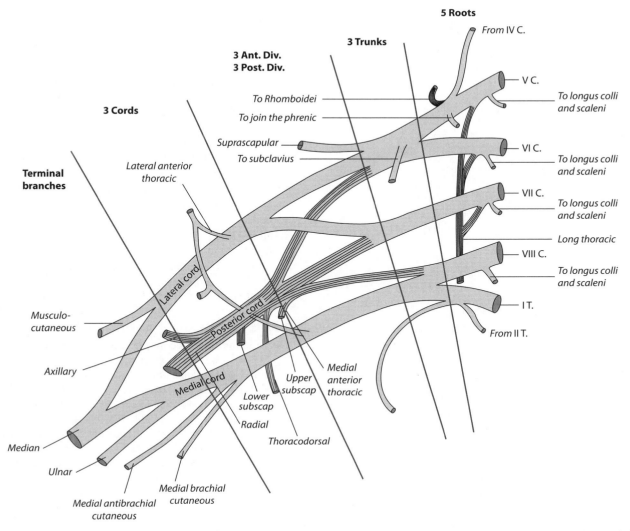

5 Roots

From IV C.

3 Trunks

V C.

3 Ant. Div.
3 Post. Div.

*To longus colli
and scaleni*

To Rhomboidei

To join the phrenic

3 Cords

Suprascapular

To subclavius

VI C.

*To longus colli
and scaleni*

**Terminal
branches**

*Lateral anterior
thoracic*

VII C.

*To longus colli
and scaleni*

Long thoracic

VIII C.

*To longus colli
and scaleni*

Lateral cord

Posterior cord

*Musculo-
cutaneous*

I T.

From II T.

Axillary

Medial cord

*Upper
subscap*

*Medial
anterior
thoracic*

*Lower
subscap*

Radial

Thoracodorsal

Median

Ulnar

*Medial brachial
cutaneous*

*Medial antibrachial
cutaneous*

FIGURE 6.2   Brachial plexus. Lewis W. *Anatomy of the Human Body.* 20th ed. Philadelphia: Bartleby.com/Lea & Febiger; 1918. Figure 807 (with permission).

hand into the interscalene groove at the level of C6. With your dominant hand, insert the block needle in between your two fingers in a direction that is perpendicular to the skin in every plane. Advance the needle as described in the Electrical Nerve Stimulation Technique section. Common responses to nerve stimulation and appropriate interventions are described in Table 6.4.[15] The goal is to obtain twitches from the pectorals, deltoid, triceps, biceps, forearm, and/or hand with 0.3 to 0.8 mA. This represents stimulation of the brachial plexus. Once that is achieved, aspirate and slowly inject with intermittent aspiration to confirm that there is no intravascular injection. Confirm that the injection is easy and painless to confirm that there is no intraneural injection.

Ultrasound-Guided Technique

Probe: High-frequency (5–12 MHz)

Probe position: Place the US probe over the interscalene groove at the level of C6. The oblique plane gives the best view of the brachial plexus. This view will show the brachial plexus at the level of the roots in cross-section. The plexus will appear hypoechoic with three of the nerve roots looking like a traffic light or snowman. If there is difficulty identifying brachial plexus at the level of nerve roots near C6, we recommend scanning the plexus at the supraclavicular level and tracking it cephalad.

Needle trajectory: This may be performed in an out-of-plane or in-plane approach.

Caveats: The block is typically performed at the upper roots (C5, 6) and spares the lower roots (C8, T1, ulnar distribution) 30%–50% of the time. Also, the C3 and C4 nerve roots (cape area) are not consistently blocked. An intercostobrachial nerve block may be needed to supplement the interscalene block for major shoulder surgery. This is performed by subcutaneous infiltration of local anesthetic from axilla to midpoint of clavicle on anterior chest.

Complications: Occasionally, there is proximal spread to the cervical plexus (C3, C4), the cervical sympathetic chain, and recurrent laryngeal nerve causing Horner's syndrome and hoarseness. In addition, it invariably

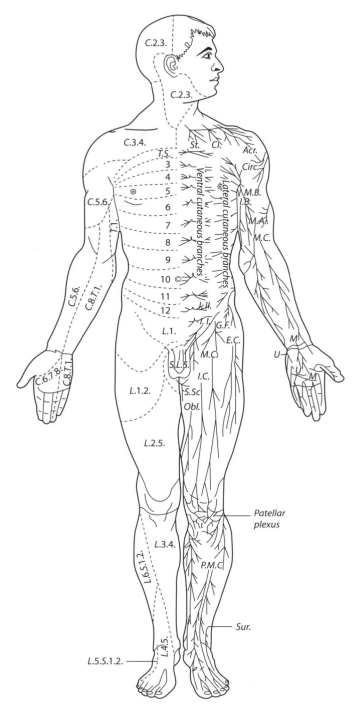

FIGURE 6.3 Dermatomes. Lewis W. *Anatomy of the Human Body.* 20th ed. Philadelphia: Bartleby.com/Lea & Febiger; 1918. Figure 797 (with permission).

causes ipsilateral hemidiaphragm paresesis due to close proximity to the phrenic nerve (C3-4-5). Patients who cannot tolerate a 30% decrease in pulmonary function should not receive this block. It follows that patients should not receive bilateral interscalene blocks. Subdural, epidural, and subarachnoid puncture/injection must all be avoided. Pneumothorax and puncture of the external jugular, internal jugular, carotid artery, or vertebral artery are other possible complications.

Infraclavicular Nerve Block

Indications: Surgery of elbow, forearm, and hand

Applied anatomy: The block is performed at the level of the cords and terminal branches. The infraclavicular nerve block is more effective than the axillary block for anesthetizing axillary and musculocutaneous nerves because it is more proximal than the axillary nerve block. It is also technically more difficult to block all of the cords.

Positioning: Supine with ipsilateral arm abducted and externally rotated. The head is turned to the contralateral side.

Landmarks: (1) The coracoid process, which is approximately 2 cm below the clavicle at the level of the (2) deltopectoral groove, near (3) the junction of the middle and lateral thirds of the clavicle. The needle insertion point is 2 cm medial and 2 cm caudad from the coracoid process.

Needle: 21-gauge, 10-cm short bevel, insulated needle

Nerve stimulation technique: Insert the needle perpendicular to skin in an anterior to posterior direction and stimulate. In adults, brachial plexus stimulation is typically obtained at 4–6 cm depth from skin. Common responses to nerve stimulation and appropriate interventions are described in Table 6.5. The goal is to obtain twitches from the wrist or fingers at 0.3–0.8 mA. This represents stimulation of the brachial plexus. Once that is achieved, aspirate and slowly inject with intermittent aspiration to confirm that there is no intravascular injection. Confirm that the injection is easy and painless to confirm that there is no intraneural injection.

Ultrasound-Guided Technique

Probe: High-frequency (5–12 MHz)

Probe position: Place the US probe on the patient's chest, just inferior to the clavicle, immediately medial to the coracoid process in a parasagittal plane, rotating the probe in a slightly oblique fashion such that the US probe is almost perpendicular to the clavicle. This view will provide a parasagittal cross-section of the muscles, vessels, and nerves. Identify the pectoralis major and minor muscles. Deep to the muscles will be the axillary artery (cephalad) and vein (caudad), which will appear like two eyes staring back at you. The brachial plexus will appear hyperechoic around the axillary artery. Usually, the lateral cord will be at the 9-o'clock position, the posterior cord at 6 o'clock, and the medial cord at 3 o'clock. However, there is significant variability.

Needle trajectory: In an in-plane approach, insert the needle next to the cephalad edge of the US probe at a 15- to 45-degree angle depending on body habitus. Advance the needle while avoiding the axillary artery and vein. Once the needle tip is immediately adjacent to the posterior cord near the 6-o'clock position, aspirate and

TABLE 6.4

Fine-tuning interscalene block

Response	Interpretation	Problem	Action
Local twitch	Direct stimulation of anterior scalene or SCM.	Needle too anterior or medial.	Withdraw and redirect 15° lateral or posterior.
Needle hits bone at 1–2 cm; no twitch	Needle hitting transverse process.	Needle too posterior or lateral.	Withdraw and redirect 15° medial or anterior.
Diaphragm twitch	Needle stimulating phrenic nerve.	Needle too anterior and medial.	Withdraw and reinsert 15° posterior or lateral.
Arterial blood aspirated	Carotid puncture (most likely) vs. vertebral artery puncture.	If carotid, too anterior and medial. If vertebral, too deep and medial.	Withdraw and keep pressure 5 minutes. If carotid, reinsert 1–2 cm posterior. If vertebral, reinsert 1 cm more shallow and more lateral.
Twitch of scapula	Stimulating thoracodorsal nerve (twitch of serratus anterior).	Needle too posterior and deep to brachial plexus.	Withdraw and redirect more anterior.
Twitch of trapezius	Stimulating accessory nerve.	Needle too posterior.	Withdraw and redirect more anterior.
Twitch of pectorals, deltoids, triceps, biceps, forearms, and/or hand	Brachial plexus stimulation.	None.	Accept and inject local anesthetic slowly with intermittent aspiration.

Hadzic, Admir. *Textbook of Regional Anesthesia and Acute Pain Management.* Columbus: McGraw-Hill; 2007. Table 25-3.

TABLE 6.5

Fine-tuning infraclavicular block

Response	Interpretation	Problem	Action
Twitch of pectoralis muscle	Direct stimulation of pectoralis m.	Needle too shallow.	Continue advancing the needle.
Deltoid muscle twitch	Stimulating axillary nerve.	Needle too inferior.	Withdraw needle and redirect more cephalad.
Twitch of biceps	Stimulating musculocutaneous nerve.	Needle too lateral.	
			Withdraw and redirect more medially.
Twitch of fingers (or wrist)	Stimulating radial nerve (extension) or median nerve (flexion).	No problem.	Inject local anesthetic slowly with intermittent aspiration.

From Navil F. Sethna.

inject the local anesthetic. The local anesthetic should spread around all three cords from 9 o'clock to 3 o'clock around the axillary artery. If it is not surrounding the medial cord, the needle may need to be redirected over top the axillary artery to reach the medial cord.

Caveats: (1) This is not a block for clinicians who rarely perform peripheral nerve blocks. (2) Use adequate sedation and generous local infiltration, as this block is uncomfortable for most patients.

Complications: (1) Hematoma: Care must be taken to avoid vascular puncture because the bleeding vessels are deeply situated and not accessible for manual compression. (2) Pneumothorax can be avoided by directing the needle laterally.

Axillary Nerve Block

Indications: Surgery of forearm and hand

Anatomy/clinical correlation: This is a block of the terminal nerves of the brachial plexus. There are two major nerves from each cord. The lateral cord divides into the musculocutaneous nerve and the lateral portion of the median nerve. The medial cord divides into the ulnar nerve and the medial portion of the median nerve. The posterior cord divides into the radial nerve

and the axillary nerve. The median, ulnar, and radial nerves travel distally with the axillary artery within the sheath. However, the musculocutaneous nerve leaves the plexus and the sheath separately within the belly of the coracobrachialis muscle. Therefore, the musculocutaneous nerve must be blocked separately.

Because of the distal location, there is negligible risk of respiratory complications due to pneumothorax or phrenic nerve blockade.

Positioning: Supine with operative arm abducted and externally rotated. If the patient is unable to abduct the arm more than 45 degrees, the patient is not an appropriate candidate for this block.

Transarterial Technique

Landmarks: (1) Axillary artery palpated as proximal in the base of the axilla as possible. (2) Biceps muscle. (3) Coracobrachialis muscle: To identify, displace the biceps muscle laterally. The coracobrachialis is the cord-like structure palpated under biceps in the upper half of the humerus.

Needle: 1.5-inch, 25-gauge thin long-bevel needle.

The primary advantage of this technique is that it does not rely on any additional technology such as nerve stimulation or imaging guidance. The disadvantage is the higher risk of accidental intra-arterial injection, nerve transfixion, hematoma, and arterial occlusion due to arterial spasm or plaque dislodgement. Needle placement within the neurovascular sheath is confirmed by arterial puncture.

Palpate the axillary artery and stabilize it with two fingers. Insert the needle in a distal to proximal fashion into the axillary artery at a 10- to 30-degree angle to skin while continuously aspirating. The needle is advanced deeper until bright red blood is no longer aspirated, indicating that the needle tip has gone beyond the posterior wall of axillary artery. Inject 0.3 mL/kg or 10–15 mL (approximately half of the total) of the local anesthetic behind the posterior wall of the artery to block the radial nerve.

Slowly withdraw the needle again while aspirating. As the needle tip reenters the artery, bright red blood is again aspirated.

Withdraw the needle until blood is again no longer aspirated, indicating that the needle tip is now superficial or medial to the artery.

Now inject 0.3 mL/kg or 10–15 mL (the other half of the total volume) of the local anesthetic to block the median and ulnar nerves.

To block the musculocutaneous nerve separately as a field block, at the level of the proximal humerus, the biceps muscle is retracted laterally and the coracobrachialis muscle is palpated medial to it. Insert the needle into the coracobrachialis muscle, aspirate and inject 0.2 mL/kg or up to 10 mL of local anesthetic.

Nerve Stimulation Technique and Ultrasound Technique

Needle: 22-gauge, 5-cm short bevel, insulated needle

Landmarks: (1) Biceps muscle. (2) Coracobrachialis muscle: To identify it, displace the biceps muscle laterally. The coracobrachialis is the cord-like structure palpated under biceps in the upper half of the humerus. (3) Axillary artery palpated immediately posterior to the coracobrachialis. Palpate the pulse as proximal in the base of the axilla as possible. Mark out the trajectory of the artery as it courses to the axilla. (4) Pectoralis major muscle. (5) Triceps muscle.

Musculocutaneous nerve block: Block the musculocutaneous first. Identify patient's bicep and displace it laterally, exposing the coracobrachialis. Insert the needle perpendicular to the arm into the coracobrachialis and stimulate (as noted earlier). The target response is elbow flexion. Then confirm negative aspiration and inject 0.2 mL/kg or 10 mL of local anesthetic slowly with intermittent aspiration.

Axillary nerve block: Redirect the needle above the arterial pulse to stimulate the median nerve (tangential to the pulse), which leads to hand and wrist flexion. Direct the needle below the arterial pulse to find the radial and ulnar nerves. Stimulating the radial nerve (deep to the pulse) results in hand and wrist extension. Stimulating the ulnar nerve (tangential to the pulse) results in hand and wrist flexion. For each nerve, stimulate as stated earlier, and then inject 0.1–0.2 mL/kg or 5–10 mL of local anesthetic slowly with intermittent aspiration.

Ultrasound-Guided Technique

Probe: High-frequency (5–12 MHz)

Probe position: Place the US probe high in the patient's axilla at the intersection of the pectoralis major muscle and the biceps muscle. This probe position will allow visualization of the artery and the three nerves in transverse view. The typical arrangement of the nerves around the artery is as follows: the median nerve lies superficial and lateral to the artery (12 o'clock), the radial nerve lies deep to the artery (6 o'clock), and the ulnar nerve lies medial to the artery (3 o'clock). The musculocutaneous nerve can be identified by following the nerves proximally and locating the musculocutaneous nerve departing the lateral cord in the proximal axilla and following it back distally between the coracobrachialis and biceps muscles.

Needle approach: This block can be performed in an in-plane or out-of-plane fashion. Block the musculocutaneous nerve first in the coracobrachialis. Advance the needle through skin with intermittent injection of sterile saline to identify the tip as the needle is advanced and being careful to avoid puncturing vascular structures (axillary artery and vein). Once the needle tip is immediately adjacent to the target nerve, aspirate and inject the local anesthetic. The local anesthetic should spread around all three nerves. If spread is inadequate, the needle should be redirected to block each individual nerve with 5–10 mL of local anesthetic.

Caveats: Nerve stimulation: (1) Elbow flexion indicates the needle is outside the neurovascular sheath near the musculocutaneous nerve. (2) Stimulation of the median and ulnar nerves produces hand and wrist flexion. (3) Median nerve stimulation causes forearm pronation and tightening of tendons in the middle of the wrist. (4) Ulnar nerve stimulation causes tightening of the tendons in the medial aspect of the wrist and flexion of the ring and little fingers.

Intercostobrachial nerve block is necessary to minimize the tourniquet pain of arm tourniquets. To perform a field block of the intercostobrachial nerve, inject 0.2 mL/kg or 10 mL of local anesthetic as a cuff subcutaneously around the upper arm as proximal as possible (e.g. at the level of the pectoralis muscle insertion onto the humerus and the inferior border of the axilla).

Complications: Inadvertent intravascular injection and hematoma.

Lower Extremity Basic Anatomy

Two major nerve plexuses, lumbar and sacral, innervate of the lower extremity. The lumbar nerve roots exit the spinal cord at one level below the vertebrae with similar spinal segments designation and divide into anterior and posterior rami. The anterior rami of L1–L4 merge to form the lumbar plexus on the anterior surface of the lumbar transverse processes within the posterior third of the psoas muscle, which inserts onto the lumbar transverse processes.

The major nerves of the lumbar plexus include: (1) ilioinguinal and iliohypogastric nerves (L1), which provide sensation to the inguinal and perineal region; (2) lateral femoral cutaneous nerve

(L2–L3), which provides sensation to the anterolateral surface of the thigh down to the knee; (3) femoral nerve (L2–L4), which provides motor innervation to the iliacus, hip flexors, and knee extensors of the thigh and sensory innervation to the anteromedial thigh, anterior knee, and medial aspect of the lower leg; (4) obturator nerve (L2–L4), which provides motor innervation to the medial thigh adductors and sensory innervation to a small part of the knee joint; and (5) lumbosacral trunk (L4–L5), which joins anterior rami of S1–S4 in the formation of the sacral plexus.

The sacral plexus is located in the lesser pelvis along the anterior surface of the piriformis muscle where the anterior rami of spinal nerves L4–S4 merge. Most of the nerves from the sacral plexus exit the pelvis through the greater sciatic foramen. The major nerves of the sacral plexus include the following:

- Sciatic nerve (L4–S3): provides motor and sensory innervation to the posterior thigh and the foot. It divides into two main branches above the knee, the tibial nerve and common peroneal nerve.
- Pudendal nerve (S2–S4): provides motor and sensory innervation to the perineum.
- Posterior femoral cutaneous nerve (S2–S3): provides sensation to the posterior surface of the proximal thigh.
- Superior gluteal nerve (L4–S1): innervates the gluteus medius and minimus muscles.
- Inferior gluteal nerve (L5–S2): innervates the gluteus maximus muscle.

Femoral Nerve Block

Indications: Surgery of anterior thigh and knee. A sciatic nerve block covers almost the entire hip, leg, and foot. When combined with popliteal fossa nerve block, it provides anesthesia to the entire lower leg and foot.

Applied anatomy: The femoral nerve is the largest terminal branch of the lumbar plexus and is formed by the dorsal divisions of the anterior rami of L2–L4. It lies lateral and posterior to the femoral artery in the region between the inguinal ligament and inguinal crease. The nerve is divided into anterior and posterior branches: (1) anterior branch provides motor innervation to sartorius and pectineus muscles and sensory innervation to anterior and medial thigh, and (2) posterior branch provides motor innervation to the quadriceps muscle and the medial surface of the lower leg via the saphenous nerve.

Positioning: Supine with operative leg straight with slight external rotation

Landmarks: (1) Anterior superior iliac spine (ASIS); (2) pubic symphysis; (3) inguinal ligament (draw line between ASIS and pubic symphysis); (4) inguinal crease; and (5) femoral artery pulse

Needle: 22-gauge, 5-cm short bevel, insulated needle

Nerve stimulation technique: Insert needle 1–1.5 cm directly lateral to the femoral artery at the level of the crease. The femoral nerve is wide and superficial, and is accessible under the skin and subcutaneous tissue usually at a depth less than 3 cm. Direct the needle cephalad toward the midpoint of the inguinal ligament with a 30- to 45-degree angle to skin and stimulate as noted earlier. The femoral nerve usually runs through the center of the inguinal ligament, which is helpful to know particularly for the obese patient. Common responses to nerve stimulation and appropriate interventions are described in Table 6.6.[16] The goal is to obtain twitches from the quadriceps and patella at 0.3–0.8 mA. This represents stimulation of the femoral nerve. Once that is achieved, aspirate and slowly inject with intermittent aspiration to confirm that there is no intravascular injection. Confirm that the injection is easy and painless to confirm that there is no intraneural injection.

Ultrasound-Guided Technique

Probe: High-frequency (5–12 MHz)

Probe position: Place the US probe in the region of the groin between the inguinal ligament and inguinal crease. Identify the femoral nerve, artery, and vein from lateral to medial in the short-axis view. Both the femoral artery and nerve usually bifurcate at the level of the inguinal crease. Therefore, it is advisable to perform the block above the level of the bifurcation.

Needle trajectory: This may be performed in an out-of-plane or in-plane fashion. When performing out of plane, position the probe with the lateral margin of the femoral nerve in the middle of the probe and advance the needle through skin, fascia lata, and fascia iliaca. As the needle tip traverses each layer, a "pop" sensation is felt. For the in-plane approach, position the probe so that the femoral nerve is on the medial edge of the probe. Advance the needle from lateral to medial so that the entire needle is visible. For both approaches, identify the needle tip with intermittent injection of

TABLE 6.6

Fine-tuning femoral nerve block

Response	Interpretation	Problem	Action
Twitch of sartorius muscle	Stimulating anterior branch of femoral nerve.	Needle tip is slightly anterior and medial to the main trunk of the femoral nerve.	Withdraw and redirect needle lateral. May need to advance several mm deeper.
Vascular puncture	Blood usually indicates puncture of femoral artery.	Needle too medial.	Remove needle and hold pressure for 5 min. reinsert needle 1 cm lateral to previous site.
Patella twitch	Stimulation of the main trunk of femoral nerve.	None.	Accept and inject local anesthetic.

Hadzic, Admir. *Textbook of Regional Anesthesia and Acute Pain Management.* Columbus: McGraw-Hill; 2007. Table 35-1.

sterile saline. Once the needle tip pierces the fascia iliaca, lateral to the nerve, confirm negative aspiration for blood and inject the local anesthetic as described earlier.

Caveats: The block will fail if the local anesthetic is deposited outside the fascia iliaca compartment. During US-guided block, the correct deposition of the local anesthetic is confirmed by observing the spread around the femoral nerve and within the fascia iliaca.

Complications: As with all lower extremity blocks, patients should not be allowed to ambulate before full recovery of sensory and motor function.

Fascia Iliaca Compartment Block Technique

When nerve stimulation or ultrasound technologies are unavailable, an alternative method is the fascia iliaca compartment block technique, which relies purely on landmarks and loss of resistance technique. The compartment contains three of the four major nerves innervating the leg, namely, the femoral nerve, lateral femoral cutaneous nerve, and obturator nerve. This block will reliably block the femoral and lateral femoral cutaneous, but frequently miss the obturator. Landmarks for this block, like the femoral nerve block, are the ASIS, pubic symphysis, and femoral artery pulse. Draw a line between the ASIS and pubic symphysis, representing the inguinal ligament. Divide this line into thirds and mark the femoral artery pulse. The puncture site will be at the junction of the lateral third and middle third of the line. Make sure that this site is lateral to the femoral artery pulse and the femoral nerve. After appropriate skin preparation and subcutaneous infiltration of local anesthetic, insert a 5-cm short-bevel or blunt tip needle at a right angle to the skin, feeling sequential distinct "pops" and loss of resistance through skin and fascia lata, and then the more subtle pop of the fascia iliaca. Aspirate to confirm the absence of blood and inject local anesthetic slowly with intermittent aspiration. There should be minimal resistance to injection.

Sciatic Nerve Block

Indications: When combined with femoral nerve block, it blocks almost the entire hip and lower extremity.

Applied anatomy: The sciatic nerve is the largest nerve in the body and is formed by the anterior rami of the L4–S3 spinal nerves. It exits the pelvis through the greater sciatic foramen, traveling under the gluteus maximus and the piriformis muscle. Distal to the piriformis muscle, it travels in the middle between the ischial tuberosity and the greater trochanter of the femur. As it descends it divides into the tibial and common peroneal nerves at a variable distant but usually around mid-thigh. However, in approximately 10% of the population the division may occur within the pelvis. It supplies motor and sensory innervation to the posterior thigh, entire lower leg, and foot, with exception to the medial aspect of the lower leg (saphenous nerve). It does not innervate any muscles in the gluteal region.

Positioning: Lateral decubitus position with operative side up and slight forward tilt. The hip and knee are flexed with ipsilateral foot positioned over the dependent leg so that twitches can be easily observed. If the patient is unable to flex the knee, the leg should be extended at the hip as far as possible.

Landmarks: There are several approaches. The classic Labat approach for adults is described here. Locate the (1) greater trochanter (GT) and (2) posterior superior iliac spine (PSIS); (3) draw a line from GT to PSIS; (4) draw a 4 cm line perpendicular to this first line distally (caudad and medial). (5) The point 4 cm distal to the midpoint of the first line is the needle insertion site.

Needle: 21-gauge, 10-cm short bevel, insulated needle for majority of patients. A 15-cm needle may be needed for obese patients.

Classic Labat nerve stimulation technique: The needle should be inserted perpendicular to the skin in all directions. Initially set the nerve stimulator at 1.5 mA to allow detection of gluteal muscle twitch and stimulation of sciatic nerve. The goal is muscle twitch of hamstrings, calf muscles, foot, or toes. The first twitches observed are from the gluteal muscles and indicate that the needle is still too shallow. Once gluteal muscle twitch disappears, plantar flexion/inversion (tibial nerve) or dorsiflexion/eversion (common peroneal nerve) typically appear. Muscle twitch at 0.3–0.8 mA indicates adequate proximity to the sciatic nerve for local anesthetic injection. If foot twitch is not obtained with the first needle pass: (1) check nerve stimulator connections, (2) reassess your needle position, (3) withdraw the needle and redirect either 5 to 10 degrees cephalad or caudad. If hamstring twitch is obtained, that is usually acceptable at this level. However, I would try redirecting the needle slightly laterally to obtain foot twitch.

Ultrasound-Guided Technique

Probe: Low-frequency (2–5 MHz)

Probe position: With patient lying in lateral decubitus, identify the GT and ischial tuberosity (IT) and draw a line connecting the two points. Place the US probe over the midpoint of this line as the sciatic nerve frequently bisects this line. This probe placement will provide a transverse view of the nerve, which will appear as a hyperechoic elliptical structure. The IT (medial) and GT (lateral) should be visible as hyperechoic structures on each side of the nerve.

Needle trajectory: This may be performed in an out-of-plane or in-plane approach.

Key points: The advantage of Labat's technique is that it captures the posterior femoral cutaneous nerve, which provides sensation to the gluteus and proximal posterior thigh.

Plantar flexion/inversion (tibial) has shorter onset for block and greater success rate than dorsiflexion/eversion (common peroneal).

With ultrasound guidance, the lateral to medial needle approach is preferred due to the presence of the inferior gluteal artery present medial to the nerve.

Complications: The sciatic nerve is confined between bony prominences and therefore at risk for external pressure injury in recumbent and sitting position. Following the block, frequent gluteal repositioning by caregiver may minimize this complication.

Popliteal Fossa Sciatic Nerve Block

Indications: Foot and ankle surgery when combined with femoral (saphenous) nerve block for ankle surgery.

Applied anatomy: This is a sciatic nerve block at the level of the popliteal fossa, which preserves hamstring function. The lateral border of popliteal fossa is the biceps femoris muscle. The medial border consists of the semitendinosus/semimembranosus muscles. The sciatic nerve typically branches into the tibial and common peroneal nerves at this level. It is lateral and superficial to the popliteal artery and vein.

Positioning: Prone with ipsilateral knee flexed with a pillow under the leg. The foot should rest freely to allow plantar and dorsiflexion during nerve stimulation and easier scanning with US probe.

Landmarks: (1) Tendon of biceps femoris (laterally) and tendon of semitendinosus and semimembranosus muscles (medially). (2) Apex of the triangle popliteal fossa is formed by intersection of the biceps femoris and semitendinosus/semimembranosus muscles and the base is the popliteal fossa crease. The patient is asked to flex the knee to accentuate the landmarks.

Needle: 22-gauge, 5-cm short bevel, insulated needle

Nerve stimulation technique: Insert the needle at a 45- to 60-degree angle to the skin approximately 7 cm cephalad and 1 cm lateral to the apex of the popliteal fossa to target the sciatic nerve before it bifurcates. Common responses to nerve stimulation and appropriate interventions are described in Table 6.7.[17] The goal is to obtain foot twitches that result in plantar flexion,

inversion, dorsiflexion, and/or eversion with 0.3–0.8 mA. This represents stimulation of the sciatic nerve. Once that is achieved, aspirate and slowly inject with intermittent aspiration to confirm that there is no intravascular injection. Confirm that the injection is easy and painless to confirm that there is no intraneural injection.

Ultrasound-Guided Technique

Probe: High-frequency (5–12 MHz)

Probe position: Place the US probe over the popliteal crease. The sciatic nerve will most likely have already bifurcated at this point. If so, identify the common peroneal and tibial nerves, which will be lateral and medial in the crease respectively. The nerves will appear as a hyperechoic honeycomb-like structure. As the probe is moved cephalad, the two branches will merge to form the sciatic nerve where the local anesthetic should be deposited for complete sciatic nerve block. The popliteal artery is located deep and medial to the sciatic nerve.

Needle trajectory: This block may be performed in plane or out of plane.

Caveats: Nerve stimulation: Foot Inversion (tibial) has the best success rate. Dorsiflexion (deep peroneal) has the second best success rate.

Ultrasound guidance: If there is difficulty identifying the sciatic nerve images, passive plantar flexion and dorsiflexion of the foot produces a back-and-forth movement of the sciatic nerve ("seesaw sign").

Complications: Vascular puncture. If no nerve stimulation occurs at 2 cm, redirect the needle laterally as opposed to deeper or more medially to avoid popliteal artery injury.

Ankle Block

When nerve stimulation or ultrasound technologies are unavailable, an alternative method to provide anesthesia and analgesia for foot surgery or injuries is the ankle block, which relies

TABLE 6.7

Fine-tuning popliteal fossa block

Response	Interpretation	Problem	Action
Twitch of semimembranosus.	Direct stimulation of semimembranosus.	Needle too medial.	Withdraw and redirect slightly more lateral.
Twitch of biceps femoris.	Direct stimulation of biceps femoris.	Needle too lateral.	Withdraw and redirect slightly more medial.
Vascular puncture.	Popliteal artery or vein puncture.	Needle too medial and likely too deep.	Remove needle and hold pressure for 5 minutes.
Redirect needle more lateral.			
Plantar flexion, inversion, dorsiflexion, eversion.	Stimulation of sciatic nerve.	None.	Accept and inject local anesthetic slowly with intermittent aspiration.

1. Hadzic, Admir. *Textbook of Regional Anesthesia and Acute Pain Management*. McGraw-Hill. 2007. Table 38-2.

purely on landmarks. Five terminal nerves innervate the foot. The saphenous nerve, a branch of the femoral nerve, supplies the medial aspect of the foot. Terminal branches of the sciatic nerve supply the remainder of the foot: (1) the sural nerve supplies the lateral aspect; (2) the posterior tibial nerve supplies the deep plantar structures; (3) the superficial peroneal nerve supplies the dorsum of the foot; and (4) the deep peroneal nerve supplies the deeper structures of the dorsum of the foot and the web space between the first and second toes. Landmarks for this block are the medial and lateral malleoli, the Achilles tendon, extensor hallucis longus (EHL) tendon, and the posterior tibial (PT) artery.

After appropriate skin preparation of the ankle, each nerve is blocked individually with a 25- or 27-gauge needle. The first set of nerve blocks includes three circumferential subcutaneous injections of local anesthetic along a line just proximal to the medial and lateral malleoli using a total of 0.2 mL/kg or 15 mL of local anesthetic. This ring block anesthetizes the saphenous, sural, and superficial peroneal nerves. Use one-third of the local anesthetic volume for each of the three nerves. To block the saphenous nerve, inject the local anesthetic subcutaneously along the line going posterior to anterior from the medial malleolus to the anterior aspect of the tibia. To block the superficial peroneal nerve, continue the subcutaneous injection going across the anterior surface of the tibia. To block the sural nerve, complete the circumferential subcutaneous injection going from the anterior surface of the tibia to the lateral malleolus. The deep peroneal nerve is blocked by injection of an additional 0.1 ml/kg or 8 mL of local anesthetic just lateral to the EHL tendon deep to the retinaculum along the same circumferential line. The EHL tendon can be identified easily by having the patient extend the great toe, which accentuates the tendon. Immediately lateral to the tendon, the needle is inserted perpendicular to the skin and advanced until it touches the tibia. The needle is then slightly withdrawn and 0.1 ml/kg or 8 mL of local anesthetic is injected after negative aspiration. The location for the posterior tibial nerve block, will be immediately posterior to the PT artery pulse or, if it is not palpable, the midpoint between the Achilles tendon and the posterior aspect of the medial malleolus. Direct the needle toward the tibia at a 45-degree angle to the skin and advance to contact bone. Then withdraw the needle slightly, and after negative aspiration, inject 0.1 ml/kg or 8 mL of local anesthetic. It is important to note that epinephrine should not be added to the local anesthetic for the ankle block because of the concern for compromising the distal circulation.

Useful Field Blocks

Ilioinguinal/Iliohypogastric Nerve Block

Indications: Surgical procedures involving the lower abdominal wall, such as inguinal hernia repairs or analgesia for Pfannenstiel incisions (e.g., caesarean section or hysterectomy)

Applied anatomy: Both the ilioinguinal (IIN) and iliohypogastric (IHN) nerves arise from the L1 nerve root. Both nerves travel between the transversus abdominis and internal oblique muscles superior and medial to the ASIS.

Positioning: Supine

Technique: Palpate the ASIS. Draw a line between ASIS and umbilicus and divide the line into thirds. The junction of the lateral and middle thirds is the puncture site. After appropriate skin preparation and infiltration with local anesthetic over the site, insert a 5–8 cm 22G Tuohy (or other blunt tip needle) perpendicular to skin. There will be increased resistance and subsequent loss of resistance when going through the external oblique and again when going through the internal oblique. After loss of resistance through the internal oblique, confirm negative aspiration for blood and inject 10 mL of local anesthetic (e.g., 0.25% to 0.5% bupivacaine with epinephrine).

Complications: Small incidence of incidental femoral nerve block, perforation of bowel, and pelvic hematoma. This emphasizes the importance of using blunt needles to detect the loss of resistance as the needle pierces the fascial layers.

Caveats: Keep in mind that this block does not provide visceral anesthesia, and therefore cannot be used as surgical anesthesia alone. If the inguinal hernia repair must be done with regional anesthesia alone, then the surgeon must supplement the block with injection of local anesthetic into the sac.

Penile Block

Indications: Release of paraphimosis, dorsal slit of the foreskin, circumcision, and penile lacerations

Applied anatomy: The penis is innervated by the pudendal nerve (S2–S4), which divides into the right and left dorsal nerves of the penis. The dorsal nerve on each side passes under the inferior ramus of the pubis and penetrates the layer of superficial fascia to supply the skin and also gives a branch to the corpus canvernosus. The nerves on each side are separated by the suspensory ligament of the penis.

Positioning: Supine

Ring block technique: After appropriate skin preparation, perform a circumferential subcutaneous infiltration around the base of the penile shaft using a 27-gauge needle. After negative aspiration to confirm no intravascular needle placement, 1 mL + 0.1 mL/kg (up to 10 mL) of local anesthetic should be enough to surround the base of the penis ventrally and dorsally.

Dorsal penile block (DPB): After appropriate skin preparation, insert a 27-gauge needle in the middle of the pubic arch at the base of the penis perpendicular to the skin and advance until it touches the pubic symphysis, giving a frame of reference for depth. The needle is then withdrawn and redirected to pass below the symphysis, 3–5 mm deeper depending on the size of the patient, and slightly to the left or right until a pop is felt as the needle enters the fascial compartment bounded superficially by Scarpa's fascia. After aspiration to confirm no intravascular needle placement, inject 5–7 mL of local anesthetic, withdraw the needle almost to the skin, and repeat the procedure on the other side.

Complications: Ischemia and/or permanent numbness are unlikely occurrences.

Caveats: DPB can miss the nerves to the frenulum. Therefore, doing both techniques together will likely give the best analgesia. Epinephrine should not be added to the local anesthetic for this block due to concerns of compromising the distal circulation and causing ischemia to the penis.

Digital Block

Indications: Minor procedures of the fingers

Applied anatomy: The digital nerves are branches of the median and ulnar nerves, which divide in the palm of the hand. The main nerves run medially and laterally along the palmar surface of the fingers.

Technique: Keep the hand mildly pronated to observe the dorsal and palmar surfaces. After appropriate skin preparation, a 25- or 27-gauge needle is inserted at a 45-degree angle into the dorsolateral webbing at the base of the finger and a small skin wheal is raised. Direct the needle toward the palmar surface of the base of the finger until the needle tip causes a slight skin bulge on the palmar aspect. Inject 0.05 ml/kg or 3 mL of local anesthetic, saving the last 20%–30% of volume to inject as the needle is withdrawn. Repeat the procedure on the dorsomedial webbing at the base of the finger.

Complications: Infection, ischemia of the digit, nerve injury

Caveats: Epinephrine should not be added to the local anesthetic for this block due to concern for compromising the distal circulation. Do not give more than 3 mL of local anesthetic on each side. Avoid multiple needle insertions.

COMMENTARY

Alexandra Torborg, South Africa

Providing regional anesthesia on global surgery trips is a worthwhile endeavor. It enables the medical team to efficiently care for many cases while working in LMICs. The advantages are well described in this chapter.

In my experience in rural hospitals in the less developed world, the success of regional anesthesia is dependent on a number of factors. First, patients must be made aware of the possibility of regional anesthesia; otherwise, they will likely expect general anesthesia. Second, as was the case in my practice as a rural doctor, anesthesia providers need to be armed with the skills to properly perform a few basic nerve blocks and field blocks. Lastly, in rural areas, anesthesia providers will benefit from being able to perform field blocks and peripheral nerve blocks using a nerve stimulator.

There will always be the potential for block failure, and this is especially true in inexperienced hands. The medical team and the patients should be prepared for this. It is necessary for anesthesia providers also to be competent at general anesthesia, airway management, and resuscitation. In my experience, nonspecialist anesthesia providers working in LMICs mainly use ketamine (sedation or anesthesia) without a definitive airway or alternatively spinal anesthesia. The result is that they are not experienced in airway management and rather choose to avoid any form of airway manipulation. This lack of experience in airway management creates a significant potential for morbidity and mortality. Furthermore, the use of ketamine for anesthesia and/or sedation as an alternative to good regional anesthesia or general anesthesia can sometimes result in poor operating conditions and poor patient outcomes.

In patients with successful regional blocks, it is important that patients understand that the block may still be working after the operation and that they need to take care not to injure the particular area that has been blocked.

There are a number of potential difficulties associated with teaching regional anesthesia during visiting surgical team trips. These include a lack of time, a lack of supervision, and an absence of ongoing training after the trip. Some of these limitations can be overcome by internet access, which is fortunately becoming increasingly possible at a number of rural hospitals in Africa. A number of rural hospitals will also have difficulty acquiring and storing drugs and needles. In HICs, ultrasound is increasingly being used for nerve localization. In some places, anesthesia trainees are being taught this technique exclusively. Ultrasound machines are becoming more advanced and more portable, making them a viable option for nerve localization for anesthetists on trips. However, I do not believe that this is currently a sustainable method to teach anesthesia providers working in LMICs. In LMIC, the vast majority of anesthesia is performed by anesthesia technicians or general practitioners/nonspecialists. There is not sufficient expertise or technical support for the majority of these practitioners to continue using ultrasound. I have heard anecdotes from colleagues of hospital storage rooms in LMICs that are filled with new equipment, including ultrasound machines, that have never been used. These machines had been kindly donated, but no one had the expertise to use them and there was no technical support in place to maintain the machines. Ultrasound machines certainly have great potential in LMICs, since they have multiple uses and are not limited to peripheral nerve blocks. The biggest limitation is the need for the training of healthcare workers, which requires money, expertise, and time. I would hope that, in the future, the use of ultrasound in LMICs will become a reality.

7

Preoperative Evaluation

Cynthia S. Tung

Introduction

Preoperative evaluation is a necessary component of facilitating a good perioperative outcome. A thorough preoperative evaluation is sometimes a challenge, even in high-income countries (HICs), due to time, financial, and other resource constraints. In low- and middle-income countries (LMICs), these resource constraints can present added problems in perioperative management. Challenges of surgical and perioperative management will vary, so it is important to tailor the preoperative evaluation to the country or region in which you serve and the unique comorbidities that exist there. An assessment of the country's health problems and needs provides valuable information in defining the problems of that particular community.[1] However, such an assessment is not always possible and there remains a paucity of data about how to best provide high-quality, low-cost anesthetic services in LMICs. Several guidelines have been developed by organizations such as the World Health Organization (WHO).[2] As a result, the anesthesiologist must gather and process a wide array of information and data regarding the patient, the local community, the region, and international guidelines. The synthesis of this information into a coherent perioperative plan is necessary to make informed decisions on providing safe anesthesia and surgical care in a given setting. The anesthesiologist must consider the demographic and epidemiologic data of the population being served, as well as the impact that service or surgery will have on the individual and the community.

Global Burden of Disease and Common Risk Factors in LMICs

Demographic and Epidemiologic Transitions

Demographic transition describes the changes in population composition over time, while *epidemiologic transition* describes the change in common causes of death over time in a given population.[3] Demographic and epidemiologic transitions are powerfully linked to the health patterns of a region. In order to better understand the common health concerns of the region or country in question, it is helpful to understand the current stage of demographic and epidemiologic transition for the given country and/or region.

In early demographic pretransition stages, fertility rates are high and common causes of mortality are infectious etiologies and poor nutrition. During this pretransition stage, the population consists of more young people and few older people.[3,4] As countries undergo demographic transition, fertility rates decline and mortality from infectious diseases and malnutrition declines. For example, the differences in population pyramids between an LMIC, such as Nigeria, and that of an HIC, such as the United States, can be seen in Figures 7.1 and Figure 7.2.[5] Countries like Nigeria are in the pre-transition phase of demographic transition and tend to have higher crude birth rates, fertility rates, and crude death rates.[6,7] Their population pyramids are wider at the bottom, illustrating an expanding, younger population. Countries like the United States are in the late stages of demographic transition and, thus, have lower crude birth rates, fertility rates, and crude death rates.[6] These countries show a typical rectangular pattern (Figure 7.2) in their population pyramids, illustrating the growth in the aging population as industrial and technological advances improve life expectancy.

Epidemiologic transition is linked to the changing age structure of a population. As a population in a country lives longer, common diseases and causes of mortality evolve from acute or infectious into chronic or noncommunicable etiologies, such as cardiovascular disease, cerebrovascular disease, and diabetes. Again, using Nigeria as an example, the major causes for disability-adjusted life years (DALYs) lost are from communicable diseases, maternal conditions, perinatal conditions, and nutritional deficiencies, accounting for about 59% of all DALYs lost.[8] Of all these causes, the top three contributors are infectious or parasitic disease, respiratory infections, and perinatal conditions. One must also consider that the human immunodeficiency virus/acquired immunodeficiency syndrome (HIV/AIDS) epidemic will also play an important role in affecting disease patterns, and respiratory infections may be a result of co-infection secondary to HIV/AIDS. The most common causes of DALYs lost for each WHO subregion (see Table 7.1)[9] can be found on The World Health Report statistical annex (see Table 7.2).[10] Referencing this statistical annex will provide a healthcare worker with a sense of the health patterns of the country in question.

Global Burden of Surgical Disease and Role of Anesthesia

A portion of the overall global burden of disease includes surgical needs that are unmet. The burden of surgical disease has been defined in the global health community as "the total disability and premature deaths that would occur in a population should there be no surgical care."[11] Some global health

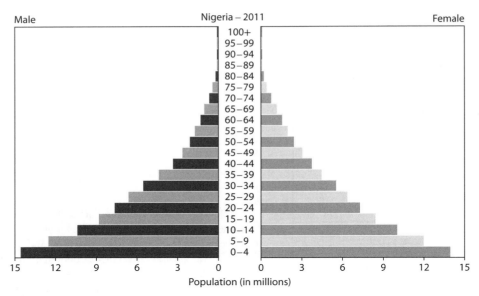

FIGURE 7.1 Population pyramid of Nigeria in 2011.
U.S. Census Bureau [Internet]. 2011 International Data Base. Available from www.census.gov

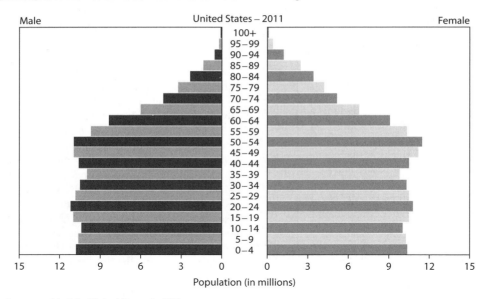

FIGURE 7.2 Population pyramid of the United States in 2011.
U.S. Census Bureau [Internet]. 2011 International Data Base. Available from www.census.gov

experts previously suggested that surgical conditions may contribute to 11% of the total global burden of disease, but other experts believe the actual surgical burden to be significantly higher.[11–13] Such surgical conditions include, but are not limited to, trauma, obstetrical care, perinatal conditions, congenital anomalies, and malignancies.[12–14]

Anesthesia services and access to these services is closely tied to this burden of surgical disease, because the lack of trained anesthesia providers, monitoring equipment, blood products, medicines, and supplies simply obstructs the facilitation of surgical care.[1,15] Little data exists that quantifies the number of anesthesia providers in LMICs and its impact on public health. Instead, global health experts infer such impact based on the number of healthcare providers per unit population and common

public health indicators, such as maternal mortality rates, child mortality rates, or life expectancy.[13] For example, maternal mortality rates in HICs like the United States and the United Kingdom range from 7 to 9.8 per 100,000 births[13,15], where the number of physicians per 10,000 people is approximately 26 and 27, respectively.[16–18] In contrast, areas of West Africa and Nepal have maternal mortality rates of 600 and 740 per 100,000 births, respectively[15], and less than one physician per 10,000 people.[16–18] The lack of anesthesia services can also impair the ability to provide safe, life-saving obstetric care, as seen by the lower rates of caesarean section in LMICs.[19] Therefore, impaired obstetric care can also impact infant and child mortality rates.[1] This is just one example of the impact that limited anesthesia care has on the global burden of surgical disease.

TABLE 7.1

WHO Member States, by region and mortality stratum

Region and mortality stratum	Description	Broad grouping	Member States
Africa			
Afr-D	Africa with high child and high adult mortality.	High-mortality developing.	Algeria, Angola, Benin, Burkina Faso, Cameroon, Cape Verde, Chad, Comoros, Equatorial Guinea, Gabon, Gambia, Ghana, Guinea, Guinea-Bissau, Liberia, Madagascar, Mali, Mauritania, Mauritius, Niger, Nigeria, Sao Tome and Principe, Senegal, Seychelles, Sierra Leone, Togo.
Afr-E	Africa with high child and very high adult mortality.	High-mortality developing.	Botswana, Burundi, Central African Republic, Congo, Côte d'Ivoire, Democratic Republic of the Congo, Eritrea, Ethiopia, Kenya, Lesotho, Malawi, Mozambique, Namibia, Rwanda, South Africa, Swaziland, Uganda, United Republic of Tanzania, Zambia, Zimbabwe.
Americas			
Amr-A	Americas with very low child and very low adult mortality.	Developed.	Canada, Cuba, United States of America.
Amr-B	Americas with low child and low adult mortality.	Low-mortality developing.	Antigua and Barbuda, Argentina, Bahamas, Barbados, Belize, Brazil, Chile, Colombia, Costa Rica, Dominica, Dominican Republic, El Salvador, Grenada, Guyana, Honduras, Jamaica, Mexico, Panama, Paraguay, Saint Kitts and Nevis, Saint Lucia, Saint Vincent and the Grenadines, Suriname, Trinidad and Tobago, Uruguay, Venezuela (Bolivarian Republic of).
Amr-D	Americas with high child and high adult mortality.	High-mortality developing.	Bolivia, Ecuador, Guatemala, Haiti, Nicaragua, Peru.
Southeast Asia			
Sear-B	Southeast Asia with low child and low adult mortality.	Low-mortality developing.	Indonesia, Sri Lanka, Thailand.
Sear-D	Southeast Asia with high child and high adult mortality.	High-mortality developing.	Bangladesh, Bhutan, Democratic People's Republic of Korea, India, Maldives, Myanmar, Nepal, Timor-Leste.
Europe			
Eur-A	Europe with very low child and very low adult mortality.	Developed.	Andorra, Austria, Belgium, Croatia, Cyprus, Czech Republic, Denmark, Finland, France, Germany, Greece, Iceland, Ireland, Israel, Italy, Luxembourg, Malta, Monaco, Netherlands, Norway, Portugal, San Marino, Slovenia, Spain, Sweden, Switzerland, United Kingdom.
Eur-B	Europe with low child and low adult mortality.	Developed.	Albania, Armenia, Azerbaijan, Bosnia and Herzegovina, Bulgaria, Georgia, Kyrgyzstan, Poland, Romania, Slovakia, Tajikistan, The former Yugoslav Republic of Macedonia, Serbia and Montenegro, Turkey, Turkmenistan, Uzbekistan.
Eur-C	Europe with low child and high adult mortality.	Developed.	Belarus, Estonia, Hungary, Kazakhstan, Latvia, Lithuania, Republic of Moldova, Russian Federation, Ukraine.
Eastern Mediterranean			
Emr-B	Eastern Mediterranean with low child and low adult mortality.	Low-mortality developing.	Bahrain, Iran (Islamic Republic of), Jordan, Kuwait, Lebanon, Libyan Arab Jamahiriya, Oman, Qatar, Saudi Arabia, Syrian Arab Republic, Tunisia, United Arab Emirates.
Emr-D	Eastern Mediterranean with high child and high adult mortality.	High-mortality developing.	Afghanistan, Djibouti, Egypt,* Iraq, Morocco, Pakistan, Somalia, Sudan, Yemen.
Western Pacific			
Wpr-A	Western Pacific with very low child and very low adult mortality.	Developed.	Australia, Brunei Darussalam, Japan, New Zealand, Singapore.
Wpr-B	Western Pacific with low child and low adult mortality.	Low-mortality developing.	Cambodia,** China, Cook Islands, Fiji, Kiribati, Lao People's Democratic Republic,** Malaysia, Marshall Islands, Micronesia (Federated States of), Mongolia, Nauru, Niue, Palau, Papua New Guinea,** Philippines, Republic of Korea, Samoa, Solomon Islands, Tonga, Tuvalu, Vanuatu, Vietnam.

* Following improvements in child mortality over recent years, Egypt meets criteria for inclusion in subregion Emr-B with low child and low adult mortality. Egypt has been included in Emr-D for the presentation of subregional totals for mortality and burden to ensure comparability with previous editions of The World Health Report and the WHO publications.

** Although Cambodia, the Lao People's Democratic Republic, and Papua New Guinea meet criteria for high child mortality, they have been included in the Wpr-B subregion with other developing countries of the Western Pacific Region for reporting purposes.

TABLE 7.2

Deaths by cause, sex and mortality stratum in WHO regions,[a] estimates for 2002. Figures computed by WHO to assure comparability;[b] they are not necessarily the official statistics of Member States, which may use alternative rigorous methods.

Cause[d]	SEX[c]						AFRICA Mortality stratum		THE AMERICAS Mortality stratum		
	Both sexes		Males		Females		High child, high adult	High child, very high adult	Very low child, very low adult	Low child, low adult	High child, high adult
	(000)	% total	(000)	% total	(000)	% total	(000)	(000)	(000)	(000)	(000)
Population (000)	6 224 985		3 131 052		3 093 933		311 273	360 965	333 580	445 161	73 810
TOTAL Deaths	57 027	100	29 949	100	27 078	100	4 634	6 144	2 720	2 691	547
I. Communicable diseases, maternal and perinatal conditions and nutritional deficiencies	18 416	32.3	9 477	31.6	8 938	33.0	3 222	4 557	167	475	233
Infectious and parasitic diseases	11 122	19.5	5 968	19.9	5 154	19.0	2 238	3 549	69	188	137
Tuberculosis	1 605	2.8	1 055	3.5	550	2.0	121	182	1	25	18
STIs excluding HIV	180	0.3	91	0.3	89	0.3	41	52	0	1	1
Syphilis	157	0.3	84	0.3	72	0.3	39	50	0	1	0
Chlamydia	9	0.0	0	0.0	9	0.0	1	0	0	0	0
Gonorrhoea	1	0.0	0	0.0	1	0.0	0	0	0	0	0
HIV/AIDS	2 821	4.9	1 532	5.1	1 290	4.8	456	1 747	14	46	43
Diarrhoeal diseases	1 767	3.1	924	3.1	844	3.1	341	354	2	33	20
Childhood diseases	1 360	2.4	679	2.3	681	2.5	426	295	0	1	6
Pertussis	301	0.5	151	0.5	151	0.6	101	71	0	0	6
Poliomyelitis	1	0.0	0	0.0	0	0.0	0	0	0	0	0
Diphtheria	5	0.0	3	0.0	3	0.0	1	1	0	0	0
Measles	760	1.3	379	1.3	382	1.4	261	178	0	0	0
Tetanus	292	0.5	147	0.5	146	0.5	64	45	0	0	0
Meningitis	173	0.3	90	0.3	83	0.3	8	12	1	8	9
Hepatitis B[e]	103	0.2	71	0.2	32	0.1	10	10	1	3	2
Hepatitis C[e]	53	0.1	35	0.1	18	0.1	4	4	5	2	0
Malaria	1 222	2.1	585	2.0	637	2.4	538	549	0	1	0
Tropical diseases	130	0.2	79	0.3	50	0.2	28	28	0	12	4
Trypanosomiasis	48	0.1	31	0.1	17	0.1	24	23	0	0	0
Chagas disease	14	0.0	8	0.0	7	0.0	0	0	0	11	4
Schistosomiasis	15	0.0	10	0.0	5	0.0	1	1	0	1	0
Leishmaniasis	51	0.1	30	0.1	21	0.1	4	4	0	0	0
Lymphatic filariasis	0	0.0	0	0.0	0	0.0	0	0	0	0	0
Onchocerciasis	0	0.0	0	0.0	0	0.0	0	0	0	0	0

Leprosy	6	0.0	4	0.0	2	0.0	0	0	0	1	0
Dengue	19	0.0	8	0.0	10	0.0	0	0	0	1	1
Japanese encephalitis	14	0.0	7	0.0	7	0.0	0	0	0	0	0
Trachoma	0	0.0	0	0.0	0	0.0	0	0	0	0	0
Intestinal nematode infections	12	0.0	6	0.0	6	0.0	1	2	0	0	1
Ascariasis	3	0.0	1	0.0	2	0.0	0	1	0	0	0
Trichuriasis	3	0.0	2	0.0	1	0.0	0	0	0	0	0
Hookworm disease	3	0.0	2	0.0	1	0.0	1	1	0	0	0
Respiratory infections	3 845	6.7	1 931	6.4	1 914	7.1	533	538	72	107	49
Lower respiratory infections	3 766	6.6	1 890	6.3	1 875	6.9	525	531	72	105	47
Upper respiratory infections	75	0.1	38	0.1	37	0.1	7	6	0	1	2
Otitis media	4	0.0	3	0.0	1	0.0	1	1	0	0	0
Maternal conditions	510	0.9	…	…	510	1.9	102	129	1	9	7
Perinatal conditions	2 464	4.3	1 368	4.6	1 096	4.0	284	270	17	132	26
Nutritional deficiencies	475	0.8	210	0.7	264	1.0	65	72	8	38	14
Protein-energy malnutrition	250	0.4	125	0.4	125	0.5	48	50	5	29	8
Iodine deficiency	7	0.0	3	0.0	3	0.0	0	2	0	0	0
Vitamin A deficiency	23	0.0	11	0.0	12	0.0	10	7	0	0	0
Iron-deficiency anaemia	137	0.2	47	0.2	90	0.3	6	11	3	7	5

Source: The World Health Report 2004.

[a] See list of Member States by WHO region and mortality stratum.

[b] See explanatory notes for sources and methods.

[c] World totals for males and females include residual populations living outside WHO Member States.

[d] Estimates for specific causes may not sum to broader cause groupings owing to omission of residual categories.

Global Burden of Disease and Anesthetic Considerations

A review of all potential disease throughout the world is beyond the scope of this chapter; however, a few common diseases and risk factors in LMICs will be discussed here. In LMICs, the top three causes of global burden of disease are lower respiratory conditions, perinatal conditions, and HIV/AIDS.[3] Acute respiratory infections and enteric infections account for a large proportion of childhood morbidity and mortality.[3] Both types of infections tend to have similar risk factors, including poverty, crowding, poor parental education, malnutrition, low birth weight, and lack of breastfeeding.[3] Because of the burden of disease associated with these infections, children who present for surgery preoperatively should be screened for recent respiratory or enteric infections and may be dehydrated with electrolyte and acid-base imbalances.

Tuberculosis (TB) is another prevalent disease among LMICs and, because of the HIV/AIDS epidemic in many countries, the incidence of new cases is projected to increase. In addition to pulmonary manifestations of TB, the anesthesiologist should also consider other sequelae from TB infection that could affect anesthetic management, such as TB meningitis or Pott's disease. In sub-Saharan Africa, the most common cause of nontraumatic spinal cord injury is TB.[20] It is possible that patients with no prior diagnosis of TB may present preoperatively with signs and symptoms of meningitis or paraplegia, for example, which may warrant a high suspicion for an existing TB infection. In LMICs, TB is diagnosed and treated based on clinical findings, sputum examination under a microscope, or chest x-ray.[3] If a patient presents for surgery with suspected TB, basic steps should be taken to prevent the spread of infection to other patients and to healthcare workers, and the urgency of the surgical procedure should be weighed along with adequate resources for perioperative care.

Malaria and other arthropod-borne diseases, such as dengue and yellow fever, also have a significant presence in LMICs. Malaria accounts for 700,000 to 2.7 million deaths per year[3], and sequelae from other parasitic infections can lead to fever, hemorrhagic fever, neurologic deficits, or heart failure. Patients may also present with dehydration or jaundice, or have liver and kidney dysfunction that may affect metabolism of certain anesthetic drugs.

Maternal and child health are undeniably linked in terms of morbidity and mortality among both populations. Birth order, maternal age, birth spacing intervals, unwanted pregnancies, and lack of breastfeeding are all factors that may affect a child's health.[3] Gestational age and size at birth are also linked to poor nutritional status in early childhood.[3] Likewise, these same factors may also affect the mother's health; for example, short intervals between the birth of one child and conception of another child may deplete the mother of her nutritional status, lead to anemia, and place the mother at increased risk of mortality during childbirth if hemorrhaging occurs.

Undernutrition at any age has many possible health consequences including anemia, iron deficiency, coagulopathies, and iodine and zinc deficiency. These can lead to infectious morbidity and mortality and poor wound healing.[2] Perioperative patients may also be at a higher risk of bleeding secondary to nutritional deficits.

As countries become more industrialized, and the population ages, chronic noncommunicable conditions such as ischemic heart disease, cerebrovascular disease, and diabetes become more prevalent.[2] In some LMICs where ischemic heart disease is present, the disease may affect younger people more than it does in HICs.[3] Thus, knowledge of demographic and epidemiologic data is important to obtain relevant preoperative information and maximize the safety of patients.

Preoperative Evaluation

In the United States, there are several means by which the preoperative evaluation is performed; for example, by the anesthesiologist who will be providing care or by a series of primary or surgical care providers before an anesthesiologist ultimately evaluates the patient on the day of surgery. In LMICs, an anesthesiologist may not have the luxury to play an active role in the preoperative evaluation; therefore, patients may be at increased perioperative risk. Sometimes, there simply may not be a preoperative evaluation system in place. Therefore, it is imperative that anesthesiologists practicing in such countries remember the calling of "first, do no harm" and perform their own preoperative evaluations, tailored to their environment, to ensure that risk is minimized and the patients are appropriate candidates for the scheduled surgery. For instance, patients may have been preselected by healthcare providers in that country with the expectation or hope that the surgery will occur. In some settings, there may be considerable secondary gain from scheduling as many procedures as possible. As a result, medical comorbidities may be overlooked given the time and resource constraints of the country or program. The anesthesiologist must then decide whether or not it is safe to proceed given the available resources. There may not be resources for common preoperative testing in many settings, such as exercise stress-tests, echocardiograms, or pulmonary function tests. The anesthesiologist must then rely significantly on the patient's history and physical examination to assess the relative risk and benefit of surgical intervention.

Another important secondary function of a thorough preoperative evaluation is the opportunity to offer basic primary care. In LMICs, the anesthesiologist must become the complete perioperative physician. This often involves administering basic primary care to those who are screened for surgery. For example, it is relatively common to detect minor, treatable infections such as mild pneumonia or otitis media. These conditions may preclude surgical intervention, but the provider can still offer treatment and facilitate a better outcome for the patient.

History

A thorough medical history provides important information for planning and providing a safe anesthetic course in any setting, but in an LMIC the history becomes even more crucial. Basic medical history and review of systems that should be obtained include, but are not limited to:

- Previous surgical history
- Medication history: prescription medications, herbal medications, local or folk medicines, illicit drug use
- Cardiovascular history: exercise tolerance, chest pain, shortness of breath, syncope, fatigue, bleeding history

- Pulmonary history: respiratory infections; reactive airway symptoms; smoking history; rural or urban dwelling location, which can suggest the level of pollution the patient is exposed to chronically
- Gastrointestinal history: reflux symptoms, abdominal pain, vomiting, alcohol consumption
- Nutritional history

For pediatric patients, additional information that could be helpful includes the child's nutrition status and history of prematurity, the mother's health and age, the ages of her other children, and the mother's pregnancy and delivery course. A history of recent pulmonary infectious processes should also be obtained, as children with recent upper respiratory tract infections are at significantly increased risk for respiratory complications when undergoing general anesthesia.[22,23] An undernourished child may be at higher risk of infections or other perioperative complications. Environmental factors such as pollution, location of domicile, smokers in the home, or poor sanitation can play a role in undiagnosed asthma, reactive airway disease, pneumonias, chronic lung disease, or gastrointestinal disease.

Some patients have lived with a symptom or disease for years without being able to seek medical care, so it may be necessary to delve further into a patient's history to elicit pieces of information that would not otherwise be apparent. For example, a patient's exercise tolerance currently may seem unchanged, but compared to 5 years ago the patient may report she could walk many more miles before becoming short of breath.

In some settings, it is also important to understand the cultural differences to overcome some barriers to obtaining a thorough history. Language can obviously be a barrier to obtaining a thorough history, so it is helpful to have interpreters well versed in medical language when possible. It is most useful to have interpreters who can translate in an unbiased manner, rather than a translator who has a vested interest in generating large numbers of cases. It is also important to ask questions in the correct cultural context. For example, in some cultures, women defer to their husbands for guidance and decision making, or it may not be appropriate to talk about a woman's symptoms in front of her family members. Pain thresholds and tolerance may also be culturally driven, and both adults and children may not explicitly express pain symptoms, so it may be necessary to specifically ask about individual pain symptoms. These and other cultural differences will influence the way information is obtained and the quality of information obtained.

Physical Exam

The physical exam is just as important as the history in LMICs, where laboratory testing is scarce or non-existent. The type of surgery, resources available, and urgency of the procedure will guide the focus and extent of the physical exam and ultimately the decision of whether to proceed with the surgery. While not an exhaustive list, basic examination findings that may be useful include:

- Vital signs, including oxygen saturation
- Airway: Mallampati class, craniofacial anomalies, neck masses, nasal masses, rhinorrhea, cough, hoarse voice, evidence for stridor, burns or scars over the face or neck

- Cardiovascular: pulse; blood pressure; heart rate and rhythm; heart murmurs; evidence of cyanosis; clubbing of nails; temperature or mottling of skin for poor perfusion; edema of extremities; lips, tongue, and skin turgor for dehydration; pallor at nails or conjunctiva for signs of anemia
- Pulmonary: auscultation and percussion of lung fields, evidence of rhinorrhea or cough
- Gastrointestinal: abdominal exam for distention, tenderness, palpable masses, palpable liver edge, evidence of jaundice

Laboratory/Diagnostic Tests

If laboratory tests are needed, one should consider the value of such testing. In many LMICs tests either are not available or the patient must travel a long distance and pay out of pocket to obtain such testing. Therefore, the anesthesiologist must ask if the information obtained from the test is going to change the management of the patient. Some helpful, but not always necessary, laboratory data could include: hematocrit, electrolytes, blood urea nitrogen (BUN), creatinine, chest x-ray, and ultrasound. In addition, there are cheap and portable devices that may be available to assess hematocrit and blood glucose.

Anesthetic Plan

After the preoperative evaluation is complete, the decision to proceed with a surgery depends, again, on understanding the country or region in question. The benefits and risks of proceeding with anesthesia and surgery on any patient must be weighed carefully. In LMICs, there are multiple factors that can affect patient care and safety, both intraoperatively and postoperatively. These factors include available types of anesthesia equipment, access to and types of medications, availability of critical care services, and the training and expertise of physicians, nurses, and other healthcare staff who will follow the patient postoperatively. The *WHO Manual: Surgical Care at the District Hospital*[2] lists some key questions to keep in mind when deciding whether to proceed with surgery:

- Can we do the procedure here?
- Is the operating room safe and fit for use?
- Are the necessary equipment and drugs available?
- Are all members of the team available?
- Do I have the knowledge and skill to perform the necessary procedure?
- Can we manage this patient?
- Is there backup or extra support available, if required?
- Can we manage the potential complications if problems arise?
- Do we have nursing facilities for good postoperative care?

(Adapted from the WHO Manual: Surgical Care at the District Hospital, 2003[21])

TABLE 7.3

International standards for a safe practice of anesthesia

Level 1 (Should meet at least HIGHLY RECOMMENDED anesthesia standards) Small hospital / health centre	Level 2 (Should meet at least HIGHLY RECOMMENDED and RECOMMENDED anesthesia standards) District/provincial hospital	Level 3 (Should meet at least HIGHLY RECOMMENDED, RECOMMENDED and SUGGESTED anesthesia standards) Referral hospital
Rural hospital or health centre with a small number of beds (or urban location in an extremely disadvantaged area); sparsely equipped operating room (OR) for "minor" procedures. Provides emergency measures in the treatment of 90–95% of trauma and obstetrics cases (excluding caesarean section). Referral of other patients (for example, obstructed labour, bowel obstruction) for further management at a higher level.	District or provincial hospital (e.g. with 100–300 beds) and adequately equipped major and minor operating rooms. Short term treatment of 95–99% of the major life threatening conditions.	A referral hospital of 300–1000 or more beds with basic intensive care facilities. Treatment aims are the same as for Level 2, with the addition of: • Ventilation in OR and ICU • Prolonged endotracheal intubation • Thoracic trauma care • Haemodynamic and inotropic treatment Basic ICU patient management and monitoring for up to 1 week: all types of cases, but possibly with limited provision for: • Multi–organ system failure • Haemodialysis • Complex neurological and cardiac surgery • Prolonged respiratory failure • Metabolic care or monitoring
Essential Procedures Normal delivery Uterine evacuation Circumcision Hydrocele reduction, incision and drainage Wound suturing Control of haemorrhage with pressure dressings Debridement and dressing of wounds Temporary reduction of fractures Cleaning or stabilization of open and closed fractures Chest drainage (possibly) Abscess drainage	Same as Level 1 with the following additions: • Caesarean section • Laparotomy (usually not for bowel obstruction) • Amputation • Hernia repair • Tubal ligation • Closed fracture treatment and application of plaster of Paris • Acute open orthopaedic surgery: e.g internal fixation of fractures • Eye operations, including cataract extraction • Removal of foreign bodies: e.g. in the airway Emergency ventilation and airway management for referred patients such as those with chest and head injuries.	Same as Level 2 with the following additions: • Facial and intracranial surgery • Bowel surgery • Paediatric and neonatal surgery • Thoracic surgery • Major eye surgery • Major gynecological surgery, e.g. vesico-vaginal repair
Personnel Paramedical staff/anesthetic officer (including on-the-job training) who may have other duties as well. Nurse-midwife.	One or more trained anesthesia professionals. District medical officers, senior clinical officers, nurses, midwives. Visiting specialists or resident surgeon and/or obstetrician/ gynecologist.	Clinical officers and specialists in anesthesia and surgery.
Drugs Ketamine 50 mg/ml injection. Lidocaine 1% or 2%. Diazepam 5 mg/ml injection, 2 ml or midazolam 1 mg/ml injection, 5 ml. Pethidine 50 mg/ml injection, 2 ml. Morphine 10 mg/ml, 1 ml. Epinephrine (Adrenaline) 1 mg. Atropine 0.6 mg/ml. Appropriate inhalation anesthetic if vaporizer available.	Same as Level 1, but also: • Thiopental 500 mg/1g powder or propofol • Suxamethonium bromide 500 mg powder • Pancuronium • Neostigmine 2.5 mg injection • Ether, halothane or other inhalation anesthetics • Lidocaine 5% heavy spinal solution, 2 ml • Bupivacaine 0.5% heavy or plain, 4 ml	Same as Level 2 with these additions: • Propofol • Nitrous oxide • Various modern neuromuscular blocking agents • Various modern inhalation anesthetics • Various inotropic angents • Various intravenous antiarrhythmic agents • Nitroglycerine for infusion • Calcium chloride 10% 10 im injection • Potassium chloride 20% 10 ml injection for infusion

Level 1 (Should meet at least HIGHLY RECOMMENDED anesthesia standards) Small hospital / health centre	Level 2 (Should meet at least HIGHLY RECOMMENDED and RECOMMENDED anesthesia standards) District/provincial hospital	Level 3 (Should meet at least HIGHLY RECOMMENDED, RECOMMENDED and SUGGESTED anesthesia standards) Referral hospital
	• Hydralazine 20 mg injection • Frusemide 20 mg injection • Dextrose 50% 20 ml injection • Aminophylline 250 mg injection • Ephedrine 30/50 mg ampoules • Hydrocortisone • Nitrous oxide	
Equipment: Capital outlay Adult and pediatric self-inflating breathing bags with masks. Foot-powered suction. Stethoscope, sphygmomanometer, thermometer Pulse oximeter. Oxygen concentrator or tank oxygen and a draw-over vaporizer with hoses. Laryngoscopes, bougies.	Complete anesthesia, resuscitation and airway management systems including: • Reliable oxygen sources • Vaporizer(s) • Hoses and valves • Bellows or bag to inflate lungs • Face masks (sizes 00–5) • Work surface and storage • Pediatric anesthesia system • Oxygen supply failure alarm; oxygen analyzer • Adult and pediatric resuscitator sets • Pulse oximeter, spare probes, adult and paediatric* • Capnograph* • Defibrillator (one per O.R. suite / ICU)* • ECG (electrocardiograph) monitor* • Laryngoscope, Macintosh blades 1–3(4) • Oxygen concentrator[s] [cylinder] • Foot or electric suction • IV pressure infusor bag • Adult and paediatric resuscitator sets • Magill forceps (adult and child), intubation stylet and/or bougie • Spinal needles 25G • Nerve stimulator Automatic non-invasive blood pressure monitor	Same as Level 2 with these additions (per each per OR room or per ICU bed, except where stated): • ECG (electrocardiograph) monitor* • Anesthesia ventilator, reliable electric power source with manual override • Infusion pumps (2 per bed) • Pressure bag for IV infusion • Electric or pneumatic suction • Oxygen analyzer* • Thermometer [temperature probe*] • Electric warming blanket • Electric overhead heater • Infant incubator • Laryngeal mask airways sizes 2, 3, 4 (3 sets per O.R) • Intubating bougies, adult and child (1 set per O.R) • Anesthetic agent (gas and vapour) analyser • Depth of anesthesia monitor are being increasingly recommended for cases at high risk of awareness but are not standard monitoring in many countries.
Equipment: Disposable Examination gloves. IV infusion/drug injection equipment. Suction catheters size 16 FG. Airway support equipment, including airways and tracheal tubes. Oral and nasal airways.	ECG electrodes IV equipment (minimum fluids: normal saline, Ringer's lactate and dextrose 5%) Paediatric giving sets Suction catheters size 16 FG Sterile gloves sizes 6–8 Nasogastric tubes sizes 10–16 FG Oral airways sizes 000–4 Tracheal tubes sizes 3–8.5 mm Spinal needles sizes 22 G and 25G Batteries size C	Same as Level 2 with these additions: • Ventilator circuits • Yankauer suckers • Giving sets for IV infusion pumps • Disposables for suction machines Disposables for capnography, oxygen analyzer, in accordance with manufacturers' specifications: • Sampling lines • Water traps • Connectors • Filters, Fuel cells

Note: Drug concentrations and quantities are indicative only. All equipment should be appropriate for patients' age and size.
(Emergency and Essential Anaesthesia and Surgical Procedures, adapted in part from WHO Manual: Surgical Care at the District Hospital 2003 and the 1992 International Standards for a Safe Practice of Anaesthesia).
* It is preferable to combine these modalities all in one unit.

Such barriers should be considered concomitantly with the patient's condition, type of surgery, and urgency of surgery. For example, even though a facility has a fully staffed critical care unit, the healthcare staff may not be accustomed to caring for a patient after a laryngotracheal reconstruction and the long follow-up care that is required for this type of procedure. One would need to consider the risks and benefits of surgical intervention versus an already stable patient, living with a functioning tracheostomy. Similarly, the threshold for proceeding with a case may be higher based on patient comorbidities, given the resources available. For example, a child with an upper respiratory infection scheduled for a circumcision in a facility where there is no access to an intensive care unit or adequate monitoring postoperatively may not be the best candidate for surgery in that particular setting.

In contrast, there may be circumstances when the threshold for proceeding is lowered, despite limited resources, because there are no other options for the patient. In cases of trauma or natural disasters, proceeding with surgery for hemorrhage in a distended abdomen despite inadequate volume of blood products may be a necessary decision given the circumstances of the patient and setting. In less emergent cases, it may be beneficial to transfer care to a referral center; however, referral centers may not be an option in certain settings or may present prohibitive costs to the patient. The financial burden on individual patients and a country's healthcare system should also be weighed carefully. One must consider the costs incurred on the patient or the health system if a patient misses his transportation home because he had an unexpected prolonged recovery room stay, or if a blood transfusion becomes necessary and a blood bank is depleted for those who are in emergent need of blood products.

Equipment Considerations

Even in the wealthiest countries, no monitoring equipment can replace clinical assessment and vigilance by the anesthesiologist. In LMICs, use of a stethoscope is essential and sometimes the only monitor available. Pulse oximetry may be the single most important and useful piece of monitoring equipment in LMICs, but may not be available because of the maintenance required and replacement parts necessary for continued use.[24,25] The World Federation of Societies of Anaesthesiologists (WFSA) created a list of anesthesia standards and essential equipment based on type of infrastructure that is available: small hospital/health center, district/provincial hospital, and referral hospital (Table 7.3).[26] Even in developing nations, it is considered outside the standard of care for foreign medical workers to proceed with elective cases without appropriate monitoring, both intra- and postoperatively. However, such standards may need to be adjusted in certain settings, such as conflict zones or disaster areas. While these standards provide guidelines for what is considered safe anesthesia practice in particular settings, judgments should be based on individual circumstances and the comfort level of the practitioner.

Conclusion

An important part to providing a safe and effective anesthetic is the preoperative evaluation. In LMICs, a technologically heavy preoperative evaluation is often a luxury, and the anesthesiologist must make decisions and anesthetic plans based on incomplete data in sometimes less than ideal conditions. Prior to working in such regions of the world, knowledge of the local health patterns and medical resources can help the healthcare provider establish anesthetic plans and goals. Many LMICs continue to struggle with communicable diseases, including HIV/AIDS, and patients may present with illnesses not commonly seen in HICs that may influence perioperative care. However, noncommunicable diseases are fast becoming common causes of mortality in developing nations and must also be considered during a preoperative evaluation. In LMICs, a thorough history and physical exam, along with clinical acumen and vigilance in the operating room, are imperative to provide the best perioperative outcomes for the patients who are served.

COMMENTARY

Francoise Nizeyimana, Rwanda
Denise M. Chan, USA

Preoperative evaluation is an integral part of perioperative care. A thorough and thoughtful preoperative evaluation reduces perioperative morbidity and mortality. In Rwanda, both time and financial resources affect the care we can provide for our patients. At one of the major referral hospitals, we have a system to ensure that every surgical patient undergoes a preoperative evaluation. An anesthesia technician or anesthesia resident visits the patient the day before the procedure, performs a focused history and physical exam, and orders laboratory investigations, radiologic studies, or blood products that may be necessary. Oftentimes these studies cannot be obtained in a timely fashion, or the patient cannot afford to pay for the studies, and we must decide whether to proceed without them or postpone surgery. Emergent cases are especially difficult, as the likelihood of obtaining adequate preoperative information, either by history or studies, is low. In addition, we do not have access to certain exams, such as cardiac stress tests

and pulmonary function tests, and as such, the importance of a solid history and physical exam is further emphasized.

As mentioned in the chapter, it is essential for the anesthesia provider to be familiar with the demographics of the country and disease profile of the population. In Rwanda, our population is transitioning from a youth-dominant demographic to an older population. We are still seeing many of our patients present preoperatively with upper and lower respiratory infections, enteric infections, malnutrition, and electrolyte imbalances, but we are also finding increasing numbers of patients with obesity and cardiovascular disease. Our scope of medical practice in Rwanda extends beyond the perioperative period, and we often provide primary pediatric and general medical care as well.

The limitation of resources undoubtedly affects our preoperative assessment of patients. However, we use what we have, namely our history-taking and physical exam skills, to minimize or patients' perioperative risk as much as possible.

8

Intraoperative Management

Terrance A. Yemen

Introduction

All operating rooms seem the same; patients undergo a variety of open and closed procedures, depending upon the needs of the patients, skills of the providers, and the resources of the community in which the work is being provided. But it is these last two factors that also make some operating rooms different. Most operating room teams coming from high-income countries (HICs) are highly skilled and are accustomed to providing their best work with unlimited, or nearly unlimited, resources.

We take for granted the many resources, both natural and human, which allow us to do the work we consider routine. However, a single visit to a field or makeshift hospital in a less developed country teaches the provider that nothing should be taken for granted. In these settings, power, clean water, basic medical supplies, and equipment become "gifts" that are cherished and vital to the success of the operating room (Figure 8.1). Healthcare providers unfamiliar with these conditions often struggle to provide even the most basic care, until they adapt to the new reality.

The purpose of this chapter is to discuss the various methods and options that may be used in providing intraoperative

anesthetic care in low- and middle-income countries (LMICs) and disaster relief areas regardless of their resources. Some of these techniques are simple and best applied to "bare bones" operations, and some require basic anesthesia equipment and skills for more elaborate scenarios. The underlying premise of this chapter is to provide safe and adaptable care under a variety of conditions with limited means.

Basic Considerations

One of the most basic considerations of intraoperative anesthesia is to know your patient(s). All anesthetics, regardless of setting, must take into consideration the health of the patient. For the purposes of this chapter, patients fall into four specific, but broad, categories.

1. Adults
2. Pediatrics
3. Obstetrics
4. Trauma

Adults

Adult patients raise a number of basic concerns that affect technique and specifically affect risk and outcome.

- Cardiovascular status: In addition to concerns about atherosclerotic and valvular heart disease, one should also screen for hypertension, possibly untreated and severe. Therefore, renal status should also be considered.
- Respiratory diseases, including infectious conditions such as tuberculosis (TB) or acquired ones such as chronic obstructive pulmonary disease (COPD), asthma, or bronchitis (not uncommonly the result of smoking, exposure to open fires for heating and cooking, and air pollution).
- Obesity, although less common in LMICs, is still a significant risk factor when present, for both technical and physiologic reasons.
- Endocrine diseases, such as hyper- and hypothyroidism and diabetes mellitus, often untreated in the poor, all may have a significant effect upon narcotic tolerance and infection rates.
- Infectious diseases such as human immunodeficiency virus (HIV); TB; and hepatitis A, B, and C; as well as

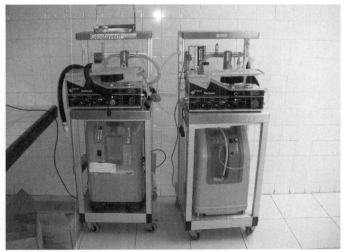

FIGURE 8.1 Two examples of the Glostavent anesthesia machine, which utilizes an oxygen concentrator and gas driven bellows ventilator, are shown. Such machines may be unfamiliar to visiting practitioners but can be quite common in many less developed nations. Thus, it is crucial that, prior to leaving on a trip, visiting anesthesiologists have a thorough understanding of the basics of such delivery systems. Image by Craig D. McClain.

a host of parasitic infections depending upon the country location. This list would certainly include malaria, typhoid, and other infectious diseases specific to the environment in question.

- Dental considerations such as loose teeth and abscesses.

Pediatrics

Pediatric patients are not simply small adults. Babies, in particular, have a number of physiologic differences that make them a higher risk for surgery and anesthesia compared to older children and adults.

- **Respiratory.** Seventy percent of adverse outcomes from surgery and anesthesia are the result of a respiratory mishap. Infants have a metabolic rate three times that of an adult. Therefore, oxygen consumption, alveolar ventilation, and respiratory rate are greatly elevated. Any interruption of normal respiration in an infant rapidly leads to hypoxia. Additionally, it is technically more difficult to maintain a patent airway in babies. This includes laryngoscopy and placement of supraglottic airways such as a laryngeal mask airway (LMA). Neonates are prone to apnea after sedation or general anesthesia due to an immature central nervous system. This risk is significantly increased in the premature infant and does not decrease until the baby is around 60 weeks' post-conceptual age. Elective surgery should be postponed until a full-term newborn is at least 46 weeks' post-conceptual age.

- **Cardiovascular.** Babies function at near maximal cardiac status even at rest because of the high metabolic rate and a limited (almost fixed) stroke volume. This means that, unlike adults, they have little or no cardiac reserve. Dehydration, blood loss, and myocardial depression are poorly tolerated, and infants rapidly decompensate as a result.

- **Hematology.** The newborn infant functions with a hematocrit in excess of 40%–45%. This is the result of the presence of fetal hemoglobin in the first three months of life. As a result, less oxygen is unloaded to the tissues for a given oxygen tension in the blood. As fetal hemoglobin is replaced with hemoglobin A, the infant develops a physiologic anemia with a hematocrit of 30% or less until erythropoietin levels rise and stimulate red cell production. This generally occurs around the second or third month of life.

- **Metabolic.** Both oxidative and reductive pathways are reduced in the infant. Additionally, many protein-bound-drugs, especially those bound by alpha 1 acid glycoprotein have a higher free (active component) fraction of drug present in the infant for any given dosage. Local anesthetics are particularly affected. Inability to effectively induce glucuronidation leads to extended effects of active metabolites and difficulty with drug elimination. Renal clearance of drugs is also reduced in the first few months of life.

- **Renal, water, and electrolytes.** The infant kidney functions with little reserve. Babies compensate poorly for water deprivation and overload. Also, they cannot adjust appropriately for salt wastage and overload. Babies are at high risk for hyponatremia that can result in seizures, cerebral edema, and death. Total body water, especially extracellular water, is increased in infants. This increase affects the volume of distribution of water-soluble drugs.

- **Heat conservation.** Infants are prone to heat loss. A large surface area, especially the head, predisposes infants to heat loss via the mechanism of radiation in the operating room. Hypothermia can result in apnea in the newborn. Shivering is poorly developed in the newborn, and general anesthesia eliminates most compensatory mechanisms. It is also important to appreciate that infants are, as a result of the aforementioned reasons, easy to overheat as well. Active heating and cooling of the infant should always be accompanied by continuous temperature monitoring.

Obstetrics

Obstetrical patients also have unique physiologic demands that affect anesthesia and intraoperative management.

- **Two patients instead of one.** The pregnant patient is really two patients, with the infant placing huge physiologic stress upon the mother while predisposing her to a number of disease states such as preeclampsia, placenta previa, placenta abruption, uterine atony, and uterine rupture. Anesthetic misadventures with the mother will result in the same or worse outcome in the fetus. Most drugs cross the placenta and therefore act upon the fetus (not always in a desired fashion). Remembering that you have two patients is important in all anesthetics involving parturients. Operations during pregnancy place the fetus at risk during the operation and after recovery. Fetal injury and premature labor are possibilities with any procedure near or involving the gravid uterus.

- **Hematology.** The pregnant patient develops a physiologic anemia with a hematocrit of 30% or less in the third trimester as a result of an increased blood volume. Therefore, there is an increased volume of drug distribution in this trimester. Lastly, blood loss during delivery can be considerable, especially during caesarean section or with uterine atony. Not only can this situation produce a shock-like state in the acute setting, but the mother also may be incapacitated by severe anemia immediately after delivery and for several weeks thereafter. Peripartum hemorrhage with inadequate resuscitation is a major cause of maternal mortality in the less developed world.

- **Respiratory.** There is a decrease in the functional residual capacity of the mother by the third trimester that encompasses the added oxygen consumption of the term fetus. As a result, the mother is at an increased risk of hypoxia when respiration is interrupted. Further, the airway becomes edematous at term. Some patients who were not originally difficult airways become difficult to manage at the time of delivery. LMAs can become invaluable, and endotracheal tubes should be downsized for an easier and better fit.

- **Cardiac.** The presence of the fetus and resultant increased metabolic demand, along with the third-term anemia, results in an increased cardiac workload for the mother. The result is a decreased cardiac reserve. This decrease in reserve, along with the increase in cardiac work demand, can precipitate a cardiac event in mothers with preexisting cardiac disease, valvular or otherwise.

- **Pregnancy-induced disease states.** A variety of conditions place the pregnant patient at risk of morbidity and mortality, especially in LMICs. These conditions include, but are not limited to, preeclampsia and eclampsia, HELLP syndrome, placental abruption, placenta accrete, premature rupture of the membranes and infection, uterine rupture, uterine atony, and cervical laceration. Blood products are a necessity for many of these conditions to be appropriately treated. Mortality for parturients with these conditions in the less developed world remains extremely high.

- **Specific anesthesia concerns.** Loss of the esophageal sphincter tone at term predisposes the mother to reflux and aspiration of stomach contents during sedation or general anesthesia. Changes in progesterone result in an increased sensitivity to many anesthetic agents.

- **Drugs.** As previously mentioned, most drugs cross the placenta and are present in the fetus. Although safe in adults, many drugs are teratogenic in the fetus, particularly during the first trimester. Some effects are minor and some devastating. No drug should be administered to a pregnant, or potentially pregnant, woman without consideration of the effects upon the fetus first.

Trauma

Trauma is responsible for 1.2 million deaths worldwide annually, with many occurring in the less developed world. Trauma patients are common in any natural disaster situation. They are also unique in terms of their needs in the intraoperative setting.

- **Blood loss and fluid resuscitation.** Many trauma patients, especially those with burns, require extensive fluid and blood products for survival. First, these patients need adequate intravenous access. Fluid and blood products are useless if you are consistently losing them faster via hemorrhage than you can get them in. Blood products are often limited in type and volume in many less developed nations and disaster situations. Often, family members serve as walking blood banks for their loved ones if there is a need for blood products. The ability to type and collect fresh whole blood in these situations is critical to success. Many places lack the facilities and financial resources to process and store components such as fresh whole plasma, packed red cells, or platelets. Thus, fresh whole blood is the most commonly available product when there is

anything available. Balance salt solutions are required in great volume but are easy to store and usually available in all but the worst of circumstances.

- **Head and neck injuries.** Many traumas involve head and neck injuries. These may be the main injuries or simply associated with more severe injuries elsewhere on the body. Fifty percent of neck injuries have a head injury and vice versa. Careful consideration must be given when providing anesthesia to patients who have significant neck injuries, stable or unknown, to avoid further compromise. Given the limited availability of definitive radiographic investigation in many of these settings, any anesthetic that avoids manipulation of the airway is desirable. In regard to head injuries, maintenance of adequate cerebral perfusion is paramount. Any anesthetic that avoids loss of consciousness or the elevation of intracranial pressure is also desirable. It is much easier to assess the neurologic status of the victim if he or she remains conscious, if at all possible.

- **Respiratory compromise.** Multiple trauma patients often have respiratory compromise, intra-operatively and post-operatively. This may be the result of direct blunt or infiltrating trauma. Also, inflammatory lung disease secondary to resuscitation with blood products can lead to respiratory compromise. These patients may benefit from short- and long-term ventilation strategies that are not available in many LMICs or disaster relief areas. The intraoperative care of these patients must reflect the resources that these patients need, and their ability to consume vast amounts of potentially limited medical equipment and supplies. The continued triage of these patients is required. Although it is often taken for granted, oxygen supplies can be inconsistent in many relief areas. Oxygen supplies should be constantly assessed and usage carefully monitored. The same can be said about electrical power as most ventilators work poorly without it. Multiple trauma patients fare poorly without either.

Intraoperative Monitoring

The intraoperative monitoring of general anesthesia has evolved significantly in HICs over the past 20 or more years. These changes have had a significant impact on the decrease in intraoperative anesthetic mortality and morbidity. The standardized monitoring of all patients, regardless of health or anesthetic technique, represents the greatest of these improvements. Most notable are the pulse oximeter and the end-tidal carbon dioxide monitor with capnograph. Practitioners should be aware that simply working in a less developed world setting is no excuse for poor monitoring. In fact, on short-term visiting surgical team trips, where expatriate caregivers are providing elective care, the same standards should apply as in the more developed world (American Society of Anesthesiologists [ASA] monitors). Certainly, purely educational trips (teaching local providers in their own environment without direct clinical care) and disaster settings will alter the paradigm of what is necessary to proceed with a case. Efforts should be made in all settings to offer the best perioperative monitoring available.

Recently, the World Health Organization (WHO) has aggressively pushed forward the adoption of many of these same standards, with the use of a pulse oximeter foremost in the recommendations. While the use of an oximeter adds greatly to the identification of perioperative hypoxia, it should not be used as a substitute for other standard monitors, which include the electrocardiogram (EKG) and non-invasive blood pressure monitor. Different monitoring modalities used together provide a more complete understanding of the patient's operative condition. Figure 8.2 shows the Lifebox pulse oximeter, which is the pulse oximeter of choice for the Global Oximetry Project.

The EKG is an inexpensive, real-time, easy-to-use monitor that can be used on anyone. It provides pulse rate and electrical rhythm and, with five leads, can be modestly used to diagnose ischemic cardiac events. Increases in conduction times and repolarization can be used as an early warning of amide local anesthetic toxicity or hyperkalemia. It is invaluable in diagnosing conduction defects and dysrhythmias. Additionally, most modern EKG monitors are integrated into larger monitors that include blood pressure and pulse oximetry. The EKG works whether the patient is cold, hypotensive, or hypoxic, and the information provided is in real time. No other modality can make that claim.

Blood pressure monitoring is critical to measure adequate fluid resuscitation and gauge the overall perfusion of patients of all ages. Both manual and automated devices are equally reliable. Many automated non-invasive blood pressure monitors are conveniently integrated with EKG and oximetry.

A variety of blood pressure cuff sizes are readily available for all types of patients and systems. Non-invasive blood pressure monitoring is particularly useful in those patients whose blood pressure is expected to vary greatly. This would be common in patients who are bleeding, dehydrated, previously hypertensive, or receiving a spinal axial anesthetic. All of the patient groups previously described eventually fall into one or more of the aforementioned states.

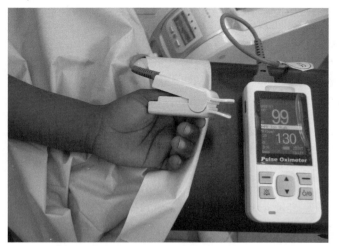

FIGURE 8.2 The Lifebox pulse oximeter is the device chosen by the Global Oximetry Project to outfit every operating room (OR) in the world that doesn't already have a pulse oximeter with a functional device. More information is available at www.lifebox.org. Semer N. Lifebox Pulse Oximeter. [Internet] Available from: http://practicalplasticsurgery.org/2011/08/lifebox-a-pulse-oximeter-for-low-income-countries/

Although blood pressure monitoring does not reflect regional differences in perfusion, it is a vast improvement over extrapolating the cardiac output from solely the pulse rate or the patient's color. If noninvasive blood pressure monitoring is not available, it is useful for the practitioner to monitor a peripheral pulse (radial, carotid, etc.) by simply placing his or her fingers on it.

The pulse oximeter allows the provider to have a beat-to-beat assessment of the patient's oxygen saturation. With this device, oxygen saturation can be measured using any pulsatile appendage, including the nose and ears. It is accurate, in general, to within 3%–5% of true values. A variety of probes are available in disposable and nondisposable forms and sizes, suitable for all ages including neonates. Most devices provide readout of signal strength with saturation values being more accurate with increased signal strength. Most pulse oximeters used in the operating room also have an audio output which, by its changeable tone, alerts the provider to the trend in saturation without having to read the actual value on the screen. This change in tone works even for those who are considered tone-deaf. This feature allows the provider to work on other issues while still knowing the status of the patient's oxygenation. By its very nature of function, the pulse oximeter provides an accurate assessment of heart rate as well. Given these features, many would argue that it is the single most valuable intraoperative monitor and should be available to all patients receiving a general, regional, or local anesthetic. It is also important to appreciate its limitations.

The pulse oximeter only works if there is a pulse. In patients who are in cardiac arrest, in shock, hypotensive, or hypothermic, the device often fails to find an adequate pulse for an accurate readout. Movement also disturbs the signal strength. Newer generation pulse oximeters have addressed these issues with incomplete success. Portable handheld devices still use relatively old technology. Direct bright light, especially red light, causes all probes to fail. Probes must be protected from direct light at all times. Electronically, these devices have been hard to isolate from electrocautery. They are prone to nonfunction during periods of extensive cautery use. In patients receiving large doses of methylene blue, the oximeter cannot distinguish between oxyhemoglobin and methemoglobin and the displayed value defaults to 85%–87%. Lastly, the pulse oximeter does not provide real-time readout of saturation, but rather is a retrospective analysis. Most pulse oximeters provide data that is 30–60 seconds old. In other words, you see where you were, not where you are or where you are going. The patient is hypoxic before the oximeter tells you so and is recovering, hopefully, before the saturation readout recovers. The pulse oximeter is the rearview mirror of monitors. Therefore, good clinical assessment skills continue to be necessary to complement modern technology.

The modern-day end-tidal carbon dioxide (CO_2) monitor provides a real-time measurement of the patient's exhaled CO_2 provided by a continuous waveform display of the exhaled CO_2. It assesses ventilation function as expressed by the exchange of CO_2 and thereby provides critical information not possible with pulse oximetry. The CO_2 values, combined with the waveform readout, allow the provider to assess adequacy of gas exchange and may also detect bronchospasm, air embolism, and leaks in the breathing system. In the operating room these monitors are essential to detect three important factors: the correct placement of the LMA or endotracheal tube, disconnection from the breathing circuit, and hyper- or hypoventilation. In the sedated patient these monitors can be extremely useful for detecting airway obstruction and apnea.

Many modern anesthesia-monitoring systems incorporate all basic monitoring, including end-tidal CO_2. However for older systems, often the case in LMICs, a separate portable monitor is the only option.

Disadvantages of end-tidal CO_2 are few. They do require calibration against a known sample from time to time, especially portable devices. Sample gas is continually removed from the system for analysis. This gas loss is significant especially when very low-flow and/or closed-circuit anesthesia techniques are utilized. Many portable anesthesia machines lack the connection to reintroduce these gases into the breathing system. This is especially true if non-rebreathing systems are being used for general anesthesia. Gases that cannot be returned to the breathing system need disposal and should be scavenged, especially if inhalational agents are being used for anesthesia. Operating rooms without regular room air turnover rapidly become sleepy, uncomfortable places.

A glucose monitor is not routinely viewed as an intraoperative monitor, but it warrants mention for two reasons: it is inexpensive and it provides another margin of safety in neonates and the obstetric patient. Infants kept without fluids and foods for surgery are at a low but real risk of hypoglycemia, especially during surgeries lasting more than two hours. Pregnant women are always at risk of gestational diabetes. Hyperglycemia only makes head trauma worse.

Handheld glucometers are easily accessible for less than 40 American dollars in any American pharmacy. Although they can become less inaccurate when blood glucose is very high or very low, they provide simple testing with a single drop of blood. For most patients they are more than adequate.

Although it would seem obvious, it is worth remarking that all of these intraoperative monitoring systems require power. A finger on the pulse, a precordial stethoscope, and a manual blood pressure cuff are the three exceptions, and everyone should have and be capable of interpreting these nonpowered monitors. Power cannot be assumed.

A few comments about the practicality and wisdom of intraoperative monitoring are worth mentioning at this time. Anesthesia safety has not been advanced solely by the development of newer monitors. The willingness of anesthesia societies and their members to adopt these monitors as standards of care has been a factor. It is their actual use in everyday practice, for all patients—general, regional, and local—that has helped reduce anesthetic mortality from 1 in 10,000 30 years ago to 1 in 100,000, or less today in more developed nations.

Recently, the WHO has adopted this approach and is now recommending adoption of these same standards for all patients throughout the world. A relatively recent study addressed this point and provided data to show how adoption of this approach in LMICs could reduce operative mortality. It is recommended that the anesthesia provider take the approach of "How can I fully monitor my patient?" rather than "What is the least I can monitor and still get away with it?" No patient ever died because he had too many monitors attached to him. The fundamental goal for anesthesiologists should be to provide the same level of care and vigilance to patients in the less developed world that they provide in the more developed world. This includes monitoring modalities. For elective procedures (e.g., a sort, cleft palate trip),

if practitioners cannot provide standard ASA monitors for all patients, the trip should probably not be undertaken in the first place. Techniques may need to be adapted to a given environment, but the days of visitors making excuses for substandard care for elective surgical procedures are (hopefully) long gone. Certainly, emergent cases, disaster situations, and purely educational trips may require adoption of slightly different standards in concert with risk/benefit assessment.

Patients at particular risk are those believed to be at low risk. The sedated patient receiving local or regional anesthesia by a sole provider is at particular risk. All patients should be monitored. Additionally, a person not involved in the surgical procedure should supervise the monitoring. This may be taxing on human resources in some settings, but it does save lives, and that is the point of the surgery in the first place.

Fluid Management

Fluid management is a basic component of intraoperative care. It has only four requirements: the ability to successfully insert an intravenous catheter, the catheter itself, intravenous tubing, and, for most situations, balanced salt solutions. One of the most significant obstacles in providing safe intraoperative fluid management is a basic lack of understanding of what constitutes a balance salt solution and why it should be used in the operating room.

Balance salt solutions are isotonic. They contain a balance of sodium salt and, depending upon the solution, other low levels of lactate, calcium, or magnesium. D5W, D5 1/4 normal saline, and D5 1/2 normal saline are all hypotonic solutions and really have no place in the operating room. Most patients become modestly hyperglycemic with surgery simply from the surgical stress. Hyperglycemia has been shown to impair wound healing and increase surgical infection rates. All dextrose should be treated as a drug and given only when the patient is hypoglycemic.

Fluid losses during surgery required balanced salt solutions. The use of hypotonic solutions leads to hyponatremia, inadequate resuscitation, and water overload. Unfortunately, this concept, while not new, is not accepted in many LMICs. Yet case reports of patients dying during or after surgery from the use of hypotonic solutions still appear in the literature. Teaching others the value of balance salt solutions in the operating room is one of the best gifts we can give, at no cost to either party.

Most commonly available balanced salt solutions include normal saline, Ringer's lactate, plasmalyte, and Hartmann's solution. In the short term, none of these solutions has been shown to be superior to another. It is reasonable to use whichever of these solutions is most readily available. The costs of these solutions are similar in most countries.

Normal saline has 154 meq/L of sodium and 154 meq/L of chloride. Because of this high load of chloride, patients given large volumes of normal saline will develop a hyperchloremic, strong ion-gap metabolic acidosis. This is particularly true in infants and young children. The long-term significance of this problem is in debate.

Ringer's lactate contains less chloride than normal saline and does not cause hyperchloremic acidosis. It can be used in all ages and is well tolerated by infants. Although there is some concern about using a lactate solution in diabetic mellitus patients (for fear of causing hyperglycemia), this concern is more theoretical than real. The amount of calcium in Ringer's lactate is not enough to interact with the chelate in stored packed red cells and cause clotting.

The use of colloid and starch solutions should be reserved for only those patients receiving very large volumes of fluids accompanied by blood loss. These solutions are vastly more expensive and often not available unless the surgical team has brought their own to a given destination.

It is beyond the scope of this chapter to talk about blood products. It is sufficient to say that if they are needed, prior planning is paramount. In many disaster situations, and in many LMICs, blood products are at a premium. As previously mentioned, fresh whole blood is often the only product available in an emergency. It takes considerable foresight to have it available when needed. It is useful to keep in mind that O negative is the universal donor blood group. In emergency situations, such as a disaster response, a healthy team member with O negative blood can offer a last-ditch, lifesaving option by donating for immediate transfusion. All team members should know their blood type prior to deployment.

A simple guideline for fluid administration is as follows.

NPO replacement fluids: 20–30 ml/kg

Maintenance fluids: Adult and pediatric, 2–3 ml/kg/hr

Fluid shifts (in addition to maintenance baseline requirements):

Superficial surgery, 2 ml/kg/hr

Thoracic, 6 ml/kg/hr

Abdominal, 8–10 ml/kg/hr

Blood loss:

Crystalloids, 3 ml for every 1 ml blood lost

Colloids and Starches, 1 ml for every 1 ml blood lost

Thus intraoperative fluid administration needs to account for baseline deficits from blood loss (i.e., trauma) or being NPO (elective cases), fluid requirements to maintain homeostasis, and insensible losses (adjusted by type of surgery). The sum of the baseline requirements and insensible losses should make up the intraoperative fluid requirements once the initial deficit has been replaced with an isotonic solution.

There are a few practical points about fluid administration that deserve mention. Small infants can be easily overloaded with any solution when 500–1,000 ml bottles or bags are used. It is advisable to use pediatric tubing that includes a measuring chamber in which one should place no more than 30 ml/kg of solution at any one time, if available. If the intravenous line is left open by accident, then the child will not receive an excessive volume of fluid, but one that will be tolerated by most children with healthy hearts.

Infants in many HICs are often kept without food or fluid far beyond the 6 hours for food, 3 hours for breast milk, and 2 hours for clear liquids that is recommended by the ASA. As such they are often dehydrated at the time of surgery, especially on long, hot days. Care should be taken to make sure these children received an intravenous line at the earliest convenience and that an adjusted and adequate amount of balance salt solution is given before proceeding with surgery.

It is important to remember that, in many intemperate climates, the operating and recovery rooms are not air-conditioned. In these hot environments, these patients will require significant increases in fluid administration to adjust for postoperative insensible losses. Extra attention needs to be paid to their fluid balance before they are discharged. This is especially true for any patient at risk of nausea/vomiting.

Airway Management

General anesthesia can be induced and maintained in a variety of ways utilizing both intravenous and inhalational drugs together as one technique or separately as another. There are pros and cons of both techniques. General anesthesia can be maintained with a natural airway, LMA, or endotracheal tube. The decision of which to use is based upon the type and length of surgery; the condition of the patient, which includes the preoperative airway assessment; the equipment available; and, not least of all, the skill and experience of the anesthesia provider.

It is beyond the scope of this chapter to have a detailed discussion of airway assessment and management. This topic is well covered in any standard anesthesiology textbook. The problem does not change just because you are in a foreign country. In fact, it may become more complicated without adequate equipment or backup strategies. See Figure 8.3 for a detailed algorithm of the difficult airway from the ASA. It works in any location and all anesthesia providers should be familiar with it.

There are a few salient points that bear further discussion. The first practical point is to examine the patient yourself. Do not proceed to induce deep sedation or anesthesia in anyone you have not personally reviewed. Everyone has his or her own capabilities, experiences, and limits. What might be a difficult airway for one person may be impossible for another. Work within your own limits. What looks bad to one provider might look good to another and vice versa.

Second, ask for help early. Often the most difficult airway is the one for which you are the only person who has any airway skills or insight in the airway disaster that is unfolding before you. Skilled assistance is invaluable. If you suspect a difficult airway, you should be asking for assistance long before you need it.

Third, understand the limitations of your personnel and equipment. In many situations the specialized equipment you may be accustomed to in your home institution may not be available in your current place. Fiber-optic laryngoscopes, glide scopes, Bullard scopes, and others are rarely available in remote locations. Your local otorhinolaryngologist may not be present to stand by and perform an emergency tracheotomy if attempts at securing the airway fail.

Fourth, patients die because we cannot ventilate them after induction, not because we cannot intubate them. Establishing a patent airway and providing some ventilation is more important than intubation. When managing a critical airway, all efforts should focus on establishing ventilation, and not obsession with intubation.

LMAs have proven to be invaluable. If it is possible to open the mouth and place an LMA, then you can ventilate, regardless of age, with rare exception. As such, in remote situations a variety of age-appropriate sizes of LMAs are extremely helpful. In patients whose mouths cannot be opened, an appropriate sized nasal airway is

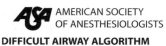

AMERICAN SOCIETY
OF ANESTHESIOLOGISTS

DIFFICULT AIRWAY ALGORITHM

1. Assess the likelihood and clinical impact of basic management problems:
   - A. Difficult ventilation
   - B. Difficult intubation
   - C. Difficulty with patient cooperation or consent
   - D. Difficult tracheostomy

2. Actively pursue opportunities to deliver supplemental oxygen throughout the process of difficult airway management

3. Consider the relative merits and feasibility of basic management choices:

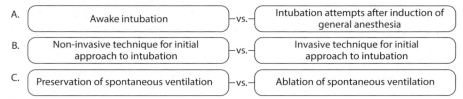

A.	Awake intubation	vs.	Intubation attempts after induction of general anesthesia
B.	Non-invasive technique for initial approach to intubation	vs.	Invasive technique for initial approach to intubation
C.	Preservation of spontaneous ventilation	vs.	Ablation of spontaneous ventilation

4. Develop primary and alternative strategies:

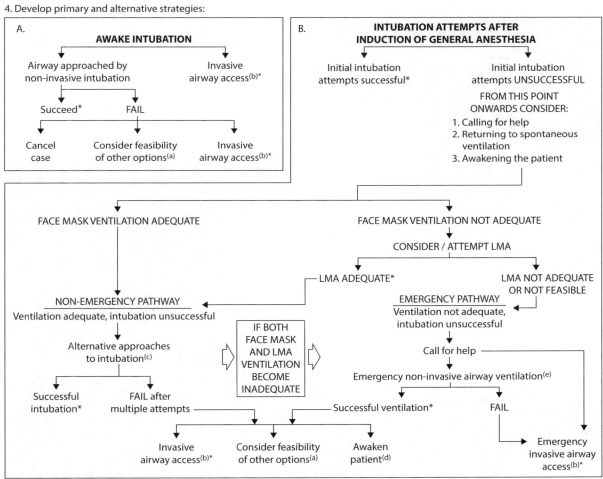

* Confirm ventilation, tracheal intubation, or LMA placement with exhaled CO$_2$

a. Other options include (but are not limited to): surgery utilizing face mask or LMA anesthesia, local anesthesia infiltration or regional nerve blockade. Pursuit of these options usually implies that mask ventilation will not be problematic. Therefore, these options may be of limited value if this step in the algorithm has been reached via the emergency pathway.

b. Invasive airway access includes surgical or percutaneous tracheostomy or cricothyrotomy.

c. Alternative non-invasive approaches to difficult intubation include (but are not limited to): use of different laryngoscope blades, LMA as an intubation conduit (with or without fiberoptic guidance), fiberoptic intubation, intubating stylet or tube changer, light wand, retrograde intubation, and blind oral or nasal intubation.

d. Consider re-preparation of the patient for awake intubation or canceling surgery.

e. Options for emergency non-invasive airway ventilation include (but are not limited to): rigid bronchoscope, esophageal-tracheal combitube ventilation, or transtracheal jet ventilation.

FIGURE 8.3 Difficult airway alogrithm. Adapted from Practice Guidelines for Management of the Difficult Airway, An Update Report by the American Society of Anesthesiologists Task Force on Management of the Difficult Airway.

often an effective intervention to establish ventilation. Figure 8.4A and Figure 8.4B display a situation where an LMA is used to facilitate management of a known difficult airway in a patient with severe burn contractures to the anterior neck and chest.

Last, never be talked into inducing a patient if you are not confident you can manage all airway contingencies. On many short-term trips, people are in a hurry but most surgeries are elective or semi-elective. Unless a case is life threatening, be conservative. Nothing is as tragic and negates trust as quickly as losing a patient whose death was not imminent because you could not manage the airway.

It is possible to manage patients for superficial surgeries, with very difficult airways, using total intravenous anesthesia. Fortunately, there are a number of anesthesia medications (e.g., ketamine) that maintain upper airway integrity and spontaneous ventilation. Figure 8.5 represents a case where ketamine was the

anesthetic used for a patient with significant post-burn scars over the anterior neck, which resulted in a difficult airway (even with modern fiber-optic equipment).

General Anesthesia

Overview

The advantages of general anesthesia are legion. Nervous, confused, or developmentally delayed patients will often not tolerate procedures under local or regional anesthesia even with some sedation. Infants and children are common examples. Many procedures are difficult to perform on an awake patient, even one who is motivated. Procedures involving the airway, intrathoracic cases, and lengthy procedures are especially difficult without general anesthesia.

General anesthesia offers the surgeon a motionless surgical field, except for the respirations of the patient. General anesthesia offers the advantage of time. Patients do not become restless because the procedure is long and/or difficult. It also offers the advantage of honest intraoperative discussions about the patient's condition—discussions that can be difficult in front of the awake patient. Last, general anesthesia is the only option when control of ventilation is required or control of the airway is necessary.

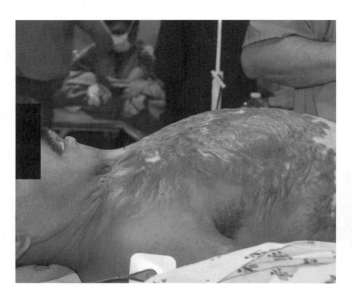

FIGURE 8.4A   Patient with severe post-burn scarring to the neck, which profoundly limited his flexion and extension, creating a difficult airway. The patient underwent a general anesthetic with an LMA, and then a scar release was performed to improve his function. The patient preoperatively. Image by Craig D. McClain.

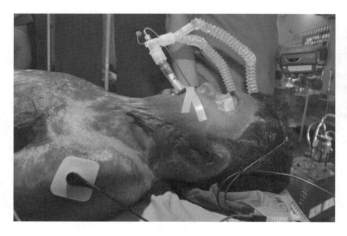

FIGURE 8.4B   Patient after uneventful induction and placement of LMA.

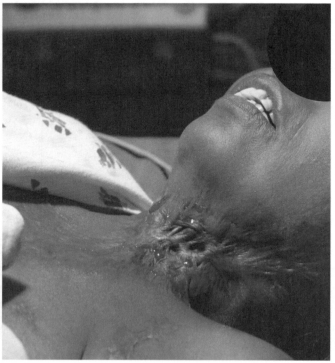

FIGURE 8.5   A patient with neck scars from an old burn injury from cooking. A ketamine anesthetic facilitated local anesthetic infiltration and a scar release. The patient maintained spontaneous ventilation and a natural airway during the procedure. Her function was significantly improved. Because of her limited neck extension and flexion, she would likely have had a difficult airway with no real opportunity for a cricothyroidotomy due to the thick scars over her anterior neck.

There are also several disadvantages of general anesthesia. General anesthesia requires specialized equipment and specialized medical personnel to deliver the care. Patients who are hypovolemic or in shock do not tolerate general anesthesia well, often requiring significant resuscitation. General anesthesia renders intraoperative neurological checks impossible. Patients recovering from general anesthesia require greater care postoperatively. This affects personnel, medication, and equipment allocation. Patients who have had general anesthesia are also more prone to postoperative nausea/vomiting as compared to those who have had local or regional anesthesia.

In the more developed world, the risk of anesthesia in healthy patients is the same for local, regional, and general anesthesia. General anesthesia may involve more risk in critically ill patients, but these patients usually have general anesthesia as a last resort and other options are not available or practical. The situation may be very different in the less developed world. There is no literature to support the assertion, but given the dramatic differences in training, experience, continuing education, and general skill level of anesthesia providers in the less developed world, local and regional techniques may be much safer than general anesthesia.

Inhalational Agents

Inhalational anesthesia has advantages and disadvantages. Inhalational anesthesia can be used for both induction and maintenance of anesthesia. This is particularly useful in patients without intravenous access, such as infants and children. It can be used as the sole agent in a spontaneously breathing patient or may be combined with muscle relaxant when necessary. In fact, one of the unique features on inhalational agents is that they provide a significant degree of muscle relaxation as part of their side-effect profile.

Most are bronchodilators and, with the exception of halothane, most have little metabolism, thereby reducing the risk of hepatic or renal failure. They are complete anesthetic agents. Newer agents such as sevoflurane and desflurane are proven safe and effective with a very high benefit/risk ratio. Neither has any significant myocardial depressant effect. They are all inflammable, thus making surgical cautery safe. For adults they remain one of the least expensive anesthesia drugs on a cost per minute basis. Another advantage, and this is not insignificant in many circumstances, some anesthetic machines require no power source whatsoever to deliver these agents to the patient. This is a decided advantage in an unstable environment.

There are some disadvantages. Inhalational anesthesia requires agent-specific vaporizers to deliver the drug into the breathing circuit. That means they require an anesthetic machine of some type. To reduce cost and waste they are best used in a semi-closed breathing system with a CO_2 absorber, better known as a "circle system."

Since newer agents are minimally metabolized, nearly 100% of the gas delivered must be scavenged or vented to avoid pollution of the operating area. Scavenging requires some type of gas collection system or the gas must be "scrubbed" by passing it through activated charcoal canisters. This is of particular concern in close environments with little room air turnover, as previously mentioned.

Although modern vaporizers control for a variety of conditions, they are best operated in temperatures between 60° and 90°F and at sea level. This can be an issue in many less developed nations with tropical climates or in mountainous regions. Inhalation agents have no prolonged analgesic effect. All, but especially sevoflurane, are associated with emergence delirium, which is most pronounced in children. Unfortunately, all inhalational agents are associated with postoperative nausea and/or vomiting.

A number of inhalational anesthetics are available throughout the world but it is noteworthy that old drugs such as halothane have become increasingly unavailable. Halothane is only available in a few remaining LMICs. It was and remains relatively cheap.

Halothane is a significant myocardial depressant, may cause halothane hepatitis in adults, and sensitizes the myocardium to endogenous and exogenous catecholamines, leading to dysrhythmias. This is particularly relevant for surgeons using epinephrine in local anesthetics for hemostasis. Care must be taken not to inject intravenously as the consequences when using halothane can be deadly. Halothane vasodilates cerebral vessels and places head trauma patients at risk of increased intracranial pressure. Halothane also requires a preservative, thymol, which eventually causes vaporizers to seize if not properly drained and maintained. Most importantly, halothane has been the single agent most associated with drug-related anesthesia deaths over the past 50 years. Undoubtedly this is due to its narrow safety margin with overdose resulting in significant myocardial depression, bradycardia, and cardiac arrest, especially in children.

Sevoflurane is the inhalational agent that has replaced halothane in most instances. Sevoflurane is not pungent, making it suitable as an induction agent for infants, children, and adults. In fact, it is no more pungent at 8% than at 1% inhaled concentration, allowing for quick inductions using maximal concentrations. It is relatively insoluble in blood, so induction and emergence are quick, even with prolonged anesthetics. It has little myocardial depressant effect, does not interact with catecholamines, and has little or no peripheral vasodilatory properties. It is not associated with bradycardia, even in infants, and is an excellent bronchodilator.

It is a desirable agent in regard to the airway. The incidence and severity of laryngospasm is less with sevoflurane than with any other available inhalational agent. It does not require a preservative. Most importantly, its use has been associated with a significant drop in drug-related anesthesia deaths in the United States.

There are also several disadvantages of sevoflurane. It unfortunately interacts with soda lime absorbers. The resultant interaction produces significant heat, and in the oxygen-enriched environment of the breathing circuit, explosions and fires have been reported. Newer absorbers have been developed which have alleviated this problem, but they may not be available in LMICs. Sevoflurane does cause some spike activity on electroencephalogram (EEG) but has not been definitively shown to cause seizures, including in patients with a history of seizures.

Sevoflurane is associated with significant emergence delirium, (25%–35% of patients), which is most pronounced in children. The significance of this problem, aside from annoyance, is still debated. Emergence delirium may be prevented or reduced by the use of propofol, 1 mg/kg, or dexmedetomidine, 0.5–1 mcg/kg, given intravenously before emergence. Although sevoflurane was prohibitively expensive when first released, generic versions of the drug have significantly reduced its cost.

Inhalational anesthesia is an excellent choice when providing anesthesia to spontaneously breathing patients of all ages, albeit artificial airways are usually needed. Additionally, inhalational anesthesia is easily converted into controlled ventilation scenarios as required by the surgical situation. The one great disadvantage of this technique is the need for airway support once anesthesia in induced. Upper airway relaxation is the norm, and few patients will breathe without significant airway obstruction unless the provider manages the airway.

Intravenous Agents

In regard to general anesthesia in less developed world settings, there are five intravenous agents that are worthy of discussion. They are propofol, sodium thiopental (pentothal), ketamine, the benzodiazepines midazolam and diazepam, and dexmedetomidine.

Propofol is a unique alcohol-based intravenous anesthetic agent. It can be used as an induction agent in all populations. Depending upon the dose, it can be used as a mild sedative (doses of 25–75 mcg/kg/min), for deep sedation (75–100 mcg/kg/min), or to provide a general anesthetic (100–300 mcg/kg/min). These doses represent a continuum taken from a fairly wide bell curve; differences in doses for a needed effect can vary significantly from one patient to another. Also, patients can easily slip from one state of consciousness, or unconsciousness, to another without a change in dose. There are no definite end-points for dosing, only continual evaluation of the patient's status. Expertise in airway management should be considered a requirement for using propofol, as airway compromise can occur rapidly across a wide range of doses.

For the purpose of using propofol as a sole anesthetic agent, best results are obtained by using a continuous infusion pump, which ultimately requires a power source. Short anesthetics can be maintained, if necessary, by intermittent boluses given by the anesthesia provider. However, such a method results in frequent under- and overdosing of the drug. Propofol can be used in all patients, including those with raised intracranial pressure and infants. Airway manipulation is tolerated with a low incidence of laryngospasm.

Propofol is not associated with nausea/vomiting when used either as a sedative or general anesthetic. In fact, low doses are associated with an anti-emetic effect. Some sedated patients describe vivid dreams, not infrequently sexual in nature. One great advantage of propofol, in some settings, is that general anesthesia can be provided without the use of an anesthesia machine.

There are some problems with propofol. Propofol is prepared as a lipid emulsion. Bottles of propofol must be handled aseptically. Open vials must be discarded within eight hours of opening. Severe sepsis has been described when open vials of propofol were used after being open to room air for greater periods of time. It must also be stored in reasonable controlled temperature settings.

Propofol is commonly painful upon injection in adults and children. A variety of methods to reduce this have been used, such as diluting the concentration or adding lidocaine to the propofol solution. These efforts have been modestly successful at best.

Propofol is not an analgesic at any dose. As a result, propofol is also poor at preventing movement during painful procedures.

Propofol is therefore commonly used in conjunction with other agents to prevent movement during surgery.

Propofol is a significant vasodilator and must be used with caution in hypotensive patients, in the presence of dehydration or shock. Tolerance to repeat anesthetics with propofol does occur and can be dramatic. Propofol is not associated with significant emergence delirium.

A toxic metabolic syndrome has been described in teenagers and young adults exposed to a continuous infusion of propofol for periods greater than 24 hours.

Sodium thiopental is a barbiturate and, like many sedative/hypnotic agents, works centrally on GABA receptors. Doses of 5–7 mg/kg will induce apnea and general anesthesia. It is commonly found in the less developed world, where it is still manufactured. It is no longer available in the United States. Thus, many younger practitioners will be unfamiliar with its use. It is generally not as "clean" a drug as propofol. Specifically, it is highly associated with postoperative nausea and vomiting (PONV), it does not cause airway relaxation as propofol does, and it must be reconstituted in an aqueous solution prior to use. Once in the aqueous form, the drug degrades rather quickly, so older ampules of thiopental may not produce the desired effect. It has a very high pH and thus some drugs such as rocuronium will precipitate when mixed with thiopental. When compared to propofol, thiopental is considered an inferior drug, but many less developed world settings will only have thiopental available and not propofol, so practitioners should familiarize themselves with this drug prior to travel.

Ketamine is a controversial drug but also an excellent one, especially in remote settings where access to anesthesia delivery machines is limited. Ketamine is very common in operating theaters in the less developed world. Practitioners should be comfortable with using ketamine for a variety of indications, including inducing general anesthesia, sedation, and analgesia. Further, it can be given orally as a sedative, intramuscularly for sedation and/or anesthesia, or intravenously for sedation or anesthesia. Patients often exhibit nystagmus when sedated with ketamine.

The great benefit of ketamine is twofold. First, when used as the sole agent, patients of all ages usually maintain spontaneous respiration with moderately well controlled upper airway reflexes. Second, it is a potent analgesic, and therefore patients remain motionless, even during relatively painful procedures. It is not a myocardial depressant nor does it vasodilate.

Its use does not require an anesthetic machine nor is an infusion pump a necessity, since ketamine is not a short-acting drug. This allows for easier manual intermittent dosing. It is the perfect anesthetic choice when one needs to perform brief painful procedures and wants to avoid having to manage the upper airway, such as setting a fracture or changing wound dressings. This is especially valuable when providing acute care in disaster relief areas. Of note is the fact that ketamine does not completely protect laryngeal reflexes, thus aspiration risk is always present. Full-stomach patients should wait until they have fasted.

Ketamine's side-effect profile also makes it a reasonable induction agent in patients whose volume status is questionable. However, it may still result in a substantial drop in pressure in those patients whose shock condition has resulted in an endogenous catecholamine depletion state.

Ketamine has several disadvantages. It is associated with delirium in all age groups, which can be partially offset by combining ketamine with a benzodiazepine or low-dose propofol. It is also associated with increased intracranial pressure, so it should be avoided in head trauma patients. Ketamine is not a short-acting agent, and patients given high doses of ketamine will sleep for a considerable time, aggravating issues in the recovery room. Its use is associated with nausea/vomiting.

Dexmedetomidine is a relatively new anesthetic agent and will therefore unlikely be available locally in the less developed world. However, it offers significant benefits in these settings and may be brought along by practitioners for use on visiting surgical team trips. It acts as an alpha 2-receptor agonist. As such it can provide sedation, anesthesia, and analgesia. Because it acts upon alpha-2 receptors, moderate to high doses can cause a drop in heart rate and blood pressure, especially in the elderly. Dexmedetomidine has been safely used in children and adults. It can be given safely as a bolus (1–3 mcg/kg) in young patients for analgesia, or it may be used as an adjunct to general anesthesia (0.5–1 mcg/kg/hr). It is safe to use in patients with head trauma and elevated intracranial pressure. It seems to have a synergistic effect when used along with opioids, so care must be taken when administering the two classes of drugs simultaneously.

One advantage of dexmedetomidine is that upper airway tone is maintained and it is not a respiratory depressant. Therefore, it is of particular use in patients at risk of intraoperative and postoperative airway obstruction and apnea. It is also an excellent adjunct to propofol when used to provide analgesia while maintaining a natural airway. It is not associated with nausea/vomiting and does not cause emergence delirium. In fact low doses (0.5–1 mcg/kg), given before emergence, prevent or ameliorate delirium.

Dexmedetomidine can be an excellent analgesic in children, protecting the upper airway and maintaining spontaneous respiration without causing delirium or nausea/vomiting. In fact, this avoids the headaches of using narcotics for pain control. One caveat is that after extubation patients, given a reasonable analgesic dose, will sleep for 20–40 minutes in the recovery room before awakening. But they are often ready for discharge upon awakening.

The benzodiazepines are not true anesthetics and are not analgesics. But they are very useful as adjuncts to patients requiring sedation for surgeries that can be done under local or regional anesthesia. By themselves they are not respiratory depressants, but used with a respiratory depressant, they become synergistic in that regard. This is where most providers make their mistake. Benzodiazepines are very safe drugs until the addition of opioids to the sedation regimen. Ideally, sedation should consist mostly of benzodiazepines and as little opioid as possible. Such a procedure depends on good local anesthetic infiltration for analgesia.

Midazolam is a water-soluble benzodiazepine with a very short effective half-life. It can be given orally as a sedative premedication in children (0.5–1 mg/kg) and intramuscular for sedation (0.3 mg/kg). Incremental doses of 1–2 mg can be given intravenously in children and adults for sedation before and during a procedure. Midazolam is a mild anxiolytic with strong amnestic properties. Because of its short half-life, it is ideal for short procedures where rapid recovery and discharge are required. It is intermittently available in the less developed world.

Diazepam is an older, longer-acting benzodiazepine. It is not water soluble and therefore often uncomfortable when given intravenously. A lipid emulsion preparation is available in many countries, which avoids this venous irritation. Diazepam can be given orally, intramuscularly, and intravenously. It has strong anxiolytic properties and is mildly amnestic. It is of intermediate duration compared to midazolam but nearly as sedating in clinically useful doses. Diazepam is the ideal drug for long sedation procedures. Dosing is less frequent, and patients, while relaxed, are less drowsy. Patients ambulate well after its use but are not nearly as alert as after the use of midazolam. One advantage of diazepam is that it is much more readily available than midazolam in many LMICs.

Muscle Relaxants

Long-acting muscle relaxants have a very limited role in general anesthesia on visiting surgical team trips. Although they are necessary in some situations, most notably in intra-thoracic and intra-abdominal surgeries, they can be a significant complicating factor. Given the limitations of resources in many remote locations, muscle relaxants are a luxury that may often not be affordable.

Muscle relaxants are associated with a number of adverse events or interactions. Succinylcholine is normally a rapid onset, short-acting muscle relaxant. It is commonly used to facilitate intubation of a patient or to abort laryngospasm. Because succinylcholine is a depolarizing agent, it cannot be used in patients who have burns, spinal cord injuries, or a variety of neuromuscular disorders. In such cases it may cause life-threatening hyperkalemia or rhabdomyolysis.

Because of these concerns, many practitioners prefer to intubate patients without a muscle relaxant, which can be done with intravenous and inhalational agents and some local anesthetic topicalization of the airway. This can be done in all age groups. Preference is to reserve succinylcholine for emergencies such as severe laryngospasm. Succinylcholine should always be available for this reason as it is lifesaving in such situations.

The details of other non-depolarizing muscle relaxants relevant to care in this environment will be discussed in the pharmacology section. When muscle relaxants other than succinylcholine are used, it may be necessary to reverse the effects with a combination of neostigmine and an anticholinergic agent (e.g., glycopyrolate). It is strongly recommended that if a provider is going to use muscle relaxants, he or she must have, and know how to properly use, a muscle twitch monitor. Problematic is the fact that the use of a muscle twitch monitor in infants is associated with a large number of false positive and false negative findings; the monitor is not very reliable in this age group.

All of the aforementioned properties and problems with muscle relaxants should make the provider aware that muscle relaxants can significantly complicate even a simple anesthetic. Given the settings of care at which this text is directed, these drugs should be used very carefully, and only when absolutely necessary.

Spinal Anesthesia

Spinal anesthesia is a popular anesthetic technique for cooperative patients undergoing procedures below the umbilicus. Spinal anesthetics have been given for patients having procedures above the umbilicus, but success of such procedures requires a highly motivated patient and a patient, motivated surgeon.

Spinal anesthetics can provide ideal operative conditions. A spinal anesthetic blocks all modalities including pain, proprioception, light touch, temperature sensation, deep pressure sensation, and motor function. The technique has the advantage of avoiding invasive airway management with minimal PONV. It can be used in patients of all ages, if they are cooperative. It can also be used to control postoperative pain if long-acting narcotics are added to the local anesthetic (albeit these patients are at risk of urinary retention, PONV, pruritus, and, most significantly, apnea and delayed respiratory depression).

The three most important aspects affecting the spread of the local anesthetics injected for a spinal anesthetic are the baricity of the local anesthetic, the position of the patient immediately after the injection of the local anesthetic, and the total dose (mg) of the local anesthetic.

The baricity of the local anesthetic can be adjusted to be hypobaric, isobaric, and hyperbaric. Hypobaric solutions have a specific gravity less than that of cerebral spinal fluid (CSF). Isobaric solutions have the same specific gravity as CSF and hyperbaric has a greater specific gravity than CSF. Mixing local anesthetics with sterile water, CSF, or 5% dextrose, respectively, can make these solutions.

Hypobaric solutions will rise against gravity, and hyperbaric solutions will move in the direction of gravitational pull. Isobaric solutions tend to stay where they are injected. As such, patient positioning has a significant effect on the spread of spinal local anesthetic in hypobaric and hyperbaric spinals, and must be considered immediately after injection. Patient positioning has little effect upon isobaric solutions.

Spinal anesthetics can produce a significant sympathetic block depending upon the dose injected and the patient positioning. The number of thoracic dermatomes (T4–T12) blocked determines the degree of the sympathetic block. The result of the sympathetic block is bradycardia and hypotension. The hypotension induced may be offset by fluid loading prior to initiation of the spinal anesthetic or through the use of vasopressors such as phenylephrine or ephedrine. The bradycardia induced by high spinals can be problematic.

Bradycardia should be treated aggressively if it occurs. Though heart rates of 50–55 beats/minute are often well tolerated in patients under general anesthesia, this is not always the case with spinal anesthetics. Numerous case reports of cardiac arrest with spinal anesthesia have taught that when significant bradycardia occurs, there can be a sudden onset of asystole and cardiac arrest. Bradycardia below 55 beats per minute should therefore be treated with ephedrine or atropine, even if the blood pressure is stable. In the event of asystole, the patient should be immediately given epinephrine, not atropine. Delays in aggressive management of this critical situation often result in death.

The addition of epinephrine to a total concentration of 1:200,000 to local anesthetics can result in a modest increase in duration in the case of lidocaine, and a very significant increase in the case of tetracaine or bupivacaine. Fentanyl (25–50 mcg) or sufentanil (10–15 mcg) can also be added to the local anesthetic mixture. Doing so has been shown to improve the overall quality of spinal anesthesia, especially for caesarean sections. The short duration of these opioids does not cause delayed postoperative respiratory depression, as in the case of morphine.

Nausea and vomiting can occur with spinal anesthetics. This is usually the result of an unbalanced parasympathetic system in the face of a reduced sympathetic tone. In general, the maintenance of the mean baseline blood pressure will prevent or alleviate this problem. Atropine can also be effective.

Absolute contraindications to spinal anesthesia include coagulopathies and patient refusal. The use of aspirin is not a concern. Infection at or near the site of injection is a relative contraindication. Spinal anesthetics should be used with caution in patients whose cardiovascular status is in question, especially trauma patients. Hypotension is expected with spinal anesthesia even in healthy patients; it will certainly occur in the under-resuscitated patient.

The overall risk/benefit of spinal anesthesia is the same as that of general anesthesia per evidence from the more developed world. However, in the less developed world, spinal anesthesia may be a safer mode for less-skilled anesthesia providers. High spinal anesthetics do not reduce the risk of anesthesia in patients with respiratory compromise. The use of spinal anesthesia in patients with hip fractures has shown to reduce the incidence of deep venous thrombosis.

Local Anesthetic Agents

Local anesthetics are commonly used in the operating room as the primary anesthetic (e.g., peripheral nerve block or neuraxial block). They may also be used as a local infiltration for minor surgery with or without sedation and postoperative pain management. The local anesthetics fall into two groups: esters and amides. Ester local anesthetics most commonly include cocaine, benzocaine, tetracaine and 2-chloroprocaine. The amide local anesthetics are commonly lidocaine, mepivacaine, bupivacaine, and ropivacaine.

Amide local anesthetics without preservatives are suitable for all blocks including spinal anesthesia. Tetracaine is the only ester anesthetic commonly used for spinal anesthesia. Cocaine and benzocaine are commonly used for topical anesthesia of mucus membranes.

Smaller nerves like sympathetic and pain fibers are blocked at lower concentrations of local anesthetics than motor fibers, which tend to be larger and heavily myelinated. By adjusting the local anesthetic concentration, the provider can reduce the motor blockade of a given block while still blocking pain fibers. The dose, site of placement, use of additives, temperature, and pregnancy directly influence the overall effectiveness of a given local anesthetic. Pregnant patients have an increased susceptibility to local anesthetics.

Various additives may be used with local anesthetics to improve the quality of the block or its duration, with epinephrine being the most common. Not only does epinephrine cause vasoconstriction, thereby slowing absorption and decreasing peak serum levels, but it also enhances block effectiveness by stimulating presynaptic alpha-adrenergic receptors. Epinephrine has little effect upon blocks with ropivacaine due to its inherent vasoconstrictor properties. Total epinephrine doses in excess of 0.25 mg are associated with cardiac dysrhythmias. Care should be taken when using epinephrine as an additive to local anesthetics when halothane is used as a general anesthetic because of halothane's ability to sensitize the myocardium to catecholamines that may result in significant dysrhythmias.

Clonidine can also be added to local anesthetics in doses of 1–2 mcg/kg. Its effect is additive but not synergistic. Clonidine provides increased analgesia and prolongs the effect of caudal and epidural blocks. It is sedative but has minimal respiratory depressant effects.

All local anesthetics can be both neurotoxic and cardiotoxic. The toxicity of local anesthetics is determined by the drug itself and also by the location of injection, with some blocks resulting in higher serum blood levels than others. The peak concentrations of local anesthetics in the serum ranging from highest to lowest are intercostal block, caudal, epidural, brachial plexus, femoral/sciatic blocks, and subcutaneous infiltration. For intercostal, caudal, and epidural nerve blocks, the maximum amount of local anesthetic that is safe to be given to infants and adults is 3 mg/kg of bupivacaine and ropivacaine, and 5–7 mg/kg of lidocaine.

Neurotoxicity (manifested by tinnitus, oral numbness, and ultimately seizures) occurs at lower levels of toxic drugs. Cardiac dysrhythmias and collapse occur at the higher end. Cardiac toxicity occurs at three times neurotoxic serum levels for most local anesthetics. Cardiotoxic reactions secondary to bupivacaine and ropivacaine are highly resistant to treatment and commonly fatal. Therefore, fractionating the dose and/or the use of intravascular markers is strongly recommended. Treatment of cardiotoxic reactions with 20% lipid emulsions is currently recommended, although its overall treatment success rate is still debated.

Many anesthesia providers believe that the use of ropivacaine relative to bupivacaine is safer regarding cardiotoxicity. Ropivacaine is less cardiotoxic than bupivacaine, but it is also less potent. When given in equipotent doses, these drugs are probably very similar in toxicity.

Allergies to the amide local anesthetics are essentially nonexistent. Most reactions to their use are the result of allergies to a preservative or an unrecognized intravascular injection. Allergies to the ester local anesthetics are well documented but uncommon.

The safe use of local anesthetics involves knowledge of the specific local being utilized, the type of block being attempted, fractionation of total dose, the use of intravascular markers, knowledge of the minimal effective dose, knowledge of the maximum dose, and the ability to recognize and treat an overdose of local anesthetic or an intravascular injection. Safe use of these drugs also requires that the patient be monitored and be directly observed by a care provider, separate from the surgeon.

Management of Postoperative Nausea and Vomiting

It is important to identify those patients at risk for PONV in order to develop a strategy for avoidance. Risk factors for adults include female; nonsmoker; history of motion sickness; previous PONV; use of inhalational agents; use of opioids; surgery over two hours in duration; laparoscopic surgery; breast surgery; and eye, ears, nose, and throat surgery. In children the risk factors include children over 3 years of age, history of PONV or motion sickness, surgery over 30 minutes, the use of inhalational agents, the use of opioids, and any surgery involving the cranial nerves. Children under 1 year of age are not prone to PONV for reasons that are not clear.

Once patients at risk for PONV have been identified, the anesthesiologist can take appropriate action to reduce or eliminate this risk. Anesthesia techniques most likely to avoid PONV are the most effective interventions. For high-risk patients this would include the use of local anesthetic or regional techniques and use of non-opioid analgesics for pain control. Inhalational agents should be avoided if possible. Additionally, the use of prophylactic anti-emetics can be added to the anesthetic regimen. The most effective techniques require the use of dexamethasone (0.15 mg/kg up to a maximum of 4 mg) and a 5HT drug such as ondansetron (50–100 mcg/kg) or droperidol (10–20 mcg/kg up to a maximum of 0.625 mg). In patients who are very high risk, the use of all three drugs is appropriate. These modalities are appropriate for both children and adults.

Management of Perioperative Pain

Post-operative pain management starts in the operating room and should be a component of every anesthetic. Studies have shown that the need to treat pain or PONV in the recovery room is the number-one reason for delayed discharge from the recovery room.

Pain can be managed by a variety of methods and drugs. They include the nonsteroidal anti-inflammatory drugs (NSAIDS), acetaminophen, opioids, dexmedetomidine, regional anesthesia, and local anesthetic infiltration. The WHO has developed a pain ladder (Figure 8.6) for escalating pain management based on pain severity. It was originally designed for cancer patients but can easily be utilized for all perioperative patients.

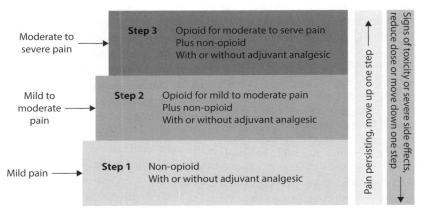

FIGURE 8.6   The WHO Pain Ladder for Cancer Pain. http://www.ccjm.org/content/78/7/449/F1.large.jpg.

NSAIDS and acetaminophen all share a number of common advantages: they provide pain relief without respiratory depression, they do not exacerbate PONV, they are non-addicting, and they are not controlled substances and therefore easy to store and transport. NSAIDS include common drugs such as aspirin and ibuprofen. They are most commonly available in oral or rectal form. Therefore, they are best administered prior to the surgery. They are potent anti-inflammatory drugs in addition to their analgesic effects, as well as anti-pyretic. They can be used alone for minor surgery or as an adjunct to other pain relief techniques. They are opioid sparing in acute pain management. Used on a regular schedule, they are highly effective analgesics and should be considered a first line of pain treatment.

The NSAIDS do have a few disadvantages. They all have an anti-platelet effect by their inhibition of thromboxane A_2. This effect is irreversible for the life of the platelet(s). They all can cause gastric upset and erosion, especially in the critically ill. Last, their use over several days has been demonstrated to impede osteoblastic activity and impair healing of long bone fractures and spinal fusions. They are probably safe in this regard if their use is discontinued within 48 hours of surgery. NSAIDs are an excellent choice in a patient with a history of PONV or in those with upper airway concerns and/or apnea.

Ketorolac is an intravenous NSAID. It is a potent analgesic. 30 mg IM of ketorolac is equivalent to 6–12 mg of morphine. It is an anti-inflammatory and is not a respiratory depressant. Like other NSAIDs, it can be used as the sole analgesic or as an adjunct to a pain treatment regimen. It does have an anti-platelet effect that is reversible after just a few hours. Its use in the short term has not been associated with impairment of long bone fractures. It should be avoided or used with caution in any patient with, or at risk of, renal compromise. In some studies its use is associated with a decrease in the incidence of emergence delirium. It is an excellent adjunct to regional anesthetic techniques.

Acetaminophen is available in oral, rectal, and intravenous preparations. It is a surprisingly effective analgesic, especially in infants and children. It is an excellent anti-pyretic despite its lack of anti-inflammatory effect. It is a reasonable choice for minor surgery or as an adjunct to a pain regimen for major surgery. Like the NSAIDs, it should be considered a first-line pain drug and may be combined with NSAIDs in the same pain regimen. It does not cause gastric irritation, inhibit platelet function, or impair bone healing. It is not a respiratory depressant. Rectal acetaminophen is commonly under-dosed. The first dose of rectal acetaminophen should be 30–40 mg/kg with subsequent doses reduced to 15 mg/kg.

For many, opioids are the most common group of drugs used in managing post-operative pain relief. They are very potent sedative analgesics with an unfortunate side effect profile that has caused as much pain in society as it has alleviated. The opioids fall into at least two categories: those derived from naturally occurring opioids, such as cocaine, morphine and heroin; and the synthetic opioids, such as fentanyl, sufentanil, remifentanil, and methadone.

The use of opioids is associated with a host of problems. All are potent respiratory depressants by shifting normal hypoxic and hypercarbic responsiveness. They relax upper airway muscle tone and can cause obstruction and apnea. Because of these side effects, all patients receiving opioids must have their respiratory status continuously monitored. The opioids are all associated with PONV, delayed gastric motility, urinary retention, sedation, tolerance, and addiction. And last but not least, they are all controlled substances and therefore difficult to store and transport.

The synthetic opioids fentanyl, sufentanil, and remifentanil are rapid-onset potent analgesics. They are, unfortunately, associated with immediate upregulation of narcotic receptors and acute tolerance. The use of these drugs results in an increased opioid requirement in the immediate post-operative period compared to patients receiving morphine or methadone. Therefore, in patients requiring post-operative opioids over several days, the choice of morphine or methadone is preferred.

The availability of opioids in LMICs can be quite variable depending on the country in question. Often, domestic drug policy results in an inadequate availability of opioid analgesics because of concerns of diversion. The WHO has advocated for easing of restriction of opioid drugs in the less developed world, but the practitioner should be comfortable with the use of multiple types of opioids as a region may only have access to a single type (e.g., fentanyl, morphine, or meperidine but not all three). Further, it should be part of the anesthesia provider's trip planning to ensure a local supply of opioid analgesics prior to departing on the trip. In general, perioperative pain management is almost nonexistent in many LMICs. This is an area where an expatriate practitioner can have a significant effect on anesthetic practice in this environment.

Dexmedetomidine has been previously discussed in this chapter. However, it is worthwhile to make a few practical points regarding its use as an analgesic in the operating room. Dexmedetomidine is an excellent analgesic in children. It does not increase PONV. Its lack of respiratory depression and preservation of upper airway muscle tone makes it a perfect choice for any child having surgery in and around the airway. These cases include eye surgery, cleft lip and palate repairs, and adenotonsillectomy. In appropriate doses (1–3 mcg/kg), it can also be used for analgesia after orthopedic and general surgery procedures. It is most effective given near or at the end of the procedure, due to its relatively short half-life. Children receiving higher doses do sleep for 20–40 minutes after its administration. Once again, it can act synergistically with opioids, so care must be taken when administering dexmedetomidine concomitantly with other classes of drugs causing respiratory depression and sedation.

The use of a regional anesthetic technique is a safe and excellent method of pain control in adults and children. Major regional techniques can be safely performed in a variety of surgical settings. Such techniques are capable of providing conditions suitable for surgery while providing prolonged pain control. Combined with sedation or a light general anesthetic, they provide for safe effective care, rapid recovery and turnover of cases, and the avoidance of PONV. These techniques are particularly useful in patients with obstructive sleep apnea and respiratory or cardiac compromise. Without these techniques, surgery can be very difficult or impossible for many patients in remote settings. The details of these techniques are discussed in the chapter on regional anesthesia.

Suggested Reading

1. Funk LM, Weiser TG, Berry WR, et al. Global operating theatre and pulse oximetry supply; an estimation from reported data. *Lancet*. 2010;376(9746):1055–61.

2. Haynes AB, Weiser RG, Berry WR, et al. A surgical safety checklist to reduce mortality and morbidity in a global population. *New England Journal of Medicine*. 2009;360(5):491–9.

3. Hodges SC, Mijumbi C, Okello M, et al. Anaesthesia services in developing countries: defining the problems. *Anaesthesia*. 2007;62:4–11.

4. Hodges SC, Walker IA, Bosenberg AT. Paediatric anaesthesia in developing countries. *Anaesthesia*. 2007;62 (suppl 1):26–31.

5. Kushner AL, Cherian MN, Noel L, et al. Addressing the Millenium Development Goals for a surgical perspective: essential surgery and anesthesia in 8 low- and middle-income countries. *Archives of Surgery*. 2010;145(2):154–9.

6. Morray JP, Geiduschek JM, Ramamoorthy C, et al. Anesthesia-related cardiac arrest in children: Initial findings of the pediatric perioperative cardiac arrest (POCA) registry. *Anesthesiology*. 2000;93(1):6–14.

7. Notrica MR, Evans FM, Knowlton LM, McQueen KA. Rwandan surgical and anesthesia infrastructure: a survey of district hospitals. *World Journal of Surgery*. 2011;35(8):1770–80.

8. Schneider WJ, Politis GD, Gosain AK, et al. Volunteers in plastic surgery guideline for providing surgical care for children in the less developed world. *Plastic and Reconstructive Surgery*. 2011;127(6):2477–86.

9. Schneider WJ, Migliori MR, Gosain AK, et al. Volunteers in plastic surgery guidelines for providing surgical care for children in the less developed world: part II. Ethical considerations. *Plastic and Reconstructive Surgery*. 2011;128(3):216e–22e.

10. Walker IA, Merry AF, Wilson IH, et al. Global oximetry: an international anaesthesia quality improvement project. *Anaesthesia*. 2009;64(10):1051–60.

COMMENTARY

Francoise Nizeyimana, Rwanda
Denise M. Chan, USA

Our operating rooms in Rwanda are basically set up like many operating rooms around the world: a space with an anesthesia machine, medications, monitors, and other equipment. However, we have a unique patient population, often presenting in late stages of disease, as well as limitations in the skills of our anesthesia providers and types of resources available. These factors undoubtedly influence our intraoperative management of patients, but we adapt our practice to best utilize our talents and resources, as there are many ways to provide anesthesia.

Two of our greatest limitations are in human and material resources. The majority of anesthetics in Rwanda are performed by anesthesia technicians, who complete a three-year certificate program after high school. Physician anesthesiologists are few; only 15 consultants are in the country (as of 2014), and all are at the teaching hospitals in Kigali and Butare with none in the district hospitals. Consequently, most anesthesia technicians practice independently and do not have physician support for complex adult patients or pediatric patients. In addition, there are no fellowship-trained pediatric or obstetric anesthesiologists in the country.

A shortage of skilled healthcare providers also means that many patients cannot receive treatment in a timely manner. For example, patients with orthopedic fractures often need surgery within minutes or hours, but they may not undergo surgery for days or even weeks. This delay obviously has an effect on how we ultimately manage these patients intraoperatively.

Intraoperative monitoring is performed using standard ASA monitors, although this often proves to be challenging, as much of our monitoring equipment is dysfunctional or missing parts. Many times we must triage our available equipment to allow the patient most in need to use a certain modality. For instance, a neurosurgical patient would take priority over others for use of the portable capnograph. Most difficult is the monitoring of neonates, as we often do not have appropriately-sized blood pressure cuffs or pulse oximetry probes. Lifebox pulse oximeters have been a wonderful addition to our operating rooms and recovery rooms, and they are now available for almost every intraoperative patient in our teaching hospitals. We hope to be able to measure intra-arterial blood pressure in the future. Our most important monitors, however, are our own eyes and ears, and we must remember to stay vigilant above all else.

Fluid resuscitation is performed with an isotonic solution; we have both normal saline and lactated Ringer's solution as choices for crystalloids. Haemacel is the colloid available in Rwanda, and we use it despite the high incidence of allergic reactions and other adverse effects associated with it. Fractionated blood products (packed red blood cells, fresh frozen plasma, and platelets) are available and used regularly. Laboratory tests cannot be performed quickly enough to help guide our intraoperative management, so we administer these blood products based on clinical judgment.

Glucose control and hypothermia are also more challenging to manage intraoperatively in Rwanda. Although the chapter mentions that glucometers are easily accessible and inexpensive in the United States, they are inaccessible in Rwanda. Without glucometers, checking a patient's blood glucose level can be nearly impossible. For this reason, we give glucose-containing solutions empirically, with an understanding that there is a potentially dangerous risk of hyperglycemia, especially in neonates. The most common scenario involves a patient who is slow to emerge from anesthesia, and hypoglycemia is thought to be one of the possible causes.

Hypothermia is a real risk to our patients, even in a sub-Saharan climate. In our main referral hospital in Kigali, we have just one radiant infant warmer in the main operating room, which we use to operate on neonates. We also have just one fluid warmer. Surgical drapes can be used to cover patients, but these quickly become wet and cold. Foreign anesthesiologists have brought plastic shower caps to cover patients' heads and trap in heat. Despite these efforts, virtually all of our patients are hypothermic by the time they reach the recovery room. However, most practitioners are not aware of this since we do not have thermometers in our perioperative area.

Perhaps the most critical intraoperative issue we face in our setting is the difficult airway, which frequently escalates into a true emergency. This is the case for both the unanticipated and the anticipated difficult airway. Unfortunately, the unanticipated difficult airway is more common than perhaps in other settings, mostly because of the inexperience of our anesthesia providers. Airway assessments are not always performed thoroughly, and as mentioned previously, the majority of our patients in Rwanda are not assessed by a physician anesthesiologist. Loss of life because of loss of airway is the consequence. When a difficult airway is anticipated, an airway management plan is made using our available tools. Most anesthesia technicians are facile with the bougie, and as these are usually available, it is our preferred device. There is also one video laryngoscope in the hospital, and a few of the physicians are becoming more accustomed to using it. The otorhinolaryngology department has a fiber-optic bronchoscope that we use only on rare occasion. In other instances, patients do not have a difficult airway, per se, but due to lack of experience of the anesthesia provider, hypoxia, bradycardia, or cardiac arrest can ensue. This especially holds true for pediatric and obstetric patients.

As you can see, a multitude of factors—patient population, number and experience of anesthesia providers, and resource availability—affect how we manage our patients intraoperatively. We will continue to learn and adapt our patient management as our country changes and resources grow.

9

Postoperative Care: PACU and ICU

Traci A. Wolbrink
Martin Zammert

Introduction

An important component to successful surgical intervention is appropriate postoperative management. It is imperative that prior to commencing surgery, one understands the capability of the hospital, including staffing, resources, and facilities available. This includes the availability of a patient recovery area or an intensive care unit, the bed capacity, the nursing staffing capabilities, and what resources are available (i.e., patient monitors, mechanical ventilators, blood products). In many hospitals in the less developed world, only ward care is available and the nursing to patient ratio is quite high. Therefore, a patient cannot be expected to receive frequent assessment or ongoing fluid resuscitation in this setting. It could possibly be the case that the capability exists to perform the procedure, but there are not appropriate staff and/or resources to safely care for the patient postoperatively. In this setting, referral may be the best and safest alternative. Many hospitals do not have a blood bank or mechanisms to separate blood products. Thus, blood is often directly donated from family members or staff when needed, and only whole blood might be available. Infection screening processes may be limited, if available at all. Thus, performing a surgery with significant expected blood loss may not be possible unless an appropriate amount of blood can be procured and stored for use during surgery and postoperatively.

The development of postanesthesia recovery units (PACUs), or patient recovery areas, and intensive care units (ICUs) has led to better outcomes in patients and the ability to care for sicker patients following surgical procedures. Some key components leading to success of PACUs or ICUs includes ensuring that healthcare providers working in these units/areas are trained to appropriately recognize and manage postoperative complications, patients are adequately monitored to identify postoperative problems early, medications and equipment necessary to manage postoperative complications are sufficiently stocked and readily available to healthcare providers, and a thorough hand-off is performed to ensure the communication of important information to healthcare providers caring for the patient. Physician and nurse vigilance is a crucial component of successful postoperative care. It is essential that any healthcare providers working in these areas familiarize themselves with the capabilities of the staff, and the location and contents of the available equipment and medications, and understand the capacity of the hospital to manage postoperative patients. This chapter will introduce the general principles of postoperative care, including a description of structural, staffing, equipment, and monitoring considerations; commonly encountered postoperative problems and their management; and criteria for discharge from a PACU or an ICU environment.

Patient Recovery Area/PACU

General Principles

Location and Size

The PACU should provide a safe environment for patients to recover from surgery and anesthesia. It should be located close to the operating theater to limit time spent between transferring patients, especially if there is a lack of portable monitoring devices. It should be large enough to accommodate the maximum number of patients expected to be recovering at one time.

Staffing

All staff members in the PACU must be able to recognize and manage common postoperative complications. In many environments, the staff may not have been specifically trained to provide postoperative care including close monitoring of postoperative patients, recognizing acute complications, appropriate delivery of medications to treat complications, and determining when a patient is safe for transfer to the wards or to be discharged home. It is important to emphasize to the staff that being vigilant and proactive will help to recognize problems early and provide better and safer patient care. It is essential to understand and respect the capabilities of the staff in order to safely deliver care in this environment.

Equipment

Essential PACU equipment includes patient monitoring devices (i.e., pulse oximeter), oxygen source with a means of delivery (face mask or manual ventilation bag), suction, emergency airway equipment (laryngoscope, blades, endotracheal tubes, manual ventilation bag, and masks of varying sizes for adult and pediatric patients), and emergency medications. Oral and nasal airways of varying sizes, a defibrillator, and end-tidal carbon dioxide detector devices would be desirable. Familiarizing oneself with the equipment and resources available at the hospital, specifically in the PACU, should be done prior to delivering any clinical care, as essential equipment may often be broken,

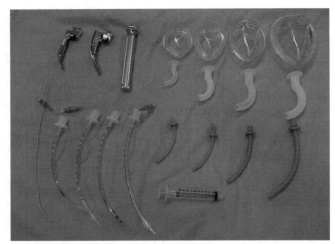

FIGURE 9.1 Photograph displaying some emergency airway equipment (not shown: manual ventilation bag) recommended to be available in the PACU. Image by Traci A. Wolbrink.

TABLE 9.1

Essential components of a safe surgical and anesthesia hand-off

1. Confirmation of patient's identity
2. Pertinent past medical history
3. Drug allergies
4. Name of procedure performed
5. Airway management
6. Surgical and anesthetic complications
7. Hemodynamic stability
8. Estimated surgical blood loss
9. Fluids and blood products administered
10. Timing and dosing of antibiotics, pain medications, or other medications given
11. Anticipated postoperative issues

misplaced, or expired in this environment. Figure 9.1 displays some recommended emergency airway equipment.

Medications

Medications should be readily available to manage the common postoperative complications, and should include pain medications, anti-emetics, reversal agents (naloxone, flumazenil, neostigmine, and glycopyrrolate), fluids, blood products, vasopressors, anti-hypertensive drugs, beta-agonists, racemic epinephrine, steroids, diphenhydramine, and medications for emergent airway management (muscle relaxants and induction agents).

Monitoring

All patients should be monitored for adequate airway patency, breathing, and circulation utilizing data from physical examination, vital signs, and basic clinical assessment. All patients should be examined upon admission and be frequently assessed.[1] Patients must also be examined prior to discharge to ensure suitability for transfer to the ward or home. If the capabilities exist, it is recommended that all patients, but especially neonatal, pediatric, and elderly patients, be placed on a continuous monitoring device (i.e., pulse oximeter) to monitor oxygen saturation and heart rate.

Hand-Off to PACU from Anesthesia Staff

An appropriate hand-off from the surgical and anesthesia staff is a necessary component of postanesthesia care. It serves to assist PACU providers in the anticipation and treatment of postoperative complications. The essential components of a safe hand-off are listed in Table 9.1.[1-3]

A checklist may be a helpful tool to ensure that the essential components of hand-off are performed following every surgical procedure, and is an essential component of the WHO Surgical Safety Checklist (Figure 9.2).[2]

Commonly Encountered Problems in PACU

Respiratory Insufficiency

A patient may be unable to adequately ventilate or oxygenate in the PACU secondary to a wide variety of postoperative causes. Upper airway obstruction, laryngospasm, airway edema, residual anesthetic drug effects, and pulmonary edema are all common etiologies for respiratory insufficiency in the PACU.

Upper airway obstruction: Upper airway obstruction can often occur as a result of the loss of pharyngeal tone related to residual anesthetic agents. A patient who is breathing against an obstructed upper airway may have evidence of suprasternal retractions and significant abdominal muscle use, and may demonstrate snoring or, in severe cases, absent breath sounds from complete upper airway obstruction. Such patients may still demonstrate chest movement but will not have adequate gas exchange because of airway obstruction. The increased respiratory effort from hypercarbia and/or hypoxia can exacerbate the process by increasing the negative inspiratory pressure, thus worsening the upper airway obstruction. Treatment includes opening the upper airway; this can be accomplished by a jaw thrust maneuver, continuous positive airway pressure (CPAP) (delivered via bag-mask ventilation or CPAP machine with 5–15 cm H_2O pressure), and/or a nasal or oral airway (nasal airway preferred in a semi-awake patient) until the patient recovers from the effects of anesthesia.[1] In severe cases, re-intubation with an endotracheal tube or placement of a laryngeal mask airway (LMA) may be necessary. Timely recognition and treatment of upper airway obstruction is essential as postobstructive pulmonary edema, hypoxemia, hypercarbia, respiratory failure and arrest, and cardiac arrest can occur quickly if upper airway obstruction is not recognized. Given this, practitioners should ensure that patients delivered to the PACU in a developing world setting have a patent airway and are at minimal risk for further airway management.

Laryngospasm: Laryngospasm occurs when the vocal cords close suddenly secondary to direct stimulation from secretions, from foreign objects, or during extubation as a patient awakens from anesthesia. This life-threatening event can present similarly to upper airway obstruction with suprasternal retractions, increased abdominal muscle use, and/or absent breath sounds evident. Often stridor is present. Treatment includes a jaw thrust maneuver and CPAP (often up to 40 cm H_2O pressure is needed) to

World Health Organization

SURGICAL SAFETY CHECKLIST (FIRST EDITION)

Before induction of anesthesia ▶▶▶▶▶▶▶▶ Before skin incision ▶▶▶▶▶▶▶▶▶▶▶▶▶▶ Before patient leaves operating room

SIGN IN

☐ **PATIENT HAS CONFIRMED**
· IDENTITY
· SITE
· PROCEDURE
· CONSENT

☐ **SITE MARKED/NOT APPLICABLE**

☐ **ANESTHESIA SAFETY CHECK COMPLETED**

☐ **PULSE OXIMETER ON PATIENT AND FUNCTIONING**

☐ **DOES PATIENT HAVE A:**

KNOWN ALLERGY?
☐ NO
☐ YES

DIFFICULT AIRWAY/ASPIRATION RISK?
☐ NO
☐ YES, AND EQUIPMENT/ASSISTANCE AVAILABLE

RISK OF >500ML BLOOD LOSS (7ML/KG IN CHILDREN)?
☐ NO
☐ YES, AND ADEQUATE INTRAVENOUS ACCESS AND FLUIDS PLANNED

TIME OUT

☐ **CONFIRM ALL TEAM MEMBERS HAVE INTRODUCED THEMSELVES BY NAME AND ROLE**

☐ **SURGEON, ANESTHESIA PROFESSIONAL AND NURSE VERBALLY CONFIRM**
· PATIENT
· SITE
· PROCEDURE

☐ **ANTICIPATED CRITICAL EVENTS**

☐ **SURGEON REVIEWS:** WHAT ARE THE CRITICAL OR UNEXPECTED STEPS, OPERATIVE DURATION, ANTICIPATED BLOOD LOSS?

☐ **ANESTHESIA TEAM REVIEWS:** ARE THERE ANY PATIENT-SPECIFIC CONCERNS?

☐ **NURSING TEAM REVIEWS:** HAS STERILITY (INCLUDING INDICATOR RESULTS) BEEN CONFIRMED? ARE THERE EQUIPMENT ISSUES OR ANY CONCERNS?

☐ **HAS ANTIBIOTIC PROPHYLAXIS BEEN GIVEN WITHIN THE LAST 60 MINUTES?**
☐ YES
☐ NOT APPLICABLE

☐ **IS ESSENTIAL IMAGING DISPLAYED?**
☐ YES
☐ NOT APPLICABLE

SIGN OUT

☐ **NURSE VERBALLY CONFIRMS WITH THE TEAM:**

☐ **THE NAME OF THE PROCEDURE RECORDED**

☐ **THAT INSTRUMENT, SPONGE AND NEEDLE COUNTS ARE CORRECT** (OR NOT APPLICABLE)

☐ **HOW THE SPECIMEN IS LABELLED** (INCLUDING PATIENT NAME)

☐ **WHETHER THERE ARE ANY EQUIPMENT PROBLEMS TO BE ADDRESSED**

☐ **SURGEON, ANESTHESIA PROFESSIONAL AND NURSE REVIEW THE KEY CONCERNS FOR RECOVERY AND MANAGEMENT OF THIS PATIENT**

FIGURE 9.2 WHO Surgical Safety Checklist.[2]

resolve the laryngospasm.[1] In severe cases, a small dose of succinylcholine (0.5–1 mg/kg IV or 4mg/kg IM) may be necessary to relieve the laryngospasm.[1,3] If succinylcholine is administered, one must be prepared to perform bag-mask ventilation or endotracheal intubation with mechanical ventilation as needed.

Airway edema: Airway edema may be related to the acute process that necessitated surgery (i.e., acute epiglottitis), an effect from surgery (i.e., removal of an airway mass), excessive airway manipulation (i.e., multiple intubation attempts or prolonged airway manipulation), swelling from positioning during surgery (i.e., prone positioning during a long surgery), or aggressive volume resuscitation. Patients with airway edema may present with inspiratory stridor, increased work of breathing, hypercarbia, and/or hypoxia. There may also be significant facial or orbital edema present in the case of prolonged prone positioning or aggressive volume resuscitation. Treatment includes medications to decrease the airway edema, including steroids, inhaled nebulized epinephrine, and/or the consideration of diuretics if hemodynamically stable. In severe cases, CPAP (delivered via bag-mask ventilation or CPAP machine with 5–15 cm H_2O pressure) or re-intubation may be necessary. Caution should be exercised in the case of re-intubation as the swollen airway may be more difficult to manage than it was initially. Children may be more significantly affected as compared to adult patients due to the smaller caliber of their airways and the markedly increased resistance to flow that occurs with small decreases in airway diameter. Understanding Poiseuille's law, which demonstrates that resistance is inversely proportional to the size of the radius: $R = 8ln/\pi r^4$ (where R is resistance, l is the length of the tube, n is the gas viscosity, and r is the radius) is key. Therefore, any decrease in the radius from airway swelling can be expected to increase the resistance of airway flow, and is much more significant in small airways.

Residual Anesthetic Drug Effects

Following surgery and anesthesia, patients may continue to experience residual effects of the anesthetic drugs given during surgery, including somnolence, hypoventilation, hypotension, or muscle weakness. An important special consideration is that neonates, infants, and elderly patients may have an exaggerated response to anesthesia and are at increased risk for residual drug effects. Often, allowing the patient time to recover while ensuring adequate oxygenation and ventilation is sufficient. However, there are times when it may be necessary to intervene and reverse the action of one or more of the anesthetic drugs. When a patient is unable to breathe effectively, this may be related to skeletal muscle weakness from residual muscle relaxants or from opiate- or benzodiazepine-induced hypoventilation. A review of the medications, including dosages and timing, may reveal the offending drug. A physical exam will also be helpful to discover the etiology. Asking the patient to lift his head off the bed and hold it up for 4 seconds, and/or examining for normal strength in his extremities can be useful to detect muscle weakness in a cooperative patient. In a patient who is extremely somnolent, a neuromuscular stimulation device can help assess if full reversal or recovery of neuromuscular function has been achieved. Full muscle function recovery is considered if all four stimuli lead to four equal contractions. If a fade in between the contractions or fewer than four contractions is detected, additional reversal agent should be administered. If residual muscle weakness from intraoperative administration of nondepolarizing muscle relaxants is suspected, the drug effect can be reversed using neostigmine (Table 9.2). If a patient has adequate muscle strength but is very somnolent, not breathing effectively, and you suspect residual effects from opiates or benzodiazepines given during surgery, you may want to reverse one or both of these drugs. Naloxone may be used to reverse the effects of opiates. Full reverse of the analgesic effects of opiates may be undesirable. Therefore, a partial reversal dose (Table 9.2) and titration to effect will hopefully minimize hemodynamic changes and prevent precipitating acute pain. In a situation of cardiopulmonary arrest, full reversal of opiates may be indicated. Flumazenil (Table 9.2) is used to reverse the effects of benzodiazepines.

Postoperative Pain

One of the most commonly encountered problems in the PACU is postoperative pain. Educating the local staff about the reasons to treat a postoperative patient's pain, and explaining that postoperative pain treatment helps to minimize the physiological stress on the patient, leading to better surgical outcomes, are essential. Prompt and appropriate treatment of a patient's pain can help minimize cardiovascular changes and prevent splinting and atelectasis. Using a combination of opiate and nonopiate medications can be quite helpful. Table 9.3 lists some commonly available drugs and their dosage.

When dosing opiates, a key strategy to success is starting with a small starting dose and titrating subsequent doses to affect. Titration is generally easier to accomplish in an awake patient in the PACU than intraoperatively in an anesthetized patient. This will facilitate good pain control while minimizing nondesirable side effects such as respiratory depression. It is crucial to titrate doses of analgesics. This will help prevent excessive somnolence in patients in the PACU or on the general wards. Given that monitoring can be limited and patient-to-nurse ratios can be high, it can be quite dangerous to have overly sedated patients in the PACU or on the wards as they may develop respiratory insufficiency or arrest if not detected and acted upon in a timely manner.

Visual analog scales can be useful in assessing and managing pain in both children and adults. In older children and adults, a numerical scale can be used. This involves asking the patient to rate his or her pain on a scale from 1–10, with 1 indicating no pain and 10 indicating severe pain. Multiple instruments exist for children. One of the more common scales is the FACES scale (Figure 9.3) in which multiple faces of smiling and crying are shown and children are asked to pick the face that best describes how they are feeling.[5]

An alternative to systemic pain therapy is the use of regional anesthetic technique. These techniques are discussed in the chapter on regional anesthesia. Even if the surgical field is not amenable to a peripheral nerve block, skin infiltration of the incision site with local anesthetics can be very helpful in reducing the need for systemic analgesia and is highly recommended. When administering local anesthetic, it is important to be aware of the maximum amount of local anesthetic that can be administered in a single dose. Table 9.4 lists some commonly used local anesthetics, their

TABLE 9.2

Names, dosages, and indications of medication used to reverse effects of opiates, benzodiazepines, and muscle relaxant[4]

Drug name	Route of admin.	Pediatric dose (per dose)	Adult dose (per dose)	Dosing interval	Indications
Naloxone*					
For reversal of postop opiates/ **(Note: this dose will partially reverse opiates)**	IV/IM/IO/SQ	1–2 µg/kg	1–2 µg/kg	Repeat Q2–3 min PRN, based on response, dose until patient can maintain a stable respiratory pattern	Used to reverse the effects of opiates (morphine, fentanyl, hydromorphone, methadone)
Flumazenil**	IV	0.01 mg/kg (max 0.2mg)	0.2 mg	Give over 15 sec, may repeat Q1 min PRN for effect up to 5 doses	Used to reverse the effects of benzodiazepines (midazolam, lorazepam, diazepam)
Neostigmine*** (use only in conjunction with glycopyrrolate or atropine)	IV	0.04–0.07 mg/kg	2–5 mg	Give atropine or glycopyrrolate prior to neostigmine	Use to reverse the effects of nondepolarizing neuromuscular blocking agents (pancuronium, vecuronium, rocuronium)
Atropine	IV	0.02 mg/kg (min dose 0.1 mg, max dose 0.5 mg in children and 1 mg in adolescents)	0.4–1 mg	Give prior to neostigmine	Give prior to neostigmine to prevent bradycardia
Glycopyrrolate	IV	0.2 mg for each 1 mg of neostigmine given	0.2 mg for each 1 mg of neostigmine given	Give prior to neostigmine	Give prior to neostigmine to prevent bradycardia

IV = intravenous, IM = intramuscular, IO = intraosseus, SQ = subcutaneous, ETT = via endotracheal tube.

* Side effects include sudden hemodynamic changes (hypertension, hypotension), cardiac instability (arrhythmias), pulmonary edema, acute withdrawal (pain, hypertension, agitation, sweating), seizures. Caution use in patients with chronic narcotic use as use of naloxone can precipitate acute withdrawal (use small titrated doses).

** Side effects include seizures. Caution use in patients with history of seizures or in patients with hepatic insufficiency (use smaller doses).

*** Side effects include cholinergic effects (salivation, sweating, urinary incontinence), cardiac arrhythmias (bradycardia), hypotension, seizures, bronchospasm. Caution use in patients with renal impairment and in elderly patients. Do not use to treat residual neuromuscular blockage from depolarizing neuromuscular blocking agents as it will prolong the duration of paralysis.

TABLE 9.3

Names and dosages of analgesic medications for adults and children in a PACU[4]

Drug name	Route of administration	Pediatric dose** (per dose)	Adult dose (per dose)	Dosing interval
Morphine	IV	0.025–0.01 mg/kg	2.5–5 mg	Q4 hr PRN
	IM	0.05–0.1 mg/kg	5–10 mg	Q4 hr PRN
	PO	0.2–0.5 mg/kg	10 mg	Q4 hr PRN
Fentanyl***	IV	0.5–1 mcg/kg	25–100 mcg	Q1–2 hr PRN
Hydromorphone	IV	0.015 mg/kg	0.2–0.6 mg	Q2–4 hr PRN
	PO	0.03–0.08 mg/kg	2–4 mg	Q4–6 hr PRN
Codeine	PO	0.5–1 mg/kg	30–60 mg	Q4–6 PRN
Acetaminophen/paracetamol	IV	10–15 mg/kg	650 mg	Q4–6 hr PRN
	PO/PR	10–15 mg/kg	325–650 mg	Q4–6 hr PRN
Ibuprofen	PO	10 mg/kg	200–800 mg	Q6–8 hr PRN
Ketorolac****	IV	0.25–0.5 kg	30 mg	Q6 hr PRN
	IM		30 mg	Q6 hr PRN

IV = intravenous, IM = intramuscular, PO = orally, PR = rectally, PRN = as needed.

* Neonatal/elderly/critically ill patients may have increased sensitivity to drugs and dosing at lower end of spectrum is recommended. Caution in patients with renal or hepatic impairment.

** Neonates should be given doses at the lower end of the dosage spectrum secondary to risk of central nervous system effects including respiratory depression and/or apnea.

*** Inject slowly as rapid infusion may cause skeletal muscle or chest wall rigidity. Elderly patients may have increased sensitivity to effects of fentanyl; therefore, dosing a lower end of dosage spectrum is suggested.

**** Do not use in patients less than 6 months old. Give half of normal dose for elderly patients or those with renal impairment.

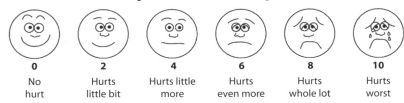

FIGURE 9.3   Wong-Baker FACES Pain Rating Scale.[5]

TABLE 9.4

Commonly used local anesthetic medications, their maximum dose, and expected duration[6]

Drug	Maximum dose (infiltration, NOT IV)	Maximum duration
Lidocaine	3–4 mg/kg (7 mg/kg with epinephrine)	1–2 hrs (3 hrs with epinephrine)
Mepivacaine	4.5 mg kg (7 mg/kg with epinephrine)	1–2 hrs (3–4 hrs with epinephrine
Bupivacaine	2.5 mg/kg	2–8 hrs (8–16 hrs with epinephrine)

IV = intravenous.

maximum dosages, and the expected duration of analgesia. The addition of small doses of epinephrine (1:200,000 dilution or 5 micrograms epinephrine/1 mL local anesthetic) can increase this dose as well as the duration of the block; however, the addition of epinephrine should be avoided in very distal nerve blocks, such as nerve blockades of single digits or in penile nerve blockades, to prevent necrosis of the skin.

Postoperative Nausea and Vomiting

Another very commonly encountered problem in the PACU is postoperative nausea and vomiting (PONV). Many of the most commonly used anesthetic drugs are emetogenic, including inhalation anesthetics and opiates. Higher risk patients are identified prior to surgery and appropriate treatment should be initiated

intraoperatively. However, many patients do suffer from PONV, and ongoing administration of anti-emetics is necessary in the PACU. Table 9.5 lists the commonly available anti-emetic drugs.

Hypotension

Hypotension in the immediate postoperative period may be related to residual effects of anesthesia, inadequate replacement of surgical losses intraoperatively, ongoing bleeding, or significant third spacing. An estimation of dehydration prior to starting surgery is important. The climate of many developing world nations is tropical, and thus patients can experience significant insensible losses preoperatively simply from living in their native environment. Patients who have been sick for a long time prior to surgery are at high risk for having significant preexisting dehydration. Diarrheal diseases are all too common in the developing world, and such patients can have tremendous fluid deficits. Adequate intraoperative fluid resuscitation will depend on appropriate replacement of surgical blood loss, preoperative fluid deficit, and intraoperative baseline requirements including insensible losses. A rule of thumb is that blood loss should be replaced using blood at a 1:1 ratio, whereas crystalloid should replace blood loss at a 3:1 ratio. A patient that remains hypotensive despite replacement of preoperative dehydration and intraoperative blood loss is likely hypotensive because of residual effects of anesthesia (often having clinical signs of sedation) or ongoing intravascular losses from bleeding or third spacing. An isotonic fluid bolus should be given as a first step when replacing preoperative dehydration, intraoperative blood loss, or ongoing intravascular losses. Lactated Ringer's solution, normal saline, and albumin are all reasonable choices. Typical

TABLE 9.5

Names and dosages of anti-emetic medications for adults and children in a PACU[4]

Drug name	Route of administration	Pediatric dose (per dose)	Adult dose (per dose)	Dosing interval
Metoclopramide*	IV/IM	0.05–0.1 mg/kg	10 mg	Q6–8 hr PRN
Promethazine**	IV/IM/PO/PR	0.25–1 mg/kg	12.5–25 mg	Q4–6 hr PRN
Ondansetron***	IV/ IM (adults only)	0.1 mg/kg (max dose 4mg)	2–4 mg	Q8 hr PRN
Dexamethasone****	IV	0.1–0.2 mg/kg	2–5 mg	Q6 hr PRN (prolonged use may generate concern for wound healing)
Droperidol	IV	10–20 µg/kg (max dose 0.625 mg)	0.625 mg	Q 6–8 hr PRN

IV = intravenous, IM = intramuscular, PO = orally, PR = rectally, SC = subcutaneously PRN = as needed.

*   Requires dosing adjustment in renal impairment. Side effects may include extrapyramidal symptoms, neuroleptic malignant syndrome, tardive dyskinesia. Caution use in pediatric and elderly patients.

**   Side effects may include altered cardiac conduction, extrapyramidal symptoms, neuroleptic malignant syndrome, anticholinergic symptoms. Caution use in pediatric and elderly patients. Contraindicated in children less than 2 years of age.

***   Requires dosing adjustment in hepatic failure. May prolong ECG interval (PR, QRS, QTc). Caution use in patients with long QT syndrome.

****   Antiemetic effect is significantly improved when given in operating room prior to completion of anesthesia.

fluid replacement as a bolus is 500–1000 mL for an adult patient, and 10–20 mL/kg in pediatric patients. Blood products can be considered for significant bleeding, if available. If hypotension is persistent and not responsive to several fluid boluses, ongoing occult surgical bleeding must be considered. Re-exploration of the surgical site may be necessary. A patient may continue to bleed after major surgery if he or she is coagulopathic. This can be due to concomitant sepsis/disseminated intravascular coagulation (DIC) or hepatic/renal failure, or if large volume blood losses were replaced with only packed red blood cells, resulting in a dilutional coagulopathy. A special consideration is the pregnant patient. The gravid uterus may compress the inferior vena cava, obstructing the adequate return of blood flow to the heart. Therefore, the initial response to hypotension in a pregnant woman should be uterine displacement by placing the patient in left lateral decubitus position.

Hypothermia

Hypothermia, defined as a core body temperature of less than 35°C (95°F), is a common occurrence during many operative procedures in the developed world, where operating rooms have lower temperatures maintained to prevent bacterial growth. In LMICs, operating rooms are often quite warm or simply not cooled. Thus, hypothermia is not seen as commonly as in HICs, although certain patients may still be at significant risk, including the very young and very old. The physiologic consequences of hypothermia may have significant negative impact on these patients.

TABLE 9.6

Description of the common physiological effects of hypothermia[7]

System affected	Physiological effects
Cardiovascular	Intraoperative hypothermia can lead to postoperative shivering, which subsequently leads to a significant increase in total body oxygen consumption (35%). In patients with cardiopulmonary diseases this can increase the risk of myocardial infarction by three times.
Coagulation	Platelet aggregation seems to be reduced as the production of thrombin, a potent platelet activator, is reduced in states of hypothermia. If the core body temperature decreases below 35°C, the activated partial thromboplastin time can be elevated by 10% compared to normal body temperature due to a decrease in the function of various clotting factors. These effects can cause increased blood loss in hypothermic patients.
Wound healing	A reduction in body temperature is known to decrease the cellular immune response as well as to cause vasoconstriction and subsequent tissue hypoxia. Hypothermia of only 2°C may triple the incidence of wound infection.
Pharmacology	As enzyme activity is highly influenced by temperature it is not surprising that the pharmacokinetic properties of many anesthetic drugs are altered by the presence of hypothermia. For example, the duration of muscle relaxants can be doubled if the temperature of the patient decreases. Also, the MAC of volatile anesthetics is decreased with a decrease in body temperature.

The three main mechanisms leading to a decrease in body core temperature in the surgical setting are convection (e.g., contact to a cold bed), radiation (heat loss from being exposed and uncovered), and evaporation (breathing cold, dry anesthetic gases). While healthy individuals can compensate for any heat loss, a patient under general anesthesia has an altered response to heat loss. Hypothermia has various significant physiological effects (Table 9.6).

The best treatment for intraoperative hypothermia is prevention. Whenever possible, the temperature of the patient should be monitored. If available, intraoperative heating devices (e.g., air blankets) are very effective in keeping the patient warm. The patient should be covered when possible. The use of low- or minimal-flow anesthetic technique is also helpful in avoiding the heat loss from cold and dry anesthetic gases. Hot-air devices or heat radiators can be used to increase core body temperature in the recovery room. However, caution should be used when applying these devices to avoid overheating or local burns of the patient.

Postoperative Shivering

Shivering, or involuntary fasciculation of the muscles, is a natural response of the human body to increase heat production and counteract hypothermia. Male gender, young adults, and longer duration of anesthesia are risk factors for the occurrence of postoperative shivering. The use of halogenated agents also increases the likelihood of shivering, whereas its incidence is lower when a propofol total intravenous technique is used. Shivering increases the patient's metabolic rate and with this the total oxygen consumption by 70%–120%, putting patients with cardiovascular disease at three times the risk for postoperative myocardial ischemia.[8] Opiates, especially meperidine, or clonidine, a central alpha agonist, can be used to treat shivering once it has occurred. Table 9.7 lists the dosing and side effects of meperidine and clonidine.

Criteria for Transfer to Wards

A patient may be considered suitable for transfer to the hospital ward when he/she is awake, extubated and breathing comfortably, following commands, not requiring aggressive ongoing resuscitation, and has adequate pain control and stable vital signs (oxygen saturation, heart rate, and blood pressure are appropriate for age). The anesthesiologist must be cognizant of the environment his or her patient will be discharged into. It may be quite likely that this patient will have little assessment on the ward. This must be taken into account when deciding when a given patient is ready for transfer out of the PACU.

TABLE 9.7

Drugs used for the prevention and treatment of postoperative shivering[8,9]

Drug	Route	Dose	Common side effects
Meperidine	IV	0.5–1 mg/kg	respiratory depression hypotension, sedation
	IM	1–2 mg/kg	
Clonidine	IV, IM	1 mcg/kg	sedation, bradycardia, hypotension

IV = intravenous, IM = intramuscular.

Hand-Off from PACU to Ward Team

A detailed hand-off to the ward team is another important component of safe surgical care. The same information that was passed on during hand-off to the PACU must be repeated to the ward team. Hand-off must also include the significant details of the PACU course, including any complications encountered and medications administered in the PACU.

ICU/High-Dependency Unit (HDU)

General Principles

An important component of successful surgical care is the capability to safely manage very sick patients postoperatively, including those requiring ongoing mechanical ventilation. Each ICU/HDU will have its own admission criteria, and one must be familiar with its size, the number of staff, the available equipment and resources, and the clinical capacity of the caregivers.

Although it is important to understand what an ICU/HDU can and cannot do, this level of care is usually unavailable in all but the best-funded locations in the less developed world. ICU/HDU care is expensive and resource intensive, and the healthcare systems of many less developed nations simply do not currently have the ability to direct resources to the development and maintenance of ICUs and HDUs. That being said, it is important to engage local providers in such care as this is where healthcare systems should be headed in order to provide complete surgical care.

Staffing

All members of the ICU staff should be trained to appropriately recognize and manage common postoperative complications in a timely manner. The nurses and physicians working in the ICU/HDU should have undergone specialized training in common postoperative complications as described previously, as well as special training in mechanical ventilation and airway management, and in neurological, cardiac, and hemodynamic problems. The nurse-to-patient staffing ratio should be higher than on the general wards due to the higher acuity of the ICU/HDU patients. Common nurse-to-patient ratios may vary from 1 nurse to 1 patient to 1 nurse to 4 patients, but clearly this depends on the size of the unit and the capability of staff. Physician and nursing vigilance, including early identification of postoperative problems and their appropriate treatments, should be highlighted and stressed as a means to provide better and safer patient care.

Equipment

The ICU/HDU should contain patient monitoring devices (pulse oximeter or patient monitor), oxygen source with patient interface device (tubing, mask, and nasal cannula), suction device, emergency airway equipment (laryngoscope, blades, endotracheal tubes, oral airways, masks and ventilation bags—all of varying sizes for adult and pediatric patients), nasal airways of varying sizes, end-tidal carbon dioxide detector, defibrillator, emergency medications (see below), and mechanical ventilators (if trained personnel are available).

Medications

Medications should be readily available to manage the common postoperative complications, and should include pain medications (narcotic and nonnarcotic drugs), sedatives (benzodiazepines and propofol), anti-emetics, reversal agents (naloxone, flumazenil, glycopyrrolate, and neostigmine), crystalloid fluids, blood products, vasopressors, anti-hypertensive drugs, beta-agonists, racemic epinephrine, steroids, diphenhydramine, and medications for intubation (muscle relaxants and induction agents).

Indications for Admission

The indications for admission into the ICU/HDU will vary between hospitals, as well as medical and surgical capabilities of the clinicians caring for the patients postoperatively. Some of the common indications for admission into an ICU/HDU are described below in greater detail. Table 9.8 includes a list of common indications for admission.

Airway Monitoring

Patients who have undergone surgery in or near the airway may be at risk for acute decompensation and loss of a patent airway. Postoperative swelling, ongoing bleeding, hematomas, or third spacing of fluid can all be important contributors to airway instability. Surgical procedures that may put a patient a risk of airway compromise may include: resection of tumor or mass in or near the airway, thyroid surgery with possible hematoma formation and expansion postoperatively, maxillofacial surgeries including cleft palate repair, or repair of facial traumatic injuries. Surgeries in the prone position and procedures requiring large volume resuscitation can also put the patient at risk for airway edema. In many of these conditions, the surgeon and anesthesiologist may decide to keep the patient intubated postoperatively until the airway swelling is resolved. As resistance is inversely proportional to the size of the radius according to Poiseuille's law (discussed above), any decrease in the radius can be expected to increase the resistance of airway flow, and is much more significant in small pediatric airways. Additionally, pregnant women often have anasarca related to hormonal changes during pregnancy, and their airway can be more swollen than normal under usual conditions. Thus, any additional increase in airway swelling from any procedures/factors as above can cause greater airway swelling than might be expected in the nonpregnant patient.

TABLE 9.8

Common indications for admission into the ICU/HDU

Airway monitoring and management
Hemodynamic monitoring and management
Neurological monitoring and management
Anticipated ongoing volume resuscitation
Mechanical ventilation and extubation
Sepsis and shock

Hemodynamic Monitoring

Patients may require admission to the ICU/HDU postoperatively for close monitoring of their hemodynamic status. Patients who may benefit from close monitoring of their hemodynamic status include patients with shock and/or sepsis, patients with significant cardiac disease, patients who have had cardiac surgery, and patients who have undergone procedures with significant and/or anticipated blood loss or third spacing. These patients should be placed on continuous cardiorespiratory monitors with vital sign monitoring performed frequently; in severe cases, arterial line placement can be considered, if possible. Mental status changes are often a late sign of hemodynamic insufficiency.

Neurological Monitoring

Patients may require admission to the ICU/HDU postoperatively for close monitoring of their neurological status, including patients with traumatic brain injury, intracranial hemorrhage, extraventricular drains in place, following intracranial operations, and patients with prolonged seizures. Patients should have frequent neurological checks performed to identify any acute changes in mental status or a neurological exam. Cardiorespiratory monitoring to look for evidence of elevated intracranial pressure (ICP) (Cushing's triad includes bradycardia, hypotension, and abnormal breathing pattern) or seizure activity (tachycardia and/or desaturation episodes often noted) should be utilized.

Ongoing Fluid Resuscitation

Patients may also be admitted to the ICU/HDU postoperatively for ongoing fluid resuscitation, including those with ongoing bleeding, sepsis and/or shock, and significant third spacing. These patients should be placed on continuous cardiorespiratory monitors with frequent assessment. Urine output, heart rate, blood pressure, fluid losses into dressings and/or drains, and mental status must be monitored closely. Arterial line placement can be considered especially for unstable patients.

Fluid Selection and Dose

The selection of fluid will be different for maintenance hydration compared to replacement of losses. Maintenance fluid is commonly administered as lactated Ringer's, normal saline, or 5% dextrose with normal saline. Potassium may be added if urine output is adequate and the patient has good renal function. In addition to matching ongoing maintenance needs, fluid may need to be administered to replace surgical losses or ongoing losses from third spacing, drains, or bleeding. In general, all fluid used to replace losses or third spacing should be isotonic. Albumin has not been proven to be better than crystalloids for volume replacement.[10] Blood should be reserved for patients with impaired oxygen delivery because of the risk of transfusion reactions and transmission of infections. For massive blood losses, it is important to replace not only packed red blood cells, but also platelets and clotting factors (fresh frozen plasma and cryoprecipitate). For massive transfusion requirements in trauma patients, a 1:1 ratio of one unit of packed red blood cells with one unit of fresh frozen plasma should be employed.[11] It is important to realize that in many places, whole blood may be the only available blood product.

The rate of maintenance fluid must be carefully calculated, especially in children. For adults, the fluid rate is generally 100–125 mL/hr to cover maintenance needs. For children, one can use the 4:2:1 rule to estimate hourly maintenance fluid needs. The 4:2:1 rule is as follows:

1. For the first 10 kg of weight, maintenance rate is 4 mL/kg/hr.
2. For the second 10 kg, maintenance rate is 2 mL/kg/hr plus the previous 40 mL/hr.
3. For any additional kg beyond 20 kg, maintenance rate is 1 mL/kg/hr plus the previous 60 mL/hr.

To demonstrate this, let's consider a 42 kg child. His hourly maintenance fluid would be:

1. 4 mL/kg/hr for the first 10 kg = 4 mL*10 kg/hr = 40 mL/hr.
2. Plus 2 mL/kg/hr for the next 10 kg = 2 mL*10 kg/hr = 20 mL/hr.
3. Plus 1 mL/kg/hr for any additional kg = 1 mL*22 kg/hr = 22 mL/hr.
4. The total is 40 + 20 + 22 = 82 mL/hr.

Urine Output

Adequate urine output can be defined as at least 0.5–1 mL/kg/hr. Inadequate urine output can be a sign of volume depletion and/or syndrome of inappropriate secretion of antidiuretic hormone (SIADH), both of which are commonly seen in postoperative patients. A fluid bolus and its response, as well as a sodium level, may be helpful to distinguish the two. In volume depletion, the sodium level may often be elevated, especially if the patient has already received a large amount of crystalloid volume. In SIADH, one would expect the patient to have a low sodium value.

Hypotension

Patients who remain hypotensive despite adequate volume resuscitation may benefit from vasopressor therapy. Table 9.9 lists the name, dosing, receptors affected, and some considerations for use. Vasopressors should be administered through a central venous line if at all possible (except in true emergencies), due to risk of severe skin necrosis with extravasation from peripheral intravenous line.

Mechanical Ventilation

Indications

The selection of which patients should remain intubated following surgery should be based on the capacity of the ICU to safely care for intubated patients, including the number of ventilators as well as staff available to manage expected postoperative problems. Table 9.10 lists common criteria for postoperative mechanical ventilation.

TABLE 9.9

Name, dosing, receptors affected, and some considerations for use of common vasopressors[9]

Name	Dosing (intravenous infusion)	Peripheral vascular effects			Cardiac effects		Physiological effects	Clinical indications
		α_1	β_2	Dopa	β_1	β_2		
Epinephrine	0.05–0.1 µg/kg/min	+++	++	0	+++	+++	Systemic vasoconstriction, tachycardia, increased cardiac inotropy, bronchodilation	Low cardiac output, anaphylaxis, cardiac arrest
	0.2–0.5 µg/kg/min	++++	++	0	++++	++++		
Norepinephrine	0.05–1 µg/kg/min	++++	0	0	++	0	Systemic vasoconstriction, tachycardia	Septic shock, low cardiac output
Dopamine	1–5 µg/kg/min	0	+	++	+	+	Increased renal blood flow, increased cardiac inotropy	Septic shock, low cardiac output, may improve renal blood flow and promote diuresis
	5–15 µg/kg/min	++	++	++	++	++	Vasoconstriction, tachycardia	
	15–20 µg/kg/min	+++	++	++	++	++	Vasoconstriction, tachycardia	
Dobutamine	0.5–40 µg/kg/min	+	+++	0	++++	++	Increased cardiac contractility, tachycardia, systemic vasodilatation and vasoconstriction	Low cardiac output states (Note: less risk of arrhythmias at lower doses)
Vasopressin	Pediatric: 0.002–0.003 U/kg/min							
	Adult: 0.01–0.04 U/min	0	0	0	0	0	Potent vasoconstrictor	Refractory septic shock
Phenylephrine	0.04–0.4 µg/kg/min	++++	0	0	0	0	Systemic vasoconstriction	Hypotension

TABLE 9.10

Common criteria for postoperative mechanical ventilation

1. Known or expected airway edema or bleeding
2. Significant lung disease, such as pneumonia or severe chronic obstructive pulmonary disease (COPD)
3. Inability to protect his or her airway because of compromised neurologic status (e.g., residual anesthesia, head injury, etc.)
4. High risk for hemodynamic complications, such as sepsis or possible bleeding
5. Requires ongoing significant volume resuscitation
6. Neonatal patients because of high risk of apnea

Modes of Ventilation

There are many different modes of ventilation, but all ventilators essentially perform the same function: provide a breath to a patient with some frequency. Goal tidal volumes should be 5–7 mL/kg for patients with lung injury or lung disease (lung protective strategy ventilation) and 6–10 mL/kg for patients with healthy lungs.

Oxygenation and Ventilation

The goals of mechanical ventilation in the postoperative period are to provide adequate oxygenation, ventilation, and airway control. A pulse oximeter can be a very useful adjunct to help guide mechanical ventilation and should be used continuously if available. An oxygen saturation of greater than 92% is appropriate in the postoperative period. Ventilation goals include a normal pH (7.35–7.40) and $PaCO_2$ (40–50 mmHg), and these can often be easily achieved with low ventilator settings. However, in patients who have significant lung disease or lung injury, it is reasonable to strive for lung protective strategies which include targeting oxygen saturations >88% and pH $\geq$ 7.25 with permissive hypercapnia.

Sedation of Mechanically Ventilated Patient

Patients who remain mechanically ventilated postoperatively will require sedation and pain control to tolerate the endotracheal tube (ETT). This can be accomplished by intermittent boluses of sedatives and analgesics or by continuous infusions. The choice of intermittent versus continuous medications will be influenced by the drugs that are available for use, the availability of medication pumps with which to deliver continuous infusions, the number of staff caring for the patients, and the caregivers' comfort with the medications and their administration. Patients who are expected to remain intubated for short periods of time are likely to be successfully managed by intermittent administration of medications. However, it is important to administer medication early in order to prevent accidental or premature self-extubation by the patient. Continuous infusions of medications can often provide a smoother course of intubation by providing constant and steady sedation and analgesia. This may be useful when a patient is expected to remain intubated for greater than two days, or when one needs the patient to be immobile. The patient on sedative or analgesic medications for long periods of time may develop tolerance to these drugs and the dosages may have to be increased over time. In addition, the patient may still move and react to the ETT on continuous infusions, so it is important to closely monitor all patients for arousal. It may be necessary to administer additional bolus doses of medications if patients are uncomfortable and/or are at risk for self-extubation. Table 9.11 lists the names and dosage of medications that may be used for sedation and analgesia of mechanically ventilated patients.

Endotracheal Tube Suctioning

Blood and/or secretions can easily block the endotracheal tube. The intubated patient should be suctioned whenever there are secretions visible or audible in the tube; at least every 8–12 hours. The suction catheter should be new, or at least cleaned and sterilized between each use, especially if it is necessary to reuse the suction catheters on different patients. It is important to remember that smaller tubes are much more easily blocked than larger tubes, and small tubes may need to be suctioned more frequently.

Extubation Readiness

An extubation readiness test, or spontaneous breathing trial, may be used to assess a patient's readiness to be extubated. Patients are often placed on a spontaneous breathing mode on the ventilator, and the respiratory rate, oxygen saturation, and tidal volumes should be monitored while breathing on minimal settings. If a patient tolerates minimal settings while maintaining a normal respiratory rate, oxygen saturation, and tidal volume, he or she may be ready for extubation from a respiratory standpoint.

Extubation Criteria

In addition to passing some form of extubation readiness testing, a patient must also meet airway and neurological criteria for extubation (Table 9.12). He or she must have had reversal of whatever factors led the patient to be intubated or remain intubated in the first place. A patient must meet neurological criteria, including being awake, being able to follow commands, and being able to protect his or her airway. In patients with a concern about airway edema, one can assess for a leak around the endotracheal tube. If the patient has an appropriately sized endotracheal tube, a leak of less than 20 cm H_2O may indicate that there is not significant airway edema. To perform this test, one must deflate the endotracheal tube cuff, place a stethoscope on the patient's neck, and listen for a coarse rush of air coming back through the airway past the endotracheal tube. This can be done while the patient is on a ventilator, as long as the peak inspiratory pressure is higher than the pressure required to leak around the endotracheal tube, or with a manual ventilation bag that has a manometer attached. Assessing for a leak is most important in pediatric patients who are at significant risk for airway edema and postextubation stridor with respiratory distress when even a small amount of subglottic edema is present.

Complications of Mechanical Ventilation

Many complications can occur as a result of mechanical ventilation. Difficulty with ventilation can occur if secretions obstruct the endotracheal tube and/or blood and can lead to a respiratory arrest. An obstructed endotracheal tube is more common in neonates and children. Ventilator-induced lung injury or pneumothorax may occur, especially if high pressures are necessary for adequate gas exchange. Patients may develop skin breakdown or pressure ulcers from prolonged time in bed and immobility, which is especially significant if they are not repositioned frequently. Patients who are not well sedated are at risk for unplanned self-extubation. Following self-extubation, a patient may have laryngeal injury from an inflated

TABLE 9.11

Names and dosages of medications used for analgesia/sedation of mechanically ventilated patients[4]

Drug	Route of administration	Pediatric dose	Adult dose	Dosing interval
Morphine	IV bolus	0.05–0.1 mg/kg	2.5–5 mg	Q1–4 hr PRN
	IV gtt	0.05–0.1 mg/kg/hr	2.5–10 mg/hr	Continuous infusion
Fentanyl	IV bolus	0.5–2 mcg/kg	25–100 mcg	Q1–4 hr PRN
IV gtt		0.5–2 mcg/kg/hr	50–200 mcg/kg/hr	Continuous infusion
Hydromorphone	IV gtt		0.5–1 mg/hr	Continuous infusion
Ketamine	IV gtt	5–20 mcg/kg/min	2–7 mcg/kg/min	Continuous infusion
Midazolam	IV bolus	0.05–0.1 mg/kg	1–5 mg	Q1–4 hr PRN
	IV gtt	0.05–0.1 mg/kg/hr	0.04/0.2 mg/kg/hr	Continuous infusion
Lorazepam	IV bolus	0.05–0.1 mg/kg	0.02–0.06 mg/kg	Q4 hr PRN
	IV gtt		0.01–0.1 mg/kg/hr	Continuous infusion
Diazepam	IV bolus	0.04–0.3 mg/kg	0.03–0.1 mg/kg	Q2–6 hr PRN
Propofol**	IV gtt	25–150 mcg/kg/min	0.3–3 mg/kg/hr	Continuous infusion

IV = intravenous, gtt = drip/continuous infusion, PRN = as needed

* These are suggested starting doses but will need to be adjusted based on clinical response. Elderly, critically ill, and neonatal patients will often have increased sensitivity to these medications and may require smaller doses and/or dosing at the lower end of dosing spectrum. Caution use in patients with hepatic or renal failure.

** Pediatric patients are at increased risk for propofol infusion syndrome; therefore, limit duration of infusion to </= 12 hours. Caution use in patients with hypotension.

TABLE 9.12

Respiratory and neurological criteria for extubation

A patient may be eligible for extubation when he or she:
- is awake
- is able to follow commands
- is able to protect his or her airway
- can sustain a head lift for >5 seconds
- has a leak around the endotracheal tube
- is spontaneously breathing
- is on minimal ventilator settings
- is not tachypneic and has good tidal volumes
- has no or minimal airway swelling
- has normal oxygen saturation

endotracheal tube cuff, may aspirate, or may require re-intubation. Finally, patients who are intubated, especially when intubated for longer periods of time, are at risk for ventilator-associated pneumonia (VAP). Interventions that are believed to reduce the risk of VAP include raising the head of bed by 30 degrees, keeping the patient's mouth and lips moist, oral care at least every 12 hours, and using sterile suction catheters with each suctioning.

Criteria for Transfer to Wards

A patient may be considered suitable for transfer to the hospital ward when he/she is awake, extubated and breathing comfortably, following commands, not requiring aggressive ongoing resuscitation, and has adequate pain control and stable vital signs (oxygen saturation, heart rate, and blood pressure are appropriate for age). The same concerns apply for transfer from the ICU to the ward as from the PACU.

Hand-Off from ICU/HDU to Ward Team

A detailed hand-off from the ICU/HDU team to the wards is essential to allow for the continuation of safe surgical care, and must include patient's identity, medical history, allergies, details of surgical course (surgery performed and surgical complications), details of the ICU/HDU course (airway and respiratory management, hemodynamic stability, and fluid resuscitation), and any anticipated ongoing postoperative problems. Direct hand-off between both nursing staff and physicians is essential.

COMMENTARY

Francoise Nizeyimana, Rwanda
Denise M. Chan, USA

Proper postoperative care, whether in the PACU or ICU, is essential to good surgical outcomes. In Rwanda, most hospitals lack the facilities and personnel to adequately monitor and care for postoperative patients. Patients who undergo minor surgical procedures and have no complications understandably have the best outcomes. Critically ill patients, however, have poor outcomes overall for a multitude of reasons. For example, in one of the main referral hospitals in Rwanda's capital city of Kigali, an ICU bed is rarely available for patients who are known to need postoperative intensive care, and is available even less often for patients whose ICU admission is not planned in advance. If a bed does happen to be available, the patient will be transferred to the ICU directly from the operating room. If a bed is not available, the surgery is postponed if possible; if surgery cannot be postponed, the patient is taken to the PACU after surgery. In the PACU, monitoring may or may not be available, and the nursing staff may or may not have the knowledge base to care for the patient. If the patient needs mechanical ventilation, there must be an available anesthesia machine to borrow from the operating room; without a ventilator, the patient remains intubated and breathing spontaneously on a T-piece. Whether or not a patient is managed by a physician depends upon the availability and other clinical responsibilities of the staff, as it is often a single anesthesiologist who is covering the PACU, operating rooms, and sometimes even the ICU. These factors contribute to the high morbidity and mortality rates in the PACU.

If a patient presents to a district hospital and needs intensive care, he or she is often transferred to one of the main referral hospitals. Transportation can be difficult to arrange, and the time to reach the next hospital may be long. As mentioned above, the referral hospital will most likely have no beds available in the ICU, and the patient will be held in the emergency room or PACU. These areas of the hospital are understaffed, and the staff's skill level may be inadequate to care for critically ill patients. The availability of physicians, equipment, and medications is variable. In addition, multidisciplinary management of complex patients is rare, although this sort of coordination of patient care would surely improve both knowledge level of caretakers and patient outcomes.

10

Resuscitation and Approach to Crisis Situations

Ann T. Hau
Craig D. McClain

Introduction

Despite thoughtful preparation, highly developed technical skills, and meticulous vigilance, perioperative crisis situations can occur and often require aggressive resuscitation. Such efforts may involve urgent but controlled stabilization of a patient's hemodynamics or respiratory mechanics. However, more hyperacute situations may occur which require emergent intervention and necessitate gaining control of a potentially chaotic situation. Treatment of conditions such as early sepsis or early respiratory failure is covered extensively in other sources as well as in Chapter 9 of this book. This chapter provides an overview of the basic principles of cardiopulmonary resuscitation (CPR) and emergency cardiovascular care (ECC) for the trained rescuer, based on the most recent recommendations at the time of publishing. There are often updates and revisions to existing advanced cardiovascular life support (ACLS) and pediatric advanced life support (PALS) algorithms based on updated research. It is essential for the practitioner to be knowledgeable of the most up-to-date protocols and current in his or her basic life support (BLS), ACLS, and PALS certification in order to provide safe care in these environments.

The International Liaison Committee on Resuscitation (ILCOR) was founded in 1992 to provide a collaborative effort among various resuscitation organizations to design protocols and guidelines for CPR and ECC. ILCOR currently includes representatives from the American Heart Association, the European Resuscitation Council, the Heart and Stroke Foundation of Canada, the Australian and New Zealand Committee on Resuscitation, the Resuscitation Council of Southern Africa, the Inter-American Heart Foundation, and the Resuscitation Council of Asia. Since 2000, the Committee has evaluated resuscitation science in 5-year cycles. Following the International Consensus Conference in February 2010, the committee released the most recent worldwide guidelines for CPR and ECC.[1] These documents are referenced below.

Components of Resuscitation

Airway, breathing, circulation, drugs, and electrical therapy—summarized by the letters *ABCDE*—describe the major components of resuscitation from cardiopulmonary arrest. The 2010 ILCOR guidelines changed the BLS sequence of steps from *A-B-C* (airway, breathing, circulation) to *C-A-B* (circulation, airway, breathing) for adults and children, excluding newborns.[2] The change was made in an effort to emphasize early and effective chest compressions. Several studies have demonstrated that chest compressions, which are the critical element in resuscitating children and adults, were often delayed with the initial tasks of opening and clearing the airway and delivering breaths. Starting with chest compressions also ensures that rescuers unable or unwilling to provide ventilations will at least perform chest compressions. The BLS algorithm is shown in Figure 10.1.

The critical initial elements of BLS include immediate recognition of sudden cardiac arrest and activation of the emergency response system, early performance of effective CPR, and rapid defibrillation, if necessary. ACLS builds upon BLS skills to treat adult cardiac arrest.[3] The basic approach to ACLS is seen in Figure 10.2. The right side of Figure 10.2 also summarizes factors that contribute to good-quality CPR, emergency drug dosing, and recommended starting energy for both monophasic and biphasic defibrillators.

Recognition and Initiation of Compressions

After recognition of an arrest, efforts to respond and stabilize the patient should begin immediately. Call for help early. A pulse check should take no more than 10 seconds. Chest compressions should be initiated immediately. Effective chest compressions are essential for generating blood flow and oxygen delivery to the brain and myocardium. Compressions should be delivered at a rate of at least 100 compressions per minute, with a compression depth of at least 2 inches/5 cm. The person performing the compressions should allow complete recoil of the chest after each compression. Care should be taken to minimize interruptions in compressions throughout the resuscitation. Correctly delivered chest compressions require much energy and effort; thus it is helpful to switch the person providing chest compressions every 2–3 minutes in order to keep people physically fresh while maintaining effective compressions.

Airway Management and Ventilation

Once compressions are initiated, efficient and rapid management of the airway should be performed. Attempts to open the

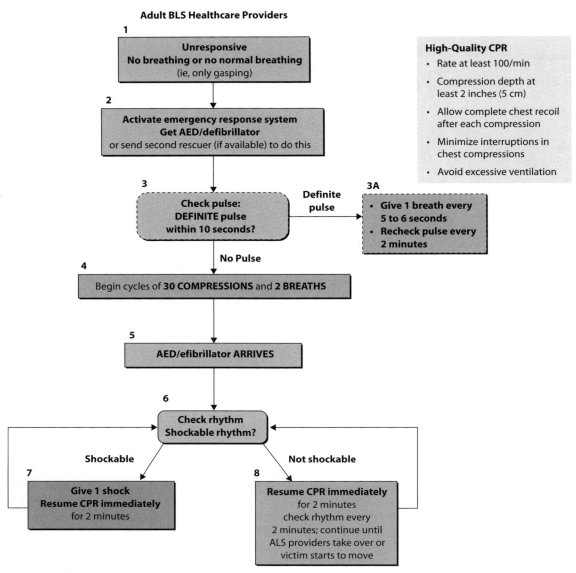

FIGURE 10.1 Adult BLS algorithm. 2010 American Heart Association Guidelines for Cardiopulmonary Resuscitation and Emergency Cardiovascular Care Science. Part 5: Adult Basic Life Support. *American Heart Association.* 2010; **122**(3): S685–S705.

airway, set up airway equipment, and ventilate should not delay the initiation of chest compressions and should interrupt compressions as little as possible. The "head tilt–chin lift" maneuver relieves obstruction by the tongue and should be used to open the airway in victims without evidence of head or neck trauma. The "jaw thrust" maneuver, in which pressure is applied behind the rami of the mandible, is also effective. Ventilation should be provided to the patient in the form of rescue breaths delivered mouth-to-mouth or by bag-mask. Breaths should be delivered over 1 second and should produce visible chest rise. A compression-ventilation ratio of 30:2 is recommended. With an advanced airway in place, compressions should continue at a rate of at least 100 per minute without pauses for ventilation. One breath should be given every 6–8 seconds (approximately 8–10 breaths per minute) via the advanced airway. Ideally, effective ventilation

should be confirmed by capnography. However, it should be noted that without effective pulmonary blood flow, there will be no expired CO_2, despite correct placement of a laryngeal mask airway (LMA) or endotracheal tube (ETT).

Early Defibrillation

High-quality CPR and defibrillation of ventricular fibrillation (VF)/pulseless ventricular tachycardia (VT) are the therapies that have been proven to increase survival to discharge from the hospital. When bystander CPR is provided and defibrillation occurs within 3–5 minutes of collapse, victims with VF have the highest survival rates. In an ideal situation, the first provider in a cardiac arrest should start CPR with chest compressions and

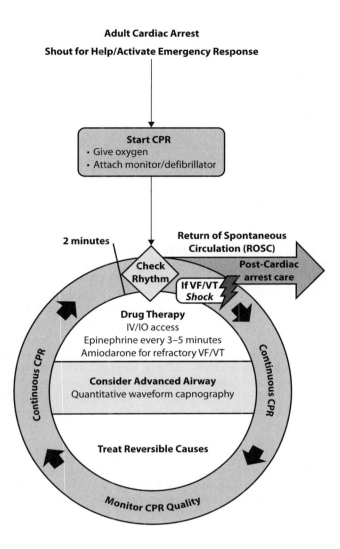

CPR Quality

- Push hard (≥2 inches [5 cm]) and fast (≥100/min) and allow complete chest recoil
- Minimize interruptions in compressions
- Avoid excessive ventilation
- Rotate compressor every 2 minutes
- If no advanced airway, 30:2 compression-ventilation ratio
- Quantitative waveform capnography
  - If P_{ETCO_2} <10 mm Hg, attempt to improve CPR quality
- Intra-arterial pressure
  - If relaxation phase (diastolic) pressure <20 mm Hg, attempt to improve CPR quality

Return of Spontaneous Circulation (ROSC)

- Pulse and blood pressure
- Abrupt sustained increase in P_{ETCO_2} (typically ≥40 mm Hg)
- Spontaneous arterial pressure waves with intra-arterial monitoring

Shock Enery

- **Biphasic:** Manufacturer recommendation (120–200 J); if unknown, use maximum available. Second and subsequent doses should be equivalent, and higher doses may be considered.
- **Monophasic:** 360 J

Drug Therapy

- **Epinephrine IV/IO Dose:** 1 mg every 3–5 minutes
- **Vasopressin IV/IO Dose:** 40 units can replace first or second dose of epinephrine
- **Amiodarone IV/IO Dose:** First dose: 300 mg bolus. Second dose: 150 mg.

Advanced Airway

- Supraglottic advanced airway or endotracheal intubation
- Waveform capnography to confirm and monitor ET tube placement
- 8-10 breaths per minute with continuous chest compressions

Reversible Causes

– Hypovolemia	– Tension pneumothorax
– Hypoxia	– Tamponade, cardiac
– Hydrogen ion (acidosis)	– Toxins
– Hypo-/hyperkalemia	– Thrombosis, pulmonary
– Hypothermia	– Thrombosis, coronary

FIGURE 10.2 The figure above graphically displays the ACLS approach to cardiac arrest. The 5 Hs and Ts are included on the right. 2010 American Heart Association Guidelines for Cardiopulmonary Resuscitation and Emergency Cardiovascular Care Science. Part 8: Adult Advanced Cardiovascular Life Support. *American Heart Association.* 2010; **122**(3): S729–S767.

the second provider should get the automated external defibrillator (AED), attach the pads or paddles, and check the patient's rhythm. Chest compressions should be resumed immediately after delivery of each shock instead of waiting for a pulse check.

After attempts to restore adequate circulation and oxygenation have been initiated, it is prudent to consider addressing the common treatable causes of the arrest. These causes include the Hs and Ts and are summarized in Figure 10.2.

VF/Pulseless VT

A rhythm check on the AED that demonstrates VF/VT requires a delivery of a shock. Biphasic defibrillators utilize a dose of 120–200 J (depending on the manufacturer's recommended energy dose) for terminating VF. Subsequent energy levels should be at least equivalent or higher, if needed. Monophasic defibrillators should be set to deliver 360 J for initial and subsequent shocks. After the patient is cleared, a shock should be delivered. Rescue providers should resume CPR as quickly as possible, continuing for a full 2 minutes before a second rhythm check is performed.

Team Organization

Modern crisis management concepts in the operating room (OR) rely on a team approach.[4] There should be a team leader who will direct the resuscitation. This leader should not be responsible for anything other than directing the team so he or she can focus on leading the resuscitation rather than other tasks such as airway management or adequate chest compressions. The team leader must maintain the "30,000-foot view." In other words, the leader must keep the big picture in focus rather than fixate on the individual components of the entire process, such as drug administration or airway management. This allows the other team members to completely direct their attention to their given task rather than having to simultaneously consider other tasks that are being performed by other individuals. Frequently summarizing the situation is helpful to keep the entire team engaged and up to date. Good horizontal communication is a hallmark of effective teams. This involves closed-loop communication (e.g., Dr. Jones says, "Dr. Smith, please give 1 mg of epinephrine now." Dr. Smith replies, "Dr. Jones, I'm giving 1 mg of epinephrine." Dr. Jones closes the loop, "OK. 1 mg of epinephrine is in."). Finally, a strong team dynamic creates an environment where members feel comfortable raising their concerns without leading to a confrontational situation. An example would be a team leader directing an unsynchronized cardioversion of a supraventricular tachycardia. Team members should be willing and able to speak up and remind the leader that the cardioversion should be synchronized. In the perioperative setting, the anesthesiologist is often the team leader, but any member of the perioperative care team should be prepared to assume the leader role if necessary. It may be quite useful to quickly go through a few crisis scenarios early in the trip to identify and address any major problems. This is also an effective method of team-building.

Pediatric/Neonatal Resuscitation

The basic principles behind adult resuscitation also apply to PALS.[5] The rate of compressions is the same as for adults, at least 100/minute. Adequate depth of compression in children is 1/3 to 1/2 the depth of the chest. As mentioned in Chapter 4, if the team is planning on caring for children, there should be an anesthesiologist who is experienced with this patient population. Any pediatric anesthesiologist will be familiar with the PALS approaches and algorithms. In the event of a pediatric patient suffering an arrest, a practitioner familiar with PALS should lead the team. In children, it should be noted that most cardiac arrests are secondary to respiratory failure or shock. Thus, unrecognized loss of airway in a child ultimately results in the predictable and (usually) avoidable consequence of cardiac arrest. One of the maxims taught by many anesthesiologists is that one does not need to be able to intubate to save a life. What is necessary is the ability to effectively bag-mask ventilate a patient. This is a skill that should be second nature to anyone providing general anesthesia, regional anesthesia, spinal anesthesia, and/or any level of sedation. If one cannot provide some degree of airway assistance, one should not be administering any drugs that may (in one way or another) result in loss of airway.

A systematic approach to caring for the acutely ill child is the guiding principle behind PALS.[6] PALS teaches a team-based, standard approach to children in distress. While some of the algorithms in the course are specifically designed for arrest situations, the overall approach can and should be applied to any acutely ill or injured child. The approach taught in PALS consists of an initial assessment that should take only a few seconds. This initial assessment should be quite rapid and include evaluation of the child's overall appearance, overall work of breathing, and quality of circulation. Following this, a true primary assessment should be conducted that involves the traditional, hands-on evaluation of airway, breathing, circulation, disability, and ensuring adequate exposure (ABCDE). Vital signs should also be obtained at this juncture. This assessment allows the caregiver to get a clearer idea of cardiopulmonary

and neurologic status. Further assessments involve obtaining more detailed medical history and laboratory evaluation that may be beneficial to aiding the child. Finally, the caregiver must include reassessment as part of the overall approach. Thus, the caregiver engages in a process of assessment, organization of problems, treatment of problems, and reassessment of the situation.

In a child, signs of increased work of breathing can include nasal flaring, retractions on inspiration, poor respiratory effort, tachypnea, or abnormal sounds (stridor, wheezing, or grunting). Evidence of poor or inadequate circulation include mottled skin, pallor, poor capillary refill (>2–3 seconds), or nonpalpable pulses (radial, brachial, femoral, and carotid). Cyanosis is easiest to appreciate in the lips or tongue in children (appearance of a bluish or purple color), although it may be more difficult to distinguish from normal skin color in darker-skinned individuals. Although certainly not a hard-and-fast rule, circulatory status leading to tachycardia is poor for adults, while bradycardia is generally bad for younger children. Small children have immature myocardium and cannot augment cardiac output through climbing the Starling curve and increasing stroke volume. Thus, cardiac output becomes directly proportional to heart rate.

In 2008, it was estimated that there were approximately 840,000 neonatal deaths due to birth asphyxia.[7] Several studies have demonstrated a decrease in perinatal mortality in the developing world when a package of neonatal care, including neonatal life support, was initiated. Other parts of the package of care introduced include thermal protection, early nutrition, and infection control. Anesthesia providers may be called upon to aid in resuscitating neonates on trips to developing world nations. Knowledge of basic neonatal life-support techniques and protocols is useful in such an event.[8] A simple algorithm for such events is illustrated in Figure 10.3. An effective location for palpation of a neonate's pulse is the base of the umbilical cord.

Challenges in LMICs

In order to follow the algorithms, certain basic equipment is necessary, including a defibrillator. In a low- or middle-income setting (LMIC) there may be no defibrillator or there may only be an older monophasic defibrillator that is unfamiliar to visiting practitioners. The presence of adequate resuscitation equipment should factor into the decisions to proceed with any cases that have a higher risk of arrest. One option is for the team to bring a portable AED. These devices are compact, portable, and can prove invaluable in the event of a VF/pulseless VT arrest. It is possible to purchase an AED for around $1,000. While this is not cheap, it is still a relatively small financial investment in the context of the total cost of trip. Further, these devices are reusable with replaceable pads, so there can be quite a bit of marginal benefit after the initial outlay.

Other equipment and physical resource limitations can become painfully apparent when a team faces an unstable or arresting patient. As stated earlier in this section, there may or may not be an oxygen source available. There may also be no intensive care unit (ICU), so it may be necessary to turn the OR into a make-shift ICU until the patient is more stable. This can have obvious consequences on the goals of the trip as far as limiting other procedures that could be accomplished and use of limited drug and

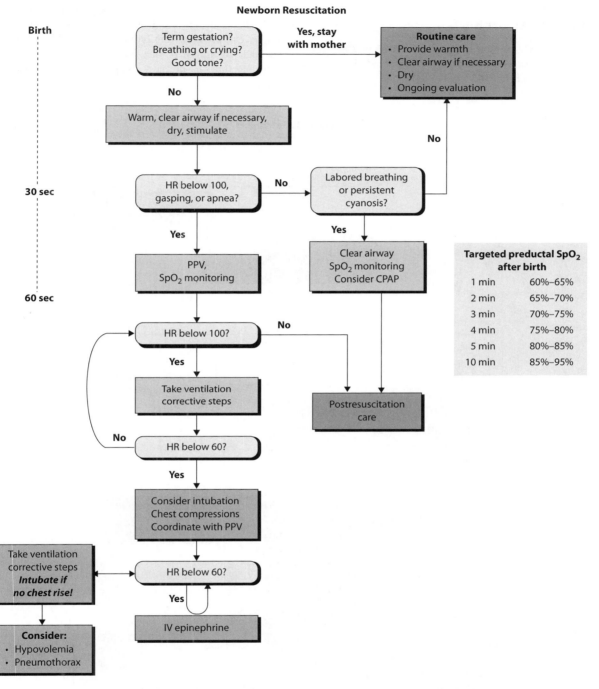

FIGURE 10.3 Basic approach to neonatal life support. American Academy of Pediatrics, American Heart Association. *Neonatal Resuscitation Textbook,* 6th edn. American Academy of Pediatrics, 2011.

equipment resources. Many of these concerns can be identified and dealt with by running through some crisis scenarios, with the entire team participating, prior to actual patient care.

In addition to the resources discussed above, human resources may be limited in number and in capacity. In particular, personnel familiar with and comfortable with resuscitation protocols may be profoundly limited. In many LMICs, there is little concept of an OR team. Rather, each service may appear to function independently, and communication may be poor or nearly

nonexistent. Surgeons, nurses, and anesthesia providers often function in their own silos and have little communication, if any, with other members of the care team outside of their specialty. Unfortunately, it is relatively common for no single anesthesia provider to be in charge of the case. Instead, there may be a rotating cast of providers who come and go without any real sign-out or transfer of care. These practice patterns create an environment where crisis situations are more likely and are more difficult to effectively deal with when they occur.

The Universal Algorithm

The European Resuscitation Council has developed the Universal Cardiac Arrest Algorithm, which is intended for resuscitation of infant, child, and adult victims of cardiac arrest, excluding newborns. CPR should begin immediately for victims with absent or abnormal breathing. Rescuers should utilize a single compression-ventilation ratio of 30:2. Efforts should be made to minimize interruptions in compressions; unnecessary interruptions in chest compressions decrease effectiveness (Figure 10.4).

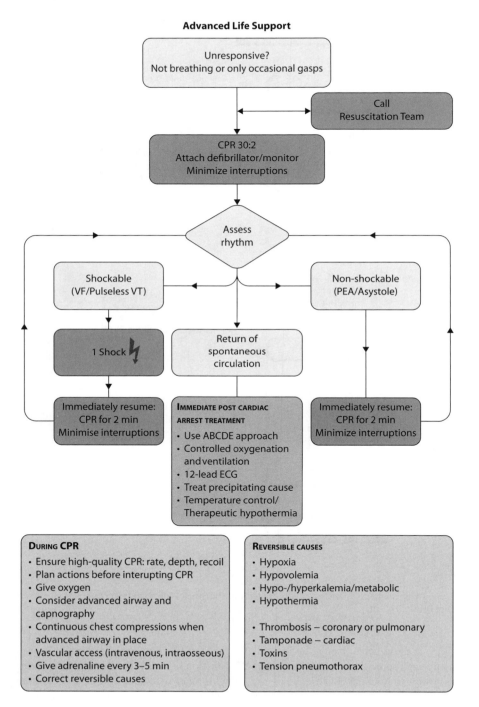

FIGURE 10.4 The Universal Life Support algorithm. Nolan JP, Soar J, Zideman DA, et al. European Resuscitation Council Guidelines for Resuscitation 2010. *Resuscitation.* 2010; **81**: 1219–1276.

COMMENTARY

Edouard Uwamahoro, Rwanda
Denise M. Chan, USA

Crisis situations arise on a frequent basis in our hospitals in Rwanda. As anesthesiologists, we are often involved in the crisis response and, if needed, the resuscitation of patients. We have come to recognize the significance of, but current deficit of, skilled medical personnel, adequate medications, and equipment required for this response.

Communication skills, task assignment, and teamwork are crucial to a crisis response. However, as mentioned in the chapter, these fundamentals are not routinely taught or emphasized in many LMICs, including Rwanda. We are attempting to build this skill set among our physicians (including anesthesiologists and surgeons), nurses, and anesthesia technicians to improve the management of crises and hopefully improve patient outcomes. For example, by implementing the World Health Organization (WHO) Surgical Safety Checklist in our operating rooms, we have strengthened communication and encouraged active participation among members of the operative team. Our simulation center has been essential to building both technical and nontechnical skills. This is where we teach and practice BLS and ACLS. We have airway and chest compression mannequins on which to practice technical skills, but more importantly, we conduct simulated crisis scenarios to practice closed-loop communication, task assignment, and leadership.

Since we are still learning and becoming accustomed to these concepts and techniques, our codes can be quite chaotic and disorganized. Often, there is no one comfortable with taking charge of the crisis, so communication falls to the wayside; and there may or may not be someone available to manage the airway, perform proper chest compressions, or operate the defibrillator (if one is available). In addition, medications and equipment needed for resuscitation may or may not be available immediately. In some of our hospitals in Rwanda, we have created resuscitation carts with many of these essential materials. Manual defibrillators and automated external defibrillators are few, but we hope to increase their availability around our hospitals soon.

Capacity for postresuscitation care is also a scarce resource in our setting. Many more critically ill patients exist than there are beds and personnel to care for them. Our recovery rooms often serve as overflow ICUs, but nursing staff are stretched thinly and proper monitoring is rarely available.

The survival rate after cardiac arrest is very low in LMICs such as ours, for a myriad of reasons, including the resource and skill limitations mentioned above. In addition, patients often present to the hospital late, and the time between cardiopulmonary arrest and initiation of resuscitation is great. While we can hope for acquisition of more equipment, medications, and other material resources to improve resuscitation of patients, what we have the power to do now is to continue improving our knowledge base, and training more of our healthcare providers in BLS, communications, and other skills essential to crisis management.

Section III

Non-Trauma

11

Chest

Abraham Lebenthal
Alexi C. Matousek

Introduction

Infectious diseases are the most frequent cause of thoracic disease in the world. The most common of these infectious diseases is tuberculosis caused by the bacterium *Mycobacterium tuberculosis*. After infectious diseases, trauma and lung carcinoma cause the most morbidity and mortality. Major thoracic diseases are accompanied by a high mortality due to the following reasons: development of drug resistance in infectious etiologies, lack of surveillance and appropriate administration of drug regimens, and lack of access to medical facilities with sufficient anesthesia and surgical capabilities to perform curative procedures. Major general thoracic surgical procedures are associated with a higher morbidity and mortality than the vast majority of nonthoracic surgical procedures, and therefore require an advanced minimum surgical capacity to perform safely.

This chapter presents some urgent and emergent procedures that can be undertaken by providers with a basic level of general surgery training and associated competencies. Appropriate caution will be indicated for procedures that may be ill-advised to perform in low- and middle-income countries (LMICs). To this end, important factors that are thought to seriously affect morbidity and mortality in thoracic patients will be highlighted. Procedures that can be performed in LMICs with a reasonable expectation of a good outcome will be emphasized.

There are a number of simple thoracic surgical procedures that if performed expediently convert life-threatening injury (i.e., tension pneumothorax) into stable non–life-threatening conditions. Pattern recognition and aggressive early treatment are crucial. Successful general thoracic procedures require a team with expertise in the perioperative management of such patients. This includes but is not limited to the following: a surgeon with general thoracic experience, anesthesia familiar with one-lung ventilation and epidural anesthesia for pain control, blood bank capability, chest imaging, continuous pulse oximetry, oxygen supplementation, and intensive care; as well as intermediate care units, dedicated nursing, physical therapy, and respiratory therapy. The fundamentals of attaining good patient outcomes depend on accuracy of diagnosis, adequate lung function, fluid restriction in the immediate postoperative period, excellent pain control, and early ambulation. Major thoracic surgery such as lobectomy, pneumonectomy, and esophagectomy should only be considered with the utmost caution and care to ensure that adequate resources are in place to allow an acceptable chance of a good outcome.

Preoperative lung function can be determined by spirometry, which can then be used to calculate the predicted post operative lung function. *Volume restriction is critical in preventing right heart failure for which there is no effective treatment.* Pain control in the perioperative period is critical in preventing atelectasis and pneumonia, which are major causes of postoperative morbidity and mortality. In the United States, in experienced hands and healthcare systems, the estimated mortality from lobectomy, pneumonectomy, and esophagectomy ranges between 1%–5%, 4%–20%, and 2%–20%, respectively.

Thus, in the setting of inexperienced surgeons, poor support systems, and limited resources, these procedures should only be done when no other therapeutic option is available. It is beyond the scope of this chapter to comprehensively describe the systems approach and steps of all thoracic surgical procedures that may be found in a standard textbook of thoracic surgery; however, we will provide simple, low-cost descriptions for how to optimize surgical success and minimize postoperative complications.

Epidemiology: Global Burden of Thoracic Surgical Disease

It is hard to estimate the global burden of thoracic surgical disease, because little has been written on this topic. Infectious etiologies affecting the lungs are common in the developing world. These include the following: complications of pneumonia (empyema and fibrothorax), tuberculosis, and parasitic infections such as amebiasis, malaria, trypanosomiasis, ascariasis, strongyloidiasis, dirofilariasis, cystic echinococcosis, and schistosomiasis. Trauma to the chest is a major cause of morbidity and mortality. When massive, it can lead to instantaneous or rapid death. Respiratory complications are significant causes of late postinjury morbidity and mortality; these can be proactively prevented with aggressive pain control and proper antibiotic coverage. Lung cancer is the leading cause of cancer death in HICs, where it accounts for more deaths than the sum of cancer deaths from breast cancer, colon cancer, and prostate cancer combined. In LMICs, increasing tobacco use is a serious problem. As life expectancy increases in LMICs, we expect to see a sharp rise in lung cancer. The incidence of esophageal cancer in LMICs is variable with a 60-fold difference between endemic regions and regions of low incidence. There is a clear male predominance. Squamous cell carcinoma is more prevalent as it is associated with tobacco, alcohol, hot tea gulping, nitrosamine, fungal mycotoxins, and human papillomavirus (HPV). There are endemic regions in Xinjiang province of China, Iran, and Transkei in South Africa. In the Western world, adenocarcinoma of the distal esophagus and the gastroesophageal junction is the most rapidly increasing solid organ tumor. It has had a six-fold increase in incidence over the last two decades. It is associated with gastroesophageal reflux disease and obesity.

Anatomy and Physiology

The thoracic cavity extends from the thoracic inlet to the diaphragm. The cavity is made up of 12 ribs anchored to thoracic vertebra posteriorly and the sternum and costochondral angle anteriorly. This mobile bony cage protects the vital structures that it houses: heart, lungs, esophagus, and great vessels. The first seven ribs are attached to the sternum directly. The first rib is flat and strong and thus requires great force to fracture. The 11th and 12th ribs are floating ribs. Rib fractures in adults are associated with additional intrathoracic injuries, such as lung contusion, even when the pleural covering is intact. The ribs of small children are more elastic than those of adults and thus moderate and sometimes severe injuries occur without fracture. Age plays an important role in the pattern recognition of associated injuries. The intercostal spaces are numbered according to the rib above it. For example, the fourth intercostal space would be the space between the fourth and fifth ribs. All ribs have a vein, artery, and nerve in the intercostal groove located on the inner, inferior rib surface. When entering the chest, injury to the neurovascular bundle of the rib is avoided by cutting along the top of the lower rib in the intercostal space. During inspiration, the diaphragm contracts and moves downward. As the rib cage expands, the sternum is pushed anteriorly, and lung volumes increase. During expiration, the diaphragm relaxes as it moves up the rib cage, and the lung volumes decrease. The lungs work under negative pressure. A healthy adult breathes approximately 12 times a minute, which is 17,280 times a day. The number of breaths a minute typically increases with injury. The disturbance of respiratory mechanics by trauma, iatrogenic or otherwise, is a major source of thoracic morbidity and mortality. It will be fully addressed in the sections on rib fractures and postoperative pain management.

The trachea enters the thoracic inlet anterior to the esophagus. It is 12 cm in length, and the carina lies directly behind the angle of Louis. The proximal third can be easily accessed from the neck, the distal third is best accessed from the right chest, while the middle third is difficult to access and can best be accessed with sternotomy. The left mainstem bronchus is 4 cm long and has an acute angle from the carina; it lies between the aortic arch and pulmonary artery. The left lung is made up of an upper lobe with its lingula and a lower lobe.

The right lung is made up of three lobes: an upper lobe with three segments, a middle lobe with two segments, and a lower lobe with five segments. The right lung accounts for 60% of lung volume and function, while the left lung accounts for the remaining 40%.

Imaging

In LMICs, the only available imaging may include ultrasound, chest X-ray, fluoroscopy, and rarely a chest computed tomography. The chest X-ray has been in use since 1895 to diagnose diseases of the chest. It is useful in assessing the lungs, heart, chest wall, diaphragm, major vessels, spinal column, and soft tissue. The lungs can be assessed for nodules or masses, cavitary lesions, and pleural and pericardial effusions. Additionally, it enables assessment of the great vessels, mediastinal structures, and chest wall. Typically, two types of exams exist:

- The PA and lateral exam consisting of two x-rays: the PA (posteroanterior), where the patient faces the X-ray film, and the lateral, with the patient turned sideways. Two views enable more precise recognition and localization of abnormalities. When only a PA view is available, consideration of anatomic landmarks, such as fissures and selective obscuration of anatomic structures, may be adequate for localizing pathology.
- The AP (anterior-posterior) exam is a single image taken with the X-ray film behind or under the patient's back. This exam is typically taken with a portable X-ray machine for a patient that cannot be safely ambulated to radiology.

Ultrasound has traditionally been of limited use in the chest because ultrasound is impaired by aerated lung. The amplification of ultrasound passing through fluid can provide superior visualization of pleural effusions as well as physiologic information regarding diaphragmatic and cardiac function. The most accurate diagnoses in the focused assessment with sonography for trauma (FAST) are pericardial and pleural effusions. Fluoroscopy can be used to assess the esophagus, great vessels, and the diaphragm. Chest CT, if available, can be used to gain a more comprehensive staging of suspected malignancy, infectious process, or other pathology.

Pulmonary Function Tests

Spirometry is a simple and highly predictive test for elective thoracic surgical procedures. The forced expiratory volume in one second (FEV1) is the most important predictive parameter that can be measured. In general, the right lung accounts for 60% of respiratory function and is divided into three lobes. The upper lobe accounts for 20% of overall lung function, the middle lobe 10%, and the lower lobe 30%. The left lung is divided into two lobes: the upper lobe, which includes the lingula, and the lower lobe. Each accounts for 20% of total lung function. The predicted postoperative FEV1 (ppoFEV1) can be calculated by taking the calculated FEV1 and multiplying it by the percentage of lung that will remain after a thoracic surgical procedure. In high-income countries (HICs), patients with a ppoFEV1 of 80%–60% are at mild risk, 40%–60% moderate risk, and 25%–40% at high risk. Patients with a ppoFEV1 of less than 800 cc should not undergo surgery and may be oxygen dependent for life.

In an LMIC, a ppoFEV1 of less than 50% should be avoided. It is important to note that in the initial postoperative period, a patient's lung function will most likely decrease below the ppoFEV1 due to postoperative pain and altered mechanics of respiration. Typically, patients reach their ppoFEV1 at approximately 3–6 months after surgery.

If spirometry is not available, a simple 6-minute walk test (preferably with pulse oximetry) can be performed. The patient should be able to walk at least 500 meters without becoming short of breath or suffering desaturation to less than 90%. Alternatively, the patient can be made to climb three standard flights of stairs. If able to do so without dyspnea or desaturation, this is predictive of good overall heart and lung capacity. These patients should be able to tolerate significant thoracic procedures, such as lobectomy or even pneumonectomy.

Management of Infectious Diseases of the Thorax

Thoracic surgery for infectious disease was by far the most common indication for chest surgery in Europe and North America in the early to mid-20th century. Today, this is likely the major indication for thoracic interventions in LMICs. Hippocrates described the presentation, physical examination findings, and treatment of empyema in 229 BC. He recommended a partial rib resection and daily packing as therapy. In 1843, Trosseau described thoracocentesis as therapy for empyema. Sedillot, a French surgeon, described thoracotomy and drainage. In 1879, Estlander described thoracoplasty, and in 1893 Fowler described decortication. In the early 20th century, mortality of empyema without drainage approached 70%. With early rib resection and open drainage, mortality was reduced to 30%. In 1918, Graham and Bell published their findings as part of the US Army empyema commission, where mortality from acute empyema was reduced to 4.3% by early closed tube drainage. Eloesser (1935) described a "flap" or valve that enabled drainage of empyema and gradual expansion of the lungs. In 1963, Clagett proposed a "window" obtained by resecting a portion of two to three ribs, that enabled daily packing over 6–8 weeks, in order to clean a chronic empyema space, facilitating eventual closure.

Today, acute respiratory infections remain an important cause of morbidity and mortality. Streptococcus pneumonia, respiratory syncytial virus, parainfluenza virus, and influenza virus are all etiologies of these infections. Appropriate prevention strategies include vaccinations and quarantine precautions, as needed. Treatment strategies include adequate nutrition, sanitation, hand hygiene, hydration, and supportive measures for symptom relief. Surgical management is indicated only when bacterial pneumonia leads to parapneumonic effusion or abscess formation in the lung.

The general surgical principle on treatment of an abscess is the same in the chest as it is elsewhere in the body. For resolution, an abscess must be completely drained, and the inciting site must be resected or repaired. The space must be clean, and healthy tissue must expand to fill the space. When the lung is compliant, it will completely fill the pleural space. If lung expansion is limited by a thick pleural rind, it must be decorticated. When the lung has been resected, a space may exist. A hemithoracic space can be obliterated by an apical pleural tent, mobilization of a tissue flap (e.g., latisimus, serratus, pectoral, or omental), thoracoplasty, temporary paresis of phrenic nerve, or pneumoperitonium (insufflation of the abdomen with air).

Tuberculosis

Tuberculosis is a treatable disease that kills approximately 2 million people per year. TB is the leading cause of death among HIV infected individuals. Drug-resistant TB causes nearly 500,000 deaths per year.[1] The emergence of multi–drug-resistant TB (MDR-TB) and extensively drug-resistant TB (XDR-TB) may lead to a resurgence of thoracic surgery for tuberculosis in the years to come.

Pleural Effusion

Pleural effusions are classified as transudates and exudates. Transudates are effusions that are secondary to increased hydrostatic pressure or decreased colloid osmotic pressure. Thus they are clear and have a low specific gravity, low protein, and elevated LDH. In contrast, exudates are the result of inflammation. They tend to be cloudy in appearance and have a high specific gravity, high protein content, and elevated LDH. Light developed criteria to help guide management between the exudative and transudate stages.[2] In HICs, transudative pleural effusions are due to heart failure, liver or kidney disease, and rarely pulmonary embolism or malnutrition. Exudative effusions are most often secondary to infection; however, the differential diagnosis includes: cancer, esophageal perforation, and rheumatoid pleuritis. Transudates can be drained for diagnosis or therapy with thoracocentesis or tube thoracostomy.

Presentation: Dyspnea, chest pain, fatigue

Diagnosis: Physical exam dullness on percussion, chest X-ray (CXR) blunting of costophrenic angle, ultrasound (US): effusion above diaphragm, can mark posterior chest for drainage

Procedure: Thoracocentesis. This is a quick, safe, and least technically demanding procedure for drainage of transudate.

Equipment needed: A 14- or 16-French intravenous (IV) cannula, an alcohol swab, drapes, IV tubing, a 500–1000 cc bottle on negative suction.

Positioning: Sitting straight up

Procedure: Prep the back in the midscapular line of the affected side with an alcohol swab. Percussion for dullness or use a prior ultrasound marked point just above the superior aspect of a rib. Insert a 14- or 16-French IV cannula, remove the needle, attach IV tubing to the cannula, and place a needle on the proximal side of the IV tubing. Insert this into a negative pressure bottle. As the lung reexpands, the patient will feel chest pain and may cough. Fluid removed should be sent for Gram stain, culture, acid-fast bacilli (AFB), glucose, pH, lactate dehydrogenase (LDH), and protein. The fluid can be spun. Cytologic examination of precipitate can rule out cancer.

Caution: The maximum fluid removed at one time should not exceed 1500 cc to minimize the risk of reexpansion pulmonary edema. This is especially important in settings without the ability to use positive pressure to assist respiration.

If bottles with negative pressure are not available, the following can be done:

1. A closed system can be made (see prior explanation) and run on wall suction.
2. Drain IV tubing down to gravity bag.
3. Use a T connector and a large syringe to manually remove fluid.

Empyema

Empyema can be caused by: bacterial pneumonia, tuberculosis, prior lung resection, trauma, or intra-abdominal processes. In the western world, over 50% of empyemas are associated with pneumonia. *Streptococcus hemolyticus* (also known as pneumococcus) is the most frequent pathogen isolated. In LMICs, tuberculosis is the leading cause of empyema. Typically, virulent, untreated or partially treated pneumonias can lead to parapneumonic effusions, which can evolve into an empyema. Typically, this is associated with three stages: an exudative phase (acute), a fibro-purulent stage consisting of bacteria and fibrin deposit, and a chronic or organized phase in which a thickened rind is formed from fibroblast ingrowth and collagen deposit.

Presentation: Chest pain, pleurisy, dyspnea, fever, malaise, weight loss

Diagnosis: Tachycardia, tachypnea, decreased ventilation, dullness on percussion

Imaging: CXR: lung volume loss, pleural thickening, blunting of costophrenic angle

Therapy: Thoracocentesis for diagnosis (Gram stain and culture), evacuation of fluid. Antibiotics are chosen with information from thoracocentesis. The optimal surgical approach (see Box 11.1) depends on the stage of empyema:

1. Exudative phase (acute): thoracostomy tube placement
2. Fibro-purulent stage: minithoracotomy and washout, thoracostomy tube drainage
3. Chronic or organized phase: thoracotomy and decortication

BOX 11.1 SURGICAL TIPS

- Surgery is "easier" and less bloody with one-lung ventilation.
- Use the rib space widest between anterior and posterior axillary line.
- If videoscopic equipment is available, attempt careful decortication with 30-degree scope and ring forceps. Will require two to three ports.
- Send pus for Gram stain and culture. Send rind for pathology and tissue culture.
- Can use hydrogen peroxide to help lyse adhesions.
- Irrigate with Betadine and/or antibiotic solution prior to closing.
- At the completion of the procedure, the lung must fully reexpand, filling the hemithoracic space.
- When operating for empyema, at the completion of surgery, leave three thoracostomy tubes for drainage: straight apical anterior, straight apical posterior, and an inferior right angle tube along the costophrenic angle.
- Anchor chest tubes with a #2 silk suture.
- If decortication results in significant raw surface and blood loss, keep patient intubated with positive end expiratory pressure (PEEP) on ventilator overnight (if available).
- A large multichamber air leak in posterolateral position with positive pressure ventilation will usually greatly diminish after turning the patient supine and extubating.

Cancer

The predominant forms of surgically treatable intrathoracic cancer in the developing world are lung and esophageal cancers. Their incidence is rising as life expectancy increases. It is important to remember that in the majority of the Western world, only approximately 25%–35% of patients with these diagnoses are operable at the time of diagnosis. This is probably due to the late stage of presentation, since the majority of patients present with stage IV disease.

In the Western world, the accuracy of diagnosis for major procedures heavily relies on imaging (CXR, chest computed tomography [CT], endoscopic ultrasound [EUS], etc.). This is especially true for cancer surgery, where successful treatment is dependent on accurate staging and the surgeon's ability to obtain a complete resection. Over the past two to three decades, the accuracy of preoperative clinical staging has greatly improved. This has resulted in a sharp decline of surgery for metastatic cancer. Modern clinical staging is based on imaging as well as minor surgical staging procedures. The information derived is typically presented in a tumor, node, metastasis (TNM) classification: T(1–4)N(1–3)M(0,1). An *X* is placed when data is not known. For the vast majority of solid tumors stages I–III, the treatment modality associated with the best survival overall survival is surgery; however, this is also associated with the highest treatment-related mortality. The perioperative surgical morbidity and mortality from complex procedures has greatly decreased in high-volume centers of excellence, where complex procedures are done repetitively by a skilled team with optimal facilities. These results often quoted in the modern surgical literature cannot and do not apply to an LMIC.

Diagnosis in LMICs

Lung cancer patients are likely to present when symptoms appear. Typically, this occurs as a result of advanced and metastatic disease. For lung cancer, symptoms may include the following: persistent cough, hemoptysis, chest pain, and paraneoplastic syndromes. Screening and early detection is by and large nonexistent. An incidental CXR finding is one typical form of presentation. A complete evaluation includes a chest CT down to the adrenals, brain CT, and bone scans. These tests may not be possible. In an LMIC, a CXR, an ultrasound of the liver and adrenal glands, and possibly a bone scan may be available. Thus, without clinical symptoms of metastatic disease (e.g., bone pain, headaches, memory loss, or other central neurologic symptom) in a young and fit patient, selection for cervical mediastinoscopy should be performed if pathology is available. Criteria include patients with central tumors and with peripheral tumors greater than 3 cm in size. Positive peritracheal or subcarinal disease confirms that the patient has at least clinical stage IIIa disease. If properly staged, the best expected survival is around 25%. If mediastinoscopy is negative, the patient would be suspected to have stage I or stage II disease. Depending on the involvement of hilar nodes, the expected survival would be 75% and 50%, respectively, for stage I and II disease. Spirometry, if available, enables an accurate risk assessment as well as prediction of postoperative lung function. If not available, the ability to climb three flights of stairs without stopping may be a good predictor of overall performance status. Surgical options could include wedge resection and hilar lymph node dissection versus anatomical lobectomy with no lymph node dissection. If pathology is not available, or results are not available in a timely fashion, careful consideration must be given to whether surgical therapy is warranted and palliative options should be seriously entertained.

Esophageal cancer patients are likely to present when symptoms of dysphasia or weight loss appear. Typically, this occurs as a result of advanced and metastatic disease. Screening and early detection is regional in nature. In endemic areas, such as Xinjiang province in China, the incidence of esophageal cancer is 60 times greater than most places. Flexible endoscopy may not be possible, due to limited resources; however, a balloon attached to a nasogastric (NG) tube can be inserted, and the balloon inflated and then deflated to diagnose an area of esophageal narrowing. Cytologic specimens can be removed, enabling pathologic diagnosis. In HICs, tissue biopsy is obtained during endoscopy. Staging involves a combination of EUS, contrast chest CT, and positron emission tomography–computed tomography (PET-CT). The majority of patients have stage IV disease on presentation. Approximately 35% are operable. (Of these cases, 10% have stage I disease, and 90% have stage II or III disease.) In LMICs, a CXR, an ultrasound of the liver and adrenal glands, and possibly a bone scan should be used if possible. Thus, without clinical symptoms of metastatic disease (e.g., bone pain, headaches, memory loss, or other central neurologic symptoms) in a young and fit patient, surgical resection or stenting should be considered. Esophageal cancer tends to spread quickly to local regional lymph nodes. Early tumors involving the mucosa may extend into but not beyond the muscularis mucosa. These are classified as T1a and are associated with <5% lymph node involvement. Tumors between the muscularis mucosa and muscularis propria are called T1b and are associated with 20%–60% lymph node metastasis, depending on the series. Tumors that invade the muscularis propria (T2) or the serosa (T3) are associated with 60%–80% lymph node involvement. Tumors can also invade adjacent structures (T4) and should not be operated on. Esophageal tumors can be divided into early T1a, late T1b–T3, N1–3, and metastatic T4 or M1. In HICs, the majority of early esophageal cancer patients are referred to surgery directly, but patients with advanced but not metastatic esophageal cancer may receive neoadjuvant therapy (i.e., concurrent chemoradiation therapy (CCRT) consisting of two cycles 5-FU and cis-platinum combined with 45 gray radiation). Patients with esophageal cancer of the upper third of the esophagus are typically treated with chemoradiation. Stenting is reserved for patients with tracheoesophageal fistulas or those who cannot control their secretions. In an LMIC, most patients with stage I–III esophageal cancer may undergo surgery as a single modality therapy if the correct level of surgical expertise and post-operative facilities and processes are available. A group in sub-Saharan Africa recently presented stenting as single modality therapy for esophageal cancer.[3]

Operative Management in LMICs

Patient selection is critical. In HICs, the majority of cancer is diagnosed in a late stage. This is even more likely to be true in LMICs. Thus the majority of operations are likely to be palliative and not curative in nature. Heroic endeavors and large surgeries should be avoided. Surgeons must take into account their training and comfort level as well as the resources available to them prior to undertaking major endeavors. In general, if the patient is an excellent surgical candidate and the surgeon is a well-trained and experienced general surgeon (without robust training and experience in thoracic surgery), a wedge or possibly a lobectomy would be the largest cancer operation that should be attempted.

A number of papers have recently been published from Africa recommending esophageal stenting as the sole palliative procedure for esophageal cancer in LMICs.[3] Self-expanding stents can be placed without the use of fluoroscopy.[4,5] The majority of esophageal cancer patients in the LMICs present with advanced squamous cell carcinoma of the mid-esophagus. In this setting, these patients have an expected 5-year survival with surgery of around 20%, and an expected surgical operative and perioperative mortality in excess of 10%. Therefore, esophagectomy should be considered only in the most carefully selected cases.

Anesthesia and Analgesia for Thoracic Surgery

The anesthesiologist is a critical member of a thoracic surgical team. Balanced anesthesia can be maintained utilizing a combined approach: inhaled gases delivered through endotracheal tube, anesthetics, and analgesics that are delivered through an IV as well as epidural catheter.

Epidural analgesia can greatly reduce the need for systemic opiates. A thoracic epidural catheter can be placed prior to surgery that necessitates a major thoracotomy. Analgesia can be given through this catheter continuously or through boluses. Usually, a mixture of local anesthetic with narcotic is given. One should remember that the thoracic epidural can be a major cause for hypotension in the thoracic surgical patient.

Operative Monitoring by Anesthesia

Monitoring during surgery should include pulse, O_2 saturation, continuous electrocardiogram (EKG), noninvasive blood pressure, and occasional temperature.

Lines and Drains

For lines, two large-bore IVs are necessary. A central line may be needed to measure or trend central venous pressure. If placed prior to surgery, the central line should be placed on the operative side. An arterial line should be placed, when possible, for large procedures, such as pneumonectomy or esophagectomy.

Additionally, a Foley catheter should be placed to actively monitor urine output. A nasogastric tube should be placed in the stomach on suction in order to decrease aspiration risk.

A mechanical ventilator with adjustable FiO2, tidal volumes, rate and PEEP is desirable. Fluid restriction is a critical component of modern effective thoracic anesthesia strategy. This can be facilitated by judicious use of intraoperative inotropic agents and pressors. Single-lung isolation and ventilation are recommended.

Thoracic procedures are frequently performed on a patient who is positioned in the lateral decubitus position and ventilated through his or her dependent lung. Endotracheal intubation and one-lung ventilation is accomplished by isolating the right and left mainstem bronchi. This can be done using a double-lumen tube (usually left-sided), a tube with a bronchial blocker, or direct intubation of the nonoperative lung with a single-lumen tube. Typically, the patient will be intubated supine, and tube placement is then confirmed. The patient is then repositioned in lateral decubitus, and tube placement is again confirmed. Confirmation of tube placement can be done utilizing a fiber-optic bronchoscope when available or by simple auscultation with a stethoscope. One-lung ventilation results in collapse of the operative lung and is critical in facilitating a workspace during chest surgery. Additionally, blood flow to the collapsed lung is greatly diminished, increasing the overall oxygenation of blood passing the lungs. This physiologic shunting is important for decreasing the blood loss during surgical procedures on the unventilated lung. Common causes of desaturation with one-lung ventilation include the following: distal migration of the endotracheal tube leading to single-lobe ventilation (especially when the left lung is ventilated through a left-sided double-lumen tube), mucus plugging, and incomplete shunting prior to full collapse of the operated lung. Anesthesia for thoracic procedures is unique in that ventilatory lung volumes must be reduced, because only one lung is being ventilated during surgery. When done appropriately, barotrauma of the ventilated lung will be prevented. This is extremely important in the postoperative period because after significant lung resection this unaffected side may account for a large proportion of the remaining lung function.

In almost all general thoracic cases requiring lung resection, the patient should be awakened and then extubated at the completion of surgery.

Nerve Blocks

Nerve blocks can be used to decrease the pain around minor thoracic procedures, such as tube thoracostomy, thoracoscopy, and thoracoscopic wedge resection. Additionally, they can be used to break or prevent the pain cycle that is associated with rib fractures. Intercostal nerve blocks are performed after the area around the desired ribs is cleaned with alcohol. Typically, 3 cc Marcaine 0.25% (bupivacaine) is injected along the inferior aspects of the ribs medial to the mid-scapular line, taking great care to avoid injection or injury to the neurovascular bundle. The maximal dose of Marcaine depends on its strength. Typically, it is safe to use 175 mg Marcaine without epinephrine or 225 mg with epinephrine 1:200,000. A total dose of 400 mg is the maximal dose that should be used over 24 hours. Marcaine should not be given to children under the age of 12.

- 0.25% Marcaine is used in epidurals or peripheral nerve blocks. This concentration will enable analgesia but does not relax muscles.
- 0.5% provides a spinal motor block but incomplete muscle relaxation.
- 0.75% provides a spinal motor block as well as complete muscle relaxation.

Surgical Technique for Thoracic Procedures

Posterolateral Thoracotomy

This procedure is the "Work Horse" of elective general thoracic surgery.

Use: Provides the best exposure to the lungs as well as hilum, distal trachea, and bronchial tree. On the right, it provides good exposure to the esophagus, azygos vein, and distal trachea.

Positioning: Full lateral decubitus. Takes time to set up. Requires lung isolation (blocker or double-lumen tube). Suboptimal in acute setting.

Skin incision extends from the anterior axillary line beyond the tip of the scapula. Typically, the latissimus muscle is divided and the serratus muscle is spared. The incision into the intercostal space depends on the planned surgery: 3rd for Pancoast tumor,

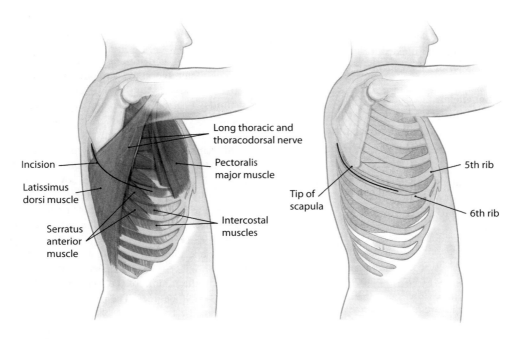

FIGURE 11.1 Standard Posterolateral Thoracotomy. The incision parallels the course of the 6th rib and wraps around the tip of the scapula. Source: Figure 2-1. Erkman CP, Ducko CT, Jaklitsch MT. Chapter 2, *Thoracic Incisions in Adult Chest Surgery*. 2009, McGraw-Hill. Page 6. Illustrated by Marcia Williams.

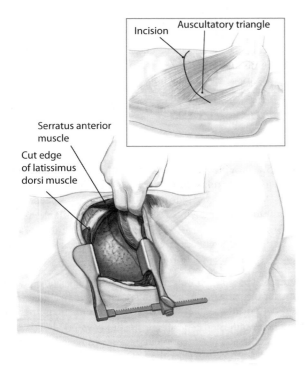

FIGURE 11.2 Operative exposure through a posterolateral thoracotomy. The incision divides the latissimus dorsi muscle and retracts the serratus anterior muscle forward. The incision is centered on the greater fissure of the lung, providing access to the pulmonary artery. Source: Figure 2-2. Erkman CP, Ducko CT, Jaklitsch MT. Chapter 2, *Thoracic Incisions in Adult Chest Surgery*. 2009, McGraw-Hill. Page 7. Illustrated by Marcia Williams.

4th for upper lobes, 5th for lower lobes, and 6th for esophagus (Figure 11.1 and Figure 11.2).

Staff Requirements

Staff should include surgeon and assistant, anesthesiologist, and two nurses or operating room technicians (one scrubbed and the other circulating).

Equipment

- Operating room, adjustable lighting, headlight (the most important light source in thoracic surgery).
- An adjustable operating room table that enables jack-knifing (lateral flexing at hips) of the patient. This fully opens the intercostal spaces enabling optimal exposure.
- Beanbag or two round pillows for lateral decubitus positioning.
- Armrests enabling arm of operated side to be placed in "swimmer's position," elevating the scapula and exposing the intercostal spaces.
- Blankets to wrap lower body and proactively prevent hypothermia.
- Strong working wall suction device.
- Alcohol or Betadine, sterile drapes.
- A major thoracotomy tray. Essential elements include a large knife, long Metzenbaum scissors, Mayo scissors, DeBakey forceps, mid and long needle drivers, multiple long straight and curved clamps, lung compression

clamp, aortic clamps (straight and curved), a large Finochietto retractor, large egg beater retractor.

- Multiple large laparotomy pads.
- Large chest tubes and/or Blakes (or soft drainage tubes). Underwater, chest tube collecting system (preferably with suction).
- **Optional but beneficial:**
  - Electrocautery, linear staplers with reloads (preferably endoGIA), and vascular (30 mm) as well as heavy tissue loads (45–60 mm).
  - Sutures and ties (open as needed).
  - Availability of monofilament 2-0, 3-0, and 4-0 for vascular ligation or repair.
  - 2-0 and 3-0 chromic or Vicryl for lung parenchymal resection.
  - Long- and medium-sized clips (if available).

- **For closure:** #1 or 2 Vicryl for rib reapproximation, 0 Vicryl for muscle reapproximation, 2-0 Vicryl for deep subcutaneous tissue closure.
- **For skin closure:** Skin stapler or absorbable 3-0 suture or 3-0 nylon, and a heavy silk suture for securing chest tube to the chest wall.

Anesthesia

Anesthesia can be general or combined. A mechanical ventilator with the ability to give oxygen at increased FiO_2 is needed.

Expertise is required to position a double-lumen endotracheal tube. Left-sided tubes are easier to position and work for the vast majority of patients. A bronchial blocker or a smaller endotracheal tube can be placed directly in the left mainstem bronchus, if a double-lumen tube is unavailable. This can enable right-sided surgery, with one-lung ventilation; however, it does not allow suctioning of the right lung in order to hasten collapse. One-lung intubation on the right (for left-sided surgery) is problematic since secure tube placement would necessitate blockage of right upper lobe and thus lead to suboptimal ventilation during surgery. Fiber-optic bronchoscopy facilitates accurate placement of the tube. Tube placement without fiber-optic guidance can be done with clinical examination; however, this is suboptimal. The endotracheal tube is placed by anesthesia in a supine position and then fixed appropriately. The patient is then turned to lateral decubitus position, and tube placement must be reconfirmed. Remember: The left main stem bronchus is long and at a sharp angle, while the right mainstem bronchus is short and the right upper lobe typically originates 5–15 mm from the carina. Identification of the right upper lobe is done when seeing three segmental bronchi that appear like a Mercedes-Benz sign. An epidural catheter can improve the ability to give balance anesthesia and decrease the need in the postoperative setting for opioids, thus significantly improving pain management. This should be used for all major general thoracic procedures, when possible.

Lines and tubes: Two peripheral large-bore IVs, a Foley catheter with urimeter, and a nasogastric tube are recommended. An arterial line and central venous pressure (CVP) are optional when needed and available. Any case that would require a Swan-Ganz catheter (e.g., marginal patient or extensive procedure) should not be done in LMICs.

Intraoperative continuous monitoring: O_2 saturation with pulse oximeter, blood pressure with noninvasive cuff on nonoperative arm, and rhythm with EKG.

IV fluids: Lactated Ringer's or normal saline. Blood products should be available, including whole blood or packed red blood cells and fresh frozen plasma.

Positioning: The operative table has a beanbag covered with a sheet in the area of the patient's chest or two Curlex rolls fully opened, folded in half, and then covered by a bed sheet. The patient is initially positioned supine. After administration of general anesthesia, placement and confirmation of the double-lumen tube, as well as of lines and continuous monitoring devices, the patient will be turned. This requires four people and is coordinated by anesthesia in order to assure that the endotracheal tube does not migrate. The patient is then moved so that the down side will be in the middle of the long axis of the operative bed and then turned 90 degrees. The patient is lifted, and an axillary roll (i.e., 1 liter IV bag) is then placed just caudal to the axilla. The beanbag is then suctioned or soft rolls are placed in the Curlex. The patient is slightly elevated, and the Curlex rolls are tied. The dependent leg is flexed; a pillow is placed between the legs, and the upper leg is the left straight. Using heavy tape extending from one side of the bed to the other, the iliac crest is taped and stabilized. The arm on the operative side is placed on an arm board and extended in a "swimmer's position." The other arm is placed on the extended arm board attached to the bed or bent upwards in a 90-degree angle. Care should be taken to properly pad all possible pressure points and avoid iatrogenic positioning injuries. The bed is now jackknifed, facilitating maximal opening of the intercostal spaces. A grounding pad is placed on the buttocks or thigh. The lower body is covered with blankets or a bear hugger, if available.

Prophylaxis

IV antibiotics are given by anesthesia to cover skin flora (cephalexin 2 grams or an equivalent) within an hour prior to skin incision. Antibiotics are redosed by anesthesia, as needed. Five thousand units subcutaneous (SQ) heparin, if available, is given for deep venous thrombosis (DVT) prophylaxis for all thoracotomies. Additionally, when available, sequential venous compression boots should be placed on the patient's legs.

Technique: The surgeon wearing a headlight stands at the patient's back. After the patient is prepped and draped as is customary, electrocautery (if available) and two large Yankauer suctions are set up, and lights are adjusted. Anesthesia institutes single-lung ventilation, thus stopping the ventilation into the operative lung. Typically, it will take 15–20 minutes for the nonventilated lung to fully collapse. The surgeon makes a posterior lateral incision using a large (22) blade to cut a lazy *S* incision along the 6th interspace from the anterior axillary line to beyond scapular tip in a line one fingerbreadth beneath the tip of the scapula and then T-ed upwards. Divide the skin and the subcutaneous tissue. When dividing the latissimus muscle, coagulate or tie vascular bundles that are encountered. Mobilize and retract the serratus, sparing the muscle. A scapula retractor is now placed under the scapula, which the assistant elevates while the surgeon counts ribs. The first rib is a flat rib that must be identified by palpation in order to assure that the count is correct. The interspace chosen is based on the pathology. The 3rd intercostal space is the best approach to Pancoast tumors and structures near the thoracic inlet (e.g., superior vena cava [SVC], subclavian artery and vein, proximal thoracic trachea, and esophagus). The 4th intercostal space is best for upper and middle lobe tumors of the lung. The 5th intercostal space is best for mid-esophageal tumors and lower lobe tumors. The 6th intercostal space is best for distal esophageal tumors and pathologies in the area of the diaphragm. It is important to cut the intercostal muscle fibers along the lower rib of the interspace and not along the upper rib to avoid injury to the neurovascular bundle. Care should be taken upon initial entrance into the thoracic cavity to avoid lung injury. In the vast majority of general thoracic cases, the incision should be made through the 4th or 5th intercostal space. A Finochietto retractor can be placed opening the chest cavity and opened slowly. If additional exposure is needed, the incision can be opened internally by dividing the intercostal muscle insertion along the lower rib medially as well as in the posterior direction. On posterior extension, care must be taken to elevate the erector spinous ligaments from the intercostal muscle so that these are not divided (Figure 11.3). The retractor is then opened further. If this is not enough, a rib can be "shingled" by removing 1 cm of posterior rib (Figure 11.4). This is done to the rib that is above or below the incision, depending on where one wishes to gain maximal additional exposure.

Modification for additional exposure

1. Incision extension
   a. Internal by medial as well as posterior division of the intercostal muscle along the rib space
   b. External by extension of the skin incision medially or posteriorly apically just lateral to the posterior scapula
2. Rib shingling
   - **Pitfall:** Transection of small arteries leading to unrecognized delayed bleeding
     - **Solution:** Meticulous hemostasis
   - **Pitfall:** Aggressive opening of rib spreader leading to broken ribs. This is usually the result of an inadequate incision size, significant tension on the retractor, or severe osteoporosis. It will cause increased postoperative pain with its possible sequelae (e.g., poor ventilation, atelectasis, consolidation, pneumonia, and even death).
     - **Solution:** Slow opening of rib spreader, attention to tension, and enlargement of incision or rib shingling, as needed
   - **Pitfall:** Injury to intercostal bundle (vein, artery, and nerve) in the interspace entered can result in chronic post-thoracotomy pain. Often due to

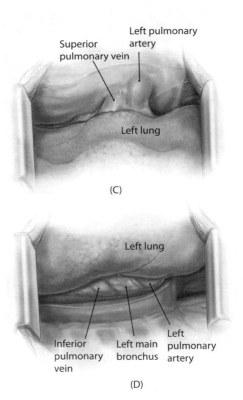

FIGURE 11.3 Anterior and posterior views of the hilum of the lung from a standard posterolateral thoracotomy. A. Anterior view of right lung. B. Posterior view of right lung. C. Anterior view of left lung. D. Posterior view of left lung. Source: Figure 2-4. Erkman CP, Ducko CT, Jaklitsch MT. Chapter 2, *Thoracic Incisions in Adult Chest Surgery*. 2009, McGraw-Hill. Page 8. Illustrated by Marcia Williams.

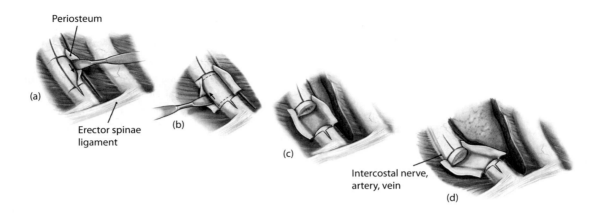

FIGURE 11.4   Rib shingling can provide extra exposure if needed. The nerve is susceptible to stretch injury. Source: Figure 2-3. Erkman CP, Ducko CT, Jaklitsch MT. Chapter 2, *Thoracic Incisions in Adult Chest Surgery*. 2009, McGraw-Hill. Page 7. Illustrated by Marcia Williams.

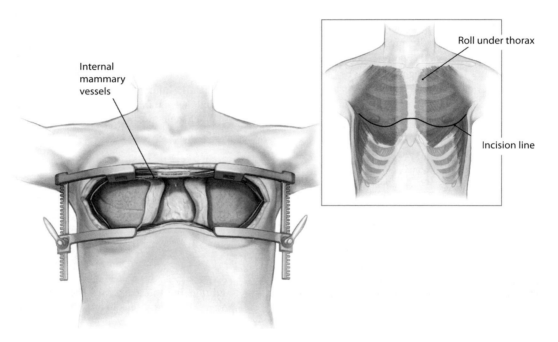

FIGURE 11.5   Clamshell incision. Source: Figure 2-9. Landmarks for placement of a clamshell (bilateral inframammary) incision and view of internal structures. Erkman CP, Ducko CT, Jaklitsch MT. Chapter 2, *Thoracic Incisions in Adult Chest Surgery*. 2009, McGraw-Hill. Page 12. Illustrated by Marcia Williams.

incision just "below" a rib and not "above" the lower rib in the intercostal space that is entered

 – **Solution:** Attention to proper surgical technique.

• **Pitfall:** Lung injury, upon entrance to the chest, can be due to continued ventilation (e.g., patient still on double-lung ventilation) or improper placement of double-lumen tube, lung adhesions to the chest wall, or slow lung collapse.

 – **Solution:** The anesthesia practitioner verifies the proper tube placement after the patient is repositioned from supine to lateral decubitus. One-lung ventilation is instituted from the time of the skin incision. The surgeon carefully

enters the intercostal space visualizing and cutting along a protective finger or Yankauer suction. The lung may need to be suctioned out by the anesthesia practitioner.

3. Clamshell (Figure 11.5)

A curvilinear incision along the 4th intercostal space (top of 5th rib), spanning between both anterior axillary lines. The mammary vessels are ligated and two Finochietto retractors are used. Provides rapid and excellent exposure to the lungs, heart, great vessels.

4. Midline sternotomy (Figure 11.6)

Extends from above the sternal notch down past the xiphoid. Classic cardiac surgery incision because it

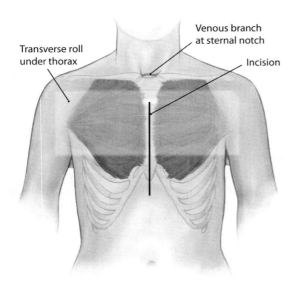

FIGURE 11.6 Midline sternotomy. Source: Figure 2-10. Landmarks for placement of skin incision for a median sternotomy. Erkman CP, Ducko CT, Jaklitsch MT. Chapter 2, *Thoracic Incisions in Adult Chest Surgery*. 2009, McGraw-Hill. Page 13. Illustrated by Marcia Williams.

provides excellent exposure to the heart, ascending aorta, aortic arch and its branches, main pulmonary artery trunk, IVC and SVC, innominate artery and vein. Its only weakness is poor exposure of the left subclavian artery.

5. Trapdoor thoracotomy

   This is a C-shaped incision that provides optimal exposure to the left subclavian artery. It involves an incision along the left clavicle and curves to midline along the superior portion of the sternum and then laterally along the 4th rib. A mini-sternotomy should be performed from the sternal notch down to the third intercostal space and then lateral division of the pectoralis and intercostal muscles along the cranial portion of the fourth rib. The block of sternum/clavicle/ribs is then retracted laterally, resembling a "trap door."

Postoperative Care Following Thoracic Procedures

The decrease in postoperative morbidity and mortality over the past two decades has been largely multifactorial. Although it is impossible to list all factors that have decreased the morbidity and mortality, the major factors are:

1. **Oxygen supplementation:** Enriched oxygen should be given through a nasal cannula in the early postoperative period. Oxygen reduces pulmonary blood pressure by dilating the capillary bed.

   Action: Humidified 100% oxygen is given through a nasal cannula and titered to a flow rate of 1–6 L/min, as needed in order to maintain a SO2 > 90%.

2. **Fluid management:** Thoracic surgery is fundamentally different from general surgery in that volume restriction is important in the postoperative period. Lung resection leads to a decrease in the size of the capillary bed through which the right ventricle pushes the blood. This decreases acutely and thus gradual compensation does not occur. Lung resection, especially bi-lobectomy and pneumonectomy, results in a relative volume overload of the remaining lung as the intravascular volume that previously flowed through five lobes now flows through two to three lobes. Thus, even in a euvolemic patient, the remaining lung sees significantly larger blood flow, which can simulate a pulmonary edema–like picture and, if severe, lead to acute respiratory distress syndrome (ARDS) or acute right heart failure.

   Action: Volume restriction to minimize IV as well as oral intake. Keep the patient dry by giving diuretics early and often.

3. **Arrhythmias:** Very common after lung resection and esophageal surgery. This is likely multifactorial but may be due to vagal mediation, linked to acute cardiac atrial distention, as well as electrolyte shifts (e.g., K^+/Mg^{++}).

   Action: Repletion of electrolytes to high normal levels ($K^+ > 4.5$, $Mg^{++} > 2.2$)

4. **Pain control:** Adequate pain control is important to facilitate deep breathing, coughing, and ambulation in order to prevent atelectasis, pneumonia, and DVT. Pain medicines should be scheduled in the postoperative period because "as needed" therapy is ineffective, leading to the development of a pain cycle that is much harder to reverse.

   Action: Utilize epidural catheters for surgery and the early postoperative period. Make judicious use of IV narcotics and pain cocktails utilizing multiple analgesics with synergistic effects (e.g., Oxycodone 5 mg every 6 hours, Ibuprofen 600 mg every 8 hours and Acetaminophen 650 mg every 6 hours).

5. **Early ambulation:** Facilitates improved lung ventilation, decreasing the risk of postoperative pulmonary complications, such as atelectasis and pneumonia. Additionally, this decreases the risk for DVT and its potentially fatal sequelae of pulmonary embolism.

   Action: Adequate pain control. Trained staff must mobilize the patient from the first postoperative day.

6. **Pulmonary toilet:** Coughing and deep breathing exercises prevent mucous plugging of remaining airways.

   Action: Aggressive chest physical therapy should be performed regularly on the patient by the treatment staff early in the postoperative period. Incentive spirometry can be as simple as a surgical glove that is fully inflated 10 times an hour by the patient who blows deeply into the glove. This provides the patient with visual feedback on his or her respiratory effort.

7. **Aspiration:** Patients are at increased aspiration risk due to postoperative somnolence (due to narcotics), as well as altered swallowing mechanism.

   Action: Judicious use of narcotics. The patient should sit out of bed in a chair for many hours in the day, eat out of bed when fully awake and fully upright, and lie in bed flexed at the hips with the head and back elevated to at least 30–45 degrees.

8. **Nutrition:** High-protein diet

   Action: When tolerated, patient should receive a volume restricted high-protein diet as long as he or she can eat out of bed, when fully awake and upright. Eggs are a concentrated and inexpensive way to provide protein as well as essential nutrients to a patient.

9. **Prophylaxis** for hypercoagulability associated with surgery, thoracic malignancy, and diminished mobility.

   Action: Early ambulation and 5,000 Units SQ heparin from the time of surgery

Summary

General thoracic surgery in LMICs is challenging. Results are dependent on optimizing cooperation in a multidisciplinary setting of providers dedicated to the care of patients with diseases of the chest. This includes surgeons trained in thoracic surgical procedures, dedicated anesthesiologists, pulmonologists, intensivists, radiologists, ICU and floor nurses familiar with the care of thoracic surgical patients, and respiratory therapists, to name a few.

For this patient population, prevention of residual lung injury during surgery, fluid restriction, pain control, aspiration prevention, and early ambulation are critical. Unlike in general surgery where most hemodynamic issues can be solved with IV fluids and then more fluids, these patients do better with fluid restriction and early diuresis.

Thoracic surgery in the setting of limited surgical training and resources should be reserved for the treatment of life-threatening conditions that can be easily treated.

Large and morbid procedures such as pneumonectomy and esophagectomy should only be undertaken with great caution.

COMMENTARY

Koffi Herve Yangni-Angate, Cote d'Ivoire

In West and Central Africa, the main topics within nontrauma thoracic surgery relate to pulmonary tuberculosis, infections of the pleura, and, less frequently, carcinoma in the lungs.

Surgery for sequela of pulmonary TB is very common in West and Central Africa; most of these cases occur in the young population. Pulmonary TB is diagnosed based on clinical and roentgenographic features, and when symptoms persist after anti-TB chemotherapeutic drugs have been administered. In Cote d'Ivoire, we have reported extensively on clinical patterns, indications for surgery, surgical procedures, and results related to surgery for pulmonary TB. The data shows a mortality rate of less than 5% in a population of over 240 patients that have undergone surgery for pulmonary TB, and similar data have been seen in Senegal.[6–9]

Pleural empyema is highly prevalent in Cote d'Ivoire. Empyema, whether acute or chronic, often requires surgery because its symptoms are severe. Symptoms may include an abundance of pus in the pleural space and/or the presence of rigid, thickened parietal and visceral pleural. Drainage and decortication are the two surgical procedures that are performed to treat empyema. Thoracoplasty is not indicated in all of our cases.[10–12]

In Cote d'Ivoire, patients with lung carcinoma present very late to clinics and are consequently diagnosed at a late stage. According to TNM classification, over half of the patients are at stage III or IV, and less than half of them are eligible for surgery. Consequently, the prognosis for these patients is poor, and the survival rate for patients who undergo surgery for lung carcinoma is very low. One year after surgery, most lung carcinoma patients are lost to follow-up; the 5-year survival rate is below 3%. Cigarette smoking is the most significant risk factor for developing primary carcinoma of the lung.[13–14]

12

Acute Abdomen

Reinou S. Groen
Adam L. Kushner

Introduction

This chapter provides an overview for treating patients in low- and middle-income countries (LMICs) who present with an acute abdomen. Included here is a general overview on diagnosis and management; however, for detailed techniques and specific organ systems, it is best to consult individual chapters.

Specific Considerations for LMICs

Patients around the world often give varying descriptions of abdominal pain. While the elements of a physical exam are mostly consistent, it is important to be aware that differences in local culture or language may hinder a proper history. Questions about length of symptoms, severity, and quality of pain may differ from location to location, and, as always, it is best to use open-ended questions, with proper translation, when obtaining a history.

Many patients in LMICs present late after often having exhausted a regimen of expectant waiting, visiting traditional healers, and ingesting ill-defined herbal medications. Due to shame or fear of disrespecting a physician, some patients will not admit to having received such care. Hints such as abdominal markings and scars and remnants of leaves or herbal preparations in various body fluids can alert the provider that the described symptoms have been going on longer than described by the patient or his caregivers. Additionally, these local preparations might be found orally, rectally, or vaginally even after several days of treatment in the hospital.

Key Pitfalls and Problems to Avoid

Due to the delayed presentation of many patients, diseases that result in an acute abdomen will often need significant attention; however, while a proper history and physical examination are needed, as in any other location, there are a number of important pitfalls to avoid when working in an LMIC.

First, before proceeding to the operating room, remember that the surgical team has only one chance, and they need to do things right the first time. Contrary to popular belief that "something is better than nothing," poorly performed initial operations will end up causing an unnecessary burden on an already stressed health system, and leaving a patient with iatrogenic morbidity will be deleterious to the economic situation of a family and, possibly, the community as a whole.[1]

Second, due to the late presentation of many diseases and the frequent long distances that patients travel before reaching a health facility, one needs to carefully assess the physical condition of the patient. Is the patient fit enough to undergo a needed operation? Will he or she survive? With abdominal conditions, the patient is likely severely dehydrated, often malnourished, and anemic, possibly ketotic and hypoglycemic, and, in the worst cases, profoundly septic. Most probably there are electrolyte abnormalities; however, frequently, there are no laboratory facilities. Correction of all these findings is a difficult task. The key is to correct as much as possible; however, too rapid a correction will be just as dangerous as too slow, especially in cases of severe anemia and sepsis. Ordinarily, if a patient survives resuscitation in the first few hours after arrival to a health facility, there is a greater likelihood the patient will survive an operation.

Third, surgical procedures and their success or failure are closely linked with a health facility's reputation. Poor surgical outcomes and intraoperative deaths will reflect poorly on a hospital's reputation and result in patients presenting even later as the community will see the health facility as the caregiver of very last resort. The same logic applies to operating without a good initial preoperative resuscitation. Even if a death was most likely nonpreventable due to the severity of the primary disease or poor physical condition, an operative death will be looked upon less favorably in the community and will negatively affect the reputation of the hospital and possibly even the safety of the surgeon.

Working With a Population With a High HIV Prevalence

Knowing a patient's human immunodeficiency virus (HIV) status is not routinely needed before performing abdominal surgery. However, universal precautions should be followed for all patients. Safe handling of sharps and instruments is mandatory and can be achieved by always passing scalpels in a kidney basin and having proper containers for sharps disposal. Double-gloving is recommended for all procedures even if gloves are in short supply.

History

In LMICs, it is imperative to have a close working collaboration with local colleagues as many patients who present to health facilities may not speak the official national language. If one is unfamiliar with the local language and customs, a detailed history may be difficult or even impossible to obtain.

When taking a history, it is best to start by asking the patient or guardian the patient's age and the chief complaint. Thereafter, for an acute abdomen, elicit more information on the nature of the abdominal pain. As much detail as possible should be sought about the pain: the quality, severity, onset, radiation, duration, location, what makes it better or worse, and the course of the pain and illness. Often, the answers will not seem totally reasonable because, as stated above, patients may be hesitant to offer a full story; however, correlation with the physical exam will help establish a differential diagnosis.

A full review of symptoms must be sought and should include a history of nausea or vomiting, including frequency; amount; color; presence or absence of blood, food, or worms; the time course; and if it is getting better or worse. Additionally, interrogation about anorexia and bowel function, including absence or presence of blood, mucus, and flatus, is imperative.

Signs of urinary frequency, urgency, dysuria, or discharge can help with some causes of abdominal pain. Decreased and dark urine can point to dehydration. All women of childbearing age should be questioned about menses and vaginal bleeding or discharge.

A history of fevers, night sweats, weight loss or gain, headaches, chills, and muscle pain or weakness is also useful in helping to form a differential diagnosis. Additionally, try to elicit any previous medical or surgical history, and any tobacco, alcohol, or local drug or herb use, although this information may often be inaccurate or difficult to interpret.

Physical Exam

Conducting a thorough physical examination has increased importance in an LMIC, where a good history can be difficult to obtain and where limited technology makes other investigations difficult to obtain or interpret. Additionally, when examining a female patient it is good practice to always have a female colleague or nurse in the room and be aware of any cultural taboos. Rectal and vaginal examination might take considerably more time to explain and possibly should be done during a second examination, sometimes after talking with a family member or guardian. If the patient is severely dehydrated, anemic, and septic, a secondary physical exam after initial resuscitation might be in order.

When examining a patient with a possible acute abdomen, it is important to measure and record the vital signs (temperature, blood pressure, and respiratory and heart rate) and include a general observation of the overall status, looking for signs of malnutrition or dehydration, an immunocompromised status, or signs of shock.

A full exam should be undertaken. Starting with the head, examine the quality of the hair and note loose strands or straw coloring that may indicate malnutrition or vitamin deficiency. Sunken eyes and cheeks can be seen with severe dehydration or malnutrition. Check for icteric sclera and see if the patient is anemic by noting if the conjunctiva are pink or pale. An examination of the mouth and tongue will point to signs of dehydration, poor dentition, or oral candida. Assess the neck for rigidity and lymphadenopathy. Auscultation of the heart and chest may reveal murmurs, rhonchi, or rales.

For the abdominal examination, begin with inspection, looking for distention, scars (surgical and from traditional healers), and possible visible peristalsis. Often, it is good to ask the patient to point with one finger to the point of maximal tenderness. Auscultate the abdomen for bowels sounds, noting their absence, presence, regularity, and pitch. Palpate the abdomen starting from the point furthest away from the pain and look for guarding, rebound, or rigidity. Rebound is best tested by simply percussing lightly on the patient's abdomen and seeing the patient's response; there is little cause to push forcefully and release quickly to cause the patient undue discomfort. Any masses identified should be described in terms of location, size, tenderness, and temperature.

All hernial orifices, including inguinal, femoral, and umbilical, should be assessed. Check for costovertebral angle tenderness. A rectal exam, noting tone, blood, stool consistency, or masses, is always indicated. For female patients, a pelvic examination noting cervical motion tenderness, blood, or discharge is often necessary. For males, a testicular exam to rule out a testicular mass or torsion may be indicated.

Additional Tests

Laboratory tests can be useful in helping diagnose and manage patients with an acute abdomen. Hemoglobin or hematocrit can often been obtained, and frequently white blood cell or even full blood counts are available. Unfortunately, electrolytes, liver function tests, amylase, lipase, arterial blood gases, lactate, and coagulation studies are rarer. A test to assess coagulation status can easily be performed at bedside: obtain 2 cc of blood in a clean test tube, keep it at body temperature (in your hands), and within 7 minutes a firm clot should have been formed. Urinalysis and stool examinations, when available, are useful. Pregnancy tests should be obtained for all women of childbearing age.

Upright X-rays of the chest and abdomen can be useful in identifying free air from perforations and distended bowel or air fluid levels from obstructions. Additionally, calculi can often be seen and pneumonia (which especially in children can present as abdominal pain) diagnosed. If available, ultrasound examination can help make a diagnosis, but knowledge of its use and the ability to interpret the images are needed; for example a target or "donut" sign might indicate intussusception, and blood in the abdomen can lead to a diagnosis of a ruptured ectopic pregnancy or ruptured spleen. In locations without ultrasound, a peritoneal tap or diagnostic peritoneal lavage can be useful if internal hemorrhage is included in the initial differential diagnosis. In locations with more resources, computerized tomography (CT) scanning or diagnostic laparoscopy can be extremely helpful.

Pre- and Postoperative Considerations

There are several questions one must consider before operating in general and, specifically, for a patient with an acute abdomen.

What is the indication for surgery?

Although a definite diagnosis might be difficult to ascertain before surgery, a clear indication and differential diagnosis for an exploratory laparotomy is warranted. Be sure the patient, guardians, and local staff understand the clinical situation and the risks and benefits. Be aware that poor outcomes will unduly burden a fragile health system, and, therefore, all operations, but especially complex elective cases, should be attempted only if there is strong local support.

Are the necessary skills and knowledge available?

Before operating, one must be familiar with the anatomy, techniques, and possible postoperative complications. Especially for an emergent case, it is worthwhile to take time to read specifics that one may not be familiar with or may have forgotten. Additionally, take into account issues such as hospital bed capacity and reliability of anesthesia or operating room staff and equipment. The timing for an operation may change based on availability of assistants, nursing support for postoperative care, or seemingly simple needs such as sterile gowns and instruments.

Is the patient fit for operation?

If a patient will not survive a resuscitation, there is little hope that he or she will survive an operation; however, there are occasions when a plan for damage control surgery will allow for a patient in severe shock to be stabilized with a rapid initial operation and a longer postoperative resuscitation. Before attempting this technique, it is important that the local staff understand what is going to happen and that there is adequate postoperative care to undertake the resuscitation.

Postoperative considerations

Clear and detailed operative notes should be written for every operation, and all procedures should be recorded in a logbook. Postoperative orders should also be clearly written and communicated to ward nurses. Of note, for tropical climates, a common cause of a postoperative fever is malaria.

Differential Diagnosis

As the differential diagnosis of the acute abdomen is very broad, an important guideline is to know the epidemiology of the local region. It is imperative to be familiar with the most common diagnoses that one is likely to encounter. Again, relying on local colleagues is imperative as they have the experience and often know the most common conditions to expect.

With late presentations, making a preoperative diagnosis can be extremely difficult. In organizing a differential diagnosis, however, it is useful to use broad categories such as obstruction, perforation, inflammation, hemorrhage, other surgical conditions, and medical conditions that can cause abdominal pain.

Obstruction

Causes of obstruction can be hernias, volvulus (midgut and colonic), ascaris, intussusception, adhesions, cancer, strictures, and foreign bodies. The patient can present with nausea and vomiting, abdominal distention, changes in bowel habits, and abdominal pain. Fever may be absent or might simply be caused by endemic malaria. Signs of shock are common with late presentations. If there is necrosis or perforation, peritoneal signs will commonly be present.

Hernia

In case of a hernia, a tender, tense, mass will be felt at a hernial orifice (e.g., inguinal, femoral, umbilical, or incisional). An attempt at reduction of the incarcerated mass is indicated if the patient reports a less than 6-hour time course and if there is no suspicion of ischemia or necrosis. If the reduction is successful, then an elective repair can be planned. If not, an urgent operation and examination of the bowel and possible resection is recommended.

Midgut Volvulus

Volvulus of the small intestine in adults and children is not uncommon. Often, patients present with a history of sudden severe cramping pain, vomiting, and an increasingly tender and growing central abdominal mass. Plain abdominal X-rays can assist to differentiate a volvulus from ascaris impaction. After careful resuscitation, a laparotomy is indicated to search for an internal band, adhesions, or internal hernia. If cases are operated on late, a bowel resection will be needed for necrotic bowel.

Sigmoid Volvulus

With sigmoid volvulus, patients will often describe previous subacute episodes of abdominal pain, distention, and lack of bowel movements and flatus. The patient will often present with extreme distension and a large, tender tympanic abdomen. Patients who present early can possibly have a sigmoid volvulus reduced by sigmoidoscopy; however, if that is not successful or if there are indications of bowel necrosis, a laparotomy is needed. For viable bowel, some options include detorsion of the sigmoid colon with a sigmoid resection at a later date or immediate sigmoid resection with an on-table bowel prep. For necrotic bowel, a resection and colostomy with a possible reanastamosis and closure after 6 weeks may be indicated. Be aware that a difficult variant, sigmoid volvulus with ileo-sigmoid knotting, is not uncommon and often requires decompression of the sigmoid before reduction can be accomplished. In severe cases or with necrosis, an ileosotomy will be needed.

Ascaris

Obstruction from ascaris can be caused by small masses of tangled worms that can individually reach 15–20 cm in length. To aid in the diagnosis, eggs can be microscopically viewed in stool specimens or adult worms can be seen grossly in stool or vomitus. Antihelminthic drugs are not recommended initially when a patient is obstructed as this may lead to worsening of the obstruction and perforation or hypermotility of the worms, which can then possibly migrate into bile and pancreatic ducts. With a complete obstruction, after initial resuscitation, close monitoring for signs of perforation, necrosis, or peritonitis is warranted. Intravenous (IV) fluids, bowel rest, and observation are usually all that are needed with the obstruction resolving within 3 days.

Surgery for obstruction from ascaris is needed in cases of necrosis, perforation, peritonitis, profuse bleeding per rectum, or if the nonoperative management fails because the patient deteriorates. Intraoperatively, the bowel should not be opened if there is no necrosis or perforation. With gentle milking, the worms can be pushed past the point of obstruction, commonly the ileocecal valve. An intestinal segment packed with worms can also become dense and twist, causing a volvulus. Additionally, the worms secrete toxic products can cause intense mucosal inflammation and with compression may lead to intestinal necrosis. If surgery is needed, levamisole or albendazole can be prescribed with a repeated dose after 15 days. Stools should be evaluated at a later date to ensure they are free of eggs.

Intussusception

Intussusception is fairly common in children who present with a history of colicky abdominal pain and "currant jelly" or bloody stools. In addition, intussusception is not uncommon in various parts of Africa due to tuberculosis, tumors, or idiopathic causes. A painful abdominal mass and an empty right lower quadrant may be seen on examination; however, using an ultrasound and seeing a target or donut sign is useful and reasonably conclusive. Although reduction by enema is common in high-income countries (HICs), in LMICs, such resources are rare or risky and a laparotomy is more common. For children, the bowel can be gently milked to reduce the obstruction, being careful not to pull as this will cause a tear; for adults, given the risk of a malignancy causing the intussusception, a resection is recommended.

Tumors

Obstruction from cancer is less common in many low-income settings; however, with changing dietary habits in many regions of the world, an increase in abdominal cancers is being seen and should be considered as part of the differential diagnosis.

Strictures

Obstructions caused by strictures may be observed with abdominal tuberculosis; however, inflammatory bowel disease, such as Crohn's disease, is rare.

Perforation

Patients with a perforation often present with a history of sudden sharp abdominal pain. They may have a fever, rebound, guarding, or a rigid abdomen. A plain upright chest or abdominal X-ray showing the diaphragm is valuable to demonstrate free air. All patients with a suspected perforation need to be aggressively resuscitated before being taken for an operation.

Peptic Ulcers

Perforation from peptic ulcers is common and should be suspected with a history of dyspepsia. Omental patch repair and abdominal irrigation can routinely be performed with therapy for *Helicobacter pylori* eradication postoperatively to prevent recurrences.

Typhoid Perforation

Typhoid perforation is common in LMICs with a typical history of headache, fever, and malaise for some weeks with dull abdominal pain, which worsened suddenly. Intraoperatively, the entire small intestine and colon should be inspected, even if an initial perforation is easily found, as there may be multiple perforations. Most commonly, the perforation(s) will be on the anti-mesenteric border of the terminal ileum. With typhoid perforation, excision of the ulcer margins and primary suture of the ileum is simple and effective; however, resection is advisable if there are three or more perforations and a right hemicolectomy may be justified with a cecal perforation. If the patient is acutely ill, the affected segment of bowel can be exteriorized. Ciprofloxacin or chloramphenicol should be given to treat the underlying *Salmonella typhi* infection.

Colon Perforation

Colon perforations caused by cancer or diverticulitis are infrequently seen in LMICs; however, perforations from amoebic colitis or trauma are not uncommon and discussed below.

Inflammation and Infection

Depending on the geographic location, patients presenting with a diagnosis of appendicitis or cholecystitis can be very common or exceedingly rare. In LMICs, when faced with a patient presenting with an acute abdomen, depending on the geographic location, one must also consider such diagnoses as abdominal tuberculosis, psoas abscess, pig bel, toxic mega-colon from Chagas disease, spontaneous bacterial peritonitis, and even pyomyositis of the rectus sheath.

Abdominal tuberculosis (TB) often presents with fever and abdominal pain and is commonly associated with HIV/acquired immunodeficiency syndrome (AIDS). Differentiation needs to be made between peritoneal TB and intestinal TB. Multidrug therapy according to local protocols should be administered for all patients diagnosed with TB.

Peritoneal TB is divided into four variants: exudative, dry, encapsulated, and poly-serositic. Exudative is the most common variety with ascites being the main feature. The encapsulated form causes tuberculous adhesions and is frequently associated with obstructions. The poly-serositic form involves the peritoneum, pleura, and pericardium. Culture or Ziehl-Neelson stains from taps of abdominal fluid are not always conclusive, and intraoperatively one might suspect the diagnosis by seeing "rice spots," granulomas, or adhesions on the intestine or peritoneum.

Intestinal or ileo-cecal TB can present with a partial or complete obstruction associated with wasting and colicky pains that worsened over weeks to months. It may also be associated with a mass in the lower right quadrant or ascites. Surgical resection is indicated in cases of intestinal stenosis, bleeding, peritoneal perforation, and visceral or external fistulae. Right hemicolectomy may be required with severe ileo-cecal involvement.

Amoebic colitis and *liver abscesses* caused by *Entamoeba histolytica* can result in an acute abdomen. The signs and symptoms of colitis can include crampy abdominal pain, bloody diarrhea with mucus, and colonic tenderness. A liver abscess is often associated with fever and diffuse abdominal pain with the maximal point of tenderness in the right hypochondrium. Frequently, there is a history of drinking quantities of locally produced alcohol. The liver in these patients is diffusely enlarged and tender, and the patient might complain of right shoulder pain. Therapy consists of oral metronidazole, but, if diagnosed by ultrasound, abscesses greater than 5 cm can additionally be drained percutaneously. Occasionally, liver abscesses may rupture into the peritoneal cavity, and a laparotomy may be necessary.

Amoebic colitis can perforate through the colon. In such cases, drainage of any abscesses and a colostomy are required in combination with an amoebicide, such as metronidazole. Stools should be checked 2 weeks after completion of the medical therapy to confirm eradication of amoebas.

Hemorrhage

Due to a high incidence of splenomegaly, blunt abdominal trauma can predispose to life-threatening conditions. A high index of suspicion, close observation, and ultrasound or peritoneal lavage will help determine the need for an exploratory laparotomy for ruptured spleen. Other causes of hemorrhage frequently include a ruptured ectopic pregnancy or hepatic tumor.

Other Surgical Conditions

Multiple other surgical conditions can also present with an acute abdomen. These include urologic and vascular conditions, and diseases associated with the gallbladder, pancreas, and female reproductive tract.

Urologic conditions, such as renal or urethral stones, urinary tract infections, or pyelonephritis may present with severe abdominal pain, nausea, and vomiting. All patients should be examined for costovertebral angle tenderness. Older males may present with severe abdominal pain from a severely distended bladder due to urethral obstruction from benign prostatic hypertrophy or prostate carcinoma. An attempt at uretheral catheterization should be attempted with sufficient lubrication; however, not infrequently a supra-pubic catheter may be indicated.

Vascular conditions such as aortic aneurysms or mesenteric thrombosis are infrequently seen in LMICs most likely because patients with these conditions die before presenting to a health facility. If patients with vascular conditions do present, there are often few therapeutic options.

Gallbladder diseases are infrequently seen in sub-Saharan Africa but more prevalent in Latin America and Asia and especially in India where gallbladder cancer is the most common cancer.

The pancreas can be affected by acute pancreatitis due to gallstones, chronic alcohol ingestion, or parasites. Pain will usually be deep and radiate to the back.

The female reproductive tract can be the source of an acute abdomen from such conditions as peritonitis from pelvic inflammatory disease or a ruptured tubo-ovarian abscess. Torsion of an ovary or an ovarian cyst, Mittelsmerz, or an ectopic pregnancy may cause severe abdominal pain. A uterine myoma can be a source of subacute pain and an abdominal mass on examination, but will have a long time course and should be detectable on pelvic exam.

Medical Conditions Causing Abdominal Pain

In addition to the multitude of surgical conditions causing an acute abdomen, there are numerous medical conditions that must be considered. Various abdominal diagnoses such as gastritis, gastroenteritis, or mesenteric lymphadenitis should be entertained, in addition to malaria, pneumonia, influenza, or a myocardial infarction. Other less frequently seen conditions include porphyria, polio, mumps, or measles. Abdominal masses due to lymphadenopathy resulting from HIV or lymphoma (including Burkitt's lymphoma) should be part of a differential diagnosis depending on the local epidemiology and immunologic status. Right upper quadrant pain may be seen in hepatitis. Generalized abdominal pain can be caused by herpes zoster or even spinal root lesions.

Diabetic-ketoacidosis can mimic an acute abdomen with a slow onset of abdominal pain and vomiting. Profound dehydration and ketone bodies in urine and on the breath are keys for making the diagnosis. Lastly, sickle-cell crisis presents with headache, fever, and painful fingers and tibias, and can be associated with symptoms such as vomiting and centralized abdominal pain. On physical exam, the patient might even have guarding or rigidity; however, laboratory blood examination will show sickle cells. The medical causes mimicking an acute abdomen can be difficult to diagnose with limited laboratory support; however, after the initial resuscitation, time will more clearly settle the diagnosis and possibly prevent a negative exploratory laparotomy.

Conclusion

Managing patients with an acute abdomen in LMICs can be challenging. With limited diagnostic and therapeutic options, often no clear understanding of the underlying condition can be definitely ascertained before going to the operating room for an exploratory laparotomy. Good preoperative resuscitation is mandatory for success, and close cooperation with local staff and colleagues is vital. Strong history taking and physical diagnosis skills, along with flexibility and a firm understanding of general surgical principles, are needed to care for patients that will present late and be prone to complications. For additional information we recommend the specific chapters in references 2 through 4.

COMMENTARY

Okao Patrick, Rwanda

This chapter comprehensively covers the acute abdomen and takes into consideration the socio-economic and cultural aspects important to overall patient management. The difficulty encountered by most patients in accessing competent practitioners contributes to late presentation; patients sometimes also present late because they first try unnecessary treatment, including local herbs, antibiotics, and laxatives.

The challenges posed by cultural differences are clearly described. The challenges impact all stages of patient management ranging from medical history, where it is a taboo to discuss some topics, to surgical procedures like colostomy, which is completely unacceptable in some societies.

It should be emphasized that practicing in LMICs involves much more than going without some investigations; practitioners also require insight on how to rationally use the limited resources and improvise for those that are unavailable. One example is seen in drawing a blood sample at the same time as inserting an intravenous catheter. An example of improvisation is using a nasogastric tube for a drain.

The discussion by the author of this chapter will be a useful guide not only for surgeons who live in LMICs, but also for surgeons who intend to work in these areas.

COMMENTARY

Louis-Franck Telemaque, Haiti

This chapter demonstrates a profound knowledge of LMICs. Indeed, treating patients under these conditions can be very challenging. Additionally, management is often complicated by the difficulties of communication, the advanced state of the disease, and the deleterious impact of previous empirical treatments. Even after obtaining the patient's complete medical history and conducting a thorough physical examination, surgeons must pay attention to detail; one example where this is necessary is in young female patients who may not disclose the abortion procedures they have undergone.

Surgeons will benefit from taking the necessary time to understand what is happening with the patient. Surgeons can take advantage of this time to prepare the patient for surgery and to get as many as possible and available paraclinical exams, particularly for patients with septic shock or acute anemia. When the window of opportunity presents itself, it is best to perform the surgery as efficiently as possible in order to achieve the best outcome.

Personally, I never hesitate to seek the advice of a colleague when I have doubts about a case. The most dramatic situations involve massive intestinal infarctions due to the constriction of the superior mesenteric artery in strangulated inguinal hernia (W) and strangulated internal hernia, even through the falciform ligament.

Intussusception in children can be concerning and warrants extra attention. The diagnosis is usually made late (fifth day) with intussusceptum at anus in a child with precarious conditions. Despite rigorous resuscitation, a heavy intervention can be unbearable. Even after a successful intervention, it is not uncommon for complications (including dehiscence) to arise, or for sudden death to occur.

Generally, if surgeons feel that the abdomen is surgical, they must arm themselves with all the elements that can help to better prepare the patient. They should also expect surprises to be faced with serenity but always in favor of saving the patient's life.

COMMENTARY

Ntakiyiruta Georges, Rwanda

The management of acute abdomen cases in Rwanda is not different from what is excellently described in this chapter. Patients are diagnosed based on medical history and physical exams; we believe that we capture at least 80% of cases with these criteria alone. Medical history is of paramount importance for diagnosing common surgical conditions, including typhoid perforations, perforated peptic ulcer diseases, and various types of intestinal obstructions. Therapeutic abdominal marks are also indicative of a diagnosis of generalized peritonitis, but patients rarely will admit to having used local herbal remedies prior to coming to the hospital.

Almost all patients with features of an acute abdomen will present late to the hospital; this occurs for several reasons. The patient will first delay at home while he or she and family are trying other means of treatment in order to avoid the hospital. When this option fails, family members take the patient to the health center, the primary healthcare level. Patients must go through the system, no matter how severe their condition, if they want to use the nationwide community healthcare insurance. Since patients with an acute abdomen are expected to be dehydrated and in significant pain, the health center personnel, usually the nurses, admit the patient and then initiate treatment. Usually, they will notice that the patient is deteriorating after 24 hours. At this point, the patient is referred to the district hospital, where there are general practitioners. The patient is admitted, put under observation, and eventually referred to the university teaching hospital to be seen by a surgeon. As a rule, patients with acute abdomen will always present late as a result of these delays.

Staged operations can be lifesaving in the very sick patients. For example, for patients who present late with severe peritonitis on perforated gangrenous bowels, minimal surgery might be sufficient in terms of resecting what needs to be resected, controlling contamination, closing the abdomen with clips, and admitting the patient in the intensive care unit(ICU) (if there is one) or in the high-dependency unit (HDU) for continuous critical care. In these cases, you need to plan a re-look surgery. These patients need either a colostomy or ileostomy, but these procedures are poorly tolerated by the population in Rwanda, and stoma bags are not easily available.

Good resuscitation is also very important. Patients' response must be monitored by clinicians, however, since specific laboratory tests are almost never available. A good urinary output is a good indicator of good resuscitation.

It is also important to note that limited resources can impact treatment plans in Rwanda. For example, while patients with gallstones are very common in Rwanda, they must be treated with biliary colics. Another example is seen in sigmoid volvulus patients, who end up having a resection and a colostomy because sigmoid scopes are rarely available.

13

Stomach

David S. Shapiro

Introduction

The surgical approach to gastroduodenal pathology includes consideration of the most frequently encountered diagnoses: bleeding, perforation, and obstruction. While other phenomena may present urgently, for example, bezoars, foreign bodies, parasitic disease, and others, they are far less commonly encountered by surgeons. The goals of therapy for any gastroduodenal procedure include cessation of bleeding, control of contamination, restoration of continuity, and the treatment of underlying etiology. Surgical complications of gastroduodenal pathology may be approached with similar respect for the functional anatomy and physiology, but will include particularities specific to the diagnosis. The high-income countries (HICs) of the world will include advanced imaging, endoscopic techniques, and nonsurgical therapies, and these are important to consider. As low- and middle-income countries (LMICs) differ in the ability to manage acute problems, however, those with differing resources at their disposal may be less facile with one component of the required care. More specifically, experience with the surgical management of gastroduodenal disease is variable. While endoscopy, imaging, and other technologies are available only sparingly, well established—albeit more invasive—management techniques are often required. Changes in the epidemiology of peptic ulcer disease have modified the approach to gastroduodenal surgery, but these changes may be less important in LMICs. The existence of gastroduodenal problems and, more specifically, peptic ulcer disease in the absence of appropriate nonsurgical and antimicrobial therapy in these areas will make useful this review of surgical management.

Primer on Gastroduodenal Disease

Pathology

Peptic ulcer disease is not the only etiology for gastric pathology, but it is the most common. This primer will provide a background for therapy. Surgical management of gastroduodenal pathology will follow.

Peptic ulcer disease was the major indication for surgery on the stomach and duodenum in the 1950s through the 1970s. The number of procedures worldwide has dropped substantially over the last 30 years, and *elective* surgery for peptic ulcers has all but vanished. There is evidence, however, to demonstrate that the incidence of perforated and bleeding ulcer disease, and therefore surgical management, is again starting to increase.[1]

The epidemiology of peptic ulcer disease has changed, likely due to identification and control of *Helicobacter pylori* infection (HPI) and the development of proton-pump inhibitors (PPIs), both of which are associated with a decrease in the need for ulcer surgery.[2] Complicated peptic ulcer disease is the most common diagnosis requiring emergency surgery on the stomach and duodenum. Ulcerations can occur in the stomach or duodenum, and can result in mucosal bleeding, perforation, and/or stricture at the pylorus, resulting in obstruction. Initial management has included nonsurgical means as a mainstay, but surgery must be considered with haste if medical management fails or if life is threatened.

Bleeding

Though patients with bleeding due to gastroduodenal pathology may present with hemodynamic instability and hemorrhagic shock, most will present with hematochezia or melena without hemodynamic abnormality. Associated symptoms of near syncope, tachycardia, or symptoms resulting from anemia are also not uncommon.[3] Intraluminal blood may act as a cathartic, so multiple bowel movements with blood may occur. These patients require the same aggressive therapy as anyone in the setting of hemorrhage—volume resuscitation, restoration of red cell mass, attention to coagulopathy and acidosis, investigations to identify etiology, and, sometimes, surgical management.

Though hematochezia, or bright-red blood per rectum, may be uncommon in gastroduodenal bleeding, its presence with the appropriate clinical history may suggest brisk active bleeding. Most patients with bleeding from the upper gastrointestinal tract—proximal to the ligament of Treitz—will present with the finding of melena; blood partially digested by gastric secretions causes the stool to become dark, tenacious, and malodorous. The frequency of bowel movements may increase with continued bleeding. Patients who suffer from acute gastroduodenal bleeding may also present with hematemesis; the vomiting of blood may be readily noticeable, or may have the appearance of coffee grounds. Whether presenting with melena or hematemesis, anemia must be considered as the source of shock, and appropriate measures taken.

Perforation

Patients with gastric or duodenal perforation often present with evolving peritonitis, though some may present with a more subtle course. The abdominal examination will often reveal distension in an uncomfortable patient. Early signs and symptoms manifest as malaise, nausea, abdominal pain, and diaphoresis. A rigid, tender abdomen may evolve, and signs of systemic inflammatory response herald concern. Typical findings also include fever, leukocytosis, and rigors. Patients immunocompromised from comorbid conditions, corticosteroid use or syndromes may demonstrate far more subtle findings.

As control of contamination is imperative to prevent and treat septic complications of the perforated viscous, surgical management is the standard of care. Perioperative fluid resuscitation, appropriate antimicrobial therapy, and expeditious exploration are important considerations. Patients with shock should be aggressively resuscitated. Although adequate volume resuscitation is of high importance, patients with blood pressure refractory to volume alone may require vasopressors early in the course of therapy. [4]

Obstruction

Though benign disease due to chronic inflammation is encountered, malignancy is the more frequent cause of cause of gastric outlet obstruction in LMICs.[5] Acute and chronic inflammatory changes in the distal stomach may result in evolving stenosis of the pylorus. Changes—perhaps related to microperforation, translocation of flora, and/or transmural inflammation near the gastroduodenal junction—may result in severe edema and fibrosis, the etiology of which may be multifactorial. Tuberculosis, immunoproliferative disorders, or peptic ulcer disease may etiologically contribute. Regardless of the etiology, patients present with nonbilious vomiting, which is usually unrelieved by antiemetics with or without nasogastric decompression. Weight loss, fatigue, and weakness are not exclusive to malignancy, as the diet is universally affected. A history suggestive of peptic ulcer disease is also nonspecific, and the wide availability of PPIs and histamine blockers has contributed to a decrease in the evolution of benign disease into gastric outlet obstruction (GOO). Though nonoperative treatment is preferred in the setting of benign disease (antibiotics for infectious etiologies, acid reduction therapies, etc.), the prevalence of malignancy should prompt endoscopic tissue sampling where possible, and surgical management to diagnose and treat the obstruction if endoscopy is impossible. Acute management includes volume and electrolyte repletion, nasogastric decompression, and supplementation of nutrition distally when possible or, if the option exists, parenterally.

Malignancy may be managed surgically by either therapeutic resection with reconstruction or palliatively with surgical decompression and bypass of the stomach and/or duodenum. These techniques are discussed below.

Though many disease states result in gastroduodenal pathology, peptic ulcer disease and its complications represent the majority of surgically managed disease. Bleeding, perforation, and obstruction, though differing in presentation, are not dissimilar in pathophysiology and are managed with similar means.

Pathophysiology

The pathophysiology of peptic ulcer disease may be divided into three distinct and most common etiologies:

1. Hypersecretion (Zollinger-Ellison syndrome [ZES], G-cell hyperplasia, and unopposed gastrin effect)
2. Physiologic aberrations due to extrinsic causes (psychological stressors, smoking, ethanol consumption, nonsteroidal anti-inflammatory medications (NSAIDs), corticosteroids, and age-related decrease in intrinsic prostaglandin production)
3. Infectious (HPI)[3]

Hypersecretory states are often associated with a gastrin-producing tumor, as in ZES. ZES is the result of duodenal or pancreatic neoplasia which secrete unregulated amounts of the hormone gastrin, stimulating gastric parietal cells to generate and pump hydrogen ions into the gastric lumen. Identification and resection of the source is curative, though localization can be difficult. Years may pass from first symptoms and diagnosis of ulcer to the diagnosis of a gastrin-producing tumor.

Adverse extrinsic effects on gastroduodenal physiology are predominantly caused by NSAIDs. Nearly half of asymptomatic patients taking aspirin may have incidentally identified asymptomatic ulcerations in the gastric mucosa. The etiology of NSAID-associated gastric ulcers is related to the inhibition of natural mucosal barriers in the lumen. The intrinsic barriers include mucus, bicarbonates, surface-active phospholipids, tight junctions, cell proliferation, microcirculation and leukocyte-mediated events. NSAIDs result in the uncoupling of mitochondrial oxidative phosphorylation, resulting in increased intestinal permeability, disabling many of the intrinsic barriers. The invasion of inflammatory agents (bile, proteolytic enzymes, microbes) result in tissue injury, causing ulcers, perforations, strictures and bleeding.[6]

HPI results in a chronic inflammatory state in the gastric mucosa. This results in decreased mucosal perfusion, decreasing gastric mucus production, and exposure of the unprotected gastric epithelium. HPI can also result in a hypersecretion of gastrin. The predominant cause of duodenal ulcer is *H. pylori*–associated hypersecretion and gastric metaplasia in the duodenal mucosa.[21] Gastric ulcers are more commonly involved with external influences rather than HPI, though an association exists. The mainstay of therapy for patients with uncomplicated HPI associated ulcer is eradication therapy including antibiotic, PPI, and bismuth subsalicylate for a duration of 2 to 4 weeks, with reassessment. Successful treatment is usually accompanied by symptom relief, but repeat endoscopy is the most important determination of success, when available. Those patients who present with bleeding, perforation, or obstruction also should be assessed for HPI and will often require post-procedural eradication therapy. HPI may be detected with a urease-based breath test, histology of endoscopically-obtained specimen, or serum antibody. It should be noted, though, that serological testing remains antibody positive even following successful eradication. Intraluminal blood may result in false-negative breath testing.

Patient History

Patients presenting with gastroduodenal pathology may present acutely or more innocuously. Gastric and duodenal ulcerative disease may also often present with similar findings. Patients may be tobacco smokers, ethanol drinkers, or chronic users of NSAIDs, corticosteroids, or aspirin. There may be a history of dyspepsia, or intermittent intolerances to food, but these are often vague. Patients will complain of historically having nausea, upset stomach, and indigestion between meals, and may report improvements immediately postprandially. Additionally, patients may present on evaluation with evidence of occult blood in the stool. In the acutely presenting patient, signs of hemorrhagic shock must be appreciated early in the bleeding patient. Similarly, malaise, confusion, signs of systemic inflammatory response, fevers, and peritoneal signs are cardinal findings indicating perforation and must be identified. Eructation, shoulder pain (Kerr's sign), and vague upper abdominal pain may be the only findings present in some. Patients with suspicion of peptic ulcer disease complications should be evaluated expeditiously.

Gastric and Duodenal Bleeding

Presentation

Bleeding may present with anemia, hematochezia, melena, and/or hematemesis, but may often present with only occult blood loss detected on stool examination. Blood in the stool may indicate foregut bleeding in addition to more distal sources. Any blood may represent an upper gastrointestinal bleed, and must be evaluated quickly. So-called coffee ground emesis represents blood mixed with gastric secretions. Melena suggests a source of bleeding higher than the ileocecal valve, as mixing of blood with digestive juices results in color, consistency, and character changes. Patients may be acutely anemic, with tachycardia, hypotension, and near-syncope, but will present along the spectrum of severity. Some present with occult, low-level bleeding, melena, chronic or acute anemia, and perhaps chronic NSAID or aspirin use. Other historical features include alcohol abuse, tobacco smoking, and possibly cirrhosis or other etiologies of portal hypertension, such as schistosomal disease. Patients may present more acutely, though, with tachycardia, hypotension, and oliguria, and should be treated as in any other source of bleeding. Ulcers and bleeding esophageal varices are the most common etiologies, accounting for greater than 80% of cases.[8,9] Other etiologies, including Mallory-Weiss syndrome, Dieulafoy's Lesion, gastric neoplasia, and hemobilia, are less frequent. History may lead the provider to the diagnosis of ulcer, including a history of episodic epigastric pain associated with social history listed above. Comorbid conditions among alcohol abusers may include hepatic insufficiency, including encephalopathy, ascites, or alcohol withdrawal syndrome in patients, and can complicate care for bleeding ulcers or variceal disease. Patients may present with splenomegaly or stigmata of liver disease on physical examination. Data endemic to the region may offer suggestions of schistosomal or other infectious or regionally more prominent etiologies.

Evaluation and Management

Assessment of the airway, breathing, and circulatory (ABC) status of the patient is of significant importance. An assessment of airway includes attention to risk of vomiting and aspiration as well as mental status, which may be diminished in the acutely decompensating patient. Tachypnea may represent significant acidosis associated with blood loss. Evidence of shock may be present depending upon the degree of acute anemia, and readily judicious crystalloid and blood product resuscitation must be considered. Patients should have large-bore venous access, cardiac and oxygenation monitoring, and, most importantly, efforts started toward control of the bleeding source. Nasogastric tube lavage is very useful in patients who have gastroduodenal bleeding as a diagnostic maneuver—as an aspiration of frank blood or blood-tinged fluid is diagnostic for bleeding above the ligament of Treitz—but it cannot be relied upon for localization. Additionally, nasogastric aspiration is nondiagnostic with absence of blood in the aspirate. Bilious fluid will successfully suggest a bleeding source distal to the ligament of Treitz in most patients. Rapid assessment, restoration of circulating volume, treatment of coagulopathy, and close monitoring are important first steps, but the mainstay of bleeding management is endoscopic.

Patients who experience intermittent hematemesis, or so-called coffee ground emesis, may be monitored in the hospital setting and should be endoscopically evaluated during that admission. Patients who arrive with any degree of shock, acute anemia, and/or evidence of exsanguinating bleed should have rapid endoscopic evaluation followed by endoscopic or surgical intervention.[4] In the absence of endoscopic management, close monitoring is paramount, and changes in vital signs should prompt urgent intervention. Waiting until patients are hypotensive or in extremis is rarely a beneficial maneuver.

Resource-limited settings may not have available endoscopy for assessment. Maneuvers to employ in the absence of endoscopy include cold gastric lavage of a noradrenalin solution (8 mg noradrenalin in 200–400 ml iced cold saline) that may result in vasoconstriction of the bleeding source, slowing or stopping it.[10] This should be aspirated and replaced every 30 to 45 minutes. When aspirated, the absence of bloody fluid suggests successful topical therapy. If the bleeding continues despite therapy for 2 hours, consider other methods.

Vasopressin may also be utilized in a similar fashion, with 20 units diluted in 500 ml saline, and may be given as lavage over 2 to 4 hours. This method may result in significant cramping, hypertension, headache, and palpitations.

Should neither maneuver be successful, or if blood loss proves brisk and is accompanied by hypotension, and transfusion products are scarce, surgical management should be endeavored early and aggressively.

When available, upper endoscopy is facilitated by adequate airway protection, sufficient sedation and analgesia, and an experienced endoscopist. Upper endoscopy should visualize the esophagus, stomach, and duodenum into the first and second portion. Though visualization is often difficult with fresh bleeding, clots can be relatively easily evacuated with lavage tubing, or with an aspiration-capable endoscope. Without an experienced endoscopist, surgical intervention may be the only option.[5,6]

In addition to procedurally based diagnostics and therapeutics, of high importance is the treatment of coagulopathy. As many patients with gastroduodenal disease present with bleeding, many have comorbid platelet abnormalities (consumptive depletion, cirrhosis, NSAID or aspirin usage, primary coagulopathies, and others) and the restoration of normal coagulation is important. Reversal or treatment of acquired coagulopathies, including administration of phytonadione (vitamin K) in the treatment of elevated prothrombin time, and cessation of antiplatelet agents is important. While useful, the utilizaton of thromboelastography (TEG) may be difficult in an LMIC.

Endoscopic treatment for ulcers includes sclerosis by injection with alcohol or epinephrine, contact thermal multipolar coagulation therapy, and/or metal clip or band ligation. Successful therapy depends upon the modality, nature of the bleeding, and the lesion treated, but is predictable.[11] Rebleeding incidence depends upon noted activity during initial endoscopy. Active bleeding or spurting has a rebleeding incidence of 55%–100%, requiring surgical intervention in more than 33% of cases. Stigmata of recent bleeding, including visualization of a nonbleeding vessel, is associated with nearly 50% incidence of rebleeding, while noting clot adherent to the mucosa is reported to rebleed in up to 30% of cases. Evidence of a clean-based ulcer or flat area of mucosa is associated with less than 10% rebleeding and rarely requires surgery. Access to endoscopic means will facilitate control of bleeding ulcer disease, gastritis, and Mallory-Weiss syndrome in the majority of cases. Evidence of variceal disease of the esophagus and cardia are treated endoscopically, but efforts to reduce portal pressures must be employed to have any effect on the recurrence of bleeding. Those patients who rebleed may be controlled by a second endoscopic procedure, but surgical consultation should be considered early. Guidelines to proceed to surgical intervention include recurrent or refractory bleeding, difficult visualization, hypotensive patients, and patients in whom more than four to six units of blood have been administered. Additionally, patients who do not respond to blood volume resuscitation should receive early intervention. Lastly, in areas with poor access to blood products or endoscopic therapy, early surgery will preclude the likelihood of progressive blood and volume losses, acidosis, and coagulopathy often associated with ongoing hemorrhage.

Etiologies of Gastroduodenal Hemorrhage

The following include etiologies commonly encountered in patients with bleeding from the stomach and duodenum. The diagnoses will be described here, and management briefly addressed. The section to follow will address specifics of surgical management.

Mallory-Weiss Syndrome

The Mallory-Weiss syndrome is characterized by gastrointestinal (GI) bleeding due to linear lacerations through the mucosa at the gastroesophageal junction or isolated to the gastric cardia. Classically, this syndrome follows retching and vomiting after acute gastrointestinal illness, alcohol imbibitions and intoxication, or other acute illness. This phenomenon accounts for between 2% and 15% of all upper gastrointestinal bleeding (UGIB) and may affect any age.[12]

Many patients with Mallory-Weiss tears may have a predisposing hiatal hernia, but often there are no identifiable associated comorbidities. Suspicion for a Mallory-Weiss type laceration is usually enough to warrant endoscopic evaluation based upon history, but it is important to avoid low-yield contrast imaging studies, which frequently demonstrate no pathology. Most bleeding associated with the Mallory-Weiss syndrome will stop spontaneously, but if discovered on endoscopic evaluation may be treated with coagulation or sclerotherapy. Epinephrine injection and contact thermal multipolar coagulation therapy are useful, and metal clip or band ligation may be of utility in some cases.

Surgical therapy is limited in necessity, but may be accomplished via a gastrotomy and single-layer oversewing and closure in special situations.

Gastritis

Gastritis is associated with alcohol abuse, NSAIDs, severe anxiety, and HPI, among other contributors. Etiologies of gastritis include eosinophilia, Henoch-Schonlein gastritis, corrosive ingestions, viral infection, and bile reflux gastropathy, among others. Gastritis may present with mild intermittent symptoms of indigestion, but occasional hematemesis and/or epigastric discomfort may occur. Changes in appetite, nausea, and bloating may be the only symptoms, and in many patients who present with nonspecific abdominal complaints, gastritis may be noted as the diagnosis.

Viral, fungal, and parasitic infections may lead to gastritis, and providers in endemic regions should be aware of the risk factors. Anisakidosis, a nematode infestation from undercooked seafood containing larvae of *Anisakis simplex,* can result in an infestation-related gastritis, and should be treated with benzimidazole antihelminthic when discovered in association with gastritis or other intestinal inflammation. Antihelminthics may not be sufficient, however, and endoscopic or surgical removal of the worm may be required. Perforations have been reported.[13]

Most gastritis is treated with identification and elimination of the etiology, most importantly considering HPI. Particular historical features can usually identify a source, and it is important to monitor anemia and hepatic and renal function, and examine stool for occult blood, ova, parasites, and evidence of larvae. Treatment is nonsurgical except in extensive or gastritis with gastric wall phlegmon, which may require resection. PPIs, treatment of HPI, and eliminating contributors to pathology (NSAIDs, ethanol, etc.) are warranted. In most unusual situations, fulminant acute diffuse gastritis may be unresponsive to medical therapy alone, and endoscopic therapy is unhelpful due to the diffuse disease. Vascular control of the stomach can be achieved by ligation of any of the gastric supplying arteries, but this should be reserved for patients in whom bleeding is uncontrollable and unlocalizable to a single lesion. Operative technique is approached judiciously and identification of each branch performed with Rumel tourniquets or vessel loops, and ligation performed in a decisive manner sequentially, with each subsequent vessel checked for continued patency. Avoiding injury to the gastroepiploic and gastric arteries is imperative to avoid inadvertent ischemic complications, though the gastric blood supply is often sufficiently redundant.

Esophageal/Gastric Variceal Disease

Intraparenchymal or intraportal obstruction of the hepatic portal system increases intraportal pressure, and transmission of that increased pressure to all tributary vessels, including those emptying into the inferior and superior mesenteric and splenic veins. Normal portal pressure is <10 mm Hg due to very low hepatic sinusoidal resistance. Increased resistance in the portal system results in increased venous pressure in the tributaries to the portal system, including the left gastric vein and the coronary vein, which travel in close proximity to the gastroesophageal junction. Perisplenic venous structures may also be affected. Transmitted portal hypertension results in increased venous pressure in these structures, with resultant dilated, thin-walled varices that may be prone to rupture with increasing size and pressure. These patients present with often exsanguinating hematemesis.

Treatment of esophageal and gastric variceal disease must include treatment for (and possible elimination of) portal hypertension. This is challenging in the acutely decompensating patient, so focus is often placed upon temporarily controlling bleeding while definitive therapies are offered. Transjugular intrahepatic porto-systemic shunts (TIPSS) are used either as primary therapy or bridge to transplantation for portal hypertension, and may offer definitive—if only temporary—treatment for variceal bleeding. The presence of experienced interventional radiology providers is paramount to the success of TIPSS. Endoscopic sclerotherapy, banding, or clipping may be of utility, and medical therapeutics have demonstrated efficacy in controlling bleeding temporarily. These include somatostatin analogues, beta-antagonists, vasopressin, others. TIPSS is contraindicated in patients with hepatic encephalopathy, as their condition is likely to worsen or become refractory to prebiotic therapy.

The use of Sengstaken-Blakemore, Linton, or Minnesota tubes for esophagogastric tamponade has fallen out of favor. Though these devices did provide some control of bleeding, esophageal ischemia, esophagogastric perforation, and the ubiquitous and effective use of endoscopic techniques to curtail bleeding have reduced the need for these balloon tamponade devices. In some situations, however, they may be lifesaving. Currently, recommendations include usage only in patients with varices who fail or who are unable to undergo medical therapeutics, and as a temporary measure. These devices contain a manometry-monitored esophageal balloon and a large gastric balloon. The esophageal balloon must be completely evacuated prior to insertion. The lubricated tube is inserted in an intubated patient, and passed transorally into the stomach to a distance of approximately 45–60 cm, and the gastric balloon inflated with 100 ml of saline or water. Careful attention to inflation is paid to avoid esophageal rupture. A radiograph confirms intragastric location of the balloon, and it is inflated to 200–500 ml of water and traction placed on the tube, with the external portion secured to either a helmet or to the bedframe, to tamponade bleeding at the gastroesophageal junction. The patient should remain in a 30-degree head-up position. Only 500–1,000 grams of traction is required, and this may be accomplished with a liter bag of IV fluid, sandbag, or other light weight. If bleeding continues above the level of the gastroesophageal tamponade, the esophageal balloon is inflated *with air* to 35–45 mm Hg as measured by manometer. Every 1–2 hours, the pressure should be deflated for 10 minutes and monitored, then reinflated. The esophageal balloon should never be continuously inflated for longer than 6–12 hours.

During balloon tamponade, or in its absence, therapies targeting control or decrease of the portal gradient should be endeavored. Control of portal hypertension can be achieved with a combination of medical therapy (beta blockers, octreotide) and portosystemic shunting (operative or transjugular stenting). Local emergent control can be achieved in some cases by endoscopic band ligation, sclerotherapy, and clip placement, but portal hypertension predisposes these patients to rebleeding. Nearly 40% of patients will rebleed, depending upon the control of the portal hypertension and degree of cirrhosis.[14,15]

Surgical management of exsanguinating variceal bleeding can be accomplished with meso-caval or portacaval surgical shunts, but encephalopathy, coagulopathy, and poor nutrition contribute to mortality in these procedures. Techniques specific to these procedures are reviewed elsewhere.[16-18]

Gastric and Duodenal Perforation

Presentation

Perforation will often present with the acute and memorable onset of abdominal pain. Patients may report fevers, chills, rigors, nausea, and epigastric or right-sided abdominal pain. Generalized peritonitis is also possible. Some patients may present only with referred shoulder pain (Kerr's sign), vague abdominal symptoms, and belching, but often the presentation is quite dramatic. Peritoneal inflammation is typical, though occasionally ulcer perforations occur retroperitoneally or into the lesser sac, with less reliable physical findings. Patients may have a quiet abdomen upon auscultation. An acute worsening of previously experienced pain is not uncommon. Signs of systemic inflammatory response or sepsis may be present, including fever, tachycardia, hypotension, and mental status changes. These are ominous signs in the patient being evaluated for pain, and must be attended to with expedience.

Evaluation and Management

Patients who are being evaluated for abdominal pain should have early intravenous access and rehydration, and those with vomiting should have nasogastric decompression. Thorough physical examination and imaging should include an abdominal series, including an anteroposterior supine film and an upright chest radiograph or left-lateral decubitus film. Gravity-dependent studies may demonstrate extraluminal intraperitoneal air, indicating perforated viscus. Computed tomography (CT) may be included in the imaging algorithm as available but is not required nor recommended for the assessment of the acute abdomen, unless operative intervention must be delayed and all other studies are without significant finding. The discovery of pneumoperitoneum is diagnostic and an indication for exploration. Upper gastrointestinal contrast imaging with contrast gastro-duodenogram may indicate free extravasation of contrast from an ulcer, but may be an unnecessary step. Sonography has little value, except to demonstrate intraperitoneal fluid, but may not be sensitive enough to evaluate luminal integrity. Peritoneal lavage has no role in the current algorithm outside of traumatically injured patients.[7,19]

Laboratory analysis should be performed to diagnose acidemia and dehydration, and a leukocyte count can be evidence of inflammatory processes. Additionally, the platelet count and coagulation studies can be important as hepatic dysfunction and cirrhosis may be comorbid conditions among those patients with peptic ulcer disease.

The diagnosis of perforation should be made without endoscopy. Free intraperitoneal air, noted in the subphrenic space on an upright chest radiograph, or along the right peritoneal border on a lateral decubitus film, is diagnostic. Peritoneal signs in the absence of radiography-demonstrated free air may provide evidence sufficient for exploration, but with caution. Contrast extravasation is similarly diagnostic. Occasionally, patients will present following a prolonged delay after the onset of symptoms, and plain imaging demonstrates "free air." If the clinical picture demonstrates a stable, well-compensated patient, and if the history is uncertain or symptoms of similar discomfort have been experienced for longer than 24 hours, it may be prudent to perform a contrast exam (contrast CT or gastroduodenogram). Extravasation of contrast is an operative indication, but occasionally patients will demonstrate a sealed leak (i.e., free air on plain films or CT, and no leak on dynamic contrast studies). This situation, in the absence of sepsis or systemic inflammatory response syndrome (SIRS), may be treated with broad-spectrum antibiotics and observation alone, but close monitoring is prudent.

Patients undergoing exploration for perforation must receive general anesthesia with measures to protect the airway from significant aspiration, as gastric emptying is often delayed in peritonitis. Once under anesthetic, a vertical upper midline incision is the best approach to the stomach and duodenum. A right subcostal can be used but may be difficult in assessing the vascular supply of the stomach, and in examining the remainder of the viscus structures.

A midline incision is created and the structures of the peritoneum examined. Succus entericus is evacuated and irrigation provided to facilitate visualization. Obvious perforations are often seen on the anterior surface of the duodenum or distal stomach. Occasionally, the perforation is not evident, and thorough exploration of the lesser sac, visualization of the entire gastric surface anatomy, and Kocher maneuver performed to visualize the entire duodenum are important. Once discovered, the leak must be controlled to avoid further contamination, copious irrigation performed and evacuated, and definitive treatment undertaken.[19]

For patients who are treated chronically for ulcer disease, or for those in whom antacid therapy is unavailable or ineffective, a definitive acid-reducing procedure must be undertaken (see below). For those with untreated disease, control of the leak is a sufficient operation provided PPI and/or control of contributing factors (cessation of NSAIDs or other medications, eradication of HPI) has been undertaken, and the therapies and compliance can be monitored.

Gastric Outlet Obstruction

Presentation

Gastroduodenal obstruction may result from either benign or malignant etiologies. Peptic ulcer disease represents the most common benign source of obstruction. With the success of medical management for ulcer disease, however, malignant etiologies represent more than half of all GOO, and malignant presentations are often more indolent.[9,20] Patients with GOO typically present with nausea and nonbilious vomiting, with emesis occasionally containing undigested food. Early satiety, fullness, or bloating often accompany history, and patients with prolonged histories are often poorly nourished and experience loss of weight. Weight loss is more common and more pronounced in patients with malignant processes. Abdominal pain is often a late finding, and may precede the symptoms of obstruction as simply the symptoms of the underlying etiology, i.e., pancreatic neoplasm or peptic ulcer disease. Patients may appear dehydrated and malnourished. Dilated stomach, manifested as tympani in the left upper quadrant and epigastrum, may be present. Electrolyte abnormalities are not uncommon and often accompany patients with vomiting due to GOO. Loss of hydrochloric acid contributes to an increase in plasma bicarbonate production to compensate for lost chloride and sodium ions. This results in a hypokalemic, hypochloremic metabolic alkalosis. The alkalosis will initiate a shift of potassium into the extracellular space, favoring sequestration of hydrogen ions intracellularly, and renal excretion of potassium increases in an attempt to preserve sodium and water volume.

Only 5%–8% of patients with complicated ulcer disease present with obstruction.[21,22] Obstruction presents in the often dyspeptic patient with vague, sometimes intermittent symptoms, and may evolve over several days, culminating in the intolerance of oral intake. Occasionally, the patient may have weight loss and malnutrition. Patients will have sometimes vigorous vomiting or retching, and may have brief episodic hematemesis representing mucosal tears related to retching (Mallory-Weiss syndrome).[23] Patients may also present with a contraction alkalosis.

Evaluation and Management

ABC should be considered in the vomiting patient and should be watched carefully. Aspiration of gastric contents adds to surgical risk and added morbidity. Clinical suspicion and a dilated stomach on plain radiography are usually sufficient to make the diagnosis of outlet obstruction, but contrast studies may provide a more definitive diagnosis. Endoscopy can reveal peripyloric or duodenal pathology contributing to the obstruction in the malignant or benign etiology. Acute inflammation and edema at the pylorus are the usual findings, but chronic changes with fibrosis may be evident in patients with long history. Contrast studies may be useful with inert or barium-based contrast materials. Upper endoscopy can be diagnostic in facile hands. Visualization is often good, given the failure of insufflated air to move quickly past the stomach. Scarring and fibrosis may be present at the pylorus, precluding transition into the proximal duodenum.

Patients presenting with gastric obstruction should be judiciously fluid resuscitated and electrolyte or metabolic abnormalities treated. The diagnosis of GOO on contrast imaging should prompt admission, nasogastric decompression, electrolyte and fluid repletion, and a monitored setting due to sometimes severe alkalosis in some patients. Patients who do not resolve despite 48–72 hours of decompression with fluid administration and antisecretory therapy may require surgical intervention. Balloon dilatation of a scarred, chronically diseased pylorus has been reported, and may be a reasonable therapy. In this setting, however, endoscopy with histology is imperative, as more than 50% of patients with GOO in the setting of peptic ulcer disease (PUD) have a malignancy.[23]

Antrectomy with truncal vagotomy is the definitive operation in this setting, with simultaneous distal jejunal feeding tube placement. Resolution of the gastric obstruction with acid-reducing maneuvers treats the primary problem while distal enteral access provides for nutritional supplementation. Occasionally, scarring at the pylorus precludes safe antrectomy, requiring only vagotomy and a drainage procedure, including loop gastrojejunostomy. Evaluation for malignancy is similarly important here.[24]

When neoplasia is the causative factor in GOO, pancreatic cancer is the most likely diagnosis. Patients presenting with a pancreatic mass and outlet obstruction may eventually be amenable to resection, but often the advanced nature of the obstructing lesion results in the need to create a surgical bypass, either with the less common duodenoduodenostomy (as in congenital lesions, annular pancreas, or other benign findings), or with a loop gastrojejunostomy. When the lesion is amenable, endoscopic stenting may be a better palliative means for therapy than open surgical bypass.[24]

Bezoar

Presentation

Patients with bezoars often present with a chief complaint of vague epigastric pain. Undigested plant material (phytobezoar), ingested hair (trichobezoar), and milk (lactobezoar) are relatively common. Pharmacobezoars may be encountered as well, comprised of undigested medications. Nausea, vomiting, anorexia, early satiety, and weight loss are not uncommon. Large bezoars can result in gastric mucosal necrosis, ulceration, and perforation in rare cases. Physical exam is often without revealing signs, though a palpable mass is occasionally discovered. Patients with history of trichotillomania (chronic ingestion of hair) may present with concurrent patchy hair loss.

Evaluation and Management

Bezoars can be demonstrated on plain films in the patient being evaluated for abdominal pain. CT scans may provide more information, though often merely an amorphous mass appears intraluminally. Contrast studies will often demonstrate filling defects, but nearly 80% of bezoars can be missed on imaging studies. Endoscopy remains the gold standard for the diagnosis, and may provide histological or physical evidence of the source.[25]

Surgical Management of Gastroduodenal Pathology

Approach to the Stomach and Duodenum

Following diagnostic and resuscitative maneuvers, surgical management can be lifesaving. Attention to patient compliance, home support, preoperative nutritional status, and functional ability all contribute to operative planning. Following a vertical, midline incision and entry into the peritoneum, the falciform ligament is controlled with clamps, divided, and ligated to allow retraction of the right hepatic lobe. The stomach and duodenum must be exposed, which is facilitated by self-retaining retractor (e.g., Balfour or Bookwalter) when possible, and nasogastric or orogastric decompression. This author prefers retraction of the right hepatic lobe with folded laparotomy sponges, and the right costal margin retracted with a body-wall retractor. Use of a headlamp is ideal, but well-positioned floor, ceiling, or handheld supplemental lighting may offer improved vision. The omentum should be first gently elevated from its position, with attention paid to pathological adhesions. The omentum may be a key component in surgical therapy and should be preserved as much as possible.[18]

The gastric anatomy should be evaluated, and the existence of a hiatal hernia, dense short gastric attachments, and other nearby anatomical variations and pathology noted. Preservation of the gastric vascular supply is prudent, with early identification of the gastroepiploic and gastric arteries.

The stomach may be manipulated easily with the surgeon's hand, but overzealous retraction before control of a perforation could increase contamination. Adequate suction evacuation is desirable. Additionally, well-intentioned instrumentation can result in further injury, especially to the duodenum, and should be avoided. The duodenum should be handled with the gloved hand alone or with a moistened sponge.

Control of Bleeding/Perforation/Obstruction

Similar approaches can be made to evaluate the stomach and duodenum. Exposure through a generous midline is usually sufficient, and a self-retaining retractor is often helpful. Subcostal incisions on the right may facilitate duodenal and distal gastric dissection, while a left subcostal approach may make hiatus and fundus procedures more accessible. This author prefers a generous upper midline approach for the vast majority of gastroduodenal pathologies.

For bleeding, access to the lumen of the stomach or duodenum must be created. Endoscopic evaluation can facilitate gastric or duodenal incision initially, as visualization can be quite specific. Without endoscopic localization, the patient's history will help to dictate the location of the enterotomy, but for most cases, the stomach is more forgiving and should be approached first. For gastric bleeding, a generous mid-to-distal body gastrotomy is performed with electrocautery or sharp incision. The gastric edges are held with stay sutures or atraumatic clamps and contamination is minimized. The gastric contents are evacuated with suction if possible, and an examination of the mucosa performed. Active bleeding can be controlled with figure-of-eight or simple suture ligation and the remainder of the stomach examined. Friability of mucosal tissues should be anticipated. Actively bleeding vessels are oversewn similarly, and suture ends left long to identify the location after control. Once bleeding is controlled, locations are evaluated. If ulcers exist, and assessment identifies chronically inflamed tissue or suspicion of tumor, wedge resection and biopsy for neoplasia should be performed. If frozen section histology is available, a malignancy can be identified early and definitive operation performed. In the acidemic, hypotensive or coagulopathic patient, prudence may suggest to control bleeding and return for definitive therapy after histological diagnosis can be obtained. Incisional biopsy should be included, with frozen-section assessment of histology performed when feasible. When contamination has been reduced and the offending event controlled, an acid-reducing procedure may then be undertaken.

If bleeding is identified in the duodenum, a pyloric incision and (subsequent pyloroplasty) may be performed to facilitate control. This is easily performed with sharp dissection, and should include 2–4 cm onto each of the stomach and duodenum. Avoiding electrocautery or other energy devices is important, as any ischemia to the pylorus and duodenal repair will increase the risk of leak or late stricture. The midpoint of the longitudinal incision, begun on the distal antrum and continued along the anterior surface to the proximal duodenum, is secured with stay sutures of long silk (Figure 13.1). Elevation of these sutures in opposite directions will facilitate visualization into the duodenal lumen, and will facilitate closure in a transverse direction. This has been described by Heineke and Mikulicz previously, and is widely reported.[20] Bleeding in the posterior duodenum from the gastroduodenal artery can be controlled with passage of a *U*-shaped stitch, encompassing the vessel's three contributors (Figure 13.2). The gastroduodenal artery courses along the posterior duodenum in a caudad direction, with a medial branch toward the pancreas, as if it were an uppercase letter *T* on its side. Careful ligation of all three branches is required for adequate bleeding control. Figure 13.3 depicts the means of closure. A two-layer closure is traditionally performed, but in the transverse direction, preventing stricture.

In the setting of perforation, warm lavage of the peritoneal cavity is an important first step, both to decrease contamination and to increase visibility. Localization of an unknown perforation will determine the operative plan. Gastric perforations may be closed primarily by direct suture, given the redundancy of gastric wall, and control is easily obtained with one or two layers. Patients with chronic ulcer or recurrent disease must raise suspicion of malignant disease, and a wedge resection with frozen-section assessment can help guide the surgical hand.[26]

For perforations in proximity (<1 cm) of the pylorus, the etiology is usually inflammatory, or acid hypersecretion (Figure 13.4). Single- or two-layer closure of a small lesion is reasonable and relatively simply achieved. Thicker, more inflamed tissue may preclude the success of simple primary closure. As mentioned, biopsy is indicated for lesions on the stomach as well as for suspiciously thickened or dense tissue, as the risk of malignancy does exist. Upon closure of the perforation, stricture is an important and morbid complication, so suture closure is always oriented

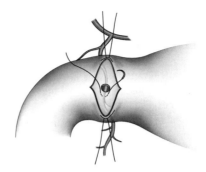

FIGURE 13.2   Once exposed, the posterior wall of the duodenum is often the site of bleeding, with the gastroduodenal artery descending behind the second portion. A U-stitch is configured by passing the suture lateral-to-medial at the inferior aspect of the ulcer, and reversing the direction at the superior aspect. This will often control bleeding and help visualization. The suture is passed full-thickness through the duodenal wall. Illustration by Jacob C. Wood.

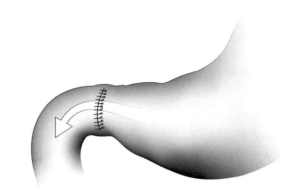

FIGURE 13.3   Closure of the pyloric-duodenal incision is completed transversely, which helps to prevent stricture. Two-layer closure is preferred. Of note, passage of an enteral feeding tube is facilitated by visualization before this closure. Illustration by Jacob C. Wood.

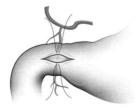

FIGURE 13.1   A longitudinal incision is made along the pylorus and extends several centimeters onto the anterior proximal duodenum. Stay sutures used in the midpoint of the incision along both sides help with exposure and can be used to assist in configuring closure. Illustration by Jacob C. Wood.

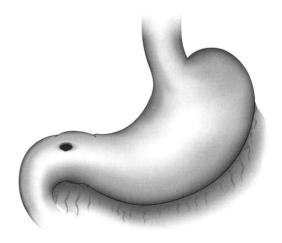

FIGURE 13.4   A pyloric channel ulcer perforation is often anterior and clearly visible upon entering the peritoneum. Illustration by Jacob C. Wood.

transversely (Figure 13.3). Additionally, for lesions of the pyloric channel, a patch of a viable segment of omentum can offer additional protection. The tongue of omentum is allowed to lie in place following vertical mattress-type suture placement, and tension is avoided. The omentum is then included in the closure, allowing for a buttressing of the sutures placed. Sutures are tied down to approximate the tissues, but avoid strangulation of the omental segment (Figure 13.6). A closed-suction drain is optional.[27]

For patients with complicated ulcer disease (bleeding, perforation, or obstruction), pyloroplasty with vagotomy should be the operative plan of choice. Resection is not required in the setting of acute perforation, as aggressive acid reduction therapy and eradication of HPI are very effective, but biopsy of suspicious lesions should be undertaken to avoid missed neoplasm. Truncal vagotomy is simply approached, and the vagus nerves are identified in their anatomic positions and divided. Often a small segment of vagus is excised for histological confirmation. Pyloroplasty can be performed in any number of means to avoid post-vagotomy pyloric stenosis.

In patients with GOO at or near the pylorus, the approach is to provide effective gastric emptying without disruption of physiology. A generous pyloroplasty must be performed to obviate recurrence, and an acid-reducing procedure performed as described. In patients with significant scarring of the pylorus due to chronic disease, it is reasonable and safe to perform definitive acid-reduction therapy with a gastric-emptying diverting procedure without resection to palliate the obstruction, but concern for malignancy must be raised. Those with outlet obstruction and concern for neoplasia may be treated with antrectomy and reconstruction. A Billroth-type reconstructive gastrojejunostomy or roux-n-Y gastric decompression may be performed. The reconstruction may include a direct gastroduodenostomy (Billroth I) or a gastrojejunostomy utilizing a loop of jejunum 20–40 cm distal to the ligament of Treitz. Both procedures have particularities of technique including leak and recurrent ulceration.[28]

Following gastroduodenal surgery, nasogastric decompression is important to prevent gastric dilatation and ischemia proximal to the repair. Nasogastric tubes should be sump-type tubes affixed to low-pressure suction or open to gravity drainage, and may be removed as early as 1 to 3 days postoperatively, according to surgeon preference and volume of drainage. Postoperatively, contrast studies are at the preference of the surgeon, though their value in the simple repair is unclear.[24,27]

Diet should be advanced as tolerated, and bowel regimen provided including gastric-emptying facilitation and/or antiemetics for comfort. Early mobilization and activity will assist with pulmonary recovery, and avoidance of excessive exertion prevents wound concerns including dehiscence and late hernia development.

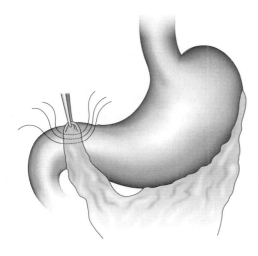

FIGURE 13.5 A strip of omentum is gently raised and, after sutures are placed in the transverse direction to closure, delivered without tension to the debrided perforated ulcer. Illustration by Jacob C. Wood.

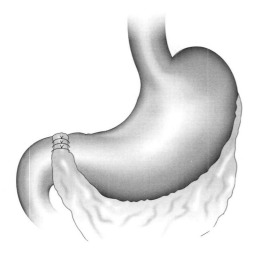

FIGURE 13.6 Sutures are then secured over the omental flap, fixating the omental patch in place. Strangulating the omentum is counterproductive. Illustration by Jacob C. Wood.

Trauma

Traumatic injuries to the stomach are repaired with the basic tenets of gastrointestinal surgery. Small (<5 cm) injuries can be managed with debridement and primary single-layer or two-layer closure. Stapling devices are successfully utilized in this setting, when available, but caution should be employed to confirm full thickness apposition. Larger defects or a significant quantity of devitalized tissue may require larger debridement or formal resection and reconstruction as previously described. Large injuries to the proximal body and fundus may be primarily closed with little concern in previously healthy patients, so long as the esophagus is uncompromised. Larger injuries in the distal stomach may be repaired primarily in addition, though pyloric injuries may require additional reconstruction or pyloroplasty. Postoperatively, nasogastric decompression is usually required, though the duration of decompression depends upon volume of drainage and should not be arbitrary.

Traumatic duodenal injuries should be repaired primarily when <1.5–2 cm, but larger wounds may require duodenal exclusion or diverticulization and requisite gastric decompression with loop gastrojejunostomy. Biliary outflow must not be compromised and repairs are often tenuous, so judicious drainage with closed systems is advocated. Distal enteral access is also highly suggested, given the duration and frequency with which patients experiencing this type of trauma must go without oral intake.[29]

Penetrating injuries to one aspect of the stomach are often accompanied by a second wound when the implement passes through-and-through the organ. Exploration must include the posterior gastric wall and the anterior body of the pancreas, as well as the mesenteric root. Nasogastric decompression of the stomach is recommended following repair.

Foreign Bodies

Foreign bodies in the stomach and duodenum may occasionally be ameliorated with endoscopic means. Failure of these means, or the need to retrieve more sinister ingestions, for example, batteries, magnets, or sharp objects, requires surgical intervention and removal.

Watchful waiting may be employed for simple, small objects, provided radiological monitoring is available to follow the object. Objects often lodge at the gastroesophageal junction or pylorus, but beyond the upper GI tract, most objects will obstruct at the ileocecal valve. Careful attention to this possibility is important. In the absence of endoscopic or radiological expectant management, operative intervention early may potentiate the avoidance of an unexpected perforation or obstruction.

Enteral Access

Decompression

Traditionally, patients with gastroduodenal pathology are treated with nasogastric tube decompression as a diagnostic and/or therapeutic maneuver. Patients with nausea from GOO, gastric dilatation, or poor emptying will often have significant relief from decompression and evacuation. Similarly, aspiration of gastric contents may be helpful in determining bile or blood content of the aspirant. Tubes used for gastric decompression may be placed transorally or transnasally, favoring the nasogastric route in patients who are awake. These tubes should be flexible, and of 16 French size or better in the adult, and should have a functional sump incorporated in their construction, as in the Salem Sump. Nonsump tubes risk adherence to gastric mucosa, inefficient evacuation, and tube obstruction. Ideally, tubes should be placed with the patient seated upright in the chin-down position. Water-soluble lubricant facilitates placement, as does having the awake patient sip water and swallow as the tube passes. Patients in the supine position should not be asked to drink liquids. Antiemetics provided prior to placement may result in a decrease in the likelihood of vomiting and aspiration. Once in place, the patient should be asked to phonate. Inability to phonate may indicate intratracheal placement. The tube should be insufflated with 20–50 ml of air while auscultating the abdomen to audibly confirm intragastric placement. Once in place, the tube should be secured at the nose with caution, as pressure on the nasal ala can result in soft tissue necrosis and loss.

Patients with gastric decompression can have losses including 1.5 liters or greater daily, and lose acid, chloride, and potassium. Repletion of these losses should be 1:1, and should include 0.45% or 0.9% sodium chloride with added potassium chloride. Careful attention to fluid losses can abate progression to a metabolic alkalosis.

Patients with signs of obstruction should be investigated and remedied of the etiology with haste. Patients can evolve a metabolic alkalosis rapidly, and coagulopathy or profound hypokalemia, can complicate surgical intervention. Fluid resuscitation, nasogastric decompression, and radiological studies should be endeavored early in the course of diagnosis and treatment. Surgical treatment for intestinal obstruction should be pursued with equal rapidity.

Feeding Access

Enteral access is often important in patients with malnutrition. Many means exist to provide access, including nasogastric, nasojejunal, or orogastric/orojejunal tube placement. Surgically achieved access should be considered in any patient with other operative indications and performed judiciously at the time of definitive therapy. Those in a damage-control setting should be considered for access, and considerations made for their severity of illness.

Many types of surgical gastrostomy tubes exist, and they vary according to manufacturer. The simplest tube is usually sufficient—it includes a balloon for intraluminal security, and a single lumen with one or more distal outlet openings and a single or double access port. Placement is easily achieved during laparotomy by introduction into the peritoneal cavity through a separate stab incision, and subsequent placement into the gastric lumen via a double or single purse-string suture around an adequate gastrotomy. The balloon is inflated within the lumen and the catheter secured with the pursestring. Once within the lumen, the gastric serosa is secured in the traditional Stamm fashion by individual sutures from the gastric wall up to the abdominal wall, in close proximity to the tube entry. This will facilitate evolution of an intact tract, allowing for long-term access, and decreasing the likelihood of leak. Longer tubes are available which permit transgastric jejunal access for nutrition and medication administration. Some contain intragastric sump ports for gastric decompression with simultaneous jejunal administration.

Caution should be observed when maintaining tubes, as narrow-lumen tubes will often form concretions of a variety of medications or nutritional supplements, occluding the lumen. Frequent attention to patency, using flushing and tube assessments, is an important consideration.

Occluded tubes can often be cleared by instillation of lytic agents, including carbonated beverages (soda water), papain-containing food-preparation agents (meat tenderizer), and even commercially available agents, but the best method is to provide frequent flushes with water and avoid clogs altogether. The use of brushes or probes risks perforation of the tube sidewall, therefore increasing the risk of gastrointestinal lumen perforation.

Summary

This chapter includes discussion of the evaluation, diagnosis, and treatment for the most common gastroduodenal emergencies, with a focus on the surgical management of these problems. Though not a comprehensive list of gastroduodenal pathologies, the most common emergencies are discussed. Care of the patient with gastroduodenal pathology will include restoration of circulating volume, acid reduction therapy, control of bleeding and contamination, and reconstitution of gastroduodenal continuity. Also important are considerations for etiology of disease, eradication of infection, and the provision of nutrition.

COMMENTARY

Ntakiyiruta Georges, Rwanda

In Rwanda, the gastric pathologies amenable to surgical treatment are dominated by perforation and obstruction. Upper GI bleeding is not very frequent, and the patient's history will help to establish a differential diagnosis, which will guide further investigations.

As a result of limited resources, variceal bleeding is very challenging to manage. There are very few interventionist endoscopists, Sengstaken-Blakemore tubes are not available, and TIPSS is not yet available. Additionally, there is no vascular surgical capacity to manage portal hypertension. However, established gastric bleeding (duodenal or gastric) that does not respond to resuscitation measures is amenable to surgical management for direct surgical hemostasis.

GOO is highly prevalent and always requires surgery. Newborns with a diagnosis of hypertrophic pyloric stenosis receive a Ramstedt operation. In adults, the gastric outflow is blocked by scarring from either duodenal ulcer or a distal gastric cancer. Pancreatic cancer may obstruct the gastric outflow, but this is not the most frequent cause of the blockage among patients in Rwanda. The insidious onset of symptoms for a gastric cancer makes the patients present late with advanced cancer. In addition to the symptoms and signs that are well discussed in the chapter, the abdominal examination will show visible peristalsis from left to right, and the succussion splash is always present.

After a well-conducted fluid resuscitation and correction of electrolytes imbalance, we also approach through an upper midline incision that may be extended depending on the operative diagnosis. In case of pyloric stenosis, many surgeons will perform either a pyloroplasty or posterior (retrocolic) gastrojejunostomy. As medical treatment to reduce gastric acid secretion is now readily available, truncal vagotomy is less frequently considered as a surgical option.

In case of distal gastric cancer, at surgery we assess the tumor resectability. If the tumor is resectable, we perform a partial gastrectomy and we reconstruct with either a Billroth I (gastroduodenostomy) or a Billroth II (gastrojejunostomy) when technically the Billroth I is not possible.

In cases of unresectable gastric tumors, we always perform a bypass with anterior (antecolic) gastrojejunostomy in order to delay local invasion of the stoma by the tumor.

14

Liver, Pancreas and Gall Bladder

Kelly Hewitt
Raymond R. Price

Biliary Disease

Introduction

More than 3,500 years ago, autopsy studies in Egypt and China provided the earliest reports of gallstones.[1] Remarkably, the first successful cholecystectomy was not performed until 1882, by Carl Langenbuch at the Lazarus Krankenhaus in Berlin, Germany.[2] In England at the beginning of the twentieth century, the surgical profession hesitated to diagnose a patient with gallstones unless the patient was jaundiced. Laparoscopic cholecystectomy revolutionized surgical treatment of the gallbladder less than 100 years later, resulting in cholecystectomy becoming the most common elective abdominal surgical procedure performed in the United States and much of the developed world. At a cost of more than $6 billion USD annually, gallbladder disease constitutes a significant health burden for the United States.

Cholecystectomy in low- and middle-income countries (LMICs) is much less common. The frequency of any surgical procedure is directly related to the disease prevalence, local social acceptance and perceived need for the procedure, appropriately trained healthcare providers, and accessibility of care for the population. Accessibility may be limited by austere environments, inadequate facilities, and limited human and physical resources. Patients tend to then present later in the course of their disease, resulting in more complex and difficult biliary operations.

Worldwide Burden of Gallbladder Disease

Identifying the true burden of gallbladder disease presents a complex interrelated conundrum. Ultrasound identification of the number of people harboring gallstones in a defined population at a specified time quantifies the prevalence of asymptomatic gallstones—of which at most 20% ever develop symptoms.[3] Autopsy studies similarly indicate a baseline prevalence of gallstones but do not address the incidence of symptomatic disease. Operative logs underestimate the true burden of gallbladder disease as they are significantly limited by access and social constraints.

Prevalence of gallstones serves as a surrogate for identifying one type of gallbladder disease. The prevalence of gallstones varies widely among various ethnic groups and localities. The Pima Indian women over age 30 in North America have the highest prevalence rate (73%), while gallstones are nearly non-existent in the Masai and Bantu tribes in Eastern Sub-Saharan Africa.[4] In South America, gallstones afflict the native Chilean Mapuche in 49.4% of their women and 12.6% of their men. Prevalence rates are fairly similar in Northern Europe and white American women (20% and 16.6%, respectively); rates drop to 11% in Italy. Intermediate rates occur in Asian populations (women 13.9% and men 5.3%).[4] In Sub-Saharan Africa, earlier twentieth-century studies reported gallstone prevalence rates of less than 5%. However, countries like Nigeria, South Africa, and Ethiopia have documented rapidly increasing prevalence rates and numbers of patients requiring cholecystectomy.[5-8]

Risk Factors

Worldwide, regardless of race or geographic location, gallbladder disease affects women more than men. A Western diet high in refined carbohydrates and fat (triglycerides) and low in fiber has been implicated in unmasking the presumably inherent genetic predisposition in American Indians and in the rising incidence of gallbladder disease in urban areas of Sub-Saharan Africa. Rapid weight loss and obesity, which is also spreading to LMICs, increase the incidence of gallstones. Disease processes such as cirrhosis (infections etiologies more common than alcoholic), Crohn's disease, cystic fibrosis, and various hemolytic anemias such as sickle cell disease (more common in some African populations) are associated with a higher prevalence of gallstones. Other risk factors include oral contraceptive use and estrogen replacement therapy.[1] Older patients with gallstones may develop symptoms up to 40% of the time compared to only 1%–2% per year in younger patients.[9]

Bile and Gallbladder Function

The liver produces approximately 700 ml of bile daily. Bile is composed of electrolytes, bilirubin, bile salts, phospholipids, and cholesterol. The gallbladder functions to store and secrete this bile into the intestines in response to stimulation from eating a meal. The gallbladder also has an absorptive capability and acts to concentrate bile through the absorption of water and electrolytes. Bile secreted into the intestines aids in the body's absorption of fats and fat-soluble vitamins and also allows for excretion of cholesterol and bilirubin. Cholecystokinin, a hormone released from the duodenum, is a major stimulant for gallbladder emptying. Following secretion into the duodenum, bile acids are reabsorbed in the terminal ileum and recycled—the cycle of enterohepatic circulation.

Types of Gallstones

Gallstones can be either cholesterol or pigment stones. Cholesterol stones clearly predominate in high-income countries (HICs) and make up approximately 70%–80% of stones seen in the United States and closer to 60% in some African countries.[10] The presence of biliary sludge (particulate material generally composed of cholesterol crystals and calcium salts) may aid in the formation of stones and can be seen in individuals who have undergone prolonged fasting, are pregnant, or have undergone rapid weight loss.[1]

Pigment stones can be either black or brown. Black pigment stones usually are formed in individuals with hemolytic or hepatic conditions and are found in the gallbladder. Brown pigment stones, the predominant type in Asia and which can originate in the bile ducts, lead to increased biliary obstruction and recurrent cholangitis resulting in dilation and stricturing of the biliary tree.[1]

Diagnostic Studies

Laboratory

Simple biochemical studies should be evaluated to assist in the diagnosis of biliary disease. A complete blood count (CBC) can identify patients with leukocytosis or anemia. Elevated liver function tests (LFTs) can help differentiate between the myriad of other causes of upper abdominal pain. An elevated bilirubin suggests choledocholithiasis and when combined with an elevated amylase or lipase indicates possible gallstone pancreatitis.

Imaging Modalities

The various modalities used to image the gallbladder and its function may be limited depending on geographic location and local resources. The most accessible and useful tool is the abdominal ultrasound (US). An abdominal ultrasound can be used to assess asymptomatic, symptomatic, benign, and malignant biliary system pathology. Ultrasonography is the gold standard for diagnosing cholelithiaisis, having a specificity and sensitivity of over 95% for gallstones greater than 1.5 mm in size. Ultrasonography provides important information about the thickness of the gallbladder wall, evidence of pericholecystic fluid, and size of the common bile duct; these findings can help identify more complex patients and can guide important preoperative and intraoperative decisions. While US is sensitive for gallstones in the gallbladder, abdominal US may miss small gallstones in the common bile duct (50% sensitive).

Other imaging modalities can aid in the visualization of the gallbladder and biliary system. Some allow for potential interventions. Unfortunately, in LMICs, most are unlikely to be available outside of teaching facilities or private institutions in urban areas. Acquisition of endoscopic retrograde cholangiopancreatography (ERCP) skills requires considerable training, but ERCP is a highly sensitive and specific method for evaluating the biliary and pancreatic ducts. While common bile duct stones can be extracted and sphincterotomies performed, complications, including pancreatitis, bleeding, and duodenal perforation, can occur up to 5%–8% of the time; the mortality rate following endoscopic sphincterotomy (ES) is 0.5%–0.8%.[11]

Magnetic resonance cholangiopancreatography (MRCP) lacks therapeutic capability but is increasingly used for its diagnostic capability. Hepatobiliary iminodiacetic acid (HIDA) scans evaluate function and cystic duct obstruction. When performed appropriately, patients can be diagnosed with biliary dyskinesia. Transhepatic percutaneous cholangiopancreatography (TPC) requires advanced equipment and interventional radiology training but can be useful in accessing, diagnosing, and treating biliary pathology when available. Limited information exists in LMICs about the use of MRCP, TPC, and HIDA scans, but they are likely to increasingly find a role as access to these diagnostic capabilities improves in LMICs.

Differential Diagnosis

Gallbladder disease may go unrecognized for many years as not all patients report the classic symptoms of right upper quadrant abdominal pain radiating either to the back or in a band-like fashion around the upper abdomen occurring particularly after fatty meals. Many of the symptoms—nausea, vomiting, diarrhea, increased gas, bloating, and burping—are nonspecific, commonly related to other disease processes including indigestion, constipation, or gastroesophageal reflux disease (GERD). The differential diagnosis includes peptic ulcer disease, pancreatitis, small bowel obstructions of various causes, amebic liver abscesses, a right basilar pneumonia, cardiac ischemia, and kidney stones.

Biliary symptoms may arise from simple biliary colic, acute cholecystitis, biliary dyskinesia, choledocholithiasis, gallstone pancreatitis, gallstone ileus, parasitic infestation, or gallbladder

---

BOX 14.1   TAILORING TREATMENT TO AVAILABLE RESOURCES

Evaluating available resources is critical in providing safe treatment for gallbladder disease in LMICs. The accessibility of preoperative imaging may be limited to ultrasound and a few basic laboratory tests. Even these basic studies can help guide decisions about the advisability of performing surgery locally or referring to a larger center. When facilities lack equipment and instruments for common bile duct exploration, and if a patient is jaundiced, has a dilated common bile duct on ultrasound, and has an elevated bilirubin, referral to a larger medical center may be more prudent rather than a biliary drainage procedure for temporary amelioration of symptoms that still requires definitive treatment. However, whether because of the clinical status of the patient, geography, or social reasons, referral may not be an option. In many instances, surgical options must be tailored to provide the best possible care given the available resources. Cholecystostomy or t-tube drainage may be required until definitive care can be provided. In hospitals that perform laparoscopic and open cholecystectomy but do not have the capability to perform laparoscopic common bile duct exploration or ERCP, surgeons should operate through an open approach to allow for the necessary common bile duct exploration at the same time.

carcinoma. Within the confines of the LMIC, a detailed history coupled with a few simple laboratory tests and ultrasound evaluation of the abdomen provides a sure compass for healthcare professionals in LMICs to correctly navigate toward the correct diagnosis and design appropriate treatment.

Surgical Anatomy

Understanding the anatomy of the gallbladder, the cystic duct, and its blood supply, along with their normal variants, is critical for successful and safe surgical care of biliary diseases (Figure 14.1). The gallbladder is a blind pouch that is connected to the liver and duodenum via ducts. The gallbladder contains up to approximately 50 ml of bile and is situated against the liver and attached by a reflection of the visceral peritoneum. The cystic duct emanates from the gallbladder and joins the common hepatic duct to form the common bile duct. The common hepatic duct is formed from the union of the right and left hepatic ducts draining bile from the liver. The common bile duct travels through the pancreas and drains into the duodenum via the papilla of Vater. The pancreatic duct can join the common bile duct at or prior to its entrance into the duodenum or may also drain into the duodenum by a separate opening.

The arterial blood supply of the gallbladder comes from the cystic artery, which usually arises from a branch of the right hepatic artery; approximately 15%–20% of the time the cystic artery may come off branches from the superior mesenteric artery (SMA). The common bile duct (CBD) receives branches from the common and right hepatic arteries supplying the marginal arteries that run parallel to the CBD on the antero-lateral portions of the duct and communicate with an epicholedochal plexus around the bile ducts. The venous drainage of the gallbladder and bile ducts empties into the portal system.

Healthcare providers operating on the gallbladder must understand the relationship of the gallbladder, cystic duct, cystic artery, and hepatic and common bile ducts. Commonly, the cystic artery is found in the center of the triangle of Calot (Figure 14.2).

However, when the cystic artery arises from branches of the SMA, the cystic artery may be encountered in a reverse fashion, posing a challenge during cholecystectomy. Recognizing the common anatomical biliary variations (Figure 14.3) and their relationship to the cystic arterial variants is crucial in preventing injuries to the bile ducts (Figure 14.4).

Gallbladder Pathophysiology

Biliary Colic

Approximately 20% of people with gallstones ultimately become symptomatic from gallstones. Of all asymptomatic individuals with gallstones, approximately 1%–2% per year develop serious symptoms or complications. Biliary colic is often the initial presentation of symptomatic gallstones defined as postprandial right upper quadrant or epigastric pain that occur as the result of transient impaction of a gallstone in the neck of the gallbladder. Biliary colic is classically thought to occur after consuming fatty foods, although this is not always the case. Pain can also be constant when the cystic duct remains obstructed. Pain generally lasts between 1 and 24 hours in biliary colic and may be severe enough to prompt seeking medical attention. Pain medicine and oral or intravenous (IV) hydration may help alleviate the acute symptoms, while avoiding fatty foods can sometimes provide longer intervals between attacks. However, elective or urgent cholecystectomy should be considered for long-term cure.

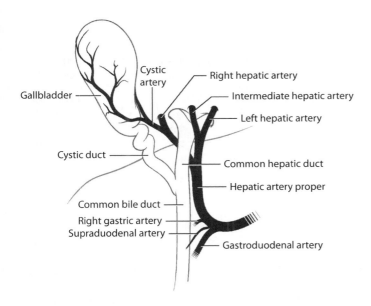

FIGURE 14.1 Normal anatomy of the gallbladder, bile ducts, and their blood supply. Illustrated by Jill Rhead. Intermountain Healthcare. Adapted from: Mulholland, et al. *Greenfield's Surgery: Scientific Principles and Practice*. Philadelphia: Lippincott Williams & Wilkins, 2006.

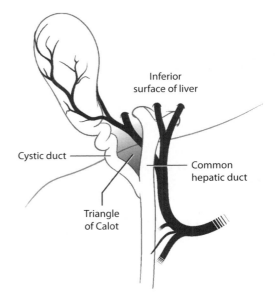

FIGURE 14.2 Triangle of Calot. Illustrated by Jill Rhead. Intermountain Healthcare. Adapted from: Norton J, et al. *Surgery: Basic Science and Clinical Evidence*. New York: Springer Publishing Company, 2008.

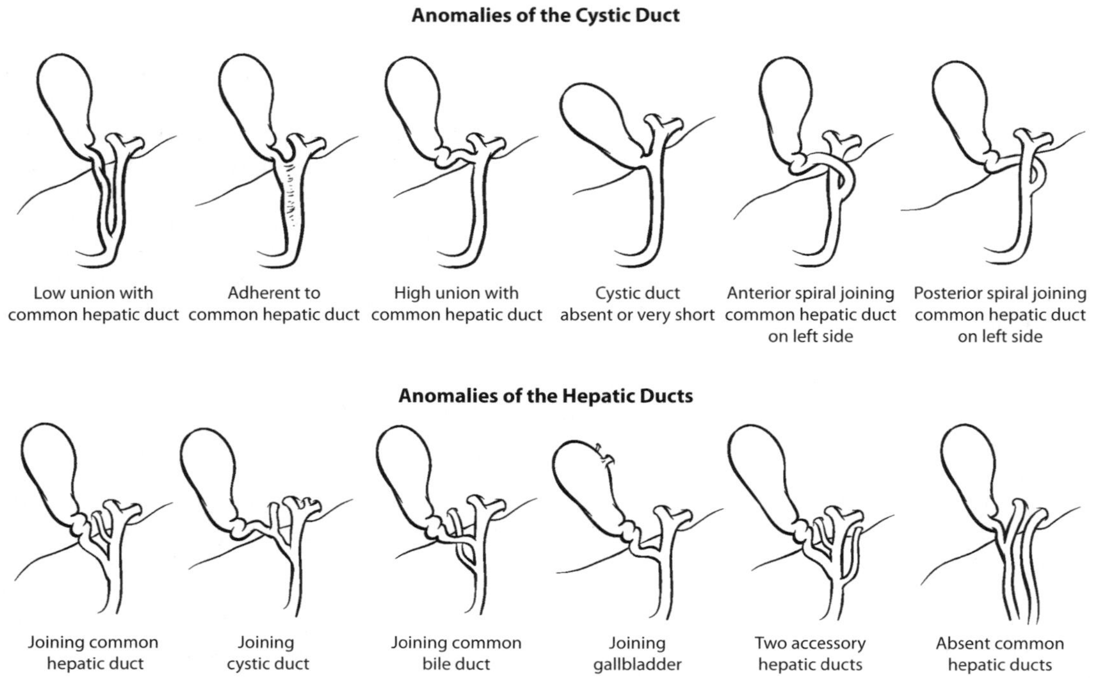

Anomalies of the Cystic Duct

| Low union with common hepatic duct | Adherent to common hepatic duct | High union with common hepatic duct | Cystic duct absent or very short | Anterior spiral joining common hepatic duct on left side | Posterior spiral joining common hepatic duct on left side |

Anomalies of the Hepatic Ducts

| Joining common hepatic duct | Joining cystic duct | Joining common bile duct | Joining gallbladder | Two accessory hepatic ducts | Absent common hepatic ducts |

FIGURE 14.3 Common anatomical cystic and hepatic duct biliary variations. Illustrated by Jill Rhead. Intermountain Healthcare. Adapted from: Mulholland, et al. *Greenfield's Surgery: Scientific Principles and Practice.* Philadelphia: Lippincott Williams & Wilkins, 2006.

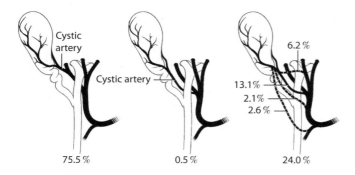

FIGURE 14.4 Common cystic artery variants and relationship to bile ducts. Illustrated by Jill Rhead. Intermountain Healthcare. Adapted from: Norton J, et al. *Surgery: Basic Science and Clinical Evidence.* New York: Springer Publishing Company, 2008.

TABLE 14.1

Tokyo guidelines for diagnosis of acute cholecystitis*

Local signs of inflammation	Systemic signs of inflammation	Imaging results
Murphy's sign	Fever	Imaging findings
RUQ mass/pain/ tenderness	Elevated CRP	characteristic of acute
	Elevated WBC count	cholecystitis

Definitive diagnosis of acute cholecystitis requires: (1) One item in A and one item in B positive (2) C confirms the diagnosis when acute cholecystitis is suspected clinically

Illustrated by Jill Rhead. Intermountain Healthcare. Adapted from: Hirota, et al. Diagnostic criteria and severity assessment of acute cholecystitis: Tokyo Guidelines. *Journal of Hepatobiliary Pancreatic Surgery.* 2007; **14**(1):78–82.[12]

* Acute hepatitis, other acute abdominal diseases, and chronic cholecystitis should be excluded.

BOX 14.2   ACUTE CHOLECYSTITIS: ULTRASOUND FINDINGS

The best imaging modality for evaluating acute cholecystitis is the abdominal ultrasound. Findings on ultrasound that may suggest acute cholecystitis include:

1. Positive sonographic Murphy's sign
2. Gallbladder distention
3. Thickened gallbladder wall >4 mm
4. Pericholecystic fluid
5. Visualization of impacted stones

While not diagnostic, these findings coupled with the correct clinical scenario have correlated well with the operative findings and increasingly complicated surgery in some LMICs.[13] This may help healthcare professionals in LMICs decide the most appropriate location and surgical team to tackle a potentially more difficult cholecystectomy.

Cholecystitis

Cholecystitis, or inflammation of the gallbladder, generally occurs as a result of prolonged obstruction of the cystic duct with a stone. Parasites can also lead to cholecystitis. Symptoms of acute cholecystitis include right upper quadrant/epigastric pain, fever, nausea, and vomiting. Patients will frequently have a history of biliary colic-type symptoms that resolved in the past. Physical exam will often reveal tachycardia and a positive Murphy's sign, or arrest of inspiration upon palpation of the right upper quadrant. If laboratory values are available, leukocytosis may also be present (Table 14.1).

The most commonly implicated bacteria causing cholecystitis are *E. coli, Klebsiella, Enterobacter, Enterococcus, Streptococcus, Bacteroides,* and *Clostridium.* The microbiology of acute cholecystitis may differ in different countries. For example, *Pseudomonas* and *Salmonella* were also frequently seen in the bile of Ghanaian patients.[14] While routine culture of bile from elective cholecystectomy is not warranted because of the infrequent presence of bacteria in the bile, when available, culturing the bile from patients with acute cholecystitis may help select appropriate bacterial coverage as the type of bacteria become more virulent with worsening cholecystitis. Healthcare professionals may then select antibiotics with broader coverage based on known regional differences.

Emphysematous cholecystitis characterized by gas in the lumen and/or wall of the gallbladder is an unusual type of cholecystitis seen worldwide. This is more commonly seen in diabetic patients; gas in the gallbladder can be visualized on a plain film of the abdomen. The gallbladder is particularly susceptible to perforation in these cases and emergent cholecystectomy should be pursued. Alternatively, cholecystostomy tube placement, aggressive antibiotic treatment, and fluid management can be offered as initial management to stabilize the patient. An interval cholecystectomy can be performed six weeks later.

Acute cholecystitis can also occur in individuals with typhoid fever and is caused by *Salmonella typhi*. The gallbladder can become colonized in those who have had typhoid fever and lead to chronic cholecystitis and gallstones.

Treatment options for acute cholecystitis include nonoperative management, cholecystostomy, and cholecystectomy. Traditionally, medical treatment for 72 hours followed by cholecystectomy was advocated. However, with the advent of laparoscopic cholecystectomy, early intervention has been found to allow for easier dissection. However, treatment with analgesia, intravenous fluid, and broad spectrum antibiotics followed with an interval cholecystectomy weeks later will be successful a majority of the time. Twenty percent of patients treated in this manner may require surgical intervention for complications, such as empyema of the gallbladder, gangrene, perforation, or cholecystoenteric fistula. These complications are more common in diabetic and elderly patients.[11] Cholecystostomy with aggressive medical management may be the safest option when the patient is too sick for more complex surgery, inflammation is too severe, or human or physical resources are inadequate.

Cholangitis

Cholangitis indicates infection of the bile ducts and can be a severe entity leading to sepsis if not recognized and treated promptly. Those at risk for cholangitis include individuals with biliary obstruction either from sludge, stones, parasites or flukes, or tumors. Stones in the gallbladder, or secondary choledocholithiasis, can also lead to cholangitis.

The classic symptoms of cholangitis were characterized by Charcot and are aptly referred to as Charcot's triad. They consist of fever, right upper quadrant pain, and jaundice. As patients' symptoms worsen they may progress to develop Reynolds' pentad, which includes Charcot's triad accompanied by altered mental status and hypotension indicating septic shock as a result of cholangitis. Typical lab findings include leukocytosis and an elevated direct bilirubin level. Imaging may reveal dilated bile ducts as well as obstructing masses or lesions. As with cholecystitis, the initial diagnostic imaging modality remains the abdominal ultrasound. Computed tomography (CT) scan can better delineate the extent of masses and adjacent organ involvement. In many areas of the world, exploratory laparotomy or diagnostic laparoscopy may be the only other diagnostic tests available.

ERCP can be an excellent diagnostic and therapeutic intervention for cholangitis caused by an obstructing stone, parasite, or mass. If ERCP is unavailable, another therapeutic option is percutaneous transhepatic cholangiography (PTC) but this requires interventional radiology capabilities.

Treatment for cholangitis includes adequate resuscitation (urine output greater than 30 ml/hour), antibiotics, and intervention to relieve the underlying cause. Antibiotic coverage should be broad spectrum with special attention to enteric gram-negative organisms as well as gram positives. With resuscitation and antibiotics for a 7- to 10-day duration, approximately 85% of patients will improve without the need for acute invasive intervention.[15] Therefore, even with minimal resources, an individual who is recognized and treated early can improve without the need for emergent endoscopic or surgical intervention. Ideally, these patients should undergo elective biliary drainage once they have recovered from the acute phase of their illness. If an individual does not respond to medical management within the first day or two, then further urgent intervention should be sought.

Gallstone Pancreatitis

The exact etiology of gallstone pancreatitis is not clearly understood, though it is believed to most likely be related to obstruction of the pancreatic duct by a gallstone. The obstruction is often transient but remains for enough time to lead to inflammation of the pancreas. Patients with pancreatitis often present with nausea, vomiting, and epigastric pain. Amylase and lipase levels will be elevated, indicating the presence of pancreatitis. These patients should initially be managed similar to any other patient with pancreatitis—with bowel rest (NPO), intravenous fluids, and pain control. Gallstone pancreatitis can cause mild, moderate, or severe clinical presentations. Initial adequate resuscitation is the critical first management goal.

A majority of common bile duct (CBD) stones pass spontaneously. At least 10% of patients require surgical or endoscopic removal of the CBD stones. Once the pancreatitis has resolved, patients should undergo either ERCP or surgical removal of the CBD stones. Surgical approaches include laparoscopic or open cholecystectomy with intraoperative cholangiogram. When CBD stones are identified, they can be removed either transcystically, through a choledochotomy, or via a transduodenal sphincteroplasty. In rare cases, drainage of the CBD with a choledochoduodenostomy or Roux-en-Y may be necessary. In LMICs where more modern treatments such as postoperative ERCP are unavailable, surgeons need to become adept at standard open surgical techniques.

Gallstone Ileus

Gallstone ileus occurs when a stone fistulizes from the gallbladder or CBD into the intestine. The stone then gains entrance to the intestine through the fistula. This can lead to cholangitis.

When the luminal intestinal diameter is less than that of the stone, the intestine may become obstructed. One presentation of a gallstone ileus is a tumbling obstruction, where a patient intermittently experiences obstructive symptoms as a large stone migrates through the intestinal tract causing obstructive symptoms in narrower areas and abatement of symptoms as the lumen enlarges. The majority of fistulas occur between the gallbladder and the duodenum; the most common site for obstruction is the ileum. The stone can sometimes be seen on plain films of the abdomen if the stone is radiopaque or it can be identified by the presence of surrounding intestinal air. A pathognomic finding is air in the biliary tree in an individual who has not had any surgical or endoscopic manipulation of the biliary system.

Gallstone ileus is treated by relieving the obstruction via surgical enterotomy and removing the offending stone. Repair of the fistula is debatable, but if there is minimal inflammation in an otherwise good surgical candidate patient and the surgeon is comfortable, then repair of the fistula can be pursued. If left unrepaired there is an approximately 5% risk of recurrent gallstone ileus.[16]

Parasitic Disease

Multiple parasites, including flukes and *Ascaris lumbricoides,* can cause infection and obstruction in the biliary system and are common in endemic areas. Flukes that are commonly found in the biliary tract include *Clonorchis sinesis, Opiesthorchi viverini, Opisthorchis felineus,* and *Fasciola hepatica.*[17] Generally, those with flukes remain asymptomatic. Flukes are common in much of Asia and Eastern Europe (Figure 14.5). In parts of Southeast Asia, millions are infected with liver flukes. Individuals become infected after consuming raw fish containing cyst-encapsulated larvae. The larvae migrate from the duodenum through the ampulla of vater and into the biliary system and then mature. The flukes prefer the smaller-sized intrahepatic ducts but can be found throughout the biliary system and can then go on to cause obstruction, fibrosis, inflammation, and hyperplasia. On imaging the flukes are generally seen as elongated filling defects that can cause biliary duct dilatation if there is an underlying obstruction. Because flukes are so thin and often asymptomatic, they are frequently challenging to visualize on imaging studies. *Fasciola hepatica* is a trematode seen in cattle and sheep that infects humans who have consumed infected water or raw plants. The trematodes then track through the liver into the biliary system where they mature and release eggs leading to cysts, abscesses, and necrosis. These trematodes are more commonly seen in developed areas such as Europe and Australia where cattle and sheep are raised.[18]

Ascaris biliary infiltration can lead to cholecystitis, cholangitis, biliary colic, and obstructive jaundice and is commonly found in tropical and subtropical areas where humans become infected after ingesting the parasites' eggs. Ascariasis infection can present as emesis or diarrhea of worms, bowel obstruction as a result of worm infestation, or biliary pathology when worms migrate through the duodenum into the biliary system. On US the larvae are visualized as echogenic structures often with a central echo-free line that is the worms' gastrointestinal tract. Ascariasis infection is surprisingly common, with potentially 1.5 billion people worldwide affected.[18] Worms can cause a wide range of hepatobiliary pathology including cholangitis, pancreatitis, cholecystitis, and liver abscess.

Biliary ascariasis can generally be managed conservatively with medical management. General treatment consists of intravenous fluids, NPO status, antihelminths, and antispasmodics. Response is measured with serial US to identify the ongoing presence of worms in the biliary system, and success is gauged by improvement in symptoms. Approximately 42%–90% of patients respond to medical therapy alone.[19] If medical management fails, the next potential intervention is dependent upon the location of the worms. If the ascaris infestation is in the ampulla, then endoscopy may be sufficient; worms further in the bile ducts may need to be extracted using ERCP. Sphincterotomy should be avoided in this situation because of the likelihood of repeat infection and easier access for future worms to migrate from the duodenum into the biliary tree. Gallbladder ascariasis should also be initially managed with medical measures. However, a significant number may go on to require

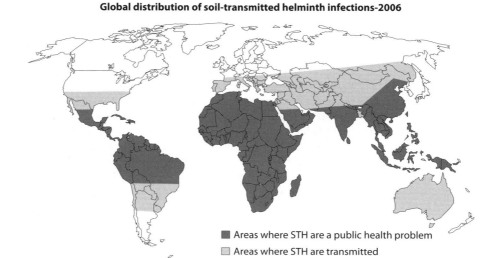

Global distribution of soil-transmitted helminth infections-2006

■ Areas where STH are a public health problem
▨ Areas where STH are transmitted

FIGURE 14.5 Global transmission of soil-transmitted helminth infections. World Health Organization. Global Transmission of Soil-Transmitted Helminth Infections [Internet]. 2006 [cited 2014 Jan 28] Available from http://www.who.int/intestinal_worms/epidemiology/map/en/index.html.[20]

surgical intervention with cholecystectomy. The progress of these patients can be followed with serial US, and if the patients fail to expel the worms within 7–10 days or symptoms worsen, then surgical cholecystectomy should be pursued.[18] Once worms are in the intestine they are increasingly susceptible to treatment with antihelminths such as mebendazole, and a 90% eradication can be achieved using these drugs.[19]

Gallbladder Carcinoma

Although a relatively rare cancer, carcinoma of the gallbladder is the most common malignancy of the biliary tract. The malignancy affects females more than males and is associated with gallstones. Although most patients with gallbladder carcinoma have gallstones, less than 1% of individuals with gallstones ever develop gallbladder carcinoma. Risk factors include a calcified gallbladder (porcelain gallbladder), gallstones greater than 2.5 cm in diameter, *Salmonella typhus* infection, an anomalous pancreaticobiliary duct junction (more frequently seen in parts of Asia), and choledochal cysts. The worldwide incidence of gallbladder cancer varies widely and it is actually the number one cause of cancer-related death in some groups of women in South America (Figure 14.6).[22] Populations that appear to have the highest incidence of gallbladder cancer are women in India, Pakistan, Ecuador, Korea, Japan, and some areas of Eastern Europe.[21,22]

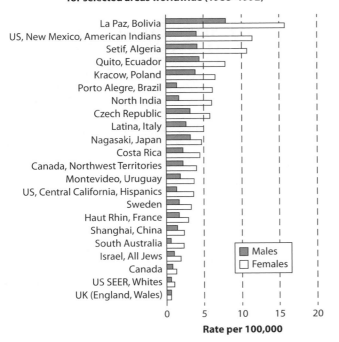

Incidence rates of gallbladder cancer for selected areas worldwide (1988–1992)

La Paz, Bolivia
US, New Mexico, American Indians
Setif, Algeria
Quito, Ecuador
Kracow, Poland
Porto Alegre, Brazil
North India
Czech Republic
Latina, Italy
Nagasaki, Japan
Costa Rica
Canada, Northwest Territories
Montevideo, Uruguay
US, Central California, Hispanics
Sweden
Haut Rhin, France
Shanghai, China
South Australia
Israel, All Jews
Canada
US SEER, Whites
UK (England, Wales)

■ Males
□ Females

0   5   10   15   20
Rate per 100,000

FIGURE 14.6 Worldwide distribution of gallbladder cancer. Illustrated by Jill Rhead. Intermountain Healthcare. Adapted from: Lazcano-Ponce EC, et al. Epidemiology and molecular pathology of gallbladder cancer. *CA: A Cancer Journal for Clinicians.* 2001; **51**(6): 349–364; Randi G, Franceschi, S, La Vecchia C. Gallbladder cancer worldwide: geographical distribution and risk factors. *International Journal of Cancer.* 2006; **118**(7): 1591–1602.

Gallbladder cancer can spread in many ways including via lymphatics, vessels, intraperitoneal seeding, neural, intraductal, and direct extension. Symptoms are nonspecific and generally include pain, weight loss, and right upper quadrant tenderness. If gallbladder cancer is suspected preoperatively, an open cholecystectomy with local hepatic resection is the operation of choice for potentially resectable cancer. Since the disease is generally identified late in its course, the 5-year survival is approximately 10%.[22] In LMICs, patients typically present with later stages of disease and even worse survival rates.[22]

Surgical Management Options

Cholecystostomy

The most common indication for placement of a cholecystostomy tube is a severely inflamed acute cholecystitis. In LMICs, where resources are scarce and local nonspecialist surgical physicians provide a majority of surgical care, a cholecystostomy provides doctors with a lifesaving temporizing option. A relative indication includes uncomplicated acute cholecystitis when identified during an exploratory laparotomy by nonspecialist surgeons.[23] Alternatively, closing the abdomen and treating medically before performing a delayed cholecystectomy is also a viable approach. Medical officers can be trained to safely perform this procedure under local, intercostals block, epidural, or general anesthesia. US or CT guidance provides a minimally invasive approach in high-income countries (HICs) to treat patients too sick for emergent surgical treatment. Occasionally, laparoscopic or open placement follows after initial surgical evaluation identifies a gallbladder encased in severe inflammation and removal is deemed unsafe or too difficult.

Various incisions may be used, including small incisions directly over the area of maximum tenderness which may be accompanied by a mass. Small incisions over the inflamed area or paramedian, subcostal, and midline incisions all provide differing exposures. At times, the gallbladder is intimately incorporated within an ill-defined mass surrounded by marked inflammation, while at other times the gallbladder is more easily identified. A cholecystostomy is performed by placing a 2–0 dissolvable purse string at the dome of the gallbladder (see Figure 14.7). Suction the bile with a syringe or a trocar drainage tube in the center of the purse string. The gallbladder can be incised with a scalpel or electrocautery and stones extracted before inserting a drainage catheter. A 20–26 French Foley balloon or Malenkot tube are ideal. Connect the catheter to a clean closed drainage reservoir (see Box 14.3).

A multitude of substitute gravity reservoirs provide adequate drainage. Plastic bags, surgical gloves, larger candy bags, and empty intravenous bags can be secured to the drain tube with rubber bands or ties (Figure 14.8).

Open Cholecystectomy

Open cholecystectomy continues to be the predominant method for gallbladder removal in the developing world.[24] Cholecystectomy has been accepted as the most appropriate treatment for biliary colic, acute cholecystitis, emphysematous or gangrenous cholecystitis, and interval resection following cholecystostomy tube placement. The traditionally midline and right upper quadrant incisions

Steps of cholecystostomy

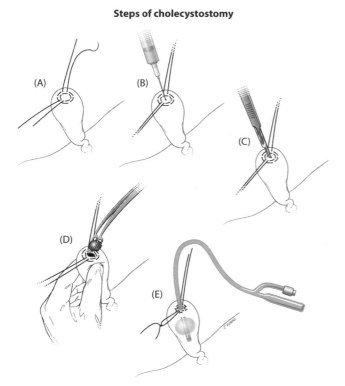

FIGURE 14.7   Cholecystostomy. Illustration by Jill Rhead. Intermountain Healthcare.

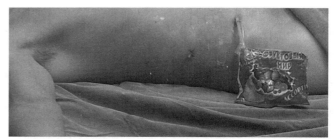

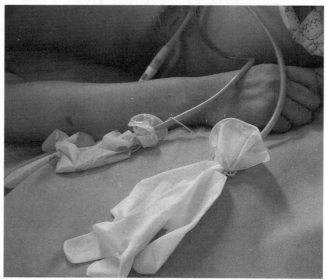

FIGURE 14.8   Candy bag and glove reservoir. Images by Raymond Price.

BOX 14.3   INNOVATIVE CATHETERS AND RESERVOIRS

Contained catheter systems such as vacuum suction drains or gravity down drains that have catheters that connect to well-fitting reservoirs are in short supply in many developing areas. Identifying appropriate substitutes requires some innovative problem-solving skills. Whereas, in a hospital with seemingly unlimited resources, a Silastic© suction tube could be cut a little shorter for patient convenience, carefully cutting the tube originally made for one patient into two equal but noticeably smaller pieces provides a second drainage tube. Rubber tubing from the hardware store can be sterilized. Nasogastric tubes, respiratory suction catheters, pediatric feeding tubes, and other tubing identified for specific uses can sometime be adapted and used as drainage catheters. Recognizing the different catheter properties, especially the stiffness, will help select the best alternative.

BOX 14.4   TECHNICAL CHALLENGES FOR CHOLECYSTECTOMY IN LMICs

Adequate lighting and exposure are two of the major technical challenges for cholecystectomy in LMICs. Electrical power is frequently intermittent. When operating lights are available, often there may be only one out of 8–12 bulbs still functioning. A long-lasting, bright headlight with the ability to focus a narrow beam becomes one of the surgeon's best tools for abdominal operations. Instruments may be antiquated. Self-supporting mechanical retraction devices are nearly non-existent. Handheld retractors are commonly inadequate for a given procedure.

previously resulted in prolonged hospital stays (4–8 days). In India, mini-laparotomy cholecystectomy identified 78% of patients appropriate for discharge on the same night of surgery, and 93% by the following morning.[24] Incisions of 5–6 cm were made in the right upper quadrant. The rectus muscle was either split or spread depending on surgeon preference. Lighted narrow Deaver retractors provided illumination and exposure. The gallbladder was removed by a top-down approach if exposure at the triangle of Calot was obscured. Titanium clips were used for occlusion of the cystic duct and artery. Others have reported

similar results using ties and other tools for exposure.[25] Same-day mini-laparotomy cholecystectomy may be a reasonable and affordable alternative to laparoscopic cholecystectomy in LMICs temporarily bridging an equity gap during further infrastructure and resource development.

Laparoscopic Cholecystectomy

Many LMICs are now gaining access to the equipment and training necessary to perform laparoscopic cholecystectomies. The laparoscopic route is safe and cost-effective, and results in faster recovery times and return to work in addition to better cosmetic results than traditional open techniques. Chapter 20 examines the issues of laparoscopy for LMICs and outlines basic infrastructure and resources necessary for successful laparoscopic surgery.

Intraoperative Cholangiogram (IOC)

Debates in HICs continue on whether routine intraoperative cholangiogram is necessary to identify CBD stones and to delineate the biliary anatomy. Common bile duct stones may be found in 6%–12% of patients with stones in their gallbladders. However, in LMICs, intraoperative radiology capabilities are extremely limited or non-existent. At times, a portable X-ray machine may be available, but contrast dye and cholangiocatheters are missing, or vice versa. Often the quality of the X-ray picture precludes any reasonable interpretation. Fluoroscopy occasionally may be found in large urban areas but many times is limited to private institutions.

Clinical evaluation becomes extremely important in identifying patients suspected with CBD stones, allowing for expeditious referral to facilities with the necessary resources. The risk of patients harboring gallstones can be clinically classified based on a complete patient history, liver function tests, and US (Table 14.2).[11]

Although the ability to stratify this risk in patients will not identify 100% of people with CBD stones, reports from LMICs have concluded that IOC is not essential to prevent missed CBD stones or, for that matter, biliary tract injuries in patients undergoing laparoscopic cholecystectomy.[26]

Common Bile Duct Exploration (CBDE)

All CBD stones should be removed. In most of the developing world, a formal CBDE remains the only viable method for treating CBD stones. This can be accomplished sometimes through a transcystic approach or via a choledochotomy. Occasionally, an open transduodenal sphincteroplasty may be required for

TABLE 14.2

Risk of harboring common bile duct stones

Low Risk (<5%)
Large stones
No history of jaundice or pancreatitis
No liver function abnormalities
Common bile duct <4 mm by ultrasound

Moderate Risk (10%–50%)
Small stones with any of the following:
  History of jaundice or pancreatitis
  Elevated live function test
  Common bile duct >4 mm by ultrasound

High Risk (>50%)
Patients with jaundice or cholangitis
Common bile duct >4 mm by ultrasound

Created by Jill Rhead, Medical Illustrator. Intermountain Healthcare. Adapted from: Ostrow B. Cholelithiasis, cholecystitis and cholecystectomy-their relevance for African surgeons. *Surgery in Africa-Monthly Review.* July 2006;16.

otherwise irremovable stones. However, access to qualified surgeons is woefully inadequate in LMICs. Even in HICs, where ERCP has replaced open techniques, many surgeons finish their training with very limited or no experience in CBD exploration techniques. The steps of a CBDE are diagrammed in Figure 14.9.

Dissolvable sutures prevent stone formation. A t-tube is ideal for drainage; however, other soft tubes such as urethral, red rubber, or other catheters directed toward the liver can be used. In a review of randomized studies comparing primary closure with t-tube drainage, Gurusamy concluded that primary closure was safer both in laparoscopic and open cases.[27,28] However, a t-tube provides access for postoperative CBD manipulation and provides surgeons with a safe alternative when faced with the need for increasingly complex operative procedures. Irrigating and sweeping a balloon catheter after it has passed beyond the CBD stone can remove a significant number of gallstones; this can be approached either through the cystic duct or through a formal choledochotomy. Instruments designed for CBD exploration such as Desjardins gallstone forceps of various angles and gallstone scoops can facilitate successful removal of stones (Figure 14.10).

Choledocoscopy can be accomplished laparoscopically or during a formal laparotomy with direct basket removal of CBD stones. However, this requires significantly more equipment and surgical skills than are available to the majority of the world's poor.

BOX 14.5   COMMON BILE DUCT STONES IN MONGOLIA

A significant number of patients in rural Mongolia suffer multiple (up to four to five) attacks of abdominal pain associated with jaundice and elevated amylase before subjecting themselves to surgical cure. Often, this is due to lack of appropriately trained surgeons, the austere geographical environment, and difficult travel. An elderly gentleman with a retained stone following CBDE in northern Mongolia refused the arduous journey to the capital city, Ulaanbaatar (UB), for an ERCP by the single qualified endoscopist in the country. Instead, he chose to wait for an open common bile duct exploration when a visiting professor from the capital and a foreign surgical training team arrived. Local surgeons learned the CBDE techniques from the visiting professors. Still, X-ray capability was limited, only one bottle of contrast dye was available, and common bile duct instruments were brought and donated to the hospital.

Millions of gazelle roam the steppe in larger herds outside Choibalsan in Eastern Mongolia. Hoof-and-mouth disease had quarantined the city and no ground travel was allowed in or out of the city. A woman had an obstructing CBD stone, but it was impossible for her to fly to UB for treatment. During open cholecystectomy and CBDE, a poor quality X-ray suggested the stone has been removed. A t-tube was left in place and a follow-up cholangiogram on better equipment showed an impacted stone at the ampulla. The t-tube temporized the acute emergency and allowed for a more elective transduodenal sphincterotomy and stone removal by a more advanced surgical team.

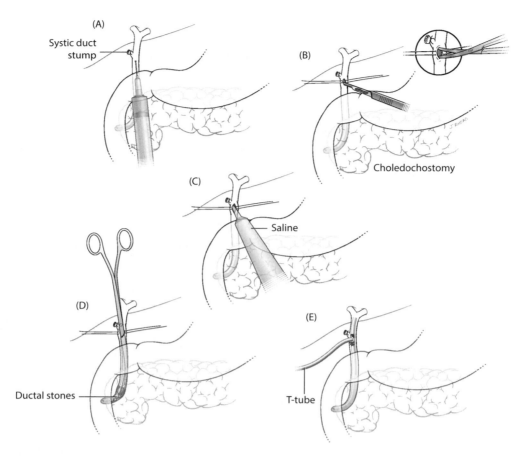

FIGURE 14.9   Steps of common bile duct exploration. Image by Jill Rhead, Medical Illustrator. Intermountain Healthcare.

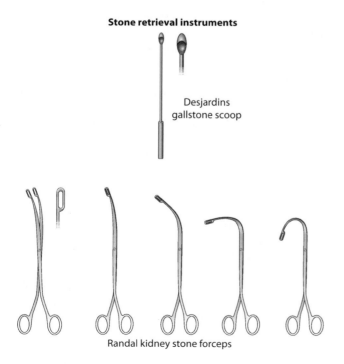

FIGURE 14.10   Gallstone forceps and gallstone scoops. Image by Jill Rhead, Medical Illustrator. Intermountain Healthcare.

Surgical Complications

Complications following cholecystectomy include wound infection, abscess, bile leak, bile duct strictures, and bile duct injury. While common bile duct injury is the most feared, wound complications present a significant problem in LMICs. Wound infections plague patients following open cholecystectomy 12% of the time in Mongolia.[29] This prompted the chief of surgery at the Health Sciences University of Mongolia to demand for the "introduction and further development of laparoscopic surgery in Mongolian surgical practice" after she demonstrated that the wound infection rate following laparoscopic cholecystectomy was dramatically lower.[29]

Patients with cystic duct leaks present with abdominal pain, fever, chills, and nausea and may or may not have an elevated bilirubin postoperatively. Cystic duct stump leaks occur as a result of inadequate ligation of the cystic duct or intraoperative injury. Imaging reveals a fluid collection in the vicinity of the gallbladder fossa that ideally requires drainage. While percutaneous drainage by radiology provides patients with a minimally invasive approach when available, surgical drainage may be the only option in LMICs. If available, ERCP with stent placement may also be performed to relieve downstream obstruction and prevent ongoing bile leakage as the cystic duct stump heals.

Bile duct injuries and strictures present a more challenging problem. The incidence of bile duct injury during laparoscopic cholecystectomy is around 0.3%–0.7%, and in open cholecystectomy it is closer to 0.1%–0.5%.[30] Injury can occur as a result of electrocautery, clip application to the common bile duct, and inability to appreciate aberrant anatomy. The major arteries to the CBD are at the 3- and 9-o'clock positions; excessive dissection of the CBD should be avoided to prevent delayed stricturing.

The management of patients with bile duct injury or stricture is a challenge. Ideally, any injury would be identified at the time of the initial operation and repaired or drained appropriately until referral to a higher level of care is possible. Unfortunately, the injury frequently goes unrecognized and presents later after patients develop progressively elevated liver function tests, jaundice, and/or abdominal pain. Patients can develop cholangitis and sepsis as a result of intra-abdominal bilomas. Prior to any intervention these patients should be appropriately resuscitated, treated with broad spectrum antibiotics, and undergo drainage procedures such as percutaneous and/or operative biliary drainage as initial management. Proximal biliary decompression and external drainage provides temporary control while patients are stabilized. It is important to note that in the setting of delayed

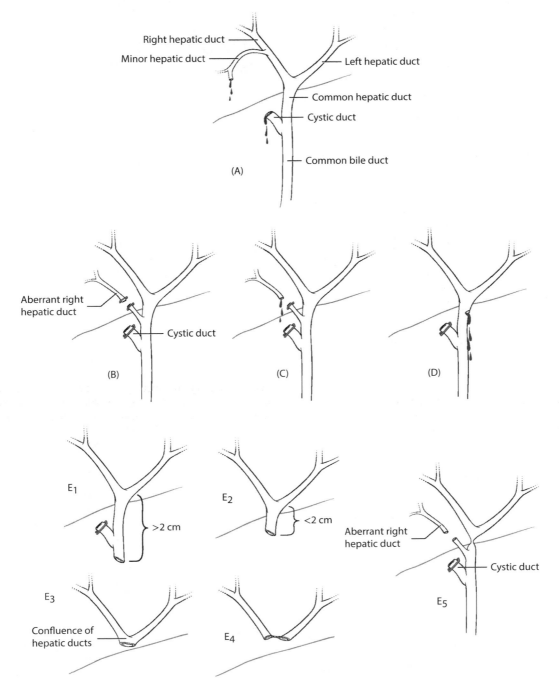

FIGURE 14.11 Types of common bile duct injuries. Created by Jill Rhead, Medical Illustrator. Intermountain Healthcare.

diagnosis of biliary injury, there is a large amount of inflammation in the area of the porta hepatis. The anatomy is hard to define and there is a significantly higher risk of causing further injury. It is best to delay definitive operative repair at this time. Once sepsis is controlled and inflammation subsides, reconstruction of the bile ducts can occur in a non-emergent fashion.

Both US and CT scan are useful diagnostic tools to evaluate an individual with a presumed bile duct injury or stricture. Exploratory laparoscopy or laparotomy may be the only diagnostic tool available in some settings. US can identify dilated ducts proximal to a ligated bile duct or stricture as well as the presence of intra-abdominal fluid collections. A CT scan can further characterize the injury or stricture location in extrahepatic bile ducts. The ideal test to evaluate a bile duct injury/stricture is cholangiography either through PTC or ERCP if they are available. PTC is better at defining the proximal biliary anatomy and useful in planning potential surgical repair. PTC can also be used to place drainage catheters to prevent the formation of cholangitis. The distal ducts are better evaluated by ERCP, and biliary stents can be inserted that combined with external drainage may provide definitive treatment for smaller partial injuries. MRCP is a noninvasive imaging modality that can also provide clear understanding of the biliary anatomy.

The classic CBD injury results from mistaking the common bile duct for the cystic duct, resulting in transaction and removal of a portion of the CBD. Understanding the various types of injuries helps guide preoperative and operative decision planning. Figure 14.11 schematically reviews the types of CBD injuries. Repair may simply require drainage and ligation of a small accessory branch or open cystic duct as in Type A. A Roux-en-Y choledochojejunostomy may be required for reconstruction for type E1 CBD injuries (see Figure 14.12) or a hepaticojejunostomy for type E4 where both right and left hepatic ducts have been injured. With any common bile duct injury, repair should be approached by an experienced biliary surgeon.[31]

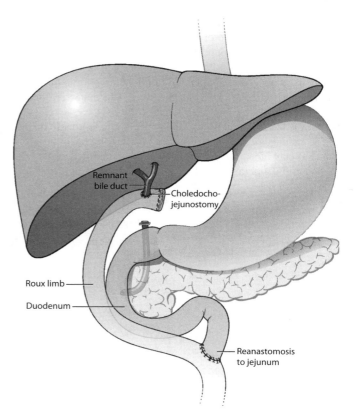

FIGURE 14.12 Roux-en-Y choledochojejunostomy for repair of type E1 common bile duct injury. Image by Jill Rhead, Medical Illustrator. Intermountain Healthcare. Adapted from: Raymond Price.

Pancreatic Diseases

Pancreatitis

Pancreatitis varies widely in its clinical presentation. Its spectrum ranges from very benign presentations in patients with only mild abdominal pain to those with massive inflammatory responses ultimately leading to intubation, surgery, and prolonged intensive care. There are multiple etiologies for pancreatitis. The two most common causes for pancreatitis worldwide are alcohol and gallstones, accounting for 80%–90% of the cases; the leading cause varies by geographic location (Figure 14.13). Causes of pancreatitis are listed in Table 14.3.

Other causes of pancreatitis are more common depending on region. Idiopathic pancreatitis, a diagnosis of exclusion, is prominent in India, China, and Singapore, where it accounts for approximately 60%–70% of cases of chronic pancreatitis.[33]

Tropical pancreatitis is juvenile nonalcoholic pancreatitis seen most commonly in LMICs in tropical regions. In some papers this entity is not distinguished from idiopathic pancreatitis. It presents with abdominal pain, steatorrhea, and diabetes. It is

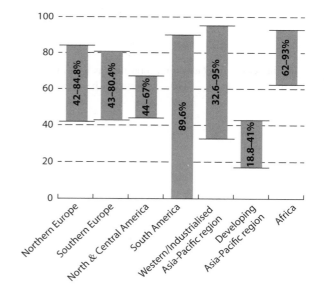

FIGURE 14.13 Percentage of patients with chronic pancreatitis in whom the cause is alcohol abuse. Image by Jill Rhead, Medical Illustrator. Intermountain Healthcare. Adapted from: Jupp J, Fine D, Johnson CD. The epidemiology and socioeconomic impact of chronic pancreatitis. *Best Practice & Research Clinical Gastroenterology.* 2010; **24**(3): 219–31.[32]

TABLE 14.3

Causes of pancreatitis

Mechanical	*Infection*
Gallstones	Viruses
Trauma	Mumps
Iatrogenic	*Coxsackie B*
ERCP	HIV
Cardiopulmonary bypass	Bacteria
Operations	*Salmonella*
Pancreas divisum	*Shigella*
Neoplasm	Hemorrhagic *Escherichia coli*
Sphincter of Oddi spasm	Parasites
Ischemia	*Ascaris lumbricoides*
Chemical	*Vasculitis*
Exogerous	Systemic lupus erthematosus
Alcohol	Poilyarteritis nodosa
Medications*	
Natural	*Hereditary*
Hypertriglyceridemia	Cystic fibrosis
Hypercalcernia	Heredutary pancreatitis
Hyperlipidemia	
Toxins	*Idiopathic*
Scorpion venom	
Parathion	

Illustrated by Jill Rhead. Intermountain Healthcare. Adapted from: Townsend C, et al. *Textbook of Surgery*. Philadelphia: Saunders Elsevier, 2012.

* Common medications include: salicylates, tetracycline, trimethoprim-sulfamethpxazole, estrogen, valporic acid, steroids.

TABLE 14.4

Ranson's criteria

At admission		Within 48 hours	
AGE	>55 years	HCT Drop	>10
WBC	>16,000/mm3	BUN elevation	>5 mg/100 ml
Blood Glucose	>200/mm3	Calcium	>8 mg/100 ml
Serum LDH	>350 IU/L	Arterial pO2	>55 mmHg
AST	>250 U/100 ml	Base deficit	>4 mEq/L
		Fluid sequestration	>6 L

Illustrated by Jill Rhead. Intermountain Healthcare. Adapted from: Townsend C, et al. *Textbook of Surgery*. Philadelphia: Saunders Elsevier, 2012.

believed to be related to malnutrition, dietary toxins, and hereditary factors.

The majority of patients follow a relatively mild and limited course. One challenge is to identify those patients that may require a higher level of care. In 1974, Ranson created criteria for identifying those with increased morbidity and mortality as a result of severe pancreatitis (see Table 14.4). These criteria are best used for cases in which pancreatitis is not due to gallstone disease and are limited to a one-time evaluation during the first 48 hours of presentation. However, the criteria provide a clinical and biochemical assessment using resources available in many rural areas. Individuals with one or two signs require minimal supportive care. Those with three to four signs have a 15% mortality, and those with five to six signs have a mortality that approaches 50%. The majority of these patients require intensive care unit (ICU) care.[34]

Initial management of patients with pancreatitis is nonoperative and consists of supportive care with fluid resuscitation, NPO, pain control, and electrolyte repletion. Patients may also require nutritional support with either nasojejunal feeds past the ligament of Treitz or parenteral nutrition. There is evidence to suggest that patients with necrotizing pancreatitis should be treated with a carbapenem antibiotic to decrease morbidity and mortality.[35] Monitoring critically ill patients in LMICs may be limited to manual vital signs and urine output with infrequent blood tests. Monitoring trends in these very basic methods allows for appropriate decision making and timely interventions. Training local staff in monitoring trends and adequate documentation may be necessary.

Operative intervention is required in a few select cases. These include the development of abdominal compartment syndrome, infected pancreatic necrosis, and cholecystectomy in the setting of gallstone pancreatitis as discussed previously. Operative management along with the intensive care needed postoperatively of severe cases may be beyond the capability of many LMICs. If transfer to other levels of care is unavailable, comfort care may be required in instances that could have been successful had more resources been available.

Pancreatic Pseudocyst

Acute fluid collections develop in 30%–50% of patients with acute pancreatitis;[36] the majority resolve on their own. In approximately 10% of patients these fluid collections enlarge, develop into pseudocysts, and become symptomatic necessitating surgical intervention. However, most remain asymptomatic and resolve over many years. A pseudocyst is usually diagnosed via either US or CT. A pseudocyst should be differentiated from a pancreatic cystic lesion based on history as well as appearance on imaging. (Septae will not be present in a pancreatic pseudocyst.) Concern for a neoplastic process increases with septated lesions or cysts identified without a history of pancreatitis. If the diagnosis is unclear the cystic fluid can be aspirated and examined further. A pancreatic pseudocyst, which communicates with the pancreatic duct, will have a high amylase content.

Surgical intervention for pancreatic pseudocysts may be pursued if the cyst has been present greater than 6 weeks in order to allow for maturation and is persistently symptomatic and/or increasing in size. However, many of these cysts resolve over time and do not require any surgical treatment. Pseudocyst drainage can be approached percutaneously, endoscopically, or surgically with surgical drainage being associated with lower recurrence rates. Internal drainage can be approached through an incision in the anterior wall of the stomach and suturing the posterior wall of the stomach to the anterior wall of the pancreatic pseudocyst (see Figure 14.14). Alternatively, a loop of jejunum can be sutured side-to-side with the pancreatic pseudocyst. In either case, where possible, a biopsy of the cyst wall may be prudent.

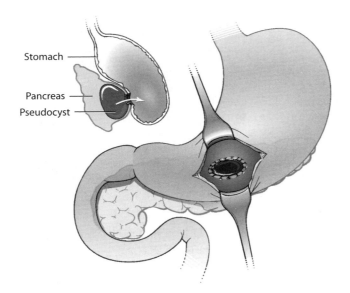

FIGURE 14.14 Cystogastrostomy for pancreatic pseudocyst drainage. Illustrated by Jill Rhead. Intermountain Healthcare.

Pancreatic Abscess

Pancreatic abscess occurs when a pseudocyst becomes infected or necrotic pancreas becomes secondarily infected and liquefied. Although there is some debate and confusion regarding terminology, some articles and texts refer to both abscesses and infected pancreatic necrosis as walled-off pancreatic necrosis (WOPN). It is a rare but morbid late complication of acute pancreatitis. Approximately 1%–9% of patients with acute pancreatitis will go on to develop WOPN generally 4–6 weeks after the initial episode of pancreatitis. Symptoms include pain, fever, and chills. Gastrointestinal flora and candida are the most commonly implicated organisms.[37] Laboratory studies are nonspecific and may include leukocytosis and elevated pancreatic enzymes, although pancreatic enzyme elevation is not always present. US, CT, and magnetic resonance imaging (MRI) can also be used for diagnosis, and air in the fluid collection is a sign of infection. The presence of either bacteria or fungus in pancreatic fluid collections aspirated via CT-guided needle biopsy is the sine qua non of WOPN. The presence of organisms either on Gram stain or culture is essential for WOPN.[37] Treatment is supportive with broad-spectrum antibiotic coverage and ultimately percutaneous or open surgical drainage (see Box 14.6).

Hepatic Abscess

Bacterial

Bacterial hepatic abscess can occur as a result of intraabdominal infection, biliary obstruction or instrumentation, hematogenous spread from dental infections or endocarditis, trauma, or secondary to chemoembolization or radiofrequency treatment.[38] Symptoms of hepatic abscesses are generally nonspecific and

---

BOX 14.6 HOMEMADE SALINE FOR IRRIGATION OF WOUNDS AND ABSCESSES

While percutaneous drainage may be ideal for many of these diseases, the reality remains that access is very limited or non-existent in much of the developing world. Still, drainage procedures combined with appropriate antibiotics provide the best chance for successful eradication of the disease. Even open treatment can be severely limited as with pancreatic abscesses that might best be treated with wide drainage, irrigation, and broad antibiotics only to be faced with limited irrigation fluid, few antibiotics, and lack of drainage catheters. Sterile saline can be made locally using the following steps.[46]

1. Clean an appropriate-sized pan and lid with soap and water.
2. Measure 1,000 ml (32 ounces) or water and pour it into the pan.
3. Add two level teaspoons of normal table salt to the water.
4. Bring the water to boiling temperature and boil for 15 minutes.
5. Remember to keep the lid on the pan to prevent evaporation.
6. Sterilize glass jars by boiling. After cooling them, poor cooled saline water into the jars.
7. Label each jar with the date the saline was made.
8. Discard any unopened jars one month after they were prepared; drain opened jars 48 hours after the jar was opened.

---

develop over the course of weeks. Individuals with diabetes are at increased risk of developing hepatic abscesses. Diagnosis may be challenging because of the vague symptomatology as is best achieved with a combination of laboratory and imaging modalities. Individuals will generally have a leukocytosis as well as an elevated CRP. Liver enzymes may or may not be elevated. US is a useful imaging tool with a sensitivity of 75%–95% while a CT scan with contrast is ideal with a sensitivity of 95%.[39,40] Multiple bacteria have been implicated in liver abscesses, including gram negatives, gram positives, and anaerobes, and it is best to obtain blood cultures on patients with a liver abscess if possible. *Staphylococcus* is the most common causative organism. The mainstays of treatment are antibiotics, drainage of pus (with percutaneous drainage preferred via CT or US guidance if available), and treatment of an underlying condition, if present (i.e., biliary obstruction, diverticulitis, appendicitis, or other instigating disease process). Broad-spectrum antibiotics should initially be used until culture results help identify the causative organisms, at which time antibiotic selection can be narrowed. Antibiotic choice can also be tailored based on local trends and suspicion of the underlying cause. IV antibiotics should be administered for 2 weeks with a further 4–6 week course of oral antibiotics for treatment.[38] If an abscess fails to respond to conservative treatment, then the next step is operative intervention.

Amebic

Entamoeba histolytica is the organism generally responsible for causing amebic liver abscesses and is most commonly seen in tropical climates. The protozoon enters through the intestinal mucosa, through the portal system, and goes on to the liver eventually forming an abscess. Ultimately, necrosis occurs and develops the "anchovy sauce" appearance. The disease is more common in young men and presents with abdominal pain and fever. Symptoms can occur 2–5 months after initial infestation. Patients will have leukocytosis with eosinophilia as well as slightly altered liver function tests. US carries a sensitivity of 90%.[38] Treatment is generally medical and consists of metronidazole followed by a luminal agent. If this fails, as is the case in 10%–15% of patients, then percutaneous drainage is the next step.[41]

Echinococcal Cyst

Echinococcal cyst occurs when humans are infected by the *Echinococcus granulosus* tapeworm. It is transmitted by canines with sheep, goats, camels, and horses serving as intermediate hosts. It is acquired by humans when they ingest parasite eggs that are released in the feces of infected hosts.[42] Infections occur worldwide. Eggs hatch in the intestinal tract, enter the circulation, and ultimately form cysts. Risk factors include unsanitary living conditions, large uncontrolled dog populations, proximity of livestock slaughter to humans and animals, as well as sheep raising.[42] Symptoms generally occur as a result of mass effect of the cyst and can also include hepatomegaly, jaundice, and cholangitis.[43] Symptomatic cysts should be treated and asymptomatic cysts observed. Infection is usually confirmed by imaging studies such as US, CT, or MRI as well as enzyme-linked immunosorbent assay (ELISA) and Western blot serology to confirm the diagnosis, if available. Traditional treatment is complete surgical removal of the cyst. According to 1996 World Health Organization (WHO) guidelines, surgery is indicated for removal of large cysts with multiple daughter cysts, single large cysts at high risk of rupture, infected cysts, or liver cysts communicating with the biliary tree or exerting pressure on other organs.[44] The traditional approach has been to remove some cystic fluid and then instill a substance to kill the germinal layer as well as any daughter cysts such as hypertonic saline or ethanol.[45] Another option is to preoperatively treat a patient with an antihelminth agent, especially if the cyst has invaded into the biliary tree as a cysticidal agent could have severe deleterious effect on the biliary system. The antihelminth agent should be given for 1–3 months preoperatively. Another option, called PAIR (puncture, aspiration, injection, reaspiration), exists as an alternative to surgical intervention. The cyst is punctured under US guidance, fluid is aspirated, and then either hypertonic saline or 95% ethanol is injected. This is allowed to sit for at least 15 minutes and then the cyst contents are reaspirated.[44] Antihelminths should also be used in combination with PAIR.

Conclusion

Clearly, minimally invasive techniques have revolutionized the approach to gallstones, pancreatic diseases, and hepatic abscesses in HICs over the last 30 years. While demands for access to similar care are resonating loudly from developing nations, many patients will continue to need access to time-honored open surgical care while infrastructure and human resource development continue to expand.

COMMENTARY

Jigjidsuren Chinburen, Mongolia

I would like to share my experience with how my team in Mongolia was trained to learn hepato-pancreato-biliary (HPB) surgery. In 2004, a Swiss surgical team visited and made significant contributions to surgery in Mongolia. Professor Gillet came with the team, and he made the first anatomical major liver resections in the National Cancer Center (NCC) in Mongolia. Since his visit in 2004, Professor Gillet has committed to training surgeons at the NCC in Mongolia. He visits twice a year, for 3 weeks at a time, to assist us in all HPB area surgeries. Four years after his visit, the number and volume of liver and pancreatic surgery has increased six times, and the complication and mortality rate is acceptable. Now, the HPBS Department of the NCC in Mongolia performs more than 250 liver surgeries annually with a less than 3% mortality rate. This illustrates how crucial it is for expert surgeons from HICs to give bench-side training over a period of time, in order to create a lasting, sustainable improvement.

When a physician is unable to address a case, it is crucial that he or she refers the patient to a specialized center. For example, a female patient from southern Mongolia presented with a lap cholecystectomy and injured CBD. A surgeon tried to fix the problem four times with an open approach and even tried to use vena safena to replace CBD. Finally, the patient referred herself by coming to my department with a biliary fistula and catheter. Her problem was solved surgically by a specialist.

COMMENTARY

Tsiiregzen Enkh-Amgalan, Mongolia

Acute conditions require immediate access to a healthcare facility. In remote areas of Mongolia, a hospital family doctor, also known as a general practitioner, is the person who initiates patient care. In most cases, the family doctor calls a surgeon from Province Center Hospital, who in turn should travel to where the patient is located, although the patient is sometimes simply transferred to where the surgeon is located. The family doctor cannot perform the surgery, so he or she organizes the patient transfer, regardless of risk to the patient.

In Mongolia, limited resources impact the quality and type of care provided, and there are many examples of this. For example, preoperative imaging is not possible in many facilities because the equipment is unavailable, or the equipment is available, but a trained, skilled specialist is not available to operate it. Without preoperative imaging, many surgeons in rural areas do not undertake CBD exploration; ERCP is not available at all. Another example is seen in laparoscopy, which is now widely available in Mongolia, although there is still a general lack of consumables, and insufficient sterilization of surgical instruments, which puts the patient at risk of infections, including hepatitis. Other examples are seen in a lack of endoscopic approach, a lack of interventional radiology (which leads to complications and longer stays), and a lack of a proper ICU.

15

Spleen

Mallory Williams
Quyen D. Chu
Selwyn O. Rogers

Introduction

The spleen is a lymphoid organ located in the retroperitoneum of the left upper quadrant beneath ribs 9 through 11. The spleen is normally not palpable on physical examination until it is enlarged. The spleen has three essential functions: filtering damaged cells from the blood, antibody production, and production of opsonins, which protect against encapsulated bacteria such as pneumococcus and other diseases such as malaria. Due to the spleen's major immunologic functions, splenectomy becomes a concern for patients living in endemic areas of malaria or other infectious diseases.

Nontraumatic diseases of the spleen can cause hemorrhagic shock and be as lethal as traumatic splenic injury. Secondary hypersplenism or splenomegaly is also a significant cause of morbidity in the world. The most common etiology is infectious disease followed by hematologic diseases and neoplastic processes. Because infectious agents play a major role in secondary hypersplenism, geography is an essential component to understanding both the epidemiology and diagnosis of these diseases. In this chapter we will focus on the infectious, hematologic, and neoplastic causes of splenic disease and secondary hypersplenism. The diagnosis and management of both splenomegaly and hypersplenism as a consequence of these diseases will be discussed.

Hypersplenism

Hypersplenism is a process that can arise out of splenomegaly. Hypersplenism is categorized as primary or secondary. Primary hypersplenism occurs when the spleen's normal filtration of damaged cells and hemolysis are increased. Normally, the spleen temporarily contains 90% of the body's platelets and 45% of the red blood cells. When hypersplenism occurs, each of these stored cell fractions are increased and the splenic plasma cells hypertrophy causing the spleen to enlarge. A decrease in one of the four blood components is present, but a pancytopenia can also occur. The anemia is caused primarily by three mechanisms: increased red blood cell pooling in the spleen, shortened red blood cell half-life, and hemodilution from increased plasma volume. Both thrombocytopenia and granulocytopenia are caused by similar mechanisms. When splenic processes become overreactive due to another disease extrasplenic process, it is called secondary hypersplenism. Sundaresan et al. estimate that only 25% of patients with splenomegaly have hypersplenism.[1]

There are four causes of splenomegaly: (1) pooling of red blood cells within the spleen due to red cell–deforming illnesses like sickle cell anemia, spherocytosis, or thalassemia; (2) antigenic stimulation from parasitic or viral infection from illnesses such as malaria or human immunodeficiency virus (HIV); (3) portal hypertension usually caused by viral cirrhosis or parasitic obstruction; and (4) space occupying lesion such as a tumor or abscess.

Hackett's classification of splenomegaly is commonly used system to document splenic enlargement (see Table 15.1).[2]

Clinical Signs and Symptoms of Splenomegaly

Splenomegaly can clinically result in compressive symptoms leading to pain in the left upper quadrant and left flank. Abdominal pain and bloating, early satiety, and gastroesophageal reflux are the most common symptoms. Most patients with mild to moderate enlargement (Hackett score 3 or less) do not have symptoms. On physical examination the spleen may be palpable beneath the costal margin. A spleen must enlarge to approximately twice its normal size to be palpable. Symptoms include fever, weakness, heart palpitations, and ulceration of the mouth, leg, and feet. Furthermore, patients may easily contract bacterial infections and bruise. This is important because patients living in endemic areas undergoing splenectomy become vulnerable to bacterial infections. In fact, fever is a common symptom when infection is the etiology of the splenomegaly. Also, spontaneous bleeding from the nose and other mucosal surfaces and gastrointestinal tract can occur. Anemia, leukopenia, and thrombocytopenia all occur and are reversible with splenectomy. The spleen can grow so large that it spontaneously ruptures into the abdomen. When this occurs, patients may present in hemorrhagic shock.

Infectious Causes of Splenomegaly

Parasites

Parasites are an important source of splenic disease in the world. Perhaps the most important parasites are malaria and schistosomiasis. Splenomegaly occurs as a result of hypertrophy, hyperplasia, and congestion. Effective treatment of these illnesses often results in shrinkage of the spleen. Rarely, spontaneously splenic rupture occurs and must be emergently managed. In this section we discuss malaria, schistosomiasis, leishmaniasis, trypanosomiasis, and hydatid disease.

TABLE 15.1

Hackett's Classification of Splenomegaly

Class	Clinical Examination Findings
0	Spleen not palpable even on deep inspiration
1	Spleen palpable below costal margin, usually on deep inspiration
2	Spleen palpable, but not beyond a horizontal line halfway between the costal margin and umbilicus, measured in a line dropped vertically from the left nipple
3	Spleen palpable more than halfway to umbilicus, but not below a line horizontally running through it.
4	Palpable below umbilicus but not below a horizontal line halfway between umbilicus and pubic symphysis.
5	Extending lower than class 4

This classification is accepted by WHO for clinical surveys and medical documentation.

Table by Mallory Williams.

Malaria

Epidemiology Malaria is endemic to most tropical parts of the world. The World Health Organization (WHO) estimates that half of the world's population is at risk for malaria. More than 200 million people develop malaria annually.[3] As many as 1.5–3 million deaths occur annually, and the majority who die are children of African descent (90%).[3] North, South, East, and West Africa; Central and South America; the Middle East; Central, South, and Southeastern Asia; the Caribbean; and the Pacific Islands all are endemic regions. North America, Europe, Greenland, Antarctica, Northern Asia, and Australia are not endemic regions for malaria. Most deaths occur in Central, East, and West Africa, and Southeast Asia. The disease is caused by the mosquito-borne eukaryotic protist, *Plasmodium*. The most severe form of the disease is caused by *Plasmodium falciparum* while milder forms are caused by *Plasmodium vivax, ovale,* and *malariae*. The vector for this disease is the *Anopheles* mosquito, the tsetse fly. Several strategies, including vector control with pesticides and environmental precautions, have been successful of limiting the impact of the illness.

There is, however, a wide variation in per capita spending on malaria control efforts, and this ultimately affects the disease's impact on people living in endemic areas.[4] One potentially fatal impact is a ruptured spleen secondary to splenomegaly from hyperreactive malaria syndrome (HMS). A cross-sectional study of 2,941 people living in rural Kenya from 1991 to 1992 found splenomegaly in 60% of children ages 2 through 9 years old.[5] This study also demonstrated that 52% of adolescents ages 10–17 years old and 38% of adults also had splenomegaly.[5] Furthermore, De Cock et al. found that of 131 patients with chronic splenomegaly in Nairobi, Kenya, 31% had HMS, 18% had hepatosplenic schistosomiasis, and 5% had visceral leishmaniasis.[6] In Northern Nigeria and Zambia, 40% of patients with splenomegaly were found to have HMS. In Kumasi, Ghana, of 21 patients with palpable spleens of at least 10 cm, the number-one etiology was HMS followed by B-lymphoproliferative disorders.

Diagnosis Diagnosis of malaria is most economically done with blood smear. The *Plasmodium* species are mostly distinct and visible inside of the red blood cells. The species *Malariae* and *Knowlesi* do appear similar and should be distinguished

if possible using polymerase chain reaction (PCR) as *knowlesi parasitemia* causes more severe disease. PCR is not widely available in low- and middle-income countries (LMICs) due to its high cost and the lack of practitioner expertise, but because *P. knowlesi* is common in Southeast Asia, clinical suspicion can also be used. Where the technology and expertise are not available to perform light microscopy, rapid immunochromatographic tests (malaria rapid diagnostic tests or antigen capture assays can be performed). The threshold for detection is 100 parasites/μl of blood with most showing excellent detection and low false positive rates at 200 parasites/μl.

Physical examination is essential to caring for both patients with malaria and patients in endemic regions. While physical examination is adequate for the diagnosis of splenomegaly, it has very low specificity for the diagnosis of malaria. *P. falciparum* is the most common cause of chronic asymptomatic splenomegaly in African children.[7] But there are many other infectious, hematologic, and neoplastic causes of splenomegaly in endemic regions. A standard approach is to evaluate the patient's abdomen for left upper quadrant tenderness and the enlargement of the spleen. Note whether the spleen is soft, firm, or hard. The spleen in acute malaria is soft and friable versus the hard spleen palpated in chronic malaria. A spleen usually has to enlarge to twice its normal size to become palpable. Then record the distance in centimeters of the spleen from the costal margin. Imaging with ultrasound may be done but usually adds little to physical examination. Standard laboratory tests will include blood films that may be negative for malaria parasites; immunofluorescent antibody test, if available; serum IgM; complete blood count; and blood cultures for bacteria. If initial studies are negative for malaria, further detailed studies such as sputum microscopy for acid fast bacteria; blood and bone marrow cultures for *Salmonellae* organisms; lymph node aspirates for trypanosomes; serological tests for HIV, leptospirosis, and visceral leishmaniasis; and splenic aspirates for leishmaniasis may be ordered.

HMS or tropical splenomegaly syndrome (big spleen disease) is a clinical condition that occurs in endemic areas secondary to chronic malarial infection. HMS is the number-one cause of splenomegaly in endemic regions.[8] Patients present with splenomegaly, anemia, neutropenia, and thrombocytopenia. HMS may present with negative blood films, but an immunofluorescent antibody test will be strongly positive and the total IgM will be increased. It must be emphasized that many tropical regions will not have access to immunological tests or broad-based laboratory support for serological examinations. Physical examination with clinical acumen guide most therapeutic regimens without comprehensive workups to rule out least likely causes of illness. Most cases of malaria are not properly identified, leading to overuse of antimalarial agents.[9]

Because of the high mortality (10%–40%) associated with severe malaria, particularly in children, some authors have proposed a grading system.[8] Utilizing the 2000 WHO criteria for malaria, Imananagha et al. retrospectively reviewed 155 children with malaria with the hypothesis that severe malaria was not a homogenous group, but a group with graded severity that can be differentiated by clinical factors on presentation that might predict overall mortality.[8] There are three grades (I–III) of severe malaria based on four major and four minor presenting clinical features (PCFs). The four major presenting clinical features are: impaired consciousness, convulsions, prostration, and respiratory distress. The four minor presenting clinical features are: cough, fever, vomiting, and anemia.

This simple system for grading severe malaria helps surgeons to understand the possible long-term impact of splenectomy in children in endemic regions who often become chronically infected.

Treatment of HMS and Splenomegaly Management of malaria begins with effective prevention strategies. Appropriate use of insecticidal nets and door spraying of insecticide is effective when possible. Chemoprevention includes effective malarial prophylaxis for the given region. In some regions the resistance profiles of Plasmodium are different. The response rates to artemisinin in Southeastern Asia are superior due to resistance of *P. falciparum* to other antimalarials. WHO recommends that malaria treatment be based on appropriate identification of the specific parasite in all cases.[10] This policy is not followed for the majority of cases being managed.

Patients with HMS who present with splenomegaly should not undergo splenectomy unless they present with hemorrhagic shock. There are no prospective data to support operative splenic salvage in patients with splenomegaly who have spontaneous rupture, although if feasible a patient with malarial splenic rupture (MSR) in an endemic region is an ideal indication. It must

be emphasized that the organ texture of a spleen in a patient with HMS is significantly different than that of a normal spleen that has been shattered from blunt trauma. In HMS the spleen is firm and hard, possibly making a splenic salvage procedure or partial splenectomy more challenging. Furthermore, the spleen is usually more than twice its normal size and compresses other abdominal organs. Conventional methods of controlling blood supply still apply but become more technically difficult. After partial resections of splenic parenchyma, hypertrophy can still occur.

There are many reports of nonoperative therapy for spontaneous splenic rupture secondary to HMS in a highly select groups of patients. Usually children with chronic malarial infection presenting with HMS will have large palpable spleens that may be symptomatic. Acutely, these patients should be resuscitated with crystalloids and blood if needed. Osman et al. described an MSR algorithm (see Figure 15.1).

Those patients responding to resuscitation with stable vital signs can be further closely observed with hemodynamic monitoring. Patients who become unstable should undergo splenectomy with consideration for some form of splenic salvage. Patients should not be put at risk for additional bleeding with high-risk partial splenectomy or splenic salvage procedures. Total splenectomy is preferred if partial splenectomy or splenic salvage is not feasible. Total splenectomy is the most often reported management for

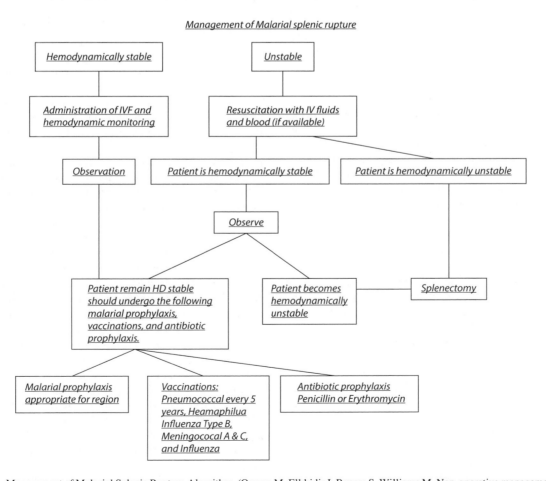

FIGURE 15.1 Management of Malarial Splenic Rupture Algorithm. (Osman M, Elkhidir I, Rogers S, Williams M. Non-operative management of malarial splenic rupture: The Khartoum experience and an international review. *International Journal of Surgery*. 2012 Dec; **46**(6): 410–415.

TABLE 15.2

Prophylactic antibiotic regimens for malaria patients

Antibiotic	Child	<12 years old
Benzathine penicillin	1.2 MU monthly IM	2.4 MU monthly IM
Phenoxymethylpenicillin	125–250 mg bid po	250 mg bid po
Erythromycin	125–250 mg bid po	250 mg bid po

Table by Mallory Williams.
Adapted from: Imananagha KK, Awotua-Efebo OE. Severe alaria in children: a proposal for clinical grading. *South African Journal of Child Health.* 2009 May; 3(1): 1–9.

these patients. Patients who continue to be hemodynamically stable will have had successful nonoperative treatment and should avoid strenuous exercise or contact to the left side of the abdomen. An algorithm for the management of these patients can be seen in Figure 15.1.[11] Effective long-term management includes treatment with antimalarial agents and lifetime prophylaxis. With effective antimalarial therapy, studies have shown a reduction in spleen size and Hackett's score.[12] All patients should be vaccinated against pneumococcus, haemaphilus influenza Type B, and *Neisseria meningitides.* Immunocompromised malaria patients should also receive both antibiotic prophylaxis and early treatment with antibiotics for infections (see Table 15.2).

The data for antibiotic prophylaxis in malaria is extrapolated from the sickle cell literature.[13,14] Compliance with these regimens declines with time. The populations that benefit the most are children less than 5 years old, patients who have had splenectomy in the past year, and patients with underlying immunodeficiency in addition to splenectomy.

Immunosuppression of Malaria Malaria simultaneously causes immunosuppression and inflammation in the host patient. T cells are stimulated by the supernatant of *P. falciparum* and produce IL-2 and promote B cell differentiation.[15] A decrease in circulating CD4+ T cells occurs with *P. falciparum* infection.[16–18] Decreases in CD4+ cells are vitally important because CD4+ cells mediate the proliferation and differentiation of B-lymphocytes. This process begins the production of immunoglobulins, which leads to immune response that ultimately is protective against infection. It has been demonstrated that non-immune patients with *P. falciparum* malaria have higher levels of parasitemia, possibly leading to decreased levels of CD4+ cells and overall immunosuppression.[19] Case series exist that demonstrate higher incidence of malaria recurrence after splenectomy.[20] Parasitemia was confirmed in 88% of these patients. In this same study, compliance with malarial prophylaxis decreased from 100% after the first year to 29% after 3 years in the splenectomy group.

Post-splenectomy or hyposplenic patients may be evaluated for splenic dysfunction. This is done by assessing the spleen's filtering function by radioisotopic methods or quantification of erythrocyte morphological abnormalities. Radioisotopic methods are expensive and not a practical use of resources in developing nations. Evaluation of erythrocyte abnormalities is more practical as it is inexpensive and less invasive. Quantifying of Howell-Jolly bodies has been proposed but is not a sensitive or specific test. Quantification of pitted erythrocytes is regarded as the gold standard for the assessment of splenic dysfunction.

Malaria patients who undergo splenectomy are susceptible to overwhelming bacterial infections. Several factors further increase the risk of overwhelming infection. Pediatric patients have higher risk (the younger the patient, the higher the risk). Patients with underlying immunocompromising diseases, such as HIV, thalassemia, sickle cell anemia, or neoplastic diseases, also are at increased risk. Patients are also at increased risk during the time period closest to the splenectomy versus many years afterwards.

Splenectomized malaria patients have increased susceptibility to overwhelming bacterial infection and recurrent episodes of malaria. For these reasons, in both selective nonoperative management and operative management the focus in decision making is on patient survival with an emphasis on splenic salvage if possible.

Malarial Splenic Rupture Malaria is the most common cause of nontraumatic splenic rupture in the world. The incidence of MSR is underreported worldwide. It is, however, interesting that only natural vector-transmitted cases of MSR have been observed. There have been no reports of transfusion-related malaria or other methods of inoculation. Imbert et al. reported 55 cases of MSR.[21] *P. falciparum* was responsible for 26 cases; *Plasmodium vivax,* 23; *Plasmodium ovale,* 2; and *Plasmodium malariae,* 2. The median age of this group was 32. The median duration of malaria symptoms before MSR was 5–6 days. Death occurred in 22% (12) of these patients. Seven of these 12 patients died from early irreversible circulatory collapse.

The mechanism of splenic rupture in malaria is unknown. Three mechanisms have been implicated in MSR. The first is increase in intrasplenic tension. That is due to cellular hyperplasia and engorgement. Second, the spleen may be compressed by the abdominal musculature during physiological activities such as sneezing, coughing, defecation, and sitting up or turning in the bed. Finally, vascular occlusion due to reticule endothelial hyperplasia, resulting in thrombosis and infarction, may lead to progressive subcapsular hemorrhage until the capsule ruptures. While splenectomy has been the management of choice historically, new evidence is building that conservative or nonoperative management may be pursued for selected patients.

Management of MSR has historically been splenectomy. Because of the increased susceptibility of patients without spleens to overwhelming infection, a more conservative approach for selected patients has been trialed. Nonoperative management in hemodynamically stable patients has been demonstrated to be successful. Furthermore, operative management aimed at splenic salvage is a useful alternative in highly selected cases.

Special Populations **HIV-positive patients.** HIV-positive patients who are asymptomatic respond well to vaccination. Patients with symptomatic disease have less positive results with vaccination. HIV-positive patients should not be given live vaccines. Malarial prophylaxis appropriate for the region should be administered.[10] HIV-positive patients presenting with hemodynamic instability from MSR should receive splenectomy.

Pregnant patients. Pregnant patients should all receive malarial prophylaxis appropriate for the region. This, however, does not occur. Pregnancy can complicate splenomegaly and lead to spontaneous rupture of an enlarged spleen. These patients are cared for using the same algorithm outlined in Figure 15.1.[11] Special attention is given to the fetus, and fetal monitoring should be done if available. Splenectomy should still be performed for hemodynamically unstable patients.

Gestational malaria also leads to low birth weight babies born to mothers with *P. falciparum.* An overall increase in parasitemia rates is seen with malarial infection and is more marked in primiparous women. Egwynyenga et al. evaluated the effect of malaria parasitemia on spleen size and anemia in approximately 2,000 pregnant women in the Jos Plateau highlands, Bauchi Savannah plains, and Ethiopia river basin of Nigeria.[22] More cases of palpable spleen were detected in pregnant woman than in nonpregnant controls. In all three study sites, parasitemic pregnant women had significantly lower hemoglobin values than malaria negative mothers, especially among primigravids. They did not find an association between higher parasite density and splenomegaly. HMS during pregnancy causes episodes of hemolytic anemia, which can be life-threatening to the both the mother and the fetus. Malaria exacerbates folate deficiency in pregnant woman. Blood transfusions are useful in the management of the anemia.

Schistosomiasis

Schistosomiasis mansoni and *japonicum* cause hepatomegaly and portal hypertension. Increased presinusoidal venous pressures lead to increase splenic vein pressures with resultant congestive splenomegaly. The second factor contributing to splenomegaly is the splenic hyperplasia that occurs as in malaria. Cell proliferation in the red pulp and germinal centers of the lymphoid follicles occurs early in schistosomiasis. Severe longstanding hepatosplenic schistosomiasis leads to splenomegaly, esophageal varices, and ascites.

Epidemiology More than 200 million people worldwide have schistosomiasis. The estimated mortality of schistosomiasis in Sub-Saharan Africa is 200,000 people per year. Different species occur in the following geographic areas (see Table 15.3).

TABLE 15.3

Geographic Regions of Schistosomiasis

Schistosomiasis	Geographic Region
S. Mansoni	Sub-Saharan Africa
	Middle East
	South America
	Caribbean
S. Haematobium	North Africa
	Sub-Saharan Africa
	Middle East
	Turkey
	India
S. Japonicum	China
	Philippines
	Thailand
	Indonesia
S. Intercalatum	Central and West Africa
S. Mekonji	Laos and Cambodia

Table by Mallory Williams.

The species that cause splenomegaly are those that lay their eggs in the hepatic presinusoidal areas. These are *S. mansoni, S. japonicum,* and *S. mekonji.*

S. haematobium also has been associated with both hepatomegaly and splenomegaly. When *S. haematobium* has been treated, regression of both hepatomegaly and splenomegaly has been demonstrated.[23] Because *S. haematobium* is mostly associated with the genitourinary system and resultant hematuria, this discussion will not focus on this species. This discussion will focus on *S. mansoni, S. japonicum,* and *S. mekonji.*

Diagnosis S. mansoni, japonicum, and *mekonji* are diagnosed by microscopy demonstrating schistosomal eggs in the stool of the patient. Concentration techniques improve detection. It has been estimated that greater than 3,000 eggs per day must be excreted to be readily visualized.[24] Determination of intensity of infection is important because complications of the infection are associated with burden of disease. Intensity of infection is evaluated by quantitative sampling of defined amounts of stool. Current infection is defined by identification of viable eggs, whereas treated infection is determined by identification of nonviable eggs. Serological tests to detect antischistosomal antibodies or schistosomal antigens are utilized for the diagnosis of schistosomiasis. These tests are not well standardized. General serology may reveal a peripheral eosinophilia in one third of patients or anemia. Radiologic studies demonstrating periportal fibrosis (Symmer's fibrosis) can be important along with clinical symptoms in diagnosing the disease. Splenomegaly, extended portal vein dimensions, and the development of venous collaterals may also be seen by computed tomography or ultrasound. It is important to understand that despite portal hypertension and periportal fibrosis, liver function remains normal in these patients. In some cases tissue biopsies of the rectum, liver, and esophagus (intervariceal) demonstrate schistosomiasis.

Treatment of Schistosomiasis and Splenomegaly Treatment of schistosomiasis is with oral doses of praziquantel. *S. haematobium, S. mansoni,* and *S. intercalatum* can be treated with a dose of 40 mg/kg (may be repeated). Recommended dose for *S. japonicum* and *S. mekonji* is 60 mg/kg in two to three doses 3 hours apart. Oxamniquine 15 mg/kg twice a day for one day is also a potent treatment for *S. mansoni.* Data from Brazil evaluated treatment of 84 patients with hepatosplenic schistosomiasis consisting of periportal thickening on ultrasound and a palpable spleen, and 50% of patients were available for 4-year follow-up.[25] A significant number of patients (68%) did not improve. Spleen size, however, decreased in 59% of patients.[25] Furthermore, in an 11-year follow-up study of schistosomiasis treatment with oxamniquine in Brazil, splenomegaly rates fell from 10% to 2%.[26] The splenomegaly regression rate increased from 43% to 91%.[26]

Patients with symptomatic splenomegaly from schistosomal disease may require splenectomy for control of symptoms or spontaneous rupture. Kamel et al. describe performance of segmental splenectomy (20%–30% remnant) in this population with a similar postoperative complication as total splenectomy patients and a low conversion rate to total splenectomy.[27] The investigators also demonstrated no growth of the splenic remnant at 4 years.

Several small studies, including prospective data, have demonstrated that treatment of pregnant women with praziquantel is safe and does not lead to increased abortions, preterm deliveries. or congenital defects.[28,29] Experts convened by WHO in 2003 issued a statement that pregnant and lactating women in endemic areas should not be excluded from receiving treatment.[30]

Visceral Leishmaniasis

Leishmaniasis is caused by a protozoan parasite, *Leishmania donavani,* transmitted by the bite of a phlebotamine female sand fly. Leishmaniasis is a disease heavily associated with poverty, malnutrition, displacement, and overall lack of shelter. Environmental factors such as deforestation and dam building have led to increased outbreaks of the disease.

Epidemiology Estimates are that 12 million people are infected with leishmaniasis. Each year 1 to 2 million new cases occur in 88 countries around the world. While the disease can be found on four continents, 90% of the visceral leishmaniasis is located in Bangladesh, India; Brazil; Nepal; and Sudan. There is a resurgence of this disease due to a growing HIV-positive population. Visceral leishmaniasis is an opportunistic infection for patients who are HIV positive. Many patients with visceral leishmaniasis do not have active disease. Concomitant infection with HIV increases the risk of developing active visceral leishmanaisis by 100 to 2,320 times. In southern Europe 70% of cases of visceral leishmaniasis in adults are associated with HIV.

Diagnosis Clinical features of leishmaniasis are prolonged fever, splenomegaly, hepatomegaly, and wasting. These are not specific. Serological studies classically show anemia, pancytopenia, low albumin, and hypergammaglobulinemia. Liver function tests are markedly elevated along with alkaline phosphatase and gamma glutamyl transferase. Serological testing for leishmaniasis is based on detection of IgG (antileishmaniasial antibodies). The tests used are indirect immunofluorescent antibody test, enzyme linked immunosorbent assay, and direct agglutination test. These tests can be expensive.

Commonly, diagnosis has been made demonstrating the parasite in spleen and bone marrow aspirates with light microscopy. The patient is placed in the supine position and given sedation. The abdomen is prepped with a sterile solution. The outline of the spleen is drawn on the patient's skin and a mark is placed where the needle is to enter the skin. A 5-ml syringe with a 21-gauge needle is used to enter the skin. Aiming cranially at a 45-degree angle as to avoid hilar vessels, the needle is introduced and withdrawn while applying suction (see Figure 15.2).

Chulay and Bryceson in 1983 developed a scoring scale for light microscopy to demonstrate overall effectiveness of treatment and distinguish slow responders from nonresponders to therapy.[31] They performed more than 500 splenic aspirations in 89 patients with only two recognized complications of intra-abdominal bleeding and intestinal perforation. Both of these complications were conservatively managed. The Chulay Bryceson Scoring System can be found in Table 15.4.

As quantities of amistogotes decreased on serial splenic aspiration, a response to therapy could be seen.

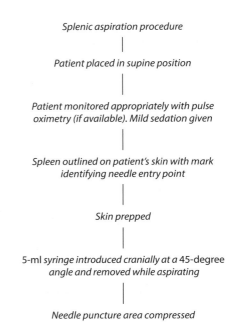

Splenic aspiration procedure

Patient placed in supine position

Patient monitored appropriately with pulse oximetry (if available). Mild sedation given

Spleen outlined on patient's skin with mark identifying needle entry point

Skin prepped

5-ml syringe introduced cranially at a 45-degree angle and removed while aspirating

Needle puncture area compressed

FIGURE 15.2 Splenic Aspiration Procedure. Illica A, Kocaoglu M, Zaybek N, Guven S, et al. Extrahepatic Abdominal Disease Caused by Echinococcus Granulosus: Imaging findings. *American Journal of Roetgenology.* 2007 Aug; 189(2): 337–343.

TABLE 15.4

Chulay Bryceson scoring system for splenic aspiration in visceral leishmaniasis

Score	Quantity of Amistogotes/oil immersion fields
6+	>100 amistogotes/oil immersion field
5+	10–100 amistogotes/oil immersion field
4+	1–10 amistogotes/oil immersion field
3+	1–10 amistogotes/10 oil immersion fields
2+	1–10 amistogotes/100 oil immersion fields
1+	1–10 amistogotes/1000 oil immersion fields
0	0 amistogotes/1000 oil immersion fields

Table by Mallory Williams.

Treatment of Visceral Leishmaniasis and Splenomegaly First-line agents for visceral leishmaniasis are sodium stibogluconate (Pentostam) and meglumine antimoniate (Glucantime). Failure and relapses occur in all forms of leishmaniaisis. The failure rate is 10%–25%. If treatment failure occurs, second-line agents are pentamidine (Lomidine) and amphotericine B (Fungizone). Resistance to sodium stibogluconate is high in India, and first-line therapy is now amphotericin B in its liposomal preparations. Amphocil 7.5 mg/kg IV over 6 days is given. Mitefosine is the first oral therapy for visceral leishmaniasis. The cure rate in phase III trials is 95%. The drug has also been shown to be effective in HIV-positive patients with visceral leishmaniasis. In resistant cases two of three patients responded to the Mitefosine. The recommended dose is 100 mg/day for 28 days.

Effective treatment of visceral leishmaniasis improves splenomegaly. There are reported cases of splenic rupture in patients with visceral leishmaniasis and they should be managed similar to the MSR algorithm. Troya et al. describe a HIV-positive subpopulation that will develop pancytopenia with recurrent relapses of visceral leishmaniasis.[32] They describe a role for splenectomy in these patients to restore the hematologic parameters and reduce the need for blood transfusions. Splenectomy in these patients does not, however, prevent relapse of the visceral leishmaniasis.

African Trypanosomiasis

African trypanosomiasis, or sleeping sickness, is caused by the protozoan parasite *Trypanosoma brucei gambiense* in West and Central Africa. The vector is the tsetse fly, *Glossina palpalis*. *T. b. gambiense* is responsible for 95% of all sleeping sickness cases. In 2009 the number of cases dropped below 10,000 for the first time in the last 50 years. The clinical symptoms of this disease are broken down into two phases. The first phase is the hemolymphatic phase. This phase consists of the multiplication of trypanosomes in the subcutaneous tissues, blood, and lymph. Clinical symptoms include fever, headaches, joint pain, and itching. The second phase is the neurologic phase, and progression to this phase can take months or years. In the neurologic phase the parasites cross the blood brain barrier and more obvious clinical symptoms occur, including confusion, change in behavior, sensory disturbances, cerebellar ataxia, pyramidal symptoms such as focal paralysis, and extrapyramidal symptoms such as rigidity and tremor. Disturbance of the sleep cycle is present, specifically daytime somnolence followed by nocturnal insomnia. Trypanosomiasis is a cause of splenomegaly in endemic regions.

Diagnosis Early diagnosis of trypanosomiasis is essential before the second phase occurs. The only serological test is for *T. b. gambiense*. The Card agglutination test for trypanosomiasis is used for screening. Diagnosis is then confirmed by locating trypanosomes in the blood, lymph nodes, or central nervous system (CNS). As many as 20%–30% of cases are missed using standard parasitological techniques.[33] Due to low sensitivity, many patients will return with later phases of the disease. The more labor-intense lymph node aspiration and microscopy can be used as well to diagnose trypanosomiasis.

Treatment of Trypanosomiasis and Splenomegaly First-line therapy for the first phase of trypanosomiasis includes intramuscular pentamidine or intravenous eflornithine. First-line therapy for the second phase of trypanosomiasis is intravenous melarsoprol 2.2 mg/kg daily for 12 consecutive days. Intravenous eflornithine may also be used in doses of 50 mg/kg q 6 hours for 14 days. If the trypansoma is resistant to melarsoprol, then eflornithine should be used or melarsoprol with nifurtimox. Patients with splenomegaly and trypanosomiasis should be treated based on the phase of their illness. Effective treatment of the disease results in improvement of the hypersplenism and regression of the splenomegaly in most cases.

American Trypanosomiasis (Chagas Disease)

Chagas disease is due to the flagellated protozoan parasite *Trypanosoma cruzi*. It is transmitted to humans through infected feces of the blood-sucking triatomine bug. The acute phase of the disease features a skin chancre (chagoma) or unilateral purplish orbital edema (Romana sign). Headaches, myalgias, cough, abdominal pain, edema in the lower extremities and face, hepatomegaly, splenomegaly, myocarditis, and meningoencephalitis are all presentations of the disease. In patients suffering from acquired immunodeficiency syndrome (AIDS), unfortunately, meningoencephalitis is the more common presentation of the disease. The chronic phase has different forms. The asymptomatic or indeterminate form can last a patient's entire life with parasites infecting target tissues such as the heart and smooth muscle of the digestive system. The cardiac form features cardiac arrhythmias and conduction problems. The digestive form features patients with megaesophagus or megacolon. There are also mixed forms.

In the acute phase, Chagas disease can be diagnosed by blood smear. In the chronic phase, serologic tests are used, such as ELISA, western blot, or indirect hemaglutination assay. Treatment for this disease is benzimidazole and nifurtimox.

Hydatid Disease (Echinococcosis)

Hydatid disease is caused by the tape worm *Echinococcus granulosis*. This parasite is found worldwide and is particularly prevalent in large grazing areas where dogs have access to feed on the dying carcasses of large stock animals. These intermediate hosts are herbivores such as sheep, horses, cattle, goats, and camels. Larval stages of cestodes reach maturity in the small intestine of humans 4–5 weeks after ingestion of feces-infected food. Human infection is characterized by long-term growth of hydatid cysts (metacestodes) in internal organs. The liver is involved in 75% of cases, with the right lobe being the most commonly involved. These cysts are unilocular fluid-filled bladders that may calcify. The cysts have two parasite-derived layers: an inner nucleated germinal layer surrounded by an outer acellular laminated layer. This outer layer is also surrounded by a host-generated fibrous capsule.

Diagnosis Diagnosis of this disease is dependent upon a combination of radiographic, serologic, and physical examinations. Ultrasound is the preferred imaging test because it is inexpensive and very sensitive for evaluating cystic lesions of the liver. Often the cysts appear as anechoic lesions on sonography (see Figure 15.3).

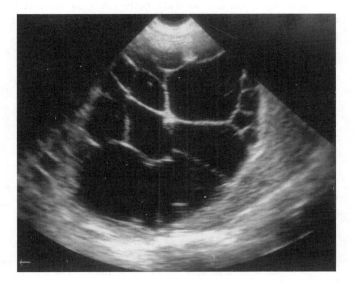

FIGURE 15.3 Ultrasound of hydatid cyst. Otal P, Escourra G, Mazerolles C, et al. Imaging features of uncommon adrenal masses with histopathologic correlation. *Radiographics*. 1999 May; **19**(3): 569–581.

Computed tomography and magnetic resonance imaging are seldom available in LMICs but also can be used (see Figures 15.4 and 15.5).

Historically, the most commonly used serologic tests due to their low cost are double diffusion and immunoelectrophoresis for the arc 5 band of Capron. These tests have very high specificity but relatively low sensitivity.[34] Cross-reactions can occur with sera from patients with cysticercosis. Better sensitivity and specificity have been reported for the enzyme-linked immuno-electrotransfer blot test (EITB).[35] Furthermore, when EITB and double diffusion tests are run simultaneously, the highest detection rates are achieved.[36] Serological tests may be negative in patients with intensely calcified cysts.[37] Serological tests are thought to be more confirmatory but not diagnostic in the modern era of managing hydatid disease.

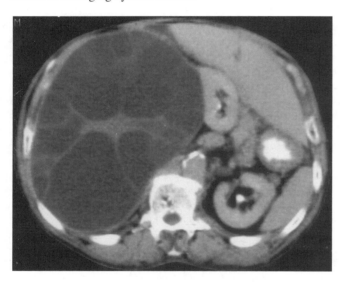

FIGURE 15.4. Computed tomography of hydatid cysts. Otal P, Escourra G, Mazerolles C, et al. Imaging features of uncommon adrenal masses with histopathologic correlation. *Radiographics*. 1999 May; **19**(3): 569–581.

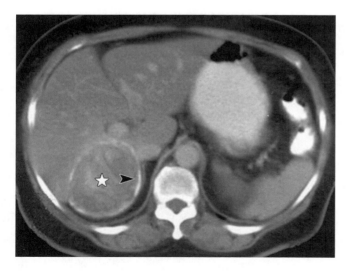

FIGURE 15.5 Computed tomography of hydatid cyst. Illica A, Kocaoglu M, Zaybek N, Guven S, et al. Extrahepatic Abdominal Disease Caused by Echinococcus Granulosus: Imaging findings. *American Journal of Roetgenology*. 2007 Aug; **189**(2): 337–343.

Treatment of Hydatid Cystic Disease of the Spleen Splenic involvement in hydatid disease is uncommon, representing less than 2% of all infestations. The most common symptoms when there is splenic involvement are the nonspecific symptoms and signs of abdominal pain, splenomegaly, and fever. Anaphylactic shock secondary to cyst rupture may also occur. Systemic dissemination and ruptured hepatic cyst account for the two major sources of splenic infestation. Franquet et al. reviewed nine patients with splenic hydatidosis.[35] The most common radiographic finding seen was splenomegaly. WHO recommends that medical therapy should be reserved for inoperable cases or to prevent recurrence.[35] Surgery is the treatment of choice. While open celiotomy remains the most common approach worldwide, laparoscopic procedures have been described. Cyst size may determine the operative approach. For larger cysts with a high risk of rupture, open procedures may be preferred. Since rupture of the cyst into the peritoneal cavity can cause both lethal anaphylactic shock and peritoneal seeding, care should be taken in manipulation of the spleen. Enucleation techniques have also been described, but splenectomy for large and multiple cysts can also be done. The surgical technique of partial cystectomy is as follows: Mebendazole or praziquantel is given preoperatively. The surgical field is surrounded by sterile laparotomy pads soaked in hypertonic saline to protect the patient from peritoneal seeding. Sterilization of the cyst is done by injection of the cysts with hypertonic saline or silver nitrates. The cyst is then carefully opened and the internal contents are aspirated using a closed suction system. Remaining cyst contents are also removed. At this time evaluation for bile leak must be done. Clean laparotomy sponges may be inserted into the cyst to check for green discoloration suggesting a bile leak. If this is found, the bile duct should be sutured closed with absorbable suture. Then capitonage is performed. The anterior walls of the cyst are sutured using absorbable sutures to the middle of the posterior wall. This prevents postoperative fluid retention in the dead space. Some surgeons choose to leave a drain, which is later removed, in the postoperative period. This is not necessary in all cases.

Other techniques include marsupialization, ablation, and radical cystectomy. These surgical procedures may be useful for individual patients. Marsupialization is a safe and quick procedure that is commonly done. The complications of this procedure are leaving a residual cavity, bile leak, peritoneal seeding, anaphylactic shock, and sepsis. Ablation is also an easy procedure that has a recurrence rate as high as 30%. More conservative approaches such as marsupialization have been reported to cause higher morbidity for patients. Skroubis et al. reported deroofing of cysts in 187 patients.[38] Complications included bile abscess in 1.5%, bile peritonitis in 0.5%, bronchobiliary fistula in 0.5%, and biliary fistula in 7%.[38] Bile leakage and fistulas were successfully treated either endoscopically or conservatively in this series of patients. Radical cystectomy usually is a more complicated procedure involving resection of hepatic tissue including the cyst and surrounding wall. Hemorrhage is the major complication to this approach.

Splenic Cyst

Cystic lesions of the spleen are classified as either primary or secondary. Primary cysts are usually parasitic but may also be congenital or neoplastic. The most common parasitic splenic cyst is *Echinococcus granulosus.* These cysts have an epithelial lining. The most common cause of a secondary cyst is trauma, and it accounts for the majority of nonparasitic splenic cysts. These cysts do not have an epithelial lining. They often will develop a calcified capsule surrounding them. Strong consideration of the infectious diseases prevalent in the geographic region should guide suspicions as to the origin of the cyst. In the absence of fever or systemic infection, neoplastic processes such as hemangioma, lymphangioma, and lymphoma should be considered.

Small cysts (< 5 cm) tend to regress and may be observed. Larger cysts (> 5 cm) may be considered for surgical resection by either cyst enucleation, partial splenectomy, or total splenectomy. Large cysts tend to recur if they are only de-roofed laparoscopically.

Bacterial Disease

Bacterial infections of the spleen are metastatic and hematogenous in etiology. Many different bacterial infections, such as brucellosis, ehrilichiosis, actinomycosis, and fusobacterium, may lead to splenomegaly. In this section tuberculosis (TB), melioidosis, and typhoid disease are discussed. Special attention is given to the management of splenic abscess.

Splenic Abscess

The true incidence of splenic abscess in the world is unknown. The often cited occurrence of between 0.14% and 0.7% in autopsy data does not include patients successfully treated with conservative and/or operative management. Case reports reported in the literature include parasites such as malaria, amoeba, and bacteria as the etiology (Table 15.5). Splenic abscesses are associated with metastatic hematogenous infections, immunocompromised individuals, and neoplastic disease.

Diagnosis

The most common clinical symptoms include fever and abdominal pain (Table 15.6). When the largest series of splenic abscesses were analyzed, fever, abdominal pain, and splenomegaly were the most common symptoms and signs on presentation. Leukocytosis is common and blood cultures may initially be positive or negative. In a Llenas-Garcia et al. review

of splenic abscesses, only 32% of cases had positive blood cultures.[39] Chiang et al. found positive blood cultures in only 24% of cases.[40] A recent review by Lee et al. demonstrated 61% of cases with positive blood cultures.[41] Splenic abscess review data from the African continent is not available, and therefore the overall impact of diseases such as malaria and HIV may be underrepresented in the literature.

Management of Splenic Abscess

Splenectomy remains the gold standard for management of most splenic abscesses. However, conservative management with intravenous antibiotics and percutaneous aspiration are viable alternatives for select patients when surgery is not an option. A Serum et al. study of percutaneous drainage of splenic abscesses demonstrates that ultrasound guided percutaneous drainage is a successful alternative to splenectomy.[42] In this study, 89% of patients (32/36) were treated successfully with percutaneous drainage. Because splenic salvage is advantageous in many regions of the world, particularly in the pediatric population, these alternatives should be considered in the appropriate patients. There have been rare reports of partial splenectomy in the setting of splenic abscess.[43]

Splenic Abscesses in the Immunocompromised Patient

Central Africa has a very high incidence of HIV-positive patients with TB. Most TB involvement of the spleen occurs in immunocompromised patients with HIV. Patients with HIV or AIDS who develop disseminated TB with splenic involvement should be treated promptly with anti-TB triple drug regimens. Reichel et al. reported two cases of AIDS patients with TB involvement of the spleen that successfully responded to anti-TB therapy and did not need surgery.[44] Bernabeu-Wittel et al. followed 32 consecutive HIV-positive patients with splenic abscesses and the etiology of the abscesses were: TB (14), visceral leishmaniasis (7), disseminated mycobacterium avium (5), salmonella (2), lymphoma (2), disseminated *Rhodococcus equi* infection (1), disseminated *Candida krusei* infection (1), and *Pneumocystis carinii* pneumonia (1).[45] Twenty-eight patients were followed for 6 months. Sixteen patients had a clinical cure and microbiological eradication. Furthermore, on follow-up high-resolution sonography, the findings were normal. In two

TABLE 15.5

Etiology of splenic abscess from case series in the medical literature

Case Series	Nation	N	Dates of Study	Two Most Common Etiologies	
Lee, et al., 2011	Korea	18	1993–2008	*Strep Virdians*	*Klebsiella pneumonia*
Llenas-Garcia et al., 2009	Spain	22	1998–2006	*M. tuberculosis*	Candidal species
Ferrioli et al., 2009	Italy	16	1979–2005	GNB	Fungal (Aspergillosis)
Yung Ng et al., 2008	Singapore	21	1996–2005	Melioidosis	*Salmonella typhi*
Chang et al., 2006	China	67	1984–2004	*K. pneumonia*	*GP cocci*
Tung et al., 2006	Taiwan	51	1998–2003	*K. pneumonia*	*E. coli* and pseudomonas
Chiang et al., 2003	Taiwan	29	1990–2001	Staphylococcal species	Salmonella, Pseudomonas, Enterococcus, Enterobacter

Table by Mallory Williams.

TABLE 15.6

Symptoms of splenic abscess from case series in the medical literature

Symptoms and Signs	Case Series in the Medical Literature						
	Lee, 2011	Llenas-Garcia, 2009	Ferraioli, 2009	Yung Ng, 2008	Chang, 2006	Tung, 2006	Chiang, 2003
Fever	28%	100%	94%	95%	85%	82%	90%
Abdominal pain	67%	50%	81%	10%	43%	71%	31%
Chills	28%	41%	NR	NR	NR	NR	41%
Constitutional symptoms	NR	36%	NR|NR	8%	NR	41%	
Splenomegaly	78%	23%	44%	29%	67%	NR	17%
Septic shock	6%	9%	N/A	NR	NR	NR	N/A
Hepatomegaly	NR	36%	NR	NR	NR	NR	7%
Leukocytosis	61%	NR	63%	NR	70%	83%	38%
Positive blood cultures	61%	95%	50%	52%	87%	8%	
NR – Not Reported							

Table by Mallory Williams.

patients the micro-abscesses persisted and 10 patients died. Patients who are immunocompromised have higher mortality but should be aggressively treated because a significant percentage will have excellent responses.

Tuberculosis

TB is a respiratory disease caused the bacteria *Mycobacterium tuberculosis*. The spread of this disease is through respiratory droplets. Although the lungs are a primary site of the disease, TB can affect all other organ systems. Healthy individuals do not become symptomatic, as their immune system is able to contain the disease. More than one-third of the world's population is infected with TB. The most rapid spread of the disease in 2008 occurred in Southeast Asia. However, the incidence rate in sub-Saharan Africa is twice that of Southeast Asia. Of the 1.7 million people who died of TB in 2009, most lived in sub-Saharan Africa.

Splenic involvement of tuberculosis is very rare. Perhaps the best evidence to support this is that among 300 cases of intra-abdominal TB, no focal splenic TB was reported. When it occurs it is usually in the miliary form as the result of hematogenous dissemination. The macro-nodular form and abscess formation are extremely rare. Llenas-Garcia et al. reported 22 cases of splenic abscess in which 8 (36%) were due to TB.[39] In all 8 cases the patients also had AIDS. The mortality for patients with splenic abscess with TB was 25%.

Diagnosis

Because splenic involvement in TB is secondary to systemic disease, clinical symptoms including fever, dyspnea, and weight loss are common. Some patients will also develop abdominal pain. Both ultrasound and computed tomography (CT) scan can be important in helping to make the diagnosis. Topal et al. reported radiologic findings for splenic abscess using ultrasound and CT.[45] If ultrasound was used, multiple hyperechoic nodules were visualized in all patients. Splenomegaly was noted in three of five patients. The most common finding on CT was multiple hypodense nodules. When CT is not available, ultrasound-guided

fine needle aspiration biopsy can provide a definitive diagnosis. Dixit et al.'s review of TB of the spleen demonstrated that 50% of patients had HIV, and more than 62% of patients had associated pulmonary TB.[46] Other findings were ascites (50%), intra-abdominal lymph nodes (37%), pleural effusion (37%), and cervical lymph nodes (12%). Ultrasound findings were multiple splenic abscesses (62%), multiple diffuse hyperechoic nodules (25%), and solitary abscess and calcified granuloma (6%).

Management of TB of the Spleen

Anti-TB medications are administered for TB of the spleen. Due to the high level of resistance seen globally, anti-TB regimens appropriate for the region should be administered. Resolution of calcification of the lesions on imaging is a sign of effective therapy. In Dixit et al.'s review, 44% of patients became asymptomatic after anti-TB treatment with complete clearance of initial sonographic abnormalities of the splenic parenchyma.[46]

Melioidosis (Whitmore's Disease)

Melioidosis is an infection caused by the bacteria *Burkholderia pseudomallei* (previously referred to as *Pseudomonas pseudomallei*). The endemic areas are tropical regions like Southeast Asia and Australia. The greatest concentration is in Vietnam, Laos, Cambodia, Thailand, Malaysia, Burma, and Northern Australia. Melioidosis is a disease of the rainy season in endemic areas. People become infected through both infected soil and water through broken skin or wounds. Person-to-person transmission can occur. The incubation period can be 1–5 days or months. More than 50% of patients present with signs and symptoms of pneumonia. Other presentations are diarrhea and septicemia. Immunocompromised patients with diabetes or renal failure and acute bloodstream infections can present with septic shock. Melioidosis does not seem to be associated with HIV infection. Diagnosis of this disease is by isolation of the bacteria in the patient's blood. Treatment of the disease is with intravenous antibiotics. *Burkholderia pseudomallei* is usually sensitive to penicillin, doxycycline, imipinem, amoxicillin-clavulanic acid, ceftazidime, ceftriaxone, and aztreonam. All cases of melioidosis should be treated with 2 weeks of intensive therapy followed by at least 3 months of oral therapy. Intensive therapy regimens include the following: ceftazidime 50 mg/kg up to 2 g IV q 6 hours, meropenem 25 mg/kg up to 1 g IV q 8 hours, and imipinem 25 mg/kg up to 1 g q 6 hours.

Splenic Disease

Melioidosis is a disease of abscess formation. Melioidosis is a very rare cause of splenic abscesses that are more commonly seen in Southeast Asia. Typically, abdominal abscesses including the liver and spleen are seen in disseminated disease. In Northeastern Thailand, Melioidosis has been reported to be the etiology of 20% of community associated septicemic cases with an overall mortality of 40%. In Yung Ng et al.'s review of splenic abscesses in Singapore, the number-one etiology was Melioidosis.[47] Apisarnthanarak et al. evaluated CT characteristics of hepatic and splenic abscesses associated with elioidosis over a 7-year period.[48] The authors found that splenic abscesses were more commonly associated with melioidosis than other etiologies and melioid intra-abdominal abscesses were smaller than non-melioid intra-abdominal abscesses. It is found that the CT necklace sign was correlated with melioidosis. The CT necklace sign was defined as an abscess with multiple, internal, rather symmetrical locules distributed in a peripheral radial fashion, similar to a pearl necklace. Concurrent hepatic abscesses also were found to be associated with melioidosis in this study focused in Central Thailand.

Typhoid Disease

Typhoid disease is caused by the bacterium *Salmonella typhi*. Typhoid disease is commonly transmitted through eating food that has been handled by a person currently shedding the bacteria. Typhoid disease is common around the world in places where hand hygiene is less common and sanitation is poor. Currently, it impacts about 21.5 million people around the world. A hallmark of the disease is a sustained fever of about 39–40°C. Clinical symptoms also include weakness with stomach pains, headache, and loss of appetite. Patients often present with upper abdominal pink papules (rose spots) that fade with manual pressure. Antibiotics that effectively treat the disease are ampicillin, trimethoprim-sulfamethoxazole, and ciprofloxacin. Patients feel better 2–3 days after taking the medication. Twenty percent of untreated patients will die from complications of the disease. There is a vaccine for the disease.

Splenic Disease

Abscess formation in abdominal and thoracic viscera can occur in *Salmonella typhi* infection. In Chiang et al.'s review of splenic abscesses, *S. typhi* was the second most common etiology. Ooi et al.'s review of 287 cases of splenic abscesses from 1987 to 1995 revealed salmonella with staphylococcus and *Escherichia coli* to be the most common organisms cultured.[49] Management of splenic abscesses due to salmonella species is similar to management of other types of splenic abscess. If the patient does not defervesce and clinically improve with appropriate intravenous antibiotics, percutaneous drainage should be performed and repeated if needed. Splenectomy should be reserved for the patient who does not improve. Sonography can be used to serially follow the abscess with good clinical correlation.

Viral Diseases

Viral diseases affecting the spleen can cause either splenomegaly through hypertrophy secondary to the immunologic response to the infection or congestion through increased portal vein pressures due to cirrhosis of the liver. Epstein-Barr virus (EBV), cytomegalovirus (CMV), and rubella cause splenic hypertrophy. Hepatitis is a cause of liver cirrhosis and portal hypertension. In this section we discuss hepatitis, EBV, and HIV.

Hepatitis

Hepatitis is caused by five different viruses (A, B, C, D, and E) that cause liver inflammation. Hepatitis B and C together are the most common causes of cirrhosis and hepatocellular carcinoma in the world. Hepatitis is the 10th leading cause of death worldwide. One third of the world, or 2 billion people, is infected with hepatitis. Hepatitis A and E are transmitted through infected water and food. Hepatitis B, C, and D are caused by exposure to infected body fluids such as blood. Approximately 15%–40% of patients will develop cirrhosis, liver failure, and hepatocellular carcinoma. Hepatitis infection can occur with minimal symptoms or major symptoms such as jaundice, dark urine, fatigue, nausea, vomiting, and abdominal pain. Vaccinations exist for the A, B, and E viruses. There is no vaccination for hepatitis C. Interferon is the most frequently used agent in the treatment of chronic liver disease with hepatitis C. Sustained virologic response to interferon improves prognosis in terms of reduction of cirrhosis and hepatocellular development.

Splenomegaly in the setting of hepatitis occurs due to vascular congestion as a result of hepatic cirrhosis; hypersplenism also occurs. Symptomatic splenomegaly and thrombocytopenia are indicators of advanced liver disease. Patients with thrombocytopenia often receive an incomplete course of interferon therapy because of continued dose reductions or discontinuation of therapy. Therefore, management of thrombocytopenia becomes essential. Historically, splenectomy has been performed. Ikezawa et al.'s study demonstrated that splenectomy could be performed safely in patients with cirrhosis and thrombocytopenia.[50] Because of portal hypertension and the well-described complication of portal vein thrombosis, splenectomy carries significant risks. Amin et al. performed a prospective study demonstrating that partial splenic embolization is effective in treating hypersplenism.[51]

Epstein-Barr Virus (Human Herpes Virus 4)

EBV is a human herpes virus. Most people become infected and gain adaptive immunity. Transmission of the virus is by contact with oral secretions. The virus infects the epithelium of the salivary glands. EBV infections are most common in early childhood with a second peak in late adolescence. Most EBV infections in infants or young children are asymptomatic or present as mild pharyngitis. However, 75% of infections in adolescents present as infectious mononucleosis. The most common symptoms are fever, malaise, and headache. The characteristic leukocytosis peaks between 10,000 and 20,000/μl during the second or third week of illness. Lymphocytosis occurs with usually greater than10% atypical lymphocytes. Liver function is abnormal in more than 90% of cases, and both aminotransferases and alkaline phosphatases are mildly elevated. Total bilirubin is also elevated. Splenomegaly occurs in 51% of cases of infectious mononucleosis.

Diagnosis of infectious mononucleosis is with the heterophile test. Heterophile tests are positive in only 40% of patients during the first week of infection and therefore repeat testing may be necessary. A titer of greater than 40-fold is diagnostic for acute EBV infection. Greater than 90% of infectious mononucleosis is due to EBV. The remaining 10% of cases are mostly due to CMV. CMV is the most common cause of heterophile-negative mononucleosis. This variant usually presents in older patients. CMV is associated with lower incidence of sore throat, splenomegaly, and lymphadenopathy.

Complications of EBV include airway compromise from hypertrophy of adenoid tissue, meningitis, hepatitis, cranial nerve palsies (especially cranial nerve VII), autoimmune hemolytic anemia, and pharyngitis. Approximately 10% of patients will develop streptococcal pharyngitis after EBV. EBV can cause cancers such as Hodgkin's lymphoma and non-Hodgkin's lymphoma that also impact the spleen.

Splenic Disease

Splenic rupture in infectious mononucleosis is one of the rare complications that can be fatal. Splenic rupture is more common in males than females with infectious mononucleosis. Splenic rupture occurs in less than 0.5% of cases. Presentation is usually with left upper quadrant pain, referred shoulder pain, hypotension, and/or tachycardia. Management of this entity is the same as the MSR algorithm found in this chapter.

HIV

The HIV virus is a retrovirus that causes AIDS. The WHO considers HIV infection pandemic. There are 38 million people living in the world who are HIV-positive.[52] Youth under the age of 25 account for more than 50% of all new HIV infections per year.[52] In 2009, HIV claimed 1.8 million lives. Sub-Saharan Africa remains the most impacted region with 23 million people living with HIV (67% of the world's total). The clinical symptoms are nonspecific and include fever, lymphadenopathy, pharyngitis, rash, and myalgia. HIV is transmitted by sexual contact, blood transfusion, or in utero. Diagnosis is made using ELISA followed by western blot if the ELISA is positive. Treatment for this disease is with highly active antiretroviral therapy (HAART). At least three drugs from at least two classes of antiretroviral are prescribed. These classes are nucleoside analogue reverse transcriptase inhibitors, protease inhibitors, and non-nucleoside reverse transcriptase inhibitors.

Splenomegaly is a frequent finding in HIV patients. Splenic rupture as a result of acute HIV infection is reported in the medical literature.[53] Solano et al. performed a prospective observational study in an attempt to determine the meaning of splenomegaly in this population.[54] Seventy patients were prospectively followed with 60 being diagnosed with splenomegaly either on physical exam or sonography. In this study splenomegaly was not predictive of any event and also not predictive of developing AIDS. However, HIV-positive patients still can be infected with malaria, schistosomiasis, leishmaniasis, melioidosis, EBV, and other infectious agents. HIV-positive patients also have a high incidence of Hodgkin's lymphoma. Therefore, HIV is commonly associated with other infections that may lead to splenomegaly or splenic disease. Bernebeu-Wittel et al. prospectively reviewed 32 consecutive HIV-positive patients with splenic abscesses.[45] TB was the most common etiology of splenic abscess in this prospective study, followed by disseminated mycobacterium avium complex (MAC). Dixit et al. reviewed clinical profiles of patients having splenic involvement in TB, and 50% of patients were found to be HIV-positive.[46] Reichel et al. reported two patients with AIDS and TB splenic abscesses and disseminated TB.[44] Either patients presented without leukocytosis or symptoms related to the splenic involvement. When evaluating HIV-positive patients with relapsing leishmaniasis, Troya et al. reported a small subset of patients who developed splenomegaly and severe cytopenias.[32] Splenectomy in this population was successful in reducing the need for blood transfusion but did not avoid the relapsing visceral leishmaniasis.

Hematologic Diseases of the Spleen

Hereditary Spherocytosis

The most common congenital hemolytic anemia requiring splenectomy for treatment is hereditary spherocytosis. The disease is caused by an autosomal dominant mutation resulting in a defective erythrocyte membrane secondary to abnormal spectrin and ankyrin proteins. The red cells are less deformable and susceptible to sequestration and destruction in the spleen; patients present with splenomegaly, jaundice, and a mild anemia. Splenomegaly is present by the time the patient is 1 year old, and 30%–60% of patients will also have pigmented gallstones. Splenectomy is generally deferred until the patient is 4–6 years of age, and cholecystectomy is also recommended if the patient has gallstones. Risk of overwhelming postsplenectomy syndrome (OPSS) should be managed with postsplenectomy vaccinations for neisseria, haemaphilus influenza, and pneumococcus. While all are essential, the most important is the vaccine against the pneumococcus, as most cases of OPSS are pneumococcal in etiology.

Sickle-Cell Anemia

Sickle-cell anemia is caused by a point mutation that replaces glutamic acid for valine at position 6 of the beta globulin chain. This disease, while protective from the deadly disease malaria, causes chronic anemia and painful complications. About 5% of the world's population carries genes responsible for hemoglobinopathies. There are more than 200,000 cases of sickle-cell anemia in Africa. Globally, there are more carriers of thalassemia than sickle-cell anemia. The prevalence of sickle-cell trait ranges between 10%–40% across equatorial African in the areas endemic to malaria to 1%–2% in northern Africa and less than 1% in South Africa. This epidemiological pattern represents the fact that sickle-cell trait confers a survival advantage against

P. falciparum in early childhood and therefore the abnormal gene is present in high numbers in areas of malaria transmission. The Indian and Arabian Peninsula as well as the Mediterranean are endemic regions.

Patients suffering from sickle-cell anemia have chronic anemia with a hemoglobin concentration of 8 g/dl. Red cells become sickle shaped and block capillaries at low oxygen tension. Painful syndromes of the hands, feet, and chest when precipitated are called crisis. Control programs for the disease are limited in developing nations. Inexpensive therapy, such as prophylactic penicillin to control infections, is not available in many nations. Prompt intravenous hydration, narcotics, and supplemental oxygen should be given. The drug hydroxyurea has decreased the rate of painful crises and improved quality of life of patients with sickle-cell anemia.

The spleen in sickle-cell patients is usually initially enlarged but then shrinks as a result of recurrent infarctions. The indication for splenectomy in sickle-cell anemia patients is hypersplenism, sequestration crises, splenic abscesses, and massive splenic infarction. Acute splenic sequestration includes splenomegaly, severe anemia, and abdominal pain. The patient can deteriorate with hypotension and tachycardia. Resuscitation with both crystalloid and blood is essential before proceeding to splenectomy. Overwhelming postsplenectomy infections are a major threat to these patients.

Thalassemia (Mediterranean Anemia)

Thalassemia is an autosomal dominant disease of deficiencies in hemoglobin synthesis. Premature destruction of red blood cells occurs. Clinical signs of thalassemia major are growth retardation, pallor, and gallstones. Patients should undergo splenectomy if they require greater than one transfusion every 30 days, have severe pain from splenic infarction, or have severe thrombocytopenia.

Idiopathic Thrombocytopenic Purpura (ITP)

ITP is the most common indication for elective splenectomy in the United States. ITP is a disease where antibodies to platelets are formed, specifically antibodies to the glycoprotein IIb/IIIa and Ia/IIa. Clinical symptoms include thrombocytopenia, petechiae, ecchymosis, purpura, and abnormal bleeding. Intracranial hemorrhage can impact up to 2% of patients early in the disease process and be lethal. This disorder in the pediatric population is often self-limiting with up to 70% of cases resolving spontaneously. In adults, therapy is often required. Oral corticosteroid therapy is initially given with infusion of immunoglobulin, if unsuccessful, splenectomy is performed. Autoimmune hemolytic anemia may also result in the need for splenectomy. Approximately 80% of patients with ITP respond to splenectomy. Even in the remaining 20% of patients, persistently thrombocytopenic post-splenectomy significant bleeding usually does not occur.

Thrombotic Thrombocytopenic Purpura (TTP)

TTP presents with the pentad of fever, thrombocytopenia, hemolytic anemia, neurologic manifestations, and renal failure. The disease results from an excess of subendothelial collagen, resulting in platelets trapping. First-line therapy should be plasmapheresis; TTP is 90% responsive to plasmapheresis. If TTP is refractory to plasmapheresis, then splenectomy can be performed with a 50% response rate. Because of the overall shortage of blood and component therapy in developing nations, persistent hemolytic anemia may be more efficiently treated with splenectomy.

Neoplastic Diseases of the Spleen

Hodgkin's Lymphoma

Hodgkin's disease is characterized by lymphoid tumor containing large multinuclear cells (Reed-Sternberg cells). Hodgkin's lymphoma is the most common lymphoma of young people in the West. Splenectomy is performed in Hodgkin's lymphoma only for symptom relief from splenomegaly.

Non-Hodgkin's Lymphoma

In developing nations non-Hodgkin's lymphoma (NHL) is the most common lymphoma. NHL is the most common malignancy involving the spleen. NHL is heavily associated with both EBV and HIV infection. NHL is an AIDS-defining illness and is the second most common cancer in HIV-positive patients. An HIV-positive patient's risk of developing NHL is 60 fold higher than the general population's risk.[55] Splenectomy is performed for patients with symptomatic splenomegaly or pancytopenia and frequent transfusion requirements. As mentioned earlier in the chapter, blood component therapy is a resource that is not readily available in most LMICs.

Chronic Myelogenous Leukemia (CML)

In CML normal bone marrow is replaced with myeloid cells. CML accounts for 30% of all adult leukemia. Splenectomy during the blastic phase of the disease has been shown to decrease transfusion requirements. Splenectomy has a palliative role in the management of CML.

The Glivac International Patient Assistant Program has been shown to be a successful partnership between the manufacturer, nongovernmental organizations, and 80 developing nations to improve overall survival by increasing access to Glivac.[56] Glivac is a tyrosine kinase inhibitor used to treat CML. It is given for newly diagnosed CML when a bone marrow transplant is not suitable or when initial treatment with interferon is unsuccessful.

Chronic Lymphocytic Leukemia (CLL)

Splenectomy is only performed in patients with symptomatic splenomegaly or hypersplenism.

Hairy Cell Leukemia

Hairy cell leukemia is a lymphocytic leukemia that presents with splenomegaly and pancytopenia. Splenectomy should be performed in patients with symptomatic hypersplenism. Interferon α and purine analogs have been demonstrated to be highly effective in this disease, and therefore splenectomy is seldom required.

Tumors of the Spleen

The most common primary tumor of the spleen is hemangioma. Hemangiomas of the spleen are typically associated with other hemangiomas of the liver. These tumors do not need treatment unless they become symptomatic. Hemangiomas can produce the Kasselback-Merritt syndrome of a consumptive coagulopathy, thrombocytopenia, and microangiopathic anemia. Hamartomas of the spleen are either solid or cystic and seldom require resection. Lymphangiomas are benign cystic lesions that may lead to hypersplenism. Like hemangiomas, these lymphangiomas of the spleen are also heavily associated with lymphangiomas of the liver. Splenectomy is performed to relieve symptoms and rarely to clarify diagnosis.

Metastatic tumors to the spleen are very rare. Tumors known to metastasize to the spleen include breast, lung, ovarian, endometrial, colonic, gastric, and melanoma.

Splenectomy Procedure

This procedure can be approached through a variety of incisions (left subcostal, transverse abdominal, or celiotomy), but most often it is approached through a celiotomy incision from the xiphoid process to the symphysis pubis. The spleen sits in the left upper quadrant just below the left diaphragmatic leaflet. The surgeon's hand can pass over the anterior portion of the body of stomach toward the greater curvature and reach the spleen, lying in a posterolateral portion of the left upper quadrant. The advantages of a celiotomy incision are exposure of surrounding organs while maintaining abdominal wall function after closure. A transverse abdominal incision can also provide excellent exposure of the spleen, particularly when it is very enlarged (Hackett's score ≥3). When the spleen is enlarged, other organs adjacent to the spleen, such as the stomach, pancreas, colon, and kidney, are displaced along with other abdominal structures. Clear visualization and careful application of vascular clamps are essential. Furthermore, the enlarged spleen may be friable and therefore tissue handling is particularly important to prevent excessive bleeding. In low-resource environments, blood transfusion capability may be limited and therefore manipulation of the spleen during the operation should be done with a focus on visualization of the hilar structures and surrounding organs while not injuring the splenic capsule.

The superior and lateral pole attachments are divided sharply or with electrocautery. These attachments are usually avascular. The splenorenal and splenocolic ligaments are also divided. Occasionally, these ligaments may be vascularized and require clamping and suture ligature. Release of these attachments allows the spleen to undergo medial rotation to the midline. In extra-large spleens there may be additional adhesions to other abdominal structures that need to be divided. The short gastric vessels are divided between clips or clamps and ligated. The approach to the splenic hilum should begin with locating the splenic vessels that run along the dorsum of the pancreas. The pancreas tail is avoided if possible. If needed the pancreas tail is gently displaced manually either medially or inferiorly to avoid injury. When the spleen is especially large, the splenic vessels can be initially approached through the gastrocolic ligament in the lesser sac at the dorsum of the pancreas. Achieving medial control of the splenic vessels may be more practical and safe in cases of splenomegaly where hilar control is difficult even after medial rotation of the spleen or in cases where there is iatrogenic injury to the capsule and ongoing bleeding. The splenic artery and vein are doubly ligated separately. The splenic bed and greater curvature of the stomach where the short gastric vessels were ligated is observed momentarily for bleeding until the patient's mean arterial pressures is above 60 mm Hg before preparation for abdominal wall closure.

Exploration for accessory spleens should be done when performing splenectomy for hematologic disease or ITP. Accessory spleens are present in 12%–20% of patients and may be the cause of inadequate response to splenectomy. The most common locations for accessory spleens are the hilum and tail of the pancreas. Drainage is not needed unless there is an injury to the tail of the pancreas.

Abdominal closure is performed with interrupted or running absorbable suture.

Complications

Early postoperative bleeding is the most common complication. This is usually due to inadequate suture ligation or inappropriate ligation of the short gastric vessels leading to sutures being dislodged from the vessel. Reoperation may be required to obtain hemostasis in environments with low transfusion resources. At reoperation, if there is a failure to identify the bleeding source, packing of the left upper quadrant can be done for 24 hours followed by a relook operation and definitive closure. This approach may also be utilized if brisk bleeding is encountered during the initial operation and there is concern about whether hemostasis has been optimally achieved.

Left lower lobe pulmonary atelectasis may result due to manipulation of the spleen in the left upper quadrant. Pain control, early ambulation, and pulmonary toilet are generally employed with success.

Injury to the tail of the pancreas, requiring drainage is thought to occur in less than 15% of cases. However, this does not reflect an MSR population. This complication is usually self-limiting when appropriate drainage is achieved

Thrombosis of the splenic vein extending into thrombosis of the portal vein and superior mesenteric vein is a rare complication. Patients with myeloproliferative disorders are at increased risk. Acute thrombosis should be treated with anticoagulation for 3–6 months with a target international normalization ratio of 2–3. If prothrombotic syndromes are diagnosed, such as paroxysmal nocturnal hemoglobinuria, antiphospholipid syndrome, protein C and S deficiencies, factor V Leiden mutation, factor II mutation, or methylenetetrahydrofolate reductase gene mutation, then anticoagulation is needed for life. Surgical management is associated with re-thrombosis. Thrombolytic therapy is complicated by bleeding in up to 60% of patients and is reserved for patients with severe disease.

Overwhelming post-splenectomy sepsis related to pneumococcal or *H. influenza* occurs most commonly in patients who are immunosuppressed or who have myeloproliferative disorders. This risk is reduced with the appropriate vaccines (see Figure 15.1).

COMMENTARY

Ndukauba Eleweke, Nigeria

In our Center at Abia State University Teaching Hospital, Aba Nigeria, splenic enlargement and traumatic rupture of the spleen are the most prevalent splenic pathologies. Chronic malarial infestation predisposes to splenomegaly. The enlarged spleen is susceptible to rupture following trauma; the trauma is most often caused by falls from heights or motor vehicle accidents. Patients with enlarged spleens present late, often with monstrous abdominal scarification marks and pancytopaenia after visiting many unorthodox treatment homes. The major challenges to treating splenic injuries are delay in presentation, lack of access to a CT scan, intervention radiologists, and a well-equipped ICU. Most of our patients are offered total splenectomy.

COMMENTARY

Ntakiyiruta Georges, Rwanda

In Rwanda, splenic diseases are largely dominated by malaria-related complications. These complications include splenomegaly syndrome (tropical splenomegaly syndrome), splenic abscesses, and neoplastic changes in cases of lymphomas.

The following causes of splenic pathology are rare: schistosomiasis, trypanosomiasis, leishmaniasis, and hydatid disease. *Schistosoma mansoni* is known to be present in Lake Kivu, although patients rarely present with clinical symptoms of schistosomiasis; praziquantel is readily available for these patients. African trypanosomiasis is present in the northeastern province of Rwanda; as a result of a national program devoted to its elimination, trypanosomiasis is now very rare. To my knowledge, I have never heard of any case of leishmaniasis in Rwanda and no case of hydatid disease.

We often see patients presenting with HMS associated with secondary hypersplenism. Some patients will present with bleeding complications, such as epistaxis, due to severe thrombocytopenia. In most cases, these patients have been treated with repeated blood transfusions. Blood therapy is not always readily available in Rwanda. In an effort to ensure safety of blood therapy, blood testing is centralized in one center in Kigali and all the hospitals have to request blood and other blood products from the central blood bank.

Patients with complicated HMS will definitely require splenectomy. Perioperative blood transfusions and, most importantly, platelets transfusion, are essential in such cases. Platelets transfusion is needed a few hours before the operation and you may require transfusing more platelets intraoperatively.

Patients with chronic splenomegaly, regardless of the etiology, are at high risk of splenic rupture as the splenic rupture is triggered by only minor abdominal injury. We do have cases of splenic abscesses, and splenectomy is our preferred option.

Sickle-cell anemia is extremely rare in the Rwandan population, and this is very surprising as it is particularly common in neighboring countries of Uganda, Democratic Republic of the Congo, and Tanzania.

COMMENTARY

Okao Patrick, Rwanda

The authors of this chapter have discussed in detail the wide range of causes of splenic diseases; this clearly conveys the complexity in the management of these conditions. It has served to simplify the approach to a patient with suspected splenic disease. Although splenomegaly is a major manifestation of splenic and other diseases, it is worth noting that not all cases of splenomegaly are associated with hypersplenism.

HMS syndrome results from abnormal immunologic response to a previously repeated malaria infection. It is therefore not uncommon for patients presenting with splenomegaly to have negative blood test for malaria infection. The response of patients with HMS to anti-malarial prophylaxis is good, but the long course of prophylaxis is associated with low compliance.

16

Appendicitis

Vladimir P. Daoud
Ibrahim M. Daoud

Introduction and Epidemiology

Appendicitis is one of the most common causes of an acute abdomen in the world and one of the most common indications for emergency abdominal surgery. Its worldwide lifetime prevalence is estimated at 1 in 7.[1] Acute appendicitis occurs most often in the second and third decades of life, with the peak incidence of approximately 233/100,000 seen in the 10- to 19-year-old population. The incidence also differs based on gender, with a male-to-female ratio of 1.4:1. Men (8.6%) have a greater lifetime incidence of appendicitis when compared to women (6.7%).[2]

While the incidence of acute appendicitis in developed nations has either remained relatively stable or has shown some signs of a decline in recent years, the incidence in low- and middle-income countries (LMICs), such as Kenya, is on the rise.[3] In many LMICs, acute appendicitis is now a leading cause of emergency department visits and/or hospital admissions.[4,5] Given the inherent lack of resources, technology, and infrastructure, surgeons in LMICs face an even more difficult task when asked to evaluate a patient with an acute abdomen or abdominal pain than their colleagues practicing in the high-income countries (HICs). Furthermore, in many LMICs such as Nigeria, the most common emergent operation performed in adults is open appendectomy (15.4%) based on a clinical diagnosis with only the addition of a urinalysis and hemoglobin level.[4] Generally, a negative appendectomy rate of 10%–15% has been deemed acceptable by Western cultures. Although the use of advanced diagnostic imaging modalities, such as computed tomography and ultrasonography, has indeed led to more accurate diagnosis of acute appendicitis in some settings, it has not been shown to reduce the rate of misdiagnosis of acute appendicitis in the general population.[6] However, in developing nations, the negative appendectomy rate is typically much higher than it is in the United States, ranging from 15.9%[4] to 46.6%.[7] Given the increase in morbidity and mortality seen with a delay in operative therapy as well as the logistical and financial limitations prevalent in LMICs, this variability is understandable. Early surgical intervention should be the norm when the clinical suspicion is high and the risk-benefit ratio falls in the patient's favor.

Appendicitis in the Pediatric Population

For a complete discussion of clinical considerations for appendicitis specific to trauma cases in the pediatric populations of LMICs, please see Chapter 31.

Anatomy and Pathophysiology

The appendix is often regarded as a vestigial organ with no known function in human beings; however, the appendix contains large amounts of lymphoid aggregates, similar to those within the Peyer's patches of gut-associated lymphoid tissue. These lymphoid nodules contain both B and T cells within their lamina propria and serve to histologically differentiate the appendix from the adjacent colon. The appendix develops as an anti-mesenteric out-pouching from the cecum and is first delineated during the fifth month of gestation.

The normal appendix can vary in length from 2–20 cm, with a mean length of approximately 9 cm. The blood supply of the appendix is from the appendicular artery, a branch of the ileo-colic artery, which itself is derived from the superior mesenteric artery. The lymphatic drainage is to the ileo-colic nodes. Often, these nodes are hyperplastic in acute appendicitis. Much like other visceral organs, the neural innervation of the appendix is derived from the autonomic nervous system as there are no somatic pain fibers within the appendix itself. Consequently, early appendiceal inflammation leads to poorly localized pain and is thus referred to the periumbilical region as the autonomic nerves follow the embryologic origin of the midgut. As the inflammation worsens, irritation of the adjacent parietal peritoneum results in the activation of somatic pain fibers and subsequent localization of signs and symptoms to the right lower quadrant.[8]

The vermiform appendix is located in proximity to the ileo-cecal valve, where the three taenia coli converge on the cecum. It is considered a true diverticulum of the cecum in that its wall contains all of the layers found in the wall of the colon, namely the mucosa, submucosa, muscularis (both longitudinal and circular), and serosa. The position of the appendix can vary greatly. In approximately two-thirds of patients, it is located in a retro-cecal position, whereas in the remaining third, it is located over the pelvic brim, occasionally descending into the pelvis.[8]

Obstruction of the appendiceal lumen is commonly noted as the primary culprit in appendicitis. However, obstruction is not required for the condition to exist. An elevated intraluminal pressure may only be seen in one-third of patients with nonperforated appendicitis.[9,10] The lumen can be obstructed by a variety of mechanisms, including fecaliths, calculi, lymphoid hyperplasia, infectious processes, and tumors, both malignant and benign. Some patients with a fecalith are later found to have a histologically normal appendix, while the majority of patients with acute appendicitis do not have a fecalith.[11]

Clinical Presentation and Evaluation of the Patient

A patient without abdominal pain is extremely unlikely to have appendicitis, as abdominal pain is the most common symptom and is present in nearly all confirmed cases.[12] The natural history of acute appendicitis is quite similar to that of other intra-abdominal inflammatory processes affecting hollow visceral organs. The clinical course involves initial inflammation of the wall of the organ (usually by obstruction leading to stretch), localized ischemia secondary to impaired venous outflow, and subsequent impedance of arterial inflow, perforation, and the potential development of either a contained abscess/phlegmon or generalized peritonitis. The chronological pattern of pain and its characteristic progression to the right lower quadrant is a direct result of the pathophysiology.

The "classic" clinical presentation of acute appendicitis includes right lower quadrant (right iliac fossa) abdominal pain, anorexia, nausea, and vomiting. The onset of abdominal pain is typically the first symptom mentioned by the patient. The pain is periumbilical in location and tends to be vague in quality. Patients, especially children, may be unable to localize the pain and may complain of something as benign as a belly ache. Initial features can be either atypical or nonspecific and include flatulence, changes in bowel habits, indigestion, and general malaise or fatigue. The pain then migrates to the right lower quadrant, becomes more severe and sharper in quality. If nausea and vomiting occur, they usually do so after the onset of pain. Fever and leukocytosis occur later in the course of the illness. Fever, a late finding typically not seen until peritonitis is present, is usually low-grade (up to 38.3°C) and generally does not progress. Moreover, the classic signs and symptoms are not very common. For example, the history of periumbilical pain migrating to the right lower quadrant may only be found in 50%–60% of patients with histologically confirmed acute appendicitis.[9,13] To complicate matters even further, the symptoms of appendicitis can vary depending on the location of the patient's appendix within the abdominal cavity[14-18] (Table 16.1).

Symptoms are markedly worse in the right lower quadrant or at McBurney's point (Figure 16.1), when the appendix is anteriorly positioned.

On the other hand, a retro-cecal appendix, seen in approximately two-thirds of patients with appendicitis, may cause minimal signs of peritonitis as the inflammation it produces is smothered by the overlying intestine.

TABLE 16.1

Physical findings and their sensitivities and specificities in acute appendicitis

	Indicative of	Sensitivity	Specificity
McBurney's Point[14–16]	anterior appendix	50%–94%	75%–86%
Rovsing's Sign[15,17]	right-sided local peritonitis	22%–68%	58%–96%
Psoas Sign[17,18]	retro-cecal appendix	13%–42%	79%–97%
Obturator Sign[18]	pelvic appendix	8%	94%

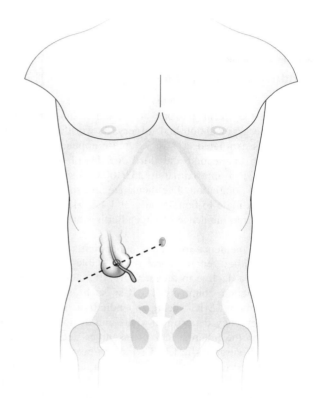

FIGURE 16.1 McBurney's point. In the right lower quadrant, approximately two-thirds the distance from the umbilicus to the anterior superior iliac spine, McBurney's point provides an anatomical landmark useful for physical examination and surgical incision. Illustration by Katherine Dunn, MD.

Differential Diagnosis

The diagnosis of acute appendicitis may be a difficult one, as many intra-abdominal processes may mimic the signs and symptoms seen in these patients. These include Crohn's disease, gynecologic conditions such as ectopic pregnancy and acute salpingitis from pelvic inflammatory disease, and diverticulitis. However, there are some other diseases to consider in LMICs.

Acute intermittent porphyria, an autosomal recessive deficiency of porphobilinogen deaminase that affects the production of heme, may present with constipation and severe, sometimes colicky abdominal pain that may or may not radiate. It is especially prevalent in women, and even more so in South Africa. Symptoms usually arise in the third or fourth decade of life with attacks of "intestinal colic" shortly after consumption of drugs (barbiturates and sulfonamides, in particular) or alcohol, or the administration of an anesthetic. Physical findings include a lack of abdominal distention, tenderness, or rigidity. Interestingly, the urine, secondary to the excretion of porphyrins, will turn dark brown upon standing.[19]

Typhoid fever is an infectious and generalized disease transmitted by the ingestion of food or water contaminated with the feces of an infected person containing the bacterium *Salmonella enterica*. It is occasionally mistaken for appendicitis due to the fact that some patients present with abdominal pain and tenderness that may or may not localize to the right lower quadrant. There are, however, more systemic symptoms that should be of assistance, such as headache, malaise, roseola, and splenomegaly.[19] Also commonly seen are diaphoresis, gastroenteritis, and a progressive fever that may reach 40°C.

Ascaris lumbricoides is a helminth infection that is commonly found in tropical climates with a worldwide prevalence estimated at 25%. Ascariasis often arises in areas of low socioeconomic status due to contamination of the soil and local water supply with human feces. Early symptoms of infection are pulmonary and include wheezing, coughing, fever, dyspnea, and chest pain. Late symptoms are abdominal pain and include nausea, emesis, and colicky pain. Mebendazole is the treatment of choice. Surgery is reserved for only the most severe cases.[20,21]

Acute gastrointestinal infection with *Yersinia enterocolitica* typically causes a somewhat transient enterocolitis. However, in some patients, it can disseminate to mesenteric lymph nodes via the terminal ileum (where it replicates), invade the Peyer's patches, and cause lymphadenopathy and right lower quadrant pain in addition to bloody diarrhea and fever. It is primarily transmitted by undercooked pork or contaminated drinking water. This "pseudoappendicitis syndrome" is more common in older children and young adults.[22]

Neutropenic enterocolitis, or typhlitis, is transmural inflammation of the cecum in the immunocompromised patient. Commonly, the inflammation involves the ascending colon and terminal ileum. International incidence rates, in countries such as India and Turkey, range from 3.5%–6.5% in adults and children, most of whom are undergoing chemotherapy regimens for leukemia, are afflicted with the acquired immunodeficiency syndrome (AIDS), or suffer from a solid malignant tumor. The common denominator among all patients is neutropenia (<1,000 cells/mm^3). The presentation very closely resembles that of acute appendicitis and tends to occur within 10–14 days of initiating chemotherapy; however, these patients may also present with other findings, including oropharyngeal mucositis and watery or bloody diarrhea. In spite of a paucity of randomized clinical control trials regarding the management of typhlitis, the following are indications for emergent operative management: perforated viscus, clinical deterioration while undergoing conservative medical management (e.g., broad-spectrum antibiotics, intravenous fluids, bowel rest), intra-abdominal sepsis or abscess formation, persistent hemorrhage, and the inability to differentiate from other causes of an acute abdomen that require surgical intervention (i.e., appendicitis). Procedures vary based on intraoperative decision making but may include cecostomy and drainage, right hemi-colectomy, total abdominal colectomy with or without a primary anastomosis, or a diverting loop ileostomy.

Appendicitis is more difficult to diagnose in females primarily due to the wider variety of differential diagnoses, including, but not limited to, pelvic inflammatory disease, Mittelschmerz, ectopic pregnancy, and ovarian cystic pathology. Pelvic inflammatory disease is seen exclusively in sexually active females, usually in their late teens to early 20s, who have either unprotected sex or a multitude of sexual partners, or both. The causative organism is primarily *Chlamydia trachomatis* and *Neisseria gonorrhea*. Although generally a nonsurgical disease, it should be treated with haste to avoid common complications, such as tubal factor infertility and the Fitz-Hugh-Curtis syndrome.

Procedure Highlights

The incision for an open appendectomy is most commonly made over McBurney's point (see Figure 16.1). The skin is incised perpendicular to the line between the right anterior superior iliac spine and the umbilicus. The minority of this incision should lie superior to that line, and the majority of it should lie below. The aponeurosis of the external oblique should be incised in a direction parallel its fibers. Blunt dissection with a Kelly clamp should be carried down to the peritoneum. The peritoneum is then elevated, incised with a scalpel or cut with scissors, and the opening enlarged with two fingers. The cecum should be identified first. Light traction on the cecum via a moist laparotomy pad will deliver both the cecum and appendix from the wound.

If the cecum cannot be identified, the surgeon must strongly consider either intestinal malrotation or an undescended cecum. After positive identification of the cecum, the taenia coli can be followed until they converge, a point at which the appendix can be found. The appendix always arises at this location, regardless of where the tip or the remainder of it may be located (retrocecal, pelvic, etc.).

In patients with a deeply buried retro-cecal appendix, it may be necessary to incise the posterior peritoneum just lateral to the cecum in order to mobilize and expose the appendix. If the surgeon is unable to expose or positively identify the appendix, intussusception should be strongly considered as congenital absence of the appendix is too rare to justify not finding it; moreover, in such cases of intussusception, a conspicuous dimple will more than likely be present at the expected site of a normal appendix. If he or she has not done so prior, the surgeon should also consider the possibility of previous appendectomy.

Evaluate and inspect the mesoappendix, divide it between two clamps, then ligate it with silk suture. After hemostasis is achieved, elevate the appendix and affix two clamps at its base, ligate the base of the appendix with chromic or catgut suture, and then remove the proximal clamp. The appendix can then be divided between the remaining clamp and the proximal suture (Figure 16.2 and Figure 16.3).

The wound must then be irrigated copiously to reduce the risk of infection and/or abscess formation, especially if there is gross spillage of pus or enteric contents into the peritoneal cavity. The layers of the abdominal wall may be closed using absorbable suture material. A recent meta-analysis of 27 studies involving 2,532 patients with gangrenous or perforated appendicitis concluded that the risk of surgical site infection was no higher with

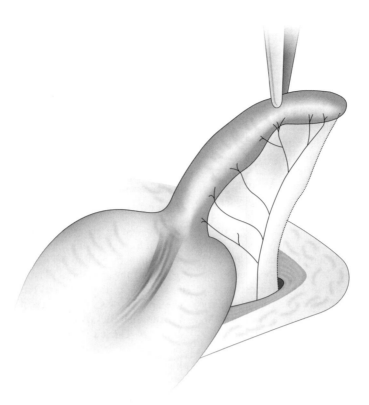

FIGURE 16.2   After delivery of the cecum from the wound, the appendix is readily identified by the convergence of the taenia coli at its base. The mesoappendix contains the appendiceal artery. Illustration by Katherine Dunn, MD.

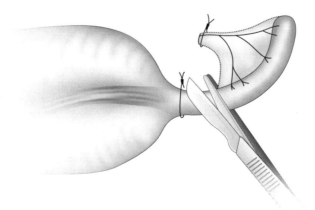

FIGURE 16.3   Placement of suture at the base of the appendix after division of the mesoappendix. The appendix can then be divided with a scalpel or electrocautery (if available) distal to the suture. Illustration by Katherine Dunn, MD.

primary closure than with delayed primary closure, insinuating that primary closure is indeed a viable option in most appendectomy patients. This has significant implications with respect to patients in LMICs in that it serves to reduce the number the patients potentially lost to follow-up in the outpatient setting and allows them to be discharged home with an intact surgical incision. The surgeon's personal preference may dictate the closure technique.

Complications

Many of the complications of acute appendicitis arise secondarily to a delay in presentation, a delay in diagnosis, a rapidly progressing disease state, or some combination of these. They include rupture, abscess/phlegmon formation, peritonitis, and subsequent sepsis. Complications following appendectomy include surgical site infection, postoperative abscess, bleeding, and enterotomy, as well as postoperative ileus. The primary purpose of early operative intervention is to prevent the risks associated with perforation of the appendix, which include the possible development of peritonitis, abscess, and/or sepsis. In children younger than 4 years of age, perforation occurs in the vast majority of cases, with rates reported as high as 80%–100%. In contrast, appendicitis in children aged 10–17 years is more common, yet the perforation rate is much lower at 10%–20%.[2,24,25]

General Considerations and Conclusions

There is no single sign, symptom, or laboratory test to reliably identify or exclude the diagnosis of appendicitis. In LMICs, the diagnosis of acute appendicitis is based primarily on some combination of the typical history of vague periumbilical pain progressing to somatic pain in the right lower quadrant, the presence of associated signs and symptoms (such as nausea, anorexia, emesis, and fever), peritoneal signs and, in some more fortunate areas, other laboratory or imaging techniques such as C-reactive protein (CRP), blood counts (neutrophilia), or ultrasound. Interestingly, serum CRP measurement does not appear to improve the accuracy in diagnosing acute appendicitis unless perforation has occurred.[26] It is, therefore, up to the clinician to determine the likelihood of appendicitis in patients with abdominal pain. There are various scoring systems noted in the literature to assist with diagnosis, two of which are described below.

The Alvarado score is a clinical scoring tool that can be a useful in attempting to diagnose appendicitis without all of the imaging techniques found in the Western world. This scoring system utilizes eight factors thought to be important in making the clinical diagnosis of acute appendicitis in patients of all ages (Table 16.2). Using data from the original work, it can be determined that the sensitivity and specificity of the original Alvarado scoring system is 81% and 74%, respectively.[27] A significant limitation to this system with respect to LMICs is that it requires the resources of a basic hematologic laboratory in order to obtain the white blood cell count and the presence or absence of neutrophilia. In addition, it neglects to stratify patients based on age; however, when utilized in children and adolescents only, the results are comparable[28,29] (Table 16.2).

It is, therefore, likely useful in children, for whom a scoring system such as this might be of utmost importance given the challenges in diagnosis. The score can then be used to qualify the likelihood of appendicitis and the subsequent appropriate management of such patients[27] (Table 16.3).

It is important to note that in the Alvarado study 34% of patients who presented with the initial complaint of abdominal pain had appendicitis, which is a relatively high prevalence of acute appendicitis even in the United States.[28] In contrast, studies from Africa have demonstrated the prevalence of acute appendicitis in patients admitted with a chief complaint of abdominal pain to be 9%–24%.[30,31] Other emergent diagnoses included typhoid intestinal perforation, nonspecific abdominal pain, acute intestinal obstruction (secondary to both hernia and adhesions), intussusception, gynecological causes of abdominal pain, and peptic ulcer disease.[30,31] Several caveats must be acknowledged with respect to the pediatric population. Leukocytosis and left shift are independently and strongly associated with appendicitis

TABLE 16.2

Alvarado score

Predictive Factor	Point Value
Localized RLQ tenderness	2
Leukocytosis* (≥10,000/L)	2
Migration of pain	1
Left shift* (≥75%)	1
Fever (≥37.3°C)	1
Nausea or vomiting	1
Anorexia	1
Rebound tenderness	1

Predictive factors and respective point values for each are noted. Factors are listed in order of clinical importance per the author of the original study.[27] Maximum Alvarado score of 10. Omitted in Kanumba et al.'s modified Alvarado score.[1]

TABLE 16.3

Alvarado score, qualitative likelihood of appendicitis, and recommended actions based on both[27]

Alvarado Score	Scoring System	Recommended Action
5–6	Compatible with appendicitis	Observe
7–8	Probable appendicitis	Surgery
9–10	Very probable appendicitis	Surgery

Maximum Alvarado score of 10.

in children aged 1–19 years. The sensitivity of an increased white blood cell (WBC) count or left shift is relatively high at 79%, but the presence of a high WBC count and left shift is very specific (94%) for acute appendicitis in children.[32] In instances where laboratories have the capability to provide a WBC count without a differential, the clinician can employ a modified Alvarado score that eliminates the need for the left-shift criterion in children admitted for the evaluation of abdominal pain. This scoring system has performed comparably to the original Alvarado score.[33]

There exists, however, a modified Alvarado score that includes only the patient's signs and symptoms that are readily available to any experienced clinician. The Kanumba modified Alvarado score eliminates the leukocyte count and the presence of a left shift. It utilizes the same cutoff score of 7 despite a maximum score of only 7; in other words, a score of 7 merits a trip to the operating room. Retrospectively, Kanumba et al. applied the modified Alvarado score to patients of all ages who underwent appendectomy for acute appendicitis at a hospital in Tanzania. The sensitivity and specificity of this scoring system were remarkably high at 94% and 90%, respectively[1] (Table 16.4).

Unlike the original Alvarado score, this modified Alvarado score eliminates the need for any laboratory studies, which is likely of great benefit to healthcare providers in LMICs with minimal effect on its clinical accuracy.

With respect to operative procedure, laparoscopic appendectomy has garnered widespread acceptance and implementation in the developed world since its inception some 30 years ago. Unfortunately, it is not only associated with a relatively steep learning curve, but it also requires a wide array of resources that are not readily available in most LMICs. Laparoscopy would require a reliable source of electricity to power the equipment, a feat not easily accomplished in many parts of the world.

TABLE 16.4

Performance of the standard Alvarado score applied to all patients, the standard Alvarado score applied to pediatric patients, and the Kanumba modified Alvarado score

Scoring System	Sensitivity	Specificity	PPV	NPV
Alvarado[27]	81%	74%	92%	46%
Alvarado (Pediatric)[29]	72%	81%	85%	65%
Modified Alvarado[1]	94%	90%	95%	88%

Furthermore, the only patients for whom laparoscopic appendectomy appears to offer any significant advantage are women of childbearing age, the obese, and patients with an unclear diagnosis of abdominal pain. Therefore, open appendectomy remains the gold standard for the surgical treatment of acute appendicitis. Laparoscopic appendectomy is associated with a lower incidence of postoperative wound infections than open appendectomy (3.5% versus 6.7%), but it is also associated with a higher incidence of postoperative intra-abdominal abscess (2.5% versus 1.1%).[34] A conglomeration of 31 randomized clinical controlled trials comparing laparoscopic versus open appendectomy has shown that the incidence of a histologically normal appendix was similar in the both groups (14.3% with laparoscopic appendectomy versus 14.8% with open appendectomy), thus potentiating the notion that laparoscopic appendectomy has not been shown to reduce the incidence of negative exploration in patients with clinically suspected acute appendicitis.[34]

Appendectomy is recommended in patients with clinically suspected acute appendicitis, even when the appendix does not appear inflamed during operative exploration.[35] The incidence of histologically normal appendiceal tissue in patients with clinical signs and symptoms of acute appendicitis is about 1 in 6, with females comprising just over two-thirds of those found to have a "normal" appendix.[36] It is important to note that appendectomy relieves symptoms in the vast majority of these patients regardless of the histological findings. A plausible explanation includes the entity of focal appendicitis, whereby polymorphonuclear infiltration is confined to a single focus, while the remaining appendix is devoid of any polymorphonuclear cells. As such, histological sectioning may fail to identify the focal inflammation, resulting in a "false-negative" appendectomy.[37]

Conclusion

When a surgeon commits to providing care in LMICs across the globe, there are several salient points that demand recognition. Surgeons may have to operate with assistants who have minimal training, if any at all, and they may have to perform various procedures from which they would admittedly shy away at their home institution. They may even have to perform some level of basic anesthesia without a trained anesthesiologist. One thing is certain: they will always have to improvise.[38] It is important to acknowledge that the clinician's experience and individual judgment with a given set of symptoms will always allow for some variability. This variability tends to become even more pronounced with the conspicuous absence of much of the objective clinical data to which physicians of the developed world are so accustomed. In LMICs, however, it is essential that all surgeons

exercise a high index of suspicion and a relatively low threshold to operate when dealing with cases of suspected appendicitis, given the higher morbidity and mortality associated with a delay in operative intervention.

Specific Considerations in Low- and Middle-Income Countries (LMICs)

- Open appendectomy remains the gold standard for the treatment of acute appendicitis.
- Use of scoring systems (e.g., Alvarado) may better distinguish operative candidates.
- Maintain a high index of suspicion and a willingness to operate urgently to reduce risk of perforation.
- Educate patients regarding expedited presentation to the hospital when the signs and symptoms are suspicious for acute appendicitis.
- Consider implementation of prehospital emergency medical care and the improvement or creation of infrastructure to decrease delay in presentation.

Potential Pitfalls and Problems to Avoid

- Acute appendicitis is difficult to diagnose in certain populations, namely adolescent females.
- Infectious causes of abdominal pain must be considered early in the differential diagnosis.
- Complications arise secondary to either a delay in presentation or a delay in diagnosis and/or therapy. As physicians, we exert the most control at the point of diagnosis and therapy.
- Symptomatology and signs of appendicitis are a function of timing of presentation; therefore, any use of scoring systems without taking into account the duration of symptoms is ill-advised.

COMMENTARY

Edgar Rodas, Ecuador
Edgar B. Rodas, Ecuador

When a patient presents with acute abdominal pain due to appendicitis, it is important to consider the availability of all resources including laboratory, imaging, surgeon, and anesthesiologist. In Ecuador, the recent creation of a trauma and acute care surgery service with an in-hospital surgeon available in a regional hospital has dramatically decreased the time delay for the diagnosis and treatment of acute appendicitis. This enables surgical intervention at earlier stages of the disease, which decreases hospital length of stay, complication rates, and overall costs. Although not applicable worldwide, this model may be replicated in secondary and tertiary hospitals that serve as referral centers. The challenge still remains in the vast majority of underserved areas, however, and telemedicine might provide some support to surgeons in these areas where new services are not yet feasible.

17

Hernia

Joaquim M. Havens

Introduction

A hernia is any area of weakness or disruption of the fibromuscular tissues of the body wall through which structures can pass from one cavity to another. They represent one of the oldest recorded human maladies, and the history of their repair parallels the history of surgery itself. Hernia repair is the most common surgical procedure performed in Western countries, with more than 1.1 million abdominal wall hernia repairs in the United States in 2003, of which 800,000 were groin hernias.[1]

The burden of disease from hernias in low- and middle-income countries (LMICs) has been, until recently, largely unstudied. The Disease Control Priorities Project, Second Edition (DCP2) concluded that 25 million disability-adjusted life years (DALYs), or 7% of those in Africa, are the result of conditions correctable by surgery.[2] Evidence suggests that inguinal hernias in Ghana are approximately 10 times as prevalent as in high-income countries. It is estimated that in Africa 175 people per 100,000 need hernia repair each year, but only a small percentage of those hernias will be repaired.[3] Of patients undergoing surgery for inguinal hernia in Ghana, their hernias were larger, more often indirect, and occurred in younger patients compared with a cohort from the United Kingdom.[4] Delay in surgical repair of hernias in Nigeria has been associated with a higher incidence of hernia morbidity and mortality, and leads to more expensive emergency care.[5] In Ghana 16% of patients undergoing hernia surgery were unable to work due to their hernia, and in a further 64% the hernia limited daily activity.[4] Overall, untreated inguinal hernias in LMICs represent a serious social and economic burden.

An overview of the diagnosis and treatment of abdominal hernias will be discussed here, with particular attention to the inguinal hernia.

Complications of Hernia

The risk of incarceration for inguinal hernias is generally greatest near presentation and tends to decrease over time. In one series of 476 groin hernias, the cumulative probability of strangulation was 2.8% at 3 months; the cumulative probability at 2 years was 4.5%.[6] However, in another study, 30% of hernias became irreducible by 10 years.[7]

Groin hernias have the highest rates of strangulation. Femoral hernias account for only 2%–4% of groin hernias but are more apt to present with strangulation and require emergency surgery and bowel resection when compared to inguinal hernias.[8]

If small or large bowel is contained within the incarcerated hernia, a complete or partial bowel obstruction may result. It is imperative to remember that in LMICs hernia is the leading cause of bowel obstruction. All cases of bowel obstruction, therefore, warrant a thorough examination for the presence of hernias.

A *sliding hernia* is present when the peritoneal lining of the hernia sac is incomplete, and an abdominal organ constitutes part of the hernia sac. The term *Richter's hernia* is applied when only a portion of the bowel wall is involved in the hernia. In the case of a Richter's hernia, local signs of strangulation may not be present and the bowel may not obstruct despite strangulation of a portion of the bowel wall.

General Principles

The ideal hernia repair will be performed using a simple and safe technique that offers low morbidity and is cost-effective. The goals of hernia surgery are to relieve pain, return any protruding organs to the appropriate cavity, prevent strangulation of organs, and prevent recurrence. The selection of procedure and type of anesthetic used to achieve these goals can vary widely and are dependent on surgeon preference, patient variables, and resources available. Basic surgical techniques for hernia repair include primary repair (suture repair), open mesh repair (tension-free repair), and laparoscopic techniques.

Primary repair has often been the only option in areas of limited surgical resources. It can usually be performed under local anesthesia, on an outpatient basis with minimal supplies. It is the preferred technique in the presence of contamination from incarcerated or strangulated intestine when avoidance of prosthetic mesh is desired. As surgical training evolves, fewer surgical trainees are exposed to primary inguinal hernia repair, making this a critical knowledge gap when Western-trained surgeons travel to LMICs.

Mesh repair has become the most popular technique for repair of inguinal hernias in the United States. This type of repair generally is technically straightforward and associated with a low postoperative morbidity and recurrence rate of approximately 1%. The European Union (EU) Hernia Trialist Collaboration meta-analysis of 2002 reported on 20 randomized trials. Compared with primary repair, patients having mesh repair had a shorter hospital stay, a faster return to normal activities, and a lower incidence of pain. A study of 26,304 groin hernias performed in Denmark found that mesh repairs had a lower reoperation rate than primary repair.[9]

While mesh repair of hernias has traditionally been limited to high-income countries (HICs), the effectiveness of using mosquito net mesh for hernia repair in LMICs shows excellent promise. Among 359 patients treated at four Indian hospitals using locally produced nylon mesh for inguinal hernia repair, Tongaonkar and colleagues found only one recurrence, no mesh rejections, and minor infections in 4.7% of patients.[10] No recurrences were observed after 6 months among 95 patients operated on in Ghana by local and European surgeons using polyester mosquito net mesh with wound complications in 7%.[11]

Laparoscopic hernia repair is widely gaining popularity in HICs. Laparoscopic inguinal and abdominal hernia repair is based on repair of the weakened posterior abdominal wall. It requires general anesthesia and significant specialized surgical instruments and supplies not available to most global surgeons.

Anesthetic options include local, regional (spinal or epidural), or general anesthesia. Most groin hernias can safely be repaired under local anesthesia. Local anesthetics offer considerable advantages over general anesthesia in terms of reduced cardiac, central nervous system, and respiratory complications.[12] They are readily available and have a low incidence of postoperative headache, nausea, and vomiting, and a lower risk of postoperative urinary retention. Local anesthesia for repair of inguinal hernia is associated with shorter hospital stay and lower overall cost with no difference in complications or recurrence rate when compared with general and regional anesthesia.[13]

General or regional anesthesia may be preferred when operating emergently for incarceration, or if significant bowel manipulation or resection may be required. General anesthesia is necessary for most ventral hernia repairs and all laparoscopic hernia repairs.

Types of Hernia

Groin Hernia

Approximately 96% of groin hernias are inguinal and 4% are femoral. Inguinal hernias occur 9 times more often in men than women, while femoral hernias occur 4 times more often in women. Inguinal hernias may be direct or indirect. The indirect inguinal hernia occurs at the internal inguinal ring through which passes the spermatic cord in males and the round ligament in females. Most indirect inguinal hernias are congenital even though they may not become evident until later in life. They are thought to result from defective obliteration of the fetal processus vaginalis. The proportion of indirect inguinal hernias is significantly higher in LMICs (82.9% in Ghana) than in HICs (60% in Europe), likely due to lack of surgical treatment of childhood hernias.[4]

Direct inguinal hernias occur as a result of a weakness in the floor of the inguinal canal. The hernia passes through Hesselbach's triangle formed by the inguinal ligament inferiorly, the inferior epigastric vessels laterally, and the rectus abdominus muscle medially. The relationship between straining or heavy lifting and direct inguinal hernias is not clear. Direct hernias are more likely to recur than indirect hernia.

Femoral hernias occur in the space medial to the femoral vessels. They occur 4 times more often in women than men, and approximately 40% will present with incarceration or strangulation. They will frequently present with bowel obstruction. Femoral hernias may present cephalad to or overlying the inguinal ligament, making them difficult to differentiate from inguinal hernias.

Abdominal Wall Hernias

There are several different hernias of the anterior abdominal wall, including umbilical, paraumbilical, epigastric, and incisional ventral hernias. The common umbilical hernia in children generally closes spontaneously and rarely requires surgery. There is a much higher incidence of umbilical hernia among children of African descent. Based on observations made in Nigeria, umbilical fascial defects continue to close until at least 14 years of age, so in the absence of symptoms, continued observation may be offered.[14] Less common is the adult paraumbilical hernia. This hernia generally occurs through a weakness in the linea alba just above or below the umbilicus rather than directly through it. These are at risk for incarceration and generally will require surgery. Epigastric hernias occur through a weakness in the linea alba between the xiphoid and the umbilicus. Epigastric hernias generally remain small and will only require repair if symptomatic. Finally, the incisional ventral hernia can occur at any site of prior procedure. Caesarean section incisions are common sites for incisional ventral hernia in LMICs. Wound infection is the strongest risk factor for development of incisional ventral hernia, but poor facial closure, malnutrition, chronic cough or constipation, as well as malignancy or systemic illness are also associated with development of hernia.

Diagnosis and Diagnostic Difficulties

History and physical exam remain the diagnostic modality of choice for identification of hernias. All indirect and sliding inguinal hernias as well as symptomatic direct inguinal hernias should be repaired due to the risk of strangulation. Remember, in areas with limited surgical resources, indirect inguinal hernias predominate. Small direct inguinal hernias in the elderly and many asymptomatic ventral hernias can be observed as their risk of strangulation remains low.

Hydroceles can be difficult to distinguish from inguinal hernias (Figure 17.1). Both will transilluminate, but the hydrocele will not reduce. A hydrocele is generally nontender and will not incite a cough reflex when palpated. If you can get above the scrotal swelling with your finger and thumb, then it does not originate above the external inguinal ring and therefore is not an inguinal hernia. In the tropics, hydrocele in adults is often a manifestation of *Bancroftian filariasis,* which will require the same surgical approach but additional therapy for the parasite. Other testicular pathology, such as testicular torsion or epididymitis, can mimic inguinal hernia. In these cases there is no normal testis in addition to the "hernia sac."

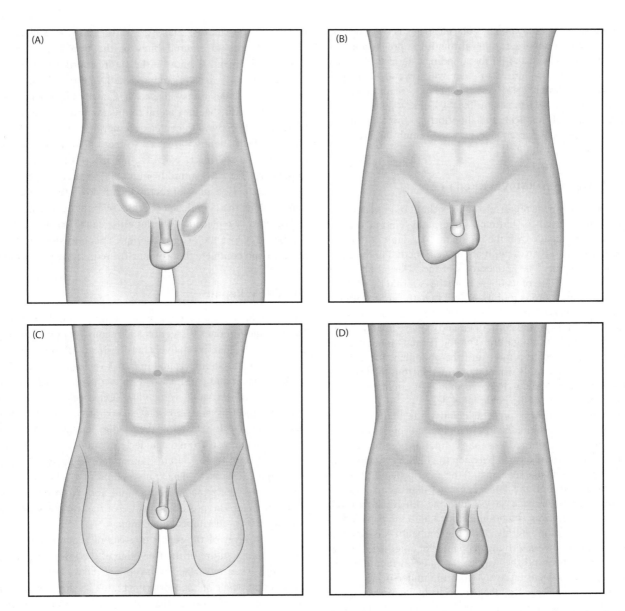

FIGURE 17.1 (A) Common location of groin hernias. The right side shows an inguinal hernia and the left shows a femoral hernia. (B) An inguinal hernia extending into the scrotum. (C) Bilateral adenolymphoceles. (D) Bilateral hydroceles. Illustrations by Alexandra Briggs.

In areas where onchocerciasis is endemic, you may encounter adenolymphoceles. In advanced cases these present as masses of edematous fibrous tissue which hang from the groins. They arise from enlarged inguinal nodes as the result of progressive lymphatic obstruction. This can be diagnosed by microfilariae in skin biopsies and should be treated medically before planning any surgical intervention.

Techniques of Inguinal Hernia Repair

Mesh Repair of Inguinal Hernia

Mesh repair is an excellent option for both primary and recurrent inguinal hernia repair. Sterilized 100% polyester mosquito net mesh can be used in place of commercially available hernia mesh. The incision is centered of the medial third of the inguinal ligament and external inguinal ring. The groin structures are exposed and the aponeurosis of the external oblique is entered in the direction of its fibers, preserving the ilioinguinal nerve. The cord structures are carefully dissected free and encircled with a Penrose drain. An indirect sac may be found anteromedial to the cord structures. If an indirect hernia sac is found, it should be separated from the cord structures all the way to the internal ring, and simply inverted into the peritoneum. The floor of the inguinal canal can be assessed by palpation. If a direct hernia defect is present, it should be dissected free and reduced into the preperitoneal space.

The mesh plug, if used, is placed into the internal ring of an indirect hernia or the fascial defect of a direct hernia so the petals unfold under the fascia and anchor it in place with several simple prolene sutures. The onlay patch is placed so as to cover the floor of the canal with the cord coming through the precut hole and the incision and tails of the mesh extending lateral to the internal ring. This patch is sutured in place with several interrupted prolene sutures. Sutures are generally placed medially at the pubic tubercle, laterally to secure the two tails together, inferiorly to the inguinal ligament, and superiorly to the conjoint tendon. The external oblique aponeurosis and remaining layers are closed in the usual fashion.[15]

Cooper's Ligament (McVay) Repair

The Cooper's ligament repair also closes the femoral canal and can therefore be used for indirect, direct, and femoral hernias. A skin incision is made over the region of external inguinal ring and continued laterally to a point about 2 cm medial to the anterosuperior iliac spine. The aponeurosis of the external oblique is entered in the direction of its fibers from the external ring for 5–7 cm. The spermatic cord is mobilized and then the entire cremasteric muscle is excised from the inguinal canal. If a hernia sac is present, dissect it from the cord, open and explore it, and close it at its neck with a suture ligature. The sac is then amputated and the stump is allowed to retract into the abdomen. Identify the external spermatic vessels where they emerge from the transversalis fascia and divide them. Remove about 4–5 cm of the vessels and ligate them again at the pubic tubercle.

If an indirect hernia is present, identify the margins of the transversalis fascia around the internal inguinal ring. If the internal inguinal ring is enlarged less than 2 cm, it is possible to close the defect with several sutures between the healthy transversalis fascia along the cephalad margin and the anterior femoral sheath at the caudad margin. If the defect is greater than 2 cm, complete reconstruction will be necessary. Incise the transversalis fascia with a scalpel beginning at a point just medial to the pubic tubercle. Carry the incision laterally with Metzenbaum scissors, taking care not injure the underlying deep inferior epigastric vessels. Continue the incision all the way to the internal inguinal ring. Sweep the preperitoneal fat away from the undersurface of the transversalis fascia. Free the deep inferior epigastric vessels so they may be retracted posteriorly together with the preperitoneal fat. A few small branches may need to be divided and ligated.

Excise the iliopubic tract adjacent to Cooper's ligament, applying two identifying hemostats to the cephalad cut edge of the transversalis fascia. Elevate the cut edge to expose the aponeurosis of the transversalis muscle. Excise the fleshy portion of the internal oblique muscle overlying the fibrous transversus arch to improve exposure.

Carefully identify the anterior femoral sheath and retract the external iliac vein and artery posteriorly using a peanut sponge retractor. To see the femoral sheath clearly, it is necessary to excise all of the overlying cremaster muscle fibers. A relaxing incision is then created by making a 7–8 cm incision in the anterior rectus sheath beginning about 1.5 cm above the pubic tubercle and continuing cephalad to a point just medial to where it fuses with the external oblique aponeurosis. The anterior belly of the rectus is exposed as downward traction is applied to the transversus arch.

The Cooper's ligament sutures are then placed by suturing the transversus arch to Cooper's ligament using atraumatic nonabsorbable sutures. Place the sutures no more than 5 mm apart and take substantial bites of the transversus arch and Cooper's ligament. Do not tie the sutures until all are in place. As the femoral vessels are approached, one transition suture is taken that includes transversus arch, Cooper's ligament, and the anterior femoral sheath. Lateral to this the transversus arch will be sutured directly to the anterior femoral sheath until the internal ring is sufficiently narrowed so that only a hemostat will fit alongside the spermatic cord. Do not insert any sutures lateral to the cord. Tie each suture from medial to lateral (Figure 17.2). Suture the incised anterior rectus sheath down to the underlying muscle along the lateral aspect of the relaxing incision.

The cord is replaced in the inguinal canal and hemostasis is confirmed. Close the external oblique aponeurosis superficial to the cord and complete the wound closure in the usual fashion.[16]

Shouldice Repair

The Shouldice repair, developed at the Shouldice clinic in Toronto, incorporates dissection and reconstruction of the inguinal floor. The repair is relatively tension-free, utilizing the opened transversalis fascia imbricated in four layers over one another.

The incision and careful isolation of the cord structures proceeds as with the McVay procedure. Once suitable exposure is achieved, the trasversalis fascia is separated from the preperitoneal fat plane by elevating the medial leaflet of the external oblique aponeurosis from the underlying transversalis muscle for a distance of at least 3–4 cm, taking care to preserve the inferior epigastric vessels. The transversalis fascia is then opened with scissors along the entire inguinal floor from intern ring to pubic tubercle. The posterior surface of the transversalis is then cleaned of its preperitoneal attachments.

The first layer of the repair consists of a continuous, imbricated, running suture of the free edge of the lower transversalis flap to the posterior surface of the upper transversalis flap and the lateral component of the posterior rectus sheath. This running suture begins medially at the pubic tubercle and is continued through the internal ring, thus tightening the transversalis fascia around the cord. This same running suture is then continued in a running fashion from lateral to medial as the second layer closing the upper transversalis flap to the base of the lower edge and the inguinal ligament. This second layer continues to the pubic tubercle where it is tied.

The third layer is again a continuous running suture that begins at the tightened internal ring and joins the conjoined tendon medially with the inguinal ligament laterally. This layer continues medially to the pubic tubercle and then returns laterally as the fourth layer, which includes the anterior rectus sheath medially and the posterior aspect of the external oblique aponeurosis laterally. This suture continues laterally to its origin at the internal ring and is tied to itself.

The cord can then be carefully returned to the new inguinal floor. The aponeurosis of the external oblique is closed superficial to the cord. You can then complete the wound closure in the usual fashion.[17]

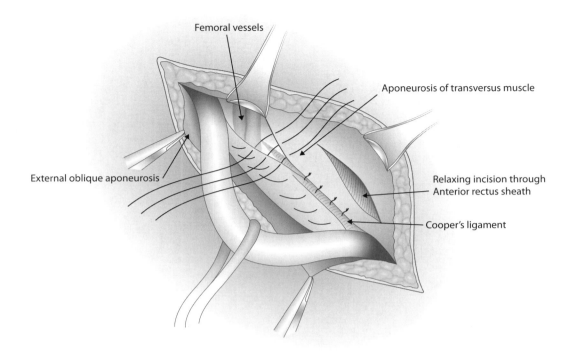

Femoral vessels

Aponeurosis of transversus muscle

External oblique aponeurosis

Relaxing incision through
Anterior rectus sheath

Cooper's ligament

FIGURE 17.2 Cooper's ligament (McVay) repair of an inguinal hernia. Illustration by Alexandra Briggs.

Difficulties With Hernia Repair

Strangulation

Whether a Richter's hernia, sliding hernia, or complete strangulated hernia, all strangulated tissue must be inspected (Figure 17.3).

This may be done by enlarging the hernia defect itself in order to deliver the bowel or other organs onto the field, incising the floor of the inguinal canal, or via a laparotomy incision. A small area of bowel injury from a Richter's hernia may be invaginated with Lembert sutures if it has not perforated and does not involve more than 50% of the bowel circumference, has clean healthy margins, and is not in close proximity to the mesentery. If bowel resection is required, then prosthetic mesh should be avoided.

Prevention of Injury to the Testis

Ischemic orchitis occurs in approximately 5% of open recurrent inguinal hernia repairs. Meticulous dissection and deliberate avoidance of injury to the cord structures is the best way to preserve testicular function. For difficult cases of recurrent hernia, the preperitoneal approach offers a reasonable alternative to decrease the risk of testicular complications. If it becomes evident that the identification and preservation of the spermatic cord will be impossible during a repair of recurrent inguinal hernia, especially in a young patient, it may be necessary to abort the anterior approach and raise a cephalad skin flap for 3–5 cm

and continue the operation by an incision through the abdominal wall using the preperitoneal approach. Repair of a large recurrent inguinal hernia in an elderly patient may be simplified by simultaneous orchiectomy if the patient is agreeable.

Loss of Abdominal Domain

Abdominal wall hernias, particularly paraumbilical and incisional hernias, can become massive, containing much of the abdominal contents. This can lead to the difficult problem of loss of abdominal domain. With much of the abdominal contents within the hernia sac, the abdominal fascia decreases in size. If the abdominal contents are then completely reduced during hernia repair, the fascia cannot be closed primarily without undue tension, leading to either failure of the repair or dangerous intra-abdominal hypertension. Intra-abdominal hypertension can be prevented by avoiding overly tight primary closure by using the technique of separation of components or placement of a prosthetic or bioprosthetic mesh.

Postoperative Complications

Recurrence

Recurrence rates vary greatly between studies, making it difficult to directly compare techniques. Recurrence overall will occur in 0.5%–15% of patients. Mesh repair of primary inguinal hernia has approximately a 2%–4% recurrence rate, which increases to

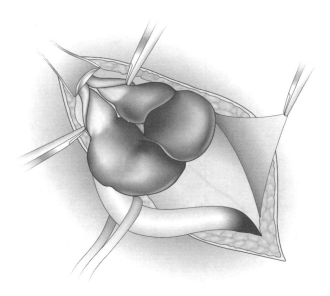

FIGURE 17.3   Indirect inguinal hernia containing strangulated bowel. Illustration by Alexandra Briggs.

greater than 10% if the repair is for a recurrent hernia. Data on recurrence with mosquito net mesh repairs is limited by small study size and short follow-up, but at up to 6 months recurrence rates were less than 1%.[10,11]

Hernia recurrence can be related to technical factors, including poor fixation, or excessive dissection leading to devascularization of tissues; patient factors such as obesity, smoking, and steroid use; and wound complications such as infection. Late recurrence (greater than 5 years) is likely due to weakening of tissue from the natural progression of the aging process.

Infection

Postoperative infection following groin hernia repair is an uncommon complication occurring in approximately 3%–4% of cases. The risk of surgical site infection increases slightly when a mesh repair is performed. In the setting of mosquito net mesh repair, the incidence of infection is reported from 1.7%–7%.[11,18] Skin flora are the most common pathogens, and most infected groin hernia repairs can be successfully treated with antibiotics. Even in the case of mesh implants for groin hernia, wound infections can often be treated with aggressive antibiotic therapy, without the need to remove the mesh. Preoperative antibiotic prophylaxis for groin hernia repair has not been shown to significantly reduce the incidence of surgical site infection, although the practice is common in the United States.

Seroma and Hematoma

Seromas or hematomas generally occur when a significant dead space was created during dissection, or when postoperative bleeding occurred. Most postoperative seromas and hematomas will resolve spontaneously or decompress through the wound. The combined incidence of seroma and hematoma following groin surgery is approximately 10%. Hematomas occurred in 4.4% of 113 patients undergoing mosquito net mesh repairs of groin hernias in Ghana.[18]

Injury to the Testis

Ischemic orchitis occurs in approximately 0.5% of primary open hernia repairs and 5% of recurrent hernia repairs. Collateral arterial blood flow to the testis is supplied by the inferior epigastric, vesicle, prostatic, and scrotal arteries. Because of its rich collateral blood supply, ischemic orchitis rarely occurs as a result of arterial injury but can occur as a result of thrombosis. Thrombosis of the spermatic veins is the most common cause of ischemic orhitis, and can occur as a result of rough handling, difficult dissection, or overly constricting repair of the internal inguinal ring. This results in painful swelling of the testis. It can be diagnosed by ultrasound, if available. Management includes systemic anticoagulation, if available; however, in the absence of imaging it can be difficult to rule out testicular torsion, which then necessitates surgical exploration. Ligation and excision of the vein is an accepted surgical therapy. There are, however, reports of worsened venous congestion and testicular ischemia following ligation and excision. Orchiectomy may be necessary if the testicle appears nonviable.

Iatrogenic injury to vas deferens generally occurs as a result of transection or compression. Diagnosis and repair of iatrogenic injury to the vas deferens generally requires referral to a center with urologic expertise.

Pain and Neuralgia

Pain following hernia surgery is often due to injury or entrapment of any of the sensory nerves within the groin. The ilioinguinal and genitofemoral nerves are the most commonly injured during open surgery, while the lateral femoral nerve of the thigh is more commonly injured during laparoscopic repairs. In one survey of almost 2,500 patients undergoing primary surgery for groin hernia, 31% reported some residual pain 2 to 3 years after their procedure, and in 6% the pain interfered with daily activities. Risk factors for postoperative pain were the presence of preoperative pain and postoperative complications.[19]

Meticulous avoidance of manipulation of nerves during dissection reduces the risk of postoperative neuralgia. Intentionally sacrificing the sensory nerves at the time of surgery also reduces the risk of postoperative neuralgia but has not been shown to be better than identification and preservation of the nerves. Nerve injury or entrapment should initially be managed by injection of local anesthetic into the area. This is useful for diagnosis and treatment, and in some cases may eliminate the pain permanently. Reexploration and neurolysis or nerve resection may be necessary.

Low- and Middle-Income Country (LMIC) Specific Considerations

- Hernias represent a serious social and economic burden of disease for LMICs.
- Hernias in LMICs tend to be larger, are more often indirect, and are in younger patients than in HICs.
- Local anesthesia is safe and cost-effective for most inguinal hernia repairs.
- Sterilized mosquito net mesh can be used for mesh repair of inguinal hernias.
- In areas where onchocerciasis is endemic, you may encounter adenolymphoceles.
- In the tropics, a hydrocele is often associated with *Bancroftian filariasis.*

Potential Pitfalls and Problems to Avoid

- Any bowel that was incarcerated must be inspected to avoid missed injury.

- If bowel resection is required, then prosthetic mesh should be avoided.
- Meticulous dissection and deliberate avoidance of injury to the cord structures is the best way to preserve testicular function.
- Hydroceles can be difficult to distinguish from inguinal hernias.
- Treat *Bancroftian filariasis* if present after repair of a hydrocele.
- Although adenolymphoceles are easy to remove, they tend to heal poorly; treat medically before planning surgery.

COMMENTARY

Edgar Rodas, Ecuador
Edgar B. Rodas, Ecuador

Over the last 20 years, we have utilized a mobile surgery unit—an operating room on a truck—to deliver surgical services to remote areas of the Andean Mountains, the Pacific Coast, and the Amazon region of Ecuador. More than 7,000 operations have been performed; herniohrraphy has been the most prevalent (23%).

During the first 5 years, we used different types of tissue repair (Shouldice, McVay, and Bassini); however, during the last 15 years, the tension-free mesh repair (Leichtenstein) has been our standard for adult patients. Thanks to donations to our program, we now utilize polypropylene mesh, so we do not have experience with mosquito mesh or other alternative materials. In children, we perform simple closure of the hernia sac.

Initially, we routinely utilized conductive anesthesia in adults and general anesthesia in children. Currently, we perform almost all cases in adults with local anesthesia with excellent results.

Patients are discharged on the same day of surgery, and follow-up is provided by any available health personnel and mobile telephone. Lately, we are also using telemedicine capabilities via a smart tablet in remote areas.

18

Colon and Rectum

Allison F. Linden
Kathryn Chu

Introduction

This chapter provides an overview of the treatment of colorectal disorders in low- and middle-income countries (LMICs). Common colorectal pathologies include trauma, infections, volvulus, diverticular disease, and neoplasm. Elective colorectal disorders such as rectal prolapse, asymptomatic colonic polyps, or carcinoma-in-situ are less common in LMICs and are not covered in this chapter.

Often patients do not have access to preventive health care and present late in their illness. A good history is invaluable. Many patients with colorectal disorders have a history of subacute or acute obstruction. Peritonitis and hemorrhage are also common. Important symptoms to ask about include fever, diarrhea, vomiting, and obstipation. There may be a history of melena or bright red blood per rectum. Comorbidities such as human immunodeficiency virus (HIV), tuberculosis (TB), and malnutrition will influence the differential diagnosis and disease progression.

Physical Exam

The physical exam is critical in making a diagnosis given the lack of imaging modalities in many LMICs. Patients are often acutely systemically ill. Depending on the etiology of their illness, they may be febrile, tachycardic, dehydrated, and have evidence of end organ failure. Palpate the abdomen for the presences of masses, rebound tenderness, and ascites. Examine the perineum and anus if rectal injury is suspected. Digital rectal exam can reveal mass lesions. In neoplasms, a longer history of early satiety, obstipation, and/or intermittent obstructive symptoms may be solicited.

Laboratory and Imaging Studies

Obtain baseline white blood cell count, hemoglobin, platelet count, electrolyte, urea, and creatinine studies if possible. A CD4 count less than 200 is a risk factor for a poor surgical outcome.[1–3] Radiographic imaging in many LMICs is limited to plain X-ray. Three-way abdominal series (including chest X-ray) are useful to look for free air, bowel dilation, and foreign bodies. Often you will perform the study yourself, especially Gastografin or

barium enemas, or stomagrams, as almost certainly the radiographer will not know how to perform these procedures. Ultrasound is less useful in colorectal disorders, but can be used to look for free fluid, intra-abdominal abscesses, or enlarged lymph nodes. Most of the time you will be expected to interpret the images without the help of a radiologist.

Differential Diagnosis

Common colorectal diseases in low- and middle-income countries (LMICs) include traumatic injuries, infectious colitis, sigmoid volvulus, diverticular disease, and neoplasms.

Trauma is covered more extensively in Chapter 38, but a few points related to colon and rectal injuries are made here. Worldwide, penetrating trauma used to be more common. As economic growth in LMICs increases, followed by greater access to roads and motor vehicles, road traffic injuries are predicted to become the third leading cause of disability-adjusted life years (DALYs) by 2020.[4] Consequently, incidences of blunt traumatic injury, of which the large and small bowel are especially vulnerable, are increasing.[5,6] The time of injury and the mechanism and velocity of injury are important. For example, a penetrating stab wound may cause more limited intra-abdominal injury compared to the broad-based injury possible with a high-velocity gunshot wound to the abdomen. If computed tomography (CT) scan and ultrasound are unavailable, have a high level of suspicion to explore the patient if bowel injury is suspected. Patient-to-nurse ratios on the wards in LMICs are usually high, and patients cannot be closely observed on the wards to see if pain is increasing or the patient decompensates. Explore the abdomen early.

Infectious Diseases

Abdominal TB should be in the differential in populations with high HIV prevalence. Symptoms may be vague and include abdominal pain, weight loss, diarrhea, fever, melena, and obstructive symptoms.[7] Patients often have low CD4 counts.[8] It is known as the "great mimicker" as its symptoms can imitate numerous other pathologies such as appendicitis, inflammatory bowel disease, and malignancy.[9] Intestinal TB most commonly affects the terminal ileum followed by the cecum and ascending colon. It often presents as an ulcerative process that can lead to perforation or fistulas or a hyperplastic reaction that can lead to obstruction due to a mass.[7] Ultrasound usually demonstrates enlarged lymph nodes.[8] Mucosal biopsies demonstrating caseating granulomas and a Ziehl-Neelsen stain revealing acid-fast bacilli gives a definitive diagnosis.[7,10] Surgical exploration is warranted if the patient has a complete obstruction or secondary to perforation or fistulae.

Infectious colitis can occur in areas of poor hygiene and contaminated drinking water. Amoebiasis, caused by *Entamoeba histolytica,* is endemic in South Asian countries and typically found in humid, low-elevation climates. It often presents with cramps, diarrhea including blood and mucus, and focal tenderness. It can also cause ulcerations, particularly in the rectum, which can mimic a neoplasm. A biopsy will demonstrate amoebas or trophozoites of *Entamoeba histolytica*. Metronidazole followed by paromycin is effective treatment. Amoebiasis can also lead to fulminant colitis resulting in intestinal perforation, which requires urgent surgical intervention.[11,12]

Volvulus

A volvulus occurs when a segment of bowel twists around its mesentery, creating a closed loop of bowel (Figure 18.1). The twisted bowel segment results in vascular occlusion and subsequent bowel ischemia. The sigmoid colon is the most commonly affected site in adults. Volvulus is a leading cause of large bowel obstruction in many LMICs, while neoplasm of the colon is the leading cause in high-income countries

(HICs).[13,14] In HICs, bedridden elderly patients are at greatest risk. However, in LMICs, this can occur in younger, otherwise healthy patients, particularly in males.[14] This condition likely develops due to redundant sigmoid colons and long mesenteries, which are more common in LMICs due to high-residue diets.

Obstruction is the predominant clinical presentation. A patient may also complain of moderate colicky abdominal pain and severe distention. There may be a history of past episodes with relief of the symptoms after passing a large amount of stool and flatus. Abdominal exam will reveal a markedly distended abdomen, often more pronounced on the left side. Rectal exam will often demonstrate an empty rectal vault. Upright abdominal X-ray will reveal a massive colonic distension in a "coffee bean" shape originating in the lower left quadrant (LLQ) and arching toward the right upper quadrant (RUQ) (Figure 18.2).

Diverticular Disease

Diverticulosis is the presence of mucosal outpouchings in the bowel wall due to weak points from the penetration of mesenteric blood vessels into the muscular layer of the bowel. It can lead to inflammation of the diverticula and bleeding. This is a common disease in HICs where there is decreased intake of dietary fiber, affecting over half of the population over 60 years of age in the United States.[15] While it is usually found in the sigmoid colon, in Asia and Africa it can present almost as commonly in the right colon.[16] While still relatively uncommon in LMICs, it should be considered when evaluating for lower gastrointestinal (GI) bleeding.

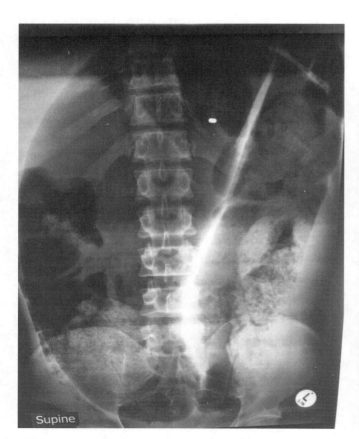

FIGURE 18.1 Radiographic appearance of sigmoid volvulus. Image by Kathryn Chu.

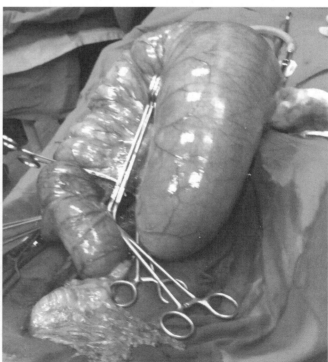

FIGURE 18.2 Sigmoid volvulus. Image by Kathryn Chu.

Neoplasms

Most colorectal cancers are adenocarcinomas. They are 5 to 10 times less common in LMICs, but the incidence is rising as wealth brings increased consumption of alcohol, red meat, and low-vegetable diets.[17,18] Screening for colorectal cancer is relatively rare in LMICs, so patients do not commonly present with asymptomatic early cancer or polyps. Instead, the presentation is usually advanced stage disease with obstruction, perforation, and/or chronic anemia.

Anal Cancer

Anal cancer should be in suspected in a patient with a firm anal mass. Rectal pain and bleeding is common. In HIV-positive individuals, anal squamous cell carcinoma (SCC) is more common due to persistent herpes papilloma virus infection. The primary treatment for anal SCC is chemotherapy and radiation, and not surgical intervention. Local recurrence is very likely after local excision and may result in a nonhealing perineal wound. Do a biopsy and refer the patient if possible. If the lesion is too debilitating or septic, do a diverting colostomy.

Lymphoma

In the HIV population with low CD4 counts, lymphoma can be a cause of intestinal obstruction. The patient is often very debilitated and unlikely to be fit for an operation. Ultrasound may reveal large lymph nodes at the root of the mesentery of the small intestine. Try not to operate on this patient if you make the diagnosis preoperatively as the outcome will be poor.

Relevant Anatomy and Physiology

The general surgeon working in LMICs needs excellent working knowledge of the anatomy of the abdomen and pelvis. The vascular supply of the large bowel comes from the superior and inferior mesenteric arteries. The ileocolic artery is a branch of the superior mesenteric artery (SMA) and is the primary blood supply for the cecum and right colon. The right colic is a branch of the SMA and supplies the ascending colon and hepatic flexure. The middle colic artery is also a branch of the SMA and supplies the transverse colon. The left colic artery is the first branch of the inferior mesenteric artery (IMA) and supplies the splenic flexure and descending colon. The sigmoid arteries branch from the IMA and supply the sigmoid colon. The IMA continues as the superior hemorrhoidal artery after crossing the left iliac vessels and is the main blood supply to the rectum.

The colon has rich collateral systems through the arcade of Riolan and the marginal artery of Drummond. The rectum receives collateral blood supply through the inferior and middle hemorrhoidal arteries.

The ureters should always be identified, especially when the pelvic anatomy is distorted with inflammation or perforation. Ureteral stents will likely be unavailable in LMICs.

Procedure Highlights

Special Considerations for LMICs

The first determination is whether the patient is fit for an operation. If the patient is unlikely to survive the procedure, do not operate. In many cultures an operative death is treated suspiciously and not seen as a heroic effort to save the patient.

Second, decide if there are any qualified anesthesia personnel at your hospital for the particular procedure. The individual does not need to be a fully trained anesthesiologist but can be a general practitioner with experienced anesthetic skills or a nurse anesthetist. If such personnel are not available, transfer the patient or give palliative care.

Minimally invasive surgery is not available in most LMICs, so diagnostic laparoscopy is usually not possible. If an operation is warranted, do an exploratory laparotomy and make a generous incision, especially if retractors, operative lights, and trained assistants are limited. The abdomen should be explored thoroughly to define the problem. Attention should be paid to the presence of free fluid, mass lesions, and liver metastasis. Large mesenteric lymph nodes are suggestive of lymphoma or TB, especially in the HIV-positive population.

General Principles

Electrocautery is not always available, so careful attention to hemostasis is needed. Temporary placement of clamps on small bleeding vessels in the subcutaneous fat controls bleeding during opening of the abdomen and saves time. Other surgical sealing devices such as Ligature and harmonic scalpels are also usually not available, so securely suture ligate named vessels. If an intestinal anastomosis is to be performed, ensure good blood supply to both ends of bowel and a tension-free anastomosis. Bowel staplers are usually not available, so plan to do a hand-sewn anastomosis in one or two layers. Be prepared for a limited choice of suture; vicryl or polydioxanone (PDS) may not be available, only catgut. Leave a drain if there is risk of postoperative hemorrhage or ureteral injury. Drains can be fashioned from Foley catheters.

Trauma

In penetrating stab wounds, the injury is usually limited in nature and can be closed primary after the wound edges are debrided and the wound freshened. In gunshot wounds, collateral damage can be extensive, so search for additional injuries even if they do not appear to be in the trajectory of the bullet. Run the entire small bowel from the ligament of Treitz to the ileocecal valve. Large bowel injuries can be hidden by hematomas; therefore, mobilize the flexures and examine the retroperitoneum if needed. Take care not to open the retroperitoneum if there is a stable contained hematoma and no evidence of bowel injury.

Infections

Intestinal TB is best treated medically unless the patient presents with sepsis from fistulae or a complete obstruction. Late strictures are best treated with surgical resection. Amoebiasis can lead to perforation requiring surgical intervention.

Sigmoid Volvulus

Nonoperative treatment of sigmoid volvulus in the LMIC is difficult. Sigmoidoscopy to reduce the volvulus is often not available. Patients usually present late with necrotic bowel. Perform an exploratory laparotomy. Consent the patient preoperatively for a possible colostomy. Gently untwist the bowel. Handle it with care as sometimes it will perforate if roughly manipulated given its dilated state and often compromised blood supply. If the patient is otherwise healthy and there is no ischemia, a primary anastomosis with resection of the redundant sigmoid can be considered. However, if the patient is immunocompromised and/or the bowel is necrotic, do a sigmoid resection with Hartmann's pouch and end colostomy. A sigmoidopexy will result in a high rate of recurrence and is not recommended.

Neoplasms

Often neoplasms will present with high-grade obstruction or perforation. In HICs, adjuvant chemotherapy, combined with radiation therapy for tumors of the rectum, is an essential part of the treatment of adenocarcinoma of the large bowel. However, in LMICs, this may not be possible. Therefore, it is essential that the surgeon perform an oncologic resection if possible. If cancer is suspected, proximal and distal bowel margins of at least 2 cm are needed. Sleeve resection is contra-indicated. For lesions in the cecum and ascending colon, a formal right colectomy is needed. Lesions in the hepatic flexure and proximal transverse colon require an extended right colectomy. Lesions in the distal transverse colon and splenic flexure require a formal left colectomy. Sigmoid lesions require a left colectomy. Even if the tumor is in the proximal to mid-sigmoid, consider making a colorectal anastomosis to the top of the rectum as this bowel has improved blood supply.[19] Ensure high ligation of the feeding vessel and remove the corresponding lymph nodes.

Rectal Cancer

Resection of rectal cancer is more challenging than colon cancer because of the confined pelvis. Reaching a distal lesion, especially in a male or an obese patient, may be difficult. Make a generous incision to the pubis and ask your anesthesiologist to fully relax the patient. A 2-cm distal margin is challenging if the rectal lesion is low. If the lesion is closer than 2 cm to the anal sphincters, do an abdominoperineal resection. If this is beyond your scope of practice, do an end colostomy and try to refer the patient. If you attempt a resection, cut across the tumor, or leave the tumor in a short rectal stump, this will make the subsequent operation more difficult. If you are able to get below the tumor with a clean margin, try to take as much mesorectum as possible as it includes the lymphatic drainage of the rectum. Staple or suture the remaining rectal stump. Attempting coloanal anastomosis in the LMIC is likely to end in a pelvic anastomotic leak. If there is any chance the patient will receive adjuvant therapy after the operation, create a stoma and avoid a primary anastomosis; the patient could develop debilitating diarrhea from the chemotherapy and/or may develop a stricture from radiation.

Special Considerations

Damage Control Surgery

If during exploratory laparotomy, the patient becomes hemodynamically unstable, acidotic, or coagulopathic, consider a damage control operation and get the patient off the operating table as quickly as possible without doing a definitive procedure. This might involve only controlling hemorrhage, oversewing a perforation, debriding devitalized tissue, and leaving the bowel in discontinuity. The abdomen should be left open and a second-look operation planned in 24–48 hours or when the patient is more stable.

Sometimes the abdomen cannot be closed due to profound bowel or abdominal wall edema. Instead, a sterile 3-liter cystoscopy or saline intravenous fluid bag can be sutured to the skin to cover the exposed bowel. This works best if the fluid is drained out and the bag is left double-sided. This is known as the Bogata bag technique.[20] In HICs, vacuum-assisted closure (VAC) dressings can be placed over the open abdomen to allow for continuous suction of abdominal ascites. In LMICs, an alternative VAC dressing can also be fashioned. The first step is to make a "sandwich" of a large transparent adhesive dressing (Opsite) folded over several abdominal pads (Figure 18.3a).

This technique prevents the abdominal pads from lying in direct contact with the bowel and abdominal organs. The abdominal pads should be completely covered with the transparent dressing except for one small section in the center of one side. The "sandwich" is tucked under the fascia, with the exposed section facing up (Figure 18.3b). A suction tube with numerous cut holes should be place in the middle of the abdominal pads (Figure 18.3c). A large-bore nasogastric tube (NGT) should be placed through the suction tubing. The suction tube/NGT combination acts as a sump and prevents the suction from collapsing. Another large transparent adhesive dressing should then be placed over the entire wound. The NGT should then be placed on continuous suction (Figure 18.3d). If the hospital does not have large transparent adhesive dressings, a suction system can also be placed under the Bogata bag. Resuscitate the patient and return to the operating room when the patient is more stable.

Stomas

Always consent for a stoma prior to any colorectal operation. Stoma creation has disadvantages in LMICs. Stomas may not be well understood by patients or their families and often have cultural stigma associated with them. There are few stomal therapists to educate patients on skin care and stoma pouching. Supplies such as stoma bags, adhesives, and skin lotions are scarce. Patients live far away from health facilities and are at risk for dehydration, electrolyte derangements, and other stoma complications such as obstruction, prolapse, and hernias. Patients may not access health facilities or a surgeon to reverse the stoma in the future.

However, these disadvantages must be balanced with the risks of a leak from a primary anastomosis. Many patients are immunocompromised, malnourished, septic, and/or have multiorgan failure on presentation. An anastomotic leak in a hospital where

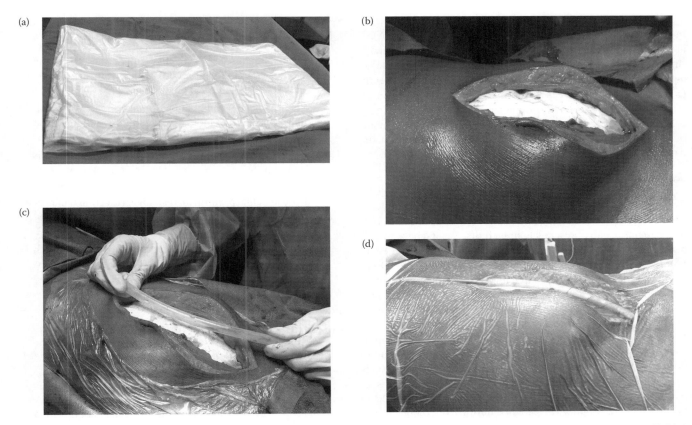

FIGURE 18.3 (a) A "sandwich" of transparent adhesive dressing wrapped around abdominal pads. (b) Place the sandwich under the fascia. (c) Place a suction tubing with holes in the middle of the wound. (d) Place a large-bore nasogastric tube through the suction tubing and cover with another layer of transparent adhesive dressing. Place the nasogastric tube on suction. Images by Kathryn Chu.

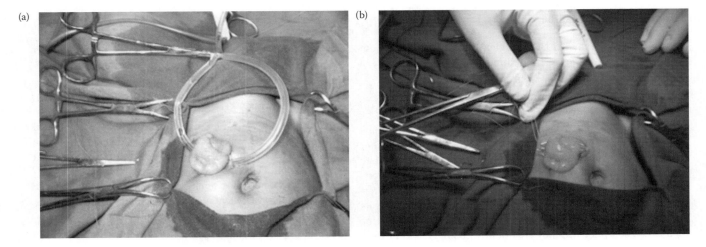

FIGURE 18.4 (a) A nasogastric tube can be used as a stoma rod. (b) The tube is trimmed to allow it to fit under the stoma bag and stitched to itself. Images by Kathryn Chu.

postoperative care is not vigilant can lead to high morbidity and mortality. The patient may not survive if he or she has to undergo a second operation. Be conservative and safe.

When maturing a loop ileostomy or colostomy, a 5-cm piece of a NGT can serve as a stoma rod. This can be stitched to itself to keep it from dislodging and placed inside the stoma bag (Figure 18.4a and Figure 18.4b).

Postoperative Management

The surgeon must be vigilant in postoperative care and watch for signs of decompensation. Vital signs and fluid balance may be poorly recorded. Nurses may not be familiar with caring for post-laparotomy patients, and good communication about the signs of wound dehiscence, infection, ileus, and anastomotic leak must be reviewed.

Most patients do not need NGT after colorectal surgery except in cases of small bowel dilation or profound ileus. If an NGT is used, intermittent wall suction is not usually available and it should instead be put to gravity drainage. Give subcutaneous heparin to prevent deep vein thrombosis and encourage early patient mobilization. Deep breathing to inflate a glove is an effective form of incentive spirometry. Removal of the urinary catheter when the fluid balance is stable will encourage mobilization as well. Postoperative antibiotics will be needed if the patient had gross fecal contamination and/or necrotic bowel.

Conclusions

Colorectal disorders are common in LMICs. Regardless of etiology, patients usually present late in their disease and have peritonitis, obstruction, or bleeding. They may have multiorgan system failure. Ensure the patient is adequately resuscitated. Order blood work if available. If you are able to safely operate, explore the abdomen through a generous incision. Resect ischemic bowel rather than attempting to oversew a perforation in the setting of sepsis. Avoid primary anastomosis if the patient is very sick. If the patient becomes hemodynamically unstable, or coagulopathic, do a damage control operation and plan on returning to the operating room once the patient is stabilized. If a neoplasm is suspected and the patient is stable, perform an oncologic resection. Postoperatively, follow the patient closely as nursing care may be limited. Monitor the patient carefully for complications, especially anastomotic leak.

LMIC Specific Considerations

- If the patient is HIV-positive, infectious colorectal disorders (i.e., abdominal TB) and certain neoplasms (anal SCC) should be in the differential.
- When exploring the abdomen, make a generous incision because retractors, good operative lights, and assistants may not be available.
- Monitor the patient intraoperatively. If the patient is decompensating, do a damage control operation and plan to return to the operating room when the patient is stable.
- If you are able, perform an oncologic resection if cancer is suspected. The patient may not get adjuvant therapy or another operation in the future.
- Monitor the patient carefully postoperatively and watch for signs of infection, wound dehiscence, and anastomotic leak.

Potential Pitfalls and Problems to Avoid

- Do not operate if you do not have qualified anesthesia personnel or appropriate postoperative care.
- Do not make a primary anastomosis if the patient is immunocompromised, malnourished, or very septic. A patient with a stoma is better than a dead patient with a primary anastomosis.

COMMENTARY

Thandinkosi E. Madiba, South Africa

In general, this chapter is comprehensive and addresses both treatment and challenges to treatment in LMICs. However, a few points to enhance the chapter are worth pointing out.

Delay in Presentation

Late presentation is a major problem in LMICs. When patients do present, they have an advanced stage of the disease. For non-trauma patients, there are a variety of reasons for the late presentation. Sometimes the personal beliefs or assumptions of the patient delay medical care; the patient may seek alternative health remedies before coming to the hospital. Patients may also feel restricted by lack of financial resources. Patients are also delayed when they are initially misdiagnosed by their primary care medical officers because they first spend time on inappropriate treatment before reaching the hospital.

Crohn's Disease and Tuberculosis

Intestinal TB and Crohn's disease have a predilection for the same area, namely the terminal ileum. In LMICs, such as many of those in Africa where Crohn's disease is not as common, when patients present with features suggestive of Crohn's disease and affecting the terminal ileum, TB must be considered. Some authorities even suggest that these patients should be treated as TB patients until proven otherwise. This is more crucial since the treatment of one condition exacerbates the other. This, together with the presentation of TB with other comorbidities, necessitates histological confirmation before treatment is initiated.

Sigmoid Volvulus

In addition to high-residue diet, there are other aetiological factors for sigmoid volvulus, such as defecation patterns, high altitudes, and use of enemas and a congenitally redundant sigmoid colon. The treatment of sigmoid volvulus is resection either as emergency or elective conditions, the advantage being low or non-existent recurrence rates.

SUGGESTED READING

Mnguni MN, Muckart DJJ, Madiba TE. Abdominal trauma in Durban, South Africa: factors influencing outcome. *Int Surg* 2012; 97:161–168

Raveenthiran V, Madiba TE, Atamanalp SS, De U. Volvulus of the sigmoid colon. *Colorectal Disease* 2010 Jul; 12 (7 Online): e1–e17.

Desai Y, Seebaran AR, Pillay CN. Crohn's Disease in the Indian population of Durban. *S Afr Med J* 1987; 25: 144–145.

Segal I. Intestinal tuberculosis, Crohn's Disease and ulcerative colitis in an urban black population. *S Afr Med J* 1984; 65; 37–44.

19

Anus and Rectum

Joel E. Goldberg

Introduction

Anorectal conditions are very common maladies that affect most people at one time or another. These disease processes include hemorrhoids, anal fissures, perirectal abscesses, fistula-in-ano, pruritus ano, and pilonidal disease. All of these conditions are frustrating to the patient and can be just as vexing for the treating physician. Anorectal disease and the complications of these disease processes remain rather straightforward in their diagnosis. However, the treatment process can often be complex and drawnout. With this in mind, the first step in diagnosing and treating an anorectal problem, whether in the most sophisticated hospital setting or the most austere environment, is having a solid understanding of anorectal anatomy and physiology. The provider must also be able to discern between the subtle and often overlapping symptoms of the anorectal disease processes. Understanding the disease processes will enable providers to develop a comprehensive treatment plan that will alleviate the suffering of the patient.

Anatomy and Physiology

The anal canal is approximately 3–5 cm in length and is the most distal end of the intestinal tract. It begins at the levator ani muscles and ends at the anal verge, which is the external-most opening of the anal canal. Externally, the first 5 cm of perianal skin and soft tissue extending outward circumferentially from the anal verge is known as the anal margin. The middle of the surgical anal canal is the dentate line. This line separates the upper half of the anal canal, which has columnar epithelium like that of the rectum, and the lower half of the anal canal, which has squamous epithelial cells like that of the anal verge. The folds in the anal mucosa that run proximally to the dentate line are called the columns of Morgagni. Anal crypts and anal glands are located between these folds in the anal mucosa. This anatomy is helpful in understanding the origin and treatment of perirectal abscess and fistula-in-ano disease.

The musculature of the anal canal is comprised of two layers of circumferential muscles. The internal anal sphincter (IAS) is the distal-most extension of circular rectal smooth muscle layer. The IAS provides approximately 25% of the muscular strength of the anal canal, which is generally involuntary muscular strength. The external anal sphincter (EAS) is made of striated skeletal muscle that provides the other 75% of anal canal

muscular strength, which is under voluntary muscular control. The upper one-third of the EAS is formed by puborectalis muscle, and the lower two-thirds is external striated skeletal muscle.

The perianal and perirectal spaces are likewise important in perianal suppurative disease. The intersphincteric space is located between the IAS and EAS, which is in direct communication with the supralevator space and the pelvic peritoneum. The ischiorectal fossa is lateral to the EAS and inferior to the levator ani musculature. On either side, the ischiorectal fossa wraps around and meets in the posterior midline connecting in the deep post-anal space. The superficial post-anal space is in the posterior midline below the level of the coccyx, and the deep space is superior to the tip of the coccyx.

There is a rich blood and nerve supply to the anal canal. An in-depth understanding of the pelvic blood supply, nerve innervation, and lymphatic drainage is important to understanding perianal disease processes. The blood supply and venous drainage is via the inferior mesenteric artery and the internal pudendal arteries, which are branches of the internal iliac arteries. The venous drainage is via both portal and systemic routes through similar above named vessels. The lymphatic drainage likewise follows the arterial and venous supply (Table 19.1).[1]

Often, when patients present with anorectal complaints, they attribute the symptoms to hemorrhoids. In actuality, the diagnosis is just as likely to be hemorrhoids as it is one of the other many anorectal maladies to be discussed in this chapter. There is considerable overlap between the symptoms experienced by patients with hemorrhoids, anal fissure, fistula, abscesses, and pilonidal disease. The symptoms that patients most often complain about include bleeding, pain, itching, leakage, perianal mass, difficulty with hygiene, difficult evacuation, and tissue prolapse. Bleeding can be either bright red blood, which is seen in fissure and internal hemorrhoids, or it can be a darker purple clot that is characteristic of a thrombosed external hemorrhoid clot with extravasation. Pain is often variable as well. It can range from a sharp, knife-like pain often described as passing glass to a sandpapery feeling to general discomfort with the passage of stool. In general, internal hemorrhoids present with discomfort or an uncomfortable feeling, whereas thrombosed external hemorrhoids are quite painful. Perianal drainage is a common complaint among all of these maladies. Purulence from an abscess or fistula or mucous leakage is associated with internal hemorrhoids or a fissure. Anal pruritus is a common symptom for all perianal disease, which varies with the amount of mucous drainage or difficulty with perianal hygiene. Finally, systemic symptoms

TABLE 19.1

Anorectal Disease Symptoms And Exam Findings

Diagnosis	Bleeding	Pain	Mass/Prolapse and Other Symptoms	Examination
Anal fissure	Small amount • Bright red • On the paper	Severe/sharp (glass or sandpaper) Worse with bowel movement	Small lesion at anal verge (sentinel pile) • Hurts when wiping Pruritus frequent	Small tear at anal verge • Best seen by effacing anal canal • Small tear inside anal canal with exposed muscle
Internal hemorrhoids	More Significant • Bright red • In the bowl • On the paper	Ranges from mild discomfort to none	Often a prolapsing mass • Can self reduce but often requires manual reduction • Tissue will be covered with pink mucosa Pruritus a common complaint	Best seen with anoscope • Unless prolapsed tissue is stuck out (grade III or IV hemorrhoids)
External Hemorrhoids (thrombosed)	Occasionally • Later in course • Clot extravasating	Severe	Usually a larger perianal mass • Does not reduce (permanently out) • Purple clot • Covered with anoderm (skin)	Large boggy/swollen anoderm • Often filled with purple clot • Tender to palpation
Perirectal Abscess	Rare	Severe	Yes and associated with systemic symptoms • Fever, chills • Malaise	Tender mass
Fistula in Ano	Frequent • Small amounts • Comes and goes	Rare unless clogs up and abscesses • Symptom free period • Increased swelling and pain • Followed by rupture and resolution of pain	Unusual/No	Small opening on anoderm/ anal margin • Often has exuberant granulation • Drainage
Pruritus Ani	Usually small amount • During excessive wiping	Uncomfortable burning sensation	No mass or prolapse Often skin tags contribute to difficult hygiene • This leads to pruritus	Excoriated perianal skin Lichenification of the skin Excess moisture
Pilonidal Disease	Occasionally • W/drainage from a chronic sinus tract	Acute abscess very painful Chronic sinus discomfort	Abscess can have systemic symptoms Often quite a bit of drainage	Usually gluteal cleft (90%)/ near anus (10%) • Very hirsute • Firm hard area off midline • Midline pits • Sometimes a chronic sinus tract

Table created by Joel E. Goldberg, MD.

of fever and malaise are almost always seen in association with perianal suppurative disease.

There are a myriad of contributing factors of perianal conditions that include constipation, diarrhea, sexually transmitted diseases (STDs) (e.g., human papilloma virus [HPV] in condyloma), and inflammatory bowel disease. Food, commercial products (e.g., scented wipes/toilet paper/powders), and clothing have all been implicated in pruritus ani. A sound understanding of the symptoms and the possible overlap between the conditions will aid in making an accurate diagnosis and treatment plan (Table 19.2).

Pruritus Ani

Pruritus ani manifests itself as burning and/or perianal itching. The symptoms can be so dramatic that patients' skin is often excoriated and there may be minor bleeding from the excoriations. The perianal skin appears lichenified and irritated (Figure 19.1).

Anal pruritus should be classified as either primary (idiopathic), which comprises 50%–90% of cases, or secondary, which comprises the balance of cases. Secondary anal pruritus is broadly attributed to infection (fungal, viral, or parasitic), dermatologic causes (psoriasis, lichen sclerosis, lichen planus, Bowen's/Paget's disease, or atopic/contact dermatitis), systemic diseases (e.g., diabetes, leukemia/lymphoma, or thyroid disease), local irritants (e.g., feces, soaps, dietary, or medications), or colorectal/anal causes (e.g., fissure, fistula, or hemorrhoids).

Fortunately, in low- and middle-income countries (LMICs), the treatment for idiopathic anal pruritus is often simple. It begins with the avoidance of the irritation by eliminating soaps, wipes, perfume, creams, and ointments. Preventing local trauma by eliminating scratching and excessive scrubbing/washing also helps. Patting the area dry after showering is recommended. Furthermore, keeping the area dry by avoiding tight-fitting

TABLE 19.2

Differential Diagnosis and Treatment of Anorectal Disease

Diagnosis	Medical Management	Nonoperative Treatment	Operative Treatment

Anal fissure	• Fiber (psyllium 30 gms/day) + H20 (80oz/day)
	• Warm sitz baths 4x/day
	• Topical anesthetic and relaxant
	  • Nitroglcerin (NTG) 0.2%
	  • Lidocaine 2% w/Nifedipine (NFP) 0.2%
	  • Diltiazem 2%
		• Botox injection	• Lateral Internal Sphincterotomy (preferred)
			  • Can be done w/block and conscious sedation
			  • Divide the internal anal sphincter (IAS) for length of fissure.

Internal hemorrhoids	• Fiber (psyllium 10 gms/day) + H20 (64oz/day)
	• Warm sitz baths 4x/day
		• Rubber Band Ligation (RBL)
		• Sclerotherapy
		  • 3 cc of 5% phenol injection into submucosa of hemorrhoid bundle
		  • 3 cc hypertonic saline (3%) into hemorrhoidal vessels
			• Hemorrhoidectomy
			  • Grade III that failed RBL or sclerotherapy
			  • Grade IV
			  • Combined internal and external disease
			  • Hemorrhoids with mucosal ectropion

External Hemorrhoids (thrombosed)	• Fiber (psyllium 30 gms/day) + H20 (80oz/day) • Warm sitz baths 4x/day	• Continued observation and medical management if symptoms improving.	• Complete excision of hemorrhoid with local anesthetic. Excise if visible clot and persistent symptoms.
Perirectal Abscess	• Only in the neutropenic patient (ANC<500) • nothing to drain since no WBCs • broad spectrum abx (GNR, GPC, anaerobes)	Same as Medical Management	• Incision & drainage: Make incision site close to anal verge to achieve adequate drainage and short fistula tract.

Fistula in Ano	• In Crohn's patient if fistula tract not bothering patient then ok to observe as repeat procedures can lead to incontinence	Same as Medical Management	• Judicious use of draining setons to control infection followed by definitive surgery:
			  • fistulotomy
			  • LIFT procedure
			  • draining and/or cutting seton
			  • endoanal advancement flap

Pruritus Ani	• Same as Nonoperative Management	• 2-inch strip shave even in asymptomatic • Curette and silver nitrate tracts and granulation as necessary	• Incise and drain abscesses • Wide local excision and marsupalization • Complex flap procedures reserved for less austere environments
Pilonidal Disease	• Elimination of causative agent • Topical agents such as Hydrocortisone cream 1% or Capsacian • Keep area dry • Avoid excessive trauma due to over aggressive cleaning • Antibiotics/antifungals for infections	• Treatment of underlying anorectal condition if present (see above other diagnoses) • Biopsy when indicated to r/o dermatologic or neoplastic conditions • Tape test to rule out pin worms	• None indicated

Table created by Joel E. Goldberg, MD.

clothes and using cotton balls, plain tissue paper, or cornstarch to absorb excess moisture also helps tremendously. Maintaining regular bowel movements by drinking plenty of water and taking a high-fiber diet aids in maintaining good anal hygiene. Moreover, eliminating certain foods, such as caffeine (e.g., chocolate, coffee, tea, soda), alcohol, spicy foods (i.e., peppers), and tomato-based products (e.g., ketchup and red sauces), may relieve the symptoms. These simple measures are usually extremely helpful in the elimination of pruritus ani. If all of this fails, then a trial of local therapy is possible with inexpensive agents such as topical capsaicin or a weak steroid cream (e.g., 1% hydrocortisone) for a few weeks. Prolonged therapy with steroid creams or stronger agents is not favored because this can lead to skin atrophy and breakdown, which makes the pruritus worse.

For the patient in the austere environment, ruling out and treating the secondary causes of pruritus ani is important. Infectious causes are often confused with perianal pruritus because of the red skin with raised borders. The most common bacterial infectious causes are *Beta hemolytic streptococcus* and *Erythrasma corynebacterium minutissimum*. Strep infections generally present themselves as moist, bright erythematous rashes with distinct borders and an absence of satellite lesions. They fail to respond to treatment with a steroid cream. On the other hand, *Erythrasma* occurs in the intertriginous areas of the body and the perianal region, and it presents as scaly patches of reddish-brown lesions that appear as coral red fluorescence when viewed under a woods lamp. *Erythrasma* is best treated with a 10-day course of erythromycin 250 mg po qid. Tetracycline is

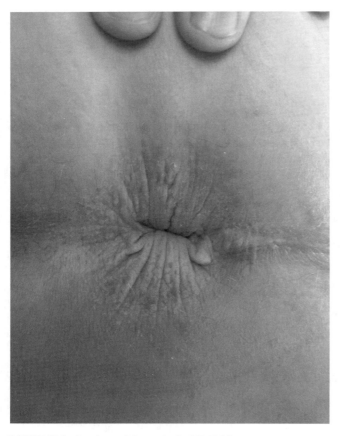

FIGURE 19.1   Pruritus ani. Image by Joel E. Goldberg.

a good alternative when erythromycin is not available or when an allergy exists.

Fungal infections account for approximately 15% of perianal infections, and they can be treated with any of the topical antifungal agents. If the patient fails to respond to the antifungal medications, then a different cause should be investigated. Parasitic causes include pinworms, scabies, and pubic lice (e.g., pediculosis pubis). The latter two are treated with topical agents. Pinworms are treated with oral antiparasitic agents. Finally, sexually transmitted diseases are more commonly associated with genital infections such as herpes, syphilis, gonorrhea, and chlamydia. These should be considered as a source for anal infection in high-risk populations. After appropriate cultures, these patients should be treated with the appropriate systemic antibiotic or antiviral agent. Testing for human immunodeficiency virus (HIV) should also be recommended.

Dermatologic conditions are common causes of anal pruritus. Psoriasis presents as scaly, red, plaque-like lesions on most areas of the skin, but in the anal region the lesions may appear less plaque-like and paler. Symptoms are best treated with a 1% hydrocortisone cream. Atopic dermatitis, a chronic inflammatory condition that is a local response to environmental allergens, is associated with asthma, hay fever, and eczema. These lesions present as dry and scaly areas on the face, neck, dorsum of the hand, and the popliteal and antecubital fossa. Contact dermatitis is another common dermatologic cause of pruritus ani, and many common items, including creams, lotions, and local

topical anesthetics, may be inciting factors. In LMICs, and even in high-income countries (HICs), treatment for these situations is to avoid the irritant and to help the skin heal by cleansing with sitz baths and keeping the area dry. The judicious use of a 1% hydrocortisone cream is also helpful.

Women are more commonly affected with a condition called lichen sclerosus that starts on the vulvar area and extends posteriorly to the perineum and perianal region. The classic physical finding is white patches around the vulva and anus with atrophy of the surrounding skin. This condition is initially treated with a potent steroid cream such as clobetasol and then maintenance therapy with hydrocortisone.

Perianal Paget's disease (cutaneous adenocarcinoma in situ) and Bowen's disease (squamous cell in-situ), also known as high-grade squamous intraepithelial legions (HSILs), are two cancers that present in the perianal region. Any suspicious erythematous, eczematous rash that fails to respond to the above-mentioned therapies needs to be biopsied to evaluate for this condition.[2-4]

Anal Fissure

An anal fissure is a tear in the anal canal skin overlying the internal anal sphincter just inside the anal verge (Figure 19.2).

In 90% of patients, the anal fissure is located in the posterior midline. In the rest, it is located in the anterior midline. Atypical fissures present laterally and are typically associated with HIV, inflammatory bowel disease (IBD), neoplasia, tuberculosis, and STDs. Appropriate cultures and directed antibiotic/antiviral therapy are indicated once a diagnosis is established.[5-7]

Affected patients usually present with severe sharp pain after defecation. This pain is caused by spasm of the anal canal and repetitive injury with subsequent defecation. Often, there is also a little spotting of blood on the toilet paper. The common misconception is that fissures are caused solely by constipation and the resulting anorectal trauma. In fact, diarrhea can also cause fissures as multiple bowel movements cause a chemical burn to the anal canal. Moreover, a hypertonic anal sphincter is seen in most patients with an anal fissure, but it is not known whether this is a cause or an effect of the fissure. The severe anal pain and spasm caused by the fissure exacerbates the hypertonic anal sphincter muscle, making the fissure more difficult to heal. All of these factors contribute to a vicious cycle of repetitive injury in the anal canal that causes the anal fissure to persist.

In both LMICs and HICs, nonoperative treatment is preferred. This includes increasing insoluble fiber (up to 10 grams daily) and fluid intake (at least 64 ounces of water daily) in the diet to bulk the stools. Controlling diarrheal illnesses also helps heal fissures, and psyllium from fiber agents is useful in absorbing excess liquid in the gastrointestinal tract. Warm sitz baths also help relieve the anal spasm. These measures have been shown to heal acute fissures in close to 90% of patients.

Topical nitroglycerin (NTG) ointment 0.2% (compounded down from 2% with Aquaphor) and topical calcium channel blockers (diltiazem 2% and nifedipine 0.2%, both compounded with lidocaine 2% and Aquaphor) applied four times daily have been shown to decrease anal sphincter resting

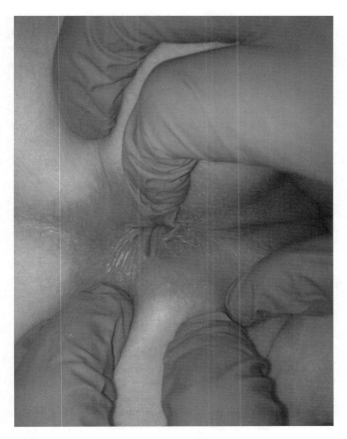

FIGURE 19.2 Anal fissure. Image by Joel E. Goldberg.

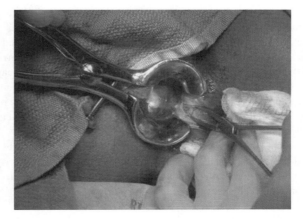

FIGURE 19.3 The internal sphincter is sharply divided, and the mucosa is eventually closed. Image by Joel E. Goldberg.

pressures and to increase healing. Unfortunately, these agents need to be made in compounding pharmacies. As a result, these compounds are often not available in many locations outside developed areas.

If these measures fail to heal the acute anal fissure, then surgical therapy is recommended. Though 90% of acute anal fissures will heal with conservative measures, chronic anal fissures do not heal as well with conservative measures. More frequently, they require the addition of topical agents and ultimately surgery. In the past, manual anal dilation was utilized, but the long-term incontinence rates were too high when compared to lateral internal sphincterotomy (LIS). Hence, the recommended surgery is an LIS. There is no need for complex anesthesia, as sphincterotomy can be performed under local anesthetic with sedation, using either the open or closed technique. The principle behind the LIS is that by dividing the internal anal sphincter for the length of the fissure, the cycle of spasm is broken and the pain resolves. In the open technique, a small incision is made in the mucosa overlying the intersphincteric groove, and then the plane between the two sphincters is developed. The internal sphincter is sharply divided, and the mucosa is eventually closed (Figure 19.3).

In the closed technique, a 15-blade scalpel is placed into the intersphincteric groove and turned toward the internal sphincter, and is used to cut the internal sphincter blindly. Both techniques work well. Surgeon preferences dictate which technique is utilized.

Hemorrhoids

Hemorrhoids are part of the normal anatomy of the human anal canal. The hemorrhoidal bundles are composed of blood vessels, connective tissue, and smooth muscle fibers. Hemorrhoids play many important roles, but the two most important are sensory function and continence. The innervated tissue in the anal canal helps distinguish between solid, liquid, and gas and when it is safe to evacuate without a toilet. The hemorrhoidal bundles also aid in the continence mechanism by helping to "plug" the anal canal when there is a Valsalva maneuver, such as coughing, sneezing, or laughing. Everyone has hemorrhoids, and they are part of the normal anatomy of the anal canal. In some patients, they become symptomatic and cause pain, discomfort, bleeding, pruritus, prolapse, and/or leakage of mucous/stool. Hemorrhoids are classified as either external or internal. External hemorrhoids have sensory innervation similar to that of the skin so they can be very painful when thrombosed, whereas internal hemorrhoids have no pain fibers, and they generally are not painful but can on occasion be described as causing discomfort.

In general, external hemorrhoids present as a painful perianal mass that sometimes bleeds when the clot extravasates. This is actually a perianal hematoma from a subcutaneous vessel that has ruptured under the external anoderm. The other complaint frequently seen in the office is difficulty with hygiene secondary to large external tags. When hemorrhoids are painless, it is best to leave them alone, particularly in an austere environment. Conservative measures of fiber, water, local anesthetics (lidocaine 2%), and nonsteroidal anti-inflammatory drugs (NSAIDs) can be applied. However, if the clot is big and visible and the patient fails to respond to the conservative measures, it is possible to excise the clot, keeping in mind that when the pain is beginning to subside on day 3 or 4 of a thrombosed hemorrhoid, that clot excision does not help as the procedure increases the pain. When treating thrombosed external hemorrhoids, some providers just "lance" the hemorrhoid, extrude the clot, and leave the area open to heal by secondary intention. This technique is messy for the patient, does not relieve the symptoms as well as complete excision, and takes a much longer time to heal. Hence, complete excision under local anesthetic is appropriate. Conversely, many patients come in to be evaluated early in the course of a "thrombosed external hemorrhoid" attack, and the exam reveals boggy edematous tissue but no visible clot. These patients should not be operated on but should receive conservative therapy only. Excision or lancing of the boggy tissue does not relieve the pain, and in fact increases the symptoms as well as leaving an open wound to heal, whereas excision of the perianal hematoma works to relieve the pain precisely because the hematoma is removed. If there is no hematoma, there is no benefit to excision.

Internal hemorrhoids, on the other hand, generally present with discomfort, bleeding, and prolapse. There is a grading system for internal hemorrhoids that aids in the diagnosis and treatment plan. The grading system is as follows:

1. Grade I: bleed but do not protrude outside of the anal canal.
2. Grade II: bleed and prolapse outside the anus; reduce spontaneously.
3. Grade III: bleed and prolapse; they require manual reduction.
4. Grade IV: bleed and prolapse, nonreducible.

The treatment of internal hemorrhoids depends upon the frequency and severity of symptoms. In all settings, most patients with grade I and grade II hemorrhoids are treated with conservative measures, including bulking of the stools with an increase in dietary fiber and/or a psyllium-containing fiber supplement to a total of 30 grams of fiber daily. Patients are also encouraged to increase their fluid intake to at least 80 ounces of water daily. Both of these maneuvers make the stool formed and bulky and easier to pass. Using these techniques to decrease constipation helps resolve the symptoms and prevent recurrence once the symptoms have resolved. There is little evidence that the multitude of over-the-counter and prescription creams and ointments do little more than temporarily relieve the symptoms that would almost surely subside on their own with time. Hence, these agents are not generally recommended. If the patients adhere to the fiber, water, and sitz bath regimen, most symptoms resolve rather quickly. These methods should be employed in both LMICs and HICs.

The conservative measures recommended for grades I and II hemorrhoids are also recommended for grade III hemorrhoids. Grade III hemorrhoids may also require surgery, such as repetitive rubber band ligation or sclerotherapy, to prevent the symptom recurrence. Grade IV hemorrhoids pose a special surgical emergency. If there is necrotic tissue (e.g., foul smell, fever, tachycardia, urinary retention, and sloughing tissue), the patient needs emergent surgical examination under anesthesia and resection of the hemorrhoidal bundles. If there is no necrotic tissue, the grade IV hemorrhoids may be reduced with a perianal block, but they generally will not stay reduced. They may require standard conservative measures of fiber, increased fluid intake, and sitz baths until the swelling has resolved, followed by definitive therapy in the clinic with sclerotherapy, banding, or other operative intervention. There are a multitude of office-based and operative procedures for hemorrhoids, including rubber band ligation, injection sclerotherapy, surgical hemorrhoidectomy, infrared coagulation, harmonic scalpel or Ligasure resection, Doppler-guided ligation, and surgical stapling with the PPH circular stapler. The mainstay

of office therapy is rubber band ligation, which is utilized for grade II and grade III hemorrhoids that do not respond to a trial of medical management alone. Patients with both internal and external components, patients who fail to respond to clinic-based procedures, those who have a prolapsed mucosal ectropion, and grade IV hemorrhoids are best treated with a surgical hemorrhoidectomy in the operating room. In all settings, this procedure can be done under local anesthetic with conscious sedation, without the use of general anesthesia.

A final tool that may be particularly helpful in the austere environment is the injection of the hemorrhoids. Injection of hemorrhoids is also known as sclerotherapy, and it is accomplished by injecting the submucosa at the base of the hemorrhoid with a few cubic centimeters (cc) of a 5% phenol solution in hypertonic saline or oil. Just like rubber band ligation, injection can be performed in the office without the use of a local anesthetic. Rubber band ligation works by causing strangulation of the excess tissue and creates a scar at the top of the anal canal that aids in decreasing future prolapse of the anal mucosa.[8-10]

Perirectal Abscess

The basic principles of treating perianal suppurative disease are the same now as they have been for centuries. The first step is to control the sepsis with incision and drainage of the abscess and then to treat the fistula while maintaining continence. Most abscesses form according to the cryptoglandular theory of abscess formation. This theory proposes that abscesses occur because the anal glands become obstructed from debris, such as undigested vegetable matter or stool. The obstructed gland then becomes infected, and the suppuration tracks along the course of least resistance into one of the many potential spaces surrounding the anorectum. Abscesses then form in these potential spaces. Perirectal abscesses are classified as:

1. Perianal
2. Intersphincteric
3. Ischiorectal
4. Supralevator

Typically, abscesses present with pain, difficulty with defecation, fever, malaise, and an indurated or a fluctuant mass. These symptoms are particularly accurate for ischiorectal and perianal abscesses, whereas intersphincteric and supralevator abscesses can be more difficult to diagnose as the suppuration is higher up in the anal canal (intersphincteric) or the pelvic floor (supralevator). The mainstay of treatment for all perianal suppurative disease is drainage of the abscess. Antibiotics are no substitute for surgical drainage but are often used as an adjunct in patients who are immunosuppressed (e.g., due to acquired immunodeficiency syndrome [AIDS], chemotherapy, or transplants), patients with diabetes mellitus, patients with artificial joints/grafts/valves, and patients with significant perineal cellulitis. Drainage of perianal suppurative disease often requires a general anesthetic as patients are uncomfortable, and local anesthetic does not work well in the acidic environment of an abscess cavity.

No discussion of perianal suppurative disease would be complete without addressing the role of Crohn's disease in this patient population. In many patients, Crohn's disease plays a major role in perianal sepsis, but a complete discussion of inflammatory bowel disease is outside the scope of this chapter. Fortunately, Crohn's disease is much less common in LMICs compared to HICs.

The most basic principles in dealing with anal disease in Crohn's patients follow:

1. Conservatively drain the sepsis.
2. Divide as little sphincter muscle as possible (preferably none).
3. Always achieve source control of the inflammatory process by medically treating Crohn's disease.
4. Judiciously use setons to prevent recurrent sepsis.
5. If perianal fistula and fissure do not bother the patient, then they should not bother the surgeon (i.e., careful observation in the asymptomatic patient is warranted).[11]

Fistula-in-Ano

One-third of patients who have an abscess drained ultimately develop a fistula-in-ano. During the operation for the drainage of the abscess, a fistula tract can be identified 80%–90% of the time. There has been much debate about whether to treat the fistula at the original setting or in a delayed fashion. Several studies support that if the fistula tract can be identified at the original operation, it should be dealt with at that time. In general, if the tract is short and superficial, it can be treated with a simple fistulotomy at the original operation with little effect on continence. Longer fistula tracts should be secured and drained with a draining seton (Figure 19.4).

Once the sepsis has resolved and a tract has formed, then the amount of sphincter involved and the trajectory of the tract can be more accurately identified, and a treatment plan can be developed. The greatest challenge in perianal suppurative disease is to treat the subsequent fistula. The main principles of fistula treatment are dictated by the following:

1. Amount of sphincter involved
2. Location of the internal opening
3. Course of the fistula tract

Anal fistulae are classified as follows:

1. Submucosal
2. Intersphincteric
3. Transsphincteric [low (distal 1/3 EAS) and (high proximal 2/3 EAS)]
4. Suprasphincteric
5. Extrasphincteric

Preoperative imaging with ultrasound and magnetic resonance imaging (MRI) has been variably advocated to help identify the course of the tract and the amount of the sphincter muscle

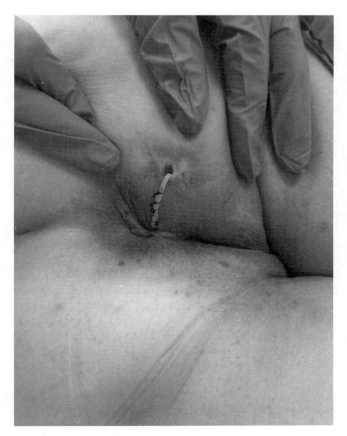

FIGURE 19.4 Fistula-in-ano. Image by Joel E. Goldberg.

involved but has no impact on the final surgical result. The biggest advantage is in identifying the internal opening and help in preoperative counseling. In an austere environment, imaging is a luxury that often is not available. In the end, a good examination under anesthesia with the injection of hydrogen peroxide or methylene blue can be just as useful to identify the internal opening and the course of the fistulous tract.

Submucosal, intersphincteric, and low transsphincteric fistulae can be treated with simple fistulotomy in the vast majority of patients who have normal continence. In patients with compromised continence, anterior fistulae in women, and/or patients with Crohn's disease, a more measured approach must be taken. (See previously mentioned rules for Crohn's disease.) Extrasphincteric fistulae do not start at the cryptoglandular level, and as a result they do not have an internal opening. Consequently, treating these types of fistulae involves treating the primary process (e.g., diverticulitis, inflammatory bowel disease, neoplasia, or rarely traumatic injury). A discussion of this magnitude is out of the scope of this chapter. Suprasphincteric fistulae and high transsphincteric fistulae are more challenging as they involve a greater amount of sphincter muscle. As a result, there is a higher risk of incontinence when treating these fistulae.

There are many surgical techniques for treating suprasphincteric and high transsphincteric fistulae. These include fibrin glue (approximate success rate of 30%–85%), collagen plug (approximate success rate of 15%–85%), and endoanal advancement flaps (approximate success rate of 75%–100%). All of these procedures have strengths and weaknesses, but the first two involve expensive materials that may not be readily available in LMICs. Moreover, recent studies suggest that the success rates in closing fistulae with either of these methods is on the lower end of the reported cure rates. The upside to these techniques is that there is little risk of incontinence, and they do not limit the ability to perform any other procedures down the road. The endoanal advancement flap has had significant success, but it is a more complex operation with a risk of incontinence. It is generally reserved as one of the last resorts for complex fistulae. The cutting seton (Figure 19.5) is probably the simplest and one of the more commonly utilized techniques to treat fistula-in-ano.

The cutting seton is low-tech and has a very good success rate. This has to be balanced with the higher rate of incontinence than seen with the plug or fibrin glue. Numerous materials, ranging from heavy sutures (e.g., #2 Silk or Ethibond) to vessel loops, pieces of surgical gloves, Penrose drains, and silastic catheters, have been used as either draining or cutting setons. If there is significant sepsis, the usual first step is to place a draining seton for several weeks to months until the sepsis has resolved and a nice, fine fistula tract has formed. Then if the fistula is a simple fistula, a fistulotomy can be performed. If it is a complex fistula, then a partial fistulotomy of the subcutaneous tissues, anal mucosa, and even a little bit of the superficial sphincter is divided, and the seton is then tied down tightly around the remnant deeper sphincter complex. The patient makes several office visits, and the seton is tightened until it completely cuts through the sphincter and

the tissues and sphincter behind the seton scar down. Finally, the LIFT (ligation of intersphincteric fistula tract) procedure has come onto the scene in the last several years (Figure 19.6).

There is a low rate of incontinence as no sphincter muscle is divided. The success rate approaches 60%. In this technique, a probe is placed through the fistula tract, and then a curvilinear incision is made over the intersphincteric groove. The fistula tract is dissected out in the intersphincteric plane and is then ligated with 2-0 silk sutures and then divided in between the sutures. This recreates the normal anatomy of the anal crypt/gland on the internal sphincter and separates it from the external tract, which is then debrided with a curette and electrocautery to open up the external tract to promote healing of the fistula external to the external anal sphincter. The sphincters are then reapproximated, and the skin is loosely closed with interrupted vicryl sutures.[12-14]

Pilonidal Disease

Pilonidal disease is a common condition that affects many patients worldwide and leads to lost time and productivity for those afflicted. In the past, it was felt to be a congenital condition, but the current accepted theory is that pilonidal disease is an acquired condition. The pathophysiology underlying pilonidal disease is repetitive trauma and a foreign body reaction to hair in the gluteal region, which form midline pits. The hair migrates into the subcutaneous space and contributes to the infectious process. Pilonidal disease

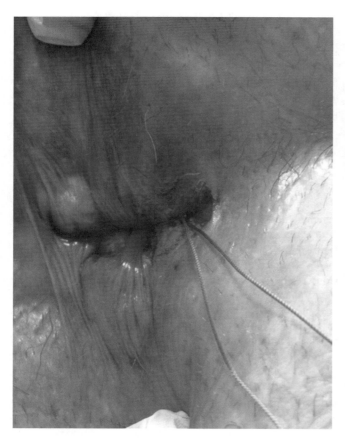

FIGURE 19.5 The cutting seton. Image by Joel E. Goldberg.

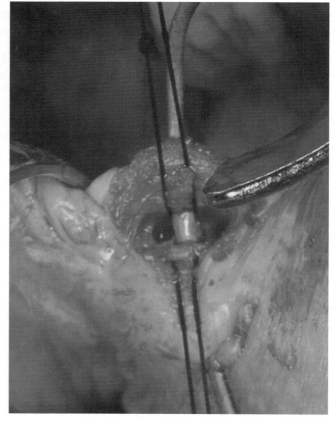

FIGURE 19.6 The LIFT procedure. Image by Joel E. Goldberg.

can present as a simple cyst, a chronic draining sinus/sinuses, or an acute abscess. A cyst causes a pressure sensation without signs or symptoms of infection, whereas a chronic sinus (Figure 19.7) presents with discomfort and drainage.

An acute abscess presents with pain, erythema, and swelling. In the overwhelming majority of patients, the gluteal cleft is excessively hirsute, and small midline holes, referred to as pits, can be seen. These holes are the route by which the excess hair gets underneath the subcutaneous skin and acts as a nidus for infection.

Treatment depends upon the activity of the disease. Patients who present with a chronic abscess need drainage, which can readily be performed under local anesthetic. The favored approach is to drain the abscess off of the midline as this promotes quicker healing due to less pressure on the incision. The patient who presents with a chronic draining sinus can more often than not be managed nonoperatively with strip shaving of the gluteal cleft (Figure 19.8) and the surrounding area of all hair for a 2-inch area from the gluteal cleft laterally.

After this is accomplished, the sinus tract can be debrided with endocervical cytet brushes (Figure 19.9) to remove chronic granulation tissue and hair (Figure 19.10) under the subcutaneous tissue within the cyst.

The tissue can then be treated with silver nitrate cautery to help control exuberant granulation tissue. In almost all instances, this technique has a high success rate in controlling disease. If the patient has a cyst alone with midline pits, then lateral drainage with excision of the midline pits is acceptable for the patient who has chronic unremitting pain. In the austere environment, this should clearly be delayed as long as possible.

Finally, for the patient with chronic multiple sinus tracts and low-grade infection, the entire area can be excised and saucerized. This technique works well in a chronic situation where complex excisions and reconstruction with advancement flaps (e.g., karydakis flap and VY advancement flaps) are not possible due to a lack of equipment, inability for long-term convalescence, and the increased possibility of infection. In the excision and marsupialization technique, the entire area is excised down

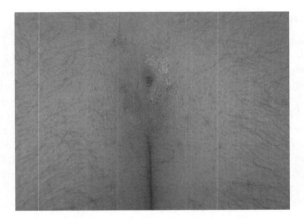

FIGURE 19.7 Pilonidal disease. Image by Joel E. Goldberg.

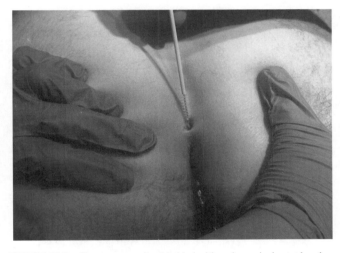

FIGURE 19.9 Sinus tract can be debrided with endocervical cytet brushes. Image by Joel E. Goldberg.

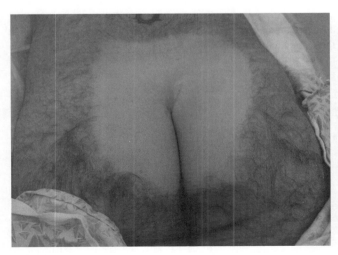

FIGURE 19.8 The patient who presents with a chronic draining sinus can more often than not be managed nonoperatively with strip shaving of the gluteal cleft. Image by Joel E. Goldberg.

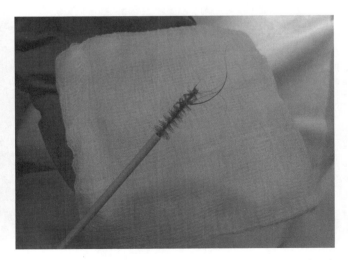

FIGURE 19.10 Remove chronic granulation tissue and hair under the subcutaneous tissue within the cyst. Image by Joel E. Goldberg.

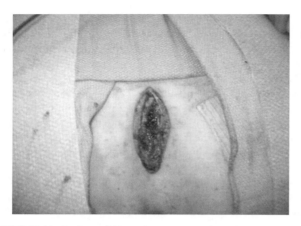

FIGURE 19.11 In the excision and marsupialization technique, the entire area is excised down to healthy tissue near the presacral fascia. Image by Joel E. Goldberg.

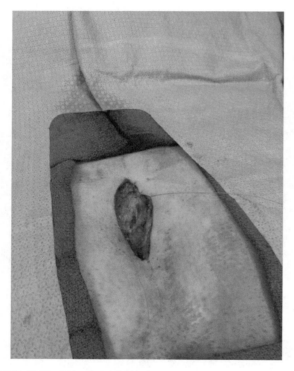

FIGURE 19.12 This closes down the wound and reduces the area that needs to heal. Image by Joel E. Goldberg.

to healthy tissue near the presacral fascia (Figure 19.11), and the skin edges are sutured down to the presacral fascia with an absorbable suture. This closes down the wound and reduces the area that needs to heal (Figure 19.12).

The wound is left open, and wet-to-dry dressing changes are utilized while the wound heals from the inside out. The upsides to this technique are fourfold: first, it cures 95% of pilonidal disease; second, it is virtually resistant to subsequent infection; third, it is easily performed under local anesthesia; and fourth, it requires little postoperative care, and the care it does require is quite simple. On the other hand, it does require a prolonged healing time, which can be quite burdensome in LMICs, and an effort must be made to keep the wound clean and as dry as possible. In the austere environment, the focus should be on controlling the symptoms with minimal surgical intervention. All patients with pilonidal disease benefit from the 2-inch strip shave to keep excess hair away from the midline pits and the subcutaneous tissues.[15-17]

Conclusions

Anorectal problems can be quite vexing in nature for the affected individual, but the solutions are often quite straightforward and amenable to medical and surgical treatment even in an austere environment. Early and correct diagnosis is critical and control of the symptoms can generally be accomplished. For anal pruritus and hemorrhoids, nonoperative management is generally preferred and is highly successful when appropriately employed. For pruritus ani, elimination of the causative agent (whether it be a particular food or external agent), treatment of infections with the appropriate antibiotics or antifungals, and identification and eradication of secondary causes are effective treatment approaches. Hemorrhoids are best managed by nonoperative medical therapy, and symptomatic relief of thrombosed hemorrhoids and banding of internal hemorrhoids can be helpful in controlling symptoms. For infectious anorectal diseases, source control of the sepsis is paramount and then judicious treatment of the fistula with preservation of the sphincter muscle is critical. Most of these procedures can be accomplished under local or general anesthesia and are often quite effective in relieving symptoms. Although these maladies are often vexing for the patient, the surgeon armed with proper knowledge can apply effective solutions in any environment.

COMMENTARY

Thandinkosi E. Madiba, South Africa

This chapter is comprehensive in addressing the treatment of anorectal disease and its challenges in LMICs.

Frequent Misdiagnosis

Anorectal conditions are frequently misdiagnosed or inappropriately treated because they are labelled "minor" anorectal conditions and, as such, are usually relegated to junior members of staff who may not have the requisite expertise to deal with them. Some of these conditions require adequate understanding of the anal anatomy, which is not the case with both junior doctors and even qualified surgeons in some instances.

Anal Fissure

Lateral sphincterotomy is the treatment of choice. Anal dilatation (Lord's procedure) and fissurectomy are no longer advisable in the treatment of anal fissure, as they lead to internal sphincteric disruption and resultant anal incontinence.

Hemorrhoids

It should be emphasised that the anal cushions, situated in the anal columns of Morgagni, are not hemorrhoids but are normal physiological entities. Hemorrhoids are a pathological entity due to the enlargement and engorgement of these cushions. Hemorrhoids used to be called internal hemorrhoids. However, the term "internal hemorrhoids" is now superfluous since there is no such thing as external hemorrhoids. What used to be called an "external hemorrhoid" is actually a thrombosed perianal vein. The terms "external hemorrhoid" and "thrombosed external pile" are misnomers, and their use should be discouraged.

Hidradenitis Suppurativa

Hidradenitis suppurativa is a chronic acneiform infection of the apocrine glands whose aetiology and pathogenesis is unclear. Hair-growing areas, like the perineum and axilla, are most commonly affected. It usually develops after puberty. There is a male predominance, and the peak incidence is between 16 and 40 years of age. The condition derives from obstruction of apocrine sweat glands with keratinous plugs, resulting in glandular dilatation, bacterial overgrowth, leukocyte infiltration, and eventual ductal destruction, which results in extensive scarring and fibrosis of the surrounding tissue and the formation of sinuses and fistulae.

The condition should be differentiated from cryptoglandular perianal fistula. In the latter, the apertures enter the anal canal at the dentate line, and the drainage tends to be suppurativa or purulent. In hidradenitis suppurativa the openings are subcutaneous and may be eccentric. Drainage tends to be thin and serous.

Management of acute disease involves incision and drainage of acute abscesses. Extensive or chronic hidradenitis suppurativa rarely responds to conservative management and requires radical excision of all affected tissue. Small wounds can be primarily closed, and for larger wounds, healing is achieved by secondary intention. Such healing is associated with considerable morbidity and historically a prolonged hospital stay, but results in a low recurrence rate.

BIBLIOGRAPHY

Slade DEM, Powell BW, Mortimer PS. Hidradenitis suppurativa: pathogenesis and management. Br J Plast Surg 2003; 56, 451–461.

COMMENTARY

Ntakiyiruta Georges, Rwanda

All the anorectal disease conditions discussed in this chapter are present in Rwanda, although the prevalence of these diseases may differ. Within our health system, patients frequently consult for chronic anal fissures (which I treat with LIS) and fistulae-in-ano, although I rarely see patients with acute anal fissures. Perianal abscesses and thrombosed external hemorrhoids are often seen at the health center level. Patients usually receive an analgesic and the perirectal abscess will progress to a fistula-in-ano; the painful thrombosed external hemorrhoid will cool down. Pilonidal disease must be extremely rare in Rwanda; I have treated only one patient. As far as I know, there are no cases of Crohn's disease in Rwandan population. High transsphincteric, suprasphincteric, and extrasphincteric fistulae-in-ano, however, are still a challenge for us. Some still add a diverting colostomy and the healing success is still low.

20

Laparoscopy

Gabriela M. Vargas
Raymond R. Price

Introduction

Laparoscopy, with its benefits of shortened hospitalizations, decreased wound infection rates, diminished pain, and improved cosmesis, has revolutionized surgical care in low- and middle-income countries (LMICs). Further expansion of laparoscopy to the 85% of the world's people who lack access has been previously limited because of several factors. Some of these factors have included: limited financial, physical, and human resources; difficult political and social conflicts; austere environments; and misconceptions of the need and abilities of the people in LMICs by those in more developed countries. Historically, surgery, especially laparoscopic surgery, has been perceived as a high-cost intervention with very little role, if any, in public health, for LMICs.

Despite these external perceptions, similar to the public demand that propelled the rapid expansion of laparoscopy in the United States and Europe, the 4 billion people at the bottom of the wealth pyramid are driving the globalization of laparoscopic surgery. Ubiquitous access to information by Internet, mobile phone, radio, and television is increasing the global community's understanding of new possibilities for improving their access to modern surgical care. The world's poor, leading a heralding charge for an equity revolution, have begun demanding access to the benefits of laparoscopic surgery. Where laparoscopic surgery is available, patients in LMICs will now often insist on this less invasive approach; where it is not available, with the mobile nature of the world's population, rather than have an open procedure, many of the more wealthy people now travel to high-income countries (HICs) for laparoscopic surgery, causing local leaders to search for ways to improve their own medical and surgical options.

Low- and middle-income countries are undergoing an epidemiologic transition of disease where deaths from noncommunicable diseases—such as trauma, cancer, and maternal and chronic diseases—are surpassing those from communicable etiologies; this has led to the recognition that surgical problems are an important public health issue and that the further development of surgical care may be an effective and cost-effective means of improving health care worldwide. Ministries of Health, medical schools and universities, local hospitals, and physicians from LMICs—recognizing these rapidly changing needs—are not merely requesting but demanding assistance in expanding laparoscopic surgery.

History of Laparoscopy

Laparoscopy, as many areas of surgery, developed through a gradual evolutionary process. Many of its earliest advances came from innovators who lived in surroundings not uncommon to the developing world today. The development of endoscopy paved the way for laparoscopy. Curiosity about unseen areas inside the body led Hippocrates and early Egyptians to inspect and visualize the natural superficial orifices of the body: the mouth, anus, and vagina. Limited technology with inadequate light and tools prevented much progress until Philip Bozzini designed his light source, the Lichtleiter, in 1805.[1]

Unfortunately, the Vienna School of Medicine chastised him for his curiosity; he also died prematurely of typhoid dysentery at age 36. Building on Bozzini's work, in 1826, Peter Segalas of Paris developed the first cystoscope, and in 1843, Antonin J. Desormeaux, the "Father of Endoscopy," performed the first successful esophagoscopy using a rigid tube. Adolph Kussmaul from Germany, in 1868, attached a tube-shaped speculum and was successful in getting a 47-cm tube with a 13-mm diameter down the throat and into the stomach of a sword swallower; this first gastroscope was not very successful due to the suboptimal illumination inside the stomach despite a gasoline lamp and a reflective lens system.[1] Better inspection and identification of pathology waited impatiently until the development of the light bulb.

The first clinically useful esophagoscope came via a collaboration of Johan von Mikulicz, a Viennese physician, and Josef Leiter, an instrument maker.[1] Through their teamwork, an endoscope with adequate light transmittal allowed doctors to accurately document pathology such as tumors, ulcers, and foreign bodies for the first time. This sentinel event not only paved the way for laparoscopy, but also now represents a collaborative model for innovation required for the sustainable advancement of laparoscopy in resource-poor areas. By the end of the nineteenth century, with the miniaturization of the lenses and improved visualization from the light bulb, endoscopy became a well-accepted common diagnostic modality and set the stage for new ventures into other cavities.

In 1901, Dimitri Ott, a professor of gynecology from St. Petersburg, Russia, passed a rigid endoscope through a posterior vaginal incision to be the first to visualize the intra-abdominal organs endoscopically.[2] In 1903, he reported on his 600 cases of "ventroscopy," or what may be the first report of natural orifice transluminal endoscopic surgery (NOTES). In the same year, Georg Kelling introduced a cystoscope into a dog's abdominal cavity to study the effect of increased pneumoperitoneum on gastrointestinal bleeding and is credited with performing the first laparoscopic procedure. But it was Hans Christian Jacobaeus, an internist, who coined the term "laparoscopy" when he recognized the diagnostic capability of the laparoscope and reported in 1910 on his initial 45 cases; patients with cirrhosis, tuberculosis peritonitis, and metastatic tumors were correctly diagnosed without the need for a more invasive laparotomy procedure.[2] Many others introduced a variety of technical innovations that advanced the capability of laparoscopy. Sharp-tipped trocars facilitated peritoneal access by eliminating the need for a significant incision. Methods for continuous insufflations maintained a steady pneumoperitoneum, replacing the need for hand injection of air. Using multiple ports facilitated therapeutic procedures. The veress needle provided easier access for insufflations. Lastly, the Hopkins' flexible glass fibers transmitted an image from one end of the laparoscope to the other thereby improving clarity, brightness, and color to the scopes and removed the light source from the tip of the scope, which decreased the risk of thermal injury. In 1946, Raoul Palmer (the "Father of Gynecologic Laparoscopy") perfected laparoscopic tubal ligation. For the next 40 years, gynecology pushed laparoscopy forward globally. Still under the Halsteadian approach that "bigger is better," and despite all the technical advancements, laparoscopy and its "keyhole" approach did not appeal to general surgeons.

Early Expansion of Laparoscopy to LMICs

Because of laparoscopy's important contributions to gynecological diagnosis and its use in fertility management, expanding laparoscopy in the developing world became a major focus of the John's Hopkins Program for International Education in Gynecology and Obstetrics (JHPIEGO), which began in 1973 with financial assistance from the Agency for International Development (AID). By 1983, JHPIEGO had 51 training centers in 34 different countries throughout Africa, Asia, South America, and the Middle East. Physicians from these countries were trained in three phases: a didactic training course, a practical training experience with successful completion of a minimum number of cases, and then local installation of laparoscopic equipment and additional training at the students' institution. From 1973–1983, 2,901 physicians received training in laparoscopy. The laparoscopic equipment installed continued to have greater than 90% usage and had required very little repair according to a follow-up survey.[3]

Diagnostic laparoscopy for medical disease was not popular in English-speaking countries in the 1970s. Conversely, reports from Africa in the 1970s and 1980s indicated that peritoneoscopy was not only safe in LMICs, but also was extremely beneficial, both in terms of decreased man-hours and a high diagnostic yield.[4] In India, diagnostic laparoscopy has been practiced since 1971 and has been found valuable in the workup of an acute abdomen and in the staging and management of abdominal malignancies, trauma, and tuberculosis.[5] In Tanzania and in Sudan, diagnostic laparoscopy has proven useful as a means of inspecting the abdominal cavity and for guided biopsies since the early 1980s.[6,7] Of note, many reports concluded diagnostic laparoscopy was much more useful in the rural setting of Sub-Saharan Africa than in HICs that had access to more modern diagnostic tools.[8,10]

Dr. Udwadia, one of the great pioneers of laparoscopy in India, reported in 1986 on his experience of 2,500 peritoneoscopy cases over the previous 14 years. As endoscopic retrograde cholangio-pancreatography (ERCP), computed tomography (CT) scans, and even ultrasound were not available when Dr. Udwadia first began laparoscopy in 1971, peritoneoscopy proved to be an invaluable diagnostic tool.[11] Developing countries found an even greater need for the laparoscope in their LMICs than most of the HICs.

Universal Acceptance of Laparoscopy: A Modern Surgical Revolution

Several sentinel innovations in the 1980s led to an explosive acceptance of laparoscopy unprecedented in the history of surgery. Dr. Kurt Semm, a German gynecologist, envisioned applying laparoscopy to a wide spectrum of conditions. In 1980, he became the first person to perform a laparoscopic appendectomy, catching the initial attention of general surgeons. But the advent of the miniature solid-state camera (or the three-chip camera) in 1986, with its ability to display video images from the scope onto a TV screen, allowed everyone in the operating room to view exactly what the surgeon was seeing; an assistant was now able to actually participate in the procedure and facilitated the surgeon's ability to operate with two hands.[2]

Although Erich Muhe performed the first laparoscopic cholecystectomy in 1985 in Europe using a galloscope, the first video-guided laparoscopic cholecystectomy was performed by Philippe Mouret in 1987 in France.[2] McKernan and Saye, and Reddick and Olsen performed their first procedure in 1988 in the United States. Initially, academic surgery in the United States did not accept laparoscopic surgery.[2] A video submission of a laparoscopic cholecystectomy by Jacques Perissat was initially rejected for the 1989 meeting of the Society of American Gastrointestinal and Endoscopic Surgeons (SAGES). A friend found Perissat a corner of free space to display the video at the meeting where many responded with skepticism when Dr. Perissat suggested that this procedure would become the future of surgery—an obvious true prediction of the near future.[12] In the United States, initially shunned by academic institutions, laparoscopic cholecystectomy was championed by the private practice sector, which initiated one of the most revolutionary advancements in general surgery—minimally invasive surgery (MIS). By 1992, a national Institutes of Health (NIH) conference declared laparoscopic cholecystectomy to be the new standard of care for gallbladder disease.[13] Since the initial introduction and acceptance of laparoscopic surgery, the

TABLE 20.1

Laparoscopic cholecystectomy in LMICs

Countries Performing Lap Chole*	Year Reported	Other Countries Performing Laparoscopy
Zimbabwe	1993	Nigeria
Mexico	1994	Vietnam
India	1995	Ethiopia
Nicaragua	1996	Laos
Bolivia	1996	Kenya
Albania	1997	Tanzania
Saudi Arabia	1998	Cameroon
Brunei	1998	Uganda
South Africa	1999	Cambodia
Mongolia	1999	Egypt
Senegal	2002	Jordan
Sudan	2002	Iraq
Thailand	2005	Iran
Tonga	2006	Turkey
Greece	2006	Ecuador
Bosnia-Herzegovina	2007	Argentina
Yemen	2008	Belize
Afghanistan	2009	Haiti
Ghana	2010	Cuba

*Non-inclusive
Created by Jill Rhead, Medical Illustrator, Intermountain Healthcare.
Adapted from Raymond Price.

practical use of laparoscopy has been extended to essentially every aspect of abdominal surgery.

Global Expansion of Laparoscopy

As demand for video laparoscopy skyrocketed, continual innovation led to an ever-increasing demand in HICs for better laparoscopes, cameras, monitors, instruments, insufflators, and energy devices; the cost for this equipment has been a major factor limiting the global expansion of laparoscopy. However, expanding surgical care in LMICs is necessarily focusing innovation and technology on sustainability, including affordability, like never before.

While many policy makers, surgical experts, and funders of international health have questioned the viability and sustainability of laparoscopy in LMICs, many of these countries, against seemingly insurmountable barriers, have established video laparoscopy. Dr. Udwadia, who was an early adopter of diagnostic laparoscopy, pioneered new advanced procedures throughout India. Searches of the English published literature identified reports from other LMICs reviewing their experience with laparoscopic cholecystectomy and are listed in Table 20.1; many other LMICs without published reports are also listed. Local pioneers in their own respective countries seeking assistance from more developed nations, industry, and global healthcare organizations have directed much of this expansion into LMICs.

Laparoscopic donor nephrectomy, splenectomy, colectomy, Nissen fundoplication, appendectomy, inguinal and ventral hernia

TABLE 20.2

Controversies surrounding laparoscopic surgery in resource poor areas

Arguments Against
• Lack of basic surgery
• Laparoscopy an additional strain to an already tenuous medical system
• Limited physical and human resources
• Limited mostly to private hospitals widening surgical gap between rich and poor
• Lack of adequate training and significant learning curve

Arguments Supporting
• Benefits local economies
• Enables patients, surgeons, and communities
• Increased worldwide demand
• Provide needed opportunities for professional advancement
• Mechanism to improve local essential and basic surgical care capabilities
• Improves access to more qualified heath care providers to the community

Created by Jill Rhead, Medical Illustrator, Intermountain Healthcare.
Adapted from Raymond Price.

repair, adrenalectomy, liver resection, and other advanced procedures are now being reported from or being performed in many HICs. Surgeons in Cuba reviewed their series of 12 transvaginal laparoscopic cholecystectomies at the 11th Cuban Surgical Congress in Havana, a recent example of the ingenuity of surgeons to successfully perform NOTES in LMICs.[14]

Controversies Surrounding Laparoscopic Surgery in LMICs

Understanding the underlying controversies about the sustainability, affordability, and accessibility of laparoscopy in LMICs engages political, financial, medical, public health, and other organizations with a vested interest in improving the health of communities in designing solutions to potential barriers (Table 20.2).

Arguments Against Laparoscopy in Developing Countries

Basic surgical services are lacking in most LMICs. Weiser et al. found that there is a disproportionate scarcity of surgical procedures performed in countries where healthcare spending was less than or equal to $100 USD per person per year.[15] One-third of the world's population falls in this low expenditure category, yet they receive only 3.5% of the operations performed worldwide. Currently, the majority of patients in low-expenditure countries undergo standard open operations when surgery is available.

In places where technical means are lacking and healthcare spending per capita is low, laparoscopy may place additional strain in an already tenuous medical system. In most LMICs, the seeming priority should be to improve traditional surgical care and access before introducing new and expensive technology. The expense of performing a single advanced laparoscopic procedure in most developing countries is often more than the surgeon's monthly salary. The overall cost savings of laparoscopy are not usually appreciated until factors such as length of stay, wound infection rate, and recovery time are taken into account; many have suggested that these are not as applicable in LMICs. In settings with already limited resources, laparoscopy may not be financially sustainable.[16]

In many parts of the world, basic amenities such as electricity and running water are unavailable, general doctors provide the majority of surgical care, and certified surgeons and anesthesiologists— when available—are few and often found only in urban areas. This makes the performance of even the most basic of operations a challenge.[17] To deal with the shortage of personnel and the growing burden of surgical disease, in some parts of Africa, training other healthcare providers, including non-physicians, to perform surgical procedures such as abscess drainage, hernia repair, and caesarean section has become a necessity.[18]

In addition, the hospitals with the infrastructure necessary to support laparoscopy are often private hospitals. Patients treated at these facilities are required to pay for their care prior to any procedure, often times being given lists of surgical supplies they must purchase before receiving their surgery; subsequently, minimally invasive procedures would only be available to those who could afford it and would not be a viable option for the majority of the population. This disparity would promote further widening of the surgical care gap between the privileged and the poor.

Most physicians in LMICs lack structured training following medical school. Surgical residencies are short, and often there are no formal continuing medical education programs. Young surgeons frequently lack mentors and are left to teach themselves. Laparoscopy requires specialized training, and there is a learning curve for mastery. The initial experience with laparoscopic cholecystectomy in HICs demonstrated that complications were higher with the minimally invasive approach than the standard open operation. One has to wonder whether the surgical workforce in LMICs has sufficient medical knowledge and resources to not only safely perform minimally invasive surgery but also to deal with the complications that may arise. Surgical innovation in LMICs regularly occurs in hospitals with little regulation regarding new procedures; consequently, patient safety may be compromised.

Arguments Supporting Laparoscopy in LMICs

Expanding laparoscopy in LMICs promotes improvements in overall healthcare delivery and enables surgeons, patients, and communities. Surgeons develop improved self-respect as they improve their skills and advance professionally; patients increase their trust and respect in the local healthcare providers and are more willing to undergo surgery earlier in the course of their disease; and communities benefit from the patients' earlier return to work, maintaining an active workforce with much less negative economic impact to families, businesses, and government (Box 20.1).

Introduction of laparoscopy in LMICs, when approached as a comprehensive program, provides a gateway for improving the medical infrastructure, medical education, and local essential and basic surgical care capabilities. Understanding the desires and motivations of the local healthcare professionals and collaboratively developing programs to address their needs elicits trust and builds lasting relationships that allows for opportunities to teach the full spectrum of surgical care. Initiating laparoscopy in these areas necessarily leads to improved infrastructure development, including power supplies, surgical instruments, and appropriate intra- and postoperative monitoring. The entire team (surgeons, nurses, anesthetists, and biotechnicians) improves their surgical capabilities, not only with laparoscopic skills, but also with many other critical components for basic and essential surgical care. Detailed preoperative evaluation and precise intraoperative training lead to improved patient selection and surgical judgment. Basic and essential surgical skills training, trauma management, anesthetic care, sterility courses, and surgical safety practices can be integrated and reinforced during laparoscopic training courses, dramatically increasing the overall impact on surgical care for these areas.

Developing the infrastructure to support laparoscopy expands the capability of the local healthcare facilities. Not only do the number of laparoscopic procedures increase as surgeons broaden their abilities and patients gain more trust in their doctors, but the volume of open procedures and the spectrum of the types of surgeries performed increases; access to basic and more advanced surgical and medical care dramatically improves (Box 20.2).

After completing a Gates Foundation–sponsored evaluation of financing healthcare in Sub-Saharan Africa, the International Finance Corporation (IFC) found that 60% of healthcare is privately funded.[25] Subsequently, the World Bank recommended a $35 billion USD investment to further develop private healthcare in Sub-Saharan Africa as a mechanism to improve healthcare for even the most underprivileged areas. The study highlighted that many of the private healthcare providers also deliver much needed care to the underprivileged areas. So if laparoscopy proves to provide avenues for professional development that help retain better-trained doctors and nurses locally, even if they work primarily in private institutions, local poorer patients may receive benefits with improved access to higher quality healthcare.

The economic impact of laparoscopy may be greater in LMICs than in HICs. Once acquired, laparoscopic equipment does not require much additional floor space or special staff for performance; additionally, laparoscopic equipment is durable. When compared to the cost of obtaining an ultrasound machine, a CT, or a magnetic resonance imaging (MRI) scanner—and the costs associated with the staff required to operate this equipment— laparoscopy may be the more affordable option. Diagnostic laparoscopy becomes a cost-effective alternative in LMICs when one factors in the 85% positive diagnosis rate.[26] In addition, providing patients with shorter hospitalizations and quicker recoveries allows each a faster return to work and decreased loss of income; this may help prevent already vulnerable populations from

BOX 20.1   BUILDING LOCAL SURGICAL CAPACITY BENEFITS LOCAL ECONOMIES

The medical systems in many LMICs face a significant decay and are faced with outdated diagnostic equipment, leading to loss of confidence in their public health system. Dr. Lkhagvaa Byradan, Medical Director, Songdo Hospital in Ulaanbaatar, Mongolia stated, "If we cannot give them [the people of Mongolia] laparoscopic surgery they will go to the other countries. Cost is one of the difficulties for us. But if somebody will not use advanced technology in our countries, the patients have to go to another country. Then the cost will be much higher!" (Personal communication, May, 2009).

The search for overseas solutions by people who live in LMICs and can afford treatment is a major loss of foreign exchange for the country. In Nigeria, gallbladder surgery is one of the many diseases for which wealthier patients seek solutions abroad.[19] Medical tourism companies, like Me Cure Health Limited, offer high-quality healthcare opportunities for Nigerian patients who can travel to India; Me Cure advertises its ability to provide solutions for average Nigerians "for who the medical treatment in Nigeria is not encouraging for life threatening disease".[20] Nigerians spend $1 billion USD each year on foreign medical services, a significant loss to the Nigerian economy.[21] To counteract this trend, reinstate public confidence in their healthcare, and reinstate this source of lost revenue, the Nigerian government and medical establishments are working to build medical and surgical capacity by improving equipment and expertise locally, including providing minimally invasive surgical care. When high-quality laparoscopic surgical care is available locally, jobs are created and the local economies improve secondarily to the retained funds.

Although multi-factorial, one reason for the continuing "brain drain" of medical personnel is a direct result of the lack of adequate opportunities for professional advancement.

Surgeons from LMICs tend to migrate to HICs seeking opportunities to learn and practice modern techniques. Establishing laparoscopy in LMICs may help decrease this trend. Basic and essential surgical training tends to focus on very general procedures that could be practiced by medical officers or other traditionally nonsurgical specialties. While basic surgical skills are arguably extremely important (simple abscess drainage, hernia repair, cataract surgery, and timely Caesarean section), surgeons and patients in LMICs now recognize quality surgical care includes access to minimally invasive surgery. Dr. Leslie Akporiye, the Medical Director of the Shawsand Medical Center in Nigeria, stated, "As we now live in a global society, it would be unconscionable for Nigerians to be denied the medical advantages of new technology."[19]

Surgeons from Mongolia to West Africa report that laparoscopic training is one of their greatest needs. In 2006 the chief of surgery from the Health Sciences University of Mongolia, Dr. Sergelen Orgoi, found that laparoscopic cholecystectomy in Mongolia carried a significantly decreased wound infection rate and decreased hospitalization.[22] In her initial report, she demanded laparoscopy be made available to all the people of Mongolia, leading a charge for further training and expansion countrywide. In West Africa, a local educational company, Trigen, surveyed the members from the West African College of Surgeons in 2010 to assess which certified courses participants would most want to attend if available and which clinical or operative skills they would find most desirable. The course most likely to be attended if offered locally was the Fundamentals of Laparoscopic Surgery (FLS) course. The top two sought after skills were endoscopic and minimally invasive skills.[23] Interestingly, open surgical skills scored the least interest (Figure 20.1). Demand for laparoscopic training in LMICs continues to increase.

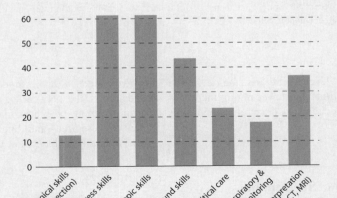

FIGURE 20.1   Most desired surgical skills—West African College of Surgeons. Created by Jill Rhead, Medical Illustrator, Intermountain Healthcare. Image by Akporiaye L. Trigen Survey: West African College of Surgeons. Port-Harcourt: Unpublished data. 2010.

BOX 20.2 TECHNOLOGY FACILITATES IMPROVED ACCESS TO SURGICAL AND MEDICAL CARE

Liver cancer is the number-one cancer in Mongolia. Surgeons at the Cancer Hospital in the capital city, Ulaanbaatar, were faced with many patients requiring liver resections but were only able to operate on one patient each day in one operating room, causing patients to enter long waiting lists while their cancers continued growing. Providing a Bookwalter retractor, a simple but robust device that attaches to the operating room bed, revolutionized exposure of the liver for resection and replaced the many assistants using inadequate handheld retractors previously required. This simple device now allows the surgeons to perform up to three liver resections per day,

which has dramatically decreased the unacceptable delay for these patients.

Similarly, in facilities that have received laparoscopic equipment and training, not only have the numbers of laparoscopic cholecystectomies increased, but the numbers of open cholecystectomies have increased even more (Figure 20.2).[24] Patients previously referred from poorly equipped rural hospitals to tertiary care centers in Ulaanbaatar now receive care in the local facilities, decreasing the financial burden on their families and communities incurred by travel and long stays in the capital city.

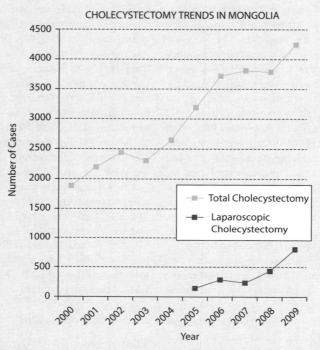

FIGURE 20.2 Cholecystectomy trends in Mongolia. Created by Jill Rhead, Medical Illustrator, Intermountain Healthcare. Image by Unusaikhan Chadraabal (Ulaanbaatar, Mongolia). Unpublished data.

falling into even lower poverty levels. Similarly, the decreased incidence of surgical site infections and fewer requirements for analgesics associated with MIS decreases hospital expenditures and promotes savings.

Fundamental Concepts for Sustainable Expansion of Laparoscopy in LMICs

For the development of laparoscopy to be sustainable, to function independently, and continue to grow after all external forces are gone requires an understanding of the global surgical ecosystem and the supportive interactions of its components. Six main components have been defined and can be examined from a laparoscopic perspective: Technology, education, community

involvement, healthcare models, business models, and interdependence or the network of disciplines[27] (Figure 20.3). While certain training programs may focus on expanding one or just a few of these areas, building successful laparoscopic programs will eventually include all of these components to some degree.

Technology

Emerging business markets in underdeveloped areas have caused a seismic shift in the approach to surgical care. Many people in HICs have been surprised at the sophistication of people in LMICs and have discounted their demands for access to laparoscopic surgery. However, the advanced technology required for laparoscopic surgery is the central component that facilitates improving education models, engaging local communities, and promoting new healthcare and business models.

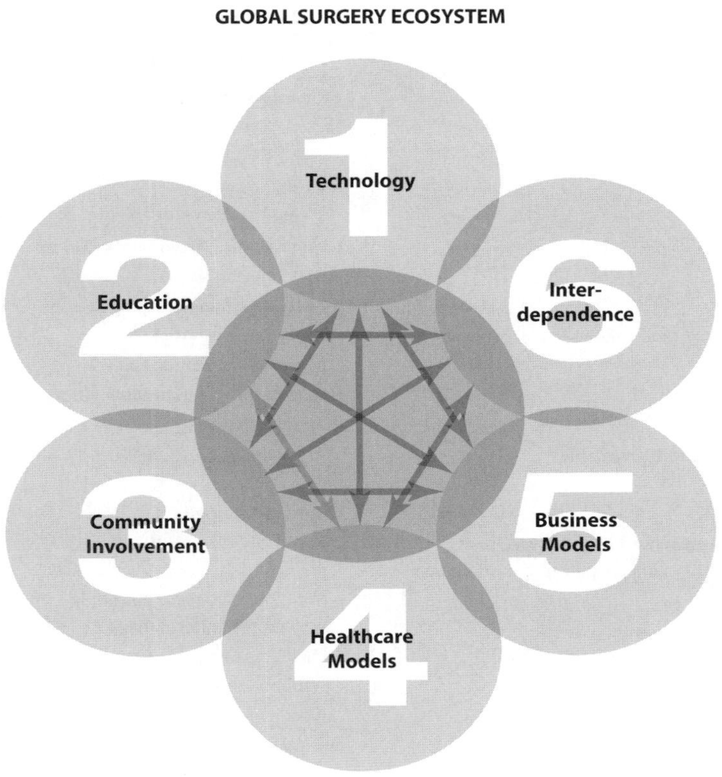

GLOBAL SURGERY ECOSYSTEM

FIGURE 20.3 Global surgery ecosystem. Image by Jill Rhead, Medical Illustrator, Intermountain Healthcare. Adapted from Raymond Price.

The physical capabilities of LMICs must be assessed when contemplating laparoscopic surgery. Baseline assessment of infrastructure, physical and human resources, and basic supplies is needed prior to embarking on any laparoscopic procedure. Laparoscopy requires a reliable electrical supply, appropriate sterilization capability, and adequate anesthesia support. Table 20.3 identifies some of these critical basic facility, equipment, and anesthetic requirements; these requirements provide a template for further laparoscopic infrastructure development when they are not initially present. As the infrastructure develops to support laparoscopy, overall access to other surgical disciplines and medical capabilities simultaneously improves.

Once adequate infrastructure exists, laparoscopic needs must be evaluated and the applicable equipment obtained. A recommended basic set of laparoscopic instruments and equipment is listed in Table 20.4. Engaging the local community will assist in identifying the most appropriate diseases for the area, which will then direct decisions about the requisite equipment to address those needs. For example, the medical community in Mongolia discovered that gallbladder disease is a significant cause of morbidity and lobbied for increased training for laparoscopic cholecystectomy; this necessarily focused equipment acquisition to support basic laparoscopic general surgical capabilities.[22,28] Further development then proceeded to support more advanced and diverse specialty procedures as needs evolved. In Nigeria, gallbladder disease is less frequent, but advanced intra-abdominal tumors can be evaluated and diagnosed by exploratory laparoscopy.[29] Female sterilization remains a major focus for improving maternal health in much of Sub-Saharan Africa. These distinct disease priorities may require other specialized equipment or simple modifications to the basic equipment.

Education

Ultimately, the goal of a training program in laparoscopy should be to impart the skills and confidence necessary for the program to be carried on and expanded by the local surgeons. Teaching laparoscopy in LMICs may be accomplished through various methods. There are, however, some general principles to consider. One of the most resourceful ways to teach is to collaborate with local universities. By incorporating the institutions responsible for medical and surgical education, laparoscopy may eventually be introduced into the standard residency curriculum, leading to a perpetual source for future laparoscopically trained surgeons. Also, cooperating with these institutions will facilitate navigating the medical system in a foreign country.

One of the greatest advantages offered by an alliance with an academic center is the ability to educate a group of surgeons rather than single individuals. Locally designed culturally appropriate laparoscopic education programs can then be instituted not only for the surgical residencies, but also for community and rural surgeons. Similar programs can be developed within private institutions. Ultimately as their experience broadens,

TABLE 20.3

Basic laparoscopic infrastructure assessment

FACILITY

Operating room

Able to accommodate:
2 laparoscopic towers each with a 1 m² footprint
Surgeon
2 assistants
Nurse
Anesthetist

Operating room table

Reverse trendelenburg, trendelenburg, and side-to-side capability

Reliable electrical supply

Back-up power supply

Minimum of 3 hours, readily available

Open set of operating instruments readily available

Electrocautery

Sterilization capability

Autoclave-Chamber dimensions sufficient for 36 cm instruments
Other (cidex, formalin chambers, etc.). Some laparoscopic equipment may not be autoclavable

Laboratory

Complete Blood Count (CBC), Liver Function Tests (LFTs)

Post-operative bed

Availability for up to 78 hours

Equipment

Ultrasound

Portable oxygen

Primary tank or source with immediately available back-up

Chest tubes

Antibiotics

DVT prophylaxis

Medical grade CO₂

Primary tank and immediately available back-up tank properly labeled

ANESTHESIA

Monitoring

End-title CO_2
Pulse oximetry
Basic vital signs

Medications

Muscle relaxants
Narcotics
Sedative hypnotics
Volatile anesthetic agents
Intravenous fluids

Endotracheal intubation

Laryngoscopes
Endotracheal tubes

Created by Jill Rhead, Medical Illustrator, Intermountain Healthcare.
Adapted from Raymond Price.

TABLE 20.4

Basic laparoscopic equipment

Trocars (reuseable)	**Light cable**
	Video system
5 mm (3)	Camera head
11 mm	Camera box
12 mm	Electronic insufflator unit
Laparoscopic Instruments (5 mm)	Monitor (2)
Metzenbaum scissors	Light source
Kelly dissecting grasping forceps (2)	Video tower (2)
Wavy grasping forceps	Slave cable 25 ft (male to male)
Maryland dissecting forceps	
Laparoscopic Instruments (10 mm)	**Electrocautery**
Spoon forceps	Generator
Tissue grasping forceps	Electrocautery cord
Clip applier	Foot activation pedal
Other Instruments	Reusable grounding pad
Verres needle	**Optional more**
	advanced instruments
Monopolar dissecting L hook	Needle drivers* (2)
Irrigating/suction catheter	Cholangiogram clamp*
Facial closure device	**Disposables**
Aspiration needle*	Clips for specific clip applier
Knot pusher*	CO_2 tubing
Telescopes	Replacement light bulb
10 mm 0°	
5 mm 0°	
5 or 10 mm 30°*	

*Beneficial but not necessary for basic set

team approach—including administrators; surgeons; anesthetists; nurses; and scrub-, bio-, and central core processing-technicians—a multidisciplinary training program engenders confidence and trust for the entire team (Table 20.5). Incorporating courses that address other basic concepts such as sterility and surgical safety in the operating room may be added to the laparoscopic curriculum. The World Health Organization "Safe Surgery Saves Lives Initiative" with its three-phase surgical safety checklist can be integrated easily (Figure 20.5). Even basic and emergency surgical courses can be easily adapted to help improve overall basic surgical and medical care in these communities. Teaching laparoscopic surgery facilitates the acceptance of a comprehensive educational program that has the ability to improve overall surgical capabilities of the facility, doctors, and nurses and should be encouraged wherever laparoscopy is implemented.

Laparoscopic surgery requires different skills not encountered with open traditional surgery. An approach to maximize patient safety while introducing laparoscopic surgery is to practice laparoscopic skills using a simulator or an animal laboratory prior to attempting the skills in the operating room. Animal labs are expensive to operate and in some regions they are outlawed; as a result, inanimate simulation trainers are an affordable alternative. The Society of American Gastrointestinal and Laparoscopic Surgeons (SAGES) developed the Fundamentals of Laparoscopy (FLS) course. Training FLS or other similar skills courses in LMICs appears to be a simple method to teach laparoscopic skills (Box 20.3). An inexpensive endotrainer may be created with a cardboard box and a webcam. The five FLS tasks (peg transfer,

the scope of their practice will expand. This global collaboration model must be envisioned as a true partnership where the goals and objectives of both local and international parties are acknowledged and valued. One model for international collaboration is depicted in Figure 20.4.[30]

Successful laparoscopic training programs are those that incorporate a comprehensive curriculum, a multidisciplinary approach, skilled instructors, and an assessment method. Since the safe performance of any laparoscopic procedure requires a

MODEL FOR INTERNATIONAL COLLABORATION

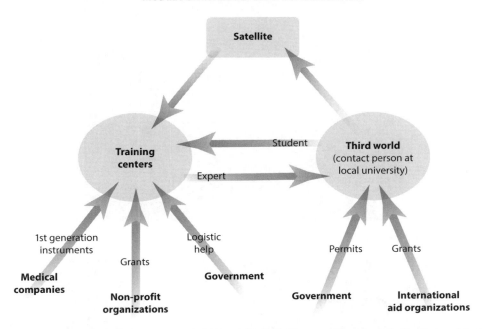

FIGURE 20.4 Model for international collaboration. Image by Jill Rhead, Medical Illustrator, Intermountain Healthcare. Adapted from: Cadiere GB, Himpens J, Bruyns J. Laparoscopic surgery and the third world. *Surgical Endoscopy*. 1996; **10**(10): 957-958.

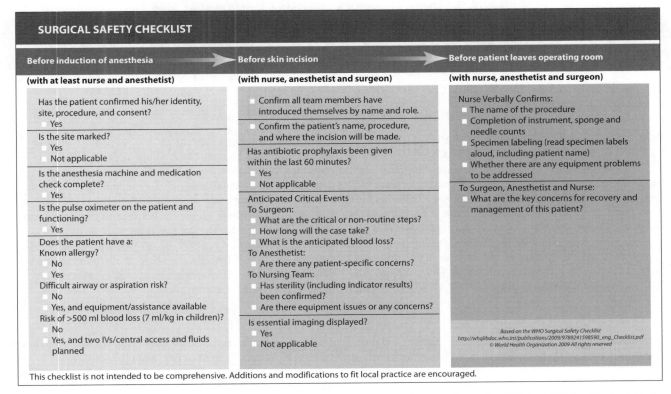

FIGURE 20.5 WHO surgical safety checklist. World Health Organization. Surgical safety checklist. [Internet]. 2009 [cited 2014 Jan 28]. Available from: http://www.who.int/patientsafety/safesurgery/en/

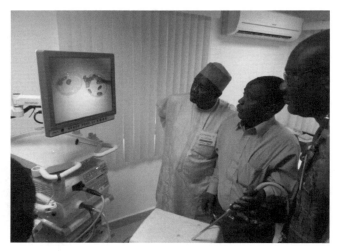

FIGURE 20.6A   Bean transfer. Image by Raymond Price.

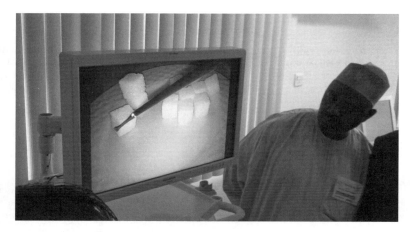

FIGURE 20.6B   Stacking sugar cubes. Image by Raymond Price.

BOX 20.3   FLS TRAINING IN BOTSWANA

In Botswana, a study to determine the feasibility and impact of a short FLS course showed that FLS was feasible; technical skills improved significantly after three days of training. Most surgeons, however, did not reach FLS passing scores, suggesting that longer courses may be necessary.[31] The authors found that the FLS program was well suited for a resource-restricted country as the simulator was light and collapsed compactly for travel. In addition, most of the equipment was inexpensive; the total cost of supplies for the course was $1,900 CAD. In a different study, the authors evaluated the effectiveness of telesimulation for teaching FLS in Botswana.

Sixteen surgeons were randomized into two different groups for an eight-week course. The first group participated in one proctored training session per week over Skype, a voice-over-Internet protocol that allowed visual and two-way communication between educators in Canada and students in Botswana. The second group did not receive proctoring but had access to FLS DVDs and practiced their skills once per week. FLS post-test scores for the telesimulation group were significantly higher than for the self-practice group, with all participants in the telesimulation group achieving scores adequate to pass the FLS certification.[32]

pattern cutting, ligating loop, extracorporeal suturing, and intracorporeal suturing) may be improvised with local materials if the exact simulation materials are not available. For example, a bean transfer or sugar cube stacking exercise may be used in lieu of the peg transfer, or cloth material may be used instead of penrose drains for knot tying (Figure 20.6a and Figure 20.6b). In instances where frequent travel to a region would not be possible,

establishing a telesimulation program may allow for continued skill building in both laparoscopic and open skills.

However, nothing can replace actual experience in the operating room. A graduated training experience in the operating room on live patients under the direct supervision of the surgical educator provides the student surgeon with the critical training opportunity to safely acquire the necessary practical

BOX 20.4   GRADUATED LAPAROSCOPIC TRAINING IN MONGOLIA

In Mongolia, a combined didactic and practical laparoscopic training course was developed in conjunction with the Health Science University of Mongolia (HSUM) and the Swanson Family Foundation (a private nongovernmental agency). Following an initial eight hours of lectures on the first day, two surgeons were selected for the practical training. Prior to the course, patients with gallbladder disease had been identified and carefully selected for laparoscopic cholecystectomy. As gallbladder disease is quite prevalent in Mongolia, 24–30 patients were able to undergo laparoscopic cholecystectomy during the subsequent eight days of practical training. The student surgeons, under the direction of the lead surgical educators, would each progress from camera holder to assistant surgeon and then to primary surgeon; each student surgeon would experience each role at least five separate times before finally operating together as surgeon and assistant forming a local surgical team. This method has been used to help expand laparoscopy safely throughout Mongolia to the major hospitals in the capital city and to five designated rural regional diagnostic centers from 2006–2011.[33] Surgeons from these trainings have now developed their own laparoscopic courses and continue to provide ongoing training for surgeons in Mongolia. In 2009, the Minister of Health awarded the Swanson Family Foundation surgical teams with the country's highest Medal of Honor presented to foreigners for their work in improving surgical care throughout Mongolia.

laparoscopic skills; a high volume of similar cases performed over a short time interval is ideal for rapid acquisition of these skills. Student surgeons gain experience gradually, progressing from camera holder to assistant surgeon and then finally the primary surgeon (Box 20.4). Ideally, the newly trained laparoscopic surgeons should continue to receive proctoring from local laparoscopic surgeons when possible.

Preoperative patient assessment and selection, intraoperative care, and postoperative management must be integral components of any laparoscopic educational program. Understanding appropriate patient selection and optimization of overall medical condition prior to surgery remain critical concepts for safe laparoscopic surgery; delaying an operation or canceling the procedure should be encouraged until significant medical problems can be addressed. Converting the procedure to an open approach should be encouraged when necessary, exemplifying clinical maturity, and should not be viewed as a failure or complication. The surgeon should already have the technical skills necessary to complete the operation open if necessary. A circulating nurse actively participating in the operating room is not a universal concept and must be included in the team educational approach as well as the specific nuances of anesthetic management and the imperative collegial working relationship between surgeon and anesthetist. Likewise, surgeons must learn to critically analyze minimally invasive surgery and decide which laparoscopic procedures provide a real benefit for their patients. Not every laparoscopic procedure will be beneficial in terms of safety, cost-effectiveness, or efficacy in all parts of the world.[26]

Any form of surgery inherently carries with it a learning curve. Safely introducing new techniques into surgical practice, whether it is in the most developed environment or in LMICs, will always be tempered by the public's interpretation of the risks and benefits; patients know quality and avoid doctors with poor outcomes. Sustainable expansion of laparoscopy in LMICs inherently encourages surgeons to obtain adequate training, to begin with less complicated cases, and to collaborate together to refine their skills. Similar constraints helped guide the introduction of laparoscopy in HICs in the early 1990s.

Community Involvement

In order for new technology to be accepted and to develop deep roots, the local community must feel the service is essential; it is imperative to identify the needs of the population. Prior experience in laparoscopic surgery, availability of local resources, the underlying character of the burden of surgical disease, and cultural influences are all factors to be considered prior to implementing a laparoscopic training course.[34] The burden of surgical disease is difficult to estimate as it can vary depending on the definition of surgery used. Hospital and procedure data from LMICs notoriously underestimate the true burden of surgical disease. For example, introducing laparoscopic cholecystectomy into Afghanistan seemed to unmask a hidden disease burden as overall numbers in gallbladder removal dramatically increased (Figure 20.7).[35] Similar effects have been found in Mongolia and other countries.

One way to maximize the success of a program is by collaborating with the local Ministry of Health and medical community. This relationship establishes a firm foundation on which strong collaboration efforts and capacity development can be built. By involving the native medical community, local physicians are more likely to take an active role in the project. These organizations can provide information on the number of certified surgeons and anesthesiologists in the region as well as the local resources. In addition, they are invaluable in providing information on the political climate in the country and advisable times for travel, and can sometimes help navigate the murky waters of customs when bringing equipment into the country. Their input may be indispensable in times of political unrest or war, as travel may be dangerous, and supplies and equipment may be difficult to obtain; even a well-developed and organized program may fail under these conditions. Additionally, many countries require licensing or special permits for foreign physicians operating locally; this licensing requires advanced planning and coordination with local governing bodies and may take several months.

Healthcare Models

The globalization of surgery is the concept of bringing the benefits of surgery, including laparoscopy, to all people regardless of race, sex, social, or economic status, geographic location, or political or religious beliefs. A sound public health strategy seeks to serve the greatest number of underserved individuals. In regions where roads are underdeveloped and transportation is cumbersome, regionalization of care may provide a solution. Community clinics in villages can provide basic primary care and refer to district hospitals, regional referral centers, or tertiary hospitals based on acuity. The 1978 Alma Ata Declaration of Health recommended that primary health care should be sustained by integrated, functional, and mutually supportive referral systems to adequately address the health needs of the community.[36] Laparoscopy can reinforce this type of system, which may provide improved care and access for patients in rural communities when laparoscopic service is provided as a partner in the continuum of care.

To establish this type of vertical healthcare in which laparoscopy becomes an integral component, governments and Ministries of Health must be engaged; cooperation must occur among the different tiers for the system to be successful. The local government must also allocate resources for improvement of transportation to facilitate transfers from one facility to another in emergent/urgent situations. Situational analyses from Mongolia, Sierra Leone, and other countries indicate that resources would not support laparoscopy in most of the rural hospitals.[37,38] But countries that are taking an active role in consolidating resources and establishing a continuum of care provide a fertile environment to expand laparoscopic surgery. Providing laparoscopy in regional centers expands access even to some of the most remote areas previously thought impossible.

Mobile surgical units present another type of healthcare model where laparoscopy has been introduced. Dr. Edgar Rodas, who served as Minister of Health from Ecuador (1998–2000), offers laparoscopic surgery in his one-room operating truck, which he drives throughout the 22 provinces of Ecuador. When not traveling, Dr. Rodas and the Cinterandes Foundation partner with local hospitals in Cuenca, Ecuador, where surgery is provided inexpensively in the truck and local hospitals provide recovery room and inpatient capability at reduced rates.[39] Neurosurgeons in Uganda treat hydrocephalus endoscopically, and gynecologists in Haiti provide laparoscopic care by transporting their laparoscopic equipment to local hospitals, providing modern surgical options for patients in some of the more resource-poor environments in their countries.

Business Models

Extreme affordability dictates sustainability in LMICs. Providing less expensive surgical care does not automatically correlate with decreased quality. In the United States, Intermountain Healthcare (IHC), a large healthcare corporation, has demonstrated that improved quality healthcare actually lowers costs; IHC provides health care at one-third the cost of similar organizations while consistently delivering excellent outcomes. Providing laparoscopy in LMICs is not just about using cheaper versions of products or unwanted older equipment from more developed markets; providing laparoscopy requires new innovative business models— ones that are more appropriate and culturally acceptable for these areas (Box 20.5). Businesses that sell replacement parts and equipment locally improve access and promote sustainability while also supporting the local economy. JNC International, a healthcare supply company in Nigeria, distributes and provides technical support for a variety of new healthcare products including laparoscopy, ultrasound machines, modern operating room suites, and more.

Businesses who design high-quality/lower-cost laparoscopic equipment and instruments provide competition in the marketplace, driving down expenses as demand increases. Some well-established companies recognizing the potential market for expansion are actively entering these markets, partnering with both visiting surgical teams and business organizations. Private healthcare models may be a viable target for laparoscopy in Sub-Saharan Africa with the IFC recommendation to invest $25–30 billion USD to improve healthcare for the poor.

Interdependence: Network of Disciplines

Similar to the early collaboration with doctors, sword swallowers, and instrument makers that helped advance early endoscopy and laparoscopy, a multidisciplinary approach for worldwide expansion of laparoscopy requires innovative partnerships with a variety of disciplines such as medicine, engineering, law, business, and social science (Table 20.5). The development of technology must be supported by local business models, accepted by

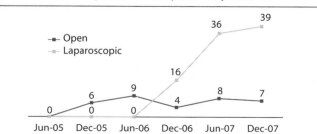

EFFECT OF LAPAROSCOPY ON THE NUMBER OF CHOLECYSTECTOMIES AT CURE INTERNATIONAL HOSPITAL KABUL, AFGHANISTAN
Total Cholecystectomies Completed Every 6 Months

FIGURE 20.7   Effect of laparoscopy on the number of cholecystectomies. Image by Jill Rhead, Medical Illustrator, Intermountain Healthcare. Adapted from: Manning RG, Aziz AQ. Should laparoscopic cholecystectomy be practiced in the developing world?: the experience of the first training program in Afghanistan. *Annals of Surgery.* 2009; **249**(5): 794–798.

BOX 20.5 NEPAL LAPAROSCOPIC BUSINESS MODEL

Previously in Nepal, an open cholecystectomy cost 800 rupees. When a small hospital introduced laparoscopy, it charged 18,000 rupees. Worried that most people could not afford this "exorbitant" price, the hospital was surprised when its clinic was inundated with patients requesting the minimally invasive surgical approach. The clinic patients usually arrived carried in baskets or on bamboo stretchers; now a new clientele arrived in expensive Land Rover and Mercedes-Benz vehicles. As word traveled quickly, patients came from throughout Nepal and neighboring countries of Bhutan and India. Ambassadors, government ministers, and even royal family members traveled long distances. The hospital's revenue skyrocketed from 8–10,000 rupees per day to 120,000 per day. The hospital, whose primary mission was to care for the poor, used the increased revenue to support its 100-bed charity hospital, which previously could barely buy the necessary medicines. The hospital was also able to repair the laparoscopic equipment and replace the reusable components, such as clip appliers and the expensive xenon light bulb. Graduated payment scales became available for poorer patients, expanding laparoscopy to all social and economic classes (Leo Vigna to Raymond Price, Personal email communication, 2008).

TABLE 20.5

Multidisciplinary laparoscopic training team

Specialty	Number
Surgeon	2
Anesthetist	1
Scrub nurse	1
Scrub technician	1
Biotechnician	1
Surgical resident	1

Created by Jill Rhead, Medical Illustrator, Intermountain Healthcare.
Adapted from Raymond Price.

TABLE 20.6

Methods of cost reduction reported for laparoscopy

- Reusable trocars and instruments
- Surgical gloves or condoms for specimen retrieval
- Angiocatheter and tie for endoclose
- Endoloops instead of staplers or clips
- Manual straw suction and irrigation
- Intracorporeal sutures or extracorporeal tying instead of titanium clips
- Bipolar coagulation (cystic artery, fallopian tube)
- Gasless laparoscopy
- Air instead of CO_2 for insufflation
- Manual insufflation with sigmoidoscopic pump
- Meticulous care of instruments and equipment
- Cleaning the scope intraoperatively by wiping on the liver

Created by Jill Rhead, Medical Illustrator, Intermountain Healthcare.
Adapted from Raymond Price.

Facilitating Laparoscopy in LMICs

Cost reduction remains one of the major obstacles for laparoscopy in LMICs. However, simple modulations in current treatment can markedly reduce many of the disposable costs both in HICs and LMICs (Table 20.6). Adaptations to equipment already present can replace more expensive tools, such as an endoclose made from a 14-gauge angiocatheter and a silk tie (Figure 20.8).

Evaluating the quality of laparoscopic equipment and supplies requires extreme vigilance. Although some of the equipment arrives new, much is used or secondhand from hospital donations after the facilities upgrade to newer equipment. Instruments, many which were intended for single use, remain in use long beyond their normal life span. With extended use, the insulation along the instruments frequently becomes damaged, and if not recognized can lead to lateral cautery damage to adjacent organs.

Laparoscopic Cholecystectomy

The following adaptations can help decrease the cost of a laparoscopic cholecystectomy:

1. 0-0 vicryl, catgut, or silk sutures may be used on the cystic duct and artery rather than titanium clips. The ties may be done either intracorporeally or extracorporeally.
2. The cystic duct can be cauterized with a bipolar cautery.
3. In cases of acute cholecystitis, the gallbladder may be removed in a condom, a rubber surgical glove, or a plastic bag rather than an endocatch bag.
4. Use reusable trocars rather than disposable trocars.
5. A pediatric feeding tube may be used as a cholangiogram catheter.
6. Ovum forceps used in gynecologic procedures are effective at extracting and crushing gallstones.
7. A 50 ml syringe serves as an adequate irrigation device.[25,41]

Many hospitals in LMICs do not have the capability to perform intraoperative cholangiograms (IOCs). One study documented the safety of performing laparoscopic cholecystectomy in appropriately selected patients in facilities without

vested communities with different social backgrounds and priorities, and engineered for extreme affordability. The innovations that will drive the global expansion of laparoscopy are not likely to originate from large institutionalized companies; the innovations will come from communities within the LMICs where local needs and resources dictate real solutions.

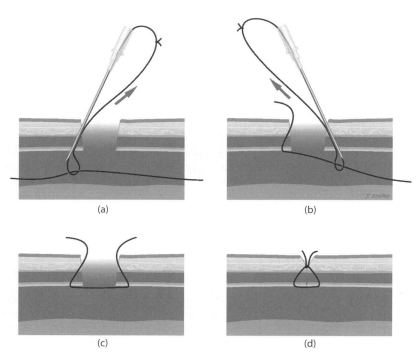

FIGURE 20.8   Homemade endoclose. Images by Jill Rhead, Medical Illustrator, Intermountain Healthcare.

IOC capabilities.[40] The conversion rate from three nonteaching rural hospitals was 1.82% over 6 years. There were no deaths and the complications were minimal. Only one patient (0.08%) suffered a common bile duct injury. A thorough workup for choledocholithiasis must be undertaken preoperatively. Appropriate interpretation of the size of the common bile duct and preoperative liver function testing help identify patients suspected of having common bile duct stones who should not be offered laparoscopic cholecystectomy where cholangiography or endoscopic retrograde cholangiopancreatography are not available.

Laparoscopic Appendectomy

Cost-saving alternatives include:

1. Catgut suture to ligate the meso-appendix, appendiceal stump, and a catgut purse string suture to bury the stump, rather than staplers, have been safe and effective.[25] A 0-0 or 2-0 PDS or vicryl tie or endoloop alone has also been used.
2. Remove the appendix in a condom, glove, or plastic bag.

Laparoscopic Hernia Repair

To create the anatomic plane necessary for an extraperitoneal repair, a low-cost balloon dissector may be created by tying a glove finger over the top of a 5-mm suction cannula with a silk suture. The balloon is distended with saline to test for any leak prior to insertion into the extraperitoneal space. The balloon is inflated with 300 ml of normal saline and remains inflated for one minute. A randomized study comparing this method with direct telescopic dissection found balloon dissection was associated with significantly reduced postoperative pain at six hours, scrotal edema, and seroma accumulation.[41]

Replacing traditional mesh with certain kinds of mosquito netting has been reported in Ghana and India and may prove to be a viable option, but needs further clinical trials.[42,43]

Diagnostic Laparoscopy

Pneumoperitoneum for a diagnostic laparoscopy can be obtained by insufflating atmospheric air using a sterilized sigmoidoscope pump.

Summary

As the field of general surgery moves toward less-invasive interventions, ingenuity and perseverance are needed to ensure the benefits of new technologies reach patients in all parts of the globe. Expanding quality laparoscopic surgical care into LMICs has become an enabling endeavor; it is a source for improved economies and poverty reduction, promotes higher quality healthcare overall, and increases the community's respect and trust in their healthcare providers. The qualities of ingenuity and innovation have no national boundaries. Patients and doctors, surgical societies, Ministries of Health, and industries provide the thrust for the current fervor leading the revolution to provide the benefits of minimally invasive surgery in LMICs. Although many obstacles continue to present themselves, solutions are being identified that negate a commonly held view that laparoscopy is too complex and expensive for LMICs. The continued growth of laparoscopic surgery globally will include development of a sustainable healthcare infrastructure, a stable economic platform, a renewable source of medical professionals, and improved communication and education with the government and the public. In the meantime, the previously neglected 4 billion people at the "bottom of the wealth pyramid"[44] are proving to be a significant engine for innovative ideas guiding the introduction and growth of laparoscopy in LMICs; the cutting edge of surgical progress is becoming available and affordable to more people worldwide than ever before.

COMMENTARY

Sergelen Orgoi, Mongolia

It is important to indicate that biliary tract diseases have the second highest incidence among surgical diseases in Mongolia. Taking a look at the history of biliary tract surgeries, it has been proven that, after the development of laparoscopy, postsurgical complications have led to an increased mortality rate. This can be explained by not having complete experience with new laparoscopic methods.

Since 2005, the Swanson Family Foundation (from the United States), in a cooperation with SAGES since 2010, has been organizing the training of professionals in laparoscopy in Ulaanbaatar and Regional Diagnosis and Treatment Centers (RDTC). Their donations have enabled laparoscopic surgeries to be performed in all state and larger private clinics in Ulaanbaatar, RDTCs in rural areas, and central hospitals in five major aimags (provinces). Studies from the Center for Health Development of Ministry of Health indicate that prior to the commencement of the laparoscopic surgery project in 2003, only 1% of 543 biliary tract surgeries were performed laparoscopically; the remaining 99% were open surgeries with a postsurgical complication rate of 0.73% and a mortality rate of 0.55%.

By 2012, there were approximately 4,440 biliary tract surgeries performed per year and 2,535 of them were laparoscopic surgeries, which decreased postsurgical complications by 0.24% and mortality rate by 0.15%. Seven cases had been shifted to open due to common bile duct injury during laparoscopic procedure.

Although improvements in biliary tract disease diagnosis reveal more gallstone cases, postsurgical complications of laparoscopic surgery are decreasing. This is because:

1. The Swanson Family Foundation and SAGES choose one or two particular hospitals every year to train about 8–10 surgeons. During the bedside training course, local surgeons perform approximately 24–30 surgeries with trainers and 10–20 surgeries on their own under their trainers' guidance.
2. The Swanson Family Foundation and SAGES donate one to two complete laparoscopic facilities every year.

Mongolian surgeons are being well-trained on laparoscopic surgeries of the biliary tract, resulting in the reduction of postsurgical complications and mortality rates. Surgeons trained under the Swanson Family Foundation and SAGES train other surgeons in Mongolia. The laparoscopic surgery course was added to the surgical residency program in 2011 in Mongolia. Since then, we have been training young residents in laparoscopic surgeries. This is one example of globalization of laparoscopic surgery, and it shows the possibilities of introducing modern technologies to LMICs.

21

Breast Cancer

Lisa A. Newman
Marcel Bayor
Evelyn Jiagge
Der Muonir Edmund
Mawuli Gyakobo

Worldwide Breast Cancer Statistics

Approximately 1.4 million breast cancers are diagnosed annually on a worldwide basis, making it the most frequently diagnosed cancer in women. As shown in Figure 21.1, population-based cancer incidence rates are highest in Western, industrialized parts of the world such as North America and Europe, and lowest in low- and middle-income countries (LMICs). It is widely assumed that "Western" lifestyle and reproductive factors (such as delayed childbearing); postmenopausal hormone replacement therapy (very popular during the 1980s and 1990s as a strategy to minimize side effects of ovarian cessation); postmenopausal obesity; increased detection rates through screening mammography programs; and probably some as-yet poorly defined dietary and environmental factors account for the notably high incidence rates of high-income countries (HICs). In contrast, delayed diagnosis and limited treatment resources result in disproportionate mortality rates; approximately 60% of breast cancer deaths occur in LMICs, and as shown in Figure 21.1, breast cancer mortality-to-incidence ratios are more than 0.5 in LMICs but only 0.2–0.3 in industrialized nations.

Compared to women from HICs, women from LMICs tend to have reproductive factors associated with fewer estrogen/ovarian cycles over the lifetime (childbearing beginning at younger ages, more pregnancies, and prolonged lactation), and these factors tend to protect against breast cancer on a population basis. Furthermore, average life expectancy is 10–30 years shorter in LMICs compared to Western populations. Since breast cancer risk rises with increasing age (average age at diagnosis for American breast cancer patients is 60–62 years), these longevity patterns also serve to limit the number of cases detected in LMICs. On the other hand, existing statistics regarding the population-based incidence and mortality rates for any cancer in LMICs must be viewed with caution, because limited financial resources can impede their efforts to generate accurate overall census data as well as cancer case volume ascertainment. As of the year 2000, it was estimated that less than 25% of the world's cancer burden and only one-third of its death certificate-linked mortality burden was accurately documented.[1]

As noted above, industrialized nations are better equipped to support large-scale mammography screening programs, contributing to early stage distribution and higher breast cancer treatment success rates. Lack of mammography screening—as well as a lack of instruction regarding self breast exams generally taught by one's ob-gyn or primary care physician—contribute to the higher breast cancer mortality rates of LMICs, but other factors account for the more advanced stage distribution that is observed as well. Because a large proportion of individuals receive their health care exclusively from herbalists and tribal practitioners, many women in LMICs do not seek conventional medical attention until later (if at all). Adding to the barrier granting access to conventional medical facilities is an overall lack of awareness, excessive distance from healthcare facilities, and lack of transportation. Availability of breast oncology specialists is quite low in LMICs, further limiting ability to diagnose and treat this disease efficiently. Many healthcare facilities that possess mammography equipment frequently lack trained radiologists, mammography technicians, and staff that are qualified to maintain the mammography equipment. For patients who are able to get to a breast clinic, they may have to endure prolonged delays waiting for surgical diagnostic biopsies because of limited operating room resources and lack of access to percutaneous needle biopsy devices.

Among those patients who do undergo biopsy, the time it takes to obtain a definitive diagnosis is often protracted because of scarcity of pathologists to read and interpret the biopsy material. Once a breast cancer diagnosis is established, the patient may not be able to afford or may not have ready access to definitive surgery, radiation, and/or systemic therapy. Indeed, immunohistochemistry resources to assess for molecular marker expression (estrogen receptor, ER; progesterone receptor, PR; and HER2/neu) are often non-existent, disabling the oncology team from making effective and optimal adjuvant therapy recommendations. Tragically, each of these junctures noted for treatment delays represents opportunities for patients to be lost to follow-up.

These multiple barriers to efficiently diagnosing and treating breast cancer in LMICs are particularly concerning in light of the fact that breast cancer incidence rates appear to be rising in these parts of the world. These increases are probably due to adoption of "Westernized" lifestyles, in particular with regard

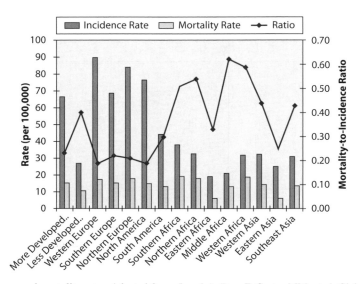

FIGURE 21.1 Breast cancer incidence and mortality rates. Adapted from: Jemal A, Bray F, Center MM, et al. Global Cancer Statistics. CA: A Cancer Journal for Clinicians. 2011; 61: 69–90. 2. International Agency for Research on Cancer. Globocan [Internet]. 2008. Accessed March 31, 2011 [cited 2014 Jan 28]. Available from: http://globocan.iarc.fr/

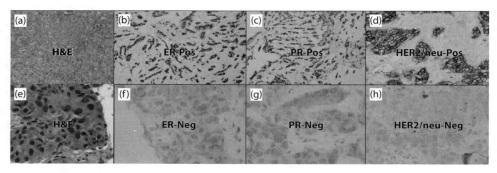

FIGURE 21.2 Photomicrograph of invasive breast cancer; triple-positive (a–d) and triple-negative (e–h); hematoxylin and eosin (H&E) stains (a and e), and immunohistochemistry stains for estrogen receptor (ER) (b and f), progesterone receptor (PR) (c and g), and HER2/neu (d and h). Image by Lisa Newman.

to diet/obesity rates. Additionally, an expanding body of literature now suggests that the multiparous childbearing pattern that is more common in LMICs may be associated with an increased risk for the so-called "triple-negative" breast cancers (TNBCs; cancers that will be resistant to endocrine and targeted anti-HER2/neu therapies), which tend to be more virulent tumors. An example of a triple-negative compared to a triple-positive breast cancer is shown in Figure 21.2. The dual issues of increasing breast cancer incidence and limited diagnostic as well as treatment resources are likely to cause worsening mortality-to-incidence ratios in LMICs.

Several other relatively unique patterns of the breast cancer burden in developing parts of the world have become apparent. Male breast cancer is more common in regions of the Middle East and Africa where liver damage from schistosomiasis/bilharzia (causing deranged hormone metabolism) is highly prevalent. Inflammatory breast cancer is seen with increased frequency in Egypt and northern Africa. Estrogen receptor-negative and triple-negative breast cancers are three to four times more common in the developing nations of continental

Africa compared to other parts of the world (Table 21.1). TNBC accounts for only 15% of the breast cancers detected in North America and Europe.

Clinical Presentation of Breast Cancer

Ideally, breast masses will be further evaluated by mammography and ultrasound imaging (Figure 21.3, Figure 21.4a and Figure 21.4b). Prompt recognition of breast cancer signs and symptoms is especially important in LMICs, where clinicians may be unable to rely upon an image-based diagnostic work-up. The standard breast exam should include the following sequential components:

1. Visual inspection of the entire chest wall with patient completely disrobed from the waist up, with arms raised over the head, and then resting on the waist. Nipple inversion, as well as areas of breast skin ulceration, puckering, and/or erythema should be noted.

TABLE 21.1

Frequency of estrogen receptor-negative and triple-negative (estrogen receptor-negative, progesterone receptor-negative, and HER2/neu-negative) breast cancer in selected LMICs.

Author, Year	Country	Number of Cases studied	Proportion of Estrogen Receptor Negative Cases	Proportion of Triple-Negative Cases
Huo et al., 2009	Nigeria, Senegal	507	76%	73%
Bird et al., 2008	Kenya	129	76%	44% (subset of 34 cases with all three markers assessed)
Stark et al., 2010	Ghana	75	76%	83% (subset of 45 cases with all three markers assessed)
Ben Abdelkrim, 2010	Tunisia	194	36%	18%
Thang, 2011	Viet Nam	249	38%	NR
Dey et al., 2010	Egypt	1759	14.8%	NR

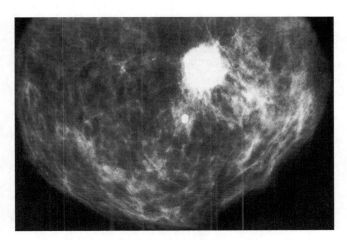

FIGURE 21.3 Spiculated mass appearance of breast cancer on mammogram, with adjacent calcified fibroadenoma. Breast cancer appears as the large, bright density, and the calcified fibroadenoma as the smaller, smooth density below it. Image by Lisa Newman.

Fixed nipple inversion may indicate the presence of an underlying subareolar tumor. Nipple-areolar eczematoid changes may indicate the presence of Paget's disease of the nipple (breast cancer cells within the areolar epidermis; this can occur with or without an associated tumor). Erythematous and/or edematous changes in the breast skin (which may be diffuse or localized in the breast) suggests the presence of cancer cells invading the dermal lymphatics caused by inflammatory breast cancer. Skin changes caused by a breast abscess and/or mastitis can mimic malignancy, but cancer must always be ruled out. Any breast abscess undergoing incision and drainage should have a concomitant biopsy of the abscess wall to rule out a necrotic tumor, and any presumed mastitis treated by antibiotics must be followed closely for complete resolution of skin changes. Suspicious breast or areolar skin changes can frequently be evaluated expeditiously by an office-based punch biopsy (discussed below).

2. Palpation of the axillary and supraclavicular nodal basins while the patient is sitting upright. Some shotty, mobile (and usually bilateral) axillary adenopathy is common and not necessarily pathologic; any fixed or dominant/asymmetric adenopathy should be considered suspicious. Supraclavicular adenopathy should always be considered pathologic. Suspicious axillary adenopathy will heighten level of concern regarding any breast findings, but occasionally breast cancer presents as isolated unilateral axillary adenopathy and an occult breast primary.

3. Gentle bimanual palpation of the breasts while the patient is sitting upright to check for nipple discharge (excessively vigorous nipple manipulation can lead to a traumatic bloody discharge).

4. Compression palpation examination of the breast while the patient is lying supine, with the arm elevated up over the head, to maximally thin out the breast tissue over the chest wall. Compression can proceed following radial lines circumferentially around each breast, or following concentric circles around the breast, as long as the examiner is consistent with the exam and feels confident that she or he is obtaining a comprehensive exam of the entire breast. Any dominant or discrete nodules should be noted, as well as any nipple discharge elicited during this exam. The mass should be characterized regarding fixation or mobility, pain, and smooth versus irregular borders. While fibrocystic breast changes (fibroadenoma, cyst, or diffuse fibrocystic mastopathy) are the most common cause of breast masses, other conditions in the differential diagnosis include diabetic mastopathy, mammary tuberculosis, or fat necrosis. It is sometimes challenging to distinguish benign lesions from a discrete or dominant malignant mass, and breast biopsy (via percutaneous needle approach or surgical/open biopsy) is necessary for definitive diagnosis of a cancer.

Breast Biopsy Options

Low- and middle-income countries must reconcile the coexisting factors of sparse finances, fewer diagnostic devices, and limited surgical and pathologic resources, as well as patients that are easily lost to follow-up because of transportation problems, inability to pay, and/or lack of breast cancer awareness. The following list presents the advantages and disadvantages of various strategies that will provide tissue for microscopic analysis, but a few basic

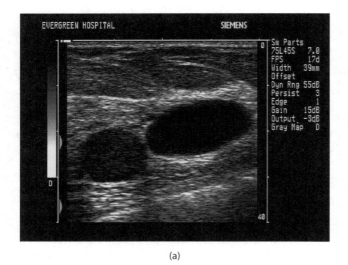

(a)

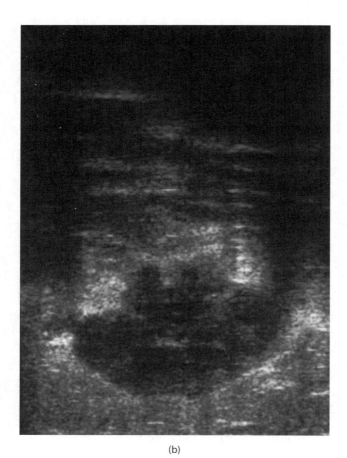

(b)

FIGURE 21.4 (a) Simple cyst (right) and adjacent complex cyst. The simple cyst is a well-encapsulated anechoic lesion; the complicated cyst is filled with debris. (b) Ultrasound image of cancer: hypoechoic mass with irregular borders; taller than wide. Images by Lisa Newman.

principles must be emphasized: (i) promptness of diagnosis is essential if a patient is at especially high risk for being lost to follow-up; (ii) biopsy results must always be concordant with the clinical impression; and (iii) if any questions remain regarding

whether or not a prior biopsy has definitively ruled out cancer, then an alternative biopsy strategy should be pursued.

Punch Biopsy

The punch biopsy device is a small handheld apparatus that has a hollow cylinder featuring a circular scalpel at its tip. It is used most commonly by dermatologists for office-based biopsy of skin lesions under local anesthesia, but it is also quite useful biopsying breast skin lesions that appear suspicious for inflammatory breast cancer or Paget's disease of the nipple. Locally advanced breast cancers with skin ulcerations or skin satellitosis may also be amenable to punch biopsy. These devices are available in various diameters ranging from 2–6 mm diameters. One disadvantage of these biopsies is that they frequently require a suture for closure of the resulting circular skin defect. The clinician should also bear in mind that occasionally the absence of dermal lymphatic invasion does not rule out the presence of inflammatory breast cancer. In the setting of any histopathologic evidence of breast cancer, the clinical impression of inflammatory malignancy is adequate to establish this diagnosis.

Percutaneous Needle Biopsy

A percutaneous needle biopsy can be performed as a fine needle aspirate (FNA) or as a core needle biopsy. Either type can be performed percutaneously or with image guidance (mammographically, usually as a stereotactic biopsy, or with ultrasonographic guidance). The FNA biopsy is easily performed with minimal local anesthetic requirements, since it is best performed using a 20–26 gauge needle and a 5–10 cc handheld syringe. The biopsy needle is passed back and forth a few times into the lesion of concern, with a constant (and limited) amount of suction applied on the aspirating syringe. The aspirate can be applied directly onto the microscope slide, and at least a portion (if not all, depending on the institutional arrangements with the local cytopathology team) washed into a special cytology preservative such as cytolyte, so that the cells can be processed and spun down for optimal microscopic analysis after appropriate staining. The FNA equipment is obviously widely available in most office, clinic, and hospital settings, but the cytolyte preservative will incur additional costs, and experienced cytopathologists are not necessarily available on a universal basis. Furthermore, the FNA will reveal scattered cells that may be diagnosed as being cancerous, but since the breast parenchymal architecture will not be present for analysis, the FNA cannot distinguish *in situ* cancers from invasive lesions. The vast majority of palpable breast masses (but not all) will be invasive tumors, but many cancerous masses will have a mixture of invasive and *in situ* components. Advances in immunohistochemical technology are such that ER, PR, and HER2/neu status can be assessed on cytologic aspirates, but these assays will not be able to document whether the markers are being evaluated on the invasive or the *in situ* portions of the pathology. The molecular marker pattern will not necessarily be the same for both components, and treatment must of course be planned on the basis of the markers identified on the invasive cancer cells. Lastly, the FNA biopsy has a higher false-negative rate compared to the core needle biopsy, because of the more limited tissue acquisition. On the other hand, an FNA biopsy that documents cancer cells within a suspicious axillary lymph node will be definitively diagnostic of an invasive cancer, because *in situ* cancers cannot metastasize to regional or distant organs.

The percutaneous needle biopsy can be performed freehand by the clinician for palpable lesions as an office- or clinic-based procedure. It can also be performed with image guidance (mammographic or ultrasonographic) for both palpable lesions and nonpalpable, screen-detected abnormalities. The false negative and sampling error rate is lower when image guidance is utilized, because the mammographic or sonographic images can confirm the trajectory of the biopsy needle into the lesion of interest. Image-guided needle biopsies of nonpalpable lesions should be accompanied by insertion of a radio-opaque clip or marker to document the biopsy site. If a high-risk lesion such as atypical hyperplasia or lobular carcinoma *in situ* is identified, then a surgical excisional biopsy is indicated as a follow-up procedure in order to rule out a coexisting cancer. High-risk lesions will be upgraded to ductal carcinoma *in situ* or invasive cancer in 15%–20% of these cases.

Open Surgical Biopsy

Open surgical biopsy to remove an entire breast lesion is the most definitive diagnostic procedure but is associated with the disadvantages of leaving surgical scars and possible breast deformity for lesions that may be benign. Furthermore, the surgical biopsy is a relatively inefficient diagnostic procedure, utilizing operating room resources that may be particularly scarce in LMICs. If a surgical biopsy becomes necessary either because of lack of needle biopsy resources or because of inconclusive or high-risk prior needle biopsy results, then the following technical points can be helpful:

1. Centrally located and circumareolar incisions are preferred because they are more readily hidden under clothes, but they are discouraged in cases of tumors located in the peripheral quadrants of the breast because excessive tunneling between the tumor bed and the skin incision can be problematic for patients that require re-excision lumpectomies for margin control.
2. Curvilinear incisions that follow the skin lines tend to heal better than radially oriented incisions.
3. It is useful for the surgeon to map out the potential location of future mastectomy incisions, because the tumor biopsy scar should be fashioned such that it could be easily encompassed within the possible mastectomy skin ellipse.
4. The biopsy cavity need not be reapproximated or drained, as the seroma accumulation will actually serve to restore the original breast shape and size.

Open surgical incisional biopsy is occasionally necessary for definitive diagnosis of large, bulky breast tumors. The incisional biopsy resects a portion of the palpable mass. The surgeon should select a portion of the mass that appears to harbor viable tumor as opposed to necrotic tissue, as the latter may yield a non-diagnostic specimen, and the skin suture closure may fail to heal.

Although LMICs are less likely to have widely available mammography screening programs, some patients will undergo mammography and nonpalpable but suspicious lesions will occasionally be identified. The biopsy maneuvers of choice would be mammographically guided (stereotactic) percutaneous needle biopsy or sonographically guided percutaneous needle biopsy (if the lesion can be confirmed by ultrasound imaging). As noted above, these procedures should be accompanied by insertion of a radio-opaque marker. If image-guided needle biopsy is not available, then the patient should be referred to undergo image-guided wire localization open surgical biopsy. This procedure involves repeat imaging on the day of surgery, and the radiologist then inserts a localizing wire into the breast to identify the anatomic site of the lesion requiring resectional biopsy. If the patient has undergone a prior image-guided needle biopsy of a nonpalpable abnormality, then the radio-opaque marker serves as the target for the localizing wire. Once the wire has been inserted, the patient is then brought to the operating room for surgery, which can be performed under local anesthesia (usually with sedation) or general anesthesia, depending on patient preference and institutional resources. The surgical incision should be fashioned to directly overlie the target, based upon the mammographic images. Mammography should always be performed on the surgical specimen itself to confirm that the target lesion and/or radio-opaque marker have been included within the resected tissue prior to submitting the specimen to pathology.

Standard Breast Cancer Treatment Options

Once an invasive breast cancer has been diagnosed, the standard treatment must address three principles: (i) resecting the primary cancer site; (ii) treating the entire breast so that microscopic/occult foci of disease in other quadrants are eliminated; and (iii) axillary surgery for staging of the cancer as well as obtaining durable regional control of disease. These principles can be addressed with a single modality when mastectomy is selected, as the breast is then removed in its entirety and axillary surgery is performed through the mastectomy incision. Breast-conserving therapy utilizes both surgery (lumpectomy plus axillary surgery) and whole-breast radiation to address these principles.

Mastectomy is the oldest form of treatment for breast cancer, and the original Halsteadian radical mastectomy (initially offered to patients at the beginning of the twentieth century) consisted of complete removal of the breast en bloc with the underlying pectoralis major and minor musculature as well as levels 1–3 of the axillary nodal basin. While this operation indeed provided local control surgery for breast cancer in a pre-screening era when most patients presented with locally advanced diseased that often involved the chest wall muscles, it is extremely disfiguring. As earlier detection of breast cancer improved during the twentieth century with heightened awareness of the disease, this procedure became largely obsolete. Furthermore, as effective chemotherapy regimens became available for breast cancer, the option of neoadjuvant treatment (see below) became a viable strategy for patients presenting with bulky tumors, improving their resectability by mastectomy with preservation of the pectoralis muscles.

A standard total mastectomy (also called a "simple" mastectomy) involves the creation of elliptical incisions superior and inferior to the nipple-areolar complex. Skin flaps are then developed using the clavicle as the palpable superior border, the lateral edge of sternum as the palpable medial border, the inframammary fold as the inferior border, and the latissimus dorsi edge as the lateral border. The breast is then dissected off of the chest wall en bloc with the fascia overlying the pectoralis major muscle. The pectoralis major and minor muscles are preserved intact. A closed system drain is usually left in place under the anterior skin flaps, and brought out to exit the skin through a separate puncture site 2–3 cm along the inferolateral aspect of the mastectomy scar. Although some centers are evaluating the feasibility of nipple-sparing mastectomy, the conventional, standard-of-care mastectomy involves sacrifice of the nipple-areolar complex.

Patients who undergo mastectomy for breast cancer may be candidates for either immediate or delayed breast reconstruction. Breast reconstruction can be performed with autogenous tissue (transverse rectus abdominis myocutaneous [TRAM] flap) or with implants or a combination of both (latissimus dorsi flap with implant). Implant reconstruction is usually performed as a staged procedure: a tissue expander is inserted subpectorally as the initial procedure and is then inflated as an office-based procedure by the plastic surgeon prior to returning the patient to the operating room for the final exchange to the permanent implant. Unfortunately, there is a definite scarcity of plastic surgeons that are skilled with breast reconstruction in LMICs, but mastectomy patients should nonetheless be informed that delayed reconstruction remains an option, even decades after a mastectomy has been performed, should the resources become available.

Breast conserving therapy for breast cancer is optimally offered to patients meeting the following eligibility criteria:

1. Patient has a personal desire for breast preservation.

2. Patient has access to a radiation facility such that daily treatment for six consecutive weeks is feasible.

3. Patient has undergone a margin-negative lumpectomy. It should be noted that there is no universally accepted definition for the optimal negative margin thickness; while it is clearly improper to transect cancer and leave overt disease in the surgical bed, the acceptable microscopically negative margins have been described as ranging from the absence of any cancer cells at the microscopic lumpectomy surface to a 10 mm negative margin. Furthermore, while a more widely negative margin tends to correlate with improved local control of disease, this benefit must be balanced against the cosmetic disadvantage of resecting a larger-volume lumpectomy.

4. Patient has a mammogram that is consistent with unicentric disease; mammograms revealing diffuse suspicious-appearing microcalcifications may be indicating the presence of diffuse ductal carcinoma *in situ* beyond the resected lumpectomy bed, and this residual disease will be poorly controlled by breast radiation. In cases where the tumor itself is associated with microcalcifications, a post-lumpectomy mammogram should be performed to confirm complete resection of all mammographically apparent sites of disease.

5. Patient has no contraindication to breast radiation, such as pregnancy, prior chest wall radiation, or scleroderma.

The lumpectomy procedure should be performed with adherence to the same surgical principles described above for the surgical excisional biopsy technique. In addition, it is helpful to leave 6–10 radio-opaque clips at the perimeter of the lumpectomy bed to facilitate planning of the subsequent radiation tangents.

Axillary surgery for invasive breast cancer has historically included an anatomically defined resection of the axillary levels 1 and 2 fat pad, located inferolateral and just deep (respectively) to the pectoralis minor muscle. This will typically yield 10–20 lymph nodes embedded in the fat pad, each of which should be analyzed pathologically for the presence of metastatic cancer. The level 3 fat pad (located superomedial to the pectoralis minor) is left intact unless palpable disease is identified in this region intraoperatively. This standard axillary lymph node dissection (ALND) serves the dual purpose of staging the breast cancer and providing durable regional control of disease. The former goal is important for prognostication and for defining the benefits of adjuvant systemic therapy; the extent of ALND is related to this goal. Removal of level 3 is unnecessary because skip metastases to the apex of the axilla (with completely negative levels 1 and 2) will only occur in fewer than 5% of cases, and routine removal of level 3 increases the risk of lymphedema. On the other hand, removal of level 2 is required (despite the risk of lymphedema) because skip metastases to the mid-axilla (with a negative level 1) can occur in 25% of cases. The latter goal of providing regional disease control is especially relevant in LMICs because the majority of these breast cancer cases will be node-positive. It should be noted that patients fortunate enough to be identified with only preinvasive breast cancer (ductal carcinoma in situ) will not require an ALND.

The technique of the ALND is very important, and the surgeon must be cautious about identifying and preserving several neurovascular structures completely intact, as a disruption of the long thoracic nerve will cause a winged scapula because of loss of serratus anterior function; disruption of the thoracodorsal nerve will denervate the latissimus dorsi muscle; and damage of the axillary vein can cause severe intraoperative hemorrhage and/or deep vein thrombosis. Patients undergoing mastectomy will have the ALND performed through the mastectomy wound, and the mastectomy plus the ALND is called a modified radical mastectomy. Lumpectomy patients have a separate incision created for the ALND at approximately the lower aspect of the axillary hairline and extending from the anterior to the posterior axillary lines. The ALND can be performed from an anterosuperior approach, with initial incision of the clavipectoral fascia and identification of the axillary vein. The thoracodorsal and long thoracic nerves are identified superiorly and traced inferiorly, with resection of the axillary fat pad lying anterior to all of these structures. Alternatively, the surgeon can incise the fascia lateral to the latissimus dorsi muscle along its inferior aspect as an initial approach, working medially to identify the thoracodorsal bundle. One of the crossing branches draining into the thoracodorsal vein is then traced further medially until reaching the serratus anterior muscle; the long thoracic nerve can be reliably identified at the junction of where this venous branch enters the muscle. The dissection then proceeds in a superior fashion, resecting all of the axillary fat lying anterior to the two neurovascular structures until the axillary vein is reached (noted by following the thoracodorsal vein until it drains into the axillary vein; at this point the thoracodorsal nerve will be seen passing posterior to the axillary vein). The inferolateral approach is particularly useful in cases of prior axillary surgery or bulky axillary disease, because the critical neurovascular structures are safely identified prior to entering nodal metastases or preexisting surgical bed. With both surgical approaches, the pectoralis minor muscle is retracted medially at the level of the axillary vein so that the level 2 contents can be extirpated and level 3 can be explored both by palpation and by visual inspection. The axillary fat pad is sent for complete pathology processing, and a closed-system drain is left in the axillary wound (with the tip cut just short of the axillary vein) and brought out to exit through a puncture site inferior to the axillary incision.

Modified radical mastectomy cases typically have two drains left in place; one to drain the axillary flaps and a second to drain the axilla. Lumpectomy cases undergoing ALND will typically have only the single axillary drain. These drains are left in place until the output volume is lower than 30 cc per 24 hours for 2 consecutive days. Wherever feasible, patients undergoing ALND should be educated regarding measures to avoid lymphedema: daily arm exercises; weight control; and avoidance of any breaks in the skin of the ipsilateral upper extremity.

The frequency of node-negative breast cancer has risen dramatically in populations characterized by successful mammographic screening, and this prompted the development of minimally invasive, lower-morbidity axillary staging procedures such as lymphatic mapping and sentinel lymph node (SLN) biopsy. Lymphatic mapping is based upon the biologic rationale that a mapping agent(s) can be injected into mammary tissue, taken up by intramammary lymphatics (replicating the pathway traversed by metastatic breast cancer), and deposited into the primary lymph nodes responsible for draining the cancerous breast. These primary (sentinel) lymph nodes are removed, and if they are negative for metastatic breast cancer, then the patient can be declared node-negative, thereby avoiding the morbidity of the staging ALND. Patients with cancerous SLNs undergo completion ALND for definitive regional control of disease and to quantify volume of axillary disease. Options for the mapping agents include blue dye (methylene blue, which can be associated with skin necrosis if injected too superficially in the skin; or lymphazurin, which is associated with 1% incidence of anaphylactic allergic reaction) or radioactive isotope (e.g., technetium-labeled sulfur colloid). The blue-stained sentinel nodes are identified by visual inspection and the radioactive nodes are identified by use of an intraoperative gamma detector. While dual-agent mapping is commonplace in HICs, the expense of the intraoperative gamma detector may preclude isotope mapping in LMICs. There is a learning curve associated with the lymphatic mapping technology. Before progressing to SLN biopsy as a stand-alone procedure to stage the axilla, surgeons developing their initial experience should perform at least 30 cases where they identify the sentinel node(s) and perform a concomitant ALND to document a false negative rate of no higher than 5%.

Indications for Adjuvant Systemic Therapy

All patients with invasive breast cancer are at risk for harboring distant organ micrometastases. Adjuvant systemic therapy can eradicate this disease and prolong survival. All systemic therapies are associated with cost and potential toxicity; their use should therefore be limited to patients with the highest risk of metastatic disease. Node-positive breast cancer patients clearly fall into this category. Node-negative breast cancers that are hormone-receptor negative and/or HER2/neu-positive are also at increased risk for requiring adjuvant systemic therapy, especially if the primary tumor is larger than 5–10 mm in size. Identification of breast cancer patients that benefit from systemic therapy is therefore highly dependent upon knowledge of molecular marker patterns. These patterns also determine choice of adjuvant systemic therapy agents. Endocrine therapy (tamoxifen at any age; aromatase inhibitors for postmenopausal patients) is indicated for hormone receptor-positive cases; trastuzumab is indicated for HER2/neu-overexpressing tumors. Chemotherapy (usually doxorubicin-based therapy with or without a taxane) is indicated for hormone receptor-negative, HER2/neu-overexpressing, and triple-negative tumors that require adjuvant systemic therapy. Determination of chemotherapy value (in addition to endocrine therapy) in node-negative, hormone receptor-positive, HER2/neu-negative breast cancer can be challenging, as tumor size is a relatively crude measure of the inherent aggressiveness of these tumors. In HICs, a comprehensive genetic profile called Oncotype DX testing can be performed, yielding a recurrence score that reliably distinguishes the biologically high-risk from low-risk tumors. A major challenge in LMICs is that immunohistochemical resources to assess molecular marker expression and financial resources usually preclude the option of genetic profiling. It should be noted that recent reports suggest that, in the presence of metastases women who respond well to chemotherapy, there is no overall survival benefit from resection of the primary mass or the related lymph nodes; however, resection for palliation may be still be required.

Indications and Applications for Neoadjuvant Systemic Therapy

Patients with inoperable breast cancer (disease that is fixed to the chest wall or axilla; disease associated with skin involvement beyond a standard mastectomy skin ellipse; or inflammatory breast cancer) are clearly candidates for primary (preoperative; neoadjuvant) chemotherapy in order to become surgical candidates. Patients with bulky but resectable breast cancer will become improved surgical candidates by virtue of disease downstaging. Extent of clinical response is an excellent surrogate marker for chemosensitivity, and patients in whom the neoadjuvant chemotherapy completely obliterates the cancer (complete pathologic response) have an optimized survival rate. Tumor downstaging is occasionally brisk enough to transform a patient into a lumpectomy candidate. In any patient where breast conservation may be ultimately desirable, it is therefore important to have a radio-opaque marker at the site of initial tumor. If the patient experiences a complete clinical response, then the marker serves as the target for a wire-localization lumpectomy following the delivery of neoadjuvant chemotherapy. Tumors associated with mammographically detected microcalcifications can have the calcifications serve as the ultimate target for image-guided lumpectomy. Patients who have diffuse microcalcifications, multicentric disease that cannot be encompassed within a single margin-negative lumpectomy, and inflammatory breast cancer patients are considered ineligible for breast conservation, regardless of extent of chemotherapy responsiveness. Clearly, mammographic services (pre- and post-neoadjuvant chemotherapy) are important for optimizing the benefits of this treatment sequence. Patients with hormone receptor-negative, triple-negative, and high-grade disease tend to have the most brisk response to neoadjuvant chemotherapy. Neoadjuvant endocrine therapy can also be offered to selected patients with bulky disease, but the pace of tumor downstaging tends to be sluggish and this approach can only be used in cases where the hormone estrogen receptor status has been definitively documented as being positive.

Indications for Extended-Field, Regional Radiation and/or Postmastectomy Radiation

Just as adjuvant systemic therapy is indicated for patients at high risk for distant organ micrometastases, some patients will be at high risk for chest wall and regional nodal recurrence because of microscopic occult disease in the soft tissues beyond the surgical field (anterior chest wall skin; internal mammary nodes; and supraclavicular and apical axillary nodes). These patients benefit from extended-field radiation treatments, which include the breast as well as apical axilla, supraclavicular nodes, and internal mammary chain for lumpectomy cases; and include the anterior chest wall as well as these nodal basins in the mastectomy cases. Standard indications for this treatment include: (i) inflammatory breast cancer at diagnosis, (ii) node-positive tumors larger than 5 cm, and (iii) tumors of any size associated with at least four metastatic lymph nodes.

Nonmalignant Causes of Breast Masses

The majority of breast masses are related to benign fibrocystic densities such as cysts, fibroadenomas, or areas of dominant nodularity. Lactating adenomas can be seen during pregnancy and in nursing mothers. Diabetic mastopathy (sometimes called granulomatous mastitis) can cause diffuse breast nodularity or a discrete mass effect, and is more commonly seen in patients with poorly controlled, insulin-dependent diabetes mellitus. Infectious problems such as mastitis or breast abscess will require management with antibiotics or incision and drainage, respectively. Clinicians in LMICs should also have a heightened awareness of tuberculosis as another cause of granulomatous mastitis. Biopsy is generally necessary to definitively distinguish benign from malignant causes of dominant, suspicious-appearing breast masses.

COMMENTARY

Ouyang Lizhi, China

In recent years, the quality of health care in China has dramatically improved as a result of economic development. However, like other LMICs, with the increasingly Western lifestyle, working environment, and diet, the incidence of breast cancer in China has soared in recent decades. According to the latest data released by the National Cancer Center and Disease Prevention and Ministry of Health of China, rough statistics on the incidence of breast cancer are 41.64 cases per 10,000 people per year. Breast cancer prevention, diagnosis, and standardized treatment have become the focus of health authorities.

In this chapter, Dr. Lisa Newman and her colleagues have provided a detailed explanation of the etiology, diagnosis, surgery, radiation therapy, and medical treatment guidelines for breast cancer. There are several breast cancer diagnostic criteria and treatment guidelines issued by various academic authorities, such as the NCCN annual cancer treatment guidelines. However, only a few are specifically designed for LMICs. The efforts and work of Dr. Newman and her colleagues in this field will greatly benefit breast surgeons in LMICs. The book provides concise, practical, and feasible policy guidance. I recommend that all health workers in LMICs read it closely and apply it into clinical practice, teaching, and scientific research.

COMMENTARY

Ruth Damuse, Haiti

Breast cancer remains a leading cause of morbidity and mortality among women in general, and this is especially true among young women in LMICs.[11] In Haiti, there is no national screening program. There only one public cancer program, which began in 2011 and offers care to cancer patients.[2] For this and other reasons, patients present late to clinics with very advanced disease. Patients have many reasons for delayed presentation: lack of education, failure to recognize a breast mass as important, lack of access to care, and fear of treatment-related costs.[22]

In Haiti, no radiation therapy is available; this changes the general approach to care for breast cancer patients. Consequently, breast-conserving surgery and oncoplastic techniques are not considered for treatment for patients with invasive breast cancer.

Furthermore, the limitations of access to a pathology laboratory influence the choice of the type of mastectomy performed. Without sentinel lymph node biopsy and the possibility of having frozen sections and assessment of margins, most of the time radical modified mastectomy is chosen over simple mastectomy. Therefore, surgical outcomes for patients are often more complicated than in countries that have radiation and pathology to guide care.

Therefore, just as in HICs, LMICs face breast cancer as a leading cause of morbidity and mortality. However, unlike HICs, LMICs lack some important components of comprehensive cancer care. We have much work to do to grow oncology care in Haiti to care for our future patients.

22

Obstetrics

Reinou S. Groen
Adam L. Kushner

Introduction

As the majority of the estimated 358,000 pregnancy-related and 5 million neonatal birth asphyxia deaths occur in low- to middle-income countries (LMICs), those who work in these settings will require a basic knowledge of emergency obstetric care.[1] As many of these deaths are preventable by appropriate and timely medical and surgical interventions, this chapter provides practical insights for clinicians who might be confronted with such issues. This chapter is organized by pregnancy period for ease of reference and describes the most essential medical problems encountered in pregnancy. It is by no means a complete reference guide for obstetrics. Aside from using this text, we encourage all clinicians to familiarize themselves with any guidelines that are locally available. For more detailed information, we recommend referring to *Primary Surgery,* edited by Maurice King, which has excellent chapters on obstetrics in remote settings.[2] Also, *Integrated Management of Pregnancy and Childbirth,* published by the World Health Organization (WHO), is a useful reference for specific detailed information.[3]

First and Second Trimester

In LMICs, every physician should be prepared to care for pregnant or lactating women as routine medical and surgical treatment often needs to be adjusted for the mother and/or the (unborn) child. Although maternal and neonatal morbidity and mortality can be significantly reduced with appropriate antenatal care, in the first half of pregnancy, a surgeon may be consulted for postabortion hemorrhage or an ectopic pregnancy, particularly if ruptured. Keep in mind that a spontaneous abortion can be a result of a number of things, including severe anemia, malaria, syphilis, or an induced abortion, so appropriate screening and treatment is vital.

Diagnosis of Pregnancy

Before 12 weeks of gestation, a pregnancy may be diagnosed with a urine-pregnancy test or ultrasound if available. Pregnancy should be considered in every woman of reproductive age who consults a physician for any reason.

Anesthesia and Surgery in a Pregnant Patient

When elective surgery is needed for a pregnant woman, if possible, delay the procedure until the second trimester and, ideally, until 6 weeks postpartum. Anesthesia and surgery increase the risk of premature labor and can have teratogenic effects on the unborn fetus between 4–8 weeks' gestation. Abdominal surgery under general anesthesia has a much greater risk than a procedure done on an extremity under local anesthesia. If major (abdominal) surgery cannot be delayed due to maternal conditions, take the following precautions noted.[4] Most of these considerations are also appropriate for patients needing a caesarean section (C-section).

1. Depending on the gestational age, prepare for the delivery of a premature neonate. A fundal height of 25 cm or more is generally believed to coincide with a viable fetus, although survival is severely dependent on the level of neonatal care. Check the fetal heart rate and maternal cervix for any evidence of dilation before the operation. To estimate gestational age by measuring the abdomen, one can use a measuring tape starting at the pubic symphysis to the fundus. For example, a symphysis to fundal height of 33 cm is ~33 weeks' gestation. The umbilicus is ~20 weeks gestational age (GA), and measurements are relatively reliable within 3 weeks GA once the uterus grows beyond the umbilicus unless growth restriction or multiple gestations is a factor. Prevent placental hypoperfusion and subsequent fetal hypoxia by positioning the patient with a left lateral tilt (to prevent vena cava syndrome) and aim to prevent maternal hypotension. This maneuver augments maternal cardiac output, 20% of which is shunted to the fetal-placental unit.

2. Be aware that the risk of aspiration is increased from the second trimester onward due to the relaxing effect of progesterone on the lower esophageal sphincter. In the third trimester, this is combined with increased intra-abdominal pressure.

3. Use local or regional (spinal) anesthesia, if possible. Ketamine and other intravenous (IV) anesthetics should be avoided as they can cause uterine hyperactivity. Of note, pregnant women usually require a reduced amount of anesthesia to be effective; this also includes spinal anesthesia.

4. Do not manipulate the uterus during surgery, if not needed. Don't touch, don't squeeze.

5. Postprocedure, secondary to monitoring the fetal heart rate, contractions should be monitored and a pelvic exam done regularly. Early labor can be silent or difficult to identify in a postoperative patient.

6. Administer and adjust a tocolytic as prescribed in the section on premature labor when the cervix shortens and contractions are observed. Indomethacin 50 mg PR × 1 postoperatively and PO q 6 hours × 24–48 hours is quite effective to stop contractions if available to be used before 32 weeks' gestation.

7. Pregnant and postpartum women are in a hypercoagulable state and are at a higher risk for thromboembolic events postoperatively. Prophylactic anticoagulation doses are safe to give at the time of surgery.

Abortion

Approximately 15% of all pregnancies will end in a spontaneous abortion. In an LMIC, most women will not seek medical attention for this condition and usually only the women who experience complications present to a health facility. Retained products of conception can be the source of hemorrhage or sepsis, and perforation of the uterus might follow an induced abortion. Treatment of the various types of abortions can include both medical and surgical interventions.

Diagnostics for an abortion include a pelvic exam, (urine) pregnancy test, and ultrasound, if available. There are several categories of abortion:

1. Threatened abortion: Bleeding and cramping but no opening of the cervical os and no complete or partial expulsion of products of conception. This pregnancy can still go to full term.

2. Inevitable abortion: Products of conception are not viable and will ultimately result in an abortion, at the time of examination, the cervical os might be open or not. Bleeding and cramping can be present.

3. Incomplete abortion: The cervical os is open and retained products of conception remain.

4. Complete abortion: All products of conception are expelled; however, there might be some cramping and scant bleeding, but the cervical os has again closed.

5. Septic abortion: Foul-smelling discharge, fever, and abdominal pain.

Categories 1 and 4 are difficult to distinguish without an ultrasound; however, both can be managed with rest and observation, if the woman is hemodynamically stable. One should keep in mind a differential diagnosis of menorrhagia, cervicitis, cervical cancer, molar pregnancy, and ectopic pregnancy. Vaginal bleeding in the second trimester can also be due to placenta previa, abruption of the placenta, or a ruptured uterus (see section on third trimester).

Category 3, an incomplete abortion, needs evacuation of the remaining conception products, either medical or surgical. This can also be initiated in case of an inevitable abortion, especially if the mother is showing signs of sepsis which can occur with cervical incompetence and prolonged exposure of the membranes to vaginal flora.

A septic abortion needs ampicillin and gentamycin or amoxicillin, metronidazole, and gentamycin IV for at least until the patient is afebrile. As the retained products are the causes of the sepsis, they need to be evacuated. Medical treatment has the preference, since an infected uterus is easily perforated. A septic abortion can be the result of an induced abortion. All locally induced abortions should receive tetanus boosters or immunoglobulin, according to their immunization status and Rhogam pending their Rh status.

Medical Treatment for Incomplete Abortion

For minimal bleeding with an incomplete abortion, a trial of misoprostol (400–800 mcg) vaginally or buccally can be given along with a nonsteroidal anti-inflammatory (NSAID). Check the patient hourly for bleeding, perform a pelvic exam every 4 hours, and repeat the misoprostol and NSAIDs every 8 hours. If expulsion of the products occurs, the patient can be sent to a general ward for 24 hours of observation. If bleeding becomes heavy or the products do not expulse after three insertions of misoprostol, surgical intervention is required.

Surgical Treatment for Incomplete Abortion

After administering prophylactic antibiotics (e.g., ampicillin 2 gram IV), the retained products of conception can be removed with curettage (Figure 22.1) or manual vacuum aspiration (MVA). The most feared complication of these procedures is perforation of the uterus, which is more likely with the curettage than with the MVA. The chance of perforation can also be reduced by knowing the position of the uterus, whether it is anteverted or retroverted, and aligning the uterus with traction on the cervix with a cervical clamp and gently using the largest curette or MVA device. MVA of retained products of conception is associated with less bleeding and a lower risk of perforation than curettage and is, therefore, the preferred method. If there is no availability of curettage or MVA, digital curettage can be attempted; however, this has a higher failure rate, since membranes are often difficult to remove. Anesthesia by sedation with diazepam and analgesics such as acetaminophen, NSAIDs, or ketamine can be used. Local cervical anesthesia with 0.5–1% lidocaine should be used, if dilatation is needed. Spinal or general anesthesia is possible but requires an anesthesiologist or nurse anesthetist, and the patient will need close perioperative monitoring.

Induced Abortion

An induced abortion can be performed with relative safety up to 12 weeks of gestation. If available, mifepristone given 48 hours prior to a dose of misoprostol (400–800 mcg) is usually sufficient after repeating the misoprostol 3 times every 8 hours; however, if this does not work, specifically in the second trimester a Foley catheter could be introduced into the cervical os and inflated with 30 cc of saline. With time, the cervical os will dilate and the catheter will fall out; soon after, expulsion of the products of conception will follow. This is uncomfortable for the patient, and analgesia is important. Inducing an abortion of

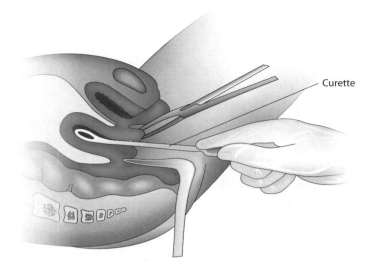

Curette

FIGURE 22.1 Curettage. Coutin AS et al. *Obstetrics in Remote Settings: Practical Guide for Non-specialized Health Care Professionals*. Geneva: Medecins Sans Frontieres; 2007, p. 167.

a healthy pregnancy is generally more difficult than for a missed abortion and more often requires surgical intervention via curettage or MVA. Knowledge of local guidelines and regulations is imperative. While some countries support abortion in cases of maternal illness, fetus malformations, or sexual violence, other countries always consider it an illegal practice. For induction of labor after 16 weeks, refer to the section on eclampsia.

Postabortion Care

The most common complications after an abortion are infection, perforation, and hemorrhage. In cases of a surgical intervention, long-term comorbidities can include cervical stenosis or Asherman's syndrome, where adhesions within the uterus prevent normal menstruation and normal conception. Additionally, Rhesus incompatibility is possible if the woman is Rh negative, but this can be prevented by giving Rh immunoglobulin postabortion (RhoGAM 300 mcg IM).

When the removed products are foul smelling or white/green-colored, or if the woman develops a fever, antibiotics should be started immediately. A broad spectrum combination such as amoxicillin-clavulanate with gentamicin or ampicillin, metronidazole, and gentamicin should be given. Oral antibiotics should continue for at least 5 days after a fever subsides. Also think about tetanus immunization, which may or may not have been previously administered based on national vaccination programs.

The most feared complication, perforation of the uterus, is most likely suspected at the time of curettage and may be the result of an improperly induced abortion. Treatment is dependent on the clinical presentation. Broad spectrum antibiotics should be administered whether or not there is a fever. Laparotomy is warranted if there is suspicion of bowel perforation, peritonitis, or intra-abdominal hemorrhage. In cases of hemorrhage, the uterus should be repaired and may need a hysterectomy. In every case of uterine perforation, the patient should be strongly counseled to

deliver any future pregnancies in a hospital with surgical facilities. Contraceptive methods should also be discussed.

Ectopic Pregnancy

A pregnancy occurring outside of the uterine endometrium is termed an ectopic pregnancy. The most common site of implantation is in a fallopian tube, but this can also occur in the cervix, in the isthmus (the entry point of the fallopian tube in the uterine cavity and termed a corneal pregnancy), or intra-abdominally.

The diagnosis of an ectopic pregnancy can be quite challenging without an ultrasound and/or diagnostic laparoscopy, since the classic triad of amenorrhea, bleeding, and severe abdominal pain may not always be present. Ultimately, the diagnosis may only be made at laparotomy (laparoscopy if available) for an acute abdomen. Pre-operative culdocentesis, aspiration of the Pouch of Douglas via a needle inserted vaginally and via the posterior fornix, might help to diagnose a ruptured ectopic pregnancy when old blood is aspirated. However, this procedure is not very sensitive. Abdominal para-centesis is sometimes better than culdocentesis, as pelvic adhesions are common. Consider an ectopic pregnancy for every woman of childbearing age with an acute abdomen.

Treatment options for an ectopic pregnancy are dependent on the gestational age, symptoms, and future fertility considerations. Methotrexate is an option in early pregnancy (an unruptured ectopic mass, with no heartbeat and total sac diameter of less than 3.5 cm) but not always available. Most ectopic pregnancies in LMICs tend to present late and ruptured. Operation is often the treatment of choice. Also remember RhoGAM 300 mcg IM if the woman is Rhesus negative.

Procedure Options for Tubal Pregnancy

Laparoscopy is the preferred method of treating an ectopic pregnancy, but the operation can also be done through a Pfannenstiel

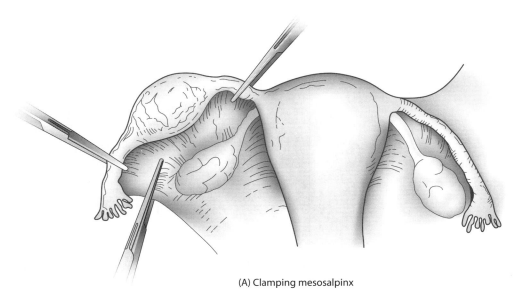

(A) Clamping mesosalpinx

FIGURE 22.2 Salpingectomy in tubal pregnancy. Mathai M et al. *Managing Complications in Pregnancy and Childbirth.* Geneva: World Health Organization; 2007, p. 362.

or lower midline incision depending on the certainty of the diagnosis. With a midline incision, one is never wrong, especially if the diagnosis appears to be of intestinal origin or if mobilization of the organs in the pelvis is challenging due to adhesions from earlier pelvic infections. Auto transfusion of the abdominal blood is possible, if the gestational sac with an embryo is still intact. The safest and easiest procedure for an ectopic pregnancy, which will most likely be found in a fallopian tube, is a tubectomy. The affected fallopian tube is identified, clamps are placed on either side of the mass containing the products of conception, the tube is cut, and each end separately tied twice, since these ends can bleed easily. If there are not too many adhesions in the true pelvis, salpingectomy, resection of the entire fallopian tube with fimbriae and products of conception, is also possible.

Similarly, both procedures can be performed in the case of a ruptured ectopic pregnancy; however, thorough cleansing of the abdomen is required to assure that all products of conception are removed. If unruptured, one can consider a salpingostomy and hydrodissection of the ectopic pregnancy, if the patient is young and future fertility is of consideration. Often, this is not a viable option as tubal distortion is greater at increasing gestational ages, making this procedure more complicated. Any patient who has undergone tubal surgery has a higher risk for ectopic pregnancy in the future.

If a tubal pregnancy is adjacent to the ampulla, one can try to squeeze the products of conception away from the uterus. This technique is not related to increased recurrences. The general recurrence rate for a tubal pregnancy is 7% to 18%.[5]

Pregnancies in the Cervix or Isthmus

These types of pregnancies are life threatening. If they are not treated in a timely manner with methotrexate, a hysterectomy is often required. If possible, consider transferring patients with these conditions to a tertiary care hospital with adequately trained gynecologists. Also note that a cervical pregnancy can mimic cervical cancer, which is much more common.

Intra-abdominal Pregnancy

An intra-abdominal pregnancy is a rare condition where a fetus develops completely outside the uterus and fallopian tubes. Aside from the risk to the fetus, many of the morbidities are due to the placenta embedding on various intra-abdominal organs. Symptoms may include abdominal pain or discomfort, rectal bleeding (due to embedding of the placenta onto a hollow viscus), bowel obstruction, or intra-abdominal hemorrhage, leading to shock and death. Signs for recognizing an intra-abdominal pregnancy include the following: easily palpable fetal parts, rectal bleeding, or a mobile small uterus on pelvic examination with a positive urine pregnancy test, and an abdominal mass. Diagnosis can be made with ultrasound or by laparotomy. The maternal mortality is as high as 10%, and fetal demise occurs in up to 90% of cases. As soon as the diagnosis is made, the fetus should be delivered by laparotomy, regardless of gestational age. The most significant problem after removal of the fetus will be management of the placenta. If the placenta is manually detached, there will most likely be brisk bleeding and injury to the underlying organ(s). Therefore, it is best to leave the placenta in place; tie and cut the umbilical cord close to the placenta, and it will eventually be spontaneously resorbed. If bleeding occurs from the placental site and it is on the bowel, a resection can also be performed for the patient's safety as expectant management in this case could lead to life-threatening blood loss. In areas with limited blood bank availability, it may be best to do a primary bowel resection, depending on the circumstances.

Molar Pregnancy

The incidence of a molar pregnancy, or a gestational trophoblastic neoplasm, can be as high as 1.2% of the total number of pregnancies. The incidence is higher for the very young or very old women.[6] In LMICs, molar pregnancies will probably present in an advanced stage, often in the second or even early third trimester, and may contain a well-developed fetus in the case of a partial molar pregnancy. Advanced gestational age carries a great risk for the mother of metastasis (most commonly to the lungs) and, therefore, it is warranted to end the pregnancy as soon as the diagnosis is made, regardless of gestational age. Be aware that molar pregnancies have a tendency to lead to uterine atony and retained products of conception and need, by definition, to be suctioned after expulsion of the fetus and molar products to prevent regrowth of the molar pregnancy or metastasis. The expulsion can be achieved in a similar manner as for an induced abortion. If there is significant hemorrhage, this can be managed as described in the section on postpartum hemorrhage.

Postexpulsion, the woman needs to be followed carefully, including pregnancy tests, sonography, and chest X-rays. The woman also needs to be counseled for contraception and followed for at least one year. As soon as a choriocarcinoma is suspected (e.g., continuous vaginal bleeding, abdominal pains, shortness of breath), chemotherapy is needed, and the woman needs to be referred to a higher level of care.

Third Trimester

In the third trimester of pregnancy, a woman has hopefully been seen in an antenatal clinic for screening and prophylactic therapy or treatment of anemia, malaria, and syphilis. At this stage of the pregnancy, she is at risk for hypertensive disorders. A pregnant woman at this time can have significant gastroesophageal reflux and constipation and is susceptible to the development of vena cava syndrome, which results in dizziness when lying flat due to the pressure of the uterus on the inferior vena cava. This can occur as early as 20 weeks' gestation.

Hypertensive Disorders

Hypertensive disorders in pregnancy can be categorized as follows:

1. Chronic hypertension
2. Pregnancy-induced hypertension
3. Preeclampsia
4. Eclampsia

A separate category is HELLP syndrome: hemolysis and elevated liver enzymes and low platelets. This complication is on the spectrum of hypertensive disorders of pregnancy and should not be managed expectantly. These patients should be delivered as they have evidence of transient end-organ damage at any gestational age. Some authors have recommended steroid administration if delivery is before 34 weeks. One needs to be mindful of the potential for rapid maternal decompensation in the interim.

Chronic Hypertension

Since most women in LMICs will not have had their blood pressure measured prior to being pregnant, few will present with a long-standing diagnosis of chronic hypertension. Physiologically, maternal blood pressure drops in the second trimester of pregnancy. Therefore, any pregnant woman prior to 20 weeks who presents with hypertension (blood pressure greater than 140/90) should be considered as having chronic hypertension. A chronic hypertensive patient is at greater risk for preeclampsia, but the treatment to lower her blood pressure should not be too aggressive, as the woman and placental perfusion are accustomed to the higher blood pressure.

Pregnancy-Induced Hypertension

Pregnancy-induced hypertension is defined as elevated blood pressure (blood pressure greater than 140/90) diagnosed after 20 weeks of gestational age. The preferred treatment for pregnancy-induced hypertension is labetalol starting at doses of 200 mg PO q 8–12 hours and can be titrated up to a total of 2400 mg daily maximum dose. Labetalol has a long-standing safety profile in pregnancy. Methyldopa starting at 250 mg bid up to 500mg tid is a reasonable alternative. If good dating is available for women with pregnancy-induced hypertension induction of labor should be considered around 39 weeks, or earlier if preeclampsia develops.

Preeclampsia

Preeclampsia is defined as pregnancy-induced hypertension with proteinuria. Severe preeclampsia manifests with a systolic blood pressure of >160 mmHg or a diastolic blood pressure over 110 mmHg and can involve symptomatic headache, visual disturbance, upper abdominal pain, and/or signs of hyperreflexia, oliguria, or pulmonary edema. For patients with preeclampsia, aggressive anti-hypertensive therapy and close monitoring of the blood pressure is warranted in order to reduce the risk of developing severe preeclampsia. For cases of severe preeclampsia, delivery of the fetus with seizure prophylaxis using magnesium sulfate is the treatment of choice (Box 22.1). The safety of the woman is given the priority in severe preeclampsia; delivery is warranted despite the gestational age. Some clinicians argue that in premature cases of less than 34 weeks, magnesium sulfate along with dexamethasone/betamethason (12 mg IM 2 days) should be used to gain an additional 48 hours of fetal maturation. This can be done with close maternal observation in the hospital ward, and the patient should be monitored for signs of worsening hypertension, end-organ effects, eclampsia, or worsening fetal status. Delivery after 34 weeks is warranted.

Eclampsia

If a pregnant woman presents to a health facility with a history of seizures or presents with a seizure, the most likely diagnosis is eclampsia. However, the differential diagnosis includes common reasons for seizures in the tropics: cerebral malaria, epilepsy, typhoid fever, and meningitis. Immediate administration of magnesium sulfate is needed with a continuation of magnesium therapy for at least 24 hours after delivery (Box 22.1). Seizures can occur more than 24 hours postpartum. Delivery should be induced immediately without waiting for additional fetal maturation. If induction of labor is not successful, within 12 hours or in case of clinical deterioration a caesarean section should quickly follow.

In cases of severe preeclampsia and eclampsia, maximal supportive therapy is needed in an intensive care unit (ICU) or

---

BOX 22.1   MAGNESIUM PROTOCOL

A. 4–6 g MgSO4 loading dose in a 20 ml 0.9% sodium chloride IV over 15–20 minutes followed by a 2 g/hour continuous infusion. This rate should be reduced or stopped if oliguria or poor renal function is present.

B. 5 g MgSO4 IM each buttock if the patient does not have IV access.

C. Followed by 5 mg MgSO4 every 4 hours in alternating buttock until 24 hours postpartum.

Antidote: Calcium gluconate 1 gram IV

BOX 22.2   TOCOLYSIS

Always for 48 hours only and accompanied by 6 mg x2 dexamethasone IM for 2 days.

Nitroglycerin

Sublingual: 10 mg every 15 min/first hour followed by 20 mg sublingual every 6 hours.

OR

Salbutamol

IV: dilute 5mg in 500ml normal saline or 5% glucose.
Start with 10 drops/min to increase every 20 min with 10 drops if contractions continue.
Do not exceed 90 drops/min; leave the infusion for at least 1 hour if the dose is effective.
If qualified personnel are not available, it is safer to administer salbutamol 0.5 mg IM 6 hourly for 48 hours.

OR

Other tocolytics

Magnesium sulfate, terbutaline, ritodrine, nifedipine, or indomethacin

---

obstetrical care unit with staff skilled in pre- and postpartum care. Good control of vital signs, recording of fluid balance and urine output, and vigilance for pulmonary edema is warranted. Administration of oxygen, antihypertensive medications, and magnesium sulfate, and toxicity screening of medications will need dedicated staff. Magnesium intoxication will manifest in an absence of reflexes, decreased respiratory rate (<16/min), and changes in mental status. To reverse these effects, calcium gluconate (1 gram) should be administered, especially if the respiratory rate decreases.

Care for an eclamptic patient might be very challenging in LMICs due to lack of trained personnel and the severity of the cases. Frequently, eclamptic patients sustain some brain injury during seizures or due to cerebral edema in severe pre-eclampsia.

Induction of Labor

Induction of labor can be done with cephalic presentation and is indicated for intrauterine fetal death, molar pregnancy, severe pre-eclampsia, eclampsia, absence of fetal movement, or oligohydramnios. If the cervix is central, soft, effaced, and open, the uterine contractions will be effective in opening the cervix so that induction with gradual increasing oxytocin has a high likelihood of success. If the cervix is stiff, long, and posterior, prostaglandins are needed to ripen the cervix. Misoprostol can be used in quantities of 25 mcg vaginally. Higher doses can give overstimulation, resulting in fetal asphyxia. Misoprostol or any prostaglandin ripening is contraindicated in women with a prior C-section who have a uterus beyond 28 weeks in size. The misoprostol can be repeated every 4–6 hours until the cervix is open or soft; then oxytocin can be started to induce contractions. If the membranes are palpable, they can be ruptured, which will give "spontaneous" contractions; however, due to the increased risk of intrauterine infection and human immunodeficiency virus (HIV) transmission, this practice is not routinely encouraged in LMICs until the cervix has dilated up to 5 cm with a cephalic presentation.

If a woman has a history of previous uterine surgery or C-section, an induction can be most safely initiated by inserting a Foley catheter into the cervix as described in the section on abortion. This method can also be used if misoprostol is not available.

Preterm Labor

Preterm labor is defined as having contractions and cervical changes before 37 weeks. Causes of preterm labor are urinary tract infection, malaria, or other infections causing fever, and all should be treated accordingly. Pregnancy-related problems such as preeclampsia, eclampsia, twin pregnancy, rupture of membranes, or polyhydramnios may also lead to preterm labor; however, take note that most cases are idiopathic.

A definitive diagnosis of the gestational age might be difficult if a patient is not certain of her last menstrual date. It is generally believed that if delivery of a viable fetus before the gestational age of 34 weeks is imminent (roughly fundal height <32 cm), attempts should be made to delay the delivery for 48 hours in order to administer dexamethasone (6 mg, 12 hourly × 4). However, it is better to let the woman deliver immediately if she is in a very poor condition with preeclampsia, eclampsia, malnutrition, sepsis, abruption, disseminated intravascular coagulation (DIC), or if her cervix is dilated more than 5 cm or if the fetus is dead.

If the patient experiences contractions without cervical changes, dexamethasone or betamethasone should be given with bed rest and close follow-up on cervical changes. If the cervix opens or is softening, tocolysis should be attempted (Box 22.2). Tocolysis may have serious side effects for the pregnant woman and indirect effects on the fetus. Nitroglycerin is an effective tocolytic but can cause flushing, hypotension, dizziness, and headache, and is not used often for tocolysis. Salbutamol can produce tachycardia, headaches, muscle cramps, and allergic reactions. Vital signs and fluid balance must be recorded hourly and medication stopped or dosages reduced if hypotension or tachycardia results. Calcium channel blockers, like nifedipine, can also be used to effectively keep maternal blood pressure in control. Indomethacin prior to 32 weeks can also be used as a tocolytic.

Premature Rupture of Membranes

Ruptured membranes before labor are treated according to the gestational age. Independent of gestational age, a primary precaution is infection. One should limit vaginal exams to those that are absolutely necessary and always use sterile gloves and, if possible, use a sterile speculum. It is important to know the fetal presentation and remember the possibility of cord prolapse. If the fetus is vertex and well engaged, cord prolapse is unlikely; however, with breech or transverse positioning, cord prolapse is a major concern. In expectant management with the possibility of cord prolapse, the woman should lie at all times on her left side or in the chest-knee position (Figure 22.3).

If the amniotic fluid is leaking after the rupture of membranes or is foul smelling or stained with meconium, the woman should be delivered, independent of the gestational age. Induction of labor should be initiated if this does not happen spontaneously. In case of maternal fever or foul-smelling liquid, IV antibiotic coverage should be initiated for 3 days (ampicillin and gentamicin) and continued with 7 days of oral amoxicillin. Other antibiotics of choice are dependent on local protocols and availability of drugs.

A woman with leakage of clear amniotic fluid at a gestational age prior to 34 weeks should be placed on bed rest and receive antibiotics compatible with pregnancy (i.e., amoxicillin for 1 week and dexamethasone 6 mg IM q 6 for 2 days or betamethasone 12 mg IM q 24 hours × 2 doses). If the woman is having contractions, a tocolytic should be administered. After 34 weeks of gestation, the management is similar but without the dexamethasone. If labor follows after 34 weeks of gestation, let the woman deliver; the risk of intrauterine infection is greater than the risk of prematurity. After 37 weeks, the contractions usually start within 24 hours of rupture; if not, labor should be induced, especially if the woman is known to be group B streptococcus positive.

Vaginitis, cervicitis, urinary tract infection, and urinary incontinence should be considered in the differential diagnosis of premature rupture of membranes.

Antepartum Hemorrhage

Bleeding in the second half of pregnancy may be due to preterm labor, cervicitis, cervical neoplasm, placenta previa, abruptio

placenta, or a ruptured uterus. Most times, the cause of the bleeding will not be found. Due to the devastating results of some causes, a thorough exam and monitoring are needed. Placenta previa, abruption placenta, or a ruptured uterus are all likely to present or end in maternal shock and fetal death and will be described here. Emergency treatment with fluid resuscitation is warranted to save the mother's life. Blood for a possible transfusion should be prepared for all cases of bleeding in the third trimester.

Placenta Previa

Placenta previa should be considered with twin pregnancies, transverse presentation, or a previous history of C-section but can also present without these classical histories. The uterus is soft and, if labor has started, will be relaxed between the contractions. The fetus will be mobile and not descended into the pelvis. Bleeding will be painless and bright red. If bleeding is heavy enough, shock will result. Preferably, start with an ultrasound examination and a sterile speculum exam. If the cervix is dilated, a digital exam could precipitate further bleeding, and you will feel the presenting placenta as a soft, spongy surface. If bleeding is scant and both mother and child are in good condition, it is safe to observe until 37 weeks of gestation. If the placenta is not covering the entire cervix, a normal vaginal delivery might be initially attempted, if the placenta can be measured >2 cm from the internal os on ultrasound. If the fetus is already dead, one can try to deliver vaginally. If the bleeding is heavy (e.g., constant blood or clots) or the mother or child is in distress, then a C-section should be performed immediately. Low-lying placentas with a history of a previous C-section should make one suspicious of a placenta accreta. For more information see the section on retained placenta in the third stage of labor.

Placental Abruption

Placental abruption, separation of the placenta before delivery of the neonate, often presents in combination with hypertension,

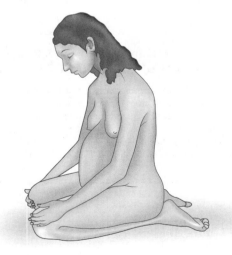
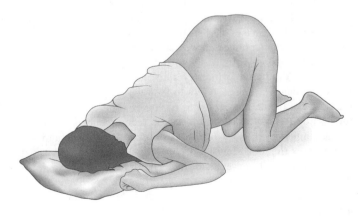

FIGURE 22.3 Chest-knee position. Mathai M et al. *Managing Complications in Pregnancy and Childbirth*. Geneva: World Health Organization; 2007, p. 79.

preeclampsia, eclampsia, or abdominal trauma. The uterus is hard and tender during and in between contractions, and the bleeding is dark red. Maternal pain seems out of proportion to "normal" early contractions. If the membranes are intact, all the blood may be retained and not visible; however, with ruptured membranes, the amniotic fluid will be blood stained.

With placental abruption, the fetus may be in severe distress (>160 bpm initially; later <100 bpm) or might be dead as the oxygen exchange will be severely diminished with decreasing placental surface area available for oxygen exchange. If the woman can be resuscitated and the fetus is dead, try letting her deliver vaginally with induction with oxytocin (Box 22.3). Once she is fully dilated, the expulsion is often fast. If the woman is in shock and the cervix is not fully dilated, resuscitate her and perform an emergent C-section, regardless of the fetal viability. Have whole blood available. Abruption of the placenta is often accompanied by rapid coagulation disorders.

Ruptured Uterus

Women with a history of a previous C-section or who are grand multiparous (>5) or present with a long obstructive labor or malpresentation are at risk for a ruptured uterus. A rupture is a sudden event after which the uterus will be soft and noncontractile. Fetal parts may be easily palpated through the abdominal wall. Bleeding may or may not be heavy due to the fetal head blocking of the pelvic outlet. Only if an emergent laparotomy is performed soon after the rupture will the fetus have a chance of survival. A midline incision is indicated whenever a ruptured uterus is suspected. For signs of pre-rupture, refer to the section on danger signs in labor.

Labor

Normal Delivery

Normal labor and delivery will hopefully be supervised by experienced nurses and midwives. A surgeon will usually be consulted only for cases of obstructed labor or the various pathological findings mentioned above and below.

A normal labor is divided into three stages. Stage 1 refers to cervical dilatation, which is split into passive and active labor (see below). Stage 2 refers to fetal delivery, and stage 3 is the delivery of the placenta. For each case where a surgeon is requested to perform a C-section, it is recommended to check the documentation, do a pelvic examination for presentation, and recheck the fetal viability preoperatively. A general consideration is that with cases of intrauterine fetal death, a vaginal delivery should be the goal.

Documentation by midwives and nurses should be done with a partogram, a useful tool to visualize the labor process and distinguish normal labor from obstructed labor. With a partogram, cervical dilatation, contraction strength, fetal heart rate, and vital signs can be easily monitored and reviewed (Figure 22.4).

First Stage of Labor

A woman in the first stage of labor (dilatation phase) should be examined vaginally at least every 3–4 hours, and the fetal heart rate checked hourly. The first stage of labor can be divided into passive and active labor, where passive labor produces cervical changes but does not result in cervical dilatation of 1 cm/ hour. This process can take up to 20 hours (mean of 8 hours) but should be monitored as well. Pain medication should be considered. Active labor generally starts at 4–6 cm of cervical dilation and ends with full dilatation. Although a nullipara will have a slower progress of labor than a multipara, the essentials of the partogram are that in active labor (after 4 cm of dilatation) progress of labor should be at least 1 cm an hour. After 6 hours of labor, dilatation should be complete. The action lines in the partogram refer to starting of oxytocin and considering instrumental delivery.

Second Stage of Labor

The second stage of labor begins with full dilatation and ends with the delivery of the neonate. If the woman is fully dilated and pushing, the fetal heart rate should be checked after each contraction or at least once every 15 minutes. Debates are ongoing about how long after full dilation a woman should be allowed to push and attempt to deliver vaginally. A rough guide is for a primipara to push up to 2 hours if there is progress and no fetal or maternal exhaustion; a multipara should deliver within one hour of the initiation of pushing.

Danger Signs in Labor

Good management of labor relies mainly on guiding and comforting the woman who actually does the delivery. But close monitoring for danger signs and symptoms is needed at all times. These signs and symptoms include the following: vaginal bleeding, maternal fever, fetal heart rate <100 or >180 bpm, severe pain between the contractions, and sudden arrest of contractions.

BOX 22.3 OXYTOCIN GUIDELINES FOR INDUCTION AND AUGMENTATION OF LABOR

Start with 2.5 IU/500ml dextrose or normal saline at 10 drops/min; augment every 30 min with 10 drops until 60 drops/min.
Continue with 5 IU/500ml at 30 drops/min until 60 drops/min.
In case of a grande multipara or C-section in history, don't augment further but deliver by C-section if there is no progress in labor.
In case of primi gravida: Continue with 10 IU/500 ml at 30 drops/ min until 60 drops/min.
Deliver by C-section if there is no progress in labor at10 IU/500 ml and 60 drops/min.
In case of hyperstimulation or fetal distress:
1. Stop oxytocin infusion
2. Salbutamol 5 mg/500ml Ringer's lactate or normal saline at 10 drops per minute (see Box 22.2).
Terbutaline 0.25 mg SC x1 can be given as an alternative to quickly slow or abate contractions.

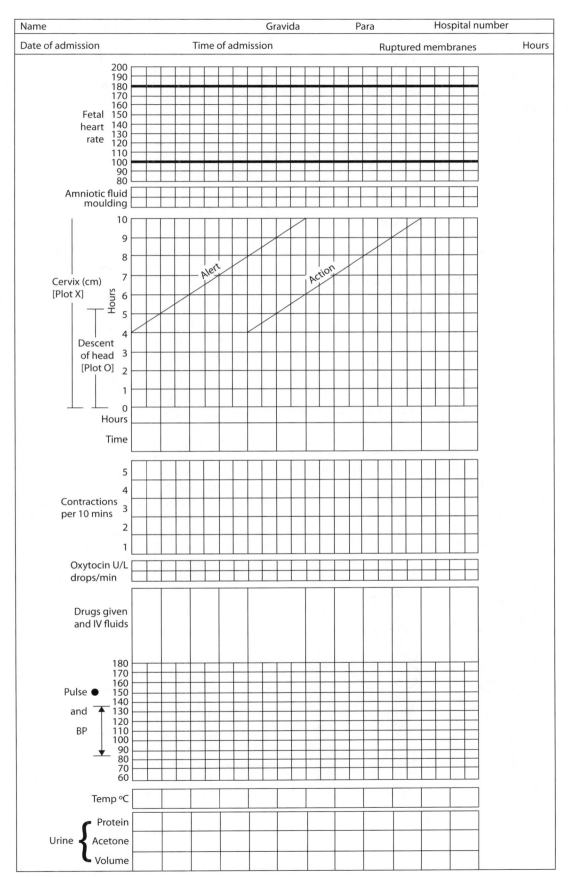

FIGURE 22.4 A WHO example of partogram. Mathai M et al. *Managing Complications in Pregnancy and Childbirth.* Geneva: World Health Organization; 2007, p. 87.

Vaginal Bleeding

Cervical dilatation might be accompanied with some bleeding during labor, but other causes should be excluded. Abruption of the placenta might result in bleeding (mainly dark, venous blood), a painful hard uterus, and no relaxation. The classic sign of pending uterine rupture is the Bandl's ring (Figure 22.5). A ruptured uterus can be diagnosed by palpating fetal parts through the abdomen, vaginal bleeding (bright red), sudden arrest of contractions, and maternal shock. More is described in the section on antepartum hemorrhage.

Maternal Fever During Labor

During labor, chorioamnionitis is a great danger to mother and fetus, and antibiotic therapy should be started. Follow local guidelines or treat with a combination of ampicillin and gentamicin. The neonate should continue with antibiotics postpartum.[3] Urinary tract infection, acute pyelonephritis, and malaria should be considered in every pregnant patient with a fever, but chorioamnionitis is much more common intrapartum.

Fetal Distress

In high-income countries (HICs) where constant fetal monitoring can be achieved, the diagnosis of fetal distress needs prolonged exposure and training of a clinician. Therefore, remember that when working with only a fetoscope and limited personnel, the detection of fetal distress can be even more difficult.

Fetal bradycardia (<100 bpm) is assumed to be a sign of fetal distress if it is prolonged (>1 minute), repetitive, and not related to a contraction. It may be accompanied by thick meconium-stained amniotic fluid. Immediate treatment consists of left lateral positioning of the woman, oxygen therapy via cannula or facemask, if available, and immediate cessation of oxytocin, if being used. If the fetal bradycardia does not improve and stays below 100/min, immediate delivery should ensue either by vacuum/forceps

or C-section, depending of the stage of labor and descent of fetal presenting part.

Fetal tachycardia (>180 bpm) can be a sign of medication use, intrauterine infection, maternal fever, or fetal anemia. One can also consider partial abruption of the placenta, which initially presents as fetal tachycardia followed with bradycardia as oxygen delivery declines. All these signs and symptoms must be carefully assessed and addressed accordingly. Generally, in the absence of maternal tachycardia, fetal tachycardia is considered a sign of fetal distress, and delivery should follow promptly.

Obstructed Labor

An arrest in progression of labor can occur for two reasons, either the contractions are not strong enough or labor will not progress due to an anatomical obstruction. Contractions during labor should be regular 3–4 per 10 minutes and last for at least 40 seconds in order to be effective. If these conditions are not attained and labor does not progress, oxytocin should be used after excluding fetal distress, malpresentation, or a malformed pelvis (Box 22.3). Large cervical polyps or myomas in the lower uterine segment may also be a reason for obstructed labor; for these conditions, vaginal delivery is contraindicated, and a C-section should follow immediately.

If labor in the active stage, even with oxytocin, does not progress with cervical dilatation, a C-section should be performed.

Artificial rupture of membranes before 5 cm of cervical dilatation is not recommended with a living fetus in a high HIV prevalence population, although the total delivery time might be reduced by as much as 2 hours.[7] Amniotomy may be necessary for an overextended uterus due to polyhydramnios, placenta previa marginalis, where bleeding can be reduced by puncturing the membranes next to the placenta, or with a fully dilated cervix and fetal distress to speed up the expulsion phase. Caution is required in all cases to avoid complications that include cervical tears, cord prolapse, and fetal injury. Absolute contraindications are transverse or breech presentation, a beating cord, and previa. These are all also absolute indications for a C-section.

Malpresentation

In settings without proper antenatal care, most malpresentations will only be diagnosed during labor. Causes of malpresentations include uterine fibroids or other uterine anomalies, twin pregnancies, placenta previa, grand multipara, and fetal abnormalities. Most are idiopathic. All these conditions should be considered before any maneuver is attempted. Hydrocephalus is a common cause of breech presentation and such cases should be delivered by C-section, if the fetus is alive. All the following described malpresentations are simplified, and one should be aware that multiple variations on these presentations occur.

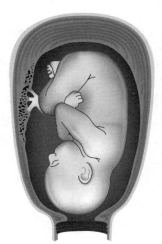
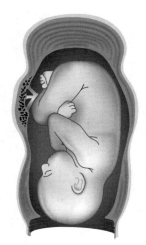

Uterine wall during contraction

Impending rupture: hourglass uterus "Bandl's ring"

FIGURE 22.5 Bandl's ring in pending ruptured uterus. Coutin AS et al. *Obstetrics in Remote Settings: Practical Guide for Non-specialized Health Care Professionals.* Geneva: Medecins Sans Frontieres; 2007, p. 43.

Cephalic Presentations

The ideal position for the fetus to be delivered is with the fetal head flexed with the chin on the chest, presenting the occiput cephalic bone. This occiput presentation is identified by the

Y- or lambda-sign of the cephalic bones, which you can feel on vaginal exam by palpating three suture lines of the cephalic bones. With an occiput anterior (Y-sign) presentation, the smallest diameter of the fetal head is presented and thereby most likely to pass the birth canal. When the occiput is posterior (lambda-sign), delivery is still feasible and rotation occurs in up to 90% of cases. By having the woman get on her chest and knees with her back up (Figure 22.3), gravity will act on the fetus and rotation can occur, which will make passage easier. When on examination the great fontanel is identified (four suture lines of the cephalic bones are palpated), the head is not flexed as it should be. Flexion can still occur (again, having the woman on all fours can be helpful and is not harmful). For multiparas, there is also the possibility that the fetus will pass in this position.

Face presentation can deliver vaginally if the chin is anterior. If the chin is posterior and the cervix is not fully dilated, one can wait for spontaneous rotation, which is more likely to happen with intact membranes in a multiparous patient. The knee-chest position is *not* helpful in this case (Figure 22.3). In any case, if labor is prolonged and/or rotation does not occur, one should proceed to a C-section.

With brow presentation, the largest diameter presents to the birth canal, and passage is nearly impossible. If the woman is in an early stage of labor and especially if the membranes are intact, the fetus might flex its head to present in occiput. In this scenario, the knee-chest position will help to change the position of the head (Figure 22.3). If the membranes are ruptured and dilatation is nearly complete, position change is less likely. In cases of prolonged labor, a C-section should be undertaken. One can attempt to change the brow presentation to a full face presentation, which has a greater chance for a vaginal delivery, by putting pressure on the forehead toward the back of the fetus while the woman is in knee-chest position. Only attempt this when the greater fontanel is anterior to achieve an anterior chin. Fetal cervical spine injuries can result from iatrogenic hyperextension.

External Cephalic Version

In case of a singleton breech presentation before rupture of membranes, one might try an attempt of external version provided that the placenta is not anterior or previa, there is a normal amount of amniotic fluid, and the woman did not have any previous uterine operations. Complications of this procedure are preterm labor, ruptured membranes, abruption placenta, and, in rare cases, a ruptured uterus. Do not perform this procedure before 37 weeks of gestational age. Prepare for an emergency C-section before the procedure in case a complication arises. Make sure the woman is comfortable on her back, and carefully explain what you are going to do and why. If the woman is guarding her abdominal muscles, the attempt of external version will definitely fail. Be sure where the head, back, and breech are. Lift the breech out of the pelvis and push the breech to the back of the fetus up to the fundus of the uterus. Some might find it easy to apply a lubricant on the maternal abdomen to help with manipulation. The head can be flexed toward the sternum of the fetus to accompany the forward roll. A backward roll can be tried as well, but manipulation on the head of the fetus due to the neck flexibility will not be helpful in this case. In case of Braxton Hicks contractions, terbutaline (250 mcg) or salbutamol (0.5 mg) IV over 5 minutes might be helpful. After the version (succeeded or not), the woman should be monitored for at least 1 hour with control of the fetal heart rate and uterine contractions.

Breech Delivery

If external version is contraindicated or fails, a woman may still be able to deliver vaginally, with the following considerations in mind: the breech is complete or frank (Figure 22.6), the fetus is not too big, the woman did not have a previous C-section for cephalic-pelvic disproportion, and her pelvis is normal on examination. Additionally, some clinicians do not advocate a vaginal delivery if the woman is shorter than 150 cm.

For a breech delivery, leave the membranes intact. If they rupture spontaneously, immediately perform a pelvic examination to exclude cord prolapse. Cord prolapse before descent of the breech, prolonged labor, or fetal heart abnormalities are reasons for an immediate C-section. If the breech presentation is malrotated and the sacrum of the fetus is posterior or if the hips (or one hip) are extended (footling breech) before full dilatation, a C-section should be done. Of note, meconium is not necessarily a sign of fetal distress in a breech presentation but rather a result of pressure on the fetal bowels.

When the cervix is fully dilated, allow the breech to descend with the sacrum lateral and anterior. The woman should be directed to lie on the very end of the labor table. Give lidocaine infiltration (0.5–1%) for a lateral episiotomy, if the descent of the breech goes through the pelvic floor. If a plateau is available, this can be placed 15 cm under the table height for the fetus to "step on" (Figure 22.7).

Check for cord pulsations and loosen it, if necessary. Touch the fetus as little as possible until the scapulae can be seen. Touching can cause extension of the upper extremities and the head. If the scapulae are seen, grab the breech with both hands with a towel by putting the thumbs on the femurs and the other fingers on the back of the fetus, make a movement sacral (to the mother's sacrum), and then flex the fetus around the pubic bone. If this fails, look for the arms, and go with your right index and middle finger over the back of the fetus and over the right shoulder to rotate the shoulder anteriorly by turning your fingers over the shoulder anterior and bringing the arm down on the abdominal side of the fetus. Do so as well with your left fingers and the left arm, if needed. During this procedure, you need to fix the legs in your opposite hand in case of unexpected fast delivery during your maneuver. After this procedure, you can let the child lie on your dominant underarm and put the index finger and middle finger on the maxilla of the child to prevent or correct extension of the head. Try again with a movement sacral and then rotate around the pubic bone. Your second hand might assist by pressure on the two shoulders but not too forcefully. An assistant might give pressure above the symphysis.

In the rare event that the head does not deliver, use Piper forceps to deliver the head. The cervix can be surgically enlarged by placing one or two fingers between the cervix and the fetus. Then bandage scissors are used to make up to three incisions on the cervix at 2, 10, and 6 o'clock (Dührssen incisions). One

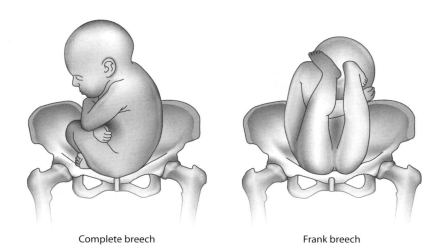

Complete breech   Frank breech

FIGURE 22.6 Breech delivery. Coutin AS et al. *Obstetrics in Remote Settings: Practical Guide for Non-specialized Health Care Professionals.* Geneva: Medecins Sans Frontieres; 2007, p. 103.

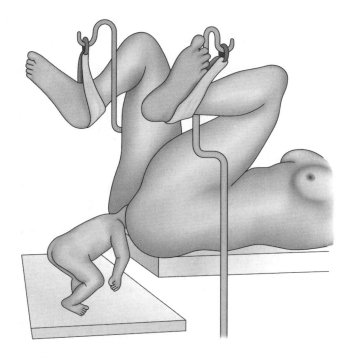

FIGURE 22.7 Breech. Coutin AS et al. *Obstetrics in Remote Settings: Practical Guide for Non-specialized Health Care Professionals.* Geneva: Medecins Sans Frontieres; 2007, p. 105.

must be careful if using these incisions to free an entrapped head as extension of the incisions into the lower uterine segment and broad ligament can occur, which can result in injury to uterine vessels and the ureter.

   If unsuccessful, perform an emergency C-section. If there was a contraindication for a vaginal breech delivery and a C-section is done, the breech is tilted out of the pelvis, after the uterine incision. The same maneuvers are applied to develop the arms and fetal head as described above.

Transverse Presentation, Arm Prolapse, or Neglected Shoulder Presentation

For a single fetus in a transverse presentation, external rotation can be attempted as with a breech presentation. The same indications and contraindications apply. If the external rotation fails, a C-section should be planned or done immediately if the woman is in labor. For a second twin in transverse presentation, an internal version can be attempted by an experienced clinician, but this is beyond the scope of this book. An arm prolapse or shoulder presentation occurs with a transverse presentation when the membranes rupture, and this always requires a C-section. An exception to this rule is a small, dead fetus, with a fully dilated cervix, where an experienced gynecologist might be able to do a destructive operation to remove the fetus vaginally.

Prolapsed Umbilical Cord

With any presentation, an umbilical cord can prolapse. When the membranes are still intact, the cord can be felt as a bounding thick vessel before the presenting fetal parts. If the cord is prolapsed or before the presenting fetal parts, the fetus will suffer from extreme asphyxia when fetal parts press the cord against the pelvic outlet during contractions or due to gravity. An immediate C-section is required. While transporting the women for the C-section, she should be on her knees and chest in an attempt to limit fetal asphyxia. Retrograde filling of the bladder with 300cc normal saline can also help lift the fetal head from the pelvis and limit fetal asphyxia. Tocolysis should be applied if the child is alive (Box 22.2). When there is a cephalic presentation, the head should constantly be pushed cranially using a sterile glove, until the fetus is delivered by C-section. If the fetus is already dead and in breech or cephalic presentation, normal delivery can proceed.

Shoulder Dystocia

The risk of shoulder dystocia is highly linked to fetal birth weight. When the head is delivered but the shoulders stay behind even after gentle downward traction of the fetal head, additional maneuvers can be needed. Flexion of the hips against the abdomen might give more pelvic space (McRobert's Maneuver), and suprapubic pressure can be applied by an assistant. Rotating the face downward can release the trapped shoulder from behind the symphysis. Alternatively, one can place a generous episiotomy and enter with the hand to reach for the posterior arm and thereafter the anterior arm. Putting the woman in knee-elbow position or a squat gives more pelvic space to develop the posterior arm.

Twin Pregnancy and Delivery

Although delivery of a twin pregnancy is not very different from a normal delivery, it is associated with more complications than a singleton delivery. Complications include preterm labor, malpresentation, placenta previa, prolonged labor, and postpartum hemorrhage. Fetal abnormalities occur at slightly higher rates as twin pregnancies tend to have higher rates of chromosomal and structural abnormalities and are associated with intrauterine growth retardation.

Ideally, one should know the chorionicity of the twins. Mono-amniotic twins are at risk for twin-to-twin-transfusion syndrome, being conjoined, and the interlocking syndrome when the first twin is breech and the second is vertex. Mono-chorionic, di-amniotic twins are also at risk for twin-to-twin transfusion syndromes. In LMICs, most often chorionicity is not known, and complications need to be addressed as they arrive. Preterm labor should be managed as described in the section on tocolysis.

Malpresentations should be addressed according to the position of the first twin. For twins where the first twin is a transverse presentation, delivery should be by C-section. If the first twin is in breech, a vaginal delivery can be attempted, and the same rules of a breech delivery apply. The position of the second twin can change after delivery of the firstborn and is, therefore, not a reason for immediate C-section.

Prolonged labor and postpartum hemorrhage should be anticipated, and early oxytocin preparation and stimulation considered in every twin delivery. An IV line should be started even with good contractions to have access in case of hemorrhage. After the first twin is delivered, the cord is clamped and cut as usual, but the placenta side of the cord is left in place. No attempt should be made to deliver the placenta until the second twin is born.

After the birth of the first twin, the position of the second twin should be checked. A previous transverse position can rotate into a more favorable position: vertex or breech. However, the opposite can also be true. If the second twin appears to be in transverse position, an external rotation can be attempted as described previously, or the fetus can be internally rotated. This should only be attempted if the second twin is estimated to be the same size or smaller than the first, and the cervix is still fully dilated. With internal rotation, the feet of the second twin are grasped intrauterinely, and thereafter the membranes should be ruptured and the twin extracted vaginally with the same maneuvers for a normal vaginal breech delivery. A C-section should be immediately available if this attempt at breech extraction is unsuccessful.

Oxytocin should be used for the same indications as in singleton delivery and the second twin should be delivered within 2 hours after the firstborn.

Third Stage of Labor and Postpartum Hemorrhage (PPH)

The third stage of labor begins after expulsion of the baby(s) and ends with the expulsion of the placenta. An active third stage of labor is effective in preventing up to 60% of the PPH and should be instituted for all deliveries (Box 22.4).

With regard to complications, PPH is the most common cause of maternal death in LMICs and is defined as a great than 500cc blood loss within 24 hours of a vaginal delivery and >1L if delivery was via caesarean. Secondary PPH is defined as more than 500cc blood loss after the first 24 hours postpartum. Severe PPH is defined as more than 1 L of blood loss; however, it is important to note that in LMICs, a woman with baseline anemia might be in shock prior to meeting the PPH criteria and, therefore, close monitoring of all postpartum women is warranted.

Causes of PPH can be categorized and anticipated for the following cases:

1. Uterine atony: most common cause of PPH and seen with prolonged labor, twin delivery, polyhydramnios, chorioamnionitis, grand multiparous women, and very quick deliveries.
2. Genital tract trauma: quick expulsion or instrumental delivery.
3. Retained placental tissue: the most common cause of secondary PPH.
4. Inversion of the uterus: home deliveries with *uncontrolled* traction on the umbilical cord.
5. Maternal bleeding disorders: common with preeclampsia, eclampsia, HELLP.
6. Ruptured uterus: as most bleeding is intra-abdominal, visible bleeding might be limited.

To assist health workers with managing PPH, every health facility should have an easy-to-understand and clearly visible flowchart with a protocol for the management of PPH.[8]

Of note is that uterine atony can be caused by urinary retention, which can be prevented by having every postpartum patient void within 2 hours after delivery. In the event of PPH, direct

---

BOX 22.4   ACTIVE THIRD STAGE OF LABOR

1. Immediate 5 IU oxytocin IV or IM after the birth of the child.
2. Massage the uterus.
3. Apply controlled cord traction with a uterine contraction, after the baby is separated.

NB: Delayed cord clamping until 3 minutes after delivery of the baby reduces neonatal anemia.

placement of a urinary catheter is important and will allow better access to the uterus and easier identification of the vaginal structures in case of a laceration.

A sample management protocol for PPH includes the following:

A. Resuscitation:
   a. Begin continuous uterine massage.
   b. Insert two large bore (if available) intravenous cannulas: one for 10 IU of oxytocin in 500L of crystalloids at 60drips/min and one for fluid resuscitation or blood transfusion, as needed.
   c. Insert a urinary catheter.
B. Inspection:
   a. Check for retained placental products.
      i. Inspect placenta.
      ii. Manually explore uterus, by removing clots and possibly retained products of conception with a gloved hand from the uterus.
   b. Check for vaginal or cervical tears and repair, if necessary.
   c. Commence 0.2 mg ergometrine IM (safe up to 1 mg), if the uterus is empty and not inverted.
   d. Add misoprostol (200–800 mcg buccal/rectal or prostaglandin 2E 0.25 mcg).
   e. Add tranexamic acid if vaginal or cervical tears identified.
C. Surgery:
   a. Go for definitive surgery as described in the procedures section if the above steps do not stop the PPH.
   b. While awaiting surgery, the uterus can be bimanually compressed (Figure 22.8), and the aorta can be compressed (Figure 22.9).

There are some other considerations in the PPH treatment. Ideally, three persons should be available to assist with a patient with PPH. One nurse or assistant should secure venous access, prepare medications, applying monitoring devices, get blood products, and so on. One nurse should massage the uterus and monitor blood loss and vital signs. The doctor or midwife should place the urinary catheter; remove retained products; identify and, if necessary, repair tears; and plan for further management.

Ergometrine is known to produce hypertension and should not be used in hypertensive patients due to the risk of intracerebral hemorrhage and myocardial infarction. It gives tetanic contraction of the uterus and will delay placenta expulsion and worsen inversion of the uterus. If there is any doubt of retained products, a manual examination of the uterine cavity should be performed first.

All women delivered at home presenting with excessive blood loss or prolonged bleeding postpartum should have the uterine cavity explored manually or digitally. Retained products are also more common in preterm delivery, a history of uterine surgery, and intrauterine fetal demise. Exploration can be done under sedation. Full sedation is preferable, but diazepam 20 mg with pain medication might be enough if there is no anesthetist available. A sterile work area and antibiotic prophylaxis is needed for every intrauterine procedure. Tetanus immunoglobulins or a booster should be considered in every home delivery with complications. Check during the manual exploration for products of conception and for uterine rupture. Products of conception should be removed, and if a uterine rupture is palpated, immediate laparotomy should follow if the patient is unstable.

Uterine Inversion

Inversion of the uterus when discovered on vaginal inspection or examination requires good sedation and tocolytics for manual reposition. Nitroglycerine works well in this setting to relax the uterus for repositioning, keeping in mind the patient may bleed more during this maneuver. Gradually, massage the edges of the inversed uterus in normal position. Central pressure will not be effective, and do not remove the placenta until the uterus is in its anatomic position. If manual reposition is not effective, a combined vaginal and intra-abdominal reposition can be tried. After complete reposition of the uterus in anatomic position, oxytocin, with or without ergometrine, should be given.

Retained Placenta

A placenta should be delivered within 30 minutes postpartum. If the placenta is retained, the woman is not bleeding, and her vital signs are stable, the clinician might consider waiting another 30 minutes, and then beginning an oxytocin drip (20–40IU in 1L NS 60 drips/min), continuing close observation of vital signs, and looking for vaginal bleeding. Saline 30cc + oxytocin 5IU can also be injected via the umbilical vein to cause separation of the placenta from the uterine wall. A final technique is manual removal of the placenta, which should not be delayed more than one hour postpartum to avoid trapping of the placenta behind the lower uterine segment (which might start to constrict). As stated above, do not give ergometrine before the placenta is delivered. Be prepared for a laparotomy if the manual removal reveals a placenta accreta. Separation of the placenta might be

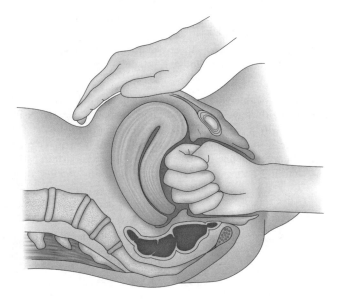

FIGURE 22.8 Bimanual compression of the uterus. Coutin AS et al. *Obstetrics in Remote Settings: Practical Guide for Non-specialized Health Care Professionals.* Geneva: Medecins Sans Frontieres; 2007, p. 148.

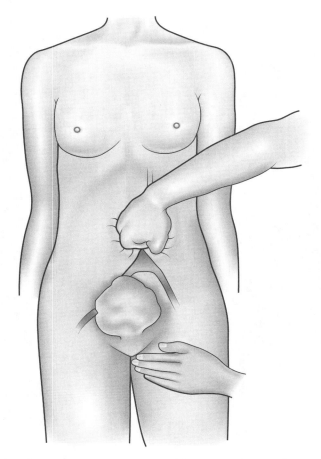

FIGURE 22.9   Aorta compression. Mathai M et al. *Managing Complications in Pregnancy and Childbirth*. Geneva: World Health Organization; 2007, p. 131

prevented in a placenta accrete due to the placenta growing through the myometrium in different degrees. Accreta, increta, and percreta, where in the last case the placenta grows totally through the uterine wall, cannot be removed otherwise except by surgery.

Procedures

For all obstetric procedures, general aseptic techniques apply. Vaginal mucosa should be cleaned and prepared with iodine rather than alcohol-based solutions. The bladder should be empty. In cases of intrauterine procedures (manual placenta removal, C-section, etc.), broad spectrum prophylactic antibiotics should be administered (e.g., a single dose ampicillin 2g or cefazolin 1g IV).

Vacuum Extraction

Indication

Maternal exhaustion or fetal distress, with fully dilated cervix, engaged head, and good uterine contractions are the indications for vacuum extraction. The membranes should be ruptured.

Contraindication

Presentations other than occiput, prematurity (<35 weeks), deformed pelvis, undescended/non-engaged head, severe caput succedaneum, or moulage, suggesting definite feto-pelvic-disproportion.

Method

Assure that contractions are efficient and augment if necessary with oxytocin (Box 22.3). Place the woman in lithotomy position, disinfect the genital area, and place sterile drapes. Inject 5–10cc lidocaine 1% in the region of a potential episiotomy. A vacuum extraction tends to be more effective if an episiotomy is not cut as the vaginal tissue helps keep the device in place. An episiotomy is recommended only if added room is necessary. A pudendal block can be given as well (Figure 22.10).

Empty the bladder. Identify by vaginal exam the junction of the parietal and occiput bones and place the vacuum cup on the midline and just ventral of this junction. Make sure that there is no vaginal tissue between the cup and the fetal head, by following the cup 360 degrees with your fingers. Pump to 100 mmHg (≈13 kPa, ≈0.2kg/cm or follow the instructions of the vacuum pump manufacturer), check again that no vaginal tissue is between the cup and the fetal head; if present, release the vacuum completely and place again. If there is no vaginal tissue between the cup and the fetal head, pump to a pressure of 500mmHg (≈67kPa, ≈0.8kg/cm). Before applying traction, check again for vaginal tissue between the cup and the fetal head. Only initiate the traction in concordance with uterine contractions and maternal pushing. Apply traction along the pelvic canal, first more sacral, and when the head descends, more caudally and ventrally if the head appears in the pelvic outlet. Traction should be applied gently and constantly. Inconsistent traction does not help and might cause lesions of the fetal skin or cup de-attachment. If the head does not follow, either the uterine contractions are not strong enough or there is fetal-pelvic-disproportion. With three tractions, the baby should be delivered, meaning three times a good contraction with maternal pushing and vacuum traction by the clinician. If there is no descent of the fetal head in this time, an immediate C-section is indicated. In the case of a failed operative vaginal delivery followed by caesarean, a low vertical uterine incision is helpful in getting the baby out safely without lateral extension into the uterine vessels. Extensions can occur into the vagina and cervix with this incision, but it can also be extended upward to make more space as delivery can be anticipated to be more challenging once a failed operative vaginal delivery has occurred.

If the baby is delivered with vacuum assistance, it should receive 30 mg of acetaminophen rectally TID for one day and be breast-fed as soon as possible due to an increased risk of neonatal hypoglycemia. Furthermore, the neonate should be handled only when necessary and continuous carrying should be discouraged for at least 2 days. Complications are mostly cephalohematoma (seen in up to 25% of the vacuum extractions), subgaleal hematoma, and anemia or jaundice secondary to the hematoma.

Considerations

The woman must be fully aware of what will happen and must cooperate fully. Sufficient explanation with good translation is

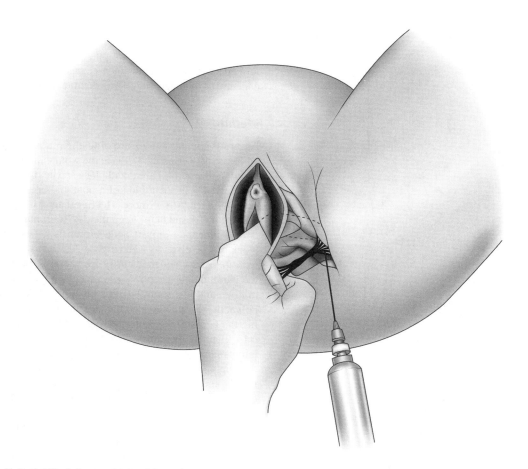

FIGURE 22.10 Pudendal block for anesthesia of the perineum. Mathai M et al. *Managing Complications in Pregnancy and Childbirth*. Geneva: World Health Organization; 2007, p. 256.

warranted. Placing the cup will be the most difficult part for the woman. To assure good positioning, she must stay calm and cooperative. Also, some gynecologists routinely perform an episiotomy as soon as the fetal head goes through the pelvic outlet to prevent a third-degree perineal tear.

Complications

The woman can suffer from perineal and vaginal tears, fistulas due to poor placement, and poor care after the procedure. Postdelivery, a thorough inspection of the cervix and vaginal canal is needed to check for tears and lacerations. In the case of an intrauterine fetal death, intrauterine manual inspection is also warranted.

Forceps Extraction

The forceps extraction has become less popular due to maternal morbidity (see considerations). If vacuum delivery is available, it will have preference in most cases. If clinicians are not familiar with the forceps extraction, it is better to deliver via an alternative way, such as vacuum or C-section. We describe the technique and considerations for being comprehensive.

Indication

Maternal exhaustion or fetal distress, with fully dilated cervix engaged head and good uterine contractions, is the primary indication. The membranes should be ruptured. The forceps has the same indications as the vacuum extraction, with the exception that the forceps might be safer in premature deliveries and can be applied to the head with a breech delivery. In experienced hands, this can also be applied to fetal heads with less descent, malrotated occiput (left/right posterior), or face presentation.

Contraindication

Presentation other than vertex occiput, deformed pelvis, no engaged head, caput succedaneum, or moulding giving the impression of definitive fetopelvic disproportion are contraindications.

Method

Make sure that the contractions are efficient, and augment if necessary with oxytocin (Box 22.3). Place the woman in lithotomy position, disinfect the genital area, and place clothes and apply a pudendal block (Figure 22.10). Empty the bladder.

The blades of the forceps are applied separately guided by the parietal bone of the fetal head (Figure 22.11). Rotation (if indicated) and tractions are applied in concordance with the mother pushing during uterine contractions. Rotational forceps have fallen out of favor because of the potential for extensive pelvic floor damage. If the fetal head does not descend after three contractions, a C-section should be performed immediately.

Episiotomy should be applied as soon as the head goes through the pelvic outlet to prevent third-degree perianal tears.

Consideration

Maternal comorbidity is the reason the forceps became unpopular, ranging from cervical lacerations, third-degree vaginal lacerations, and an increase in postpartum hemorrhage due to uterine prolapse from insufficient perianal strength and widening. Thorough inspection of the cervical and vaginal canals is necessary after the procedure. Signs of neonatal morbidity includee facial palsy, cervical neurological damage, cephalohematoma, subgaleal hematoma with associated anemia, and neonatal jaundice.

Destructive Operation/Craniotomy

Indication

For an intrauterine fetal death, a vaginal delivery should be attempted. If a vacuum-assisted delivery is not effective or there is fetopelvic disproportion (e.g., hydrocephalus or extreme young age of the mother), destructive operation is an alternative. Although not an elegant option, considering the maternal benefits in an LMIC with high parity, it is encouraged.

Contraindications

Discussion with the local staff is mandatory before attempting the procedure for cultural reasons and one's own safety so as not to be accused of feticide. Let your staff confirm fetal death and discuss together the best delivery method. If there are clinical signs of a ruptured uterus, one should not attempt vaginal delivery but first inspect the uterus via a laparotomy.

Methods

Perform this procedure in the operating room with adequate anesthesia (general if possible) and good assistance. Always double glove. Pudendal block or spinal anesthesia with light sedation can be considered as well. Place the woman in lithotomy position, disinfect the genital area, and place sterile drapes. Empty the bladder. If a transurethral catheter cannot pass due to the obstructing descended head, a suprapubic puncture of the bladder should be done to empty the bladder, and a urinary catheter placed after delivery of the fetus.

To accomplish the craniotomy, punch through the sutures of the cranial bones in vertex presentation and intracephalic structures and cerebral fluid will come out and allow more moulding for the head to be extracted. Next, grasp all the cranial bones with 4 Kochers and pull gently downward. The cranial bones can be sharp, so protect the vaginal walls with retractors and wear double gloves.

If a breech delivery attempted at home results in a stuck head (often seen with hydrocephalus), the fetus needs to be rotated with the back to the upside. Then one can pinch trough the foramen magnum by following the cervical spine up to the caudal part of the skull. After the shrinkage of the size of the head, delivery can follow. Destructive operations for transverse presentations should be left for experienced hands, since the complication of a ruptured uterus is more likely. Other complications of destructive operations are cervical and vaginal tears and retained placenta. Always do a manual inspection of the uterine cavity after a destructive operation for retained products and uterine integrity.

Considerations

Vesico-vaginal fistulas might be a complication due to the prolonged obstruction and subsequent necrosis of vaginal tissue. Place a urinary catheter for at least three days and do a methylene blue test with any suspicion of a fistula. See the section on fistula prevention. If shoulder dystocia is present in the case of macrosomia and fetal demise in a diabetic mother, one can purposefully fracture the fetal clavicles with a Kelly clamp to reduce the bi-acromial diameter and deliver the shoulders. This can be done urgently for a live fetus but is not recommended as an early option to relieve dystocia.

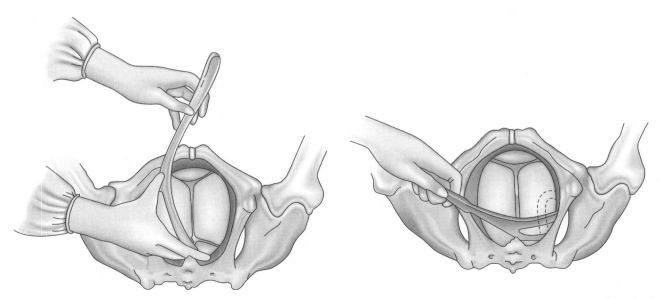

FIGURE 22.11 Applying forceps. Mathai M et al. *Managing Complications in Pregnancy and Childbirth*. Geneva: World Health Organization; 2007. P. 285

Symphysiotomy

Indications

Symphysiotomy is a quick and very useful procedure for obstructed labor in the second stage of labor due to a small pelvis in a young adolescent. A second indication is for an arrested head in breech delivery where the head is not able to follow with the above-mentioned maneuvers. Symphysiotomy can be applied in combination with a vacuum extraction, if this procedure is well indicated. The great advantage is that the next pregnancy and delivery will not be complicated with a scarred uterus, and the pelvis will be permanently enlarged.

Contraindications

Gross pelvic abnormalities, gross fetal abnormalities (e.g., hydrocephalus), conjoined twins, or fetal death are contraindications. Local guidelines might be implemented regarding the practice of symphysiotomy. Most countries state that symphysiotomy should only be applied if C-section is not available or is contraindicated. If a woman is not able (socially or economically) to rest in bed for 6 weeks after delivery or she has a heavy workload, symphysiotomy is not an option due to the high risk of a disabling unstable pelvis.

Method

Place the woman in lithotomy position and clean and disinfect the genital area. Secure her hips and legs well and place a sheet under her sacrum and lower back. Clip or shave her pubic hair and disinfect the pubic area. Feel for the junction of her pubic bones and infiltrate 1% lidocaine into the periosteum and the overlaying skin. Insert a Foley catheter and push the urethra away from the midline with your nondominant hand. Simultaneously, cut the skin overlaying the symphysis (the pubic junction) longitudinally up to the articulation and open the fibers of the articulation on the anterior side. You will feel the pelvis open 2–3 cm. Do not cut so deep that you reach the fibers on the posterior side. The neonate can now be delivered, if needed with the help of a vacuum extraction while leaving the woman in the same position. After the delivery, the pelvis needs to be fixed like a pelvic (open book) fracture by tying the sheet from behind her sacrum and lower back. You need to put this on before the intervention. She should remain at bed rest for 6 weeks with fixation of her pelvis.

Considerations

Due to the long immobility after this procedure, the woman should be very motivated and understand the need for bed rest. In-bed activity to prevent thrombosis should be explained and guided by the nurses on a daily basis. If low-molecular-weight heparin is available, it is surely indicated. Complications of the procedures are temporary and include leg and pelvic pain, stress incontinence, and pelvic instability.[9] A rare complication of late osteomyelitis can also occur.

Episiotomy and Vaginal and Cervical Tears

Definition

Vaginal or perineal tears are classified from first to fourth degree. A first-degree tear only involves the skin or mucosa; second-degree involves the underlying perineal muscles; third-degree involves the anal sphincter; and fourth-degree involves the anal sphincter and the rectal mucosa.

Indication

An episiotomy is placed to prevent a third-degree tear or to enlarge the perineum when it is not allowing rapid delivery for fetal distress.

Method of Episiotomy

An episiotomy is made from the posterior fusion of the labia toward 4 or 8 o'clock posteriorly. In case of infibulation (a type of female genital mutilation or female circumcision), an anterior cut should be made in the line of the physiological introitus. Timing of the cut is very important since the pelvic floor is highly vascularized and will bleed considerably if done before the fetal head provides compression.

Contraindications

There are no specific contraindications to an episiotomy; however, the previous standard that it be done for all nulliparas has since been stopped. With the current HIV epidemic, there is also the desire to limit the neonate to additional maternal blood exposure. Additionally, healing of a perineal tear is better with a first- or second-degree tear than with an episiotomy.

Method of Repairing the Episiotomy or Genital Tears

In every case of vaginal bleeding or an episiotomy, good cleaning, good lighting, and starting from high in the vaginal canal are the key points. Cervical tears are less likely in spontaneous delivery but should be ruled out in cases of PPH. Give a pudendal block or infiltrate the torn skin with 0.5–1% lidocaine. Tamponade any bleeding with gauze high in the vagina. At the same time, spread the vaginal walls so a clockwise inspection can be done. Absorbable sutures should be used for the full tear. Suturing of high vaginal tears should be started just above the actual tear since the blood supply, which comes cranially, will then be adequately blocked. Muscle should be separately repaired from the vaginal mucosa, and the outer skin is best repaired last by starting from posterior to anterior.

In case of rectal mucosal involvement, this layer should be addressed before approximating the rectal sphincter. Make sure to decontaminate every layer before suturing, using sterile water and Betadine after identifying the structures to reapproximate as the discoloration due to Betadine might make identification more difficult. The fibers of the rectal sphincter will be retracted into the wound and need to be pulled out with clamps. Since the fibers are easily torn, an overlapping approximation of the fibers will give the best results.

For the cervical tear, an assistant is warranted to have good exposure. Take two round clamps and follow the full circle of the cervix step wise until the tear is found. This might be harder than expected. The same principles of starting high and suturing caudally apply.

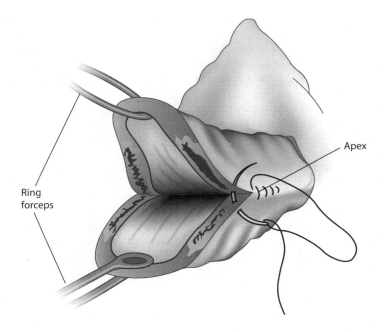

Ring forceps

Apex

FIGURE 22.12   Cervical tear. Mathai M et al. *Managing Complications in Pregnancy and Childbirth*. Geneva: World Health Organization; 2007, p. 333.

Considerations

After the repair, one should control the patency of the rectum as deep tears might come very close to the rectum mucosa. This should not be included unintentionally in the sutures. A postrepair rectal exam should be performed to ensure no sutures have traversed the rectal tissue, which could result in fistula formation. In all cases, the woman should have easy passage of stools, and she should have a high fiber diet and drink enough to prevent fecal impaction. Antibiotics are not needed, unless there is evidence of infection. An infected perineal tear should be opened, cleaned, and inspected daily for signs of necrotizing fasciitis. Antibiotics should be given if deeper layers and muscle are affected. After the daily cleaning, the wound should be kept dry for secondary healing. Delayed secondary suturing is worth attempting, although success rates are unknown.

C-Section

Indications

Fetopelvic disproportion, abnormal fetal presentations, placenta or tumor previa, fetal abnormalities (hydrocephalus), fetal distress without a fully dilated cervix, cervical dystocia, abruption of the placenta, prolapsed umbilical cord, active genital herpes, and impending maternal death are all indications for C-section.

Contraindications

A vaginal delivery can be attempted. Relative contraindication: fetal death.

Method

A C-section can be performed under general, spinal, and local anesthesia. In all cases, the woman needs to be closely monitored by personnel other than the surgeon as the delivery will result in considerable hemodynamic changes. A third person is needed for direct neonatal care.

Position the patient in a left lateral position to prevent an inferior vena cava syndrome. Prep the skin and genital area and place a urinary catheter. Do not use an iodine-based solution in the vagina with a face presentation. A low abdominal midline incision is advised for all medical doctors who are not familiar with a Pfannenstiel incision. The transverse Pfannenstiel incision is preferred due to low risk of an incisional hernia, faster wound healing, and better cosmetics, but potentially can hinder access to the upper abdomen and cannot be extended like an infra-umbilical midline incision. Definite indications for a midline incision are prerupture or rupture of the uterus, lower uterine fibroids or tumors, transverse lie with the back down, malformations such as hydrocephalus or conjoined twins, placenta previa with high vascularity in the lower uterine segment, and severe adhesions from previous uterine surgery. In all these cases, with the exception of uterine rupture, a classical vertical uterine incision is needed and thereby a midline laparotomy incision to give good access to the full uterus is recommended.

Lower Uterine Segment Incision

A lower uterine segment incision is recommended for entry into the uterus as this incision is less likely to rupture in subsequent pregnancies and associated with less intraoperative bleeding. After opening the abdomen with care not to injure the bladder, the loose peritoneum over the lower uterine segment is identified and opened transversely with scissors. The peritoneum and accompanying bladder are pulled caudally and protected with a retractor. A 3-cm transverse incision is then made in the uterus down to the membranes, after which the incision is enlarged sideways by putting two fingers in the opening and pulling gently caudally and cephaladly. One should be careful of pulling sideways as lateral extension could result in bleeding from the uterine vessels or development of a broad ligament hematoma. If sterile bandage scissors are available, these can be used as well to further extend the uterine incision in a controlled fashion. The opening should be crescent shaped with the edges directed cranially to prevent a cervical tear. Next, puncture the membranes and slide a hand over the presenting part of the fetus into the pelvis and lift it out through the uterine incision while removing the bladder retractor. Then continue like a normal delivery and deliver the breech as described for a vaginal breach delivery; for a transverse lie, search for the feet or the hips and deliver the baby in breech.

If the fetal presenting part was too engaged and cannot be extracted, an assistant, using sterile gloves, should push the presenting part cranially from the vagina.

After delivery, the umbilical cord is clamped and cut and the neonate is handed to an assistant. Prophylactic antibiotics and oxytocin (5IU IV) should now be administered, and the placenta delivered with controlled cord traction. Rounded clamps or gauze can be used to remove any remaining membranes. Manual removal of the placenta is discouraged because it is associated with increased bleeding. The edges of the uterine incision will bleed and should be clamped with atraumatic clamps like ring forceps or Babcocks as soon as the baby is delivered. The uterine cavity should be inspected and cleaned with gauze to remove any remaining placenta or membranes. Place clamps on the edges of the uterus to identify the inferior part of the incision and replace the bladder retractor. Check for patency of the lower uterine segment by following the identified uterine edge caudally to be sure not to close the lower uterine segment to the posterior side. Close the uterine incision with interlocking sutures (0 chromic catgut or polyglycolic). Assure adequate hemostasis. Closure of the peritoneum has no proven benefits and is no longer recommended.

Vertical Uterine Incision

For a classical vertical uterine incision, identify the midline of the uterus by identifying the round ligaments. A pregnant uterus might lie a bit toward one side. Make a 12-cm longitudinal incision from the fundus toward but not past the lower uterine segment and deliver the neonate as described earlier. The uterus should be repaired in three separate layers. After this incision, a woman should never be allowed to labor due to the high risk of uterine rupture.

In case of difficulty in delivering the fetus, a uterine atonicum might be used, such as salbutamol 0.5 mg IV. Since this gives uterine relaxation, more hemorrhage will occur after delivery of the baby, and oxytocin is needed in larger quantities than without salbutamol administration. Extension of the lower uterine segment incision is occasionally needed and can be performed either on the side as a J-shape or in the middle as an inverted T-shape, the latter not being the first choice due to difficulties in healing and increased risk of postoperative bleeding. Women with these types of incisions are also not advised to enter in active labor with future deliveries.

Similar strategies for addressing PPH apply for C-sections as for vaginal deliveries, with uterine massage and compression

being easier to apply. Medications include oxytocin (IV 10–60IU in RL), ergometrine (0.2mg IM) and misoprostol (400–800ug rectally). Do not close the abdomen until the uterus is well contracted and there is good hemostasis. Refer to the section on surgery in PPH for more surgical options.

Considerations

Plan the incisions carefully considering the fetal presentation and specific anatomical variations.

Carefully counsel the woman before, if possible, and definitely after a C-section. All future pregnancies should preferably be delayed for 2 years, and the woman should deliver in a facility with surgical capacity and with a planned C-section in case of a classical (vertical) uterine incision.

Postoperatively, if the woman is febrile, she should receive antibiotic such as ampicillin 2 g IV 6 hours, gentamicin 5 mg/kg body weight IV 24 hours, and metronidazole 500 mg IV 8 hours.

In the case of prolonged obstructed labor, the woman risks a vesico-uterine fistula. Check the fistula prevention part in the section on puerperium.

Complications of C-Sections

Endometritis, wound infection, hemorrhage, aspiration, atelectasis, urinary tract infection, thrombophlebitis, and pulmonary embolism are common complications. Long-term complications for the mother include placenta accreta, ruptured uterus with fetal death, and high risk of maternal hemorrhage and death.

Surgery in Postpartum Hemorrhage

There are three options to treat PPH surgically:

1. Artery ligation
2. Compressing sutures
3. Hysterectomy

The options will be tried only when medical treatment is insufficient. Nonsurgical techniques of Foley balloon or Bakri balloon placement to tamponade the uterus or uterine vessels can be quite helpful in avoiding surgical interventions for areas that have these available.

Artery Ligation

Artery ligation of the uterine, ovarian, or hypogastric arteries is the first choice in surgical treatment for PPH during a caesarean (Figure 22.13). Although artery ligation is theoretically the fastest and easiest procedure, good anatomical knowledge with the pregnant uterus and good visualization is needed to prevent neurological damage or renal failure by ligation of the ureters. O'Leary stitches (uterine artery ligation) are the quickest option to control bleeding as those vessels are easily accessible and do not require much dissection.

Compressing Sutures

B-Lynch suture, Hayman compression suture, Cho's square suture, and U-sutures (Figure 22.14, Figure 22.15, Figure 22.16, and

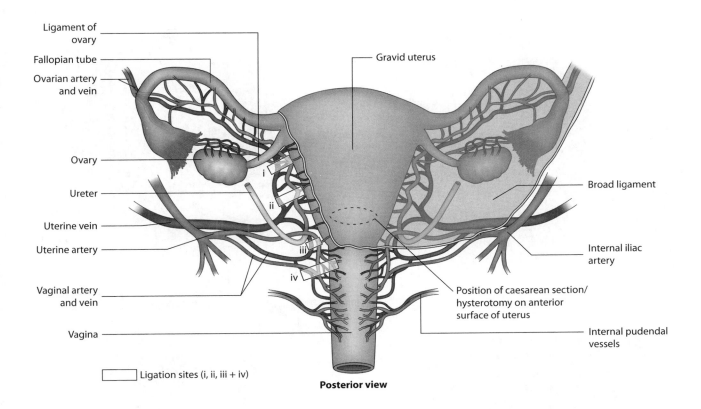

Ligament of ovary

Fallopian tube

Ovarian artery and vein

Gravid uterus

Ovary

Ureter

Uterine vein

Uterine artery

Vaginal artery and vein

Vagina

Broad ligament

Internal iliac artery

Position of caesarean section/ hysterotomy on anterior surface of uterus

Internal pudendal vessels

Ligation sites (i, ii, iii + iv)

Posterior view

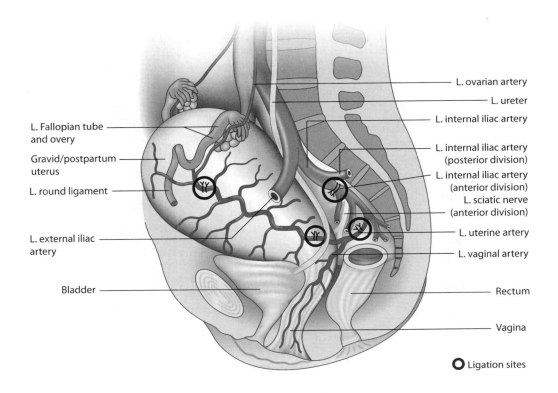

L. Fallopian tube and overy

Gravid/postpartum uterus

L. round ligament

L. external iliac artery

Bladder

L. ovarian artery

L. ureter

L. internal iliac artery

L. internal iliac artery (posterior division)

L. internal iliac artery (anterior division)

L. sciatic nerve (anterior division)

L. uterine artery

L. vaginal artery

Rectum

Vagina

Ligation sites

FIGURE 22.13 Sites for uterine and uterine-ovarian ligature of arteries in case of a PPH. Mathai M et al. *Managing Complications in Pregnancy and Childbirth.* Geneva: World Health Organization; 2007, p. 352.

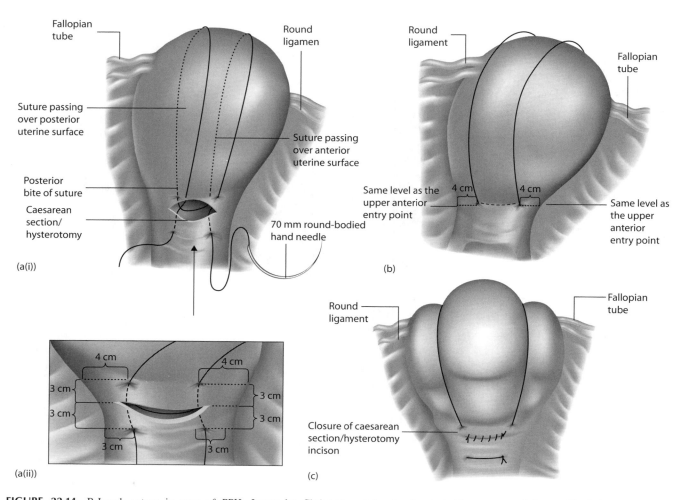

FIGURE 22.14 B-Lynch suture in case of PPH. Image by Christopher B-Lynch. *Surgical Management of Intractable Pelvic Hemorrhage* (Fig. 13a-c Summary of the application of the B-Lynch procedure). [Image on Internet] 2005. [updated 2008; cited 2014 Jan 28]. Available from: http://www. glowm.com/section_view/heading/Surgical%20Management%20of%20Intractable%20Pelvic%20Hemorrhage/item/49

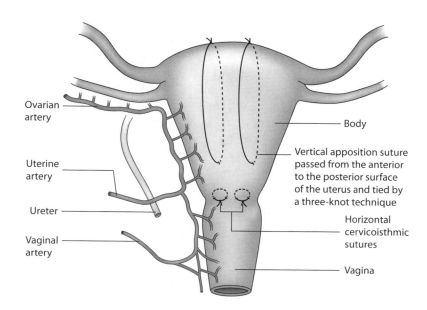

FIGURE 22.15 Hayman uterine compression suture. Image by Christopher B-Lynch. *Surgical Management of Intractable Pelvic Hemorrhage* (Fig. 16 The Hayman uterine compression suture without opening the uterine cavity). [Image on Internet] 2005. [updated 2008; cited 2014 Jan 28]. Available from: http://www.glowm.com/section_view/heading/Surgical%20Management%20of%20Intractable%20Pelvic%20Hemorrhage/item/49

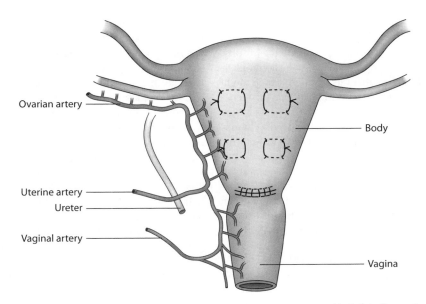

FIGURE 22.16 Cho square suture. Image by Christopher B-Lynch. *Surgical Management of Intractable Pelvic Hemorrhage* (Fig. 17 The Cho multiple square sutures compressing anterior to posterior uterine walls). [Image on Internet] 2005. [updated 2008; cited 2014 Jan 28]. Available from: http://www.glowm.com/section_view/heading/Surgical%20Management%20of%20Intractable%20Pelvic%20Hemorrhage/item/49

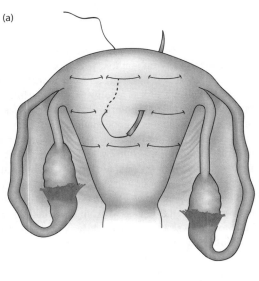

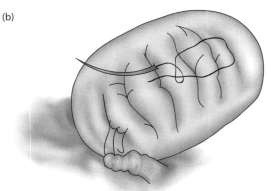

FIGURE 22.17 U-suture. Mathai M et al. *Managing Complications in Pregnancy and Childbirth*. Geneva: World Health Organization; 2007, p. 333.

Figure 22.17) are all based on the principle that compression of the uterine cavity will stop the bleeding. Success rates are high, and fertility remains intact. Although a rare complication, pyometra may occur where, due to inadequate drainage, the uterine contents cannot be expelled, and an intrauterine abscess results. A pyometra is probably more common with the U-sutures and square sutures than with the B-Lynch or Hayman compression suture.[10] These compression sutures may also make antibiotic penetration to those tissues more difficult in the setting of postoperative endometritis.

Postpartum Hysterectomy

Indications

PPH not responding to medications and other surgical techniques or devastating uterine rupture.

Method

Postpartum, the uterus can be fully or partially resected. With partial resection, the cervix (lower uterine segment in the fully dilated phase) will be left in place. The partially or so-called supracervical hysterectomy is easier, faster, and has less chance of ureteral complications and will be described here. The principles of the hysterectomy are the same as in the procedure for gynecological reasons, but there will be greater difficulties with visualization, more bleeding due to the increased vascularization of the uterus immediately postpartum, and possible coagulopathy (primary or secondary). An attempt at ligation of the uterine arteries can be helpful to increase visibility, before performing an actual hysterectomy.

The first step is to identify the lower uterine segment and decide where to resect. Clamp and tie the round ligament bilaterally. Clamp and tie the tubes and their vascular pedicles bilaterally in the first third of the tubes from the uterine cavity. Open the broad ligament (which is a continuation of the peritoneum around the uterus) from cranial to caudal on the anterior and posterior side of the uterus on both sides toward the identified lower uterine segment. This ligament is avascular, but the big uterine veins postpartum are easily torn and thus should be handled carefully.

Within the broad ligament, retroperitoneally, one should identify the ureter on both sides to be sure of its location, which might be slightly different from a nonpregnant position. Once the uterus is free of the ligamentum latum on either side, the assistant is able to pull the uterus quite far out of its position in the pelvis. Clamps can then be applied to the vessels on the sides of the lower uterine segment, and the now-devascularized uterus will become pale. It is essential to assure that both ureters are not involved. Place a stitch caudal of these clamps on both sides taking also some cervical tissue for stability of the suture. Leave these sutures long, so you can use them as identification. Do not use them for traction as arteries are involved. Cut cranially of the clamps, at the side that will be removed with the hysterectomy. If the lower uterine segment is really thin, you can use the clamp and cut method also for the dissection through the lower uterine segment. If not, just dissect with big scissors, and use Allis clamps or round clamps as soon as you enter the cervical cavity to prevent bleeding and when the cervix retracts into the pelvis. Close the cervix with interrupted sutures or, in case of bleeding with locking sutures, using a 0 or 1 chromic catgut or polyglycolic. Ensure that endocervical tissue is not exposed into the abdomen by either inversion of the tissue toward the vagina or placing a second layer of suture inverting the first layer. Check for bleeding, especially on the edges of the cervix, the edges of the ligamentum latum, the round ligament, and cut-through of the tubules. Let an assistant clean vaginally to check for bleeding. Close the abdomen if no bleeding is demonstrated.

Puerperium

Immediate postpartum should be seen as a danger period for both mother and child. Most hospitals will let the woman stay for a period of 24 hours. Anti-D should be given to Rhesus positive mothers. In this time, the woman can be observed for bleeding and fever and can be helped with neonatal care and breast-feeding. Most postpartum problems, however, start later than 24 hours postpartum.

Endometritis

Fever, abdominal pain, and foul smell from the vaginal pads are signs of endometritis. A broad spectrum antibiotic should be administered, and the uterus should be scanned with the ultrasound to make sure that no placenta or membranes are left behind to cause an infection. Puerperal sepsis, caused by endometritis, is one of the four main causes of maternal mortality.

Fistula Prevention

Prolonged labor is the case for obstetrical fistulas. Due to the continued pressure of the fetal head against the pelvic outlet, vaginal tissue gets necrotic, and the fistula will easily arise. Primary prevention of fistulas consists of family planning and appropriate timely obstetrical care. Secondary prevention can be done when fresh leaking of the urine is noticed. This should be treated immediately to enhance good re-epithelialization of the urethra.

After a known obstructed labor, a urinary catheter should be left in place for at least three days postpartum. A vaginal examination with methylene blue retrograde through the catheter should be done before removal of the catheter. In case of blue leakage, the woman should continue with the catheter and be seen every month. To prevent urinary tract infection, she should be trained to drink at least 3 liters of water a day. After 3 months, re-epithelialization is hardly possible. If the methylene blue test stays positive and there is leakage in the vagina of methylene blue, the woman should be referred for surgical fistula repair, which should be done by a specialist. First failure will give a high chance for secondary failure.

If there is no leakage with the methylene blue test, then the bladder might be dysfunctional due to the obstructed labor or urine retention in the prolonged labor. Training the bladder with gradually prolonged clamping of the catheter should be applied, in combination with an antispasmodic agent. This training should be considered before removal of a catheter.

Breast Problems

Up to three days postpartum, a woman can have painful, swollen breasts with a fever of 38°C. This breast engorgement is bilateral and is a sign of transition between colostrum and breast milk. Frequent breast-feeding should be encouraged, and the pain often subsides as breast-feeding becomes more comfortable. If after 5 to 10 days one breast becomes greatly enlarged, this is most likely the result of lymphangitis, which is inflammation of the ducts without infection and will subside if milk continues to be expressed. If direct breast-feeding is too painful, manual expression should be applied regularly. Warm compresses can be helpful, and acetaminophen is a good analgesic.

After two weeks, unilateral breast pain and engorgement is likely to be mastitis due to *Staphylococcus aureus*. The breast will be red, warm, tender on palpation and lactation, and pus might accompany the expression of milk. The woman may also be febrile. She should cease breast-feeding from that affected side and throw away any milk expressed from that side. Cloxacillin 1 gram b.i.d for 7 days or another effective anti-staphylococcal antibiotic should be prescribed, along with acetaminophen and regular checks for pockets of pus, which should be drained as soon as possible.

If the nipple is painful or has crusts, washing it with cold water before and after breast-feeding may relieve the symptoms. Persistent nipple pain can be due to a superficial bacterial or candidal infection coexisting orally in the neonate, so both mother and child should be treated.

In case of a fetal or neonatal death, the breasts should be bandaged tightly with a cloth or sheet, and nipple stimulation should be avoided to diminish breast engorgement and lactation. Acetaminophen or NSAIDs can be given for analgesics. Cabergoline can be given if lactation does not stop with these suggested maneuvers.

Family Planning

There are some specific considerations for family planning in the postpartum period. Predelivery counseling on family planning is essential for understanding of a contraceptive method.

Especially in complicated pregnancies with maternal morbidity, uterine scars, and other risks, women are served well by timely counseling.

Breast-Feeding

Breast-feeding has a preventive effect on ovulation, but only if done regularly every 3–4 hours day and night. Safer methods do exist and should be offered.

Tubal Ligation

If a woman has expressed a wish for a definitive contraceptive solution before labor, she can sign consent for tubal ligation postpartum. When it is necessary to perform a C-section, tubal ligation can be done immediately thereafter or postpartum within 48 hours via a small umbilical incision. Immediate ligation postpartum is associated with less infectious risks but a slightly higher chance of re-epithelialization. Figure 22.18

illustrates the quickest method: the Pomeroy method of tubal ligation. Different techniques are described. All are based on discontinuation of both tubes. If one side of the tube is buried in the broad ligament, there is a reduced chance of re-epithelialization occurring, but operative time will be longer and more suture will be needed. With each method used, be sure that the tubes and not the round ligament are ligated. The anatomy of the postpartum uterus can be confusing, but if fimbriae are identified, one can be certain of dealing with the tubes.

Intrauterine Device

An alternative for the definite tubal ligation is insertion of an intrauterine device (IUD). Theoretically, this can be inserted directly postpartum or immediately postabortion. Some clinicians prefer to wait 48 hours to exclude maternal fever and thereby endometritis before inserting an IUD and when spontaneous expulsion is less likely.

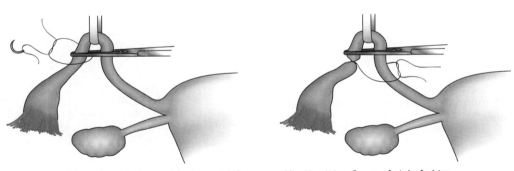

(a) Holding up a loop of the fallopian tube

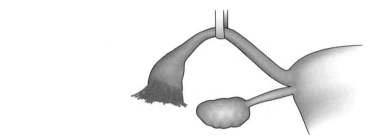

(b) Crushing the base of the loop with forceps and ligating it in a figure-of-eight fashion

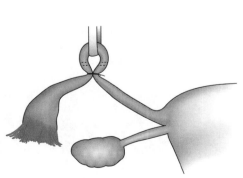

(c) Crushed area (with line of resection indicated by dotted line)

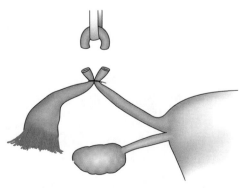

(d) Excising the loop of the fallopian tube

FIGURE 22.18 Tubal ligation: The Pomeroy method.

Progesterone-Only Methods

Other considerations regarding postpartum family planning are progesterone-only methods, most often started 6 weeks after birth. These methods are Depo-Provera at 3 monthly IM injections, a patch renewed each month, or Implanon insertion of 2 rods, which releases progesterone over a period of 3–5 years and can be removed thereafter or if the woman wants to become pregnant again. Although side effects are different per methods, most progesterone-only methods will give spotting in the beginning of the use and can result in temporary amenorrhea after 3–6 months. Although in settings with epidemic anemia the amenorrhea is medically defendable, it might not be preferable to the woman or the culture she lives in.

Neonatal Care

Midwives or obstetrical ward nurses should be capable of providing neonatal resuscitation. Key points include cleaning the mouth and nose with gauze, keeping the baby warm and dry, covering the head as soon as possible, and providing stimulation. Stimulation by simply rubbing the baby dry is usually sufficient. Ninety-five percent of neonates will be fine with this initial care. If the baby is not crying within 30 minutes after birth, suction the nose up to 1 cm and the mouth up to 4 cm and start ventilation after the suction. Make sure the baby stays warm. With good ventilation, the neonate might recover and start breathing spontaneously. For more detailed resuscitation remarks, we refer to the Integrated Management for Pregnancy and Childbirth WHO 2007.[3]

Standard postdelivery care for the neonate is 1 mg vit K IM, which is not provided in breast milk; tetracycline ointment on the conjunctiva to prevent neonatal conjunctivitis; and the umbilical cord should be wiped clean, well tied, and kept dry, to fall off by itself in about 7 days. Breast-feeding should begin within 2 hours postdelivery to prevent neonatal hypoglycemia. Special attention for this morbidity is warranted in cases of large neonates with a suspicion of gestational diabetes, prematurity, instrumental delivery, and neonatal distress.

COMMENTARY

Bomi Ogedengbe, Nigeria

The major challenges associated with abortion have largely been resolved by the discovery of the oxytocic properties of misoprostol with its stability and the many options of effective routes of administration. In addition, the safety of MVA for uterine evacuation (as endorsed by WHO over and above curettage), would have a positive effect on the reduction of maternal mortality. The benefits of both cannot be overemphasized.

However, mifepristone is too expensive for use in our environment, so surgically induced abortion remains the most popular method. Abortion still remains illegal in Nigeria except to save a woman's life. Therefore, unsafe abortion and complications from unsafe abortion remain leading causes of maternal mortality.

By institutionalizing Post Abortion Care (PAC) with its five elements in collaboration with Ipas all over Nigeria, efforts are being made to lower maternal mortality rates from induced abortion.

Ectopic pregnancies usually appear in the late stage having ruptured, and the women are seen in extremis and moribund. Autotransfusion is invaluable as transfusion facilities are not widespread. Laparoscopic evaluation of a woman with abdominal pain is rarely available. Our women have a high pain threshold, so early diagnosis is uncommon.

The availability of ultrasound for use in the first trimester of pregnancy, though widespread, is not generally useful, since the sonographer is usually unskilled in interpreting the findings.

Eclampsia appears to have a seasonal variation, being more common in the rainy season. There is often delay in bringing the patient to hospital. One reason for late presentation is a patient's wiliness to first try an alternative remedy, such as cow urine, at the advice of her local doctor; the patient suffers many fits before finally presenting to the hospital with a worsened prognosis. The advent of magnesium sulphate, which is stable and can be administered intramuscularly, has improved the prognosis for these women, though eclampsia still remains a major cause of maternal mortality.

Hemorrhage is the leading cause of maternal mortality in our environment. The lack of available and accessible blood for transfusion causes many women to lose their lives. We have not developed the culture of blood donation, and many of those who may be willing to donate are unfit to give blood due to anemia or transmissible diseases. The anti-shock garment, where available, has assisted by diverting blood to the essential areas such as the brain, heart, lungs, etc., in prolonging life until blood transfusion is available.

The lack of blood and specific products in cases of DIC also leads to many unnecessary deaths. Thus, for example, a vaginal examination should not be done if placenta previa is suspected unless immediate C-section is possible. Similarly, in abruptio placenta, the uterus must be emptied as soon as possible to prevent a coagulopathy.

There seems to be an increase in the incidence of ruptured uteri. Many occur in women with a previous C-section who want to avoid a repeat section. They go to traditional healers and faith-based providers who promise them a vaginal delivery, but they end up with a ruptured uterus.

The inappropriate use of oxytocin and now misoprostol by such and other untrained medical personnel also contributes to this rising incidence of uterine rupture.

The rising rate of C-section we are experiencing is partly due to the loss of competence with the obstetric forceps and destructive operations, specifically craniotomy for fetal demise. There is nothing worse than scarring the uterus for a dead fetus. This also indirectly contributes to the increase rate of repeat sections as well as the ruptured uteri.

Challenges faced in our environment still continue to relate to contraception. Women, no matter how educated, remain culturally averse to family planning, believing that if one has tubal ligation, they will be sterile when reincarnated. Husbands fear that their wives may become promiscuous if allowed to use contraception. Breast-feeding is almost universally accepted, but its contraceptive effect is poorly understood. Where there has been fetal demise, cabergoline is found to be far too expensive a drug to use for suppression of lactation, especially following an unsuccessful pregnancy. The women are advised to wear a firm brassiere and restrict their fluid intake.

Prevention of vesico–vaginal fistula from prolonged obstructed labor continues to be a major challenge in our environment. It persists in certain parts of the country, particularly the Northern states and the South-South. It is strongly linked to cultural practices such as early marriage and childbearing. Many young girls do not have a menarche before their first child. The lack of universal accessibility to comprehensive healthcare facilities providing emergency obstetric care is responsible for the obstructed labor and subsequent fistulae. When necessary changes involve cultural beliefs, it becomes very difficult to address.

Finally, there is a dearth of anesthesiologists in Nigeria even at the tertiary level. This makes interventions such as manual removal of placenta, repair of third-degree episiotomies, or cervical lacerations, which ideally should be done under anesthesia, more cumbersome. It is fortunate that many of our women have high pain thresholds (which often leads to a delayed presentation) and accept that pregnancy and childbirth must be associated with pain.

23

Gynecology

Felicia Lester
Sierra Washington

Introduction

Maternal mortality is defined as death of a woman while pregnant or within 42 days of the termination of pregnancy, irrespective of the duration and the site of pregnancy, from any cause related to or aggravated by the pregnancy or its management.[1] Maternal mortality is one of the leading causes of death for young women in low- and middle-income countries (LMICs); this includes death from both obstetric and gynecologic etiologies. As a region, sub-Saharan Africa accounts for 62% of maternal deaths worldwide and has a regional maternal mortality estimated at 510 per 100,000 live births, resulting in a one-sixteenth lifetime risk of dying of a pregnancy-related cause in this region.[1,2] Gynecologic mortality and morbidity are often overlooked when in fact in sub-Saharan Africa, at least 14% of maternal mortality is thought to be caused by the sequelae of unsafe abortion and one-sixth from sepsis, with ectopic pregnancy also contributing significantly to this burden of disease. This results from the fact that little attention is given to the gynecologic care of women in LMICs and few women access the healthcare system unless they are seeking prenatal care. Therefore, there is significant gynecologic pathology encountered when working in these settings and many conditions present emergently. Often, patients present with severe bleeding and hemorrhagic shock, or they present with septic shock from infectious conditions such as septic abortion or pelvic abscesses. Understanding good surgical technique for core gynecologic procedures such as manual vacuum aspiration, dilation and curettage, laparotomy for pelvic abscesses, treatment of ectopic pregnancies, and hysterectomy is critical to reduce maternal mortality and mortality.

The link between maternal and infant health has been carefully studied; with the death of a mother an infant is 10 times more likely to die within 2 years of the mother's death.[3] When a woman suffers from serious morbidity regardless of the cause, the entire family structure is jeopardized. Although this chapter deals exclusively with gynecologic surgical technique, it is important to recognize that gynecologic causes of morbidity and mortality will have the same effects on family structure and infant mortality as will obstetrical causes of morbidity and mortality. For example, hemorrhage due to hormonal imbalance, large fibroids, or cervical malignancy can cause significant anemia and resultant loss of productivity or lead to death.

Working in a resource-poor operating theater increases the surgical risk to both patients and the physicians. Maintaining sterility can be challenging without adequate supplies. Performing safe surgery can be difficult when the correct instruments are not available. In such a setting, good surgical technique is paramount to reduce perioperative morbidity in women. This chapter explains in detail the steps to core gynecologic procedures including: manual vacuum aspiration, dilation and curettage, laparotomy for ectopic pregnancy, salpingo-oophorectomy, drainage of tubo-ovarian abscess, myomectomy, and hysterectomy. Because pregnancy itself poses such a high risk to patients, interval, elective tubal ligation is also covered. Long-acting reversible contraception is also highly effective for preventing unintended pregnancy and can be accessed through most family planning programs. Complex fistula repair will not be covered in this chapter; there are detailed surgical manuals for fistula repair. These surgeries are most successful when performed by well-trained fistula surgeons at centers that can offer excellent postoperative care and support for community reintegration. All procedures covered in this chapter have been described in other texts; however, this chapter aims to take into account instruments or equipment that may be lacking in a resource-poor operating theater and provides suggestions for safe and creative alternatives.

Abnormal Uterine Bleeding

Menstruation is typically characterized by the menstrual interval or cycle length, which averages 28 days but can range from 21–37 days and still be considered normal. The duration of flow should be 7 days or less, and the amount ranges from 20–80 mL. The length of the menstrual cycle can change for a woman throughout her reproductive life. Variation is more frequent in teens close to menarche and later in the reproductive years when a woman is approaching menopause. Fluctuations in weight can affect the menstrual cycle as well. Changes are categorized as:

- Menorrhagia: Heavy bleeding at regular time intervals.
- Menometrorrhagia: Heavier bleeding at irregular time intervals.
- Amenorrhea: The absence of menses for 6 months or longer.
- Oligomenorrhea: Infrequent menstruation (menstrual cycles that are longer than 6 weeks).

Abnormal uterine bleeding includes any bleeding which is not normal in its degree or timing. In all women with abnormal uterine bleeding, a careful history and physical exam to assess for signs of anemia, and a pelvic exam to rule out obvious anatomic or pathologic causes should be performed (e.g., cervical cancer, cervical polyp, large uterine fibroids, or prolapsing fibroids). Ruling out pregnancy-related bleeding is needed as a first step toward evaluating the cause of the bleeding.

Abnormal uterine bleeding (AUB) should be classified using the PALM-COEIN (polyp; adenomyosis; leiomyoma; malignancy and hyperplasia; coagulopathy; ovulatory dysfunction; endometrial; iatrogenic; and not yet classified) classification system for abnormal uterine bleeding, which has been approved by the International Federation of Gynecology and Obstetrics (FIGO). AUB-N is defined as any condition of abnormal uterine bleeding without a known cause. The most common cause of AUB is anovulation, and patients will often present with a history of oligomenorrhea with heavy menses when they do menstruate. They may or may not have premenstrual symptoms such as moodiness and breast tenderness with this bleeding. Lack of symptoms can be an indication that the bleeding is anovulatory. These patients have unopposed estrogen causing stimulation of the endometrium with consequent irregular shedding of the uterine lining. Polycystic ovarian syndrome (PCOS) is the most common cause of anovulation in North American and European populations. In sub-Saharan Africa, more often severe malnutrition, anorexia, and severe immunological suppression are causes of anovulation. Thyroid dysfunction, hyperprolactinemia, hormonally active tumors, and Cushing's disease can also cause anovulation. Morbidly obese women can also suffer from this condition in which unopposed estrogen converted from peripheral fat stimulates the endometrium. Prolonged exposure to unopposed estrogen from whatever source can cause endometrial hyperplasia and endometrial cancer over time. Therefore, women who have this condition should be treated with either exogenous progesterone (oral progestin pills, depo-medroxy progesterone acetate, oral progesterone-only contraceptive pills, an implanted progestin, a progesterone-impregnated intrauterine contraceptive device [IUCD]) or combined oral contraceptives to prevent prolonged exposure to unopposed estrogen. In some women, it may be wise to sample the endometrium to rule out malignant causes of abnormal uterine bleeding. This can be done with an endometrial biopsy pipelle, or a manual vacuum aspirator (MVA) cannula size 4, if an endometrial pipelle is not available. However, a trained pathologist must evaluate the tissue, and this service is often lacking in many LMICs so empiric treatment may be reasonable.

Pregnancy-related bleeding is discussed elsewhere, but some of the techniques described below are also used for uterine evacuation for pregnancy-related causes.

Postmenopausal Bleeding

Post-menopausal women who present with bleeding need to be fully evaluated to assess the source of the bleeding. The first step is to rule out rectal or urinary bleeding. Vaginal bleeding in a post-menopausal patient can result from uterine or vaginal atrophy, but serious conditions such as vaginal, cervical, or endometrial cancer must be considered and thoroughly investigated. If the bleeding is caused by vaginal or cervical cancer, a thorough vaginal and speculum exam may reveal a fungating or erosive lesion. If pathology is available, take a simple biopsy of this lesion to confirm the diagnosis. These lesions tend to bleed profusely if incised, so try to bluntly remove a small piece if possible, in order to reduce the risk of bleeding. Ensure that you have plenty of cotton-wool or gauze to pack the vagina should heavy bleeding ensue after biopsy. You may find a cervical polyp, which is usually benign; its removal should resolve the problem. However, this is less common in the postmenopausal patient. If a speculum exam does not reveal the cause of the bleeding, either an ultrasound or an endometrial biopsy can be done. With a transvaginal ultrasound, an endometrial stripe >5 mm in a postmenopausal woman warrants further investigation with an office endometrial biopsy or dilation and curettage. However, an endometrial biopsy or dilation and curettage should only be done for diagnostic purposes, if there is access to a trained pathologist who can make the diagnosis when provided with a specimen. An MVA with a 4-mm cannula or a 3-mm endometrial biopsy (EMB) pipelle can be used. If no ultrasound is available, one can go straight to a biopsy. If an MVA or EMB pipelle is not available, a dilation and curettage (D&C) should be done. A dilation and curettage can be both diagnostic and therapeutic for some conditions; therefore, it is a good option if other instruments are unavailable.

Procedures for Uterine Sampling and Evacuation

Prior to any procedure that involves entering the uterine cavity, a bimanual exam is necessary to assess the uterine position. Proper assessment of uterine position is extremely important prior to the procedure to help decrease the risk of uterine perforation. Make sure that the patient is in lithotomy position with her buttocks over the edge of the table by a few centimeters to prevent the exam table from interfering with the speculum placement. Before placing the speculum, perform a bimanual exam to assess uterine position and feel the cervix for any irregularities. The "no-touch technique" should be used for all transvaginal procedures; the technique involves using sterile gloves but not touching the end of the sterile instruments that enter the uterus. Care must be taken to meticulously avoid contamination of these instruments. The routine use of antibiotics for EMB or D&C is not necessary, but for pregnancy-related uterine evacuations, prophylactic antibiotics should be used. Typically, one dose of a second generation cephalosporin or two doses of doxycycline will provide sufficiently broad antibiotic coverage for prophylaxis. Treatment of a septic abortion will be covered separately.

Endometrial Biopsy Technique

Place the speculum and visualize the cervix. Use Betadine or other antiseptic solution to clean the cervix. If you are using a paracervical block, draw 10 mL of 1% or 2% lidocaine into a syringe, ideally with a spinal needle, for length, attached to the syringe. Inject 2 mL of the 1%–2% lidocaine into the anterior lip of the cervix. Place the tenaculum at the site of the injection, either horizontally or vertically, being sure to grasp sufficient tissue (1–2 cm) to exert traction on the cervix. Use the remainder of the anesthetic agent to inject half at the cervicovaginal junction at 4 o'clock and 8 o'clock, making sure to avoid the cervical blood vessels at 3 o'clock and 9 o'clock and making sure to withdraw prior to injecting to avoid intravascular injection. If not using a paracervical block, simply place the tenaculum on the anterior lip of the cervix. Take care to close the tenaculum slowly and silently to avoid startling the patient. After the tenaculum is placed, the pipelle or 4 mm cannula is inserted through the cervical os. If using an EMB pipelle, the obturator is pulled back to generate suction, and the pipelle is moved back and forth and rotated to get a representative sample for approximately 10 seconds. If an MVA cannula is used, the syringe is used to create suction and locked in place prior to insertion. Once the cannula is inserted, the suction lock is released thus generating a vacuum, and the sampling proceeds as described above. In either case, the sample must be analyzed by an experienced pathologist to determine the diagnosis.

Dilation and Manual Vacuum Aspiration Technique

MVA has been shown to be safer for patients and provide a more complete uterine evacuation than a classical D&C. Therefore, if MVA equipment is available, then this procedure should be used preferentially over D&C.

The technique for MVA for therapeutic, incomplete, or spontaneous abortion is the same as the MVA technique for treatment of menorrhagia or diagnostic assessment of postmenopausal or abnormal uterine bleeding.

MVA should be done for diagnostic purposes only if there is a trained pathologist who can make a pathological diagnosis. Otherwise, it should be used for treatment.

To begin, place the speculum and visualize the cervix. Use Betadine or other antiseptic solution to clean the cervix. If you are using a paracervical block, draw 20 mL of 1% or 40 mL of 0.5% lidocaine into a syringe, ideally with a spinal needle attached to the syringe. Inject 2 mL of the lidocaine solution into the anterior lip of the cervix. Place the tenaculum at the site of the injection, either horizontally or vertically, being sure to grasp sufficient tissue (1–2 cm) to exert traction on the cervix. If using the 20 mL solution, use the remainder of the anesthetic agent to inject half at the cervicovaginal junction at 4 o'clock and 8 o'clock, making sure to avoid the cervical blood vessels at 3 o'clock and 9 o'clock and making sure to withdraw prior to injecting to avoid intravascular injection. If you are using the 40 mL solution, inject approximately 10 mL at 2 o'clock, 4 o'clock, 8 o'clock, and 10 o'clock. If not using a paracervical block, simply place the tenaculum on the anterior lip of the cervix. Take care to close the tenaculum slowly and silently to avoid startling the patient. While placing gentle traction on the tenaculum to help move the uterine corpus to the axial position (whether retro or anteverted), a uterine sound is used to provide further information about the size and position of the uterus. The uterus can be sounded using the smallest size of flexible plastic cannula that can pass through the cervix.

During dilation, the greatest resistance is at the level of the internal os. A metal uterine sound is not used in a pregnant uterus to avoid perforation of the soft myometrium. The cervical canal can be dilated gently with sequential Pratt dilators or sequentially increasing sizes of flexible plastic cannulas. Hegar dilators are not recommended as they require more force to dilate the cervix and thus are associated with higher rates of uterine perforation. The position of the uterus and the angulation of the cervical canal and the uterine cavity must be respected during dilation to avoid perforation. It is important to hold the dilator or flexible cannula gently between the index finger and thumb in the middle to avoid

contamination of the end that will enter the uterus and to avoid using overzealous force. If more than the force obtained with two fingers is necessary, stop the procedure and consider cervical preparation using 200 mcg of buccal, vaginal, or rectal misoprostol to reduce the risk of cervical injury or uterine perforation. This should be administered 3 hours prior to reach maximal efficacy, but as little as 90 minutes can be useful (Figure 23.1).

For most MVAs, dilation from 8–10 mm is typically sufficient to accomplish the procedure for diagnosis or treatment of abnormal uterine bleeding. Depending on the type of dilator you are using, to obtain this level of dilation you will have to go up to a correspondingly sized dilator. The Pratt dilator is measured in French, which is 3 times the millimeters of dilation (e.g., a 21 Fr Pratt dilator corresponds to 7 mm of dilation). Alternatively, flexible cannulas are numbered according to the size of dilation—e.g., a 7 flexible cannula achieves 7 mm of dilation. You can use smaller sized flexible plastic cannulas to dilate the cervix to the desired size of cannula to accomplish the goal. If the MVA is being performed for pregnancy termination or treatment of an incomplete or spontaneous abortion, the size of dilation with a flexible cannula should be equal to the weeks of gestation, but if the cervix is widely dilated from passage of clots, a larger cannula can be used as needed to maintain a vacuum seal.

Whether the flexible cannula is attached to a manual or electric suction, the technique is similar. If using a manual device, the self-locking syringe is loaded by compressing the pinch-valve and drawing back on the plunger and locking it in place. If the pinch valve is correctly placed, you should feel some resistance while drawing back and creating the suction. After the syringe is attached to the cannula, the cannula is inserted up to the uterine fundus. This is the second point of resistance. Once the fundus is reached, one should not advance further for risk of perforation. Once the cannula is at the fundus, the pinch valve is released to create the vacuum. The cannula should be rotated and moved back and forth to empty the uterus. When the syringe is full or the suction is lost, the device should be removed from the uterus, and the cannula is detached from the syringe. The cannula is kept sterile, using the no-touch-technique, while the syringe is emptied and the vacuum reattached in the syringe by repeating the steps above. The plunger should never be advanced while the cannula is within the uterus to avoid air embolism. It may take several passes with an MVA device to completely empty the uterus. Once there is no further return of tissue and the uterine walls feel gritty, the procedure is complete. A gentle torque is applied on the flexible cannula to evaluate if the uterine walls feel gritty. To ensure a systematic approach to curettage, perform one motion from fundus to internal os for each position on the clock-face circumferentially to evaluate for a gritty sensation. Once you are satisfied that the uterine cavity has been emptied, remove all instruments and evaluate for bleeding from the cervical os and the tenaculum site prior to removing the speculum (Figure 23.2).

If the procedure is being performed for pregnancy termination, missed abortion, or incomplete abortion, it is important to confirm that the products of conception have been removed by straining the tissue under water to remove blood and clots. A glass dish is then useful for examining the tissue floating in water Using a light box, such as an X-ray box, can help with tissue identification. At less than 9–10 weeks of gestation, fetal parts will not be visible, but a gestational sac and villi

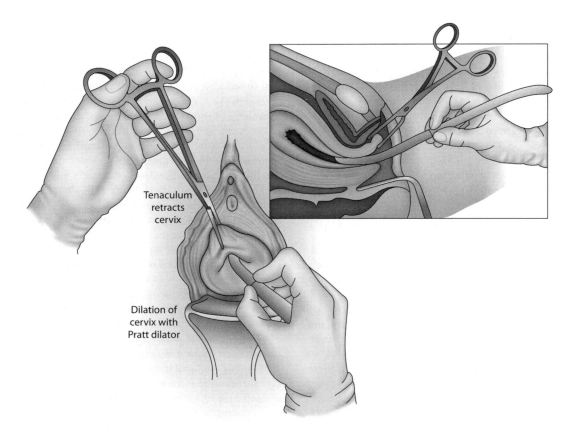

FIGURE 23.1   Dilation and curettage (D&C). Stovall DW. Cervical Dilation. [Image on Internet]. 2014. Available from: http://goo.gl/wDiciu.

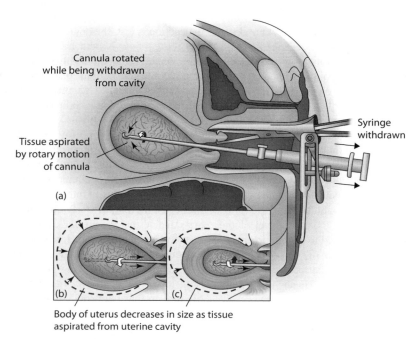

FIGURE 23.2   Dilation and curettage (D&C). Ling FW. Procedure for suction curettage pregnancy termination. [Image on Internet] 2014. Available from: http://goo.gl/fLikWU.

should be seen. Villi appear feathery and can be attached to the transparent, filmy, thin sac. This should be distinguished from decidua, which is thicker, more opaque, and shaggy. If pregnancy tissue cannot be identified, it is important to rule out an ectopic pregnancy, but a completed abortion is also possible; thus, getting a detailed history is important in such cases.

Dilation and Curettage Technique

The technique for D&C for therapeutic, incomplete, or spontaneous abortion is the same as the D&C technique for treatment of menorrhagia or diagnostic assessment of postmenopausal or abnormal uterine bleeding.

D&C should be done for diagnostic purposes only if there is a trained pathologist who can make a pathological diagnosis. Otherwise, it should be used for treatment.

After cervical analgesia is administered and dilation accomplished as described above, a sharp curette is used to systematically curette the uterine walls. A gentle but firm motion is used to scrape the curette from the fundus to the internal os along the anterior, right lateral, posterior, and left lateral quadrants. Cradle the curette in thumb and fingers and exert a torque force against the uterine wall as the curette is drawn out. To ensure a systematic approach to curettage, ensure one motion from fundus to internal os for each position circumferentially. When the uterine wall feels gritty and you can hear a gritty sound; that is usually a sign that the uterus is empty. The sample should be sent to pathology, if available.

Septic Abortion

Septic abortion is a term used to describe postabortion endometritis with associated vital sign instability. It is usually the result of patients seeking unsafe abortion services or the result of long-standing incomplete abortion that has been left untreated. Unsafe abortion and resulting sepsis accounts for approximately 1 in 5 maternal mortalities worldwide and thus is a common cause for admission to the gynecologic ward. Septic abortion is a gynecologic emergency.

Septic abortion patients present with fever, abdominal pain, vaginal bleeding, foul discharge, and sometimes pus from the vagina. Signs of sepsis include fever, tachycardia, and low blood pressure, with or without mental status changes. Patients with possible septic abortion merit a careful abdominal and bimanual pelvic exam to evaluate for signs of acute abdomen or abdomino-pelvic abscess.

If the patient presents with signs of a septic abortion, which can be determined by history and exam, proper resuscitation with intravenous (IV) fluids and broad-spectrum IV antibiotics should be initiated immediately. Low urine output in these cases is due to intravascular depletion from sepsis and volume resuscitation is of paramount importance. If the woman is bleeding or has a infected tissue left inside her uterus, evacuation must occur promptly. An infected uterus is very soft, and care must be take to avoid perforation. If ultrasound is available, a guided technique is preferable. It is best to use an MVA in this instance instead of a D&C. If you suspect pelvic abscesses, you must consider uterine and/ or bowel perforation, and a laparotomy with bowel repair/resection and possibly hysterectomy may be necessary to stabilize the patient. Generally, a second generation cephalosporin or carbapenem for Gram-positive and Gram-negative coverage, an antibiotic for anaerobic coverage such as metronidazole or clindamycin, and doxycycline to cover atypical bacteria should be started and continued for at least 10–14 days.

Prolapsing Fibroid or Polyp

Occasionally, when evaluating for abnormal uterine bleeding, a speculum exam can reveal a cervical polyp, prolapsing endometrial polyp, or prolapsing fibroid. A polyp can usually be removed quite easily by grasping the polyp with a ring forceps and twisting while applying gentle traction until it releases. There is not usually significant bleeding associated with a polypectomy, and it often treats the patient's bleeding symptoms promptly. This procedure can be done in clinic. The vast majority of polyps do not represent carcinoma, and it is typically not necessary to send these to pathology. A pedunculated fibroid within the uterine cavity can grow very large, up to 15 cm in largest diameter, and then prolapse through the cervix, causing cervical dilation. As the fibroid gradually tries to "deliver" through the cervix, the blood supply can be compromised, causing it to become necrotic and infected. A prolapsing fibroid can cause cramping, pelvic pressure, and bloody or watery foul-smelling vaginal discharge. Prolapsing fibroids pose a risk of hemorrhage and severe infection. Preoperatively, broad-spectrum antibiotics and treatment of anemia should be undertaken. A small prolapsing fibroid should be grasped with an instrument, such as a ring forceps or allis clamp, and removed by twisting it free of its attachment. A larger myoma should be grasped, and if the pedicle can be identified, it should be clamped and suture ligated as high as possible; however, too much downward traction should be avoided to prevent uterine inversion.

If the stalk cannot be easily identified, the myoma can be morcellated by removing it in small pieces. There is typically not severe bleeding, but it is always best to identify and ligate the stalk, whenever possible. Cervical dilation can be employed to try to access the stalk of the fibroid. If bleeding is encountered, a 30-mL Foley can be inserted through the cervical os and overfilled with 60–80 ml of fluid to tamponade any bleeding.

Abdominal Myomectomy

Fibroids can cause heavy vaginal bleeding resulting in life-threatening anemia. In addition, when they get very large, they can result in pelvic pressure symptoms, urinary frequency, and constipation. Abdominal myomectomy is indicated for a woman of reproductive age who suffers from these symptoms due to her fibroids and is interested in preservation of fertility. Large fibroids can also cause lower extremity edema if they get large enough to compress the inferior vena cava or iliac veins. Submucosal myomas are best treated with hysteroscopic myomectomy where available.

For symptomatic, large myomas in a woman who has completed her childbearing, a hysterectomy is the operation of choice because an abdominal myomectomy can result in severe intraoperative bleeding and may necessitate a blood transfusion and/

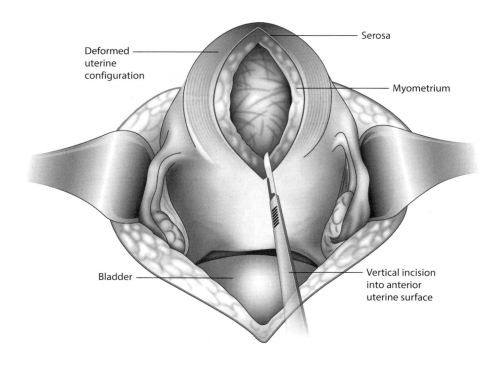

FIGURE 23.3   Abdominal myomectomy. Mann W. Abdominal Myomectomy. [Image on Internet] 2014. Available from: http://goo.gl/yDqSuz.

or emergency hysterectomy. In addition, most fibroids will recur within 5–10 years and will require repeat treatment. In some cultures, a woman may feel very strongly about retaining her uterus for cultural or social reasons. In those cases, a myomectomy may be the only option to treat symptomatic fibroids and avoid a hysterectomy. Preoperatively, the patient should be counseled that if severe hemorrhage is encountered intraoperatively, a hysterectomy may be necessary to avoid death. General principles of pelvic surgery are applicable. Greatest among them is adequate exposure, good lighting, and retraction. A single dose of prophylactic antibiotics should be administered at least 30 minutes prior to surgery to ensure tissue levels of antibiotics. A second generation cephalosporin can provide adequate coverage for prophylaxis. If patients are allergic to penicillins, gentamycin can be used as a substitute. To begin, prep the abdomen with Betadine or another antiseptic solution. A Pfannenstiel incision is usually adequate for many myomectomies, but a vertical incision may be necessary for uteri greater than 20 weeks' size. After the peritoneal cavity is entered, adhesions should be taken down to expose pelvic anatomy, and the bowel packed into the upper abdomen with sponges. Exposure can be improved by placing the patient in Trendelenburg position. The uterine serosa can bleed easily, and care should be taken to avoid the use of traumatic graspers and instruments, such as a uterine screw, tenaculum, or other penetrating instruments. The uterus should be evaluated for the location and number of fibroids, with attention to the location of the uterine vessels, fallopian tubes, and cervical canal. As this

procedure is considered fertility-sparing, the goals are to remove all fibroids, while avoiding compromise to these structures.

To avoid excessive blood loss during surgery, start by creating a window in the broad ligament bilaterally, and then use a JP drain tube or Foley catheter tube stretched tightly around the lower uterine segment to tourniquet the uterine vessels. A large mayo clamp can be used to obtain a tight tourniquet. This maneuver can vastly reduce intraoperative bleeding. We recommend this approach if you are performing this procedure with limited access to blood and blood products for transfusion. In addition, the use of dilute vasopressin (20 units in 100 mL of normal saline) injected into the myometrium and serosa where the incision is to be made can also reduce intraoperative blood loss. There have been case reports of cardiovascular collapse following myometrial injection of vasopressin, so limiting the amount of vasopressin injected is prudent. Some surgeons suggest a maximum dose of 6 units of vasopressin, or up to 30 mL of the vasopressin solution described above. An alternative is to use lidocaine 1% with epinephrine if vasopressin is unavailable. Care should be taken to avoid intravascular injection.

Once the incision site for the myomectomy has been decided, the serosa and myometrium should be injected with the dilute vasopressin or epinephrine. Blanching should be observed before making a generous incision into the uterus. Incisions on the anterior uterus are preferable to posterior incisions. If multiple myomas can be accessed through the same incision, this is preferable to making multiple incisions. The steps are described below:

1. A vertical incision is made over the myoma.
2. The incision is extended into the substance of the myoma.
3. Identify and dissect the plane between myoma capsule and the myometrium. This can be achieved with gauze covering the index finger or closed mayo scissors.
4. Remove as many myomas as possible through the same incision.
5. The base of the myoma can be vascular, and sharp dissection is sometimes necessary to remove it from the base.
6. Running sutures in layers with delayed absorbable suture are used to obliterate the dead space and reapproximate the myometrium to achieve hemostasis. Once the dead space is closed, the serosa is closed with a "baseball" suture or subcuticular suture (Figure 23.3).

If the endometrium is entered or if a deep incision is made in the fundal region of the uterus, the patient should be counseled to avoid labor and to undergo an elective cesarean section between 36–38 weeks. The timing of delivery should take into consideration the accuracy of gestational age dating, the risk of prematurity, and the related risk of neonatal death in your setting weeks to avoid uterine rupture.

The peritoneum need not be closed routinely, although some surgeons feel that this reduces adhesion formation. The fascia is closed using a running number 0 or number 1 delayed absorbable suture. If subcutaneous fatty tissue is greater than 2 cm in depth, we recommend closing this layer using 2-0 or 3-0 plain gut or chromic suture. The skin can be closed in the routine fashion.

Hysterectomy

Simple hysterectomy is indicated for women who have completed or do not desire childbearing with symptomatic uterine fibroids, abnormal uterine bleeding that does not respond to hormonal management, hemorrhage from any cause that is not responsive to standard treatment, endometrial hyperplasia, endometrial cancer, cervical cancer stage 1A and less, and various other conditions. When possible, a vaginal hysterectomy is less invasive and thus preferable to an abdominal hysterectomy, but this is often not possible when fibroids are greater than 14 weeks' size, as is often the case in LMICs. Vaginal hysterectomy requires special training and should not be attempted without extra training. In most cases, the ovaries should be left in place in women under age 60. Oophorectomy can cause premature surgical menopause and has been associated with higher all-cause mortality compared to patients who have ovarian conservation at time of hysterectomy.

Washing the Patient

In addition to prepping the abdomen with Betadine or another antiseptic, the vagina should be prepped as it will be entered for a total hysterectomy. An unprepped vagina can contaminate the surgical field. Even when the vagina is washed, a single dose of prophylactic antibiotics should be administered at least 30 minutes prior to surgery to ensure tissue levels of antibiotics. A second generation cephalosporin can provide adequate coverage for

prophylaxis. If patients are allergic to penicillins, gentamycin can be used as a substitute.

Patient Positioning

Most hysterectomies can be accomplished in the supine position. However, some surgeons prefer the use of Allen stirrups for low lithotomy positions to help with uterine manipulation and cystoscopy, if needed.

Incision Choice

After general anesthesia is induced, the bimanual exam should be performed, and a decision about the proper position should be made. Usually, a Pfannenstiel incision can provide adequate exposure. If the uterus is larger than 20 weeks' size or nonmobile, a vertical midline incision is preferable for adequate exposure.

Exposure

It is imperative to obtain excellent exposure in order to accomplish a hysterectomy safely. A self-retaining retractor is preferable, and the bowel should be packed in the upper abdomen with moist lap sponges with care to account for all sponges with care to account for all sponges at the beginning and the end of the case. Trendelenburg position can also be helpful. For obese patients, a 0-silk suture can be used to sew excess peritoneum to the abdominal wall to improve exposure. Number 1 or 0 delayed absorbable suture is used throughout the surgery.

Surgical Steps

1. The round ligaments and utero-ovarian ligaments are grasped with large Mayo, Kocher, or Kelley clamps, and the uterus is elevated out of the pelvis. The uterus is retracted to the side opposite of the main operator to stretch the round ligament. A stitch is placed and tied under the round ligament approximately halfway along its length with care to capture the small artery of Sampson, which runs within the round ligament. A second suture is placed and tied just medial to the first. Both are elevated while the surgeon divides the round ligament with the Metzenbaum scissors, thus opening the retroperitoneal space below the broad ligament (Figure 23.4).
2. The peritoneal incision is extended down the anterior leaf of the broad ligament toward the bladder reflection in preparation for dissecting the bladder off the cervix and exposing the uterine artery, but do not dissect the bladder yet, as bleeding may be encountered and this step is not necessary yet (Figure 23.5).
3. Steps 1 and 2 are repeated on the contralateral side.
4a. If the ovaries are to be left in the woman, a window is made in the peritoneum of the broad ligament just below the fallopian tube and between the uterus and the ovary. A heavy clamp (large Mayo, curved Kocher, Heaney, or Zeppelin clamp) is used to clamp across the utero-ovarian ligament with its tip in the newly created window. The clamp that was originally placed on the round ligament

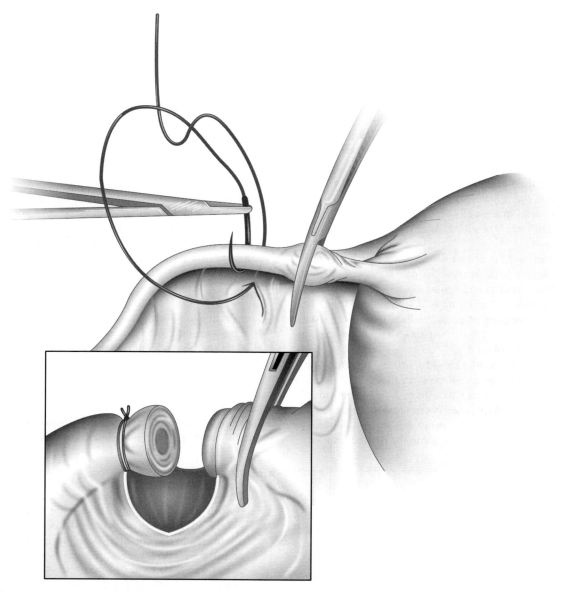

FIGURE 23.4   Dividing the broad ligament. Stovall TG, Mann WJ. Suture ligation of the round ligament during hysterectomy. [Image on Internet] 2014. Available from: http://goo.gl/sxojSK.

and fallopian tube is repositioned with the tip in the window to prevent back bleeding and then the utero-ovarian ligament is transected (Figure 23.6). The utero-ovarian pedicle is doubly ligated, first with a free tie and then a second transfixion suture is placed between the free tie and the clamp, while the assistant removes the clamp. The same steps are repeated on the contralateral side.

4b. If the ovaries are going to be removed with the uterus, the incision is brought to the posterior leaf of the broad ligament, lateral to the ovary and parallel to the infundibulopelvic (IP) ligament. The IP ligament is not a ligament at all, but rather the vascular supply to the ovaries. Once the anterior and posterior leaves of the broad ligament are dissected, the loose areolar tissue of the retroperitoneum can be dissected by gently pushing with the index finger or the back of a dissecting forceps

in the superior and inferior direction in order to identify the key structures in the retroperitoneum. The goal is to identify the external iliac artery on the psoas muscle up to the bifurcation of the common iliac artery where the ureter can be seen crossing the pelvic brim on the medial leaf of the peritoneum. Once the ureter is identified, a hole can be made in the peritoneum below the IP taking care to stay above the ureter. The IP is then doubly clamped with the tips of the clamp in the hole. The IP is divided between the two clamps, and the pedicle is doubly ligated, first with a free tie, and then a second transfixion suture is placed between the free tie and the clamp, while the assistant removes the clamp entirely.

The specimen side of the IP can be left clamped or ligated with a free tie. The ovary, which is now freed from its vascular supply, can then be tied to the

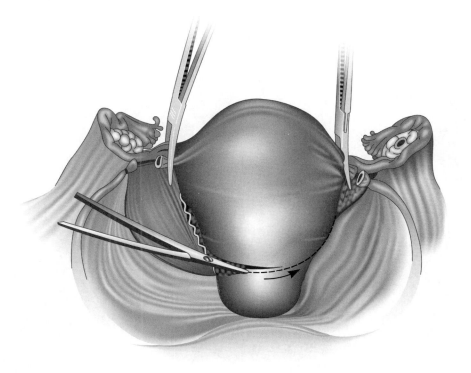

FIGURE 23.5 Developing the vesicouterine fold during hysterectomy. Stovall TG, Mann WJ. Developing the vesicouterine fold during hysterectomy. [Image on Internet] 2014. Available from: http://goo.gl/mmHxzH.

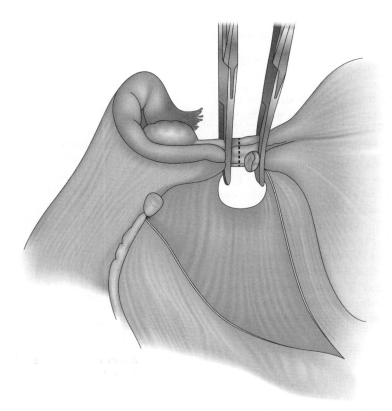

FIGURE 23.6 Dividing the utero-ovarian pedicle. Stovall TG, Mann WJ. Hysterectomy without oophorectomy. [Image on Internet] 2014. Available from: http://goo.gl/o8W7aI.

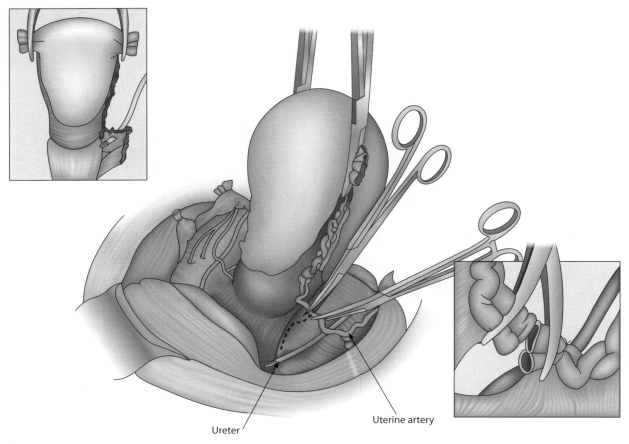

FIGURE 23.7 Abdominal hysterectomy and the relationship of the uterine vessels. The ureters usually lay 2 cm lateral to the uterine artery, but may be closer. Care must be taken during the ligation of the uterine arteries to avoid the ureters. From Uptodate Abdominal Hysterectomy, 2011 Stovall TG, Mann WJ. Ligation of uterine artery during hysterectomy. [Image on Internet] 2014. Available from: http://goo.gl/NOgjl8.

ipsilateral uterine clamp to prevent it from obscuring the surgical field. The same steps are repeated on the contralateral side.

5. The bladder must now be dissected off the cervix and lower uterine segment. Sharp Metzenbaum scissors or blunt dissection with a sponge can be used to push the bladder down. The uterus is elevated during this dissection to help with countertraction. This dissection should take place centrally over the cervix, because if it is done too far laterally, bleeding from perforating arteries of the bladder can ensue. The bladder should be dissected off the cervix below the cervicovaginal junction. When this is accomplished, the surgeon should be able to place one hand on either side of the uterus antero-posteriorly and feel only vagina between his or her extended fingers.

6. The uterine vessels are then skeletonized by dissecting the connective tissue adjacent to the lower uterus while the uterus is retracted to the opposite side. The uterine artery is found just lateral to uterus at the level of the internal os. Clearing the uterine vessels of the surrounding tissue or "skeletonizing" them allows them to be securely grasped and tied without the inclusion

of unnecessary tissue. A heavy, curved clamp (curved Kocher or curved Heaney clamp) is used to clamp the uterine vessels immediately lateral to the uterus and at a right angle to the uterus. A straight Kocher clamp should be placed vertically along the side of the uterus to prevent back bleeding. The uterine vessels are then cut with a knife or scissors and the pedicle is doubly suture-ligated, and the clamps are removed. The same steps are repeated on the contralateral side (Figure 23.7).

7. The bladder is checked to make sure it has been dissected off the anterior cervix and is well below the cervicovaginal junction. The rectum rarely has to be divided off the posterior cervix, but if necessary, this should be done. If this is difficult due to dense adhesions, and the hysterectomy is being done for benign indications, a supracervical hysterectomy should be considered. Once the dissection is complete anterior and posteriorly, the attention is turned to freeing the uterus and cervix from cardinal and uterosacral ligaments. The uterus is again placed on tension for exposure and to help pull the lower uterine segment away from the ureter. The bladder can be retracted anteriorly

with a malleable retractor or a narrow Deaver retractor. A series of straight clamps (straight Kocher or straight Zeppelin clamps) are used to successively clamp the remaining ligamentous connections by placing the clamp vertically along the lateral portion of the cervix, with each clamp placed immediately adjacent to the previous pedicle. The clamp is placed such as to slide off the firm cervical tissue and slide snugly against the lateral wall of the cervix. It is important that the clamp fits snug against the cervix because the ureter can lie as little as 1 cm lateral to this location. With snug placement of clamps, the risk of injuring the ureter is minimized. A knife or heavy scissors is used to cut away each pedicle close to the cervix and the tip of the transfixion suture is placed at the tip of the clamp. Usually one or two bites are taken on each side before moving to the opposite side and then back again until both sides are dissected free to the level of the cervicovaginal junction.

8. Once again, the surgeon should check that the bladder and rectum are well below the cervicovaginal junction and the anterior and posterior vaginal walls are freely palpable. Angled large Zeppelin clamps, curved Heaney clamps, or large curved Kochers are used to clamp across the vagina, fitting snugly just below the cervix, including tissue from the uterosacral ligament posteriorly, the cardinal ligaments laterally, and the anterior and posterior vagina. The clamps are placed from each side with the tips meeting in the middle. A knife or heavy scissors is used to amputate the specimen. A Heaney transfixion suture is placed on each lateral clamp, incorporating the uterosacral ligament with the second bite to provide support for the vaginal cuff. The latter step prevents postoperative vaginal prolapse. As these sutures are tied, the clamps are removed, and a figure-of-eight suture is placed in the center of the vaginal cuff. If the vaginal cuff is very wide and placing clamps that incorporate the anterior and posterior vagina below the cervix as described above would shorten the vagina excessively, the vagina can be entered anteriorly with scissors and then cut circumferentially around the cervical-vaginal junction. In this case, straight Kocher clamps are used to grasp the vaginal edges, and the cuff is closed with a series of figure-of-eight stitches with care to incorporate the uterosacral ligaments, which helps with apical support and prevents cuff prolapse.

9. In some cases, a total hysterectomy cannot be accomplished. If a supracervical hysterectomy is to be done, the technique is similar to that described above except that when you reach the level of the uterine arteries, you must ensure that the bladder and rectum are advanced far enough so that the cervix can be visualized anteriorly and posteriorly and the uterine vessels are ligated as described above. If you have electrocautery, that is best used to amputate the uterus just above the level where the uterine arteries were ligated with a shallow cone-shaped cut. If you do not have electrocautery, the same thing can be done using a knife, but more sutures may need to be placed for hemostasis. It is helpful to remove the endocervix so that the patient doesn't experience spotting in the future. Clamps are placed on the anterior and posterior cervix to bring the two edges together with care to avoid the bladder. The first stitch is placed on the lateral cervical edge close to the uterine artery pedicle. These stitches are held on either side, while the rest of the stump is closed. Hemostasis can be best achieved, especially if electrocautery was not used, by placing figure-of-eight stitches deep in the anterior and posterior cervix while including the posterior peritoneum (avoiding the rectum).

10. After the cuff is closed, the pelvis is irrigated with warm saline, and the pedicles are all carefully inspected for hemostasis.

11. The peritoneum may or may not be closed, depending on surgeon preference. The fascial closure is typically done with a running number 0 or number 1 delayed absorbable. For vertical incisions, mass closure can be used instead. A mass closure includes peritoneum and the anterior and posterior leaves of rectus abdominus fascia abdominus fascia, all in one stitch.

12. If subcutaneous fatty tissue is greater than 2 cm in depth, we recommend closing this layer using 2-0 or 3-0 plain gut or chromic suture. The skin can be closed in the routine fashion.

Drainage of TOA

Tubal ovarian abscesses (TOAs) can occur as a result of untreated pelvic inflammatory disease from sexually transmitted infections, such as gonorrhea or chlamydia, but are more often polymicrobial. Pelvic abscesses can also occur after septic abortions, appendicitis, or any other generalized peritonitis. Tuberculosis is an important cause of pelvic abscesses in LMICs. Broad-spectrum antibiotics should be used to treat pelvic abscesses. Generally, a second generation cephalosporin or carbapenem for Gram-positive and Gram-negative coverage, an antibiotic for anaerobic coverage such as metronidazole or clindamycin, and doxycycline to cover atypical bacteria should be started and continued for at least 10–14 days.

If there is no clinical response within 24–48 hours and the patient is very ill, it may be necessary to drain the abscesses surgically. Surgical drainage is also sometimes necessary for large abscesses (greater than 5 cm) as the abscess wall can become quite thickened and difficult for antibiotics to penetrate. Depending on the location, pelvic abscesses can be drained through a posterior colpotomy or abdominal incision. Percutaneous drainage is difficult unless ultrasound guidance is available. A transabdominal drain can be placed under ultrasound guidance.

Transvaginal Approach to Abscess Drainage

An abscess that can be accessed through the vagina should be able to be palpated in the midline on rectovaginal exam. On bimanual exam, the abscess should feel cystic and fluctuant.

Prepare the patient by placing her in high lithotomy position after spinal anesthesia is administered. Perform a bimanual and rectovaginal exam to confirm that you can access the abscess vaginally. Prep the vagina and cervix with Betadine or other antiseptic solution. Visualize the cervix with a short speculum or two right-angle retractors. Place a tenaculum on the posterior lip of the cervix and pull up to expose the posterior fornix. To confirm that you are in the right place, place a large bore needle in the suspected abscess cavity and aspirate to see what kind of fluid comes out (Figure 23.8). If the aspirate is bloody, then the operator should be concerned for a possible ruptured ectopic pregnancy or a ruptured hemorrhagic cyst. Purulent aspirate confirms the diagnosis and location of the abscess. To make a colpotomy, use curved Mayo scissors to make a transverse incision just below the cervicovaginal reflection. Widen the incision to a least 2 cm. If you have not punctured the abscess cavity with your colpotomy incision, a Kelly clamp is then used to puncture the abscess wall, and pus should drain out. Open the clamp as you remove it to make the opening wide enough for the pus to drain. Use your index finger to explore the cavity and break up any loculations carefully, with attention to avoid bursting through the abscess cavity and entering into the peritoneum or causing injury to the bowel. A drain should be placed in the abscess cavity and secured with a stitch. It should be left in place for several days, and antibiotics should be continued.

Abdominal Approach to Abscess Drainage

For large abscesses, a low midline incision is necessary. Depending on the extent and location of the abscesses, a Pfannenstiel incision may be necessary. For LMICs, if laparoscopy is available, this is the preferred approach. Position the patient in low lithotomy position if you think you may place a drain that exits the vagina. Prep the abdomen and vagina with Betadine or another antiseptic solution. Make an adequate incision for good exposure. As much as possible, the upper abdomen should be isolated from the pelvis with large moist sponges or towels to avoid contamination with pus, which will often spill during the dissection. The decision as to the extent of the necessary surgery is extremely dependent on the future childbearing desires of the patient, the extent of the abscesses and attendant adhesions, and the skill of the surgeon. If large abscesses are found but the woman wants to preserve childbearing, the tubes can be incised longitudinally and drained of all pus, the abdomen can irrigated, and the woman can be continued on broad-spectrum antibiotics. The likelihood of her having a successful pregnancy is extremely low if bilateral tubes are involved. Her risk of an ectopic pregnancy is very high, but her wishes to preserve future fertility must be taken into account.

If the woman is willing to undergo the indicated surgery, including a hysterectomy and removal of tubes, preservation of ovaries may be done. The exploration and dissection is usually best started at the round ligament, which helps orient the surgeon. There is risk of injury to ureters, bowel, and vessels, if dense adhesions are present and care must be taken to avoid these structures. The positioning in the low-lithotomy position also allows for cystoscopy to evaluate the bladder and ureteral orifices, if necessary after the surgery. Blunt dissection with your fingers can be used for the soft, fresh adhesions, but the use of

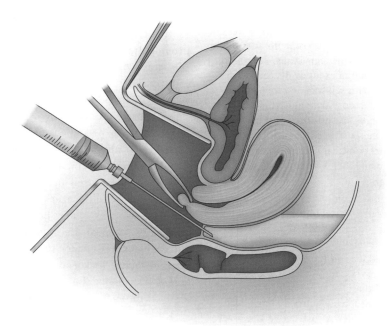

FIGURE 23.8   Culdocentesis. Webb MJ. Culdocentesis. *Journal of the American College of Emergency Physicians.* 1978 Dec; 7(12): 451–454

Metzenbaum scissors or scalpel may be necessary for the more dense adhesions. If the retroperitoneum can be entered, the ureters can be identified, allowing for safer dissection thereafter. If there are tubo-ovarian abscesses or complexes, it can be difficult to locate the ovary separate from the abscess. If the mass must be removed, the patient may lose one or both ovaries. If both adnexa must be removed, a hysterectomy should be considered if there is concern for uterine involvement. If this is done, a drain can be placed through the vaginal cuff, thus leaving it open for drainage and subsequent easy removal of the drain. Alternatively, a drain can be brought up through the abdominal wall if the vaginal cuff cannot be accessed. If the disease is unilateral, the normal ovary and tube should be left, unless the woman is postmenopausal. The uterus should be left in place to preserve fertility as long as it is not too extensively involved in the infectious process.

Regardless of the surgery, all abscess cavities should be drained, removed, and copiously irrigated. Copious irrigation is the mainstay of abscess treatment. Drain placement is indicated if there is a concern for reaccumulation or incomplete drainage. A drain can be brought out through a posterior colpotomy, the vaginal cuff, or the abdominal wall, depending on the extent of the dissection. Continuation of at least 10–14 days of broad-spectrum antibiotics is critical to achieve a cure.

Oophorectomy/Ovarian Cystectomy/Detorsion

Ovarian surgery may be indicated if a patient presents with severe abdominal or pelvic pain and ovarian torsion is suspected, a patient is taken for exploratory laparotomy and ovarian masses are found, or a large ovarian mass is suspected but not felt to be ovarian cancer. Suspected ovarian cancer should be referred to a hospital that is capable of performing intensive chemotherapy because ovarian cancer is almost never cured by surgery alone once it has become symptomatic, and primary surgery without access to chemotherapy is not necessarily indicated as it will not prolong life and may increase suffering.

Once surgery has been initiated and an ovarian mass is found, the surgeon must decide if he or she is going to perform an oophorectomy (remove the entire ovary), an ovarian cystectomy, or a simple drainage. A simple drainage is almost never the surgery of choice. The age and reproductive future of a patient must be taken into account, as removal of both ovaries will sterilize the patient, put her into acute menopause, which results in problematic symptoms, increases morbidity and mortality, and may cause social strife. Early menopause puts patients at risk for extreme vasomotor symptoms, vaginal dryness, loss of libido, mood changes, and osteoporosis, not to mention infertility. It is generally recommended to attempt to preserve ovarian tissue in any young woman who wants future childbearing, and at least one ovary should be preserved in premenopausal women unless they are close to menopause and/or malignancy is suspected.

Ovarian torsion can strike at any age and is typically seen with ovarian masses >5 cm in size, but can happen in the setting of normal ovaries as well, especially in girls less than 15 years old. This diagnosis is often suspected when a patient presents with sudden onset lower abdominal pain and an ovarian mass is palpated. The patient can have peritoneal signs and the pain can be associated with vomiting. A patient can have pain that comes and goes if the torsion is intermittent. It usually results when the enlarged ovary twists on the infundibulopelvic (IP) ligament and can cause the ovary to lose its blood supply and necrose if it is not treated promptly. Suspected torsion is considered a surgical emergency because "time is tissue" and saving the ovary is of the utmost importance, particularly in young women and girls. Surgery should be undertaken as soon as the diagnosis is suspected and certainly within 24 hours of the torsion for the best chance of saving ovarian tissue. In the past if the ovary looked purple after it was untwisted, oophorectomy was performed because it was felt that the ovarian tissue could not be salvaged and there was risk of peritonitis if the necrotic ovary was left in place. It has now become a standard of care to leave the ovary in place even if it continues to look purple because the ovary may regain function and the risk of peritonitis and thrombus is low. This has become our practice, and the default in young women should always be ovarian conservation in these cases.

If torsion is present, it is usually the case that the ovary is twisted around the IP ligament, but isolated fallopian tube torsion can occur. The first step is to untwist the ovary and wait to see how the ovary responds to reperfusion. If a cyst is present and the ovary can be salvaged, an ovarian cystectomy should be undertaken, as described below. If no cyst is present, particularly in children, pexy of the ovary may be considered. This can be achieved by shortening the utero-ovarian ligament, suturing the utero-ovarian ligament to the ipsilateral utero-sacral ligament, or suturing the ovary to the pelvic sidewall with care to avoid vascular structures and the ureter.

Oophorectomy

After entry into the abdomen, assess the pelvis and upper abdomen for evidence of malignant implants. If malignancy is suspected and there is access to a pathologist, obtain washings by using a syringe to squirt 50–100 cc of fluid into the pelvis and then suck it back up with the syringe. To perform the oophorectomy:

1. Identify the IP ligament and the ureter, which should be visible on the sidewall just below the pelvic brim.
2. Incise the peritoneum parallel to the ovarian vessels in order to enter the retroperitoneum. An alternative method is to divide the round ligament to enter the retroperitoneal space. The image below depicts the approach that incises the round ligament (Figure 23.9).
3. The loose areolar tissue of the retroperitoneum can be dissected by gently pushing with the index finger or the back of a dissecting forceps in the superior and inferior direction in order to identify the key structures in the retroperitoneum. The goal is to identify the external iliac artery on the psoas muscle up to the bifurcation of the common iliac artery where the ureter can be seen crossing the pelvic brim on the medial leaf of the peritoneum. Once the ureter is identified, a hole can be made in the peritoneum below the IP, taking care to stay above the ureter. The IP is then doubly clamped with the tips of the clamp in the hole. The IP is divided between the two clamps and the pedicle is doubly ligated, first with a free tie and then a second transfixion suture is placed between

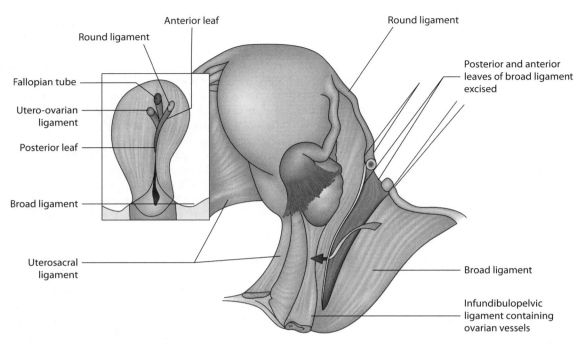

FIGURE 23.9 The round ligament is divided and the retroperitoneal space entered. Valea FA, Mann WJ. Open oophorectomy. [Image on Internet] 2014. Available from: http://goo.gl/oKzJ4i

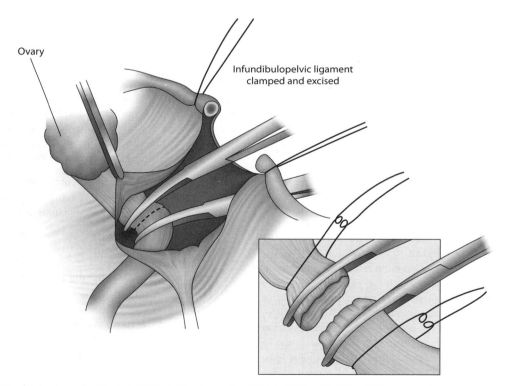

FIGURE 23.10 After the ureter is identified, the IP is doubly clamped and divided. Valea FA, Mann WJ. Open oophorectomy. [Image on Internet] 2014. Available from: http://goo.gl/Sphhyy.

the free tie and the clamp while the assistant removes the clamp entirely. The specimen side of the IP can be left clamped or ligated with a free tie (Figure 23.10).

4. If the tube is to be left in-situ, the ovary has to be freed from the utero-ovarian ligament and vessels (the ovarian branches of the uterine artery) and the broad ligament.

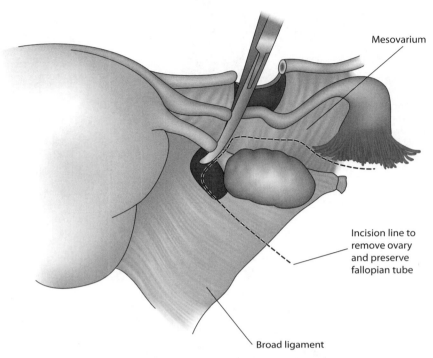

Utero-ovarian ligament and
fallopian tube clamped and excised

Mesovarium

Incision line to
remove ovary
and preserve
fallopian tube

Broad ligament

FIGURE 23.11 Oophorectomy with and without salpingectomy. Valea FA, Mann WJ. Open oophorectomy. [Image on Internet] 2014. Available from: http://goo.gl/oKzJ4i.

Sequentially clamp, cut, and tie the broad ligament below the tube and above the ovary until reaching the utero-ovarian ligament. Doubly clamp, cut, and tie this pedicle, using a free tie and a transfixion suture (Figure 23.11).

5. If the tube is to be removed, the tube and utero-ovarian ligament are clamped, cut, and ligated parallel to the cornua (Figure 23.11).

Ovarian Cystectomy

For a cyst that lies within the ovarian stroma, make a slightly curved incision over a thin portion of the ovarian cortex (Figure 23.12).

Take care to avoid the fimbria and fallopian tube to prevent fertility problems in the future. Keeping the cyst intact is helpful both to avoid spillage of potentially caustic or malignant material (sebaceous material from a dermoid, or blood from a hemorrhagic cyst, or potentially malignant cells) and to make it easier to identify the plane between the cyst wall and the ovarian stroma. In the event that spillage does occur, steps should be taken to contain it (packing the area and suctioning the contents) and copious irrigation with at least 3 liters of warm saline should be used to avoid a chemical peritonitis. Using closed Metzenbaum scissors, a finger, or the back of a knife handle, develop the plane between the cyst wall and the ovarian stroma, which should be relatively easy to define and develop using traction-countertraction. The base of the cyst may contain a vascular pedicle, and this area may be more

difficult to separate. If this seems to be the case, it is wise to clamp it prior to transection and tie it with a transfixion suture. If the ovarian tissue is not hemostatic, you may need to close the deep ovarian stroma and ovarian incision with 3-0 delayed absorbable suture, but in many cases, it is hemostatic and does not need to be closed. Do not trim the ovarian stroma, even if it appears attenuated, because it may contain immature follicles and viable ovarian tissue. If multiple cysts are present, try to use the minimal number of incisions possible on the ovary to remove the cysts, and try to avoid oophorectomy in young women whenever possible. Even small amounts of remaining ovarian tissue can be functional hormonally and lead to future pregnancy.

Large ovarian cysts may be difficult to identify separate from the ovary and may necessitate an oophorectomy. Cysts can become enormous and take over the entire abdominal cavity. These cysts may require very large incisions and may need to be drained to avoid these large incisions. In these cases, to minimize spillage, a purse-string suture can be sewn in the ovarian surface prior to making a small needle puncture to perform a controlled aspiration using a large syringe or suction tubing. Because large cysts, especially if they are adherent, can pull the ureter into the operative field, care must be taken to avoid clamping the ureter during removal of the cyst. Typically large cysts are partially drained, using the above technique, and the ovary is delivered through a small abdominal incision. The remainder of the cystectomy is performed once the ovary is external.

(a)

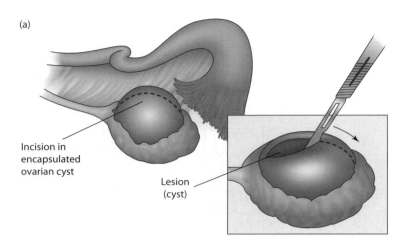

Incision in
encapsulated
ovarian cyst

Lesion
(cyst)

(b)

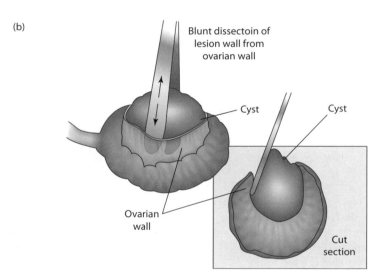

Blunt dissectoin of
lesion wall from
ovarian wall

Cyst

Cyst

Ovarian
wall

Cut
section

FIGURE 23.12   Ovarian cystectomy. Valea FA, Mann WJ. Open ovarian cystectomy. [Image on Internet] 2014. Available from: http://goo.gl/JsBV3v.

Ectopic Pregnancy

An ectopic pregnancy refers to a pregnancy that occurs anywhere outside of the uterine cavity, most commonly in the fallopian tube. However, ectopic pregnancies can also occur in the abdomen, in the cornua of the uterus, in a caesarean delivery scar, and in the cervix.

Ruptured ectopic pregnancy is a surgical emergency that must be recognized quickly and should be suspected in any woman of reproductive age presenting with severe abdominal pain, with vaginal bleeding; and/or signs or symptoms of shock. The classic symptom triad is considered amenorrhea, vaginal bleeding, and abdominal pain. To confirm that the patient has a ruptured ectopic, you can do a culdocentesis by placing a large bore needle in the posterior fornix and aspirating to make sure blood comes out. Although blood may also be aspirated if the patient has a ruptured hemorrhagic cyst, this technique can

be helpful if the diagnosis is suspected, but definitive management should not be delayed if there is high suspicion for a ruptured ectopic.

Although unruptured ectopic pregnancies can be treated with methotrexate or surgery, in places without reliable access to quantitative serum human chorionic gonadotropin (HCG), ultrasound, and close follow-up, nonsurgical treatment is not usually an option.

Surgical treatment can be accomplished with laparoscopy, though this is not an option in many settings. If it is not available, a mini-laparotomy through a Pfannenstiel incision is usually adequate to find and treat the ectopic pregnancy. If the patient is in severe shock and IV access cannot be obtained, it may be necessary to do a cut-down, but if this is not an option, local anesthesia can be used to gain entry into the peritoneal cavity, injecting the anesthetic agent at each of the levels—cutaneous, fascial, and peritoneal. The peritoneum is very sensitive, and with entry into the peritoneum, the patient may awake in pain,

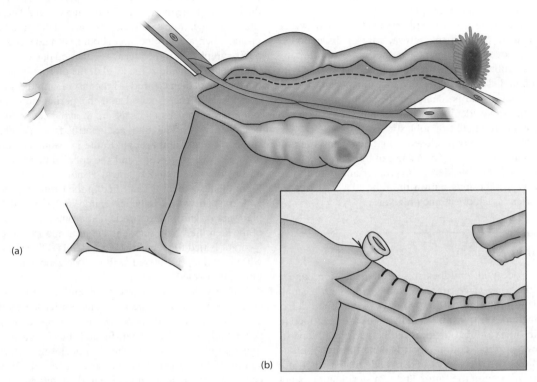

FIGURE 23.13 Salpingectomy. Tulandi T. Total salpingectomy. [Image on Internet] 2014. Available from: http://goo.gl/6He4Gg.

so make sure there are adequate personnel to hold the patient down until the ectopic is grasped and the bleeding tamponaded. Collection of the blood and clots in the abdomen for autotransfusion is possible if the pregnancy sac can be removed intact, but if products of conception are mixed with the blood and clots, this should not be done.

If a ruptured ectopic is identified, salpingectomy must be performed. After the incision is made, the surgeon should reach his or her hand into the pelvis and evacuate any blood and clot encountered. Next, the surgeon should feel for the fundus of the uterus and find the ruptured tube. The tube is then brought to the incision, and the thumb and forefinger are used to compress the blood vessels in the broad ligament to stop the bleeding.

Salpingectomy

Place a clamp across the mesosalpynx and another across the proximal portion of the tube close to the cornua. The clamps should meet in the midline and a suture ligation performed with 2.0 or 3.0 delayed absorbable suture as each clamp is slowly removed; 1.0 catgut suture is also adequate. Additional stitches can be thrown to obtain complete hemostasis (Figure 23.13). If products of conception are extruded, care should be taken to find them and remove them from the pelvis.

If the cornual region is involved (as with an interstitial pregnancy), a wedge resection of the cornual region may be necessary and hemostasis can be more difficult to achieve. Consider injecting dilute vasopressin, as with a myomectomy, to decrease

blood loss. After resection, the myometrial bed must be closed in layers, similar to the technique used following a myomectomy. The patient should be counseled about possible risk of uterine rupture in future pregnancies, though this risk is not quantified.

Salpingostomy

If an ectopic pregnancy is identified prior to rupture, a salpingostomy is an alternative to salpingectomy, but is generally not indicated as it can predispose the patient to a future ectopic pregnancy on that side. In large studies, salpingostomy does not lead to higher future fertility rates but does increase the risk for future ectopic pregnancy; therefore, it should only be done if it is the only chance to retain any fertility options for the woman and she insists that everything be done to preserve any chance of pregnancy even after understanding the increased risk of ectopic pregnancy and therefore death with any future pregnancy. Salpingectomy should be done if the patient is hemodynamically unstable, there is a recurrent ectopic in the same tube, the tube is very damaged, the tubal pregnancy is greater than 5 cm, the woman has completed childbearing, or the contralateral tube appears normal. However, if she is sure she wants to retain her fertility, and she understands it may predispose her to a future life-threatening ectopic, and her contralateral tube looks abnormal or she has already had a salpingectomy in the contralateral tube, a salpingostomy is an option.

A salpingostomy is performed by creating a 10–15 mm longitudinal incision on the antimesenteric side of the tube just above the bulge where the ectopic is suspected. Hemostasis can be aided by first injecting dilute vasopressin (0.2 IU/ml of saline) into the serosa of the tube where the incision is to be made. Once the incision is made through the serosa, careful dissection is undertaken to remove the pregnancy tissue while minimizing the damage to the tube. Hydrodissection can be undertaken with a syringe and blunt dissection with a fine instrument can be used. Once the pregnancy tissue is identified, it can be grasped and removed from the tube. Ideally the gestational sac is removed intact to prevent any retained trophoblastic tissue.

The tubal defect should not be closed, and if hemostasis cannot be achieved with pressure and minimal use of fine sutures, then a salpingectomy should be considered. It is important to minimize suturing to prevent adhesions within the tube that will further increase the patient's risk of ectopic pregnancy.

Interval Tubal Ligation

If a woman is done with childbearing, a tubal ligation can be performed at the time of cesarean section or through a small infraumbilical skin incision within two days of a vaginal delivery. These immediate postpartum tubal ligations are described in Chapter 22. An interval tubal ligation can be performed laparoscopically; however, more commonly it is done through a mini-laparotomy. Make sure the patient understands that she will not be able to have children in the future and that sterilization is not reversible. In some communities, the woman and her husband may need to be involved in the conversation. You must also confirm that she is not pregnant prior to surgery.

Interval midline mini laparotomy in LMICs is usually performed under local anesthesia and verbal reassurance. Operating under local anesthesia can be challenging, although with proper technique, surgery can be well tolerated by patients. It is important that the surgeon uses decisive yet gentle surgical technique while simultaneously offering verbal reassurance to the patients (verbo-caine). The advantages of operating under local anesthesia are that generally patients can have this procedure done in an outpatient primary health center or dispensary and thus they can avoid the cost and time associated with transfer to a larger hospital for inpatient admission.

This procedure is less challenging if a uterine manipulator is placed into the uterus via the cervix to bring the uterine fundus to the incision. To begin, a bimanual exam should be performed to assess the size of the uterus. Then a speculum exam should be performed. A cervical block as described above should be administered to decrease discomfort of uterine manipulation. A Hulka uterine manipulator should then be placed trans-cervically. Next, 20 mL of 1% lidocaine or an alternative local anesthetic should be used to inject along the skin of the proposed incision. This injection should be carried both superiorly and inferiorly along the course of the inferior epigastric nerves and lateral to the incision. The injection should also be carried down to the level of the fascia. Then a 3-cm incision should be made 2–3 cm above the pubis symphysis. If the uterus is enlarged due to fibroids, the incision should be made at the level of the uterine fundus. The subcutaneous fat is then cleared off the fascia with the surgeon's finger. The fascia is then incised and the peritoneum entered sharply using tissue forceps and scissors to avoid excess pain with blunt peritoneal entry. The tubes are identified using a tubal hook or the surgeon's finger and brought to the incision. The tube is grasped with a Babcock forceps and the tubal fimbria are identified to ensure that the round ligament is not inadvertently grasped. A 2-cm tubal segment is identified in the isthmus region of the tube and grasped with a Babcock clamp and elevated. A 0-0 or 2-0 plain gut or chromic suture is tied around the tube on either end of the identified 2 cm segment, creating a loop. A second suture of 3 catgut is tied for security (Figure 23.14). Then, the mesosalpinx within the loop is entered with the Metzenbaum scissors and the tube is transected.

The surgeon should carefully examine the transected ends to ensure hemostasis before it is released back into the abdomen. This procedure is then performed on the contra-lateral side. After both tubes have been ligated, the fascia is closed with a figure-of-eight suture and the skin is closed with a subcuticular suture. If the surgeon economizes suture, the entire procedure can be accomplished with one length of suture.

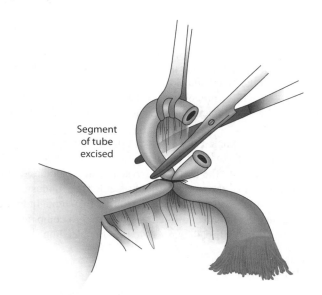

Segment of tube excised

FIGURE 23.14   Tubal ligation. Stovall TG, Mann WJ. Pomeroy tubal ligation C. [Image on Internet] 2014. http://goo.gl/2HZOAJ.

COMMENTARY

Tarek Meguid, Tanzania

No discussion of gynecology should start without mentioning the importance of quality of care. At several points in this chapter, patients are described as more than just bearers of problems; it is most important to emphasize and promote agency of patients as much as possible, especially when they have to undergo surgery. For this reason alone I find it very useful to think of the patients I am trying to serve as individual women and girls rather than as members of one or other culture. At the same time, showing respect for any culture will increase the chances of actually respecting the patient and allowing her to say what she wishes, especially concerning treatment, including surgery, involving her reproductive organs. This will dramatically increase the chances for a good outcome.

The following comments loosely follow the issues raised in the chapter.

Surgery in LMICs is a high-risk undertaking, even when the diagnosis seems clear. Both diagnostic and therapeutic options are limited, and patients tend to present late in the course of their illness. One of the most challenging problems is severe chronic and undiagnosed anemia. It is therefore very important to look at the patients holistically to avoid avoidable calamities.

The cardinal sign of vaginal bleeding is important to understand, and this chapter assists in this. The old saying that "every woman is pregnant unless proven otherwise" is still relevant and should never be forgotten.

A woman who has suffered a miscarriage and presents with a closed cervix is in need of adequate pain relief when dilation is attempted. At a minimum she should receive a paracervical block. If available, IV sedation or spinal anesthesia should be offered. Adequate pain control helps to control erratic patient movement during the procedure and makes the procedure safer.

The most effective and least expensive way of reducing fear and subsequent pain is information. Adequate information given in a caring way will go a long way to prevent complications such as uterine perforation during evacuation in local anesthesia (when the cervix is not closed).

When evacuating a uterus due to miscarriage, it is important, particularly for the inexperienced surgeon, to realize that if bleeding increases significantly during an otherwise unremarkable procedure, the curettage needs to be continued, not terminated, until the uterus is empty. While it is very clear to all health workers that a heavily bleeding patient is an emergency, this is not clear to all when the bleeding is less severe. It is important to consider each and every bleeding miscarriage, even when the bleeding is minimal, as an emergency situation and to "not allow the sun to rise or set over a miscarriage."

Myomectomies are very common in Africa, and the choice for the laparotomy incision should exclusively depend on the size and location of the fibroids and the experience of the surgeon. If in any doubt, a midline incision is preferable. A Cohen incision is a reasonable alternative to a Pfannenstiel since it allows for much more exposure. The use of vasopressin to reduce blood loss is controversial, and it is not always available. I prefer not to use it because I feel I can see where it is bleeding and trust my hemostatic sutures much more.

Names of surgical instruments are very confusing and differ from country to country and sometimes from hospital to hospital, and even from surgeon to surgeon. For this reason we like to have a picture of the instruments we use in each set together with the common name for each in our setting.

When discussing drainage of an abscess, I feel it is important to stress the necessity of draining abscesses whenever possible. If all else fails, it is also a good idea to perform a second-look laparotomy when in doubt and no other diagnostic possibilities exists.

Discussing the management option of salpingotomy with a patient suffering from a tubal pregnancy is very difficult. It is easy to underestimate the pressure under which some patients are to fall pregnant and the difficulties they might have to seek adequate help in case of a ruptured ectopic pregnancy in the future. Usually, ectopic pregnancies come to the attention of health workers far beyond the stage where salpingotomy would be an option, so this dilemma is not very common.

Performing surgery is a highly technical activity that requires special skills, but surgery is just one modality of treatment and treatment need to be imbedded in what the patient needs and wants. This is true for all patients, regardless of socioeconomic status.

24

Genitourinary Surgery

Marc D. Manganiello
Jill Buckley

Introduction

Urology comprises a wide spectrum of pathology. This ranges from elective office-based procedures to quality-of-life interventions to complex oncologic diseases and reconstructive operations. The field of urology is rapidly evolving to include and utilize minimally invasive methods such as endoscopy, laparoscopy, and robotics. However, the resources for these procedures, in terms of equipment, operating space availability, and staffing personnel, make these techniques unavailable in impoverished settings.

There are, however, many urologic conditions that may be treated with instruments from a basic surgical kit. In the chapter that follows, several common urologic operations and their indications are described. Some of these procedures, such as vasectomy and hydrocelectomy, are performed as quality-of-life measures. Circumcision has been shown to reduce the risk of human immunodeficiency virus (HIV) infection by up to 60%; however, when performed incorrectly, it may have devastating consequences. Bladder outlet obstruction in terms of benign prostatic hyperplasia or urethral stricture may ultimately lead to infection, stone formation, and renal failure. Urologic disease is common, and an understanding of the basic pathology and associated interventions is important for any surgeon practicing in low- and middle-income countries (LMICs).

Vasectomy

Vasectomy is the elective sterilization in the male. A segment of the vas deferens is isolated and removed through the anterior upper scrotum. This procedure is generally irreversible. However, it does not guarantee sterilization as the vas may recanalize spontaneously. A semen sample may be obtained 6–8 weeks after the procedure to document the absence of sperm.

Procedure: With the patient in supine position, the genitals are shaved, prepped, and draped in a sterile fashion. The left vas deferens is palpated at the level of the lateral scrotum and spermatic cord and brought up under the left anterior upper scrotal skin. Care is taken to keep the vas from falling back into the scrotum, as it is extremely difficult to identify and re-isolate the vas through the same incision. The area overlying the vas is infiltrated with 2% Xylocaine. A 1/4-inch incision is made over the left vas deferens and carried down through the skin and dartos muscle. The left vas deferens is grasped with a vasectomy clamp (or artery forceps) (Figure 24.1). A segment of the

vas is carefully freed up, attempting to preserve the veins surrounding it as these may bleed excessively (Figure 24.2). The segment of the isolated vas deferens is then excised (Figure 24.3). The cut ends of the vas are occluded with surgical clips or ligation techniques. The ends of the vas as well as the lumen are lightly electrocauterized, separated, and allowed to drop back into the hemiscrotum. The skin incision is closed with 4-0 chromic catgut suture. An identical procedure is performed on the right side for right vasectomy.[1]

The most common complication is scrotal hematoma, resulting from torn veins during the vas isolation. Chronic discomfort from congestion and/or granulation formation is rare but can occur.

Circumcision

In 2007, the World Health Organization (WHO) and Joint United Nations Programme on HIV/AIDS (UNAIDS) stated that "countries with high prevalence, generalized heterosexual HIV epidemics that currently have low rates of male circumcision consider urgently scaling up access to male circumcision services".[2] Studies from Africa have demonstrated that male circumcision reduces the risk of HIV infection by up to 60%. However, properly trained medical personnel and clean equipment are usually lacking. Traditional techniques of circumcision result in much higher rates of complications, such as bleeding, infection, postoperative pain, and erectile dysfunction (35.2%) compared with those circumcisions performed in a clinical setting with sterile technique (0.3–3.8%).[3] Therefore, adequate access and technique are of utmost importance in the promotion and performance of male circumcision. Additional indications for circumcision include prevention of phimosis, irreducible paraphimosis and balanoposthitis, as well as recurrent urinary tract infections secondary to redundant foreskin and poor hygiene. The risk of developing squamous cell carcinoma of the penis is practically eliminated after circumcision.[4] If congenital urethral or penile abnormalities are noted (i.e., hypospadias), circumcision should be deferred until the patient has been evaluated for corrective surgery as the foreskin may be used at the time of repair.

In the acute setting of paraphimosis or for patients who do not require a cosmetic result, a dorsal slit may be performed (Figure 24.4). A dorsal penile nerve block is initially placed by injecting 2% Xylocaine at the dorsolateral 10-o'clock and 2-o'clock position in the base of the penis. Once adequate anesthesia

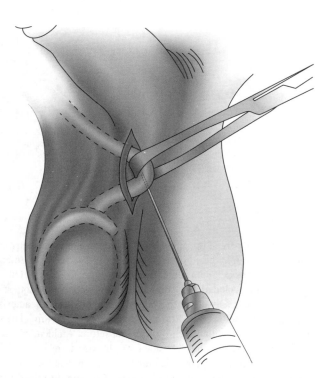

FIGURE 24.1 Isolate vas deferens. World Health Organization. *Surgical Care at the District Hospital.* Geneva: World Health Organization; 2003. Figure 9.55.

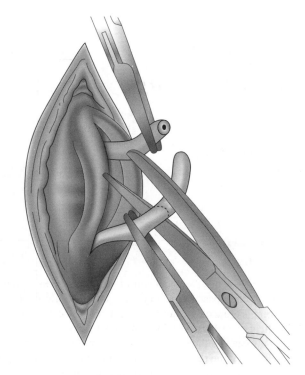

FIGURE 24.3 Excise vas deferens. World Health Organization. *Surgical Care at the District Hospital.* Geneva: World Health Organization; 2003. Figure 9.57.

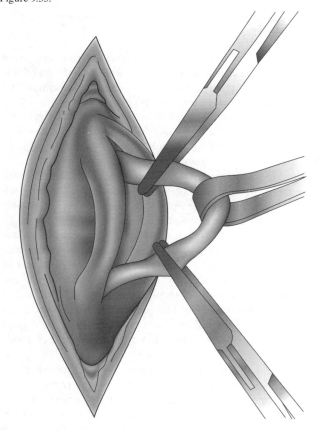

FIGURE 24.2 Dissect vas deferens. World Health Organization. *Surgical Care at the District Hospital.* Geneva: World Health Organization; 2003. Figure 9.56.

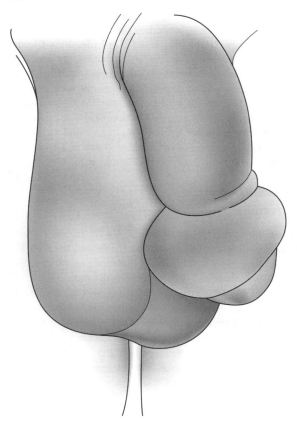

FIGURE 24.4 Paraphimosis. World Health Organization. *Surgical Care at the District Hospital.* Geneva: World Health Organization; 2003. Figure 9.35.

has been obtained, adhesions are taken down between the glans and prepuce. A Kelly clamp is slid along the dorsal aspect of the foreskin and clamped at the 12-o'clock position. This helps with hemostasis, crushing the small capillaries. The clamp is removed and the line is incised, exposing the glans penis (Figure 24.5). Chromic sutures are used in a running fashion along the incised edges, beginning at the apex of the incision.[7]

A Gomco clamp or plastic disposable device may be used in neonates. Adhesions between the prepuce and glans are taken down, and the prepuce is then pulled through the ring in the clamp. The clamp protects the glans from injury. When using the Gomco clamp, the excess foreskin may be excised and an absorbable suture placed for hemostasis. However, with the plastic clamp, the excess foreskin is typically allowed to necrose and falls off within 3–7 days.[7]

In adults, surgical excision of the foreskin is performed. Begin by prepping and draping in a sterile fashion. Local anesthesia is obtained through a dorsal nerve block, injecting at the lateral bases of the penis with 2% Xylocaine as well as circumferential injection of superficial layers at the base of the penis. Begin by taking down all adhesions between the glans and foreskin. This is an extremely important step. Retract the foreskin and with a marking pen, draw the outline of the incision circumferentially. Make sure to leave a 1–2 cm preputial cuff and go straight across the frenulum. Incise through the skin down to the dartos layer. This is the distal margin of the repair. Next, reduce the foreskin. Again, use the marking pen to outline the corona, drawing a *V* at the frenulum. Begin by making a dorsal incision down the prepuce to the coronal marking (Figure 24.6). Extend the incision circumferentially along the premarked outline, through the skin down to the dartos fascia. With the proximal and distal incisions made, dissect under the dorsal skin sleeve and incise across. Either with electrocautery or sharply, divide the skin from the dartos fascia circumferentially. Tie off (or coagulate) bleeding vessels with absorbable sutures, paying close attention to the frenular area. Place an initial suture ventrally and dorsally for control and close the remainder of the incision with interrupted absorbable suture (Figures 24.7 and 24.8). Careful hemostasis is important prior to closure to prevent large penile hematomas and wound dehiscence (Figure 24.9).[5]

Complications include bleeding, infection, glans hyperesthesia, penile hematoma, or cosmetic changes occurring from the removal of too much skin. Rarely, if the urethra is included in the Gomco clamp, a fistula may occur.

Hydrocele

Hydroceles are abnormal fluid collections within the tunica vaginalis of the scrotum. The fluid may obscure palpation of the testes and/or epididymis. Transillumination of the scrotum will not demonstrate any shadows and will appear homogenous. Ultrasonography may also be used to differentiate a hydrocele from other pathology. A reactive hydrocele may form as a result of inflammation, infection, trauma, or tumor. If the scrotal enlargement feels like a bag of worms or does not transilluminate, it is unlikely to be a hydrocele. A patent processus vaginalis may represent a hernia and hydrocele. Signs and symptoms may be described as a reducible mass that varies in size over the course of the day, and expands with a cough. A workup for hydrocele should be performed for other causes of scrotal swelling including hernia, neoplasm, pyocele, varicocele, hematocele, etc. Lymphatic filariasis is endemic in roughly 80 countries with an estimated 120 million cases. Close to 85% of these are located in Southeast Asia and Africa. Over 25 million of these cases result in hydrocele, making filariasis the most common cause worldwide for the development of a hydrocele.[6]

Surgical intervention is indicated when the hydrocele interferes with the patient's ability to work, urinate, have sexual

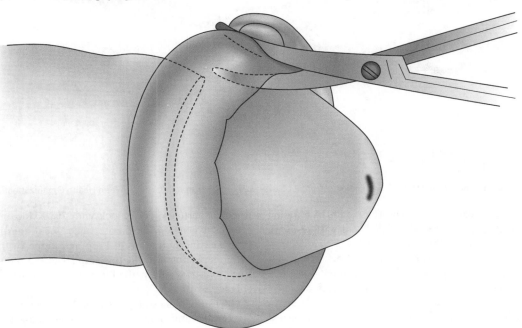

FIGURE 24.5 Dorsal slit. World Health Organization. *Surgical Care at the District Hospital.* Geneva: World Health Organization; 2003. Figure 9.40.

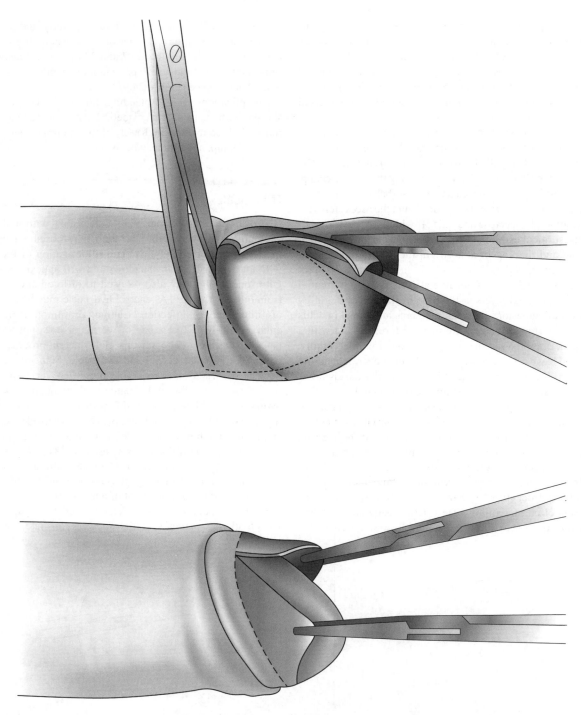

FIGURE 24.6   Dorsal incision. World Health Organization. *Surgical Care at the District Hospital*. Geneva: World Health Organization; 2003. Figure 9.30.

intercourse, or if it is causing discomfort or pain. Aspiration of the hydrocele fluid is not recommended and will result in re-accumulation and risk possible infection.[6]

Procedure: The surgical approach to hydrocelectomy is either a midline incision along the median raphe (contains fewer blood vessels) of the scrotum for bilateral hydroceles or a vertical paramedian scrotal incision for unilateral hydroceles. An inguinal approach should be used if there is a suspicion of testicular cancer; this is described later in the section on orchiectomy. Hydrocelectomy may be performed under local anesthesia

using a spermatic cord block with 2% Xylocaine, spinal anesthesia, or general anesthesia. Inject local anesthetic along the proposed incision as well. Prep and drape in the usual sterile fashion, placing a sterile towel under the scrotum. Make a midline or vertical paramedian incision depending on the hydrocele (Figure 24.10).

Cut through the skin, dartos, and spermatic fascia layers to the level of the tunica vaginalis. This may be thickened and fibrotic from inflammation and infection. Dissect the plane between the hydrocele sac and the internal spermatic fascia in order to

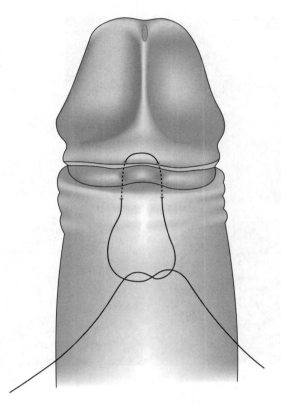

FIGURE 24.7 Ventral anastomosis. World Health Organization. *Surgical Care at the District Hospital*. Geneva: World Health Organization; 2003. Figure 9.31.

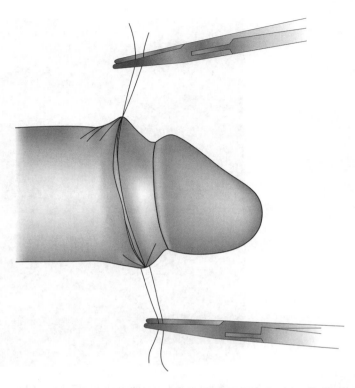

FIGURE 24.8 Initial sutures. World Health Organization. *Surgical Care at the District Hospital*. Geneva: World Health Organization; 2003. Figure 9.32.

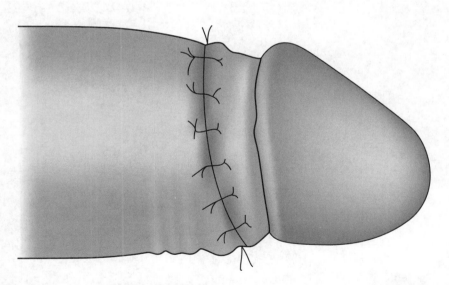

FIGURE 24.9 Completed anastomosis. World Health Organization. *Surgical Care at the District Hospital*. Geneva: World Health Organization; 2003. Figure 9.34.

identify the spermatic cord. Avoid injury to the spermatic vessels and vas deferens by using Penrose drains or vessel loops (Figure 24.11).

Open the hydrocele sac anteriorly, away from the testis and spermatic cord. Collect the hydrocele fluid for analysis. The testis and epididymis are everted through the sac incision. The parietal layer of the tunica sac is excised, leaving a 1-cm margin (Figure 24.12 and Figure 24.13).

The sac edges may then be oversewn with a running absorbable suture. The sac edges may also be sewn together behind the spermatic cord itself (Jaboulay bottleneck procedure) with running absorbable suture, but care must be taken to ensure the suture line does not compress to cord structures (Figure 24.14).

Tunical sac excision reduces re-accumulation of fluid. Meticulous hemostasis should be obtained as postoperative hematomas can readily occur. A Penrose drain may be placed

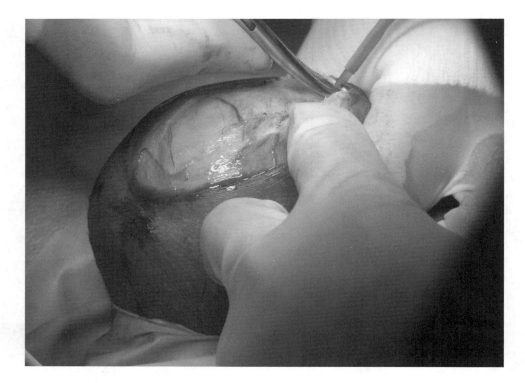

FIGURE 24.10　Skin incision. Image by Nelson Bennett, MD, Lahey Clinic, Institute of Urology.

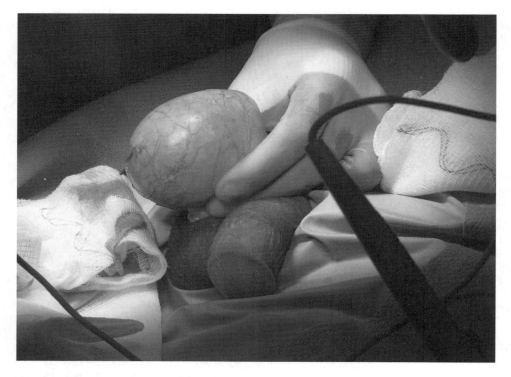

FIGURE 24.11　Complete delivery of hydrocele. Image by Nelson Bennett, MD, Lahey Clinic, Institute of Urology.

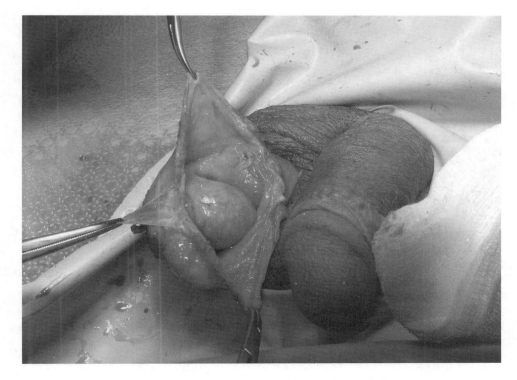

FIGURE 24.12 Hydrocele sac defined #1. Image by Nelson Bennett, MD, Lahey Clinic, Institute of Urology.

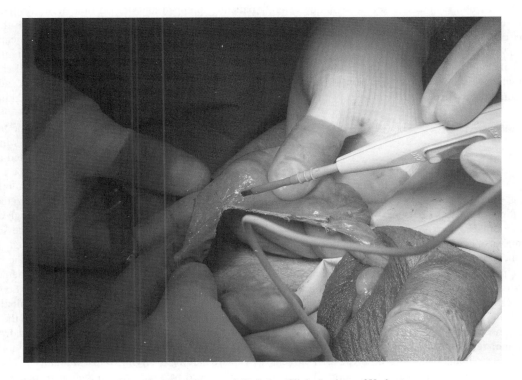

FIGURE 24.13 Excision of hydrocele sac. Image by Nelson Bennett, MD, Lahey Clinic, Institute of Urology.

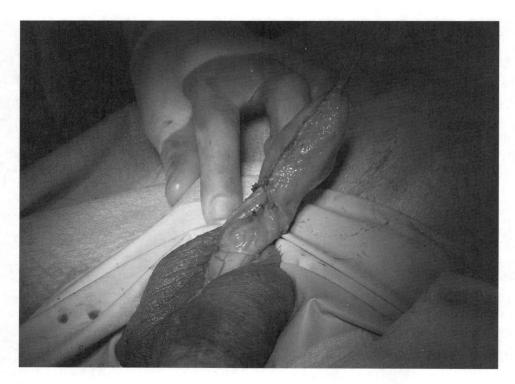

FIGURE 24.14   Jaboulay procedure. Image by Nelson Bennett, MD, Lahey Clinic, Institute of Urology.

dependently in the scrotum; however, some techniques caution against this, as patients may not return to have the drain removed. Close the dartos and skin layers with continuous absorbable suture.[1,5,6]

Complications include injury to structures within the spermatic cord (testicular vessels, vas deferens), scrotal hematoma, wound infection, and recurrence of the hydrocele.

Orchiopexy

Undescended testes, or cryptorchidism, is the most common pediatric urologic problem. The testes do not migrate farther than the inguinal ring and are usually found in the inguinal canal, although they may also be present in a high scrotal position, superficial inguinal region, or intra-abdominally. The most common associations of cryptorchidism are prematurity and low birth weight. Indications for surgical correction include preservation of fertility, protection against testicular torsion and inguinal hernia, restoring cosmetic appearance, and allowing access of screening for testicular tumors.[7] Patients with cryptorchidism have an increased risk (3.6 relative risk) for the development of testicular cancer (most commonly seminoma), and orchiopexy allows for thorough, regular examination. Preoperative radiologic studies are low yield and usually of little value. Treatment should be performed around 6 months of age. Surgical correction depends on the location of the testes and whether they are palpable or not.[5]

Procedure: Examination of the patient after the induction of anesthesia may reveal the location of previously nonpalpable testes as guarding is absent and the patient is relaxed. Once the patient is prepped and draped in a sterile fashion, a transverse inguinal incision is made and carried through the skin, subcutaneous tissue, and Scarpa's fascia. The testis can be outside or within the inguinal canal. If it is within the inguinal canal, the external fascia is opened through the external ring. The ilioinguinal nerve may be injured here. Cremasteric and gubernacular attachments are divided away from the internal oblique muscle, the testis, and the spermatic cord (which are within the tunica layers). The goal is to completely mobilize the testis and cord. Once this is performed, the tunica vaginalis is incised over the testis. The processus vaginalis is then dissected away from the spermatic cord, with extreme care taken not to compromise the vascularity of the cord structures. The mobilization of the processus vaginalis will extend just cephalad to the internal ring where it is ligated. This should allow for enough cord length for tension-free placement of the testes within the scrotum; otherwise, retroperitoneal dissection may be required. The testis may then be placed within a dartos pouch, under the scrotal skin. A transverse mid-scrotal incision is made, and a hemostat is used to develop a pouch in the inferior, dependent portion of the scrotal skin. A hemostat is then passed from the inguinal incision, over the pubic symphysis, through dartos fascia, to the medial aspect of the scrotum. A second hemostat is passed from the scrotal incision into the inguinal incision and takes hold of the testis by the remaining overlying tunica vaginalis and brought through the developed passageway into the dartos pouch. Torsion of the testicle is avoided. Absorbable sutures are used to pex the tunica vaginalis of the testis to the dartos layer.[5]

Complications include testicular atrophy due to vascular injury, vas deferens injury during dissection, scrotal hematoma, or inadequate positioning of the testis.

Orchiopexy for Testicular Torsion

Testicular torsion is a surgical emergency that presents as acute onset of severe testicular pain. Patients with cryptorchidism or a "Bell-clapper deformity" (absence of the normal posterior testicular attachment) are predisposed to torsion as the testis twists on itself, cutting off its blood supply. This is most common is males ages 12–18 but may occur at any age. Patients have an extremely tender, firm testis that may be high riding or demonstrate a horizontal lie. The cremasteric reflex may be absent. Diagnosis is usually clinical; however, if surgical exploration is not delayed, a Doppler ultrasound of the testis will generally show minimal or absent blood flow. This is in contrast to acute epididymitis, which will demonstrate increased blood flow compared to the contralateral testis. Generally, the testis will survive if blood flow is restored within 6 hours. If the testis appears nonviable upon exploration, orchiectomy should be performed.

Procedure: After standard prepping and draping, a transverse incision is performed in the affected hemiscrotum. This is carried down to the level of the tunica vaginalis, and the testis is mobilized. The cord is untwisted, and the testis is inspected for viability. It may be wrapped in warm saline wraps. If the testis appears viable, it is fixed by placing 5-0 or 6-0 permanent sutures through the tunica albuginea (transparenchymal sutures may cause an inflammatory response in the testis). The contralateral testis is also secured in the same fashion as these patients are predisposed to bilateral torsion.[1,5]

Complications are similar to those of orchiopexy for cryptorchidism.

Orchiectomy

Indications for orchiectomy include excision of a testicular mass concerning for cancer, need for hormonal ablation via castration (advanced prostate cancer or symptomatic benign prostatic hyperplasia without medical treatment available), or nonviable testes secondary to prolonged testicular torsion or chronic infection. In the case of a concerning testicular mass, an inguinal approach is performed so as not to disrupt the normal lymphatic testicular drainage, as well as to avoid the spread of disease to the scrotum during a trans-scrotal approach.

Procedure: The goal is radical orchiectomy is to obtain a pathologic diagnosis and local control of the testicular tumor. There is minimal morbidity associated with this procedure, and it may be performed under general, spinal, or local anesthesia. The patient is supine and the scrotum is prepped and draped within a sterile field. An inguinal incision is made, roughly 2 cm above the pubic tubercle. Dissection is carried down through Scarpa's to the external oblique fascia. This is divided to the internal ring, and the spermatic cord is isolated with a Penrose drain. Injury to the ilioinguinal nerve is avoided. The testis is then brought up out of the scrotum by blunt dissection and into the wound. The cord blood vessels and the vas deferens are each ligated with silk sutures just cephalad to the internal ring. The external oblique, Scarpa's, and skin incisions are closed in standard herniorrhaphy fashion. The most common postoperative complications are scrotal or retroperitoneal bleeding.

Benign Prostatic Hyperplasia

Epithelial and stromal enlargement of the prostate gland may cause an obstruction to the flow of urine from the bladder. Benign prostatic hyperplasia (BPH) is normal in the aging male and may present with lower urinary tract symptoms of decreased force of stream, hesitancy of urination, nocturia, incomplete bladder emptying, straining, frequency, and urgency. These symptoms may progress to urinary retention. As the obstructive process worsens, the bladder compensates by becoming thicker in some areas and weaker in others. This anatomic remodeling is known as trabeculations and is an effort to increase contractility. Ultimately, the bladder's ability to generate force weakens and its walls become less compliant. Post-void urine levels increase, with a resultant risk of urinary tract infection, stone formation, retention, and deterioration of renal function.

The differential diagnosis of BPH is large, and includes cystitis, prostatitis, bladder cancer, prostate cancer, neurogenic bladder, urethral stricture, bladder foreign bodies (stones), etc. If available, a urinalysis, urine culture, and prostate-specific antigen may be obtained. A digital rectal examination should exclude suspicious areas of induration, asymmetry, nodularity, or tenderness. A urine flow study and post-void residual measurements may be performed; however, these do not differentiate between outflow obstruction and poor bladder contractility. Urodynamic testing may be useful but is generally unavailable in an LMIC. Cystoscopy will help to identify pathology such as urethral strictures, bladder tumors, and other foreign bodies within the bladder (i.e., stones). Medical management for BPH includes treatment with alpha-1 receptor blockade and 5-alpha reductase inhibitors. Alpha-1 blockade reduces smooth muscle tension in the prostate gland and decreases outflow resistance; 5-alpha reductase inhibitors block the conversion of testosterone to dihydrotestosterone and inhibit prostate growth. Indications for surgical treatment of BPH include persistent hematuria due to the enlarged prostate, deterioration of renal function secondary to outlet obstruction, persistent urinary tract infections, bladder stones, and urinary retention.

Procedure: Open prostatectomy, when compared with transurethral resection of the prostate, has a lower re-operation rate as well as the advantage of more complete removal of the prostate gland. However, this procedure is associated with higher risk of postoperative hemorrhage and a longer hospitalization. Open prostatectomy may also be the procedure of choice for large glands (>75 grams), or those with concomitant bladder diverticula or bladder stones. If there is a suspicion of prostate cancer (based on a digital rectal exam), a biopsy of the prostate should be performed if the equipment is available. Prior to surgery, urinary tract infections should be treated and anticoagulant medications discontinued. Open prostatectomy may be performed through a retro pubic approach (direct exposure and incision of the prostatic capsule) or a suprapubic approach (extraperitoneal, transvesical approach). The supravesical approach is described here.

The patient is placed supine and the abdomen and pelvis are prepped and draped in the usual sterile fashion. A large catheter is used to drain the bladder. Then 250 cc of saline are instilled into the bladder and the catheter is clamped.

A midline incision is performed from the umbilicus to the pubic symphysis. This is carried through the subcutaneous tissue and the linea alba, so that the rectus abdominis may be brought laterally. The space of Retzius is entered and the prevesical space is entered and extended. The peritoneum is swept cephalad and care taken not to enter the peritoneum. Two 3-0 vicryl sutures are placed on both sides of the midline of the anterior bladder wall and a vertical cystotomy is made. This is carried down to 1 cm from the bladder neck. The locations of the ureteral orifices are noted. Exposure is very important and may be obtained through the placement of sutures in the anterior midline cystotomy. A circular incision is performed in the bladder mucosa at the level of the bladder neck (distal to the trigone). Using scissors, followed by blunt dissection, the plane between the prostate parenchyma and the prostate capsule is separated. This is carried out from the base of the prostate to the apex, as well as circumferentially. Once the apex is reached, the prostate may be pinched off, with care taken not to injure the urethra or sphincter muscles. Two 0-chromic sutures are used for figure-of-eight hemostatic sutures at the 5-o'clock and 7-o'clock positions to bring the incised bladder tissue into the prostatic fossa. Electrocautery or suture ligation may be used for further hemostasis. A large urethral catheter (22 French) is used with 50 cc of saline in the catheter balloon. A 22 French Malecot suprapubic tube is also placed. A Penrose or Jackson-Pratt drain is placed lateral to the bladder and on the contralateral side of the suprapubic tube. The cystotomy is closed in two layers, the first of which is with running an absorbable suture gathering mucosa and detrusor muscle. The second layer incorporates the detrusor muscle and serosa also in a continuous fashion with absorbable suture. The urethral and suprapubic catheters are irrigated to ensure good bladder closure. The midline incision is closed in standard fashion. Should there be significant hematuria, both catheter traction and continuous bladder irrigation are used. Postoperatively, the urethral catheter is removed once the urine is clear. If the pelvic drain has minimal output, this may be removed on postoperative day three. The suprapubic tube may be removed on postoperative day five if the patient does not have problems with postvoid residual urine volume.

Complications of the procedure include postoperative hemorrhage requiring reoperation or transfusion, urinary leak, irritative urinary tract symptoms (frequency, urgency, etc.), urinary incontinence, erectile dysfunction, bladder neck contracture, urethral stricture, and other medical complications such as postoperative pulmonary embolus, deep venous thrombosis, and myocardial infarction.[5]

Open Cystotomy

Symptomatic bladder calculi may require open surgical access to the bladder. Historically, this was an extremely morbid procedure and initially accessed through a perineal incision. In the 1700s, a long nail was inserted through the urethra and into the bladder, at which point a blacksmith's hammer was used to strike the nail and break the stone. Fortunately, treatment has evolved to safer, more effective procedures. Bladder calculi usually form in the presence of urinary stasis (from outlet obstruction, infections, anatomic anomalies, neurogenic bladder, or diverticula); however, they may also be idiopathic in nature. Bladder calculi remain a common problem in LMICs. Diet and nutrition may contribute to stone formation, as do schistosomal infections and the presence of foreign bodies within the bladder (catheter balloons, stents, sutures, etc). Workup includes obtaining a urinalysis and urine culture and sensitivity. Hematuria is likely present as are nitrites and leukocyte esterase. Bladder calculi are frequently composed of uric acid and therefore may not be visible on plain film X-rays. A cystoscopy, cystography, or intravenous pyelogram may demonstrate filling defects within the bladder or the calcified stone itself. The pH of urine in a patient with uric acid stones will be acidic. Indications for treatment include suprapubic discomfort, irritative and obstructive urinary tract symptoms, recurrent urinary tract infections, hematuria, and urinary retention. The cause of urinary stasis or metabolic abnormality associated with the formation of calculi should also be addressed. Medical treatment includes alkalinization of the urine in order to dissolve uric acid stones. Endoscopic procedures (the preferred approach when resources are available) are used to break the stone into fragments that may be removed through a cystoscope. These techniques include pneumatic or electrohydraulic lithoclasty, manual lithotripter, or laser lithotripsy. These options are rarely available in LMICs.

Procedure: Advantages to open cystotomy are that it is quick, affords easy access and visualization of the bladder, and that several, large, dense calculi may be removed at once. General, spinal, or local anesthesia may be used. The patient is in the supine position and his abdomen, pelvis, and genitalia are prepped and draped in a sterile fashion. A midline incision is performed 2 cm above the pubic symphysis. This is carried through the subcutaneous tissue and the linea alba, so that the rectus abdominis may be brought laterally. The space of Retzius is entered and the prevesical space is entered and extended. The peritoneum is swept cephalad with care taken not to enter the peritoneum. A large, distended bladder will be easily palpated. Two 3-0 vicryl sutures are placed on both sides of the midline of the anterior bladder wall and a vertical cystotomy is made, suctioning urine out of the bladder (Figure 24.15). The bladder mucosa is explored by palpation and any stones removed. The cystotomy may need to be enlarged for removal of large stones. Place a catheter into the cystotomy and inflate the balloon (Figure 24.16). Place a purse-string absorbable suture around the catheter, including bites of bladder mucosa (Figure 24.17). The bladder is closed as described in the BPH in the extraperitoneal, transvesical approach (Figure 24.18). Close the midline incision in standard fashion.

Complications include urinary tract infection, sepsis, hemorrhage, hyponatremia from use of irrigation fluids, and bladder perforation.[1]

Urethral Stricture

Stricture disease may result from a wide variety of etiologies, including prior perineal/pelvic trauma, prior surgery (radical prostatectomy), malignancies, congenital abnormalities, or infections (gonorrhea). Indications for treatment include

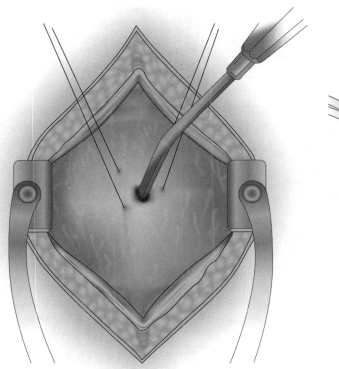

FIGURE 24.15 Stay sutures, cystotomy. World Health Organization. *Surgical Care at the District Hospital.* Geneva: World Health Organization; 2003. Figure 9.15.

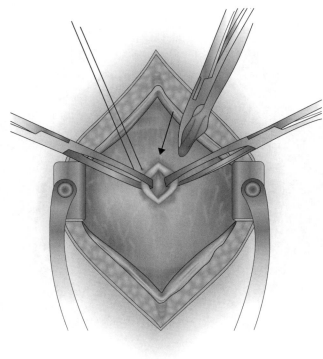

FIGURE 24.16 Placement of catheter. World Health Organization. *Surgical Care at the District Hospital.* Geneva: World Health Organization; 2003. Figure 9.17.

patients with bladder calculi, urinary retention, lower urinary tract obstructive symptoms, or recurrent infections. Prior to treatment, it is recommended to treat existing infections and biopsy suspicious lesions to exclude malignant causes. Workup may include both endoscopic and radiologic evaluation to determine the location and extent of the stricture. A retrograde or antegrade (if the patient has a suprapubic tube) urethrogram may be performed by injecting 10–15 cc of contrast into the fossa navicularis or distal urethra. A radiograph is obtained simultaneously.

Urinary retention due to a urethral stricture may be relieved with a sterile attempt at passing a Foley catheter. After well lubricating the urethra, place the penis on stretch and pass the catheter into the urethra. Gentle pressure may be required to pass the catheter across the urethral sphincters. Advance the catheter completely into the bladder, noting return of urine with additional advancement prior to inflation of the catheter balloon. This avoids improper insertion of the catheter balloon in the prostatic urethra. If the catheter is fully advanced but no urine has returned, irrigation of the catheter may be performed in order to confirm placement in the bladder. If the initial Foley catheter is unsuccessful, a coude catheter may be used. The curve of the coude catheter should be facing anteriorly (12-o'clock) to follow the course of the urethra.

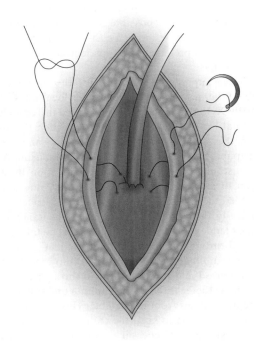

FIGURE 24.17 Pursestring closure around catheter. World Health Organization. *Surgical Care at the District Hospital.* Geneva: World Health Organization; 2003. Figure 9.19.

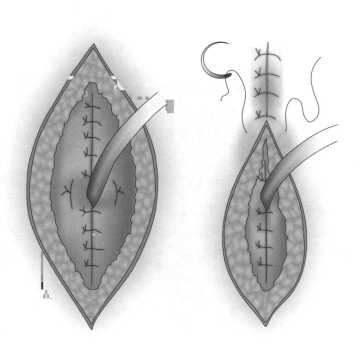

FIGURE 24.18   Two-layer bladder closure. World Health Organization. *Surgical Care at the District Hospital.* Geneva: World Health Organization; 2003. Figure 9.20.

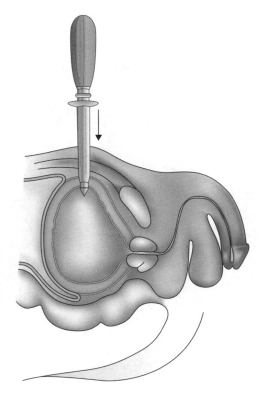

FIGURE 24.19   Trocar placement. World Health Organization. *Surgical Care at the District Hospital.* Geneva: World Health Organization; 2003. Figure 9.8.

If this is unsuccessful, a urethral dilation may be attempted with a number of dilating devices (filiform and followers, male sounds, and, if available, balloon dilators over a wire). If urethral catheterization is not possible, suprapubic catheterization via a suprapubic puncture or open cystotomy may be required. Open cystotomy is preferred if the patient has had abdominal surgery in the past.

Procedure: Suprapubic puncture for the placement of a suprapubic tube may be performed under local anesthesia by injecting 2% Xylocaine. The patient is placed in Trendelenburg position to allow the bowels to drop away, then prepped and draped in the standard fashion. Palpate the bladder 2 cm above the pubic symphysis and make a skin incision. A spinal needle is useful to identify the correct location by aspirating as you locate the bladder and to estimate the necessary depth needed to enter the bladder. Guide the trocar and cannula vertically through the incision and subcutaneous tissue toward the bladder (Figure 24.19). Care must be taken to avoid through-and-through perforation of the bladder, as the rectum will be injured. Once they have passed into the bladder, the trocar is removed and urine will drain through the cannula. Advance the catheter through the cannula and inflate the balloon once urine flows from the catheter (Figure 24.20). Insert water into the balloon to keep the catheter in place. A suture at the entry site is not necessary. Connect the catheter to a gravity drainage bag and remove the cannula. The catheter may require irrigation with saline so that it does not become blocked.[1]

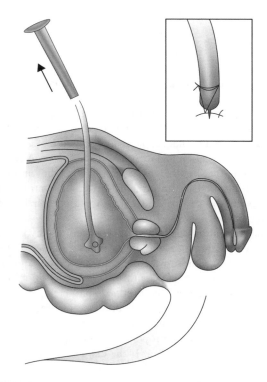

FIGURE 24.20   Catheter placement. World Health Organization. *Surgical Care at the District Hospital.* Geneva: World Health Organization; 2003. Figure 9.10.

COMMENTARY

E. Oluwabunmi Olapade-Olaopa, Nigeria

Urologic diseases are quite common in sub-Saharan Africa (SSA) and often require surgical treatment. In our hospital in Nigeria, half of the new referrals to the urology unit are urethral and prostatic (benign and malignant) bladder outflow obstruction, and infertility.[1] The surgical procedures that provide investigation and treatment of these diseases account for 60% and over 90% of procedures done in the main operating rooms and outpatient theaters, respectively. The most common elective and emergency open procedures done in the main operating rooms are: varicocoelectomies, orchidectomies, pediatric circumcision, suprapubic cystostomy, orchidopexies, and open prostatectomy and urethroplasties. A surgeon competent in these procedures would therefore be able to treat the vast majority of cases that present in SSA.

This chapter adequately describes several surgical procedures that are as effective as minimally invasive procedures in the treatment of genitourinary surgical diseases. The ability to do these procedures is therefore an important skill set that the surgeon practicing in LMICs must acquire. From our experience, additional important genitourinary surgical procedures for the SSA region would be varicocoelectomies and urethroplasties. Varicocoelectomies are done mostly for the treatment of male infertility, as child-bearing is a major cultural demand in SSA. This operation is commonly done via the supra-inguinal and inguinal approaches due to the lack of magnifying loupes, but a few centers/surgeons with that equipment use the sub-inguinal method. Also in SSA, urethroplasties are done more commonly for infective strictures (which are mostly multiple and affecting long segments) than for traumatic strictures (which are mostly short segment). The two-stage procedure is the preferred method, as it is proven to give good long-term results. However, one-stage substitution/patch urethoplasties are beginning to gain ground with training of the younger surgeons and the retraining of the older ones in modern methods.

Open prostatectomy remains the preferred method of surgical excision of the prostate gland in SSA. This is mainly because of the level of expertise and equipment available, and the size of the glands. It has the major advantage of being the best option for a once-and-for-all treatment of benign prostatic enlargement, and for patients with concurrent bladder abnormalities requiring surgery. Facilities and expertise for both open and (monopolar) endoscopic treatment are available at our center, but 75% of glands are larger than 80 g and therefore unsuitable for transurethral resection of the prostate (TURP). For this, and also training purposes, most of prostatectomies are done via the open method. In the subcontinent, the most-feared surgical complications of the procedure are hemorrhage, infection, and bladder neck contracture. Infections can largely be avoided by careful preoperative assessment with the reduction/elimination of risk factors for infection, and judicious use of antibiotics. We have also reduced the occurrence of the other two complications significantly by modifications to our surgical technique.[2] Almost all open prostatectomies done in our center are done using a modified version of Millin's retropubic prostatectomy. Our modification is to do the capsulotomy just below the bladder neck (i.e., higher than described by Millin). This combines the advantage of giving a better view of the operation wound and having the incision in the relatively avascular and immobile prostatic capsule, both of which reduce intra- and postoperative bleeding (and indeed pain). We reduce intraoperative bleeding further by reconstructing the trigone (trigonotomy/trigonectomy) and by the careful placement of "deep lateral sutures." This formal reconstruction of the trigone has the added advantage of reducing the risk of bladder neck contracture.

Urologists practicing in SSA continue to increase their repertoire of procedures (both open and minimally invasive). This process is being hastened by the collaborative efforts of local and international experts in organizing training workshops in the different subspecialties across the subcontinent. With these efforts the standard of genitourinary surgery, and thus urologic care, in SSA will improve significantly in the near future.

REFERENCES

1. EO Olapade-Olaopa, SA Adebayo, OJ Ajamu, A Ukachukwu, OB Shittu and LI Okeke. British training and urological practice in Sub-Saharan Africa. BJU International: 105 (10), 1353–1355, 2010

2. EO Olapade-Olaopa, Retropublic/Suprapubic Prostate Enucleation (Webcast). Presented at the SIU 2013 Congress, Vancouver, Canada.

   http://academy.siu-urology.org/siu/2013/vancouver/34740/e.oluwabunmi.olapade-olaopa.pp03.retropublic.suprapubic.prostate.enucleation.html?history_id=485167

COMMENTARY

Thaim Buya Kamara, Sierra Leone

In Sierra Leone, urological surgery is usually performed using traditional methods. Cystourethroscopy is the only endoscopic procedure available in my practice. Therefore, nearly all my procedures are done via open surgery. Prostatectomy, urethroplasty, and hydrocelectomy are the most common operations I perform. Prostatectomy is done by the suprapubic transvesical route, and to avoid suprapubic bladder drainage, I use a three-way Foley urethral catheter. Urethral strictures in our environment are commonly caused by infectious agents, and patients usually present with urinary retention and complications such as periurethral and/or perineal abscesses or fistulae. After evaluating these patients, I treat them in stages: I place a suprapubic cystostomy and allow the fistulae to heal before tackling the stricture. It may take several months to a few years before such patients are able to void. I also offer intermittent metal bouginage to some of my patients as necessary. Hydroceles that I see here are usually quite big, and are sometimes associated with scrotal skin ulcers or scrotal elephantiasis; they pose great surgical challenge. Although most boys are circumcised in this country, less than 10 circumcisions are done in our hospital; most circumcisions are done at home by untrained individuals. The most common complications arising from this practice are: urethrocutaneous fistulae, peno-glanular skin bridge (with or without smegma stone), and, rarely, amputation of the glans penis. Orchiectomy for testicular torsion is rare because the condition is often misdiagnosed and patients present with complications of (bilateral) testicular torsion long after it has happened.

25

Neurosurgery

Benjamin C. Warf

Introduction

Although conventionally understood to be impractical in low- and middle-income countries (LMICs), occasions for basic neurosurgical treatments are common in these contexts. Many of the resources currently available for neurosurgical diagnosis (such as neuroimaging with magnetic resonance imaging [MRI], computed tomography [CT], or angiography) and treatment (such as operating microscopes, power drills, cranial fixation, and even bipolar electrocautery) are typically unavailable in many regions of the developing world. Nonetheless, there are conditions requiring urgent treatment that can be managed with the most basic of surgical skills, instruments, and resources. This chapter will review the diagnosis and treatment of common conditions that both require and are amenable to urgent treatment in an LMIC.

For the purposes of this chapter, we will assume the reader is a physician with basic surgical training practicing in a developing world setting, at a hospital possessing the basic resources for general surgical procedures (such as a government district hospital or mission hospital). We will also assume that referral to a neurosurgical consultant is difficult and would not be possible within a few days. We will here consider selected treatable conditions unrelated to trauma that can present for emergency neurosurgical management; the management of neurosurgical trauma is considered in Chapter 44.

The common themes here will be emergency decompression of the brain or spinal cord and treatment or prevention of central nervous system infection. As is true in much of surgery, it is often equally important to know when to refrain from intervention. Some conditions are simply not amenable to diagnosis and treatment outside of a neurosurgical center. These include intracranial and intraspinal tumors, aneurysms and vascular anomalies of the central nervous system, and complex congenital anomalies such as encephaloceles and spinal cord lipomas. Attempted surgical intervention in such cases is unwarranted, and arranging for these patients to be evaluated at a neurosurgical center is imperative. However frustrating or humbling, it is sometimes necessary for a surgeon to say, "There is nothing I can do."

History and Physical Examination

A thorough history and thoughtful physical examination have, unfortunately, lost their luster in the context of ever-improving diagnostic imaging modalities. But these skills remain essential to the armamentarium of the clinician practicing in the setting of a developing country. Thus, the importance of a working knowledge of the neurological examination cannot be overstated. Particular focus should be placed on physical findings that suggest the location of the pathology, such as distinguishing an upper from a lower motor neuron lesion, dermatomal patterns of sensory loss, and abnormal eye movements and pupillary responses.

Imaging

Although access to CT or MRI imaging may be limited, many basic hospital facilities will have X-ray and ultrasound capabilities, which should be utilized to their full potential. Plain X-ray studies of the skull and spine can provide an enormous amount of information useful in the diagnosis of tumor, infection, and congenital anomalies by virtue of primary and secondary associated changes in the bone. For infants, cranial ultrasound can provide invaluable imaging of the intracranial contents, clearly demonstrating pathologies such as hydrocephalus, cysts, tumors, abscess cavities, congenital anomalies, and intracranial hematomas. This modality can be similarly employed for intraspinal imaging in newborns. After the natural sonographic windows of infancy close, ultrasound can still be enormously helpful in the operating room once the bone has been opened. This can be accomplished by encasing the ultrasound probe within a sterile lubricant-containing surgical glove and draping off its cable with a sterile surgical drape. This can provide guidance toward intracranial masses such as abscesses and hematomas, and aid in the localization of intradural spinal masses after laminectomy.

Congenital Anomalies

Because of the population distribution, high birth rates, and limited longevity in the developing world, much of the neurosurgery that should be done presents itself in infants and children. Although many congenital anomalies do not require urgent intervention, the most common ones that require neurosurgical care typically do require urgent treatment because of the risk of central nervous system infection from leakage of cerebrospinal fluid (CSF) or elevated intracranial pressure (ICP). This section will cover the urgent management of hydrocephalus as well as that of myelomeningocele.

Hydrocephalus

Hydrocephalus is the final result of obstruction to the normal outflow of CSF from the ventricles into the subarachnoid spaces or its subsequent circulation and absorption. It has a number of etiologies, both congenital and acquired, and can develop at any time of life from infancy to adulthood. It is the most common neurosurgical condition seen in infants and young children. In the developing world, infant hydrocephalus is often acquired as a result of neonatal infection.[1] However, we will consider hydrocephalus from acquired and congenital causes together, given the similarities in pathophysiology, clinical course, and management.

Pathophysiology

CSF is produced by the choroid plexus within the ventricular system as a filtrate of the blood and from water exchange across the ventricular walls, from which it exits via the fourth ventricular outlet foramina, and circulates in a pulsatile fashion throughout the subarachnoid spaces around the brain, spinal cord, and cauda equina (Figure 25.1). It ultimately returns to the vascular system through specialized invaginations of the subarachnoid space (arachnoid granulations) into the superior sagittal sinus as well as through periventricular capillaries in the brain (which appears to be the dominant mechanism for infants). Interference with the complex balance of CSF production, circulation, pulsatility,

and absorption can lead to enlargement of the ventricular system with the accumulation of CSF under pressure. Causes of hydrocephalus include: 1) congenital (such as aqueductal stenosis or abnormal anatomy in association with other anomalies like myelomeningocele or the Dandy-Walker malformation); 2) infection (i.e., meningitis or ventriculitis), which can lead to obstructions of CSF flow either inside or outside the ventricular system; 3) hemorrhage (in the ventricles or the subarachnoid spaces); and 4) obstructing mass lesions (such as tumors or cysts).

In the infant, whose cranium is capable of rapid growth, the enlarging ventricles initially lead to abnormally accelerated head growth with an increase in volume more than pressure. With time, signs and symptoms of elevated ICP develop: a tense anterior fontanel, distended scalp veins, "sunsetting" of the eyes, vomiting, and irritability or lethargy (Figure 25.2). Later symptoms can include apnea and bradycardia and, ultimately, even death. In the older child or adult who develops hydrocephalus, the situation is more urgent since the intracranial pressure can rise quickly in the noncompliant cranium with no compensatory increase in intracranial volume. The classic signs and symptoms in these patients are progressively severe headache, vomiting, and a progressive deterioration in the level of consciousness that ultimately leads to coma and death. Sustained elevation in ICP often results in papilledema, which can be noted on fundoscopic examination.

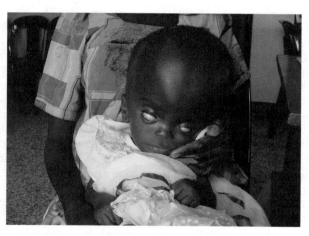

FIGURE 25.2 Infant with advanced hydrocephalus demonstrating macrocephaly and severe sunsetting of the eyes. Image by Benjamin C. Warf.

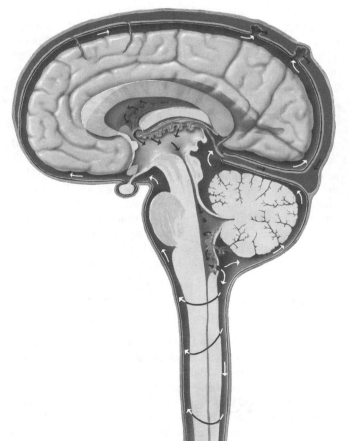

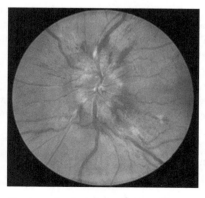

FIGURE 25.1 Normal CSF circulation. Netter F. *Atlas of Human Anatomy.* Philadelphia: Elsevier; 2010, p. 109.

FIGURE 25.3 Fundoscopic photo demonstrating papilledema. Waller E. A. et al. *Mayo Clin Proc.* 2008;83:1251-1261.

Diagnosis

For infants, a clinical diagnosis of hydrocephalus with the signs noted above is typically straightforward. CT scan or cranial ultrasound via the anterior fontanel confirms the presence of a dilated ventricular system (Figure 25.4). Although it may also suggest an etiology for the hydrocephalus (such as a mass lesion, aqueduct stenosis, or ventriculitis), this is unlikely to influence treatment given limited resources and access to neurosurgical specialty care. There is no sonographic window in the older child or adult, thus necessitating neuroimaging by CT or MRI.

Treatment

Ventricular Puncture

Emergency treatment for symptomatically elevated ICP may be necessary as a lifesaving intervention if urgent neurosurgical referral is not possible. Temporary treatment of the macrocephalic infant who is very ill with a tense fontanel can be accomplished emergently by a percutaneous ventricular puncture. This is done at the bedside as a sterile procedure with a 20- or 22-gauge spinal needle or angio-catheter. The entry point is at the right lateral corner of the anterior fontanel at the intersection of a sagittal plane through the right mid-pupillary line and a coronal plane just anterior to the tragus of the right ear (Figure 25.5). After prepping the scalp, the needle punctures the skin at an angle that is perpendicular to the plane that is tangent to the entry point. Spontaneous flow of CSF should be encountered at a depth of 5 cm or less, depending upon the size of the ventricles. Once brisk flow is encountered, sufficient CSF should be drained to decompress the fontanel until it is soft and flat or slightly sunken.

External Ventricular Drain Placement

In the older child or adult who has become severely lethargic or comatose, emergency placement of an external ventricular drain may be necessary. However, in the absence of an imaging study, this would be a purely clinical decision based upon a history that indicates a possible cause of hydrocephalus (such as a prior history of shunted hydrocephalus suggesting shunt malfunction, a clinical picture or recent history consistent with meningitis, or other suggestive clinical history) and typical signs and symptoms that warrant an emergency intervention (headache, vomiting, lethargy or coma, apnea, bradycardia, sixth nerve palsy with in-turning of one or both eyes, or abnormal posturing movements of the extremities). Without imaging, however, unknown circumstances such as anatomic distortion from a mass lesion might lead to technical failure of attempted ventricular drainage. Despite this, under life-threatening clinical circumstances, such intervention is worth the risk of failure.

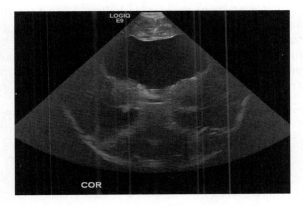

FIGURE 25.4 Coronal cranial ultrasound in infant showing ventriculomegaly. Image by Benjamin C. Warf.

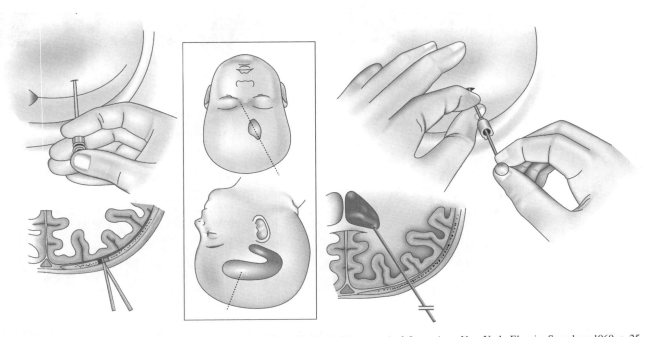

FIGURE 25.5 Percutaneous ventricular puncture. Shillito J. *An Atlas of Pediatric Neurosurgical Operations.* New York: Elsevier Saunders; 1969, p. 25.

The basic approach to ventricular drain placement is the same as the ventricular puncture for infants, with the important exception that a burr hole for access will need to be created in the skull. After clipping hair and appropriately prepping and draping the scalp in the area, local anesthesia (such as 0.25% Marcaine with 1:200,000 epinephrine) is used to infiltrate the incision site. A 1–2 cm incision is made, centered at the intersection of a sagittal plane through the right mid-pupillary line and a coronal plane just anterior to the tragus (or just anterior to the coronal suture, which can be palpated) (Figure 25.6). It is important to avoid making the opening near the midline, which is the location of the superior sagittal sinus. The skull is penetrated with a hand drill, such as a twist drill or Hudson brace and bit. Care must be taken to prevent "plunging" of the drill as it penetrates the inner table of the skull. The force applied must be primarily that of twisting the drill bit, and not of pushing downward. The bit should be allowed to "carry itself" through the bone. Penetration of the inner table as the bit turns through it can be felt distinctly. When in doubt, stop and look at the depth of the hole from time to time. The inner table is reached after the diploic space has been fully penetrated and the marrow elements give way to pure white bone. Additional edges of bone may be removed with a small curette, and bleeding from the bone edges can be controlled by pressing bone wax into the bleeding spaces. The dura at the base

of the burr hole can be penetrated by touching it with the tip of a hemostat while applying monopolar electrocautery (e.g., a Bovie) to the hemostat. This will create a small dural opening with cautery that is unlikely to bleed. After this, a ventricular catheter or a spinal needle can be passed into the ventricle. As with the ventricular puncture in the infant, the needle or catheter is directed at an angle perpendicular to the plane that is tangent to the point of entry. The ventricle should be entered with spontaneous egress of CSF at a depth of around 5 cm. The catheter should not be passed deeper than 6 cm, and if no CSF is encountered it is withdrawn fully, redirected slightly, and passed again. If available, it is best to use an external ventricular drain (EVD) and leave this in place for continuous drainage. While maintaining the position of the catheter in the ventricle, the other end should be tunneled to a separate exit site a few centimeters away, brought out through a stab incision, and anchored to the scalp with a series of tacking stitches that are snug, but do not occlude the catheter. An EVD must be connected to a sterile closed drainage system. EVD drainage systems are available. If this is not an option, then drainage into a vented empty intravenous (IV) bottle can be constructed with IV tubing. The point at which the droplet of CSF forms at the end of the tubing prior to dropping into the chamber should be placed about 5–10 cm above the level of the patient's ear. The drain should not be allowed below the level of the head.

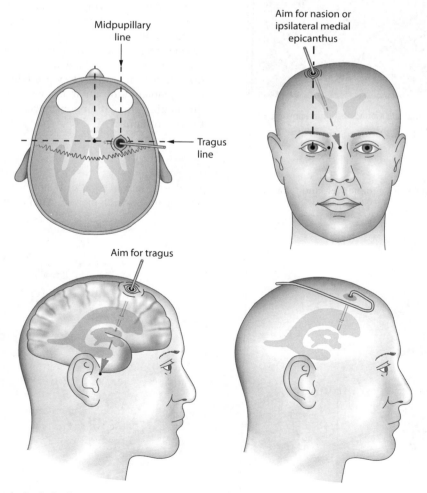

FIGURE 25.6   External ventricular drain placement. Winn R. *Youmans Neurological Surgery, 6th Edition.* New York: Elsevier Saunders; 2011, p. 3432.

Ventriculoperitoneal Shunt Placement

The above measures provide urgent but only temporary treatment for hydrocephalus. Although long-term dependence upon a ventriculoperitoneal shunt is not ideal in this context, and can often be avoided by the use of specialized neuroendoscopic techniques like endoscopic third ventriculostomy (ETV),[2] shunting is the most practical solution under the circumstances assumed here. Ideally, this should be performed by a surgeon who has training and experience with shunt placement. However, it is not so technically or conceptually difficult as to be an obstacle to treatment if such is not available. We describe here a right frontal approach since it uses the same landmarks as described above for a ventricular puncture and it affords a reliable catheter placement, although there are many variations among neurosurgeons. In addition, expensive North American or European shunts do not need to be used. We demonstrated that a shunt manufactured in India could be used with the same results as a shunt used in the United States at 5% of the cost.[3]

The patient is positioned supine with the head turned to the right and resting in a "doughnut" with a blanket or towel roll placed transversely beneath the shoulders to achieve modest neck extension (Figure 25.7). A strip of hair is clipped from the right frontal, parietal, and occipital scalp. The ventricular catheter burr hole placement (or access through the right lateral corner of the anterior fontanel for an infant) is the same as that described above for ventricular puncture or EVD placement. After prepping and draping the scalp, neck, chest, and abdomen, a *C*- or curved *L*-shaped incision is made in the scalp centered around the entry point for the ventricular catheter (described above) having the base of the scalp flap hinged posterior-laterally with one 1-cm limb of the incision in the parasagittal and the other 1-cm limb in the coronal plane. The skull is exposed and the scalp flap is tacked back to the drapes with a stitch. A burr hole (if necessary) is made and the dura penetrated as described above. A second 5-cm transverse linear incision is extended from the abdominal midline laterally at about one-third the distance between the umbilicus and the xiphoid. A shunt passer is tunneled subcutaneously from the abdominal incision to a scab incision in the right parietal scalp. This can be a risky maneuver, and great care must

be taken to remain subcutaneous, and not enter the chest cavity, by keeping a finger over the tip of the instrument. Shunt passers are of different designs, but generally have an outer sheath through which shunt tubing is passed after removing the trochar; or a long 0 silk suture is tied through a hole in the tip of the passer, pulled back through the subcutaneous tunnel, and then used to pull the tubing through the tract. A long hemostat, such as a Schnitz or tonsil dissector, is then passed from the frontal scalp incision to the parietal stab incision to grasp and pull through the shunt tubing. A short loop of tubing is left extending out of the stab incision temporarily.

After this distal shunt tubing has been passed subcutaneously, the ventricular catheter is passed into the right lateral ventricle as described for the EVD. The catheter length should generally be around 5 cm, and the excess catheter trimmed. Depending upon the type of shunt available, the valve (which may be a separate device or may be "unitized" with the distal tubing as a single component) is connected to the ventricular catheter and secured with a 2-0 silk tie. Some ventricular catheters come with a reservoir that can be interposed between the catheter and valve. Some shunts have a distal slit valve at the terminus of the abdominal tubing rather than an in-line valve immediately distal to the ventricular catheter. The distal tubing is grasped at the level of the stab incision to pull the valve down into a subcutaneous pocket beneath the scalp and eliminate any redundancy in the tubing. The tubing is then grasped at the level of the abdominal incision to similarly pull the tubing from the stab incision inferiorly into the subcutaneous tract and eliminate any redundancy. There should be no curves or kinks in the tubing. Spontaneous CSF flow is established through the distal tubing.

The anterior rectus sheath is then exposed and sharply incised through the abdominal incision. With a hemostat, the rectus abdominis muscle is bluntly spread to expose the posterior rectus sheath and hold the exposure with a small retractor. The posterior sheath is grasped multiple times medially and laterally with two fine hemostats and, while elevating it with these, is then sharply incised along with the underlying peritoneum to open into the peritoneal cavity. A probe (such as a #4 Penfield dissector) should pass easily into the space. If not, it is important to verify the peritoneum has been incised. After entry into the peritoneal cavity, the distal shunt tubing is passed with a nontoothed forceps to its full length into the cavity. It should pass easily with little resistance, and should not superficially fold up on itself. Stitches are placed beside the tubing to close the posterior and anterior sheath. Following this, the incisions are irrigated with Bacitracin solution and closed in layers.

Shunt Malfunction

Patients with shunt malfunction present with the symptoms and signs of untreated hydrocephalus. Infants will have a return of abnormally accelerated head growth, bulging anterior fontanel, sunsetting of the eyes, irritability or lethargy, poor feeding, or vomiting. Ultrasound in infants can reveal recurrent enlargement of the ventricles. Older children and adults typically present with headache, vomiting, and lethargy. In the final stages, there may be bradycardia, apnea, and ultimately coma and death.

Shunt malfunction is a life-threatening emergency. If clinically warranted in the infant or adult, an intraoperative shunt

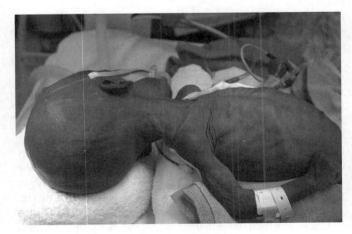

FIGURE 25.7 Infant positioned for VP shunt placement. Note towel roll beneath shoulders to effect moderate neck extension in order to facilitate passage of shunt tubing from abdominal incision to scalp incision. Image by Benjamin C. Warf.

exploration is advisable. The patient is positioned and prepared for surgery as noted above for a shunt placement. The scar from the prior scalp incision is incised, and the skin flap is retracted to reveal the ventricular catheter entry point and its connection with the reservoir and/or valve. The ventricular catheter is disconnected from the valve to check for spontaneous CSF flow. If this is absent, the catheter must be changed. IV tubing (or a manometer) filled with sterile saline is connected to the proximal port of the valve. The fluid column is allowed to run down into the valve. If the flow is good and the column halts at an acceptable height (closing pressure, which is typically between 5 and 15 cm), then the ventricular catheter is changed. If there is poor flow, the valve is disconnected from the distal tubing and the process is repeated down the distal tubing. If the flow is rapid down to around zero, the valve will need to be replaced. If the flow is still poor, a new peritoneal catheter will need to be placed, and the function of the valve will need to be similarly checked to determine whether it should be replaced as well.

Myelomeningocele

The infant or child with a myelomeningocele (open spina bifida) is an emergency only from the perspective of infection risk. Patients who have not been treated may epithelialize the skin defect, effectively sealing over the exposed neural elements and eliminating CSF leak. These patients do not require surgery in the context assumed here. Exposed neural elements and active or threatened CSF leak pose a high risk of meningitis and/or ventriculitis for these infants, which can be fatal or cause significant morbidity. Thus, closure in these instances is not elective. It should also be noted that more than half of these infants develop hydrocephalus, either present at birth or—more often—becoming obvious after the back is closed. If it is elected to place a shunt, it is best to wait as long as possible after the back is closed in this context because of the high likelihood of preoperative CSF contamination and the subsequent increased risk of shunt infection.

Pathologic Anatomy

Myelomeningocele is a neural tube defect in which the tube fails to close at one point, leading to a domino effect of failed posterior closure of the dura, posterior spinal elements (the spina bifida defect), muscle, fascia, and skin. The non-neurulated spinal cord (the placode) is open like a book, with nerve roots exiting laterally (what should have been posterior roots) and ventrally (the motor roots). The opened-out dura is fused laterally to the fascia and skin defect. The margins of the placode are fused with an epithelium connected to the edge of the skin defect. There is typically an accompanying meningocele sac beneath the epithelium, which may be ruptured at the time of presentation. Occasionally, there is no sac, but the lesion is flat and flush with the surrounding skin (sometimes referred to as "myeloschisis"). Although the malformed neural elements lead to varying levels of paralysis, the immediate threat after birth is that of meningitis and ventriculitis.

Operative Closure

The main purpose of the closure is to prevent infection. The key elements are a watertight reconstruction of the dura and a viable skin closure. After the induction of general anesthesia, the infant is positioned prone on small chest rolls with all pressure points adequately padded. The skin surrounding the defect can be washed with Betadine scrub, but the myelomeningocele itself is only prepped with the Betadine paint that is also used on the skin. A generous field is prepped and draped from well above the defect to the buttocks and laterally as far as is practical in case relaxing incisions or rotation flaps are needed.

The sac is incised and entered inferiorly, and a dissection guide, such as a hemostat, is passed superiorly and laterally to protect underlying nerve roots. The placode is circumscribed to separate it from its attachment to the surrounding epithelial tissue. After this, any small pieces of epithelium still attached to the placode are trimmed to prevent the future development of a dermoid cyst. Many pediatric neurosurgeons at this point will bring the lateral margins of the placode together medially with a few interrupted stitches through the pia.

Dissection of the dura to reconstruct the sac can be challenging. At the superior (cephalad) margin of the spina bifida skin defect, a small vertical incision is made, and blunt dissection should occur down to the epidural space, which can sometimes be identified by the epidural fat overlying the dura. This epidural space is bluntly dissected inferiorly and laterally, and the dura is incised as far laterally as possible at its lateral attachment to the skin and underlying fascia. This is done bilaterally, then the entire sheet of tissue is dissected medially from off the lumbodorsal fascia until the epidural fat is exposed beneath the floor of the dura within the spina bifida defect. Hinging the dural closure medially is key to a tension-free closure. The dura is closed with a running suture (such as 4-0 neurolon or vicryl or 5-0 prolene on a small noncutting needle). Once this is accomplished, the anesthetist provides a valsalva maneuver to check the integrity of the closure and look for points of CSF leakage. Small pinpoint leaks can be closed with a single figure-of-eight dural stitch.

Finally, the skin must be closed in a way that avoids tension and ischemia at the suture line. Some surgeons advocate swinging in a flap of lumbodorsal fascia as an extra layer of closure over the dura. Though this is optional, it can be helpful especially if the dural closure is tenuous. The skin is bluntly undermined circumferentially around the defect. Care should be taken to preserve the surrounding columns of tissue that may contain its blood supply. As much skin should be mobilized as possible by laterally undermining. The skin edges are then brought together with interrupted 3-0 or 4-0 vicryl stitches through the relatively tough layer at which the dura, fascia, and skin had been originally fused. A small, round Jackson Pratt drain can be placed subcutaneously that exits through a distant stab incision to be connected to bulb suction. This prevents fluid accumulation beneath the flap that can compromise wound healing. After the skin edges are approximated, redundant (and especially abnormal) skin and "dog ears" are trimmed, and the skin is closed with a 4-0 monofilament on a cutting needle. The wound is covered with a dry dressing and the infant kept prone or on the side for several days in the postoperative period to avoid pressure on the closure that can compromise its vascular supply.

Sometimes, a local skin flap advancement or rotation is necessary to accomplish a relatively tension-free closure. A suture line that is under too much tension is doomed to dehiscence. If closure of skin is technically impossible, which is rarely the case, relaxing incisions lateral to the defect in the flank regions can be created. This allows closure of the defect over the dura. The relaxing incisions can then heal in by secondary intention with wet-to-dry dressing changes.

Often, infants presenting late may have an infected myelomeningocele (Figure 25.8). These should be mechanically debrided and thoroughly irrigated with antibiotic solution until all inflammatory and purulent material is eliminated. The closure can then proceed as described above, although the tissue planes are often compromised and thickened. These wounds are more likely to dehisce in the days following closure. In the event of wound dehiscence, as long as there is no CSF leak, we have found dressing changes that employ raw (unprocessed) honey to be particularly effective in stimulating granulation tissue. Standard wet-to-dry dressing changes with sterile saline are an alternative.

Management of Progressive Hydrocephalus

Most infants with myelomeningocele will have some accelerated head growth and a fullness of the anterior fontanel after the back closure. About one-half to two-thirds of these will continue to manifest progressive hydrocephalus and require treatment. However, shunt placement should be delayed as long as possible, because in the developed world setting with delayed myelomeningocele closure, shunt placement soon after closure carries a very high risk of shunt infection and ventriculitis. Head circumference should be monitored and tracked on a growth chart. If it continues to increase, the fontanel is full, cranial ultrasound or CT shows enlarging ventricles, and if any clinical signs of elevated pressure develop (vomiting, irritability, lethargy, sunsetting of the eyes, or stridorous breathing), then a shunt should be placed. It is wise, however, to perform a ventricular puncture and obtain CSF for cultures, cell count,

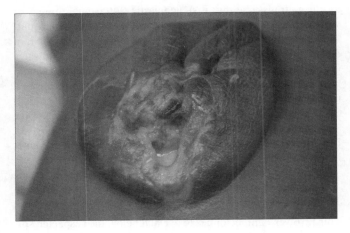

FIGURE 25.8 Infected myelomeningocele. Image by Benjamin C. Warf.

glucose, and protein to rule out infection prior to proceeding with the shunt placement.

Neurosurgical Infections

Shunt Infection

Most, though not all, shunt infections occur within 6 months of a shunt operation. In the context of an up-country hospital in a developing country, the rate of infection can, unfortunately, be expected to be anywhere from 10% to as high as 50%. Shunt infection should be expected when fever, irritability, or lethargy, with or without overt signs of shunt malfunction, present within a few months of a shunt operation (placement or revision). The diagnosis can be made by obtaining CSF for culture via a shunt tap in which, employing meticulous sterile technique, a 22-gauge needle is passed percutaneously into the shunt reservoir or valve. After obtaining CSF, treatment with broad spectrum IV antibiotics that have good central nervous system penetrance should be instituted until the culture and Gram stain results are available. A positive Gram stain or subsequent culture result should prompt urgent operative treatment to remove the shunt and replace the ventricular catheter with an EVD (described above). For infants with open fontanels, a subcutaneous reservoir attached to a new ventricular catheter can be used for daily removal of CSF to avoid the nursing challenges of an externalized drain. A Rickham reservoir is ideal for this, but a tapping reservoir can also be created by using a shunt valve with its distal tubing tied off and amputated. A minimum of one week of antibiotic treatment (tailored, if possible, to the culture and sensitivity results) is required. One week of consecutively negative CSF cultures is desirable prior to shunt replacement. The new shunt can be replaced at the prior location.

Brain Abscess, Epidural Abscess, and Subdural Empyema

Diagnosis

These infections are more common in the developing world but are very difficult to diagnose without neuroimaging. Cranial ultrasound can, however, diagnose and localize a brain abscess or subdural collection in an infant. Furthermore, if there is a strong clinical suspicion and there are lateralizing neurological signs, a small craniotomy can be created on the suspected side and intraoperative ultrasound can be employed to localize an abscess or subdural empyema in an older child or adult as described above. An epidural abscess may be encountered at the time of bone removal.

Patients with brain abscess may present with fever, but up to half may not. Subdural empyema is likely to be associated with an ill-appearing febrile patient. Other symptoms include headache, altered mental status, seizure, vomiting, papilledema, and focal neurological signs that depend upon the location of the lesion. Neurological signs are more likely to have developed more recently than expected for a brain tumor, but this is certainly in the differential diagnosis. A clinical picture of infection can be helpful in making the distinction. Neurological examination can guide the diagnosis. Pupillary asymmetry may point to a temporal lobe lesion on the side of the dilated pupil due to transtentorial third nerve compression. (See Chapter 44.) Hemiparesis or a focal motor seizure suggests a lesion in the parietal lobe on the contralateral side. In a patient with gaze palsy, the eyes may be deviated toward the side of the affected frontal lobe. These are only examples, and some knowledge of neuroanatomy and the ability to perform a basic neurologic examination is essential. In an infant, in addition to these signs, a full or tense anterior fontanel can result from the overall elevation of intracranial pressure. Transfontanel ultrasonography will suggest the diagnosis.

Treatment

These are life-threatening lesions and should be treated as such. The basic essential treatment involves drainage of pus for decompression, organism identification, and appropriate antibiotic treatment. In the infant, intraoperative ultrasound through the fontanel can guide needle aspiration of a brain abscess or drainage of subdural pus either through the corner of the fontanel or through a burr hole (described above).

In the older child or adult, the definitive diagnosis may need to be made at the time of exploratory surgery. If the suspicion is strong, and there are lateralizing neurological findings, a small craniotomy or craniectomy can be performed over the most likely location on the suspected side. The technique for making the burr hole and enlarging it into a small craniectomy are described in Chapter 44. Intraoperative ultrasound is used to image the lesion as previously discussed. If found, an abscess can be reached by using a spinal needle guided to the abscess cavity and the pus withdrawn with a syringe until no further pus is produced. If there appears to be an undrained abscess on the ultrasound, the needle should be repositioned as necessary to drain everything possible.

If a subdural collection is noted on the intraoperative ultrasound, or if the dura appears tense, a small exploratory durotomy should be made over the collection. If pus is encountered, the dural opening should be lengthened with scissors, being careful to protect the underlying cortical surface. Aerobic and anaerobic cultures should be obtained if possible. An opening of sufficient size needs to be made to obtain specimens and to wash out the collection. Irrigation with Bacitracin (or Gentamycin) and saline solution is ideal. A catheter can be gently passed in all directions in the subdural space beyond the exposure to irrigate as widely as possible. This should be done until the effluent is clear. At times, purulent material may be adherent to the underlying arachnoid or cortical surface. No attempt should be made to mechanically debride this, as this can damage the underlying cortex. The operation is complete when all liquid pus has been evacuated. If possible, the dura should be closed with a running 4-0 suture. The patient should be placed on available broad-spectrum antibiotics that include Gram-positive and Gram-negative, aerobic and anaerobic organisms until the treatment can be tailored to the microbiology laboratory results. If the suspected abscess or empyema is not encountered, then the wound is closed and the process can be repeated on the opposite side.

If an epidural abscess is encountered at the time of bone removal, this should be similarly washed out with antibiotic solution, but the dura should *not* be opened unless there is imaging evidence of a subdural empyema. The bone flap can be washed thoroughly in antibiotic solution and replaced.

In each case, the appropriate intravenous antibiotics should be administered for 6 weeks if at all possible. In addition, it should be noted that it is not unusual for reoperation to be necessary for reaccumulation of pus until the infection is fully treated.

Both the surgeon and the patient must be aware that a negative exploration or finding a tumor mass that is not amenable to aspiration are possibilities. This type of exploratory procedure should only be undertaken when 1) there is strong clinical suspicion, 2) the condition of the patient warrants it, 3) there is no reasonable way to acquire CT or MRI imaging of the patient, or 4) there is no way to refer the patient to a neurosurgical center.

Spinal Epidural Abscess

Diagnosis

In the absence of imaging, this is a clinical diagnosis. Although myelography can demonstrate the level of a block, this may not be an option in many settings. This clinical entity may or may not present with a febrile illness or accompanying back pain. Plain X-ray is indicated to rule out other possibilities, such as vertebral destruction from tuberculosis (TB) or tumor. The initial treatment for spinal TB (Pott's disease) is medical. Spinal cord compression from a vertebral column tumor should be referred to a neurosurgical center. In the patient presenting with recent onset of paraparesis and possibly urinary incontinence or retention, a detailed history and thorough neurological examination are imperative. There is a differential diagnosis in terms of both location and pathological process. The patient with spinal cord compression will most likely have a spastic paraparesis with increased muscle tone and exaggerated deep tendon reflexes. Clonus and Babinski's sign may be present. In contrast, with compression of the cauda equina, there is typically a flaccid paraparesis with decreased or absent reflexes, low muscle tone, and no clonus or Babinski's sign. The spinal cord level lesion is more likely to produce a distinct sensory level defect. Thus, a patient with a few days' history of progressive spastic paraparesis and decreased sensation below the level of the nipple line is likely to have a spinal cord lesion around the level of the 4th thoracic vertebra. The pathological process may be infectious (e.g., epidural abscess), inflammatory (e.g., transverse myelitis), neoplastic (intraspinal tumor), or vascular (e.g., epidural hematoma or spinal cord vascular malformation, both rare). In the face of new onset paraparesis in a deteriorating patient in which neurological examination indicates the likely level for operative exploration, such intervention should be undertaken unless the patient can be rapidly transferred to a neurosurgical center. Again, the possibility of a negative surgical exploration (which will be the case for transverse myelitis or for an intramedullary spinal cord lesion) must be accepted by all. However, this is worse than missing the opportunity to prevent a lifetime of paralysis from a curable disease.

Treatment

This involves laminectomies above and below the suspected spinal level of the lesion based upon the physical examination. After induction of general anesthesia the patient is positioned prone on chest rolls with all pressure points padded. The spinal level can be determined by counting up and down from defined anatomic landmarks. The top of the iliac crest is typically level with the L3–4 interspace. In a thin patient, the 12th rib can be palpated in the back and followed posteriorly and superiorly along to its junction with the 12th thoracic vertebra (T12). The most prominent spinous process in the neck is C7 at the junction of the neck and upper back. Counting up and down from these landmarks helps confirm the proper level. If available, an intraoperative lateral spine X-ray can also be used to confirm the spinous process of L5 by placing a marker at this level and counting up from there.

After identifying the desired level, the back is prepped and draped to include three to four spinous processes above and below the suspected level. After infiltration with local anesthetic, the skin is incised from one spinous process above to one below the suspected level of the lesion. The fascia is exposed and self-retaining retractors are positioned. Using a combination of monopolar electrocautery and a periosteal elevator, a subperiosteal dissection is carried out to expose the laminae on both sides at all three levels, and the retraction is deepened. The three spinous processes are removed down to the level of the lamina with a large rongeur, and the edge of the middle lamina on one side is carefully defined with a curette. Bleeding from cut bone edges should be controlled by the application of bone wax. A Kerrison rongeur is used to nip away the lamina on one side and then the other, after thinning the bone with a small drill if this is available. The lateral boundary for the laminectomy is the facet joint, which must be preserved in order to avoid spinal instability. If an epidural abscess is present, it may decompress spontaneously as soon as the epidural space is entered. If there is no abnormality, epidural fat covering the underlying dura should become evident once the laminectomy is completed. Epidural veins should be cauterized with bipolar electrocautery if available; otherwise, grasp these with a nontoothed forceps and apply monopolar electrocautery. The control of epidural venous bleeding can sometimes be problematic, but it can virtually always be controlled quickly by compression. This can be accomplished by the placement of cotton patties or cotton balls or even the edge of a sponge into the epidural space beneath the bone laterally. Surgicel or gelfoam, if available, is preferable and can be left in place.

If there is no abnormality, the laminectomy is continued first up one level and then, if normal, down one level. If the underlying dura and epidural fat look normal and there is no hint of dural compression underlying the nonlaminectomized levels above and below, then the wound is irrigated and closed. If pus is encountered, it should be thoroughly irrigated and debrided away after taking specimens for aerobic and anaerobic cultures. If another mass, such as a tumor or hematoma, is encountered, this, too, should be removed as much as possible to accomplish dural decompression. In the case of tumor, specimens should be saved for pathology if such is available. In sub-Saharan Africa, Burkitt's lymphoma can present as an epidural mass with spinal cord compression. Correct diagnosis can lead to curative chemotherapy if the patient is referred to the appropriate treatment center. If pus or other mass continues to extend above or below the exposure, the skin incision should be extended appropriately and additional laminectomies performed until the majority of dural compression has been relieved. For liquid pus, it may not be necessary to extend the laminectomies if the pus can be removed by washing and aspiration and the dura is seen to reexpand dorsally. The dura should not be opened, as this would cause contamination leading to meningitis. In the event that an abscess was evacuated, appropriate antibiotic coverage needs to be instituted for a period of 6 weeks.

Conclusion

This chapter has provided an overview of the diagnosis and management of some common conditions that both require and are amenable to urgent neurosurgical treatment in an LMIC. When possible, patients should be referred to a neurosurgical center. When doing so is not possible in a timely way, it is hoped that the foregoing will be helpful.

Further Reading

Principles and Practice of Pediatric Neurosurgery (Albright A, Pollack I, Adelson D, eds), Chapters 8, 21, 71–75, Thieme, 2008.

COMMENTARY

John Mugamba, Uganda

This chapter is a well-written, simplified text that will be understandable for physicians and general surgeons who are trained in Uganda; they will be able to follow this text to carry out lifesaving procedures. It comes at a time when capacity building is on paper, but there is little to show on the ground. The training of neurosurgeons in our region is taking off, but it is going to take time to have an impact. It is with this in mind that I think the ideas expressed in this chapter are worth trying out. Bringing it closer to home, ours is a children's hospital, and over the past 13 years our young patients are increasing in numbers and growing in age. Aware of the complications, we have questioned ourselves as to who is to inherit these patients as they transition to adulthood. We also wonder how feasible it is going to be to access one of the very few neurosurgical centers in good time before irreversible changes in the brain occur. As I reflect on Dr. Warf's chapter, I would like to think that a partnership with general surgeons and physicians is the most practical strategy for now. The techniques can be mastered by refreshing their memories if they spent some time in a place like Cure Hospital, Mbale, or if the neurosurgeon was to spend time in a given regional, district, or mission hospital.

26

Otorhinolaryngology

Robert M. Boucher

Introduction

Scope

The purpose of this chapter is to serve as a practical guide for healthcare providers serving in resource-constrained low- and middle-income countries (LMICs) in the assessment and management of common ear, nose, and throat problems.

Assumptions

The discussions assume that the reader has minimal or limited formal training in otolaryngology—head and neck surgery.

Organization

Chapter organization is by head and neck anatomic areas.

Procedures

This section presents procedures commonly performed by otolaryngologists that may also be performed by non-otolaryngologists providing the practitioner has some clinical or technical experience as well as access to the basic equipment and support staff as discussed for each procedure. Some procedures, due to their nature and attendant risk (e.g., extraction of obstructing aero-digestive foreign bodies), should, with rare exceptions, only be attempted by a clinician experienced in that area and are not presented in detail here.

The Ear

Infection

Acute Otitis Externa

Definition and Clinical Considerations

Otitis externa describes a variety of acute, subacute, or chronic inflammatory processes of the external auditory canal. The most common presentation is as an acute process (e.g., "swimmer's ear") due to maceration of the ear canal skin. The most common determinant of acute infection is excessive instrumentation of the ear canal (a cotton-tipped applicator being the most notorious offender). Instrumentation can remove protective cerumen and injure ear canal skin; underlying ear canal moisture may soften the skin, making maceration and subsequent infection more likely.

Symptoms include ear canal pruritus and tenderness as well as fullness and hearing loss. A history of instrumenting the ear canal is frequently obtained; patients often give a history of prior otitis externa.

Relevant Physical Examination and Anatomy/Physiology

Examination often shows tenderness with posterosuperior displacement of the auricle; ear canal erythema, edema, and purulence are variably present. Examination may be limited due to discomfort or ear canal edema. The infection is typically polymicrobial (e.g., pseudomonas aeruginosa, proteus mirabilis, staphylococcal and streptococcal species); fungal mycelia may be seen. Cultures are unnecessary in uncomplicated cases.

Treatment

In the absence of significant ear canal edema and debris, an otic drop alone for 5–10 days usually suffices (e.g., neomycin/hydrocortisone/polymyxin or fluoroquinolone with or without corticosteroid). Debris such as desquamated skin may be gently removed. When ear canal edema is extensive, a wick should be placed, followed by otic drops. The wick may be removed after the edema subsides. The patient should be instructed to keep the ear dry. Oral antibiotics are seldom necessary; however, in more advanced cases, or in patients with diabetes mellitus or a compromised immune system, a short course of an oral fluoroquinolone may be beneficial. Patients with extensive infection should be followed closely; those with unremitting infection should be referred for otologic evaluation.

Acute Suppurative Otitis Media

Definition and Clinical Considerations

Uncomplicated acute suppurative otitis media (AOM) is common in young children but can occur in any age group. It often accompanies an upper respiratory infection. Although the inciting infection is usually viral, secondary bacterial growth in the middle ear space often occurs. The most common bacterial pathogens are streptococcus pneumoniae, nontypable haemophilus influenza, and moraxella catarrhalis.

Young children may present with fever, fussiness, tugging at the ear, or refusal to eat. Older children and adults complain of earache and hearing loss.

Relevant Physical Examination and Anatomy/Physiology

Examination typically shows a normal ear canal and a red, bulging tympanic membrane that does not move with otoscopic insufflation. The contralateral ear is usually normal. Importantly, AOM is very *unlikely* in the presence of a clear eardrum that insufflates readily. Patients may also present with a perforated tympanic membrane and associated purulent or bloody discharge; tympanic perforation may occur after treatment begins. Tympanic perforation in AOM usually relieves otalgia. Tenderness and swelling behind the ear is unusual and, if present, may indicate acute mastoiditis. Rarely, AOM may present with facial paralysis.

Treatment

AOM with or without tympanic rupture is treated similarly. Usual treatment for AOM is a course of an oral antibiotic such as amoxicillin, amoxicillin/clavulanate, or second-generation cephalosporin; in penicillin-allergic patients, a macrolide antibiotic may be substituted. Oral analgesics should be used as necessary. Although clinical improvement typically occurs over 3–5 days, residual middle ear fluid may persist for weeks. Tympanic perforations in those without a significant prior history of middle ear infections usually heal spontaneously; persistent perforations should be referred to an otolaryngologist. Patients presenting with facial paralysis or suspected mastoiditis should be started on antibiotic therapy and urgently referred to an otolaryngologist. Urgent myringotomy may be beneficial but should only be attempted by experienced clinicians.

In some patients the acute infection resolves but a middle ear effusion remains, resulting in *serous* or *mucoid* otitis media. Middle ear effusions should be followed to ensure resolution, which can take many weeks or longer. Treatment of persistent effusions varies depending upon chronicity, type (i.e., serous or mucoid), unilateral versus bilateral, and effect on hearing. Persistent middle ear effusion should be evaluated by an otolaryngologist.

Chronic Middle Ear Disease

Definition and Clinical Considerations

For the purposes of this section, chronic middle ear disease refers to significant recurrent or persistent middle ear pathology. A history of recurrent ear problems over many months to years is often obtained. Patients typically have associated hearing loss with or without variable otalgia or otorrhea. The following are the most common pathologies, occurring alone or in combination: persistent middle ear effusion (often viscous or mucoid); significant tympanic retraction; nonhealing tympanic perforation (either wet or dry); and cholesteatoma (i.e., skin in the middle ear space) with or without obvious tympanic perforation.

Relevant Physical Examination and Anatomy/Physiology

The underlying pathophysiologic basis of almost all chronic middle ear disease is persistent eustachian tube dysfunction, which impairs normal middle ear ventilation. Chronic eustachian dysfunction produces lack of proper middle ear ventilation with variable tympanic retraction (with or without middle ear effusion) or in nonhealing tympanic perforation; cholesteatoma formation may be the long-term outcome. On physical examination, the tympanic membrane is variously abnormal and may be retracted, extensively scarred, or perforated; otorrhea may be present. Severe, persistent tympanic retraction can cause marked attenuation of the membrane with adhesions to the middle ear mucosa and ossicles. Persistent perforations also allow skin to migrate into the middle ear space with resultant cholesteatoma formation. Left untreated, cholesteatomas can expand destructively, causing ossicular damage and hearing loss; rarely, intracranial complications occur.

Persistent tympanic perforations are associated with recurrent or persistent otorrhea. The otorrhea of chronic otitis media can be profuse, purulent, and foul-smelling, or serous and scant. Although such discharge often represents a polymicrobial infection (organisms may include various staphylococcal and streptococcal as well as pseudomonal and proteus species), consideration in LMICs should be given to tuberculous middle ear disease; specimens for AFB and culture should be obtained.

Treatment

Overall, definitive treatment of chronic middle ear disease is surgical and in the purview of the otolaryngologist. Surgical options include: ventilation tube placement (for tympanic retraction, with or without effusion); tympanic membrane reconstruction (for non-healing perforations or tympanic atelectasis); and removal of cholesteatoma (with or without tympanic membrane and ossicular repair, or mastoidectomy).

The most common complication of chronic middle ear disease requiring medical therapy is otorrhea from a perforated tympanic membrane.

The otorrhea is typically painless and often fetid. Therapy with broad-spectrum topical antibiotics (fluoroquinolone-based otic drops are favored) and water avoidance are usually helpful. When profuse otorrhea prevents otic drop use, oral antibiotic therapy may be helpful and should be culture-dependent.

For persistent otorrhea in spite of otherwise reasonable therapy, specimens for culture and sensitivity as well as acid-fast bacillus (AFB) staining and culture should be obtained.

Foreign Body of Ear Canal

Diagnosis and Clinical Considerations

Consider inappropriate organic or inorganic material lateral to the tympanic membrane. Always examine contralateral ear as well. Removal is generally elective; exceptions include live insects and button batteries.

Relevant Physical Examination and Anatomy/Physiology

Most foreign bodies (FBs) are evident as such on visualization; nonetheless, they must be differentiated from ear canal anomalies such as osteomas, exostoses, cholesteatomas, granulomas, or neoplasms.

- Ear canal osteomas (single) and exostoses (multiple and bilateral) are bony growths that may partially obscure the ear drum; gentle palpation with a wax loop confirms the diagnosis. They are generally asymptomatic and no further evaluation is usually warranted.

- Ear canal cholesteatomas are usually adjacent to the tympanic membrane and appear as pearly white, soft tissue masses on palpation.
- Granulomas appear as discrete, reddish-brown, friable masses.
- Neoplasms may appear as either discrete, well-circumscribed, fleshy masses or as friable soft tissue lesions.

Any non-FB lesion of the ear canal, with the exception of osteomas or exostoses, should be evaluated by an otolaryngologist.

Treatment

Refer to the section on infectious inflammatory diseases later in this chapter for additional discussion and treatment.

Tumors/Masses

Patients presenting with tumors or masses of the auricle or external ear canal should be referred to an otolaryngologist for evaluation. The following are common entities, with a brief discussion of salient clinical considerations.

- **Keloids** are trauma-related (e.g., ear-piercing) hypertrophic scars. Keloids characteristically appear as lobular, fleshy, painless masses arising from the lobule or other pierced or injured site. Biopsy is unnecessary. There is a high likelihood of recurrence and unskillful resection can result in significant residual ear deformity; therefore, treatment is best left to otolaryngologists and surgeons familiar with plastic and reconstructive techniques.
- **Malignant neoplasms of the auricle:** The most frequent malignancies are squamous and basal cell carcinomas. They are more common on the superior aspect (i.e., most sun-exposed) of the auricle. Presentation is variable; when advanced, they may be quite friable. A simple incisional or punch biopsy usually confirms the diagnosis.
- **Soft tissue masses in the ear canal:** Differential diagnosis includes cholesteatoma, polyp/granuloma, and malignancy. Ear canal masses may represent a "tip of the iceberg" phenomenon, as the underlying process may be quite extensive within the middle ear space and temporal bone. Facial weakness with an ear canal mass is an ominous sign and warrants urgent otolaryngologic evaluation. Ear canal masses may be associated with suppuration or bleeding regardless of etiology. The presence of squamous debris suggests cholesteatoma. Polyps and granulomas of the ear canal may also reflect chronic middle ear disease. Squamous carcinoma can occur in the ear canal and may present as a friable mass with erosion of cartilage and bone. While it is not unreasonable to gently suction the ear canal for diagnostic considerations (e.g., to rule out a foreign body), primary care practitioners should generally not attempt to remove soft tissue lesions due to the risk of bleeding and inadvertent injury to middle ear structures. Patients should be referred for otolaryngologic evaluation.

Auricular Hematoma

Refer to the section on auricular hematoma later in this chapter.

Nose and Paranasal Sinuses

Epistaxis

Anterior/Uncomplicated

Definition and Clinical Considerations

Most episodes of epistaxis represent anterior nasal septal bleeding (90%–95%) and are self-limited. Etiologies include blunt or digital trauma, mucosal drying or inflammation, effects of intranasal sprays (especially steroids), or underlying nasal deformities (septal deviation or perforation). Epistaxis may also occur with anti-platelet or anti-coagulant drugs, or coagulopathies; in these cases, adjusting the offending medication or treating the underlying coagulopathy is usually necessary.

Relevant Physical Examination and Anatomy/Physiology

Initial assessment includes ruling out a foreign body or discrete mass and confirming, if possible, the primary bleeding site, which can be challenging in the presence of active bleeding. The anterior nasal septum is the most common site and attention should be focused accordingly. Gentle suctioning of the anterior nasal cavity is often all that is needed to confirm the bleeding site.

Treatment

Refer to the section on nasal packing for epistaxis later in this chapter.

Complex

Definition and Clinical Considerations

For this discussion, complex epistaxis is defined as bleeding from the posterior nasal cavity, profuse bleeding where a specific site cannot be identified, or failure of epistaxis control measures discussed in the section on nasal packing for epistaxis later in this chapter.

Relevant Physical Examination and Anatomy/Physiology

Potential posterior nasal cavity bleeding sites include the posterior septum, posterior lateral nasal wall, or superior nasal cavity. The management techniques discussed in the section on nasal packing for epistaxis generally control bleeding from posterior septal, lateral nasal wall, or superior sites.

Treatment

Refer to the section on nasal packing for epistaxis later in this chapter.

Nasal Cavity Foreign Body

Definition and Clinical Considerations

Most intranasal FBs are in young children, although individuals with developmental delay, cognitive impairment, or psychiatric history may also present.

Relevant Physical Examination and Anatomy/Physiology

Purulence and a fetid odor may be present if the FB has been present for days or longer. Unilateral nasal purulence in a child represents a FB until proven otherwise. Bloody nasal discharge and repetitive sneezing may also be present. The differential diagnosis includes nasal polyps, papillomas, pyogenic granulomas, and other benign or malignant neoplasms.

Treatment

Refer to the section on removal of foreign bodies later in this chapter.

Sinonasal Infections and Inflammatory Processes

Definition and Clinical Considerations

The most common sinonasal infectious and inflammatory disorders are viral rhinitis (e.g., "common cold"), allergic rhinitis (seasonal or perennial), and sinusitis (acute or chronic). With the exception of chronic sinusitis, patient history and examination alone are usually sufficient to make the diagnosis. Clinical presentation may include acute onset of nasal congestion, rhinorrhea, disturbance of smell sensation, nasal itching, and midfacial pain or pressure.

Uncommon conditions include fungal sinusitis (superficial or invasive), nasal sarcoidosis, unusual infections (e.g., rhinoscleroma or syphilis), and neoplasia mimicking inflammatory disease (e.g., various lymphomas and leukemias).

Patients with diabetes, human immunodeficiency virus (HIV)/acquired immunodeficiency syndrome (AIDS), or immunocompromised status are at greater risk of developing complications of sinonasal disease (e.g., ocular or intracranial involvement) and should be monitored very closely.

Relevant Physical Examination and Anatomy/Physiology

Patients with "colds" or allergic rhinitis are usually afebrile. For common conditions, the nasal mucosa is edematous, and may be variably erythematous (with infections) or pale (with allergies). Purulence is more common with infectious than allergic conditions. Tenderness to palpation over the maxillary or frontal sinuses, particularly with fever and purulent rhinorrhea, suggests acute sinusitis. Sinus transillumination is unreliable; sinus radiographs may be helpful but are generally unnecessary in uncomplicated presentations.

Computed tomography (CT) imaging of the sinuses is the "gold standard" for assessing chronic complaints and unusual presentations. Such presentations include intranasal masses, particularly when associated with expansive disfigurement of the nose and paranasal structures; proptosis with or without visual loss; or friable tissue, with or without erosion of nasal structures. Unusual presentations or refractory disease should be referred for otolaryngologic evaluation.

Treatment

Effective therapies for symptomatic allergic rhinitis include inhaled nasal corticosteroids and various antihistamines, either singly or in combination. Viral rhinitis and uncomplicated acute sinusitis in healthy patients are usually self-limited. Supportive treatment with nasal saline sprays, cool mist humidifiers, oral decongestants, or short-term topical nasal vasoconstrictors (e.g., oxymetazoline, or Neo-Synephrine) may be helpful. Intranasal cultures are not indicated in uncomplicated acute sinusitis. Empirical antimicrobial therapy may be considered in patients with persistent fever, purulent rhinorrhea, and significant facial pain. Oral antibiotics commonly used for nonresolving acute sinusitis (and chronic sinusitis) include amoxicillin, amoxicillin/clavulanate, second generation cephalosporins, macrolides, and fluoroquinolones. Refractory disease, unusual presentations, or disease extending beyond the sinonasal spaces warrants otolaryngology referral.

Intranasal Polyps and Masses

Definition and Clinical Considerations

Most intranasal polyps are benign hyperplastic manifestations of chronic mucosal inflammation. Most commonly patients present with variable bilateral nasal obstruction and decreased smell sensation. Extensive polyps may protrude from the nares. An exception is an antral-choanal polyp, so called because it originates in the maxillary sinus (antrum) and prolapses into the posterior nasal cavity (choana). An antral-choanal polyp typically presents as a unilateral, lobular, glistening mass variably obstructing the nasal cavity and prolapsing into the pharynx. It may occur in older children or adults; allergic rhinitis may be present.

Polypoid masses can represent other inflammatory processes (e.g., allergic fungal rhinosinusitis) as well as a variety of soft tissue neoplasms, either benign (e.g., pyogenic granulomas, papillomas, or hamartomas) or malignant (e.g., squamous carcinomas, lymphomas, or neuroepithelium-based).

Relevant Physical Examination and Anatomy/Physiology

Common nasal polyps are usually bilateral, often extensive, and variably obstructive. Antral-choanal polyps are usually unilateral; they can often be partially visualized in the oropharynx.

Common polyps notwithstanding, most intranasal masses are unilateral. Pyogenic granulomas tend to occur in the anterior nasal cavity, are friable, and are most common in children and pregnant women. Common papillomas usually occur in the nostril with the characteristic appearance of a common wart.

Extensive papillomatous masses may harbor foci of squamous carcinoma. Hamartomas and neoplasms, either benign or malignant, can present as extensive, obstructing masses variably distorting the external nose and surrounding midfacial structures. Associated proptosis, visual disturbance, or severe headaches are ominous findings and suggest spread beyond the sinonasal cavities.

Treatment

Common nasal polyps may improve with topical or oral corticosteroids. Antihistamines and decongestants are usually ineffective. Extensive benign polypoid disease can be treated surgically for symptomatic relief (and diagnostic confirmation) but often recurs over time.

Symptomatic antral choanal polyps require surgical removal.

All intranasal masses should be referred for otolaryngologic evaluation; referral urgency depends upon the patient's history and clinical presentation.

Oral Cavity and Upper Aerodigestive Tract

Infection

Stomatitis/Pharyngitis

Definition and Clinical Considerations

Stomatitis and pharyngitis describe inflammatory processes of the oral cavity and pharyngeal mucosa, respectively. The diagnosis is based on a thorough history and physical examination. The processes discussed below often manifest in both anatomic areas; in such cases, treatment considerations are generally the same.

Stomatitis: Notwithstanding odontogenic infections, aphthous stomatitis, viral infections (e.g., herpes simplex), fungal infections (e.g., candidiasis), and various granulomatous (e.g., Wegener's granulomatosis or Crohn's disease) and other inflammatory processes (e.g., pemphigus, pemphigoid, lichen planus, or erythema multiforme) comprise the majority of presentations. HIV/AIDS-related stomatitis may involve any of the above infectious entities as well as a variety of other opportunistic pathologies. HIV disease should always be considered when a patient presents with extensive oromucosal lesions.

Pharyngitis: Common upper respiratory and influenza viruses are the most common cause of pharyngitis. Other viral pathogens (e.g., herpes simplex, Epstein-Barr, cytomegalovirus, HIV, or measles) can present as pharyngitis. Group A beta-hemolytic streptococcus infection (i.e., "strep throat") is the most common cause of bacterial pharyngitis and a common cause of tonsillitis. Staphylococcal species occasionally cause purulent pharyngitis. Other bacterial entities include gonococcal pharyngitis and primary (as a solitary chancre) or secondary syphilis (generalized pharyngitis). In the non-immunized, *Corynebacterium diphtheriae* and *Bordetella pertussis* can also cause pharyngitis. Pharyngeal candidiasis, usually associated with compromised local or systemic immunity, is the most commonly occurring fungal variant. Granulomatous and other inflammatory entities causing stomatitis may also manifest as pharyngitis. Mucosal irritants (e.g., gastric secretions, caustic liquids, alcohol, tobacco, and certain medications) should also be considered in the differential diagnosis.

Relevant Physical Examination and Anatomy/Physiology

Stomatitis: Aphthous ulcers and oral herpes simplex (HSV) lesions may be visually indistinguishable as superficial mucosal ulcers; however, HSV lesions initially occur as vesicles (which eventually ulcerate) and are usually multiple. Aphthous lesions frequently present singly. Either lesion can occur on any oral mucosal membrane; both entities typically present with oral pain and lesional erythema; both often recur. Acute HSV infections may have associated fever, malaise, headache, and cervical adenopathy; cytologic smears can aid the diagnosis.

Oral candidiasis usually presents as painless or mildly sore white mucosal plaques ("thrush") easily removed with a tongue blade; patient history and characteristic oral findings are usually satisfactory for the diagnosis in most cases. Patient history, HIV status, comorbidities, and potentially offending medications are important considerations in evaluating unusual stomatitis presentations. Bullous and erosive lesions are difficult to definitively diagnose, even with biopsy and special stains.

Pharyngitis: Uncomplicated viral "sore throat" does not require diagnostic testing; bacterial staining and cultures may be helpful when purulence is present. Consider overall medical history, HIV status, comorbidities, and potentially offending medications when assessing unusual presentations.

Treatment

Stomatitis: Aphthous and primary HSV infections are self-limited and generally require only supportive measures. Recurrent HSV infections may require antiviral therapy (e.g., acyclovir). Uncomplicated oral candidiasis typically responds to topical therapy (e.g., nystatin) and, when indicated, discontinuation of offending medication; various systemic antifungals (e.g., fluconazole) are available for more extensive disease. Therapy for non-HIV granulomatous and ulcerative processes varies with the specific disorder; referral to a specialist (e.g., rheumatologist) may be necessary. Although corticosteroids are frequently used in these cases, steroidal therapy prior to biopsy may confound diagnosis. Oral lesions in HIV/AIDS patients are myriad; the need for cultures, special staining, or biopsy to guide treatment should be made on a case-by-case basis. Specialist referral for unusual, treatment-resistant, or recurrent lesions is recommended.

Pharyngitis: The treatment approaches discussed above for stomatitis generally apply to pharyngitis as well. Rapid testing for streptococcal pharyngitis is helpful in avoiding unnecessary antibiotic use; however, empiric therapy with a penicillin-type or macrolide antibiotic is justified by a suggestive history and physical examination in the absence of a culture. Antimicrobial treatment of less common types of pharyngitis (e.g., gonococcal and syphilis-related) should be guided by appropriate staining and culture results. Notable exceptions include diphtheria for which antitoxin is the mainstay of therapy (antibiotics have a supporting role) and pertussis, the course of which is not affected by antibiotics. (The acute phase of diphtheria often presents with extensive upper aerodigestive mucosal necrosis requiring emergent, intensive airway management.)

Oropharyngeal Abscesses (Peritonsillar, Floor of Mouth/Submandibular Space, Retro- and Parapharyngeal Spaces)

Definition and Clinical Considerations

This section describes the more common abscesses that originate in oropharyngeal structures. All are generally manifestations of advanced, often polymicrobial, infections of adjacent sites such as tonsils, adenoid, or dental structures. Important clinical questions include: What is the patient's airway status? How sick is the patient? Is the process acute or chronic? Has the patient received antibiotics?

Most infections are polymicrobial with both aerobic and anaerobic pathogens. Various streptococcal, staphylococcal,

Neisseria, Klebsiella, and *Haemophilus* species comprise the more common aerobes; various bacteroides and anaerobic streptococcal species comprise the more common anaerobes.

The most common abscess is of the peritonsillar space ("quinsy tonsillitis"), usually a complication of streptococcal tonsillitis. Patients often have a prior history of tonsillitis.

Floor-of-mouth (Ludwig's angina) and submandibular abscesses are most frequently complications of odontogenic or submandibular gland infections.

Retro- and parapharyngeal space infections are usually suppurative complications of infections involving the retropharyngeal lymph nodes (e.g., from nasopharyngeal or sinonasal sites) or parapharyngeal space (e.g., from a tonsillar or pharyngeal site), respectively.

Potentially fatal complications of untreated or ineffectively treated infections include airway obstruction, bacteremia, deep cervical vascular injury (e.g., carotid artery and jugular vein), or mediastinitis.

Relevant Physical Examination and Anatomy/Physiology

Presentation varies and may be affected by prior antibiotic therapy. There is often a history of recent sore throat, upper respiratory infection, or dental disease. Overall, patients may present with fever, pain, swelling, odynophagia, trismus, or drooling; respiratory difficulty is an ominous sign. Airway assessment is the most important part of the initial examination. Every effort is made to secure the airway prior to proceeding with definitive evaluation and therapy.

Patients with peritonsillar abscesses often have a "hot potato voice" and variable drooling and trismus. Typically, the involved tonsil and peritonsillar area is full and erythematous, although frank exudate may not be present. The swelling often pushes the soft palate and uvula to the contralateral side (refer to the section on peritonsillar abscess later in this chapter). The diagnosis may be confirmed by needle aspiration of the involved area.

Patients with Ludwig's angina typically present with tender swelling of the floor of mouth and submandibular areas, often in the presence of frank dental infection. The sublingual and submandibular fullness is often firm and board-like rather than frankly fluctuant (refer to the section on submental space [Ludwig's angina] later in this chapter).

Where the diagnosis of peritonsillar abscess or Ludwig's angina is clear, definitive management takes precedence over imaging studies.

Patients with retropharyngeal abscesses often have limitation of cervical motion; lateral neck radiographs often show abnormal fullness of the prevertebral soft tissues.

Parapharyngeal space infections usually present with fullness and tenderness more lateral than midline and may not have a clear origin. In urgent situations, definitive therapy (i.e., surgical incision and drainage) should proceed absent radiographic studies, particularly in LMICs.

Treatment

The airway should be assessed and secured first; the most appropriate, definitive means of securing the airway is utilized. The technical decision (e.g., nasopharyngeal airway, laryngeal mask airway, endotracheal intubation, or tracheotomy) should be individualized to the situation, taking into account the patient's overall condition, abscess location, available equipment, staff experience, and facilities to manage the process and patient. It is essential to choose a method with a low likelihood of loss of airway; it is usually best to do this with the patient awake or mildly sedated. Historically, tracheotomy is the gold standard; it has the highest likelihood of achieving and maintaining a secure airway until the infection resolves.

After the airway is secured, therapy should be individualized depending upon the overall clinical picture. Specimens for blood culture should be obtained; needle aspiration for cultures and treatment can be performed. Empiric, broad-spectrum parenteral antibiotics that cover the common aerobic and anaerobic pathogens discussed above should be administered along with fluid resuscitation. If the patient is otherwise stable, treatment with antibiotics alone for 1–3 days is reasonable; surgical drainage should be used for patients with advanced infections, impending complications, and those not responding to antibiotic therapy (refer to the sections on peritonsillar abscess, submental [midline submandibular] space abscess, and lateral neck abscesses later in this chapter).

Foreign Bodies

Definition and Clinical Considerations

Ingested upper aerodigestive foreign bodies (FBs) may lodge in the pharynx or esophagus; inhaled FBs generally lodge in the larynx, trachea, or a bronchus. The most commonly aspirated objects are edible (e.g., peanuts or candy), followed by pieces of toys. Coins are more often ingested than aspirated and may lodge in the cervical esophagus. Ingested or inhaled FBs can cause catastrophic airway obstruction. Young children are most susceptible, and events are often unwitnessed. Presentations vary and are determined by size, nature, and location of the offending object. Signs and symptoms include variable stridor, swallowing difficulty, coughing, or wheezing. In the absence of frank air hunger, a high index of suspicion is often necessary to make a correct, timely diagnosis.

Relevant Physical Examination and Anatomy/Physiology

As noted, object size and anatomic location are the main determinants of presenting symptoms and signs. A child with a pharyngeal FB may present with gagging and unwillingness to swallow. Objects in or about the larynx and trachea may present with variable stridor or frank airway obstruction. Coughing or wheezing without stridor are more commonly seen with bronchial than laryngotracheal FBs. For bronchial FBs, chest auscultation may show diminished breath sounds with wheezing. X-rays are variably helpful; organic foreign bodies are usually not apparent, but secondary findings (e.g., unilateral hyperinflation or atelectasis) may suggest the diagnosis.

Treatment

Significant airway compromise must be managed expeditiously by experienced clinicians using proper equipment. The possibility of making a partial airway obstruction complete by inexpert manipulation must be considered. While relief by tracheotomy is always an option, it is inherently more complex in young children and, if necessary, best undertaken by a surgeon familiar with the pediatric airway.

Children with esophageal foreign bodies can often be managed expectantly; e.g., coins may be followed with serial radiographs as many pass spontaneously. However, objects with a high likelihood of causing mucosal injury (e.g., button batteries and sharp objects) should be retrieved.

Tumors/Masses

A wide variety of congenital, developmental, benign, or malignant growths can occur in the oropharyngeal region, and a detailed discussion is beyond the scope of this chapter. However, as a general rule, any lesion compromising the airway should be managed urgently. Additionally, ulcerating or locally destructive oropharyngeal masses and those with associated cervical adenopathy are ominous and should be managed expeditiously. Given the myriad diagnostic and treatment possibilities, oropharyngeal masses should be appropriately referred (e.g., otolaryngologist, dentist, or oral surgeon). Below are some of the more common benign and malignant lesions for consideration.

- Torus mandibularis and palatinus
- Odontogenic cysts and tumors (e.g., ameloblastoma)
- Reparative/pyogenic granuloma
- Papilloma
- Squamous carcinoma
- Minor salivary gland carcinoma (e.g., adenoid cystic carcinoma)
- Sarcomas (e.g., Kaposi's in HIV/AIDS patients; rhabdomyosarcoma)
- Lymphoma (Hodgkin's and non-Hodgkin's)
- Lingual thyroid; cystic hygroma (children)

Neck

Deep Space Infections

Definition and Clinical Considerations

This section further describes the neck manifestations of advanced oral and pharyngeal infections initially discussed in the section on oropharyngeal abscesses earlier in this chapter.

Deep space infections of the neck refer to abscess formation in one or more of the cervical anatomic spaces (e.g., submental, submandibular, or lateral) and generally represent spread of infection from primary oral, pharyngeal, or sinonasal sites. (A notable exception is infection from cervical intravenous drug abuse.) As such, deep neck abscesses are usually polymicrobial and reflect the pathogens responsible for infection at the primary site (refer to clinical and management considerations in the section on oropharyngeal abscesses earlier in this chapter).

Submental Space (Ludwig's Angina)

Ludwig's angina describes a fulminant floor-of-mouth and submental space infection with diffuse, tender induration and phlegmonous type cellulitis with or without a true abscess cavity. Most presentations show associated lingual edema and superoposterior tongue displacement with variable oral airway obstruction (Figure 26.1A and Figure 26.1B).

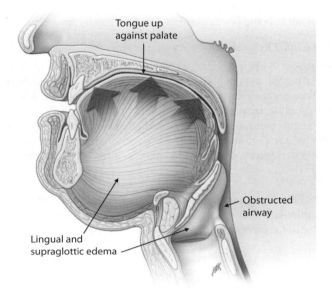

FIGURE 26.1A Advanced Ludwig's angina. Diffuse floor-of-mouth swelling with lingual and supraglottic edema; retro-displacement of the tongue contributes to airway obstruction. Illustration by John W. Karapelou, CMI.

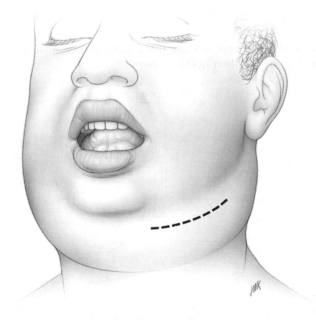

FIGURE 26.1B Associated submandibular swelling from extensive phlegmonous-type cellulitis and abscess formation. Note orolingual edema. Illustration by John W. Karapelou, CMI.

Submandibular and Lateral Deep Neck Infections

The cervical fascia separates the structures of the neck into a series of potential spaces containing adipose tissue, blood vessels, and lymphatics. Although microorganisms can invade these potential spaces by direct or hematogenous spread, the most common infectious path is via lymphatics. Lymph node suppuration can lead to abscess formation. The most common abscess locations are the submandibular triangle and lateral compartment deep to the sternocleidomastoid muscle. All extensive deep neck infections should be managed as potential airway emergencies.

Relevant Physical Examination and Anatomy/Physiology

Advanced Ludwig's angina usually presents with extensive, tender floor of mouth and submental/submandibular induration. Tongue edema with variable posterior displacement is present as are drooling, trismus, and dysarthria.

Patients presenting with advanced lateral neck abscesses usually have tender, fluctuant fullness in the submandibular triangle or along the sternocleidomastoid muscle of the involved side.

Treatment

Incision and drainage is the gold standard for treatment of fulminant abscesses. Options for less advanced infections include intravenous antibiotics and expectant management,

with or without therapeutic and diagnostic needle aspiration (Figure 26.2). Less invasive options may be considered in select patients with limited infections and stable airways (refer to the sections on peritonsillar abscess, submental [midline submandibular] space abscess, and lateral neck abscesses later in this chapter for incision and drainage procedure).

Masses and Neoplasms

The neck is an anatomically rich conduit for complex, vital neurovascular and lymphatic structures. As such, a host of infectious, inflammatory, congenital, and neoplastic processes can manifest there. The neck is anatomically divided into central and lateral compartments. By convention, the sternocleidomastoid muscle subdivides the lateral compartment into anterior and posterior triangles; the submandibular triangle is a subdivision of the superior anterior triangle. Following is a brief discussion of the more common pathologic entities causing a neck mass.

Cervical Lymphadenopathy

Definition and Clinical Considerations

The cervical lymphatics reflect lymph drainage from head and neck structures. Lymphadenopathy encompasses a range of

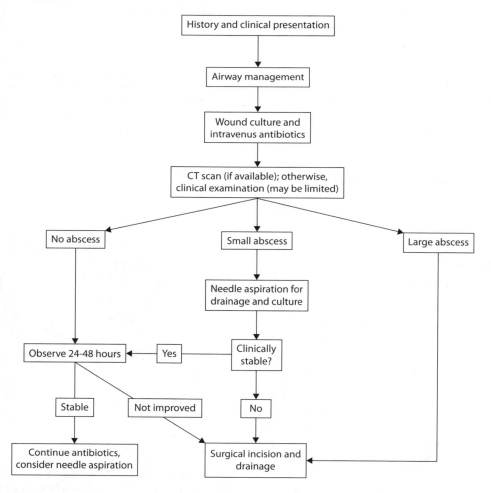

FIGURE 26.2   Management algorithm for deep neck infections. Image by Pratik Patel and Robert M. Boucher.

pathologic entities including primary and secondary infectious/inflammatory processes (lymphadenitis) as well as primary and metastatic malignancies.

Cervical lymphadenitis is most commonly a secondary (i.e., "reactive") process due to otherwise uncomplicated viral or bacterial infections of the upper aerodigestive tract. Noteworthy exceptions include primary mycobacterial infections, atypical mycobacterial adenitis, cat scratch disease, and adenitis due to systemic manifestations of HIV/AIDS, Epstein-Barr virus (EBV), cytomegalovirus (CMV), measles, hepatitis B, and dengue fever. Cervical lymphadenitis may also be caused by fungal (e.g., histoplasmosis, coccidioidomycosis, or cryptococcosis), protozoal (e.g., toxoplasmosis or leishmaniasis), spirochetal (e.g., Lyme disease or secondary syphilis), and atypical (e.g., actinomycetes) organisms. Notable non-infectious, inflammatory causes of secondary cervical lymphadenitis include Kawasaki disease (children) and sarcoidosis (adults).

Cervical lymphadenopathy is also a common manifestation of primary and metastatic neoplastic diseases. Squamous cell carcinoma and other mucosal cancers of the upper aerodigestive tract frequently manifest first as metastatic disease in cervical lymph nodes. Various major and minor salivary gland as well as thyroid and parathyroid malignancies can also metastasize to neck nodes; Hodgkin and non-Hodgkin lymphomas are relatively common primary malignancies of cervical lymphatics.

Relevant Physical Examination and Anatomy/Physiology

History and physical examination are the most important determinants in narrowing the differential diagnosis. Age is relevant as the majority of pediatric neck masses are either inflammatory or congenital processes. An indolent lateral neck mass in adults is considered malignant until proven otherwise. Other important considerations include length of time the mass has been present, constitutional symptoms (e.g., fever, chills, sweats, or weight loss), and history of tobacco and alcohol use. Chronic masses (a year or longer) with little change are more likely benign; constitutional symptoms may be seen with mycobacterial infections or lymphomas; and tobacco and alcohol use increase the risk of head and neck cancers.

Linking specific symptoms (e.g., pain, dysphagia, or hoarseness) and a sign (e.g., a discrete mucosal lesion) to an anatomic site often explains the neck mass. However, the absence of such findings does not rule out malignancy, as pharyngeal and supraglottic laryngeal cancers often present as asymptomatic neck metastases. A thorough examination of all upper aerodigestive mucosal surfaces is essential when evaluating cervical adenopathy.

As a general rule, the following describes the relationship between cervical lymphatic compartments and the anatomic structures they serve.

- Submandibular triangle: oral cavity and submandibular gland
- Anterior triangle: parotid gland, pharynx, and larynx
- Posterior triangle: nasopharynx and posterior scalp
- Central compartment: larynx, thyroid, and parathyroid

Special note is made of supraclavicular adenopathy as this is often a manifestation of extra-cervical primary disease (including thoracic, abdominal, pelvic, and retroperitoneal malignancies).

In LMICs, CT and ultrasound (US) are frequently the only available imaging modalities. Both have value: contrast CT informs location, extent, vascularity, and effect on adjacent structures; US is non-invasive, shows relationship of mass to adjacent structures, and may be very useful for guided needle biopsy.

Treatment

Lymphadenitis due to common head and neck infections (e.g., viral upper respiratory) generally resolves spontaneously or with antimicrobial therapy for the primary site infection (e.g., streptococcal pharyngitis). Non-infectious inflammatory adenitis (e.g., sarcoidosis) responds to systemic therapy for the primary condition. Cervical adenopathy in the presence of biopsy-proven upper aerodigestive malignancy can generally be assumed to be metastatic; comprehensive treatment plans for head and neck cancers typically address both the primary site and metastatic cervical adenopathy.

If the diagnosis is unclear after thorough initial evaluation, fine needle aspiration biopsy (FNAB) of the neck mass is indicated. While FNAB is often helpful for suggesting or supporting diagnoses, it should be used and interpreted judiciously due to inherent limitations. Whenever possible, definitive therapy should be guided by histopathologic results from surgical biopsy.

Congenital Cysts and Neck Masses

Definition and Clinical Considerations

Congenital cysts and neck masses may manifest at any age. The two most common cystic lesions are branchial cleft and thyroglossal duct cysts (TGDCs). A variety of other congenital lesions, including vascular anomalies, teratomas, dermoids, and thymic cysts, also occur in the neck.

Branchial cleft anomalies may present as cysts, fistulas, or sinus tracts. Branchial cleft cysts occur laterally in the neck and are classified as first, second, third, or fourth depending upon their embryologic origin. Second-cleft cysts are the most common, while first, third, and fourth cysts are rare. Laterally in the neck, first-cleft cysts present anterior to the ear or about the angle of the mandible; second-cleft cysts present just anterior to the sternocleidomastoid muscle (SCM) below the angle of the mandible; third-cleft cysts usually present deep to the SCM; and fourth-cleft cysts present in various neck and upper mediastinal locations. The cysts may present as an acutely infected mass or as a fistula with mucoid or purulent discharge from a sinus tract opening in the lateral neck.

TGDCs usually present as anterior midline masses between the hyoid bone and thyroid cartilage. They are often asymptomatic but may become infected during an upper respiratory illness.

Vascular anomalies include hemangiomas and various other malformations which encompass a wide variety of anomalous arterial, venous, or lymphatic channels. Hemangiomas in infants often regress without specific therapy. Vascular malformations are variably extensive lesions typically presenting as soft, ballotable masses.

Teratomas consist of all three germ cell layers and typically present in the first year of life as complex cystic masses in various head and neck locations. Large masses may cause symptomatic aerodigestive obstruction.

Congenital dermoid cysts are due to entrapped epithelium and typically occur as nontender midline masses.

Thymic cysts develop as rests of thymic tissue along its usual midline embryologic path of descent into the anterior mediastinum.

Relevant Physical Examination and Anatomy/Physiology

The presenting locations for branchial cysts and sinuses are discussed above. The most salient anatomic consideration for all types is that they are structurally complex with a variably meandering subcutaneous course in the neck, which has implications for safe and complete surgical resection. They are in close proximity to the facial nerve (first type) or carotid sheath (second, third, and fourth type). Any of the cysts or sinuses may occur bilaterally.

TGDCs are structural remnants of thyroid gland organogenesis and its tract as it descends from tongue base to anterior trachea during fetal development. TGDCs usually present as compressible midline masses between the hyoid bone and thyroid cartilage; they move up and down with tongue thrusting, which helps distinguish them from other anterior neck masses.

Treatment

Complete surgical resection of a branchial cleft cyst or sinus is curative; recurrence is uncommon and usually due to incomplete removal. Surgical treatment of acutely infected cysts should be deferred until treatment with a broad spectrum antibiotic covering head and neck pathogens is completed. Whenever possible, incision and drainage should be avoided as it may result in scar formation that makes later definitive resection problematic.

Treatment guidelines for TGDCs follow those for branchial cleft lesions with the exception that it is reasonable to confirm the presence of a thyroid gland with US prior to TGDC resection.

Complex or nonresolving hemangiomas (i.e., those associated with bleeding or airway compromise) can be treated with glucocorticoid or laser therapy.

Surgery is preferred for vascular malformations causing significant deformity or impaired function as well as for teratomas, dermoids, and thymic cysts.

Thyroid Nodules

Definition and Clinical Considerations

Thyroid nodules and goiterous enlargement are common worldwide. Thyroid nodules encompass a host of benign (e.g., multinodular goiter, Hashimoto's thyroiditis, or colloid cysts, adenomas) and malignant (e.g., papillary, follicular, medullary, and anaplastic carcinomas) entities.

The most important diagnostic consideration is exclusion of malignancy, which occurs in ~5% of all nodules. The likelihood of cancer is higher in children, young adults, those over 60 years of age, patients with a family history of thyroid cancer, and those with a history of head and neck radiation exposure. Clinical features suggesting malignancy include rapid growth; a hard, fixed mass; obstructive symptoms; hoarseness; and cervical adenopathy.

Serum thyroid stimulating hormone (TSH) should be assessed in all patients; a low TSH suggests a hyperfunctioning nodule, which carries a lower malignancy risk than a hypofunctioning

nodule. Elevated TSH is both an indicator of hypothyroidism and an independent risk factor for thyroid cancer.

The two most important studies in assessing thyroid nodules are US and FNAB. Thyroid US should be performed on all patients with nodular thyroid disease. US provides more detail about the thyroid and adjacent neck structures than physical examination alone. Thyroid US can distinguish cystic (more likely benign) from solid nodules, locate nodules within a specific lobe or the isthmus, demonstrate lymphadenopathy (which increases likelihood of malignancy), and identify nonthyroidal lesions such as parathyroid adenomas, vascular abnormalities, or congenital cysts.

FNAB is the best diagnostic test to determine which patients with discrete lesions confined to the thyroid gland should undergo surgical exploration.

Relevant Physical Examination and Anatomy/Physiology

Solitary nodules can present anywhere in the gland. Multinodular changes can be unilobular or involve the entire gland diffusely. Large solitary masses by palpation are often found on US to be multiple adjacent nodules. Very large thyroid goiters may cause obstructive aerodigestive symptoms; patients with very slowly progressive goiters over many years likely have benign disease. Malignancy is suggested by hard, fixed masses, adenopathy, and hoarseness.

Treatment

Treatment is generally guided by clinical presentation, US, and FNAB findings. However, FNAB is of limited utility when surgery is indicated for disfiguring or obstructing goiters; US remains valuable for demonstrating the extent of the mass and informing surgical planning.

Benign nodules by FNAB can be followed by periodic follow-up with US. FNAB may be repeated serially for nodules enlarging by US. Nodules indeterminate by FNAB but with a low likelihood of malignancy based on patient history and US assessment can be judiciously followed. Surgical resection is indicated when FNAB shows neoplasia with cellular atypia, lesions with frank malignant change, and indeterminate lesions associated with risk factors for malignancy.

The main risks of thyroid surgery include bleeding, vocal cord dysfunction (weakness or paralysis; unilateral or bilateral; transient or permanent) due to recurrent or superior laryngeal nerve injury, and hypoparathyroidism (transient or permanent) due to parathyroid gland injury or excision.

Other Neck Masses

Definition and Clinical Considerations

Other lesions to consider in the differential diagnosis of neck masses include paragangliomas (i.e., carotid body and glomus tumors), schwannomas (nerve sheath tumors), lipomas, and various skin-related cysts (e.g., epidermoid inclusion cysts, dermoids), and skin appendage tumors (e.g., pilomatrixomas).

Relevant Physical Examination and Anatomy/Physiology

Paragangliomas are associated with structures in the carotid sheath and typically present as lateral neck masses. They are often pulsatile with an associated bruit on auscultation. About

10% of patients have a family history; 10%–20% have multicentric tumors; and about 10% of tumors are malignant.

Neck schwannomas usually arise from the vagus nerve or sympathetic chain and present as firm lateral neck masses. Neurologic deficits consistent with the neural origin often occur (e.g., vagal schwannomas may cause hoarseness or aspiration; sympathetic tumors may cause Horner's syndrome).

Lipomas may occur anywhere as soft, mobile, asymptomatic masses.

Epidermoid inclusion and skin appendage cysts can occur virtually anywhere in the head and neck as firm, discrete nodular lesions.

Treatment

Paragangliomas are usually excised surgically; radiation therapy is an option for controlling advanced skull base disease, in patients who are poor surgical candidates, and for tumors otherwise considered unresectable.

Small, uncomplicated schwannomas may be managed expectantly; resection is recommended for preventing further growth or neurologic impairment.

Lipomas are resected if disfiguring or causing functional impairment.

Epidermoid and skin appendage lesions can be excised to prevent infection or for diagnostic purposes.

Major Salivary Glands (Parotid, Submandibular, Sublingual)

Inflammatory diseases (Sialadenitis)

Infectious

Definition and Clinical Considerations

Common infections of the major salivary glands can be subgrouped into three broad categories: viral, bacterial, and mycobacterial.

Mumps is the quintessential and most common viral infection of the parotid gland, and occurs more often in children than adults. Less common viral infections include cytomegalovirus, coxsackievirus A, echoviruses, and influenza A. Viral sialadenitis usually presents with fever and acute onset of pain and swelling of one or both parotid glands, often following a prodrome of malaise, headache, and myalgia.

Bacterial salivary gland infections typically manifest as either acute suppurative processes (parotid more commonly than submandibular) or chronic, recurring infections. Salivary stasis, with or without ductal obstruction, is a precondition in both processes. Acute suppurative infections are more common in older patients and those with preexisting risks such as dehydration, use of diuretic or anticholinergic medications, chronic illness, or salivary ductal obstruction (from ductal calculi or strictures).

Mycobacterial infection of the salivary glands is common and can be caused by either *Mycobacterium tuberculosis* or atypical mycobacteria. *Mycobacterium tuberculosis* is more common in the parotid gland; atypical mycobacterial infections of the submandibular gland are increasingly common in young children. Both *M. tuberculosis* and atypical mycobacterial infections can present as acute, subacute, or chronic processes.

Relevant Physical Examination and Anatomy/Physiology

The involved gland(s) are typically enlarged and variably tender to palpation; symptoms may worsen with eating.

In acute suppurative parotitis, massage of the gland will often result in purulent saliva from Stensen's duct (which may be sent for Gram stain and culture). Various aerobic and anaerobic bacteria can cause acute parotitis and include *Staphylococcus aureus*, *Streptococcus pneumoniae*, *Escheria coli*, *Haemophilus influenzae*, *Bacteroides*, and microstreptococcal species.

Obstructing calculi are more likely in submandibular than parotid disease; the more distal the calculus in the salivary duct (i.e., the closer to the ductal orifice), the more likely it can be seen or palpated intraorally.

If mycobacterial infection is suspected, an acid-fast salivary stain is warranted. Purified protein skin testing is variably helpful; its predictive value is affected by the patient's past medical history, prior tuberculosis (TB) or atypical mycobacterial exposure, or vaccination with *Bacillus Calmette–Guérin*.

Plain radiographs may be helpful in identifying a calculus; US or CT is helpful in ruling out a parotid abscess.

Treatment

Treatment of viral infections is supportive and includes hydration, analgesics, and antipyretics as necessary. (Young children should not receive aspirin.)

The mainstays of therapy for acute suppurative sialadenitis include hydration, glandular massage, sialogogues, and antibiotics (an oral or parenteral penicillinase-resistant anti-staphylococcal drug, pending outcome of cultures, is reasonable). Patients with an abscess or who are unresponsive to the above measures should be urgently referred for surgical evaluation as incision and drainage may be indicated. Obstructing calculi near the ductal opening can often be removed transorally by one familiar with the technique. Ductal calculi more proximal to the gland may require excision of the gland for definitive therapy.

Chronic, recurring sialadenitis may be a manifestation of a ductal stricture, recurring calculi, or non-infectious disorder (discussed below). Patients should be evaluated for potentially treatable predisposing factors, including strictures and stones. For symptomatic flare-ups, treatment is as for acute suppurative disease. Patients with unremitting recurrences should be referred for otolaryngologic evaluation.

Primary salivary TB is treated with an appropriate multidrug regimen in the manner of any acute TB infection. Mycobacterial infections resistant to antimicrobials should be referred for excision of the gland, which is usually curative.

Non-infectious

Definition and Clinical Considerations

The two most common non-infectious salivary inflammatory entities are sarcoidosis and Sjögren's syndrome. Salivary sarcoidosis may manifest as uncomplicated acute or subacute parotitis, or as uveoparotid fever (Heerfordt's syndrome) with parotid swelling, uveitis, and facial weakness. Salivary sarcoidosis may present with multiple glands involved or with other indicators of sarcoidosis.

Sjögren's syndrome is an autoimmune inflammatory exocrinopathy often associated with progressive xerostomia. It is more common in women and middle-aged and older adults. Primary Sjögren's syndrome is limited to the exocrine glands alone, while a secondary syndrome is associated with other rheumatologic inflammatory disorders such as rheumatoid arthritis. Salivary manifestations are typically very gradually progressive over many years.

Relevant Physical Examination and Anatomy/Physiology

Salivary sarcoidosis often presents as an acute or subacute, variably tender, nonsuppurative swelling of one or more major salivary glands, with the parotids more commonly affected than the submandibular glands. Facial weakness may be present. Patients with uveoparotid manifestations also have fever, malaise, weakness, and night sweats. Biopsy of an involved gland often shows characteristic noncaseating granulomas, which, in the presence of other manifestations of sarcoidosis, such as hilar adenopathy on chest radiographs, confirms the diagnosis.

Patients with symptomatic Sjögren's syndrome typically have indolent recurring or chronic nonsuppurative fullness or enlargement of the parotid glands associated with progressive xerostomia and dry eyes. A variety of laboratory tests are available to support the diagnosis, and patients with a suggestive history should be referred for rheumatological evaluation.

Treatment

The mainstay of treatment for salivary sarcoidosis is corticosteroid therapy. With the exception of diagnostic biopsy, surgical therapy is rarely indicated.

Salivary manifestations of Sjogren's syndrome are treated supportively, usually with saliva substitutes and attention to dental care. Biopsy or surgical excision should be considered in patients who develop a discrete mass, as salivary non-Hodgkin's lymphoma may occur. Systemic Sjogren's syndrome may require treatment with anti-inflammatory and/or anti-neoplastic drugs.

Neoplasms and Masses

Solitary tumors and discrete masses of the major salivary glands occur frequently. The majority are benign and usually present as slowly enlarging lesions. Hemi-facial weakness or cervical adenopathy in conjunction with a parotid tumor are ominous findings and warrant urgent evaluation. Tumors are more common in the parotid than submandibular glands. Of the lesions listed below, none are common in the sublingual gland with the exception of salivary retention cysts (also known as mucoceles or ranulas). All should be referred for evaluation by a specialist familiar with managing such disorders; imaging studies, fine needle aspiration, and incisional or excisional biopsies are often used to confirm the diagnosis. Most commonly, surgical resection of the gland is the mainstay or a key part of the definitive therapeutic plan.

The more common types of malignant and benign lesions are listed below in order of frequency. Therapies beyond surgical resection, especially for malignancies, vary widely and are beyond the scope of this chapter.

Malignant

- Mucoepidermoid carcinoma
- Adenoid cystic carcinoma
- Squamous cell carcinoma
- Malignant pleomorphic adenoma
- Lymphoma

Benign

- Pleomorphic adenoma (benign mixed tumor)
- Warthin tumor (papillary cystadenoma lymphomatosum)
- Hemangiomas and lymphangiomas
- Lipomas
- Benign lymphoepithelial lesions
- Congenital and acquired cysts

Selected ORL Procedures

Removal Foreign Body

External Auditory Canal

Relevant Anatomy and Clinical Considerations

The external auditory canal (EAC) is an hourglass-shaped, cartilage (lateral) and bone (medial) channel narrowest where the cartilage and bone meet. The cartilaginous canal has modest elastic properties which admit various speculae and instruments; by contrast, the bony canal is narrower and covered by thin, tender, easily injured skin. The EAC has vagal innervation; instrumentation can provoke coughing or vasovagal responses (e.g., bradycardia, hypotension, or syncope) in susceptible individuals.

Procedure Highlights and Considerations

- Proper illumination, magnification, and equipment are essential.
- Young children unable to cooperate are often better managed with sedation or general anesthesia than with restraints.
- Satisfactory local anesthesia is difficult to achieve.
- The best opportunity for success is the first attempt; repetition increases the likelihood of ear canal bleeding and pain.
- Prior to extraction, live insects can be immobilized with solutions such as isopropyl alcohol, mineral oil, or topical lidocaine. (Use only on patients with an intact tympanic membrane [TM].)
- Instruments: A right-angle hook is best for beads and round objects; an alligator forceps works well for soft materials (e.g., cotton or foam) and firm objects with a graspable edge (Figure 26.3A). Organic FBs may be removed with a suction cannula (Figure 26.3B); some FBs (e.g., dirt or gravel) may be gently irrigated. However, use caution when irrigating if tympanic membrane integrity can't be confirmed visually.
- Pitfalls include pushing the FB further into the EAC, lacerating the ear canal skin, or TM perforation.

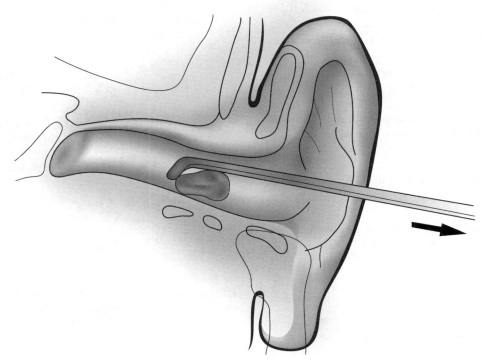

FIGURE 26.3A Removal of ear canal foreign body with right-angle hook. *Surgical Care at the District Hospital*. World Health Organization; 2003, p. 5-17. Figure 5.27.

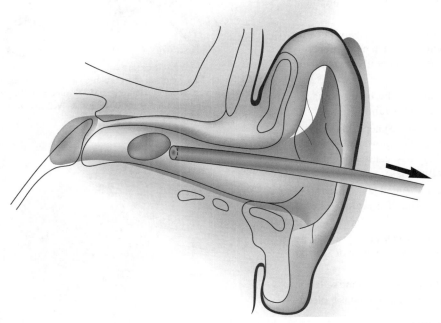

FIGURE 26.3B Suction cannula for removal of organic foreign body. *Surgical Care at the District Hospital*. World Health Organization; 2003, p. 5-17. Figure 5.25.

Recommended Equipment

- Otoscope head with moveable magnifying lens
- Largest ear speculum the ear canal comfortably accepts
- Right-angle hook, alligator forceps, 5- or 7-gauge suction catheter
- For irrigating, an 18-gauge angiocatheter with 10 cc syringe
- If a headlight is available, a nasal rather than ear speculum may be used, which may permit better visualization and room for removal of lateral canal objects.

Postremoval Management

- Visually ensure the integrity of the EAC and TM.
- For atraumatic removals, no additional treatment is necessary.
- For EAC injuries, an otic drop applied twice daily for a few days is reasonable; refer to ENT if TM integrity is uncertain.

Nasal Cavity

Relevant Anatomy and Clinical Considerations

Most FBs are found in the anterior nasal cavity; the junction of the anterior nasal septum (medially) and anterior aspect of the inferior turbinate (laterally) acts as a check valve in most instances. A nasal FB is, by definition, an airway FB; appropriate management is essential to prevent aspiration (Figure 26.4A).

Procedure Highlights

- Given the aspiration risk, removal should be attempted only in a controlled setting with proper equipment and support.
- Inexpertly managed anterior FBs may easily become posterior FBs, where extraction is much more problematic; stable posterior FBs should generally be removed by an otolaryngologist.
- Children unable to cooperate may be better managed with sedation or anesthesia than restraints.
- Topical vasoconstrictor (e.g., Neo-Synephrine or oxymetazoline) or anesthetic (e.g., lidocaine) drops should be used with caution as they may cause coughing or choking and increase aspiration risk.
- A headlight is highly recommended as it permits a bimanual approach (one for the nasal speculum, one for a forcep or suction catheter).
- Additional equipment: nasal speculum, Fraser-type suction cannula, right-angle hook, alligator or similar grasper, bayonet forcep.
- Keys to success: illumination, visualization, sedation (if necessary), and gentleness (nasal mucosa bleeds easily).
- Irregular and soft objects (e.g., paper, rubber) may be grasped with an alligator-type or cupped forcep (Figure 26.4B).

- Round or firm objects can be removed by placing a right-angle hook gently behind the object and pulling anteriorly (Figure 26.4C).
- After extraction inspect both nasal cavities for additional FBs.

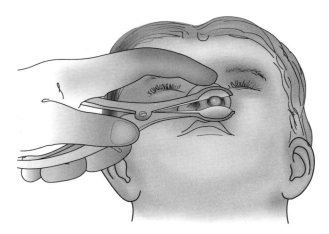

FIGURE 26.4A Visualizing nasal cavity foreign body with nasal speculum; note proper orientation of speculum. King C, Henretig FM. *Textbook of Pediatric Emergency Procedures.* 2nd ed. Lippincott Williams & Wilkins; 2008, p. 624. Figure 59.3.

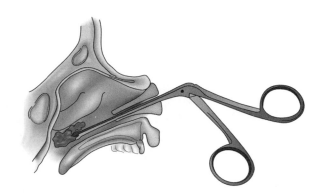

FIGURE 26.4B Removal of irregular-shaped nasal foreign body with fine grasping forcep. King C, Henretig FM. *Textbook of Pediatric Emergency Procedures.* 2nd ed. Lippincott Williams & Wilkins; 2008, p. 624. Figure 59.3 (c).

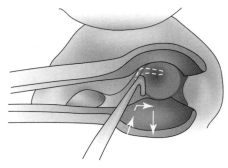

FIGURE 26.4C Use of right-angle hook for removal of round object. King C, Henretig FM. *Textbook of Pediatric Emergency Procedures.* 2nd ed. Lippincott Williams & Wilkins; 2008, p. 624. Figure 59.3 (a).

Postremoval Management

No specific therapy is required.

Nasal Packing for Epistaxis

Anterior/Uncomplicated

Relevant Anatomy and Clinical Considerations

Spontaneous nasal bleeding most commonly originates from the anterior nasal septum (known as Little's area or Keisselbach's plexus) (Figure 26.5).

The anterior location lends itself to relatively easy inspection for diagnostic and treatment purposes. However, brisk bleeding may render initial assessment challenging. Nonetheless, reasonable attempts to identify the precise site of bleeding should be made as in most cases bleeding can be controlled with limited, local measures. Additionally, confirming that Little's area is *not* the site of bleeding usually indicates a more posterior source, which may be more challenging to control. Regardless of site, patients with active bleeding usually have blood in the pharynx, some of which may appear in the contralateral (nonbleeding) nasal cavity as swallowing pushes pharyngeal blood into the opposite nasal cavity.

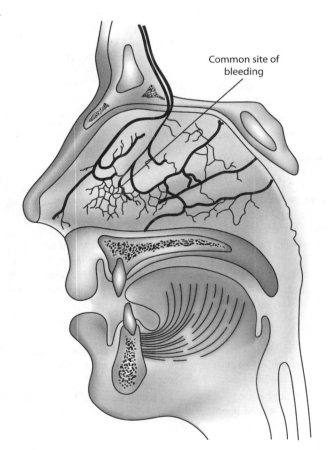

Common site of bleeding

FIGURE 26.5 Nasal septal vasculature. The most common site of bleeding is Keisselbach's plexus, anteriorly. *Surgical Care at the District Hospital.* World Health Organization; 2003, p. 5-8. Figure 5.16.

Procedure Highlights

- Presentation with exsanguinating hemorrhage is rare; active bleeding may appear impressive and is troublesome, but there is usually ample time to manage the problem in an orderly fashion.

- The patient should be in an upright position; all participants should wear protective garments and eyewear.

- Headlight illumination is optimal and frees both hands for instruments.

- **Equipment and supplies:** Nasal speculum; Frazier suction for nasal and Yankauer suction for oral cavities, respectively; bayonet forceps; cotton-tipped applicators and cotton balls; topical anesthetic (e.g., lidocaine or 4% cocaine solution [cocaine vasoconstricts, as well]); topical vasoconstrictor (e.g., oxymetazoline 0.05% or phenylephrine 0.25%); silver nitrate sticks; absorbable hemostatic material (e.g. Gelfoam); compressed, expandable sponge-type nasal tampon (e.g., Merocel); and Vaseline (½- by 72-inch strip) or other ribbon-type gauze which can be treated with antibiotic ointment (e.g., mupirocin) prior to application.

- **Treatment without packing:** Using the nasal speculum for visualization, gently suction blood with the Frazier cannula taking care not to abraid the nasal mucosa. Using cotton-tipped applicators, gently but firmly apply topical anesthetic and vasoconstrictor solutions in sequence to the bleeding site and hold in place for several minutes. If the applicator tip is too small for the bleeding site, a cotton ball soaked with vasoconstrictor solution can be used. Once bleeding is controlled, the site can be cauterized with a silver nitrate stick (Figure 26.6).

- If silver nitrate controls the bleeding, nothing additional is required, although some favor additional application of antibiotic ointment (e.g., mupirocin) or absorbable hemostatic material.

- **Anterior nasal packing:** When the above steps are unsuccessful, packing with either an expandable nasal tampon or ribbon gauze is usually necessary. As these measures are generally more uncomfortable, additional

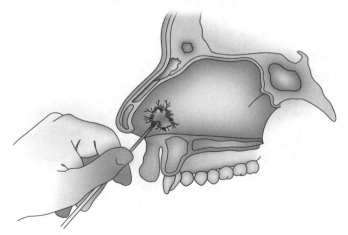

FIGURE 26.6 Silver nitrate stick cautery of bleeding nasal septal vessel. Myers EN. *Operative Otolaryngology Head and Neck Surgery.* Philadelphia: Elsevier Saunders; 1997, p. 7, Figure 1-5.

topical anesthetic before proceeding is usually required; light intravenous sedation and analgesia may be necessary. Expandable nasal tampons come in various sizes and can be trimmed as necessary for best fit (Figure 26.7).

A dessicated tampon should be coated with a thin film of antibiotic ointment, grasped digitally or with a bayonet forceps, and fully advanced directly posterior into the nasal cavity in the open space between the septum and inferior turbinate. As the tampon expands on contact with blood and secretions, it will cover the nasal septum and lateral nasal wall; active bleeding usually stops within minutes although a bloody drip may continue for a while. For Vaseline or ribbon gauze, coat the material with a thin film of antibiotic ointment and, using bayonet forceps, firmly layer the material from posterior to anterior, first along the nasal floor and then, gradually, superiorly. The first pass should be a loop (placed posteriorly, so the leading edge of the gauze is readily visible in the naris) to minimize the likelihood that the free end of the ribbon will dangle in the patient's pharynx (Figure 26.8).

Management after Packing

Residual bleeding typically abates over several minutes; it is important to leave well-enough alone as such bleeding is usually self-limited. If packing is left in the nasal cavity, prophylactic antibiotics covering *Staphylococcus aureus* should be used until the material is removed. Absorbable materials typically require no additional management; a tampon or ribbon-type packing is typically left in place for 3 days.

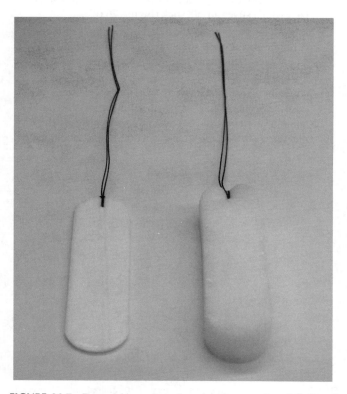

FIGURE 26.7 Expandable sponges for epistaxis: as packaged (left) and after hydration (right). Image by Pratik Patel.

Posterior/Complex Epistaxis

For significant, persistent bleeding in spite of the above measures, it may be necessary to pack the entire nasal cavity. Two options are prepackaged intranasal double balloon devices (e.g., Epi-Stat) or placement in the nasopharynx of a Foley catheter in conjunction with gauze packing of the nasal cavity. Use of judicious intravenous sedation and analgesia is often warranted with these techniques.

Prepackaged double balloons should be coated with antibiotic ointment and placed and inflated according to package directions (Figure 26.9A, Figure 26.9B, and Figure 26.9C).

In the Foley catheter technique, the 30-cc balloon is passed into the posterior nasal cavity and inflated in the choana (Figure 26.10); this acts as a buttress against which ribbon gauze packing can be placed anteriorly (Figure 26.8), thereby totally occluding the entire nasal cavity.

This technique is best done with two practitioners. The catheter is passed along the floor of the nose until the tip can be visualized in the oropharynx. The 30-cc balloon is filled with air or saline until the catheter cannot be pulled anteriorly, indicating that the filled balloon is anchored in the nasopharynx. With an assistant placing firm anterior traction on the catheter, the nasal cavity is packed with layered, antibiotic ointment-coated, ribbon gauze in the same manner as illustrated in Figure 26.8. Once the gauze fills the cavity and nasal vestibule, a small C-clamp or other device is secured to the catheter just anterior to the gauze, thereby preventing migration of the catheter into the nose. It is important to ensure the C-clamp does not put excessive pressure on the nasal rim, as necrosis of the nasal skin and cartilage may result. Systemic anti-staphylococcal antibiotics and fluid resuscitation should be administered. Patient monitoring should include pulse oximetry, if available. Ear, nose, and throat (ENT) evaluation should be obtained as soon as practicable.

Incision and Drainage

Auricular Hematoma

Relevant Anatomy and Clinical Considerations

Auricular hematoma may occur after direct blunt trauma to the ear (e.g., with a hand slap or similar mechanism of injury). Rarely, an insect bite may cause similar findings. In blunt trauma the force of the blow causes the lateral auricular skin and perichondrium to separate from the underlying cartilage; blood or serous fluid then accumulates in the resulting dead space. Left untreated, chondritis and fibrosis result in a thickened, misshapen auricle (so-called cauliflower ear).

Procedure Highlights

- Non-epinephrine–containing local anesthetic may be infiltrated into the skin of the posterior auricle but should be avoided in the scaphoid fossa.
- Acute hematomas or seromas may be aspirated with a large-gauge needle followed by application of a conforming pressure dressing.
- For subacute collections or when needle aspiration fails, a wide incision with a #11 or #15 scalpel may be required to permit complete evacuation; after

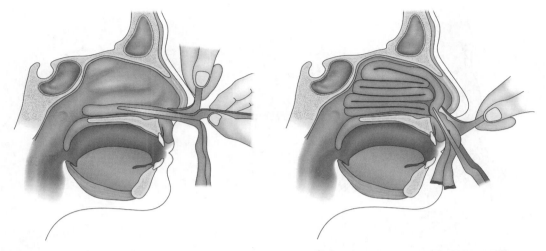

FIGURE 26.8 Proper technique for nasal packing with ribbon-type gauze; note the anterior location of the free ends of the gauze. Bailey BJ and Johnson JT. *Head & Neck Surgery-Otolaryngology.* Philadelphia: Lippincott, Williams and Wilkins; 2006, p. 509, Figure 36.3.

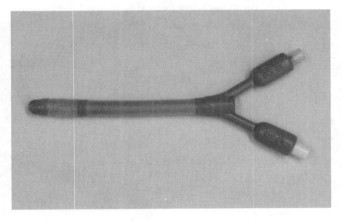

FIGURE 26.9A Double balloon epistaxis device as packaged. Image by Pratik Patel.

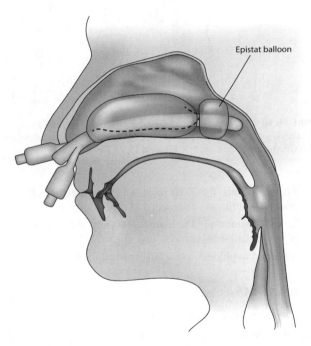

FIGURE 26.9C Device properly positioned in nasal cavity and inflated. Illustration by John W. Karapelou, CMI.

evacuation, place one or two dental sponges, buttons, or other suitable material on the scapha and skin of the ear behind the scapha, securing with one or two through-and-through mattress sutures of 3-0 monofilament suture (Figure 26.11A and Figure 26.11B).

- Pressure satisfactory to close the dead space is all that is required; undue suture tension across the bolster can cause necrosis of the ear cartilage.

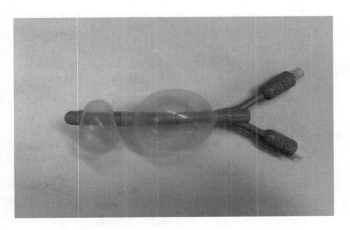

FIGURE 26.9B Balloon device as inflated. Image by Pratik Patel.

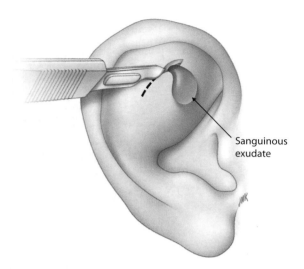

FIGURE 26.11A Incision location for drainage of auricular hematoma. Illustration by John W. Karapelou, CMI.

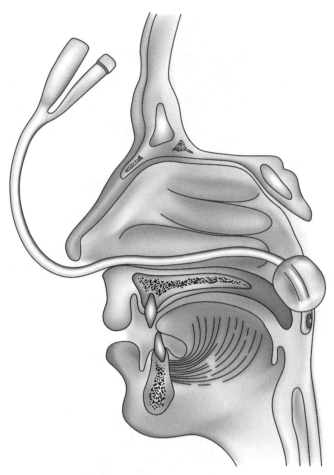

FIGURE 26.10 Foley catheter positioned in nasopharynx prior to placement of anterior gauze pack. *Surgical Care at the District Hospital.* World Health Organization; 2003, p. 5-8. Figure 5.17.

Posttreatment Management

- Leave bolsters for 7–10 days, checking periodically; coat with antibiotic ointment 2–3 times daily.

- Leave ear uncovered to assess adequacy of blood supply to auricular helix.

- Systemic antibiotics are usually not required.

Peritonsillar Abscess

Relevant Anatomy and Clinical Considerations

Peritonsillar abscess is a complication of acute tonsillitis and almost always unilateral. The abscess develops in the space between the tonsil and pharyngeal musculature; patients present variably with fever, foul breath, trismus, odynophagia, "hot potato voice," drooling, pain radiating to the ipsilateral ear, and tender cervical adenopathy. Most abscesses appear as a bulge in the superior tonsillar fossa, with the tonsil itself displaced medially; the soft palate and uvula are usually displaced to the opposite side.

Procedure Highlights

- Treatment options: Needle aspiration; incision and drainage; tonsillectomy (Figure 26.12A, Figure 26.12B, and Figure 26.12C).

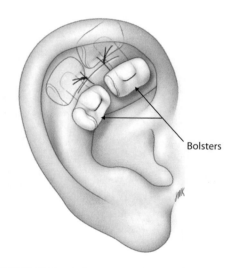

FIGURE 26.11B Bolster placement to prevent hematoma recurrence. Illustration by John W. Karapelou, CMI.

- Use penicillin (or suitable beta-lactam alternative) or clindamycin.

- Patients unable to cooperate should be treated under general anesthesia.

- If trismus prevents satisfactory visualization, mild intravenous (IV) sedation and analgesia may be helpful.

- Patient should be sitting with the head supported.

- Local anesthetic may be sparingly infiltrated into the overlying mucosa.

- Equipment: Headlight illumination, tongue depressors, Yankauer suction, long 18-gauge needle with a 20 cc syringe (abscesses are often more than 10 cc and it is very difficult to relocate the abscess cavity once the needle has been withdrawn), #11 scalpel with long handle, hemostat, and collection basin for the patient.

- Depress the tongue and gently palpate the area of greatest prominence to confirm fluctulance. Perform

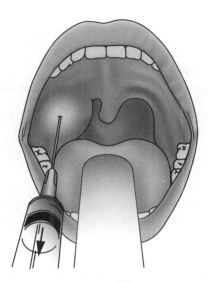

FIGURE 26.12A Drainage of peritonsillar abscess: technique for aspiration. *Surgical Care at the District Hospital.* World Health Organization; 2003, p. 5-23. Figure 5.35.

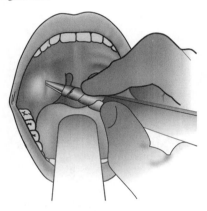

FIGURE 26.12B Incisional technique; note mucosal entry at most prominent aspect of abscess. *Surgical Care at the District Hospital.* World Health Organization; 2003, p. 5-23. Figure 5.36.

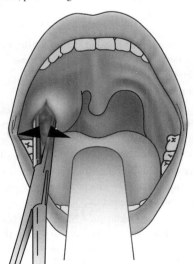

FIGURE 26.12C Abscess cavity dilated with hemostat for effective drainage. *Surgical Care at the District Hospital.* World Health Organization; 2003, p. 5-23. Figure 5.37.

needle aspiration at this site; more than one pass may be required to locate the abscess.

- Do not insert needle too lateral in the tonsillar fossa as the carotid artery can be injured.
- If aspiration is unsuccessful, incise the most prominent aspect of the mucosa with the #11 scalpel; spread the hemostat in the abscess cavity.
- The cavity may be gently suctioned and lavaged with saline.

Posttreatment Management

- Use warm saline gargles; continue antibiotics for 7–10 days.
- Avoid aspirin and nonsteroidal anti-inflammatory analgesics until it is clear that urgent tonsillectomy is not required.

Submental (Midline Submandibular) Space Abscess (e.g., for Ludwig's Angina)

Relevant Anatomy and Clinical Considerations

The sublingual space has superficial and deep compartments. Infections of the superficial compartment manifest as tender, erythematous fullness of the floor of mouth. If untreated, the infection advances into the deep sublingual compartment, submental tissues, and lateral submandibular spaces, causing posterior tongue displacement and airway compromise.

Procedure Highlights

- Equipment: Basic dissection set (scalpel, tissue forceps, scissors, retractors, hemostats) and Penrose drain.
- Secure airway and induce general anesthesia.
- Identify and sharply incise the most prominent or most fluctuant aspect of the mass horizontally (Figure 26.13A).
- Proceed with the subcutaneous dissection in the midline transversely through the platysma to the mylohyoid muscle midline raphe (Figure 26.13B).
- Incise the midline raphe sharply and retract the mylohyoid bellies laterally, thereby exposing the abscess cavity.
- Open the cavity widely with a hemostat; obtain cultures and evacuate purulent contents (Figure 26.13C).
- Irrigate with sterile water or antibiotic solution.
- Place Penrose drain and loosely close wound with rapidly absorbable sutures in all layers but the skin (Figure 26.13D).

Posttreatment Management

- Use broad spectrum antibiotics to cover oral aerobes and anaerobes for 7–10 days.
- If the infectious source is identified (most commonly odontogenic), treat definitively while patient is hospitalized.
- Leave Penrose drain in place until the infection resolves.
- If tracheotomy has been performed, leave in place until infection resolves and all related treatments completed.

Lateral Neck Abscesses

Relevant Anatomy and Clinical Considerations

For submandibular abscesses, make a horizontal incision 3–4 cm inferior to the body of the mandible to avoid injury to the mandibular

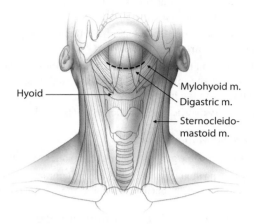

FIGURE 26.13A   Incision and drainage of midline submental/submandibular abscess: the planned incision. Illustration by John W. Karapelou, CMI.

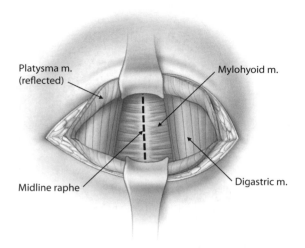

FIGURE 26.13B   The platysma and midline raphe exposed. Illustration by John W. Karapelou, CMI.

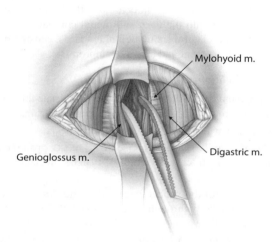

FIGURE 26.13C   The midline incised and abscess cavity entered with a hemostat. Illustration by John W. Karapelou, CMI.

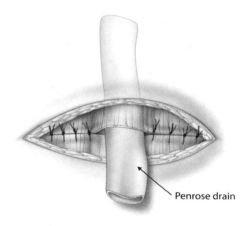

FIGURE 26.13D   Layered closure over Penrose drain in abscess cavity. Illustration by John W. Karapelou, CMI.

branch of the facial nerve (which provides motor innervation to the corner of the mouth). For abscesses deep to and along the course of the SCM, either a horizontal (preferred) or vertical incision over the abscess that allows identification of the anterior edge of the SCM is reasonable.

Procedure Highlights

- Surgical awareness of the location of the carotid sheath and its contents is essential to ensure safety.
- Equipment: Basic dissection set (scalpel, tissue forceps, scissors, retractors, and hemostats) and Penrose drain.
- Secure the airway and induce general anesthesia.
- Identify and incise the most prominent or fluctulent aspect of the mass (Figure 26.14A).
- Carry the dissection through the platysma.
- **For submandibular abscesses:** Continue the dissection as inferior as possible (to avoid injury to the

marginal branch of the facial nerve) while maintaining an otherwise direct approach to the abscess.
- Identify the anterior SCM edge as the posterior dissection landmark.
- **For abscesses along the SCM:** Identify the anterior SCM edge lateral to the most prominent aspect of the infection; dissect vertically and medially along the SCM edge to access the abscess cavity just deep to the muscle.
- Take care to remain in a direct plane to the abscess to avoid unnecessarily deep dissection, which may encounter the carotid sheath.
- If tissue edema and induration obscure the plane of dissection, use a needle and syringe to locate the abscess cavity; the needle can be left in place as a guide for dissection to the cavity (Figure 26.14B).
- Once identified, incise the abscess for a short distance to confirm the cavity; insert and gently spread a hemostat (Figure 26.14C).

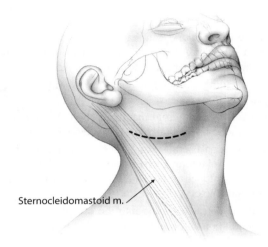

FIGURE 26.14A   Incision and drainage of lateral neck abscess: the planned incision. Illustration by John W. Karapelou, CMI.

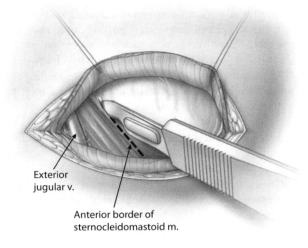

FIGURE 26.14B   Anterior border of sternocleidomastoid identified; incision through fascia for entry into abscess cavity. Illustration by John W. Karapelou, CMI.

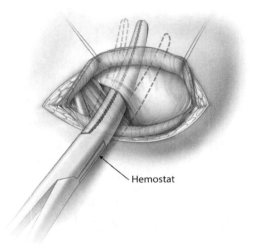

FIGURE 26.14C   Abscess cavity entered and spread with hemostat for complete drainage. Illustration by John W. Karapelou, CMI.

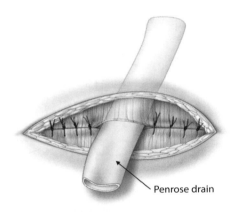

FIGURE 26.14D   Layered closure over Penrose in abscess cavity. Illustration by John W. Karapelou, CMI.

- Obtain cultures and evacuate contents.
- Irrigate the wound with sterile water or antibiotic solution.
- Place the Penrose drain and loosely close the wound with rapidly absorbable (Figure 26.14D) sutures in all layers but the skin.

Posttreatment Management

Refer to the section on submental (midline submandibular) space abscess, above.

Tracheotomy

The primary indications for tracheotomy are upper airway obstruction, inability to obtain an airway by other means, prolonged ventilatory support, pulmonary toilet, and adjunctive management of head and neck disease.

Tracheotomy, whether elective or emergent, is best performed in a controlled environment by an experienced practitioner with appropriate support staff, lighting, and equipment. In emergencies, cricothyroidotomy is preferred over traditional tracheotomy as it is simple, quick, and can be performed with minimal equipment by individuals with little surgical experience.

Cricothyroidotomy ("Emergency Tracheotomy")

Relevant Anatomy and Clinical Considerations

The key anatomic landmarks are the thyroid and cricoid cartilages, and the membranous structure between the two, the cricothyroid membrane. These structures are usually readily identifiable and palpable in most individuals. The trachea is entered through the cricothyroid membrane; the thyroid cartilage (Adam's apple) is immediately above, and the cricoid cartilage, the most superior and prominent of the tracheal cartilages, lies immediately below.

Procedure Highlights

- Surgical equipment (minimum) includes a scalpel (#11 or #15 blade) and hemostat; if possible, have available a basic dissection set with suction catheter, retractors, tissue forceps, tracheal dilator, and tracheal hook.
- Position the patient with a shoulder roll, extending the head and neck on the chest, thereby accentuating the thyroid and cricoid cartilages.
- If time permits, mark the midline with a surgical pen, drawing a vertical line from the thyroid cartilage (superiorly) to the cricoid prominence (inferiorly), a distance of ~3 cm (Figure 26.15A).
- Use the thumb and index finger of the nonscalpel hand to spread and stabilize the skin directly over the cricothyroid membrane.
- In a single motion make a vertical incision from the thyroid cartilage prominence superiorly to the cricoid cartilage inferiorly, penetrating deeply enough to encounter both structures (Figure 26.15B).

- Be assertive but not overly aggressive: too deep an incision risks injury to the thyroid cartilage and vocal cords; cricoid injury can cause subglottic stenosis; overly exuberant cricothyroid membrane incision can injure the posterior tracheal wall and esophagus.
- Some bleeding occurs but does not usually require urgent attention.
- Confirm the cricothyroid membrane by palpation and sharply incise horizontally, making a modest opening.
- Insert and open a hemostat or tracheal dilator, enlarging the cricothyroidotomy incision satisfactory to accept an endotracheal tube (for adults a #6 endotracheal tube is usually satisfactory) (Figure 26.15C).
- Pass the endotracheal tube into the opening and confirm ventilation and proper tube location by chest auscultation (Figure 26.15D).

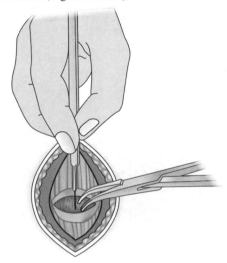

FIGURE 26.15C   Cricothyroid opening is dilated in preparation for endotracheal tube placement. *Surgical Care at the District Hospital.* World Health Organization; 2003, p. PTCM-5. Figure 3.

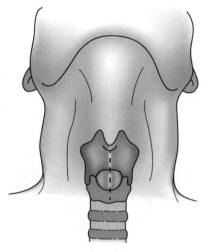

FIGURE 26.15A   Cricothyroidotomy: anatomic landmarks. *Surgical Care at the District Hospital.* World Health Organization; 2003, p. PTCM-5. Figure 1.

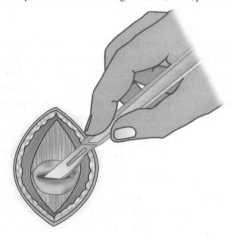

FIGURE 26.15B   Note vertical skin incision and midline dissection to cricothyroid membrane; horizontal incision is made through cricothyroid membrane to enter airway. *Surgical Care at the District Hospital.* World Health Organization; 2003, p. PTCM-5. Figure 2.

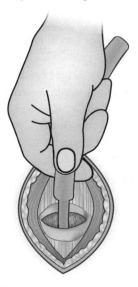

FIGURE 26.15D   Endotracheal tube placed through cricothyroidotomy opening. *Surgical Care at the District Hospital.* World Health Organization; 2003, p. PTCM-6. Figure 5.

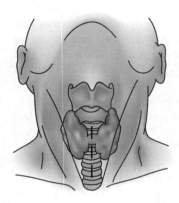

FIGURE 26.16A Elective tracheotomy: anatomic landmarks. *Surgical Care at the District Hospital.* World Health Organization; 2003, p. 16-11. Figure 16.14.

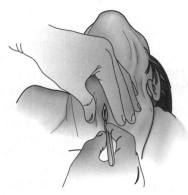

FIGURE 26.16B Skin incision; may be vertical or horizontal (horizontal preferred); note extension of head and neck. *Surgical Care at the District Hospital.* World Health Organization; 2003, p. 16-11. Figure 16.15.

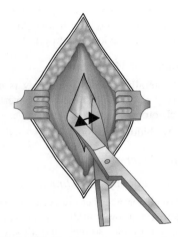

FIGURE 26.16C Incision and spreading of strap muscles in midline. *Surgical Care at the District Hospital.* World Health Organization; 2003, p. 16-11. Figure 16.16.

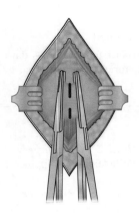

FIGURE 26.16D Thyroid isthmus may be divided for exposure, if necessary. *Surgical Care at the District Hospital.* World Health Organization; 2003, p. 16-11. Figure 16.18.

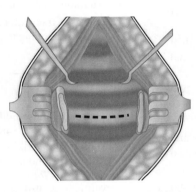

FIGURE 26.16E Tracheal exposure with planned tracheotomy incision between 2nd and 3rd cartilage rings. *Surgical Care at the District Hospital.* World Health Organization; 2003, p. 16-12. Figure 16.20.

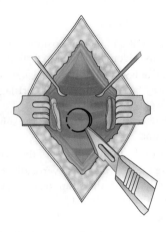

FIGURE 26.16F Tracheotomy incision: anterior segment of one tracheal ring may be removed to facilitate cannulation. *Surgical Care at the District Hospital.* World Health Organization; 2003, p. 16-12. Figure 16.21.

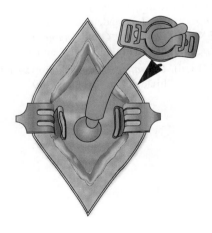

FIGURE 26.16G Insertion of tracheotomy tube. *Surgical Care at the District Hospital.* World Health Organization; 2003, p. 16-13. Figure 16.23.

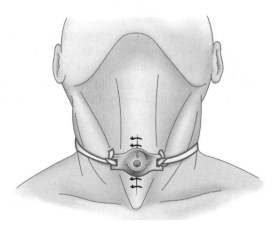

FIGURE 26.16H Closure of incision with tube and tracheotomy ties in place; suturing of tracheotomy tube flanges to skin is recommended initially. *Surgical Care at the District Hospital.* World Health Organization; 2003, p. 16-13. Figure 16.25.

- Once in proper position, the tube must be held firmly while being secured to the skin of the neck; the skin edges can be loosely closed.

Posttreatment Management

- Generally, cricothyroidotomy is considered a temporary airway and should be converted to a standard tracheotomy as soon as practicable.
- Antibiotics are not routinely used.

Elective Tracheotomy

Relevant Anatomy and Clinical Considerations

The main differences between cricothyroidotomy and formal tracheotomy are a lower midline neck incision, the need (often) to section the thyroid isthmus, and airway entry between tracheal rings rather than through the cricothyroid membrane. The rationale for the lower approach is avoidance of laryngeal injury, either acutely or with long-term tracheotomy tube placement. Key anatomic landmarks are the cricoid cartilage and suprasternal notch.

Procedure Highlights

- Equipment and patient positioning are the same as for cricothyroidotomy (Figure 26.16A).
- Make a horizontal skin incision with a #15 scalpel midway between the cricoid cartilage and suprasternal notch (Figure 26.16B).
- Carry the incision through the subcutaneous fat and platysma.
- Identify the midline raphe of the strap muscles.
- Incise the midline raphe vertically, and undermine and laterally retract the strap muscles exposing the thyroid isthmus (Figure 26.16C).
- Incise the peritracheal fascia just below the cricoid cartilage and insert a tracheal hook immediately below the cricoid; use the hook to retract the trachea superiorly.
- The thyroid isthmus is usually now visible; if the isthmus rises too superior to allow appropriate tracheotomy, incise the peritracheal fascia just inferior to the isthmus and carry the dissection to the trachea (Figure 26.16D).
- Bluntly undermine and dissect the isthmus off the trachea; secure the isthmus between clamps and transect; secure each side with suture ligatures.
- Identify the space above the 2nd, 3rd, or 4th tracheal ring and horizontally incise with a #11 scalpel, long

enough to accept the tracheotomy tube, taking care not to injure the posterior tracheal wall (Figure 26.16E).

- If necessary for an adequate opening, an anterior section of the tracheal ring below the incision can be resected: grasp the ring with a clamp and make vertical incisions in the ring ~1.5 to 2 cm apart with a scissor; remove the section of cartilage by incising its inferior attachment (Figure 26.16F).
- Place the preselected tracheotomy tube (a #6 is satisfactory for most adults) into the trachea using a tracheal spreader to gently dilate the tracheal opening, if necessary (Figure 26.16G).
- Confirm proper tube positioning and secure to the skin of the neck with sutures and circumferential tracheotomy ties (Figure 26.16H).
- To avoid subcutaneous emphysema, pneumomediastinum, or pneumothorax, do not tightly close the skin incision.
- A tracheotomy dressing is usually unnecessary.

Posttreatment Management

- Antibiotics are generally not required.
- Leave the tracheotomy tube in place for at least 5–7 days prior to changing to permit maturation of the stoma.

Suggested Reading

Bailey BJ and Johnson JT (eds): *Head & Neck Surgery – Otolaryngology*, 4th ed. Philadelphia, Lippincott Williams & Wilkins, 2006.

Bailey BJ and Calhoun KH (eds): *Head & Neck Surgery – Otolaryngology*, 3rd ed. Philadelphia, Lippincott Williams & Wilkins, 2001.

King C and Henretig FM (eds): *Textbook of Pediatric Emergency Procedures*, 2nd ed. Philadelphia, Lippincott Williams & Wilkins, 2008.

King M, Bewes PC, Cairns J, Thornton J (eds): *Primary Surgery (Non-Trauma)*. Oxford, Oxford University Press, 1990.

Loré JM and Medina JE (eds): *An Atlas of Head & Neck Surgery*, 4th ed. Philadelphia, Elsevier Saunders, 2005.

Myers EN (ed): *Operative Otolaryngology: Head and Neck Surgery*, 2nd ed. Philadelphia, Saunders, 2008.

Myers EN (ed): *Operative Otolaryngology: Head and Neck Surgery*. Philadelphia, Saunders, 1997.

COMMENTARY

Wakisa Mulwafu, Rwanda

In Malawi, improvisation is the key to performing otolaryngologic surgery. Appropriate equipment and materials may not always be available. An otoscope is an essential instrument; it is very difficult to improvise a substitute for it. However, there is a real challenge of getting a functional, quality otoscope as you move farther away from the larger hospitals.

For nasal packing for epistaxis, first-aid measures like pinching the nose for 5 minutes should be attempted, since expandable nasal tampons like Merocel may not be easily found. Anterior epistaxis is the most common form of epistaxis, and nasal packing is the most effective method of treatment. Packing is often done with vaselinated gauze, which is inexpensive and readily available.[1,2] For posterior epistaxis, a Foley catheter is easily available as compared to pre-packed balloon devices.

Proper training of non-ENT physicians is required for them to be able to perform ENT procedures adequately. In Malawi, we provide 18 months of training for clinical officers, and they qualify with a diploma in ENT and Clinical Audiology. After training, they are gradually introduced to more advanced procedures like tonsillectomy and tracheostomy.

REFERENCES

1. OA Sogebi, EAOyewole, OA Adebajo Epistaxis in Sagamu. *Nigerian Journal of Clinical Practice* March 2010 Vol. 13 (1):32–36.
2. O.V Akinpelu, Y.B Amusa, J.A.E Ezeyi, C.C Nwawolo. A Retrospective Analysis of Aetiology and Management of Epistaxis in a South-Western Nigerian Teaching Hospital. *West African Journal of Medicine*. Vol 28. No 3. May 2009.

27

Thyroidectomy

Robert M. Boucher

Introduction

The purpose of this section is to familiarize readers with the two most commonly performed thyroid operations: thyroid lobectomy and total thyroidectomy. The standard surgical techniques and overall operative sensibility applied to thyroid lobectomy form the basis for virtually all thyroid procedures. As such, the major portion of the discussion that follows addresses excision of a thyroid lobe.

This section is not presented as a definitive discussion of all aspects of thyroid-related operative procedures; it is intended, rather, as a primer for occasional or less experienced thyroid surgeons working in low- and middle-income countries (LMICs). Therefore, the discussion is based upon traditional surgical techniques using standard, generally available surgical instruments and does not address emerging surgical approaches, technology, or tools such as video-assisted endoscopic resection, ultrasonic dissection, or laryngeal nerve monitors, respectively, which are usually unavailable in LMICs. As with other organ-specific surgery, there are various well-accepted operative techniques and maneuvers which have been described to accomplish the same intraoperative goal(s). To the extent that this section occasionally expresses a preference for one approach over another, it reflects the author's successful experience with the technique in question both in well-equipped high-income countries (HICs) and under-resourced LMICs operating theaters.

Additionally, this section is limited to surgical considerations of and operative techniques for disease confined to the thyroid gland. For operative considerations when disease is extra-thyroidal, as with metastatic thyroid carcinoma, readers should consult a definitive atlas of head and neck surgery.

The clinical evaluation of thyroid nodules is discussed elsewhere in this textbook.

General Considerations

- Ultrasonography (US) is usually available in LMICs and may be of value in assessing thyroid size, location and character of discrete nodules, as well as lateral neck compartments. Cervical lymphadenopathy in the presence of nodular thyroid disease increases the likelihood of metastatic thyroid carcinoma and should be assessed with fine needle aspiration biopsy (FNAB) whenever possible.

- Benign goiterous thyroid disease is endemic in many LMICs and frequently an indication for thyroidectomy. Large goiters generally do not require US or FNAB evaluation.

- Every attempt should be made to evaluate solitary nodules with FNAB, especially when the nodule is hard or fixed, which increases the likelihood of malignancy.

- Computed tomography (CT) is of limited value and should not be routinely obtained during pre-operative assessment. However, it may have utility in ruling out laryngotracheal involvement in patients with presumed thyroid malignancy presenting with hoarseness and signs of airway compromise.

- Thyroid function studies, including a thyroid stimulating hormone level, should be measured preoperatively to identify patients with hyperfunctioning glands, for which medical rather than surgical management may be indicated. Baseline calcium and phosphorous levels should also be obtained.

- Although not routinely done in the developed world, vocal cord mobility should be assessed prior to thyroid surgery whenever possible. However, it is essential to assess the vocal cords in patients presenting with thyroid disease and hoarseness; when hoarseness is due to vocal cord immobility, injury to the contralateral recurrent laryngeal nerve during thyroid resection can result in airway obstruction from bilateral vocal cord weakness.

Surgical Principles

- Perioperative antibiotics are unnecessary.
- Orotracheal intubation is virtually always possible, even when large goiters displace or compress the trachea.
- The patient's first thyroid operation is generally the most straightforward as the planes of dissection, laryngeal nerves, and parathyroid glands have not been previously disturbed. Therefore, surgeons should take advantage of this opportunity to perform the most definitive procedure justified by the surgical indication. For example, when disease is confined to one lobe and the diagnosis remains uncertain, it is usually prudent to remove the entire lobe

as this obviates the need for a repeat dissection of the same side if a malignancy is found and only a partial lobectomy was performed initially. Similarly, when the surgical indication is a diffusely enlarged goiter involving both lobes, a total thyroidectomy is usually justified as this greatly reduces the likelihood of recurrence (which is not uncommon when a subtotal resection is performed) and the need for further thyroid surgery later.

- In LMICs, perioperative cyto- and histopathology expertise are often not readily available. While most thyroid surgery will ultimately be for benign disease, surgeons will occasionally encounter disease suspicious for malignancy for which no immediate histopathologic opinion is available. Unless timely and appropriate clinical follow-up can be ensured if partial thyroid resection is considered, surgeons are justified in performing a total thyroidectomy.

- Satisfactory exposure is essential. When planning the skin incision, cosmetic considerations are always trumped by the need for a safe and sufficient resection; specifically, less experienced thyroid surgeons should err on the side of an incision that may, in retrospect, be somewhat longer than was required, or be prepared to lengthen the incision as necessary during the procedure. As a wise surgeon once said, "The incision heals side-to-side, not end-to-end." Additionally, in cases of exceptionally large goiters sectioning the strap muscles may greatly improve exposure, and surgeons may proceed accordingly.

- Whenever available, bright headlight illumination should be used to supplement standard operating room (OR) lighting. Headlights are very helpful when working deep in the surgical bed and facilitate identification of key structures such as the laryngeal nerves and parathyroid glands.

- Optic magnification with surgical loupes greatly aids identification and preservation of key structures such as the recurrent laryngeal nerves and parathyroid glands, and should be used whenever available. Additionally, magnification is very helpful in localizing and more discriminately controlling small vessel bleeding around key structures.

- Preservation of the recurrent laryngeal nerve, external branch of the superior laryngeal nerve, and parathyroid glands is paramount. Every attempt should be made to identify the recurrent laryngeal nerve and at least one parathyroid gland when performing a thyroid lobectomy. While positive identification of the external branch of the superior laryngeal nerve may not be essential, it is necessary for surgeons to understand the anatomic relationships of the various structures around the superior pole of the lobe in order to avoid injury to the nerve. Similarly, it is important for surgeons to appreciate that "dissecting on the capsule of the gland" to obviate the need for identifying key structures does not ensure a safe operation. Dissecting as close to the gland as practicable is clearly desirable; nonetheless, it is equally important to understand the key anatomic

relationships in the thyroid bed and sort them appropriately while avoiding indiscriminate maneuvers or working distal to the gland.

- There are various well-accepted ways of dissecting a thyroid lobe; the two most common variations are the superior-to-inferior and inferior-to-superior approaches, respectively. Each has putative advantages (discussed below). It is especially prudent for occasional and less-experienced thyroid surgeons to develop an approach based on one of the above techniques, and replicate and improve their approach over time. Even so, there will likely be scenarios, e.g., with huge goiters, when a somewhat more ad hoc approach is warranted, which is all the more reason for surgeons to have a solid grasp of the key anatomic relationships in the anterior neck.

- Surgeons-in-training who intend to become proficient in thyroidectomy should consult a variety of surgical atlases that address the topic as well as assist as many experienced thyroid surgeons as practicable to best learn how to safely and sufficiently complete resections.

Operative Considerations: Thyroid Lobectomy

a. Relevant Anatomy
   i. Recurrent Laryngeal Nerve (RLN)
      - The RLN arises from vagus nerve and ascends in the tracheoesophageal groove medial to carotid artery.
      - The left RLN generally runs fairly parallel to the trachea, while the right RLN runs a more angular course from lateral to medial as it approaches the tracheoesophageal groove.
      - Relational variability between the RLN, inferior thyroid artery (ITA), and inferior parathyroid gland is common; however, the RLN more often than not lies in a plane relatively posterior (i.e., deep) and medial to the ITA and inferior parathyroid gland.
      - Notwithstanding the above, the ITA occasionally lies deep to the RLN, or gives off multiple branches around the RLN; it is generally best, therefore, to identify the RLN and dissect the ITA until it clearly enters the thyroid before ligating.
      - The RLN generally runs just posterior to the dorsal surface of the thyroid lobe as it approaches the larynx. However, the RLN may occasionally lie within the thyroid capsule, so it is important to keep the RLN under constant direct vision as dissection proceeds along the thyroid capsule.
      - The main trunk of the RLN generally lies immediately posterior to the thyroid suspensory (Berry's) ligament. However, the RLN may be adherent to the ligament or RLN branches may pass through the ligament on their way to the cricothyroid membrane. Such

variability places the RLN at risk if the ligament is indiscriminately retracted or dissected from its tracheal attachments. To prevent RLN injury here, it is imperative that any and all RLN branches about the ligament be judiciously dissected and followed until they are observed to enter the cricothyroid membrane.

ii. Superior Laryngeal Nerve (SLN)

- The SLN originates from the vagal trunk and descends medial to the internal and external carotid arteries. It courses anteriorly toward the larynx and gives off internal (sensory) and external (motor to cricothyroid muscle) branches.

- The external branch of the SLN generally lies posterior (i.e., deep), but in close proximity, to the superior thyroid artery (STA) and enters the cricothyroid muscle posteriorly.

- The STA should be positively identified, isolated, and followed to its entry into the superior pole of the thyroid lobe before it is individually ligated in order to avoid injury to the SLN.

iii. Parathyroid Glands: Location and Vascular Supply

- Although there may be variability, both inferior and superior sets of glands generally lie posterior (i.e., deep) to the dorsal surface of the thyroid lobes.

- Glands may also lie well above or below the poles of the thyroid lobe; infrequently, glands may lie within the thyroid parenchyma.

- The superior glands are generally found in a somewhat more posterior plane than their inferior counterparts.

- The inferior glands are usually proximal to the dorsolateral aspect of the inferior pole, lying in a somewhat more anterior plane than the RLN and ITA.

- The ITA and its branches provide the blood supply to the inferior glands as well most superior glands; superior glands occasionally are supplied by a plexus of branches from both inferior and superior thyroid arteries.

- The best way to avoid devascularizing the parathyroids is to individually ligate the ITA as close to the thyroid capsule as possible.

b. Thyroid Lobectomy, Inferior-to-Superior Pole Dissection: Theoretical Advantages

- This procedure permits early, continuous visualization of the RLN nerve prior to any branching; there is a greater likelihood that any/all branches will be identified and preserved as dissection proceeds superiorly toward the larynx.

- It allows early identification of the ITA, which can be used to locate and preserve the inferior parathyroid gland.

- The surgeon has the option of identifying either the RLN or the ITA first; the putative advantage of identifying the ITA first is that the ITA can be used to locate and preserve the inferior parathyroid gland, which usually lies in a more anterior plane than the RLN. Once the inferior parathyroid is preserved, dissection can proceed more deeply to locate the RLN without fear of devascularizing the inferior parathyroid. Alternatively, if the first goal is identification of the RLN, it is best not to ligate the ITA until the inferior parathyroid is also identified and preserved.

- As the inferior and mid lobe are mobilized and retracted away from the thyroid bed, it becomes relatively easy to individually identify the superior pole vessels (and, often, the superior laryngeal nerve), thus allowing ligation as they enter the gland, which minimizes risk to the nerve.

- If it is clear that the superior pole vessels can be individually isolated and ligated as they enter the superiorly retracted lobe, positive identification of the superior laryngeal nerve becomes unnecessary.

c. Thyroid Lobectomy, Superior-to-Inferior Pole Dissection: Theoretical Advantages

- This procedure emphasizes early identification and preservation of the external branch of the SLN with mobilization of the superior pole, which may be advantageous when the gland lies low in the neck or a substernal goiter is present.

- Once the superior pole is mobilized, dissection proceeds with relative ease laterally and inferiorly, which permits retraction of the lobe medially and identification of inferior pole vessels and parathyroid glands on the dorsal surface of the lobe.

- Proceeding with lateral to medial dissection to identify the RLN may lessen the likelihood of "skeletonizing" nerve, as may occur when dissection to identify the nerve proceeds from the superficial (anterior) to the deep (posterior) plane.

Step-by-Step Thyroid Lobectomy

a. Patient Positioning

- Appropriate extension of the neck is very important as it helps bring the thyroid gland more fully into the operative field. After the airway is secured, a soft bolster of the surgeon's choice should be placed under the patient's shoulders to extend the neck; a donut-type gel ring or other suitable head-holder is placed so as to secure the head extended on the neck with the chin aimed at the ceiling. While the goal is maximal extension, care must be taken not to overextend the neck; the surgeon should ensure the patient's head is firmly in the headrest before proceeding.

- Positioning is completed by tucking both arms (to facilitate access of both surgeon and assistants) and placing the table in modest reverse Trendelenburg (i.e., table tilted head up) to reduce venous congestion in the operative field. A decision to place a Foley catheter should be made based on the expected length of the procedure as well as individual patient considerations (e.g., older males may be better served with a catheter than young females). Anti-embolism devices should be applied to the legs if available.

b. Incision

- The incision should be planned and marked prior to extending the neck. Whenever possible, the incision should be placed in a natural skin fold. When a natural crease is not present, momentarily flexing the head and neck usually facilitates identification of a suitable fold, which can be marked with a surgical pen prior to repositioning the patient (Figure 27.1).
- In most cases the incision can be planned in a fold roughly midway between the cricoid cartilage and suprasternal notch; this will generally permit ready access to both inferior and superior poles of the gland.
- Placing the incision lower in the neck is more likely to result in an unsightly long-term cosmetic result as the scar tends to migrate inferiorly toward the clavicles, becoming more difficult to camouflage over time.
- The length of the incision is generally guided by the size of the lobe or gland to be removed. In most cases, a length of ~5 cm (the distance between the anterior borders of the sternocleidomastoid muscles) is sufficient. For larger glands it may be prudent to mark, but not initially incise, a greater length in the event the incision needs to be extended later in the case. Ultimately, the best incision is the one that permits adequate exposure to ensure a safe and relatively struggle-free resection.
- The planned incision is marked with a surgical pen and can be infiltrated with a local anesthetic with epinephrine for improved hemostasis.

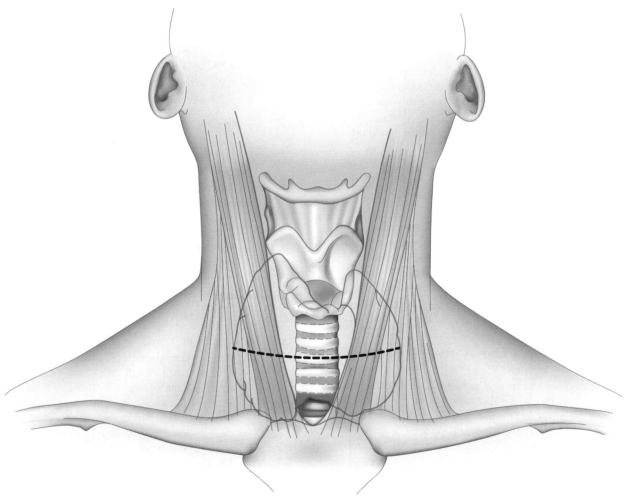

FIGURE 27.1   Incision. Illustration by John W. Karapelou, CMI.

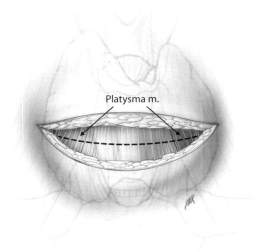

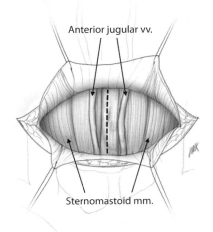

FIGURE 27.3   Exposure. Illustration by John W. Karapelou, CMI.

FIGURE 27.2   Illustration by John W. Karapelou, CMI.

- The skin is sharply incised down to the platysma. Judicious use of monopolar electrocautery helps achieve hemostasis in the subcutaneous tissues. Once hemostasis is satisfactory, the platysma is incised with care taken to avoid deep subplatysmal dissection (Figure 27.2).

- The subcutaneous and platysmal edges of the upper and lower incisions are sequentially grasped with suitable forceps (Allis, Leahy, or Kocher forceps work nicely) and retracted perpendicular to the wound as upper and lower flaps are developed in the immediate subplatysmal plane. The flaps are elevated to the thyroid notch superiorly and suprasternal notch inferiorly. The flaps can be developed using a variety of techniques; cutting electrocautery works particularly well. Skillful dissection in the subplatysmal plane preserves the anterior jugular and associated veins, which helps minimize postoperative wound edema.

- Securing the flaps to the surgical drapes with 2-0 or 3-0 silk sutures obviates the need for a wound retractor.

c. Exposure
- The midline raphe of the strap muscles is identified and exposed from suprasternal notch to thyroid notch (Figure 27.3).

- The midline raphe is bluntly undermined with a hemostat from the suprasternal notch toward the thyroid cartilage taking care not to lacerate the underlying thyroid isthmus. Monopolar electrocautery can then be used to incise the raphe along its length over the hemostat separating the strap muscles in the midline (Figure 27.4).

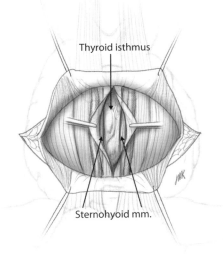

FIGURE 27.4   Illustration by John W. Karapelou, CMI.

- In most cases it is possible to preserve one or both anterior jugular veins, which lie parallel and just lateral to the midline raphe. If an anterior jugular vein must be sacrificed, it should be securely clamped and ligated.

- The strap muscles are gently undermined with blunt dissection and retracted laterally from the anterior and lateral aspects of the thyroid gland with the assistance of an army-navy or other suitable retractor (Figure 27.5).

- With very large goiters it may be necessary to incise the strap muscles to gain satisfactory lateral exposure of the gland. This is best done with electrocautery; the muscles can be reconstituted with absorbable sutures after the gland is removed.

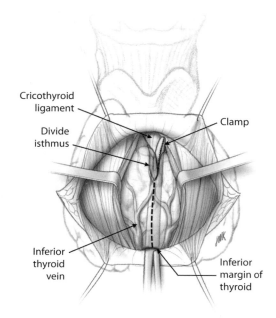

FIGURE 27.5   Illustration by John W. Karapelou, CMI.

- Now exposed, the entire gland should be palpated; this is a particularly important step to rule out more extensive disease when the preoperative plan is for lobectomy only.
- The extent of the thyroid isthmus as well as its relationship to the trachea inferiorly and superiorly should be established.

d. Excision
- The isthmus can be isolated and transected as either an initial step or after the lobe has been dissected. The author prefers to transect the isthmus first as it facilitates mobilization of the lobe during dissection.
- The inferior margin of the isthmus is identified and the thin fascia tethering it to the trachea is bluntly dissected down to the midline trachea. If the inferior margin of the isthmus lies low in the neck and is difficult to access, a cricoid hook can be used to gently retract the trachea (and thyroid) superiorly. A curved clamp is gently insinuated in the plane between the isthmus and trachea; the tip of the clamp is used to further develop the plane between the isthmus and trachea until the tip of the clamp is visible at the superior margin of the isthmus (Figure 27.5). The isthmus is transected with electrocautery (using the underlying clamp to guard against inadvertent tracheotomy); if the procedure is a lobectomy only, the edge of the remaining isthmus may be oversewn with a 2-0 silk suture. Alternatively, the isthmus may be doubly suture ligated and divided between the ligatures.
- The inferior thyroid pole is identified with blunt dissection; a moist gauze sponge is used to grasp the pole, which is gently retracted

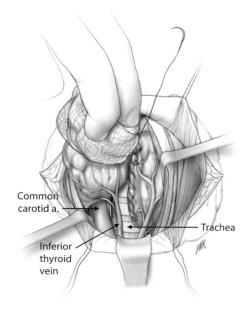

FIGURE 27.6   Excision. Illustration by John W. Karapelou, CMI.

superiorly. The use of a grasping clamp should be avoided as it may lacerate the lobe (Figure 27.6).
- As it more often than not lies in a plane ventral to the RLN, the ITA is identified first using blunt dissection. The ITA and any branches are traced toward the inferior pole. If the inferior parathyroid gland is not readily encountered, judicious dissection with a Kittner sponge about the retracted inferoposterior aspect of the lobe may demonstrate it. The parathyroid is generally small, bean-shaped, and tan, and usually found in loose areolar tissue in this area; occasionally it is loosely attached to the undersurface of the lobe (Figure 27.7).
- If the parathyroid gland is identified, the ITA branches serving it are carefully preserved. After the parathyroid is preserved, or after a reasonable effort fails to locate it, the main trunk of the ITA may be doubly ligated with 3-0 silk suture and transected at its entry into the thyroid lobe. (If the surgeon elects to identify the RLN first, care must be taken to avoid indiscriminate dissection and sacrifice of inferior pole vessels as this increases the risk of devascularizing the parathyroid glands.)
- If the parathyroid is later found to be devascularized, the gland should be thinly sliced and placed in a pocket within the sternocleidomastoid muscle and marked with a permanent suture or clip.
- The RLN is then identified in the triangle bounded laterally by the carotid artery, medially by the trachea, and superiorly by the inferior border of the thyroid lobe; the apex of the triangle points inferiorly toward the thoracic

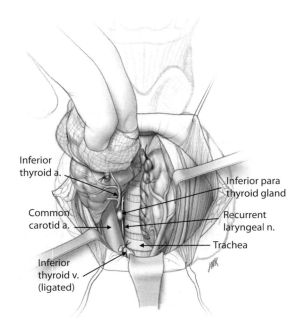

FIGURE 27.7   Illustration by John W. Karapelou, CMI.

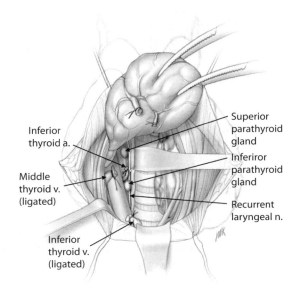

FIGURE 27.8   Illustration by John W. Karapelou, CMI.

inlet. As the ITA and inferior parathyroid gland occupy the same triangle, and are usually more lateral and ventral to the RLN, prior identification of the ITA and parathyroid may help narrow the search for the RLN. Additionally, the tracheo-esophageal groove can be used as a dorsal land-mark, as the RLN seldom lies deep to this plane.

- Once the RLN is identified, dissection of the lobe, adhering to the capsule, proceeds along the dorsal and lateral surfaces; the middle thyroid vein is isolated and ligated. At this point the supe-rior parathyroid gland may be identified either in close proximity to the dorsal surface of the retracted gland, it which case it can be gently dis-sected from the capsule with a Kittner sponge, or it may be observed in the paratracheal areolar tis-sues somewhat lateral to the RLN (Figure 27.8).

- The lobe is retracted superiorly and dissected from its bed using fine-tipped instruments and Kittner sponges while continuously visualiz-ing the RLN.

- Suction about the RLN should be used cau-tiously; judicious use of a micro-bipolar cautery may be helpful to control discrete bleeding when pressure alone fails. Monopolar cautery should not be used in close proximity to the RLN.

- Moving superiorly along the RLN, the pos-terior suspensory ligament (of Berry), which tethers the thyroid to the trachea, is encoun-tered about the upper trachea and cricoid car-tilage. Dissection here must be done carefully as close proximity of the RLN to the ligament, as well as the dense connective tissue of the ligament itself, predispose the nerve to injury during manipulation (Figure 27.9).

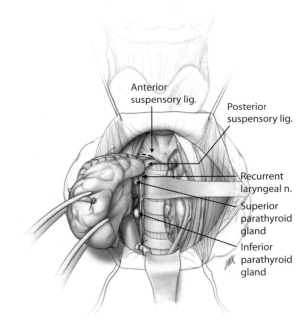

FIGURE 27.9   Illustration by John W. Karapelou, CMI.

- The RLN usually passes just deep (poste-rior) to the ligament. However, the RLN may directly pierce the ligament, or give off branches that do; all branches should be pre-served. The ligament is more resistant to blunt dissection than the pericapsular areolar tis-sues; nonetheless, care must be taken to dis-sect the ligament entirely from the nerve (a fine-tipped mosquito-type clamp works well). Once the RLN (and any branches) are free of the ligament, and can be seen to be enter-ing the posterior larynx, the ligament can be sharply incised, keeping the RLN under direct vision throughout.

• Bleeding from small vessels at this site may initially be controlled with gentle pressure; more troublesome bleeders may be controlled with judicious use of a micro-bipolar cautery or suture ligature. Indiscriminate use of cautery or clamps risks injury to the RLN.

• Transection of the suspensory ligament significantly frees the gland from its tracheal attachment; the lobe, which can be readily retracted superiorly, is now tethered only by its superior pole attachments (Figure 27.10).

• Each superior pole vessel should be bluntly exposed and dissected to its entry into the superior pole, where it is individually ligated with 2-0 silk suture. (The superior artery should be doubly ligated.) This technique ensures that the external branch of the superior laryngeal nerve is not inadvertently injured, which can occur if all of the superior pole structures are clamped and ligated as one. If these steps are followed, it is not necessary to positively identify the external branch of the superior laryngeal nerve.

• The entire lobe is passed from the field and sent for histopathologic assessment.

e. Closure

• The thyroid bed is inspected for bleeding which, depending upon the size and location of the vessel, may be controlled with bipolar cautery or suture ligatures.

• The wound is irrigated taking care not to place suction directly on the RLN or parathyroid glands.

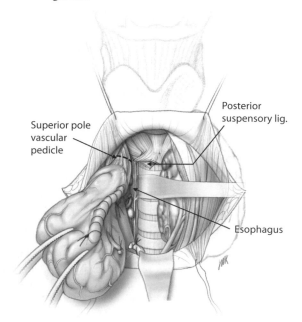

Superior pole vascular pedicle

Posterior suspensory lig.

Esophagus

FIGURE 27.10   Illustration by John W. Karapelou, CMI

• A single suction drain is placed posterolaterally in the bed so as to avoid contact with the RLN or parathyroid glands. The drain may be brought out either directly through the surgical incision or through a small adjacent skin incision.

• The strap muscles are reconstituted in the midline with absorbable suture; if they have been transected for access, the incised edges are repaired with interrupted absorbable sutures incorporating the fascia.

• The platysma and subcutaneous soft tissues may be closed individually with absorbable suture (advisable in obese patients) or as a single layer. Approximating the platysmal edges helps restore a surgical landmark that may be important in the event of future neck surgery. Regardless of technique, it is important that wound closure results in well-approximated skin edges for a good cosmetic result.

• The subcuticular skin may be approximated variously with rapidly absorbing sutures or a single pull-through monofilament suture. Tincture of benzoin, or similar adhesive, and Steri-Strips are applied; a dressing is usually not necessary.

• It is prudent to apply manual pressure to the wound during emergence from anesthesia as the patient coughing or straining prior to extubation increases the risk of bleeding or hematoma.

f. Early Postoperative Care

• The head of the bed is elevated 30–45 degrees; the patient should begin ambulation with assistance the evening of surgery.

• The diet is advanced as tolerated over 24 hours.

• For thyroid lobectomy alone, postoperative laboratory studies are generally unnecessary.

• No specific wound care is required.

• Occlusive dressings are discouraged as they may mask development of a hematoma.

• The drain is kept on suction and may be removed the following day if there has been no significant discharge over the previous 8–12 hours.

• Most patients may be discharged the day after surgery with instructions to return in one week.

• While there is a trend in HICs to perform otherwise uncomplicated thyroid lobectomy as a same-day procedure, often without use of a surgical drain, this practice cannot generally be recommended in LMICs where constraints such as lack of adequate infrastructure and emergency transportation render this option problematic. Therefore, patients in these settings should be observed until it is clear there is a very low risk of urgent complication after clinic discharge.

Total Thyroidectomy: Specific Considerations

- Completing a total excision of the gland is an exercise in replicating the preceding steps on the contralateral side.

- It is important for the surgeon to approach the contralateral dissection with the same step-wise discipline and attention to technique as on the previous side, especially if there is uncertainty regarding the status of the RLN or parathyroid glands. When dissection of the first lobe has gone well, and exposure is excellent, surgeons should resist any tendency to hurry resection of the remaining gland as this increases the likelihood of inadvertent injury to key structures.

- Which side of the patient to stand on to complete the thyroidectomy is the surgeon's choice; while some advocate switching sides, this requires the surgeon to reorient to the thyroid bed. Rotating the OR table along its axis toward the surgeon rather than switching sides is a satisfactory option. Bottom line, the surgeon should feel comfortable working in the neck regardless of which side of the table is chosen.

- As with thyroid lobectomy, any devascularized parathyroid tissue should be finely minced and placed in a pocket developed in the sternocleidomastoid muscle.

- Wound closure and care are the same as for thyroid lobectomy. Generally, a single suction drain is satisfactory; however, in cases of very large or substernal goiters, leaving a drain on each side of the thyroid bed is prudent.

- If resources permit, intact parathyroid hormone level can be measured early postoperatively and used to guide calcium supplementation, if necessary. As this assay is usually not available in LMICs, calcium and phosphorous levels should be checked 24–48 hours after surgery. Symptomatic hypocalcemia does not usually manifest within the first 24 hours; patients should be checked for Chvostek's sign and asked about symptoms such as circumoral or digital paresthesias, all of which are reliable hypocalcemia indicators.

- As total thyroidectomy results in hypothyroidism, patients treated for benign disease may be started on thyroid hormone replacement in the immediate postoperative period. Management of patients with presumed carcinoma varies and is beyond the scope of this chapter.

Major Complications of Thyroid Surgery

a. Airway Obstruction

- Airway obstruction may occur from either compressive hematoma or bilateral recurrent nerve injury.

- Hematoma is usually readily identifiable based on neck examination and assessment of the suction drain. Treatment is immediate opening of the incision at the bedside with evacuation of the hematoma. The airway is secured as necessary. Oral endotracheal intubation is usually the best choice as a laryngeal mask airway may not overcome airway resistance; safe tracheotomy in a blood-filled neck is problematic. Once the airway is secured and the hematoma evacuated, the patient is returned to the OR for orderly examination of the wound, control of bleeding, irrigation, and meticulous reclosure. Prophylactic antibiotics are justified in this scenario.

- Significant airway obstruction due to bilateral RLN injury typically manifests immediately after extubation. Patients have variable inspiratory stridor; true air hunger with inability to maintain satisfactory blood oxygen saturation requires definitive airway management, usually with urgent re-intubation. Even if the surgeon is confident that both RLNs have been preserved and that the injury is likely neuropraxic, it is most prudent to perform a tracheotomy prior to leaving the OR. This definitively addresses the acute airway obstruction and allows the surgical team to assess and manage the airway and vocal cord weakness in a controlled manner. For example, bilateral RLN neuropraxia usually resolves, although resolution may take weeks to months. Patients with tracheotomies can be discharged and followed by the ENT service until decannulation is feasible or other treatment is required.

b. Hematoma

- Management of hematoma is discussed above. This is best avoided by meticulous attention to all bleeding sites, no matter how minor-appearing, prior to wound closure. Temporarily increasing intrathoracic pressure prior to closure may unmask venous bleeding, which can then be addressed.

- Hematoma is also avoided by thorough preoperative assessment of the patient's overall medical condition and current pharmacotherapy. Although routine measurement of coagulation studies is unnecessary, complete blood count with platelet levels should be checked in all patients, especially older patients and young women, who have a higher likelihood of underlying anemia. Patients who chronically use anti-coagulant or anti-platelet drugs should have surgery deferred as necessary to reduce the likelihood of associated coagulopathy.

- If surgical bleeding occurs out of proportion to the dissection, coagulation studies and platelet count should be assessed.

c. Laryngeal Nerve Injury

- Airway obstruction due to bilateral RLN injury is discussed above.

- Nerve injuries are usually due to errors in technique, which include inadvertent clamping or cutting; inappropriate use of electrocautery; or excessive direct or indirect traction of the nerve. The risk of RLN injury is much greater if the nerve is not positively identified and followed along its course into the larynx.

- There are surgical scenarios which, with respect to the RLN, clearly increase the risk of harm to the patient. These include completion thyroidectomy in a patient with known vocal cord paralysis from prior surgery, and dissection of the contralateral lobe during planned total thyroidectomy when it is clear the RLN on the first side has been injured. Regarding the first scenario, it is best to have the completion procedure performed only by an experienced thyroid surgeon. In the second scenario, if the surgeon is relatively inexperienced and the indication for the procedure permits, it is reasonable to discontinue the procedure and arrange for later management with a more seasoned surgeon. If that is not possible, or if the attending surgeon is, in fact, experienced, the contralateral dissection must be undertaken in a very considered fashion. For example, it may be prudent to perform a subtotal contralateral lobectomy so as to reduce the risk of RLN injury. As any contralateral dissection in this circumstance increases the risk of bilateral RLN injury, the surgeon should have a heightened awareness that tracheotomy at the conclusion of the thyroidectomy may be necessary.

- Unilateral injury to a RLN or the external branch of the SLN results in variable dysphonia. A RLN injury is generally more obvious and disabling than injury to the SLN.

- Unilateral RLN injury typically produces breathy dysphonia without airway compromise; however, some patients, particularly those older or debilitated, may have associated tracheal aspiration of secretions and thin liquids (manifested by coughing), and are at risk for aspiration pneumonia.

- Unilateral vocal weakness due to RLN injury can generally be managed expectantly, as some proportion of patients will recover full function, or satisfactorily accommodate to the weakness over time. Persistent, problematic vocal cord weakness can be managed with various injection or medialization techniques performed by otolaryngologists, and patients should be referred accordingly.

- The external branch of the SLN is a tensor of the vocal cord; injury may result in the inability to modulate vocal pitch, as with singing. This injury is usually more apparent to the patient than the listener. As with RLN injury, some proportion of patients will recover function over time. Unlike unremitting RLN weakness, there is no specific intervention to restore function.

d. Hypoparathyroidism

- Hypoparathyroidism is decidedly unlikely when the initial thyroid procedure is lobectomy alone.

- Symptomatic hypocalcemia after thyroidectomy implies significant parathyroid gland compromise, either from excessive gland excision or devascularization.

- Treatment of symptomatic hypocalcemia varies based on severity: rapid intravenous infusion of 10% calcium gluconate is used emergently; moderate symptoms may be treated with continuous calcium gluconate infusion. Oral calcium carbonate is also given and, depending upon response, vitamin D (in the form of Rocaltrol) may be added. Oral therapies are modified as necessary on an outpatient basis.

- Depending upon the nature of the insult, hypocalcemia often improves or completely resolves over time as remaining viable parathyroid function improves. In the hands of experienced thyroid surgeons, the risk of permanent hypocalcemia after total thyroidectomy is 1%–2%.

SUGGESTED READING

Clayman GL: Thyroid lobectomy and isthmusectomy. In Cohen JI and Clayman GL (eds): *Atlas of Head and Neck Surgery,* 1st ed. Philadelphia, Saunders Elsevier, 2011.

Myers EN: Thyroidectomy. In Myers EN (ed): *Operative Otolaryngology: Head and Neck Surgery,* 2nd ed, vol I. Philadelphia, Saunders Elsevier, 2008.

Loré JM, Farrell M, Castillo NB: Endocrine Surgery, The Thyroid Gland. In Loré JM and Medina JE (eds): *An Atlas of Head & Neck Surgery,* 4th ed. Philadelphia, Saunders Elsevier, 2005.

The Neck. In Hollinshead WH: Anatomy for Surgeons, vol I: *The Head and Neck,* 3rd ed. Philadelphia, Lippincott, 1982.

COMMENTARY

Emmanuel R. Ezeome, Nigeria

In Nigeria, the challenges to performing thyroidectomies are no different from those in other LMICs. Most of the thyroidectomies are performed by true general surgeons who, although adequately equipped to deal with the general surgical problems of their communities, may have less experience than specialized thyroid surgeons. Patients often present very late because they lack financial resources and they are not aware that they need medical attention at a hospital. For this reason, the goiters are commonly large; some are truly giant goiters. Many patients are unable to access available treatments either due to cost or due to the remoteness of their residences. The healthcare industry is still on a cash-and-carry basis. Health insurance is either nonexistent or in its infancy. Sometimes, basic surgical equipment may not be available, and surgeons are forced to either improvise or abandon the surgery. Evaluation of patients may be limited so that even a basic thyroid function test may not be available. Surgeons may sometimes rely on only Lugol's iodine and propranolol for preoperative preparation of thyrotoxic patients. Patients may not come for regular follow-up appointments, so procedures that require constant and regular checkups may not be feasible.

Diagnosis

While pathologists are increasingly available in many centers, experienced cytopathologists are still hard to find. The value of FNAC in diagnosis of thyroid malignancies is therefore limited. Surgeons in Nigeria frequently perform total thyroidectomy for thyroid malignancies based on clinical suspicion alone. In the absence of a thyroid function test, surgeons depend on an electrocardiogram (ECG), sleeping pulse, and the patient's clinical parameters to decide on adequacy of medical control of thyrotoxicosis.

Operative Procedure

Availability of anesthesia should not be taken for granted. It is important to be able to do thyroidectomy under local anesthesia and regional nerve blocks.

Deciding on a Surgery

While total thyroidectomy has gained acceptance as the standard of care for benign goiters involving both lobes, surgeons in Nigeria do not perform total thyroidectomies as often as surgeons in HICs. L-Thyroxin availability is not assured in many places, especially for patients coming from remote villages. Lifelong intake of such drugs and compliance issues must also be considered. In addition, many of the surgeons who do these surgeries may have the experience of only 15 to 20 thyroidectomies per year. Therefore, the advantages of high volume and frequency of involvement in thyroidectomies may be limited even for the very senior surgeons. Some surgeons may not have been trained to locate and preserve the RLN and the parathyroid gland. Total thyroidectomy is therefore used selectively by surgeons who have the skill and experience necessary to do it.

A skilled and experienced surgeon, with proper adaptations, should be able to carry out most forms of thyroidectomy with morbidity and mortality figures similar to those of surgeons in HICs.

28

Ophthalmology

Matthew C. Bujak
Geoffrey Tabin

Introduction

The general surgeon may not be comfortable with ophthalmic surgery. Certainly, intraocular surgery should be reserved for ophthalmic specialists; however, surgical repair of the eyelids and certain emergent intraocular procedures may be required of the nonspecialist.

Eyelids

The function of the eyelid is primarily protection and lubrication of the globe; it is integral for preservation of good vision and ocular health. Small procedures such as chalazion incision and debridement are easily performed and provide the patient with good cosmesis and comfort. Other eyelid procedures, such as tarsorrhaphy and entropion repair, are slightly more involved but are powerful tools that can preserve vision and save a compromised eye.

Chalazion

A chalazion is a lipogranulomatous inflammatory lesion that occurs when the sebaceous glands of the eyelids are blocked and lipid secretions infiltrate into surrounding tissues (Figure 28.1). They generally present as firm, subcutaneous nodules within the eyelid with surrounding swelling, erythema, and mild tenderness. Although they may spontaneously perforate, they are not typically associated with ulceration, nor are they associated with loss of eyelashes (madarosis). Ulceration, vascularization, and madarosis are concerning for malignancy and require a different approach.

Differential Diagnosis

Preseptal cellulitis: Eyelid erythema, edema, and warmth are more prominent. Often, a periorbital skin abrasion or laceration is evident.

Sebaceous gland carcinoma: Usually develops in older patients and should be considered in the elderly with thickening of both upper and lower lids, unilateral blepharitis, or loss of eyelashes.

Pyogenic granuloma: A deep red, vascular lesion associated with trauma or surgery to the eyelid.

Kaposi's sarcoma: Presents as a purple-red, nontender nodule of either eyelid skin or conjunctiva and is associated with immunosuppression.

Treatment

Most chalazia respond to warm compresses for 15 minutes, four times daily, with light massage. A topical antibiotic such as erythromycin or bacitracin ointment can be applied twice daily. If the chalazion does not resolve after 3–4 weeks of conservative treatment, incision and curettage can be used to remove it. A steroid injection can rarely be used (0.2–1.0 mL triamcinolone 40 mg/ml) but may be inappropriate in Africans or Asians due to risk of atrophy and depigmentation of the skin.

Chalazion Incision and Curettage

The eye is prepped with topical anesthesia (e.g., amethocaine drops) and 5% povidone iodine. The center of the chalazion is marked on the eyelid skin with a marking pen prior to instillation of 2% lidocaine with epinephrine subcutaneously. If available, a chalazion clamp is secured tightly over the lesion. This ensures hemostasis during the incision and is simultaneously used to evert the eyelid to expose the inner conjunctival surface of the lid. A #11 blade is used to make a 2–3 mm vertical incision in the lesion through the conjunctival surface. When the incision is made correctly into the lesion, white lipogranulomatous material will likely express from the incision (Figure 28.2). If available, a small curette is used to scrape out any residual material from inside the chalazion cavity. No sutures are required. The eyelid is rotated back into normal position and the clamp is released. At this point there may be slight bleeding, which can easily be controlled by placing antibiotic ointment in the eye and patching it closed.

Postoperative Care

This minor procedure requires minimal follow-up. The patient should receive an antibiotic ointment twice daily for 2 weeks. The patient should be seen at postoperative week 1 to ensure proper healing.

Pitfalls

Sebaceous cell carcinoma: Recurrent chalazia in the elderly should be sent for pathology as they may rarely be malignant sebaceous cell carcinoma. Malignancy should be particularly considered if a chalazion is accompanied with loss of eyelashes.

Kaposi's sarcoma: In areas of high human immunodeficiency virus (HIV) prevalence, consider Kaposi's sarcoma in the differential diagnosis.

Full thickness incision: When incising the chalazion from the inside, through the palpebral conjunctiva, be sure not to make a full-thickness incision through the entire eyelid.[1]

Exposure Keratopathy

Exposure keratopathy is the result of incomplete eyelid closure (lagophthalmos) during blinking. It is a relatively common problem with potentially devastating consequences in both the developed and developing world. With incomplete closure of the eyelids, the tear film is not spread over the ocular surface. The ocular tear film is the most important refractive surface of the eye; thus, vision is diminished. Moreover, the tear film serves to mechanically maintain the integrity of the underlying corneal epithelium, provide nutrients, and protect with immunoglobulins. A breakdown of the natural epithelial barrier of the eye and a reduction of the lacrimal immunoglobulin A (IgA) exposes the eye to significant infectious risk. This risk is further compounded if the patient has concomitant hypesthesia of the cornea.

Lagophthalmos is caused by a number of etiologies and can be grouped into the following categories: neuroparalytic, reduced muscle tone, mechanical, and abnormal globe position. Facial nerve palsy—particularly Bell's palsy—remains one of the most common causes of significant lagophthalmos in both the developed and developing world. Fortunately, it tends to have a self-limited course with spontaneous resolution. Leprosy may cause progressive facial nerve palsy and should be considered in regions where it is prevalent.[2] It is particularly worrisome due to its association with concomitant cranial nerve V neuropathy. Herpes zoster

is another worrisome entity with a higher prevalence in low- and middle-income countries (LMICs) (Figure 28.3). Patients who are immunocompromised due to HIV are at particular risk of developing severe episodes of herpes zoster. The resultant scarring of periocular skin can cause a cicatricial foreshortening of

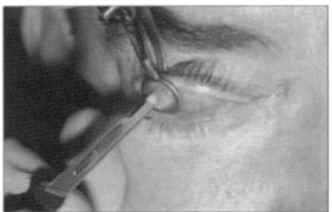

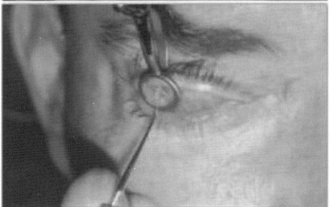

FIGURE 28.2 Chalazion incision. In the above photograph, a vertical incision is made through the palpebral conjunctiva into the chalazion. Note how the chalazion clamp helps to both evert the lid and secure the lesion. Once the chalazion is opened, a curette can be used to fully express the contents of the affected gland, as seen in the photograph below. Long, John A. "Chalazion." *Oculoplastic Surgery*. New York: Saunders Elsevier, 2009. p. 128.

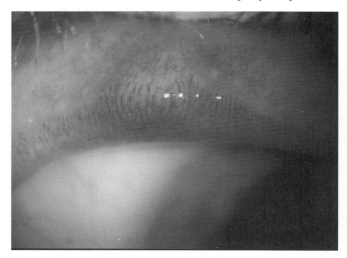

FIGURE 28.1 Chalazion. Note the appearance of an inflamed nodule arising from the glands just beneath the palpebral conjunctiva. Image by James Gilman.

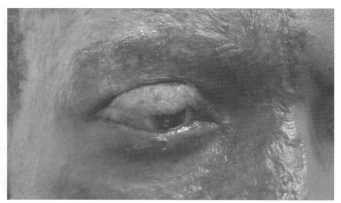

FIGURE 28.3 Extensive cicatricial changes from a Herpes zoster infection in a patient with human immunodeficiency virus (HIV) may limit eyelid closure. Image by Matthew Bujak and Geoffrey Tabin.

the eyelids that limits eye closure. As in the case of leprosy, herpes zoster may be compounded by concomitant corneal hypesthesia (Figure 28.4). Trauma, burns, and proptosis from orbital disease (e.g., thyroid orbitopathy or tumors) are other common causes of lagophthalmos.

Lagophthalmos can be observed by asking the patient to gently close the eyes as if sleeping. With the head slightly upturned, small gaps in lid closure can be observed. The corneal sensation should always be compared between the two eyes with a cotton swab or tissue. Irritation and drying of the ocular surface can be visualized with fluorescein staining under a cobalt blue light. The protective Bell's phenomenon, an upturning of the eye upon attempted closure of the eyelids, should be assessed. As in the case of corneal hypesthesia, its absence poses increased risk in the setting of lagophthalmos.

Management

Mild lagophthalmos can be managed with lubrication using a carboxymethylcellulose 1% eyedrop, or equivalent, four times daily. If required more frequently, a preservative-free lubricant is preferred but may be difficult to find in the developing world. Nocturnal lagophthalmos can be managed with nightly application of thicker liquid paraffin and lanolin ointments. The eyelids can also be taped closed at night, though this may be somewhat uncomfortable for the patient. Occasionally, cautery of the lacrimal puncta may improve ocular lubrication by reducing the outflow of tears from the fornix of the eye. These techniques may be helpful in managing mild or moderate lagophthalmos, but significant exposure needs to be managed definitively with surgical closure of the eyelids (tarsorrhaphy). Tarsorrhaphy can be performed as a temporary procedure for transient conditions such as Bell's palsy; alternatively, it can be made permanent for cicatricial causes, or for unremitting diseases such as leprosy.

Temporary Lateral Tarsorrhaphy

As the name implies, temporary tarsorrhaphies last only a finite period of 2 weeks and, as such, are ideal for transient conditions or as a temporary trial before choosing a more definitive permanent tarsorrhaphy. A double-armed 5-0 polypropylene suture is preferable if the tarsorrhaphy needs to be in place for less than 4 weeks, while a thicker 4-0 suture should be used if it needs to be in place longer. Polypropylene is preferable as it causes less inflammation, but a silk suture may be used if the former is not available.

Topical anesthetic eyedrops (e.g., proparacaine) are instilled in the eye. The periocular skin and eye are prepped with povidone iodine, and 1%–2% lidocaine with epinephrine (dilution,

1:100,000) is injected both subcutaneously and subconjunctivally on either side of both the upper and lower eyelids. Once the lateral aspect of the eyelids is well anesthetized, both arms of the double-armed suture are passed through both ends of a small 3-mm bolster. Trimming to size the foam that comes within a suture package can form an easy, makeshift bolster. Alternatively, a 3-mm segment of fine intravenous tubing can be cut and transected in half, forming a semicircle. Once passed through the bolster, the two arms of the suture are passed through the skin 5 mm above the upper eyelid margin. They travel subcutaneously and exit just posteriorly to the lashes in the grey line. The sutures are then passed through the grey line of the lower lid and exit out of the eyelid skin in a similar configuration, 5 mm below the lower lid margin. The needle is once again passed through a bolster and tied firmly with a 3-1-1 surgical knot, effectively completing the horizontal mattress suture. At the conclusion of the procedure, the lateral third of the eyelids should be firmly apposed. Antibiotic ointment (e.g., erythromycin) is instilled into the eye and onto the sutures before patching the eye closed.[3]

Permanent Lateral Tarsorrhaphy

Permanent tarsorrhaphies may be left indefinitely but may also be reversed, with minimal residual scarring, with a minor procedure. The permanent tarsorrhaphy closely resembles the aforementioned procedure. The main difference is that the edges of both upper and lower lid margins are excised with fine scissors or a #15 Bard-Parker blade. The excision should extend from the lateral corner of the eyelid (lateral canthus) for a length of 8 mm and should not include the lashes. The suture is then passed in a similar horizontal mattress fashion. But, instead of exiting through the intact grey line, it now exits through the debrided surface of the eyelid margin, thereby joining it to the debrided surface of the other eyelid. Removing the two adjacent epithelial layers thus facilitates permanent scarring of the eyelids together (Figure 28.5, Figure 28.6, and Figure 28.7).[3] This bolstered suture is left loose while three or four additional deep single interrupted sutures are used to firmly adhere the eyelids. Finally the bolstered suture is tied secure in a 3-1-1 manner.

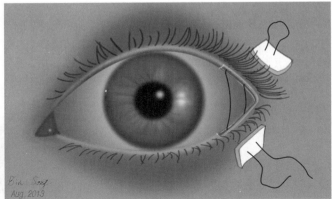

FIGURE 28.5 Tarsorrhaphy. The same method of horizontal mattress suturing—in this case, using a bolster on the lids—applies to both temporary and permanent procedures. Image by Bin Song. Adapted from: Hersh PS, Zagelbaum BA, Cremers SL. *Ophthalmic Surgical Procedures*, 2nd ed. New York: Thieme Publishing, 2009.

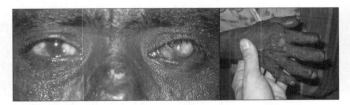

FIGURE 28.4 Characteristic features of leprosy; subsequently, this patient was at significant risk for corneal exposure from facial nerve paresis and demonstrates corneal scarring and opacification. Image by Matthew Bujak and Geoffrey Tabin.

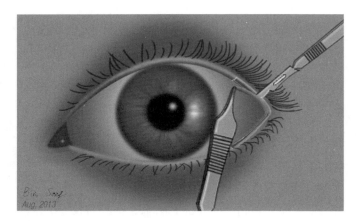

FIGURE 28.6 Permanent tarsorrhaphy. The tissue from the lid margin is carefully excised using fine scissors or a blade, taking care to avoid the globe at all times. Image by Bin Song.

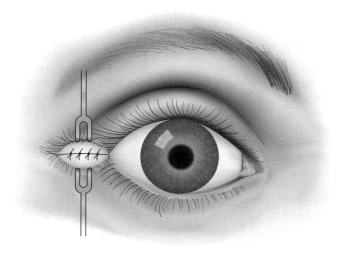

FIGURE 28.7 Permanent tarsorrhaphy: deep, interrupted sutures are used to close the tarsorrhaphy. Image by Bin Song. Adapted from: Hersh PS, Zagelbaum BA, Cremers SL. *Ophthalmic Surgical Procedures*, 2nd ed. New York: Thieme Publishing, 2009.

Postoperative Management

The eye is examined on postoperative day 1 to check for infection and patient comfort, and to ensure adequate closure of the eye. The probability of eyelid infection is very small due to the abundant blood supply of the eyelid, but the eye should be rechecked at postoperative week 1 to ensure no infection has developed.

Pitfalls

Loosening of the tarsorrhaphy: The sutures in a tarsorrhaphy need to be tightened firmly, as they have a tendency to loosen with time.

Corneal irritation from sutures: Proper placement of sutures is critical, particularly in patients who have concurrent corneal anesthesia and may not complain of postoperative irritation. The sutures should not go full-thickness through the eyelid, and they need to exit in the proper position at the grey line, just posteriorly to the

eyelashes. If the sutures exit too anteriorly, inturning of the lid margin may cause the lashes to rub against the cornea. Periodically, the surgeon should examine a temporary tarsorrhaphy, as the sutures themselves may abrade the cornea once they loosen.

Ocular examination: A tarsorrhaphy can make the eye more difficult to examine. One should be sure to examine the eye closely through the narrowed palpebral fissure. Pay particular attention to increased pain or discharge, which may be signs of ocular infection.

Trachoma

Trachoma is the eighth most common blinding disease and the leading infectious cause of blindness worldwide.[4] Trachoma is a disease of poverty and poor sanitation. With improvement in sanitation and health care, it has been virtually eliminated from high-income countries (HICs). The World Health Organization (WHO) and the alliance for the Global Elimination of Trachoma (GET 2020) have made significant strides toward the elimination of trachoma in low- and middle-income countries (LMICs). In 1981, WHO estimated that 500 million people worldwide had active trachoma; however, recent statistics from 2008 estimate that the world prevalence of trachoma has been reduced to 40 million. Nevertheless, trachoma remains a significant epidemiologic concern. It is endemic in more than 50 countries, predominantly in sub-Saharan Africa, the Middle East, and Asia.[4]

Trachoma is a chronic recurrent keratoconjunctivitis caused by four ocular serovars (A, B, Ba, and C) of the bacteria *Chlamydia trachomatis*. The genital serovars of chlamydia (D to K) can also infect the conjunctiva of both infants, causing ophthalmia neonatorum, and of adults, causing adult inclusion conjunctivitis. Yet, they usually cause isolated infections that do not lead to blindness. Trachoma, on the other hand, causes repeated episodes of conjunctivitis that eventually lead to conjunctival and corneal scarring, with subsequent blindness (Figure 28.8).[5]

Depending on the prevalence in a specific region, trachoma can be acquired in infancy or later in childhood. It is a disease of poor hygiene, with clustering of disease within villages and the family as the principal unit of transmission. It is spread by three means: direct contact, fomites, and eye-seeking flies. Infection begins with bilateral conjunctivitis, crusting of the eyelids, and a marked papillary (tiny blood vessel tufts) or follicular (white lymphocytic aggregates) response of the conjunctiva.

The conjunctival response is most marked in the superior tarsal conjunctiva and can be appreciated when the upper eyelid is everted with a cotton-tipped applicator. With chronicity, a linear fibrous band of scarring—known as an Arlt's line—appears on the superior tarsal conjunctiva (Figure 28.9).[6]

Follicles may also appear at the limbus; when they recede, they leave characteristic depressions known as Herbert's pits. During the acute phase, a marked ocular immune response is mounted to the pathogen, leading to resolution of the primary infection. Repeated cycles of infection and inflammation lead to corneal pannus, a downward growth of blood vessels over the corneoscleral limbus. And, of greater consequence, scarring of the eyelids develops, with eventual inturning of the eyelid margins (entropion).[6]

When the entropion is severe, the upper eyelashes can abrade the cornea (trichiasis), causing discomfort and breakdown of

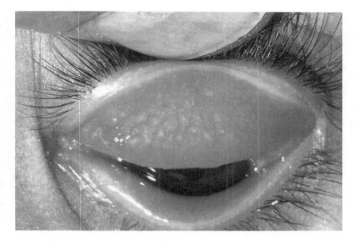

FIGURE 28.8 Trachoma grading: trachoma grade TF. World Health Organization. Trachoma [Internet]. 2013 [cited 30 Jan 2014].available from: http://www.who.int/blindness/causes/priority/en/index2.html≥

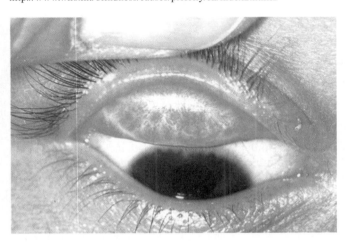

FIGURE 28.9 Trachoma grading: trachoma grade TS. Note the linear band of scar tissue across the upper palpebral conjunctiva (Arlt's line). World Health Organization. Trachoma [Internet]. 2013 [cited 30 Jan 2014]. Available from: http://www.who.int/blindness/causes/priority/en/index2.html≥

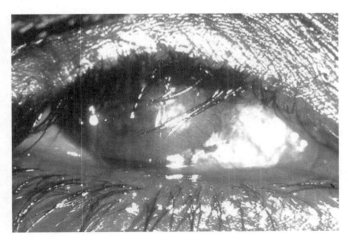

FIGURE 28.10 Trachoma grading: trachoma grade TT, with clear inturning of the eyelashes to contact the ocular surface (trichiasis). World Health Organization. Trachoma [Internet]. 2013 [cited 30 Jan 2014]. Available from: http://www.who.int/blindness/causes/priority/en/index2.html≥

the corneal epithelium (Figure 28.10). When the integrity of the epithelium is compromised, the avascular and relatively immunocompromised cornea becomes susceptible to potentially catastrophic bacterial and fungal infections. If the eyelid position is not surgically corrected, chronic irritation will eventually lead to scarring and opacification of the cornea.

Differential Diagnosis

Trachoma: Bilateral, chronic, or recurrent conjunctivitis with secondary scarring and inturning of eyelids; occurs in clusters within endemic regions.

Bacterial conjunctivitis: Typically unilateral but may be bilateral, and usually with prominent purulence. This disease may be chronic, but it does not cause inturning of the eyelids.

Adenoviral conjunctivitis: Typically bilateral with acute onset of follicular conjunctivitis, usually preceded by a viral prodrome, and occurs in epidemics with a self-limited course. Again, this disease does not cause inturning of eyelids.

Herpes conjunctivitis: Recurrent unilateral conjunctivitis that may cause corneal scarring but does not cause inturning of eyelids.

Vernal conjunctivitis: Perennial allergic conjunctivitis that is more severe in children in tropical climates; it may cause scarring and, rarely, inturning of eyelids. The predominant symptom is itching.

Management

WHO, in conjunction with GET 2020, have developed an approach to trachoma composed of four steps, termed SAFE:

- **S:** surgery for trichiasis
- **A:** antibiotics to treat inflammatory disease
- **F:** face-washing, particularly in children
- **E:** environmental changes, including provision of clean water and improvement of household sanitation

Antibiotics are typically administered in periodic mass treatments of endemic regions. Individual treatment may be effective in the short term, but if the cluster is not treated, recurrence is likely. A single 1g dose of oral azithromycin is recommended; alternately, tetracycline 1% ointment can be used twice daily for 6 weeks.[6]

Entropion should be managed surgically if the eyelashes abrade the cornea (trichiasis). This can usually be seen on direct examination, but further confirmation can be obtained by examining the cornea with a cobalt blue light for fluorescein staining. Trichiasis can be managed by epilation, electrolysis, cryoablation, and entropion repair.

- **Epilation:** Patients themselves can remove eyelashes with forceps. This strategy may be effective for mild trichiasis but is usually insufficient for significant scarring. Lashes tend to regrow in 6 weeks and may be thicker than before.
- **Electrolysis:** The follicle of the eyelash is destroyed with fine wire probes and low-voltage electric current. Although electrolysis is more effective for long-term control than epilation, eyelashes may recur.

- **Cryoablation:** The eyelash follicle is destroyed by freezing with a cryoextractor tip. It may not be as effective as manual epilation, but eyelashes are less likely to recur. It may cause depigmentation in pigmented individuals.
- **Entropion repair:** Significant trichiasis is managed with definitive entropion surgery. Although numerous techniques exist, WHO recommends the bilamellar tarsal rotation procedure due to its efficacy and decreased chance of recurrence. As with any surgical procedure, proper patient selection is critical for success. If only several lashes turn in, one of the aforementioned less-invasive procedures may be sufficient. The patient should be examined closely to ensure proper lid closure. Bilamellar tarsal rotation is contraindicated in the setting of incomplete eyelid closure; in these cases, a more involved lid lengthening procedure may be required (Figure 28.11).[7]

Bilamellar Tarsal Rotation for Cicatricial Entropion

This procedure is the treatment of choice for the management of trichiasis in trachoma but can also be used effectively for other causes of cicatricial entropion, such as severe chemical injury, Stevens-Johnson syndrome, and ocular cicatricial pemphigoid. Stevens-Johnson syndrome is particularly prevalent in certain parts of Africa due to its association with HIV. Treatment of entropion should be reserved for when the disease is stable and inflammation has subsided. The following surgery is described in reference to the upper eyelid, as it is much more commonly affected in trachoma than the lower lid. However, a similar mirror-image procedure can also be performed on the lower eyelid, if needed. If both upper and lower eyelids of the same eye need to be treated, it is recommended that this be done in two separate procedures several weeks apart.[7]

The surgeon operates seated at the head of the patient, who lies supine on the table. Several drops of topical anesthesia (e.g., tetracaine eyedrops or equivalent) are instilled into the eye (Figure 28.12). The patient's face is cleaned with povidone iodine 10% solution. A maximum of 5 ml of lidocaine 2% is injected subcutaneously into the upper eyelid about 3 mm above the eyelid margin. The needle should lie over the tarsal plate and should slide easily from the lateral to the medial aspect of the eyelid as the anesthetic is injected. In the bilamellar tarsal rotation procedure the eyelid is fixed, incised through all layers parallel to the lid margin, and then resutured to rotate the margin outward away from the eye.

Fixing the Eyelid

Two hemostats are placed perpendicular to the margin at both the medial and lateral ends of the eyelid. The hemostats should not extend more than 5 mm from the lid margin, as this will make it difficult to evert the lid margin. Due to concerns of eyelid tissue ischemia, the hemostats should not be left closed over the lid for more than 15 minutes at a time.[7]

Incising the Eyelid

The hemostats are held downward with the eyelid closed as a #15 blade is used to make a horizontal incision through the skin and underlying orbicularis muscle (Figure 28.13). The incision is placed 3 mm above the lid margin, then extended parallel to the lid margin for the full horizontal length of the lid from one hemostat to the other. The eyelid is everted with the hemostats, and a similar horizontal full-length incision is made 3 mm above the lid margin through the conjunctiva and tarsal plate (Figure 28.14). The eyelid is elevated away from the eye with the hemostats. Closed scissors are placed in the conjunctiva-tarsal plate, through the remaining intact muscle, and out through the skin-muscle incision. The scissors are opened to separate the remaining muscle, creating a full-thickness hole (Figure 28.15). The hemostats are removed and bleeding is stopped with firm pressure with gauze. Toothed forceps are used to grasp the eyelid margin, and scissors are used to extend the full thickness incision both medially and laterally through the portions of the eyelid

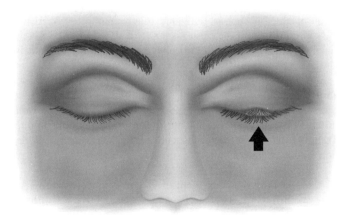

FIGURE 28.11 Incomplete eyelid closure when the patient gently closes the eyes (black arrow) is a contraindication to the "Bilamellar Tarsal Rotation Procedure" and may warrant evaluation by an ophthalmologist for definitive surgical treatment. Adapted from: Reacher M, Foster A, Huber J. *Manual: Trichiasis surgery for trachoma-The bilamellar tarsal rotation procedure.* World Health Organization, 1998. figure 21, p 44.

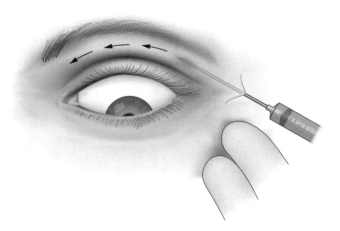

FIGURE 28.12 Bilamellar tarsal rotation procedure: subcutaneous injection of anesthetic. Reacher M, Foster A, Huber J. *Manual: Trichiasis surgery for trachoma-The bilamellar tarsal rotation procedure.* World Health Organization, 1998. figure 6, p 17.

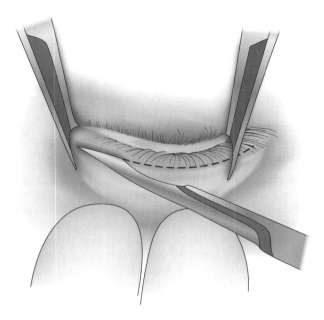

FIGURE 28.13 Bilamellar tarsal rotation procedure: initial partial thickness incision while hemostats stabilize eyelid. Note the position of the hemostats at the medial and lateral canthi. Reacher M, Foster A, Huber J. *Manual: Trichiasis surgery for trachoma-The bilamellar tarsal rotation procedure.* World Health Organization, 1998. figure 9, p. 20.

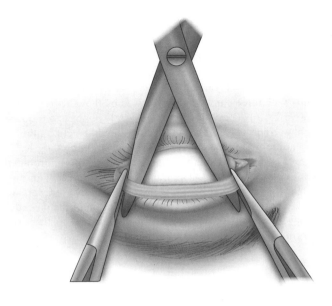

FIGURE 28.15 Bilamellar tarsal rotation procedure: the anterior and posterior lid incisions are united using blunt dissection with scissors. Reacher M, Foster A, Huber J. *Manual: Trichiasis surgery for trachoma-The bilamellar tarsal rotation procedure.* World Health Organization, 1998. figure 11, p. 22.

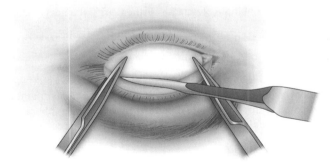

FIGURE 28.14 Bilamellar tarsal rotation procedure: the eyelid is everted and the incision is completed from inner conjunctival side. Reacher M, Foster A, Huber J. *Manual: Trichiasis surgery for trachoma-The bilamellar tarsal rotation procedure.* World Health Organization, 1998. figure 10, p. 21.

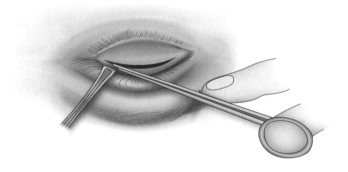

FIGURE 28.16 Bilamellar tarsal rotation procedure: incision is completed medially and laterally. Reacher M, Foster A, Huber J. *Manual: Trichiasis surgery for trachoma-The bilamellar tarsal rotation procedure.* World Health Organization, 1998. figure 12, p. 23.

previously held by the hemostat (Figure 28.16). One should not extend the cut much beyond the medial edge of the tarsal plate, as the marginal artery may be cut. A full-thickness horizontal incision should now extend 3 mm above the margin with a remaining connection at both ends.[7]

Suturing the Eyelid

Sutures are then placed to reattach the distal fragment (lid margin) to the proximal fragment (lid base) in an everted position, so that the eyelashes no longer rub the cornea. This is achieved by anchoring the sutures to the conjunctival surface of the proximal segment, then passing them just anterior to the tarsal plate of the distal segment to exit near the eyelashes (Figure 28.17). With

tension on the sutures, the eyelid margin is rotated outward and upward. Three double-armed 4-0 silk sutures are recommended.

The proximal portion of the eyelid is grasped with toothed forceps and a suture is passed on the inner surface of the eyelid through a 1-mm bite of the tarsal conjunctiva and one quarter-thickness of the tarsal plate, near the middle of the eyelid. The other end of the needle should be passed in a similar manner 2 mm lateral to the other end. Both needles thus emerge from the cut edge of the tarsal plate, forming a loop of suture on the inner conjunctival surface of the proximal segment.

A hemostat is placed on the two strands of sutures to secure them in place, while the other two sutures are placed in an identical manner on either side of the initial suture. The three double-armed sutures in the proximal fragment are now secured to the distal lid margin. Forceps stabilize the distal segment while the two arms of the sutures are successively passed along the front surface of the tarsal plate to emerge through the skin about 1 mm above the eyelashes. The entry point should correspond with the site of the suture in the proximal eyelid fragment so as to not cause distortion of the eyelid. The central suture is tied firmly with three single knots, followed by the other two sutures (Figure 28.18). They should be tied firmly enough to produce a slight overcorrection. The suture ends should be cut 3 mm from the knot to permit easy removal without irritating the eye. Two or three skin sutures are then placed without tension through the skin to close the defect. The final result should show an eyelid with a slight overcorrection and the eyelashes everted well away from the eye (Figure 28.19). At the conclusion of the procedure, tetracycline ointment is instilled in the eye and to the wound margin, and a pad is placed over the eye.[7]

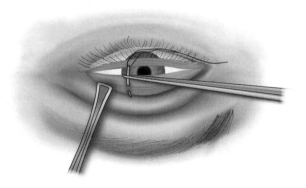

FIGURE 28.17 Bilamellar tarsal rotation procedure: double-armed suture passed partial thickness through inner conjunctiva and out wound. Reacher M, Foster A, Huber J. *Manual: Trichiasis surgery for trachoma-The bilamellar tarsal rotation procedure.* World Health Organization, 1998. figure 13, p. 24.

Postoperative Care

Tetracycline ointment is applied to the eye three times daily for 7 days. The patient is seen on postoperative day 1 to check for infection and proper positioning of the eyelid. If the eyelid is irregular, the rotation too severe, or there is incomplete eyelid closure, then one or more of the sutures can be removed and replaced. Both the skin sutures and the tarsal rotation sutures are removed on postoperative day 8.

Pitfalls

Bleeding: If the initial incision is extended too far medially, the marginal artery can be severed. The blood will be seen emitting from a single source, and this can be closed with a hemostat and tied off. Alternately, the area can be under-sewn with a suture.

Excessive rotation of the tarsus: Excessive external rotation of the tarsus can occur if the distal fragment is too big (incision more than 3 mm from lid margin), if there is excessive tension on the tarsal rotation sutures, or if the sutures emerge within the lashes instead of above them.

Incomplete lid closure: This is a serious complication that should not be left unattended. The patient should have complete closure of the eyelids when gently closing the eyes, as if in sleep. This complication can occur with improper selection of patients who, preoperatively, had an inability to close the eye (lagophthalmos), or it can occur as a result of overcorrection. In this situation, the sutures should be removed and the eyelid massaged downward. If this does not improve lid closure, the patient should be referred to an ophthalmologist for further surgical management.

Cornea

The cornea is a 540-μm-thick tissue that provides a significant portion of the focusing power of the eye, while maintaining transparency through a tight arrangement of collagen fibers and a lack of vascularity. This avascularity, however, predisposes a

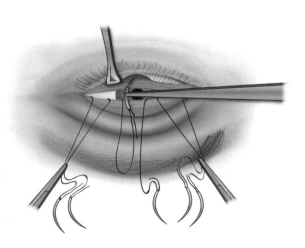

FIGURE 28.18 Bilamellar tarsal rotation procedure: the sutures are passed through the distal segment and tied just above the lashes. Reacher M, Foster A, Huber J. *Manual: Trichiasis surgery for trachoma-The bilamellar tarsal rotation procedure.* World Health Organization, 1998. figure 17, p. 27.

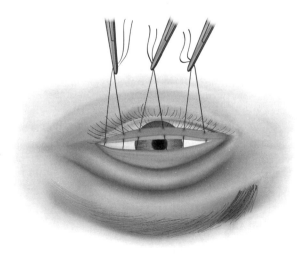

FIGURE 28.19 Bilamellar tarsal rotation procedure: all three sutures have been passed through distal margin and are now tied to evert the eyelid margin. Reacher M, Foster A, Huber J. *Manual: Trichiasis surgery for trachoma-The bilamellar tarsal rotation procedure.* World Health Organization, 1998. figure 18, p. 28.

relatively immunodeficient cornea to infection. Disruption of corneal collagen fibers, whether through trauma, infection, or inflammation, causes opacification and limits vision potential.

Corneal Abrasions

The cornea has the second highest density of nerve endings in the body; hence, corneal abrasions are characteristically quite painful. The sharp pain is accompanied with tearing, photophobia, blurred vision, and conjunctival injection. Examination of the abrasion can be facilitated with topical anesthesia; however, anesthetic should not be used as a treatment, as it can delay healing, promote erosion, and even lead to full corneal perforation. Most corneal abrasions occur as a result of mild trauma, but they can also happen spontaneously in people who have had a previous abrasion or in those with a common dystrophy termed map-dot-fingerprint dystrophy. The abrasion can sometimes be visualized with direct illumination, but can be appreciated more readily using fluorescein stain under a cobalt blue light (Figure 28.20). Abrasions are distinguished from corneal ulcers by the absence of an opaque infiltrate. An opaque white infiltrate in the corneal stroma is concerning, as an infection may be present. In HICs, corneal abrasions are occasionally patched. However, this is not a preferred practice in the developing world due to lower levels of sanitation and higher incidence of fungal corneal ulcers from horticultural injuries. Corneal abrasions are best treated with prophylactic topical antibiotics (e.g., moxifloxacin ophthalmic eyedrops) four times daily with close observation until the defect heals. Corneal abrasions typically heal within 48 to 72 hours.

Corneal Ulcers

A corneal ulcer is an infection of one or more layers of the cornea with loss of the overlying corneal epithelium. A white opacification of the cornea is concerning, as it may represent a corneal ulcer. This is in contrast to a corneal abrasion, where the cornea remains relatively clear. Corneal ulceration frequently accompanies trachomatous entropion and trichiasis. Other risk factors for corneal ulceration include inability to completely close the eye (lagophthalmos), decreased corneal sensation (e.g., ocular herpes simplex virus), and corneal abrasion (particularly if it involves organic matter). In HICs, bacterial infections are by far the most common cause of infectious corneal ulcers. In contrast, in the developing world, particularly in tropical or semitropical rural communities, fungal infections are more common. It can be difficult to clinically distinguish a bacterial corneal infection from a fungal one. Fungal infections are often preceded by an abrasion with plant matter and tend to follow a prolonged, slowly progressive course. Bacterial infections typically present with a more acute, rapidly progressive course. The most common bacterial pathogens are *Streptococcus, Staphylococcus, Haemophilus,* and *Moraxella.* When an acutely purulent response is noted, coliform bacteria such as *Pseudomonas* and *Klebsiella* should be considered. If the response is hyperacute with copious purulent discharge, *Neisseria gonorrhoeae* may be the responsible pathogen and should be treated both topically and systemically. Progression or resolution of the ulcer can be gauged by changes in the patient's subjective pain, vision, size of the corneal infiltrate, and—if present—height of the layered intraocular pus (hypopyon) (Figure 28.21). If an ulcer progresses despite two days of maximal treatment, a fungal etiology should be considered. A corneal scraping with appropriate cultures and stains may be instrumental in identifying the bacterial or fungal pathogen in these complicated cases.

Differential Diagnosis

Sterile ulcer: A white corneal ulcer may be present in the absence of an active infection. Etiologies may include rheumatoid arthritis or other collagen vascular disease, vitamin A deficiency, vernal keratoconjunctivitis, or an old scar. In these situations, the conjunctival injection is either absent or less prominent, and the conjunctiva overlying the infiltrate may be intact.

Herpes simplex/herpes zoster keratitis: Both herpes simplex and zoster may cause a unilateral injected eye with corneal opacity. There will usually be a history of recurrent episodes. In the case of zoster, old skin lesions in the V1 distribution of the trigeminal nerve may be noted. Corneal sensation can be compared

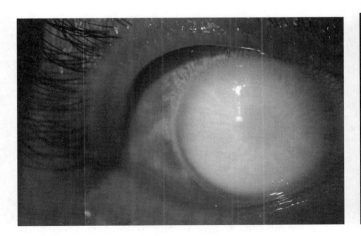

FIGURE 28.20 Corneal abrasion. The large central area of epithelial loss can be made evident by fluorescein staining and cobalt blue light in an office setting. Image by James Gilman.

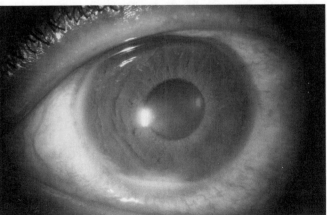

FIGURE 28.21 Corneal ulcer with layering of inflammatory cells (hypopyon) within the anterior chamber. Image by Matthew Bujak and Geoffrey Tabin.

between the two eyes with a cotton swab or tissue, as herpetic infections are often characterized by corneal hypesthesia.

Staphylococcal hypersensitivity: Peripheral corneal infiltrates can be present where the lid margins contact the conjunctiva. These lesions are the result of an immunologic reaction to staphylococcal inflammation of the overlying lid margins. They follow a more benign and indolent course, with less pain, less inflammation, no hypopyon, and an epithelial defect that is smaller than the active white corneal lesion (Figure 28.22).

Residual corneal foreign body: a corneal foreign body can cause opacification, significant inflammation, and even hypopyon formation in the anterior chamber.

Management

Corneal ulcers may progress quickly and are best managed by an ophthalmologist. If, however, access to an ophthalmologist is limited, then management may need to be initiated and continued by a comprehensive physician. If possible, the patient should be hospitalized for treatment and close observation. Cefazolin (100 mg in 0.5cc) can be injected daily into the subconjunctival space with a 25-gauge needle. Alternatively, fortified cefazolin (25 to 50 mg/ml) can be administered topically every hour. If cefazolin is not available, gentamicin 0.5 cc is widely available and can be substituted for the subconjunctival injection, although it is not particularly effective against *Streptococcus pneumoniae*. Following the subconjunctival injection, tetracycline 1% or sulfacetamide 10% should be administered hourly. Atropine 1% can be applied daily to improve patient comfort and to reduce the likelihood of intraocular scarring. When available, staining, cultures, and lab sensitivities should ideally guide the choice of antibiotics.

If the infection continues to progress despite 48 hours of treatment, particularly in hot, moist climates and in injuries with vegetable matter, a fungal etiology should be considered. Ocular antifungal drugs can be expensive and difficult to obtain. If they are not available, a buffered nystatin solution for topical ocular use may be prepared with powder from nystatin tablets or

vaginal suppositories dissolved in sterile and pH-balanced solution. A pharmacist can assist in preparing the 1% concentration that should be applied hourly to the affected eye. If an antifungal is not available, a drop of 5% povidone iodine solution can be instilled every 12 hours. Even with use of proper antifungals, fungal infections often take a full month to resolve. Periodic debridement of the corneal epithelium by scraping with a surgical blade may be required to facilitate intraocular penetration of the topical antifungal. While re-epithelialization of bacterial infections is a sign of resolution, fungal infections may progress in spite of epithelial healing.

Irrespective of fungal or bacterial etiology, if the ulcer continues to progress despite medical management, transposition of a conjunctival flap over the corneal ulcer should be considered. This procedure, known as a Gunderson flap, is particularly helpful in emergent situations with significant corneal thinning or in small infectious perforations. By covering the corneal ulcer with vascularized conjunctiva, a mechanical barrier is placed over an impending or already perforated cornea; more importantly, a blood supply with its immunologic benefits is placed within closer proximity of the normally avascular corneal ulcer.

Modified Gunderson Conjunctival Flap for Corneal Ulceration

Preparation

After topical anesthesia (e.g., proparacaine), the eye and periocular skin is prepared with 5% povidone iodine and an eyelid speculum is inserted. A cotton-tipped applicator is used to manually remove the loose epithelium between the diseased portion of the cornea and the adjacent limbus. The epithelium should be entirely denuded for an area up to 2 mm beyond the corneal lesion. A cotton-tipped applicator soaked in povidone iodine is touched to the lesion and allowed to absorb without rinsing. Approximately 1 ml of 1%–2% lidocaine with epinephrine (dilution, 1:100 000) is injected subconjunctivally as close to the corneal lesion as possible, and the cotton-tipped applicator is rolled over the inflated conjunctiva to spread the anesthetic agent.

Creation of Conjunctival Flap

Fine Westcott scissors are used to make a crescentic perilimbal incision of approximately 3 clock-hours in the conjunctiva. Care should be taken to separate the conjunctiva from the underlying Tenon's capsule. The conjunctiva can be easily undermined with blunt dissection of the conjunctiva from the Tenon's capsule. If a full thickness corneal ulcer is present, both the conjunctiva and the Tenon's capsule should be transposed together. Dissection should extend to the firm sclera and Tenon's capsule should be undermined from the underlying scleral surface. Depending on the distance of the corneal ulcer from the limbus, an appropriately sized area of conjunctiva should be mobilized to cover the entire corneal ulcer and the intervening, unaffected corneal surface. A second outer incision parallel to the initial conjunctival peritomy should be made distal to the first incision. This second, parallel incision mobilizes a strip of conjunctival tissue for transposition. At this point, a crescentic flap of conjunctival tissue

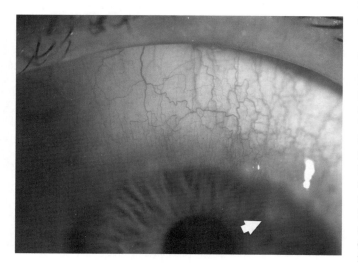

FIGURE 28.22 Staphylococcal marginal disease: note the inflammation of the corneal limbus, with a characteristic corneal lesion with a clearing between the lesion and the limbus (white arrow). Image by James Gilman.

(with or without underlying Tenon's capsule), with its own blood supply, should be freely mobile to cover the corneal ulcer. Fine-toothed forceps are used to pull the conjunctiva over the lesion. If the flap cannot extend to fully cover the lesion, the conjunctiva can be further undermined, or the two crescentic incisions can be extended to involve more than 3 clock hours.

Securing Conjunctival Flap over Corneal Ulcer

The suturing technique is one of the most crucial steps and the key to success in this procedure. The flap is secured to the cornea using 8-0 Vicryl sutures. The first four sutures are placed at the limbus where the tractioned conjunctiva overlies the cornea. Single interrupted sutures are placed half-thickness through the cornea, taking care not to incorporate any surrounding corneal epithelium. Each individual bite incorporates 0.5 mm of the conjunctival flap and 0.5 to 1 mm of peripheral corneal tissue (Figure 28.23). The knots should be tied in a 3-1-1 manner and then buried into the cornea or conjunctiva. Two more interrupted sutures are placed in a similar manner on either side of the flap, for a total of eight sutures. Antibiotic ointment and a cycloplegic drop are applied prior to patching the eye closed.[8]

Postoperative Care

The patch is removed on postoperative day 1 and the flap is examined to ensure proper coverage over the corneal ulcer. Appropriate antimicrobial topical medications are continued on an hourly basis. They are gradually tapered over the course of many days until the infection heals. If the sutures become loose, they can be removed 10 days to 2 weeks postoperatively. Otherwise, they can be left in place until they dissolve or cause irritation. Clinical improvement should be evident within the first postoperative week.

Pitfalls

Retraction of conjunctival flap: The flap over the cornea should be neither too tight nor too loose. A tight flap will retract and tear away from the corneal lesion, while a loose flap will not heal and may come off during the postoperative period. The patient should be instructed not to rub the eye, and a shield (or even a Styrofoam cup cut transversely in half) can be placed over the eye if there is a concern. The conjunctival flap should be watched closely for retraction over the first 2 postoperative weeks, as scarring tends to occur during this period.

Progression of corneal ulcer: Infections in the developing world tend to follow an aggressive course and may progress despite appropriate medical treatment and the use of a Gunderson conjunctival flap. If the lesion continues to progress, the patient should be referred to an ophthalmologist for further management with keratectomy, corneal transplantation, or evisceration of the globe.

Autoimmune peripheral corneal ulcers: Immune-related corneal ulcers typically assume a crescentic shape adjacent to the limbus. The associated intraocular inflammation is less severe, and an inflammatory hypopyon is very unlikely. A Gunderson conjunctival flap should be avoided in these situations, as the improved vascularization may worsen the autoimmune process.

Retained corneal foreign body: The cornea should be examined closely for a retained foreign body, especially if the history is consistent with projectile trauma. In this case, a conjunctival flap should not be used. Instead, the foreign body should be removed with a 27-gauge needle and appropriate prophylactic topical antibiotics should be instilled until the epithelial defect heals completely.

Acute Angle Closure Glaucoma

Most cases of glaucoma are characterized by an insidious, asymptomatic onset with gradual progressive loss of peripheral vision. These require medical management with topical and, occasionally, oral medications. If medical treatment fails in these chronic conditions, surgery is best performed by an ophthalmologist experienced in glaucoma filtration surgery. In contrast, acute angle closure glaucoma (Figure 28.24), as its name implies, typically has an acute or sub-acute onset of pain with blurred vision, colored halos around lights, and frontal headache. It usually occurs in small, hyperopic eyes with mature cataractous lenses, and it can be precipitated by dim lighting, accommodation during reading, mydriatics, or medications with anticholinergic properties, such as antihistamines and antipsychotics. On examination, the conjunctiva will be injected, and the pupil will be fixed and in mid-dilation. If a slit lamp or surgical loupes are available, prominent shallowing of the anterior chamber can be appreciated through the somewhat hazy and oedematous cornea. If an intraocular pressure (IOP) measuring device is available, the IOP will typically measure greater than 40 mmHg (normal range is 8–21 mmHg). If such an instrument is not available, the IOP can be estimated and compared between both eyes by balloting the superior aspect of each individual eyeball through closed eyelids with the index fingers of both hands. As one finger presses the eye, the adjacent finger alternately senses the fluctuation in the globe pressure. In acute angle closure glaucoma, a marked difference should be noted between the affected and unaffected eyes. Acute angle closure glaucoma is a surgical emergency. The pain is usually intolerable with secondary diaphoresis, nausea, and vomiting. If left untreated, scarring of the peripheral angle of the anterior chamber can lead to permanent angle closure glaucoma and eventual blindness. The elevated pressure can damage the optic nerve, cause corneal decompensation, and occasionally lead to retinal vein or retinal artery obstruction.

Differential Diagnosis

Secondary angle closure glaucoma: Angle closure glaucoma can occur from an inflammatory or neovascular membrane pulling the anterior chamber angle closed. Neovascularization typically occurs with significant ocular ischemia either from advanced diabetes or from ischemia resulting from obstruction of the central retinal vein (Figure 28.25). In the latter situation, neovascular angle closure will classically be preceded by a sudden loss of vision 2–3 months prior. If angle closure is caused by an inflammatory membrane, the patient will usually give a history of recurrent red eye and photophobia consistent with intraocular inflammation (uveitis), although uveitis can sometimes be relatively asymptomatic.

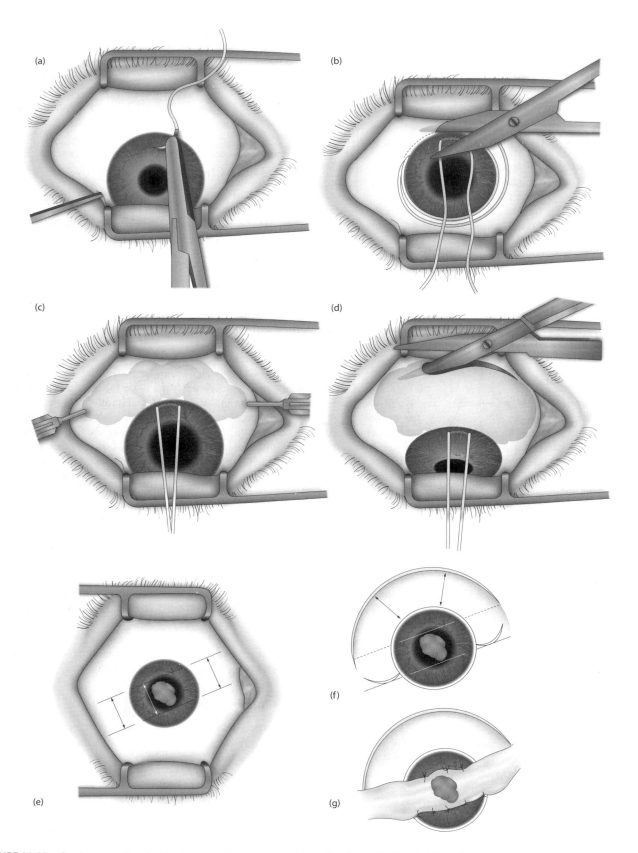

FIGURE 28.23 Gunderson conjunctival flap for corneal ulcer. Adapted from: Krachmer JH, Mannis MJ, Holland EJ. *Cornea: Surgery of the cornea and conjunctiva—Volume 2*, 3rd ed. Philadelphia: Mosby Elsevier, 2013. P. 1643 fig 145.2, fig 145.3).

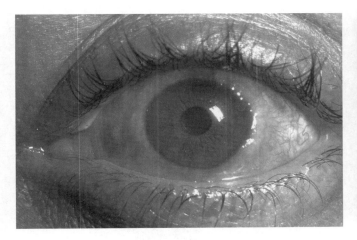

FIGURE 28.24 Angle closure glaucoma: note especially the shallow appearance of the anterior chamber. Image by James Gilman.

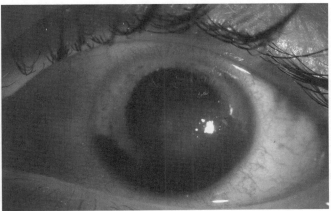

FIGURE 28.26 Hyphema: note the consolidation of the blood in the anterior chamber. At any time when blood is pathologically present within the eye, there is a risk of trabecular outflow obstruction and subsequent glaucoma. Image by James Gilman.

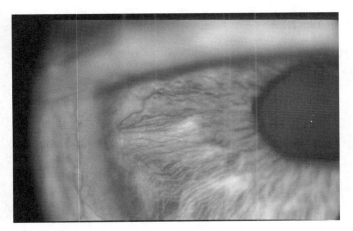

FIGURE 28.25 Neovascularization of the iris. Image by James Gilman.

Traumatic (hemolytic) glaucoma: With a history of trauma, red blood cells may be noted in the anterior chamber on close inspection with a slit lamp (Figure 28.26).

Pigmentary or inflammatory open angle glaucoma: An open anterior chamber angle is seen upon examination. Also, pigmentary or inflammatory precipitates can be noted on the endothelial layer of cornea.

Management

The urgency of treatment depends on the severity and duration of the attack. Severe, permanent damage may occur within several hours. If vision is hand motion or worse, treatment should be started immediately and should include all available glaucoma medications, administered topically and orally, as well as a cholinergic drop, and anti-inflammatory drops:

- topical ß blocker (e.g., timolol 0.5%)
- topical alpha agonist (e.g., brimonidine 0.2%)
- topical carbonic anhydrase inhibitor (e.g., dorzolamide)
- oral or parenteral carbonic anhydrase inhibitor (e.g., acetazolamide 500 mg PO or IV)
- topical steroid (e.g., prednisolone acetate 1%)
- topical cholinergic x 2 doses (pilocarpine 1 to 2%): do not use if patient has had cataract surgery or is aphakic (no lens)

If IOP and vision do not improve within 1 hour, then repeat all topical medications and give intravenous mannitol 1–2 g/kg IV over 45 minutes (a 500-ml bag of 20% mannitol contains 100 g of mannitol).

Recheck IOP and vision 1 hour later. If there is no improvement after this second course of treatment, then surgical peripheral iridectomy should be performed to reestablish a connection between the posterior and anterior chambers of the eye. Some surgeons advocate prophylactic iridectomy in the fellow eye several days later.

Surgical Peripheral Iridectomy

Topical anesthetic (e.g., proparacaine) is instilled in the eye. The periocular skin is prepped with povidone/iodine 5% and several drops are instilled into the eye. A lid speculum is placed. A 15-degree blade is used to make a full-thickness, 45-degree stab incision through the peripheral cornea at the 2-o'clock (superonasal or superotemporal) position. The conjunctiva is excised for 2 clock hours just adjacent to the limbus at the 10-o'clock position (Figure 28.27). Hemostasis is achieved with cautery.[3]

A 2- to 3-mm-long groove is made in the mid-anterior limbus at the 10-o'clock position. The incision should be perpendicular to the cornea at a two-thirds-thickness depth. Preplace two 9-0 silk, 7-0 Vicryl, or 10-0 nylon single interrupted sutures through both sides of the groove, looping out of the wound (Figure 28.28). Clamps can be placed on the sutures and the assistant can place traction on the two sutures, thus gaping the wound for better exposure.

A microsurgical blade is used to carefully scratch down at the base of the groove to obtain controlled entry into the anterior chamber. The wound should be perpendicular to the cornea (not

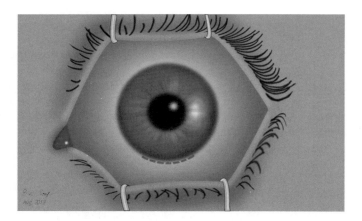

FIGURE 28.27 Surgical peripheral iridectomy: limited conjunctival peritomy at the site of planned incision through the limbus. Image by Bin Song.

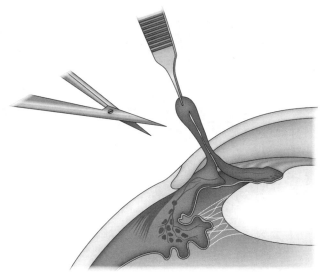

FIGURE 28.29 Surgical peripheral iridectomy: forceps are used to grasp the iris as it prolapses through the wound. Image by Bin Song. Adapted from: Hersh PS, Zagelbaum BA, Cremers SL. *Ophthalmic Surgical Procedures*, 2nd ed. New York: Thieme Publishing, 2009.

Alternatively, preservative-free Miochol (cholinergic) can be injected with a fine cannula through the original sideport incision placed at the 2-o'clock position. Inspect the pupil to ensure it is round and there is no iris incarceration in the wound. The anterior chamber should be deep and a defect should be visible in the iris. The preplaced corneal wound sutures can be used to close the wound with two single interrupted sutures tied in a 3-1-1 knot. If the anterior chamber is shallow, the eye can be reinflated through the 10-o'clock sideport wound. The eye can be palpated with the index finger to ensure proper intraocular pressure. If done correctly, the sideport incision is small and self-sealing and does not need to be sutured. If there is any concern that it is leaking, a single interrupted nylon suture can be placed. Topical antibiotic and steroid ointment is placed in the eye and a patch and shield are applied.

Postoperative Care

Cycloplegic eyedrops (e.g., cyclopentolate 1%) instilled twice daily for 2 weeks should be given. Steroid drops (e.g., prednisolone acetate 1%) are used four times daily for the first week and twice daily for the second week. IOP is monitored closely in both eyes during the follow-up period.

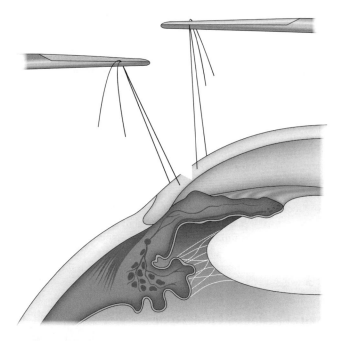

FIGURE 28.28 Surgical peripheral iridectomy: pre-placed sutures surrounding the corneal entry wound. Image by Bin Song.

Pitfalls

Chronic angle closure glaucoma: If the angle closure glaucoma has been chronic, it may not respond to surgical iridectomy, as permanent scarring of the anterior chamber angle may be present.

Intraocular mass: Rarely, angle closure glaucoma can be the result of a posterior, "pushing" mechanism from the vitreous, such as an intraocular tumor. Prior to performing a surgical iridectomy, a fundus exam should be attempted. Due to corneal

shelved) and about 2 mm in length to facilitate prolapse of the iris. Either traction on the sutures or gentle pressure on the posterior lip of the incision is used to prolapse the iris out through the wound (Figure 28.29). If the iris does not prolapse with these maneuvers, smooth-tipped forceps can be used to grasp the iris, with careful attention not to grasp the underlying lens or zonules. After the iris is prolapsed, fine 0.12 mm forceps are used to grasp the iris while Vannas or de Wecker scissors make a full thickness cut of the iris. Ensure that the specimen is full-thickness by examining the resected specimen for dark iris pigment epithelium on the posterior side and by directly visualizing a full thickness defect in the remaining iris.[3]

The iris is reposited back into the anterior chamber by irrigating the main wound with balanced salt solution on a fine cannula.

edema, the visibility may, however, be compromised. Although it may be slightly diminished, a red reflex should still be present. In a dark environment, a penlight can also be placed on the sclera to transilluminate the globe. Intraocular tumors may cast a dark shadow. The other eye can be transilluminated for comparison.

Lens damage: Care must be taken not to damage the underlying lens or zonules while performing the iridectomy.

Iris bleeding: Hemorrhage can occur from the cut iris. When the eye is closed at the end of the case, the normal IOP serves to tamponade the bleeding. The anterior chamber blood will typically resorb within a week or two. If the blood layers out to completely fill more than 50% of the eye, or if the IOP remains elevated, the patient should be referred for tertiary care by an ophthalmologist.

Incomplete iridectomy: The surgeon must ensure that the iridectomy is patent by visualizing pigment on the excised iris. The red reflex should be visible through the iris defect on retroillumination (Figure 28.30).

Cataract Surgery

Cataract is the leading cause of blindness worldwide; the developing world shoulders 90% of the burden (Figure 28.31).[9] Manual small incision cataract surgery (SICS) is one of the most successful surgeries performed, with a cost-effectiveness equivalent to immunization.[10] This technique involves minimal equipment and can be performed in less than 10 minutes by an experienced ophthalmologist. Despite its high success rate, cataract surgery is a complicated microsurgical procedure that involves incising the cornea, opening the lenticular capsular bag, and removing the mature cataractous lens, followed by replacement with an artificial lens. As such, it is a procedure potentially fraught with significant complications and should only be performed by an ophthalmologist proficient in appropriate microsurgical techniques.

Pterygium Surgery

Pterygia are fibrovascular overgrowths that extend over the cornea in a wing-shaped manner from the adjacent medial or lateral conjunctiva. These growths are common in the developing world where people have high exposure to environmental irritants and ultraviolet radiation. The slow progression of these lesions can lead to eventual vision loss. Pterygium surgery should be performed by an ophthalmologist experienced in complete resection of pterygia with subsequent placement of conjunctival autografts. Improper surgical technique often leads to more aggressive recurrence and possible restriction of ocular motility. If the patient reports progression of the pterygium, and the lesion extends more than 3 mm from the limbal margin onto the cornea, referral to an ophthalmologist should be sought. Once the pterygium begins to encroach on the central cornea, the resultant scarring and astigmatism can cause irreversible vision loss (Figure 28.32).

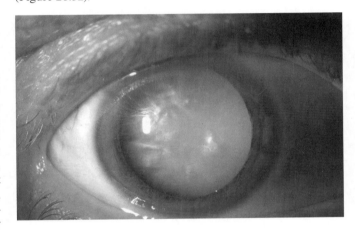

FIGURE 28.31 Mature cataract: dense opaque cataracts are commonly found in regions where access to ophthalmic care is limited. Image by Matthew Bujak and Geoffrey Tabin,

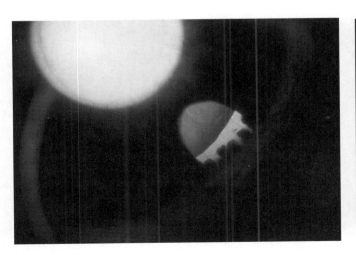

FIGURE 28.30 Slit lamp retroillumination shows patent surgical iridectomy. Underlying structures such as the lens, its zonules, and the ciliary body are visible. Care should be taken not to damage these structures during surgical iridectomy. Image by Matthew Bujak and Geoffrey Tabin.

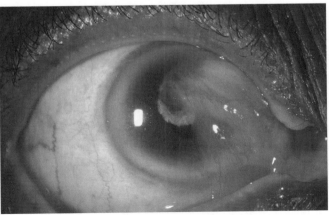

FIGURE 28.32 Severe pterygium crossing the central visual axis: although this pterygium can still be surgically removed, it would have ideally been excised prior to entering the central 3mm of the cornea, as some of the vision loss will now be irreversible, due to corneal scarring and irregular astigmatism. Image by Matthew Bujak and Geoffrey Tabin.

COMMENTARY

John Nkurikiye, Rwanda

This chapter is well written and easy to understand, even for those who do not specialize in ophthalmology. Conjunctivitis was not covered in this text as it is not a condition that is managed surgically. Vernal conjunctivitis however is a leading cause of morbidity in tropical climates and as such the the primary healthcare professional whether surgeon or comprehensive physician should be familiar with its differential diagnosis and management.

It is also helpful for the reader to note that some topics are covered in a lot of detail while others are summarized, so I will comment on several of them. With regard to eyelids, styes or internal hordeola should be mentioned; both are very common and present as localized swelling of the eyelid, but styes are painful and chalazia usually are not. With regard to trachoma, I think it would be helpful for readers to consider the complete WHO grading scale instead of focusing on TF and TS; it is good to remember signs and complications. The section on corneal ulcers is well covered, but I want to mention quinolones eyedrops, which are now readily available at local markets. They are inexpensive and have become the first line of treatment for corneal ulcers, even in some HICs.

29

Dentistry

Joel S. Reynolds
Robert P. Horne

Introduction

Proper understanding of oral and dental anatomy is of utmost importance when treating issues involving the oral cavity. The maxillary and mandibular teeth are shown in Figure 29.1. Figure 29.2 shows an overview of intraoral anatomy. Teeth are composed of enamel, dentin, and pulp tissue and surrounded by the periodontium. The periodontium consists of the gingiva, periodontal ligament, and connective tissue fibers (Figure 29.3). The most common system used to identify teeth is the universal numbering system. The teeth are numbered 1 through 32 starting with the right maxillary third molar, continuing to the left maxillary third molar, down to the left mandibular third molar, and continuing to the right mandibular third molar (Figure 29.4). While the universal numbering system may be the most universally employed system, there are still other numbering systems used by dental professionals, such as the Federation Dentaire Internationale (FDI). Understanding of dental and oral terminology will also facilitate communication regarding issues of the oral cavity.

Local Anesthesia

Armamentarium

The typical armamentarium used when providing local anesthesia for procedures in and around the oral cavity consists of three main components: the syringe, the needle, and the local anesthetic. Many syringes used in dentistry and oral and maxillofacial surgery accept dental cartridges of local anesthetic, which are usually 1.7 mL in volume (Figure 29.5). This is not a requirement for administration of local anesthesia in the oral cavity; a disposable or nondisposable syringe in which the local anesthetic must be aspirated is acceptable as well.[1]

Syringes that accept dental cartridges of local anesthetic usually consist of a thumb ring, a finger grip, a barrel, a piston with harpoon, and a needle adaptor. These come in disposable and nondisposable forms.[1]

Most needles will consist of a bevel, shaft, hub, and syringe adaptor (Figure 29.6). Syringes used with dental cartridges will also have a cartridge-penetration end. Disposable, presterilized stainless-steel needles are recommended.[1]

Choices to make when selecting a needle include the gauge and length. The most common gauges of needle used in dentistry

are 25-, 27-, and 30-gauge. The 25-gauge needle will exhibit less deflection than a 27- or 30-gauge needle, and is something to keep in mind especially when administering local anesthesia through a larger thickness of soft tissue. Larger gauge needles are also less prone to breakage and are easier to aspirate. There does not appear to be any significant difference in pain upon needle insertion among these three gauges.[1]

Needle length is another variable to consider. Most needles used for dental anesthesia come in either long or short forms, usually corresponding to around 22 and 32 mm, respectively. One should avoid inserting a needle to the hub, as this is the weakest point and most prone to breakage. A long needle can be used for most injections as long as one keeps in mind the appropriate depth of insertion. Some practitioners may feel more comfortable using short needles to avoid over-insertion. Short needles are generally acceptable for most injection techniques with the exception of the infraorbital nerve block, maxillary nerve block, inferior alveolar nerve block, and Vazirani-Akinosi mandibular nerve block, which require a long needle to reach the appropriate depth of insertion.[1]

Dental cartridges containing local anesthetic are commonly used and consist of a glass tube with a stopper, aluminum cap, and diaphragm (Figure 29.7). Many different types of local anesthetic are available in dental cartridges, including but not limited to: articaine, bupivacaine, lidocaine, mepivacaine, and prilocaine (many available with or without epinephrine). Cartridges should not be used if any signs of damage or tampering are present (rust, cracked glass, large bubbles in cartridge, etc.).[1]

Proper loading of the cartridge-type syringe consists of five steps:

1. Retract the piston fully.
2. Place the cartridge in the syringe barrel, rubber stopper end first, with the diaphragm toward the needle adapter.
3. Engage the harpoon by gently pushing the piston until the harpoon is engaged in the plunger.
4. Attach the needle to the syringe by screwing the needle onto the needle adapter of the syringe. Use gentle pressure to push the needle toward the syringe while screwing it onto the needle adapter.[1]

General Technique

General principles should be followed when administering local anesthetic in the oral cavity. After correctly loading the syringe, extrude a small amount of local anesthetic from the needle to ensure adequate flow and correct loading. The patient should then

Eruption (year)

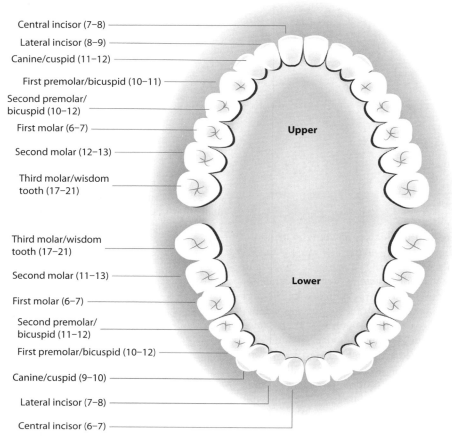

Central incisor (7–8)
Lateral incisor (8–9)
Canine/cuspid (11–12)
First premolar/bicuspid (10–11)
Second premolar/bicuspid (10–12)
First molar (6–7)
Second molar (12–13)
Third molar/wisdom tooth (17–21)

Third molar/wisdom tooth (17–21)
Second molar (11–13)
First molar (6–7)
Second premolar/bicuspid (11–12)
First premolar/bicuspid (10–12)
Canine/cuspid (9–10)
Lateral incisor (7–8)
Central incisor (6–7)

Upper

Lower

FIGURE 29.1 Maxillary and mandibular teeth. Guniita. Adult Dental Chart [Internet]. 2010 [cited 2014 Jan 28]. Available from: http://www.dreamstime.com/stock-images-adult-dental-chart-image18926014≥.

be positioned correctly; generally, supine or beach-chair positioning is preferred depending on the area to be anesthetized (Figure 29.8).[1]

Proper communication with the patient as to what to expect from the injection can help to alleviate his or her fear and anxiety prior to and during the local anesthetic administration. The needle and syringe should also be kept out of the patient's line of sight if possible. If topical anesthetic is to be used, the tissue at the injection site should be dried prior to administration, and the anesthetic given 1 to 2 minutes to achieve topical anesthesia prior to injection. Establishing a hand rest or finger rest helps to steady the needle before and during injection. The tissues at the site of injection should be made taut by retraction using a finger or other retractor. The needle can now be gently inserted into the mucosa and slowly advanced toward the target.

Aspiration should be performed once the needle has reached the intended site of injection to ensure that the tip of the needle does not lie within a blood vessel. This is done to avoid intravascular injection of local anesthetic. Slight backward pressure using the thumb ring of the syringe supplies enough negative pressure to allow inflow of blood into the anesthetic solution should the needle lie in a blood vessel. If any blood return is noted, the needle should be repositioned and negative aspiration confirmed before local anesthetic is deposited. Repeated aspiration should be performed before and during injection. After proper placement of the tip of the needle is confirmed with negative aspirations, the local anesthetic solution should be deposited slowly, at a rate of 1.0 mL per minute. This helps to diminish discomfort associated with anesthetic deposition. The needle is then slowly withdrawn and recapped once outside the mouth.[1]

Preventing needle stick injuries is of paramount importance. To this end, there are two commonly used techniques for injury prevention. The first involves a formal needle cap holder. In the absence of a needle cap holder, the needle cap can simply be scooped up with the needle. At no time should two hands be used to recap the needle. Three major types of local anesthetic injections are possible in the oral cavity; local infiltration, field blocks, and nerve blocks. Local infiltration involves anesthetizing small terminal nerve endings in the area of interest. Field blocks anesthetize larger terminal nerve branches allowing for a greater area of anesthesia. A nerve block is achieved when local anesthetic is deposited near a main nerve trunk, usually at a distance away from the area of treatment.[1]

Maxillary Anesthesia

Local Infiltration

Pulpal anesthesia of the maxillary dentition is most commonly obtained by local infiltration of local anesthetic into the maxillary labial mucosa at the root apex region of the tooth of interest. Deposition of approximately 1.0 mL of anesthetic is

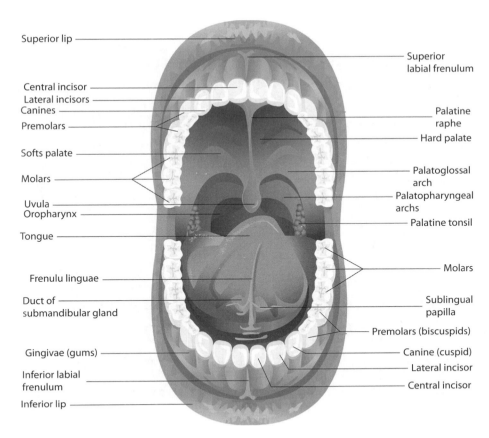

FIGURE 29.2 Intraoral anatomy inspected during examination. Legger. Cross Section of a Typical Tooth [Internet]. 2012 [cited 2014 Jan 28]. http://www.dreamstime.com/stock-photo-cross-section-typical-tooth-image24880250≥.

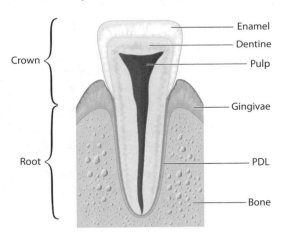

FIGURE 29.3 Anatomy of molar tooth. Stockshoppe. Mouth Anatomy [Internet]. 2012 [cited 2014 Jan 28]. Available from: http://www.dreamstime.com/stock-photo-mouth-anatomy-image24267570.

usually adequate. This anesthetizes the maxillary tooth and labial mucosa/gingiva.[1]

Posterior Superior Alveolar Nerve Block

A posterior superior alveolar nerve block will provide anesthesia to the maxillary first, second, and third molar teeth and associated buccal soft tissues. This injection is performed by inserting the needle at the height of the mucobuccal fold above the maxillary second molar, and advancing it approximately 16 mm at

45 degree angles superiorly, inward, and backward. Then 0.9 to 1.7 mL of anesthetic is deposited (Figure 29.9).[1]

Anterior Superior Alveolar Nerve Block

An anterior superior alveolar nerve block provides anesthesia to the maxillary incisors, canine teeth, and usually premolars on the side of injection. The labial soft tissue associated with these teeth and the lower eyelid, lateral nose, and upper lip will also be anesthetized. Palpation the infraorbital foramen (intended injection site) extraorally can help orient the operator prior to injection. This injection is performed by inserting the needle at the height of the mucobuccal fold over the first premolar and advancing the needle approximately 16 mm. Then 0.9 to 1.2 mL of anesthetic is deposited (Figure 29.10, Figure 29.11, and Figure 29.12).[1]

Palatal Anesthesia

Palatal anesthesia of the maxilla can be achieved by two injections; the greater palatine and nasopalatine nerve blocks. The greater palatine nerve provides innervation to the posterior hard palate to the midline, usually to the level of the first premolar anteriorly. The anterior hard palate is innervated by the nasopalatine nerve, and a nerve block will achieve anesthesia of the anterior hard palate on both sides of the midline.[1]

Greater Palatine Nerve Block

The first step in performing a greater palatine nerve block is locating the greater palatine foramen. This can be performed by

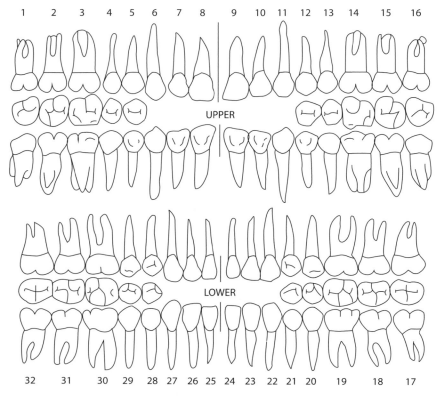

FIGURE 29.4 Universal tooth numbering system. Image by Costas Bougalis.

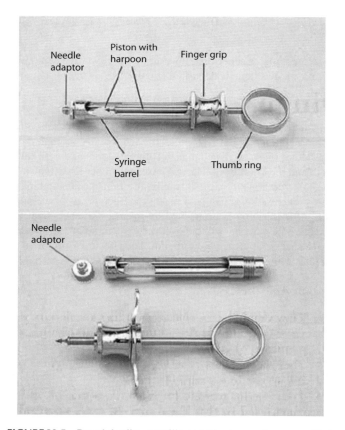

FIGURE 29.5 Breech-loading, metallic, cartridge-type syringe; assembled, and disassembled local anesthetic syringe. Malamed. *The Handbook of Local Anesthesia*, 5th ed. London: Elsevier, 2004.

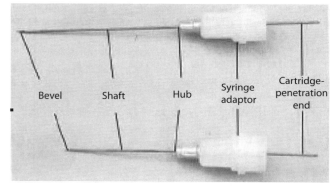

FIGURE 29.6 Components of dental local anesthetic needle. Long needle (top), short needle (bottom). Malamed. *The Handbook of Local Anesthesia*, 5th ed. London: Elsevier, 2004.

placing a cotton swab or blunt instrument at the junction of the hard palate and maxillary alveolar process. A depression can be located at the area of the greater palatine foramen using the swab or instrument. The needle is advanced in this area until bone is contacted, and approximately 0.5 mL of anesthetic is deposited.[1]

Nasopalatine Nerve Block

The main landmark for the nasopalatine nerve block is the incisive papilla. The site of injection is just lateral to the incisive papilla, at a 45-degree angle. The needle is inserted until bone is contacted, and approximately 0.2 to 0.45 mL of anesthetic is deposited.[1]

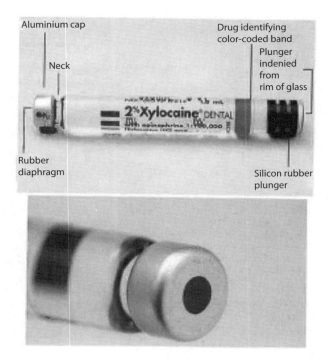

FIGURE 29.7 Components of the glass dental local anesthetic cartridge. Malamed. *The Handbook of Local Anesthesia*, 5th ed. London: Elsevier, 2004.

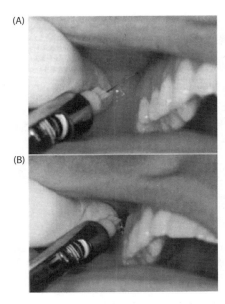

FIGURE 29.9 (A). With a "long" dental needle (>32 mm length) in an average-sized adult, the depth of penetration is half its length. Use of "long" needle on posterior superior alveolar (PSA) nerve block increases risk of over-insertion and hematoma. (B). PSA nerve block using a "short" dental needle (~20 mm length). Over-insertion is less likely. Malamed. *The Handbook of Local Anesthesia*, 5th ed. London: Elsevier, 2004.

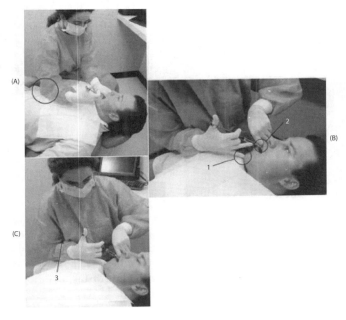

FIGURE 29.8 (a) Use of the patient's chest for stabilization of syringe during a right inferior alveolar nerve block (circle). (b) Use of the chin (1) as a finger rest, with the syringe barrel stabilized by the patient's lip (2). (c) When necessary, stabilization may be increased by drawing the administrator's arm in against his or her chest (3). Malamed. *The Handbook of Local Anesthesia*, 5th ed. London: Elsevier, 2004.

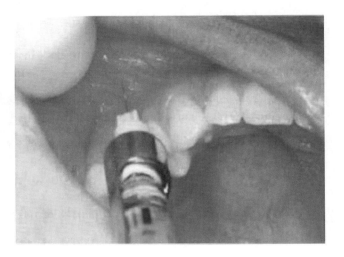

FIGURE 29.10 Insert the needle for anterior superior alveolar (ASA) nerve block in mucobuccal fold over maxillary first premolar. Malamed. *The Handbook of Local Anesthesia*, 5th ed. London: Elsevier, 2004.

innervate the mandibular teeth to the midline on that side, as well as the labial and lingual soft tissues with the exception of the buccal tissue posterior to the premolars (which is innervated by the long buccal nerve).[1]

Inferior Alveolar Nerve Block

To administer an inferior alveolar nerve block, the thumb should be placed on the anterior border of the ramus intraorally, with the rest of the fingers on the posterior border of the ramus extraorally. The site of local anesthetic deposition should be halfway between the anterior and posterior borders of the ramus. Intraorally, the distal border of the pterygomandibular raphe approximately

Mandibular Anesthesia

Anesthesia of the mandibular dentition is most commonly obtained using an inferior alveolar nerve block. This nerve block anesthetizes both the inferior alveolar and lingual nerve, which

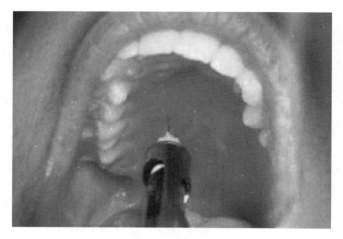

FIGURE 29.11   The cotton swab is removed when the deposition of solution ceases. Malamed. *The Handbook of Local Anesthesia*, 5th ed. London: Elsevier, 2004.

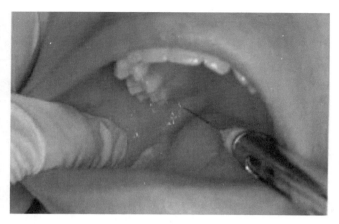

FIGURE 29.13   Notice the placement of the syringe barrel as the corner of the mouth, usually corresponding to the premolars. The needle tip gently touches the most distal end of the pterygomandibular raphe. Malamed. *The Handbook of Local Anesthesia*, 5th ed. London: Elsevier, 2004.

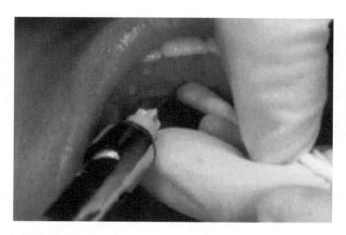

FIGURE 29.12   Pressure is maintained until the deposition of solution is completed. Needle penetration is just lateral to the incisive papilla. Malamed. *The Handbook of Local Anesthesia*, 5th ed. London: Elsevier, 2004.

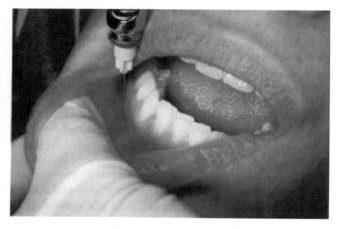

FIGURE 29.14   Mental nerve block- needle penetration site. Malamed. *The Handbook of Local Anesthesia*, 5th ed. London: Elsevier, 2004.

6–10 mm above the occlusal plane marks the usual site of insertion (Figure 29.13). Insert the needle 20–25 mm until bone is contacted. If no bone is contacted, withdraw slightly and reorient the needle. (Do not remove the needle from the intraoral tissues.) Once bone is contacted, withdraw slightly, aspirate, and inject approximately 1.5 mL of local anesthetic. Failure to achieve anesthesia commonly occurs when the anesthetic is deposited too inferiorly or too far anteriorly.[1]

Vazirani-Akinosi Closed-Mouth Mandibular Nerve Block

A variation of the inferior alveolar nerve block can be administered to a patients suffering from severe trismus. The Vazirani-Akinosi closed mouth mandibular block provides anesthesia to the same areas as the inferior alveolar nerve block. This block is performed by inserting the needle parallel to the maxillary occlusal plane at the level of the mucogingival junction of the maxillary second or third molar. Upon reaching the depth of insertion of approximately 25 mm, 1.5 to 1.8 mL of local anesthetic is deposited.[1]

Long Buccal Nerve Block

A long buccal nerve block can be administered to achieve anesthesia of the buccal soft tissue in the molar region. When used along with the inferior alveolar nerve block, anesthesia of one entire side of the mandible is achieved. The needle is inserted just distal and buccal to the most distal tooth until bone is contacted. Approximately 0.3 mL of local anesthetic is deposited.[1]

Mental Nerve Block

The mental nerve provides sensory innervation to the labial mucous membranes and skin of one side of the lower lip anterior to the mental foramen. The site of injection is the mental nerve where it exits the mental foramen, usually located between the apices of the first and second premolars (Figure 29.14). Insert the needle at the depth of the mucobuccal fold between the two premolars to a depth of 5–6 mm. Deposit approximately 0.6 mL of local anesthetic.[1]

Odontogenic Infections

Odontogenic infections are a common problem that can lead to serious morbidity and even death. Early identification of carious teeth and subsequent treatment is a simple and effective way to avoid odontogenic infection. When carious lesions have progressed to pulpal necrosis and subsequent infection, caries will be obvious. Teeth with large amounts of decay and tooth structure missing are easy to find. Brown or black discoloration and shadowing under the enamel of the tooth can also be indicative of caries. Teeth causing odontogenic infections will typically be sensitive to percussion, which can be determined by tapping the back end of a dental mirror or other blunt instrument against the tooth (Figures 29.15 through 29.18). Palpation of the soft tissue near the root apex of the tooth will also usually illicit a painful response.[2]

Imaging

A useful adjunct to clinical exam is relevant imaging (Figures 29.19 through 29.22). Computed tomography (CT) as well as panoramic and periapical dental radiographs are useful when treating odontogenic infections. CT scanning should be reserved for severe or rapidly spreading infections and should be done with contrast if possible. CT scans can be very helpful in identifying fluid collection(s) in different anatomic spaces and can help guide surgical drainage technique (Figure 29.22). Small

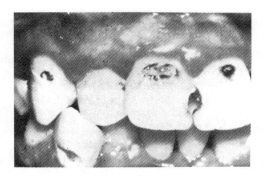

FIGURE 29.17 Cervical and occlusal surface caries (respectively). Sturdevant, Roberson, Heymann, Sturdevant. *The Art and Science of Operative Dentistry*, 3rd ed. London: Elsevier, 1995. Figure 3-51a (p. 122), and Figure 3-51b (p. 122), respectively.

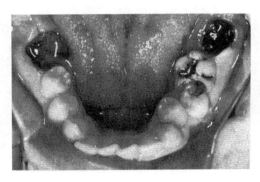

FIGURE 29.18 Cervical and occlusal surface caries (respectively). Sturdevant, Roberson, Heymann, Sturdevant. *The Art and Science of Operative Dentistry*, 3rd ed. London: Elsevier, 1995. Figure 3-51a (p. 122), and Figure 3-51b (p. 122), respectively.

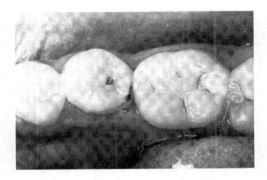

FIGURE 29.15 Occlusal surface caries. Sturdevant, Roberson, Heymann. *The Art and Science of Operative Dentistry*, 3rd ed. London: Elsevier, 1995. Figure 3-25a (p. 82), and Figure 3-25c (p. 82), respectively.

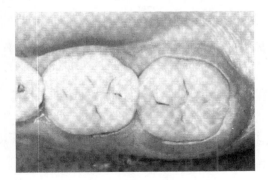

FIGURE 29.16 Occlusal surface caries. Sturdevant, Roberson, Heymann. *The Art and Science of Operative Dentistry*, 3rd ed. London: Elsevier, 1995. Figure 3-25a (p. 82), and Figure 3-25c (p. 82), respectively.

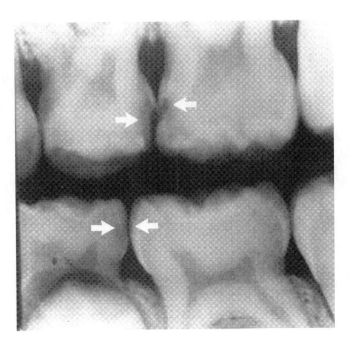

FIGURE 29.19 Radiograph demonstrating interproximal caries. White, Pharoah. *Oral Radiology: Principles and Interpretation*, 4th ed. London: Elsevier, 2000. Figure 15-2, p. 273.

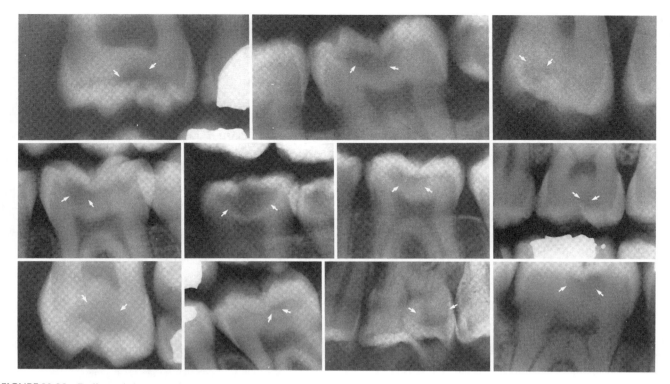

FIGURE 29.20   Radiograph demonstrating interproximal caries. White, Pharoah. *Oral Radiology: Principles and Interpretation*, 4th ed. London: Elsevier, 2000.Figure 15-4, p. 275.

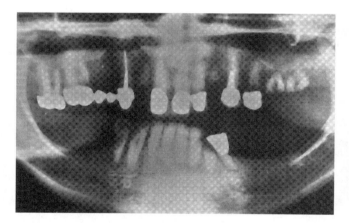

FIGURE 29.21   Panorex showing multiple decayed teeth and root tips with periapical lesions. White, Pharoah. *Oral Radiology: Principles and Interpretation*, 4th ed. London: Elsevier, 2000. Figure 15-17, p. 287.

vestibular infections and mild infections in low-risk areas do not warrant CT scanning. Plain films like a Panorex or periapical films are sufficient and will likely show periapical radiolucency around the root apex of the causative tooth. This can help to identify the offending tooth when there is question about the origin of the infection.[2]

Management

Dr. Larry Peterson developed eight sequential steps in the management of odontogenic infections that have led to a high level of success.[2]

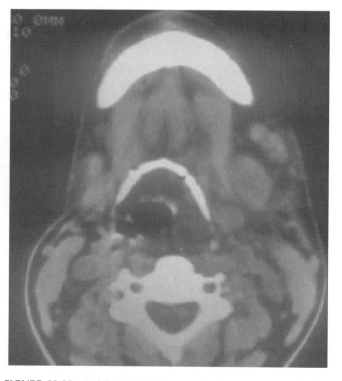

FIGURE 29.22   Axial computed tomography image at the level of the hyoid bone, demonstrating a cellulitis of the left lateral pharyngeal space that is deviating the airway to the opposite side and spreading into the retropharyngeal space. Peterson, Ellis, Hupp, Tucker. *Contemporary Oral and Maxillofacial Surgery*, 3rd ed. London: Elsevier, 1998. Figure 15-5, p. 282.

1. Determine the severity of infection.
2. Evaluate host defenses.
3. Decide on the setting of care.
4. Treat surgically.
5. Support medically.
6. Choose and prescribe antibiotic therapy.
7. Administer the antibiotic properly.
8. Evaluate the patient frequently.

The severity of the infection is determined by the anatomic location, rate of progression, and airway compromise. The borders of the anatomic spaces of the head and neck are outlined in Table 29.1.[2]

Anatomic Location

The likely cause of each type of fascial space infection, the relationships of these spaces, the anatomic structures found within each space, and the approaches for incision and drainage of these spaces are listed in Table 29.1.[2]

Infection Severity

Infection severity can be determined by airway compromise as well as the risk to associated anatomic structures. Low-risk spaces include the buccal, subperiosteal, and vestibular infraorbital spaces. Moderate-risk spaces include the submasseteric, pterygomandibular, superficial, and deep temporal spaces; and the submandibular, submental, and sublingual spaces. High-risk spaces include the lateral pharyngeal, retropharyngeal, mediastinum, and the danger spaces (between the alar and prevertebral fascia).[2]

History

Obtaining a thorough history from the patient should give a large amount of information regarding the rate of progression of the infection as well as an initial evaluation of the patient's host defenses. Rapidly spreading infections, especially in high-risk anatomical spaces, warrant prompt treatment usually requiring hospital stay with administration of intravenous antibiotics. Immediate attention should be given to the airway if there is any question of airway security. Prompt airway management followed by surgical treatment can help to avoid poor outcomes.[2]

TABLE 29.1

Borders of the deep spaces of the head and neck

Space	Anterior	Posterior	Superior	Inferior	Superficial or Medial*	Deep or Lateral†
Buccal	Corner of mouth	Masseter m., pterygomandibular space	Maxilla, infraorbital space	Mandible tissue and skin	Subcutaneous	Buccinator m.
Infraorbital	Nasal cartilages	Buccal space	Quadratus labii superioris m.	Oral mucosa	Quadratus labii superioris m.	Levator anguli oris m., maxilla
Submandibular	Ant belly digastric m.	Post, belly digastric. stylohyoid, stylopharyngeus mm.	Inf. and med. surfaces of mandible	Digastric tendon	Platysma m., investing fascia	Mylohyoid, hyoglossus sup. constrictor mm.
Submental	Inf. border of mandible	Hyoid bone	Mylohyoid m.	Investing fascia	Investing fascia	Ant. bellies digastric m.†
Sublingual	Lingual surface of mandible	Submandibular space	Oral mucosa	Mylohyoid m.	Muscles of tongue*	Lingual surface of mandible†
Pterygomandibular	Buccal space	Parotid gland	Lateral pterygoid m.	Inf. border of mandible	Med. pterygoid muscle*	Ascending ramus of mandible†
Submasseteric	Buccal space	Parotid gland	Zygomatic arch	Inf. border of mandible	Ascending ramus of mandible*	Masseter m.†
Lateral pharyngeal	Sup. and mid. pharyngeal constrictor mm.	Carotid sheath and scalene fascia	Skull base	Hyoid bone	Pharyngeal constrictors and retropharyngeal space*	Medial pterygoid m.†
Retropharyngeal	Sup. and mid. pharyngeal constrictor mm.	Alar fascia	Skull base	Fusion of alar and prevertebral fasciae at C6-T4	—	Carotid sheath and lateral pharyngeal space*
Pretracheal	Sternothyroid-thyrohyoid fascia	Retropharyngeal space	Thyroid cartilage	Superior mediastinum	Sternothyroid-thyrohyoid fascia	Visceral fascia over trachea and thyroid gland

Borders (column group header spanning Anterior through Deep or Lateral)

Adapted from Flynn TR.[5]

ant. = anterior; inf. = inferior; lat. = lateral; m. = muscle; mm. = muscles; med. = medial; mid. = middle; post = posterior, sup. = superior.

*Medial border;

†lateral border.

Peterson, Ellis, Hupp, Tucker. *Contemporary Oral and Maxillofacial Surgery,* 3rd ed. London: Elsevier, 1998. Table 15-1, p. 278.

Systemic Considerations

Immunocompromised patients and patients with limited systemic reserve also may require special considerations, and inpatient stay should be given more consideration. Diabetes, steroid therapy, malnutrition, alcoholism, and malignancy are some common conditions associated with compromised immune systems. Stress placed on the body from severe infection can deplete diminished systemic reserve in unhealthy individuals. Odontogenic infections can also upset previously stable conditions such as chronic kidney disease and diabetes. Attention should be given to appropriate fluid resuscitation and proper medical management pre- and postoperatively.[2]

Setting of Treatment

Many odontogenic infections can be treated in an outpatient setting; however, some do require admission and treatment in a hospital setting. Indications for hospital admission are listed in Table 29.2. Similarly, some infections require the operating room and general anesthesia; the indications for an operating room setting are listed in Table 29.3.[2]

Treatment

Incision and drainage of odontogenic infections is the mainstay of surgical treatment. Basic technique consists of a small incision followed by blunt dissection into the abscess cavity. Care should be taken not to place incisions in areas that contain vital structures. For example, incisions in the neck should be made approximately 2 cm below the inferior border of the mandible to avoid damage to the marginal mandibular branch of the facial nerve. Incision site placement for various fascial space infections is illustrated in Figure 29.23. Blunt dissection into any loculations of the abscess should also be performed to avoid inadequate drainage and residual abscess (Figure 29.24). A hemostat

TABLE 29.2

Indications for hospital admission

- Temperature > 101°F (38.3°C)
- **Dehydration**
- Threat to the airway or vital structures
- Infection in moderate or high severity anatomic spaces
- Need for general anesthesia
- Need for inpatient control of systemic disease

Peterson, Ellis, Hupp, Tucker. *Contemporary Oral and Maxillofacial Surgery*, 3rd ed. London: Elsevier, 1998. Table 15-6, p. 283.

TABLE 29.3

When to go to the operating room

- To establish airway security
- Moderate to high anatomic severity
- Multiple space involvement
- Rapidly progressing infection
- Need for general anesthesia

Peterson, Ellis, Hupp, Tucker. *Contemporary Oral and Maxillofacial Surgery*, 3rd ed. London: Elsevier, 1998. Table 15-7, p. 284.

can be used for blunt dissection by inserting into the incision with the beaks closed, and opening the withdrawing the instrument with the beaks open. Never close the beaks of the hemostat blindly within the wound as this may damage vital structures. Purulent material as well as tissue should be obtained and sent for culture and sensitivity testing if possible. Penrose or Jackson-Pratt drains can be placed into the abscess cavity to allow for further drainage. These drains should be removed once drainage ceases, usually around the third or fourth postoperative day. If an abscess is to be approached both from an intraoral as well as an extraoral approach, a drain can be placed that extends from inside the mouth, through the abscess cavity, and out the external skin incision site. Follow the same guidelines with these through-and-through drains although drainage is not expected to cease completely, as saliva from the oral cavity will also continuously drain.[2]

Medical Considerations

Medical care for patients with odontogenic infections centers around hydration, nutrition, and fever control. Hydration requirements may be increased in febrile patients. Attention should also be given to control of previous systemic disease in the perioperative period.[2]

Antibiotics

Antibiotic therapy for odontogenic infections is largely empirical but can be based on culture and sensitivity testing when applicable. Empiric antibiotic therapy for odontogenic infections is listed in Table 29.4.[2]

Follow-Up

Patients with odontogenic infections need frequent reevaluation to determine if the infection is resolving. Improved dyspnea, dysphagia, odynophagia, decreased edema, decreasing white blood cell count, and lack of fever are all signs of improvement. Failure to respond to treatment of odontogenic infections can occur; the common causes are listed in Table 29.5. Repeat CT scans can be considered if warranted and may show residual fluid collection, for which further surgical treatment may be necessary.[2]

Exodontia

Prior to extracting a tooth, the provider must understand the shape of the tooth being removed, specifically the number of roots the tooth has (Figure 29.1). All teeth have at least one root; mandibular molars have two roots, and maxillary molars have three roots. Molar root configuration can range from fused and conical to extremely divergent. Root length can be extremely variable as well. The easiest way to visualize root form is with either a periapical film or a Panorex film; CT scans are not necessary for this procedure. Traditional cephalometric films are of little use in extractions due to the amount of overlap with adjacent structures.

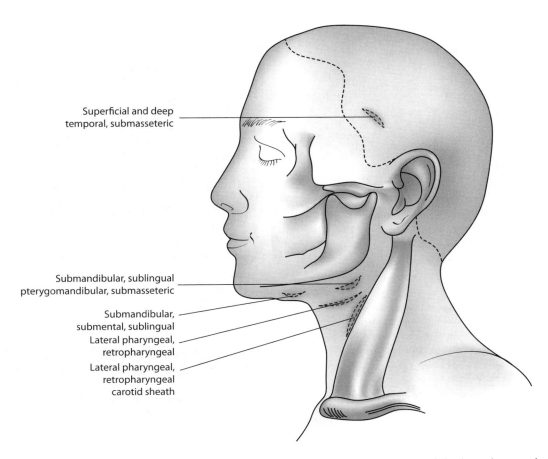

Superficial and deep
temporal, submasseteric

Submandibular, sublingual
pterygomandibular, submasseteric

Submandibular,
submental, sublingual

Lateral pharyngeal,
retropharyngeal

Lateral pharyngeal,
retropharyngeal
carotid sheath

FIGURE 29.23 Incision placement for extraoral drainage of head and neck infections. Incisions at the following points may be used to drain infections in the indicated spaces; superficial and deep temporal, submasseteric; submandibular, submental, sublingual; submandibular, sublingual, pterygomandibular, submasseteric, lateral pharyngeal, retropharyngeal; lateral pharyngeal, retropharyngeal, carotid sheath. Adapted from Flynn TR. Peterson, Ellis, Hupp, Tucker. *Contemporary Oral and Maxillofacial Surgery*, 3rd ed. London: Elsevier, 1998. Adapted from Flynn TR. Figure 15-6, p. 285.

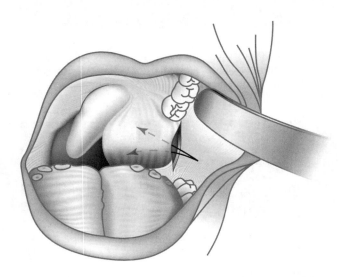

FIGURE 29.24 Intraoral incision placement for drainage of the anterior compartment of the lateral pharyngeal space (curved arrow) and the ptery-gomandibular space (straight arrow). Adapted from Flynn TR. Peterson, Ellis, Hupp, Tucker. *Contemporary Oral and Maxillofacial Surgery*, 3rd ed. London: Elsevier, 1998. Adapted from Flynn TR. Figure 15-7, p. 285.

Most teeth are surrounded by both bone and gingiva, though in the presence of severe periodontal disease there may be little or no bony support. Either way, the provider must anticipate separating the tooth from both structures.

The armamentarium required for both simple and complex extractions can be overwhelming at first. However, the basic setup is universal; it is explained in Figure 29.25.

In addition to items shown in Figure 29.25, the provider must have the correct armamentarium to administer local anesthesia as described earlier in this chapter. Also, many different types of elevators and forceps exist. The aim of this chapter is not to review each type but rather to explain the use of the most basic types. Figures 29.26 through 29.28 show pictures of three universal extraction forceps.

Extracting a tooth can range from extremely easy to surprisingly difficult. This chapter will briefly focus on uncomplicated extractions as well as removal of impacted teeth with the aid of a surgical handpiece. Factors that influence the difficulty of an extraction include root form, presence of impaction, remaining clinical crown, bone density, history of root canal treatment, and the presence of ankylosis, to name a few. The best way to approach extracting teeth is to think of it as if you were trying to untie a very tight knot in rope; brute force will not get you

TABLE 29.4

Empiric antibiotics* of choice for odontogenic infections

Severity of Infection	Antibiotic of Choice
Outpatient	• Penicillin
	• Clindamycin
	• Cephalexin (only if the penicillin allergy was not the anaphylactoid type; use caution)
	• Penicillin allergy:
	– Clindamycin
	– Moxifloxacin
	– Metronidazole alone
Inpatient	• Clindamycin
	• Ampicillin + metronidazole
	• Ampicillin + sulbactam
	• Penicillin allergy:
	– Clindamycin
	– Third-generation cephalosporin IV (only if the penicillin allergy was not the anaphylactoid type; use caution)
	• Moxifloxacin (especially for *Eiketiella corrodens*)
	• Metronidazole alone (if neither clindamycin nor cephalosporins can be tolerated)

* Empiric antibiotic therapy is used before culture and sensitivity reports are available. Cultures should be taken in severe infections that threaten vital structures. IV = intravenous.
Peterson, Ellis, Hupp, Tucker. *Contemporary Oral and Maxillofacial Surgery,* 3rd ed. London: Elsevier, 1998. Table 15-8, p. 288.

TABLE 29.5.

Causes of Treatment Failure

• Inadequate surgery
• Depressed host defenses
• Foreign body
• Antibiotic problems
  – Patient noncompliance
  – Drug not reaching site
  – Drug dosage too low
  – Wrong bacterial diagnosis
  – Wrong antibiotic

Adapted from Peterson LJ.[32]
Peterson, Ellis, Hupp, Tucker. *Contemporary Oral and Maxillofacial Surgery*, 3rd ed. London: Elsevier, 1998. Table 15-9, p. 290.

anywhere. Rather, selective, controlled force in several directions will eventually loosen the knot enough to finally untie it. Extracting an unimpacted tooth is quite similar. The goal is to loosen the tooth within the dental alveolus with dental elevators and forceps until the dental alveolus is ready to "let go" of it.

As mentioned earlier, proper imaging should be available before attempting extractions. A periapical or Panorex film allows the provider to examine not only root form, but also potential proximity to structures such as the mandibular canal and maxillary sinus (Figures 29.29 and 29.30).

Figures 29.31 and 29.32 show how a dental elevator and forceps are employed. Figures 29.33 and 29.34 show how to use an elevator

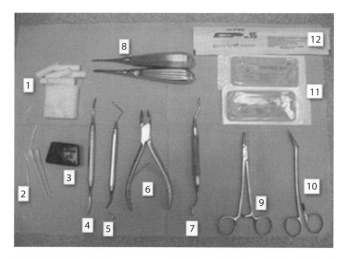

FIGURE 29.25 (1) Cotton gauze. (2) Floss and Q-tips. (3) Mouth block. (4) Periosteal elevator. (5) Curette. (6) Rongeurs. (7) Bone file. (8) Dental elevators. (9) Needle driver. (10) Suture scissors. (11) Suture material. (12) Scalpel. Image by Dr. Jeffrey Dorfman.

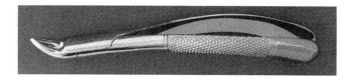

FIGURE 29.26 This forcep is a #150, which is used to grasp maxillary teeth. Peterson, Ellis, Hupp, Tucker. *Contemporary Oral and Maxillofacial Surgery*, 3rd ed. London: Elsevier, 1998. Figure 6-47B (p. 116).

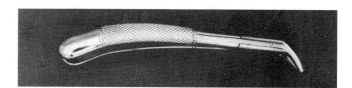

FIGURE 29.27 This is a #151 forcep, which is used to grasp mandibular teeth. The #151 has a more angulated tip than the #150. Peterson, Ellis, Hupp, Tucker. *Contemporary Oral and Maxillofacial Surgery*, 3rd ed. London: Elsevier, 1998. Figure 6-55B (p. 122).

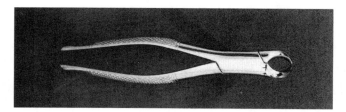

FIGURE 29.28. This forcep is a #23, or a "cowhorn," because of the way its beaks approximate. The #23 is used exclusively for mandibular molars. Peterson, Ellis, Hupp, Tucker. *Contemporary Oral and Maxillofacial Surgery*, 3rd ed. London: Elsevier, 1998. Figure 6-60A (p.125).

and forceps to extract an uncomplicated tooth. However, many symptomatic teeth will be impacted or so decayed as to require surgical exploration to identify the remaining tooth structure. At this point, the completely inexperienced provider should consider

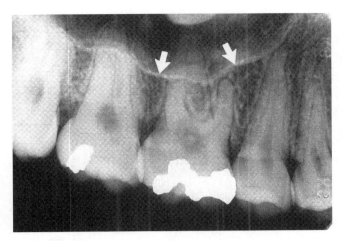

FIGURE 29.29 Arrows in the film indicate the maxillary sinus. Note proximity of root apices. White, Pharoah. *Oral Radiology: Principles and Interpretation*, 4th ed. London: Elsevier, 2000. Figure 9-30 (p. 181).

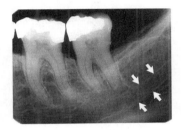

FIGURE 29. 30 Arrows in the film indicate the mandibular canal. Note the proximity of root apices. White, Pharoah. *Oral Radiology: Principles and Interpretation*, 4th ed. London: Elsevier, 2000. Figure 9-49 (p. 187).

referral, if possible. However, if this is not an option, we will discuss the bare essentials of completing a surgical extraction.

A surgical extraction begins with an incision through the gingiva overlying the dental alveolus, followed by the creation of a mucoperiosteal flap with the periosteal elevator. Developing a full thickness, mucoperiosteal flap will allow for the necessary visualization of the remaining tooth structure. Figure 29.35 provides an example of the type of flap that can be used. The first incision is typically along the crest of the alveolus or immediately adjacent to the tooth. One or two releasing incisions can be used as well.

If it is necessary to remove bone or section the tooth to allow for a favorable path of draw, the provider must have access to a handpiece with a cross-cutting bur and irrigation (Figures 29.36 and 29.38). A traditional dental handpiece that expels air in the forward direction cannot be used for surgical extractions as the pressurized air can cause air emphysema that can potentially lead to mediastinitis. It is recommended that a Hall handpiece, Impact Air handpiece, or any type of electric handpiece be used. The diagrams below give a limited example of how the provider must frequently section the tooth prior to being able to remove it.

As with any surgical procedure, postoperative complications should be expected. Symptoms can include pain, swelling, infection, bleeding, and alveolar osteitis ("dry socket").

Any patient who has a surgical extraction completed should be sent home with a prescription for antibiotics. Postoperative bleeding can usually be controlled with adequate suturing intraoperatively and biting on gauze postoperatively for several hours.

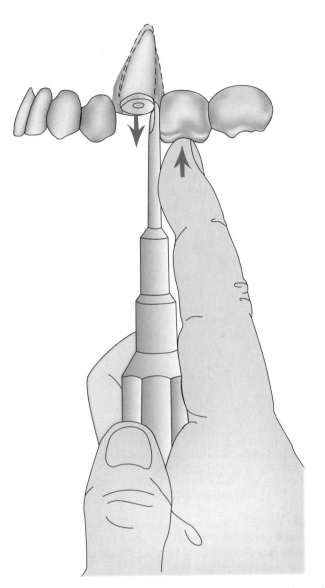

FIGURE 29.31 Dental elevators are designed to wedge into the periodontal ligament space between the tooth and alveolus. Careful insertion and twisting loosens the tooth by widening the periodontal ligament space. Completing this prior to using the forceps will help to prevent root tip fracture. Peterson, Ellis, Hupp, Tucker. *Contemporary Oral and Maxillofacial Surgery*, 3rd ed. London: Elsevier, 1998.

Biting on tea bags in the place of gauze can facilitate hemostasis as well due to the tannic acid in the tea leaves. Assuming the patient can tolerate nonsteroidal anti-inflammatory drugs (NSAIDs), Motrin is a great analgesic to prescribe. It is not uncommon to prescribe narcotics such as Vicodin and Percocet as well. If the patient returns complaining of pain around postoperative day 3 that is not controlled with the prescribed analgesics, the provider should irrigate the extraction sockets and visually inspect the area for exposed bone. If any is observed, the socket should be packed with iodoform gauze that is impregnated with eugenol. This dressing may have to be changed every 2 to 3 days until the site heals by secondary intention. If pain persists for weeks despite several eugenol dressing changes, osteomyelitis should be considered.

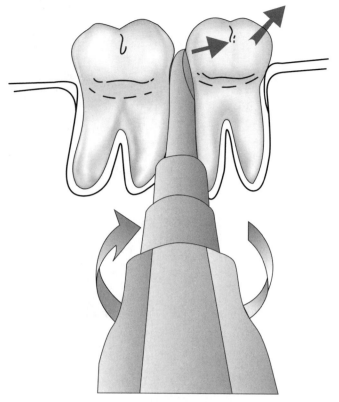

FIGURE 29.32 Dental elevators are designed to wedge into the periodontal ligament space between the tooth and alveolus. Careful insertion and twisting loosens the tooth by widening the periodontal ligament space. Completing this prior to using the forceps will help to prevent root tip fracture. Peterson, Ellis, Hupp, Tucker. *Contemporary Oral and Maxillofacial Surgery*, 3rd ed. London: Elsevier, 1998.

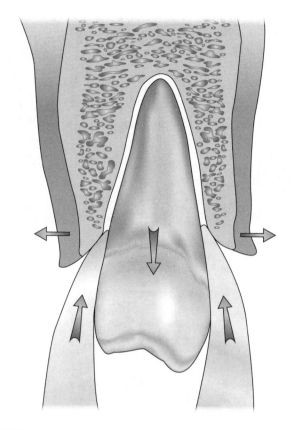

FIGURE 29.33 Dental extraction forceps are best employed when firm controlled pressure is used in all directions, including apically. Peterson, Ellis, Hupp, Tucker. *Contemporary Oral and Maxillofacial Surgery*, 3rd ed. London: Elsevier, 1998.

Due to the proximity of some maxillary teeth roots with the maxillary sinus, the potential for development of an oroantral fistula exists. These usually heal with time, antibiotics, decongestants, and sinus precautions.

When extracting posterior mandibular teeth whose roots are near the mandibular canal, it is possible for the inferior alveolar and/or lingual nerve to be injured. If these nerves are irritated, the patient will notice ipsilateral inferior alveolar nerve paresthesia and potentially ipsilateral lingual paresthesia as well. Lingual paresthesia is much rarer, but it manifests not only as a lack of sensation, but also a lack of taste. At no time should motor nerves to the muscles of facial expression be at risk during any extraction.

Oral Pathology Uncommon in HICs

Describing a comprehensive guide to oral pathology is beyond the scope of this text. There are volumes of books dedicated to this subject. However, this book is presumably being written for practitioners in remote, undeveloped areas—areas that are subject to diseases not commonly encountered in the developed world. Many of these serious diseases can have oral manifestations that can alert the astute practitioner to a possible early diagnosis. This chapter will highlight only a few examples of rarely encountered diseases. However, all practitioners should be on alert for signs of intraoral cancer, including ulceration, leukoplakia,

and/or erythroplakia. Even though cancer is certainly not limited to the developing world, it is important to mention that a thorough cancer screening should be part of every intraoral examination.

An intraoral examination should be part of every physical examination; the mucosa of the mouth should be carefully examined for anything abnormally white, red, painful, enlarged, or ulcerated. This can be completed with a simple tongue blade and flashlight. A dental mirror is extremely helpful in completing an intraoral examination, if available. The dental mirror allows not only for indirect vision of all areas of the mouth, but also helps with illuminating specific areas as well. Remember to examine the floor of the mouth and sides of the tongue in addition to the buccal mucosa.

Biopsy Technique

Should the practitioner find any lesion that is suspect, he or she should not hesitate to biopsy it. Small lesions are usually appropriate for excisional biopsy while large lesions should have an incisional biopsy to allow for margin identification during any potential ablative surgery. Brush biopsies, while simple, may not provide the amount of tissue needed to accurately diagnose the specimen, so we recommend using a #15 scalpel and removing an ellipse of tissue, followed by closure with resorbable sutures. Figures 29.39 and 29.40 show examples of both an incisional and an excisional biopsy.

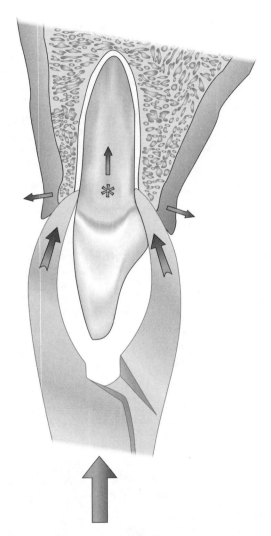

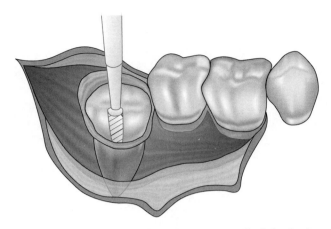

FIGURE 29.36 Example showing necessary removal of alveolar bone, followed by sectioning of the tooth, in order to allow for a path of draw to extract the tooth. Peterson, Ellis, Hupp, Tucker. *Contemporary Oral and Maxillofacial Surgery*, 3rd ed. London: Elsevier, 1998. Figure 8-3 (p. 146).

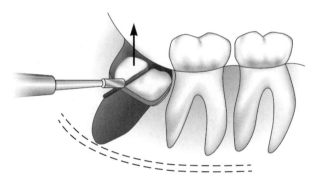

FIGURE 29.37 Example showing necessary removal of alveolar bone, followed by sectioning of the tooth, in order to allow for a path of draw to extract the tooth. Peterson, Ellis, Hupp, Tucker. *Contemporary Oral and Maxillofacial Surgery*, 3rd ed. London: Elsevier, 1998. Figure 8-4b (p. 147).

FIGURE 29.34 Dental extraction forceps are best employed when firm controlled pressure is used in all directions, including apically. Peterson, Ellis, Hupp, Tucker. *Contemporary Oral and Maxillofacial Surgery*, 3rd ed. London: Elsevier, 1998.

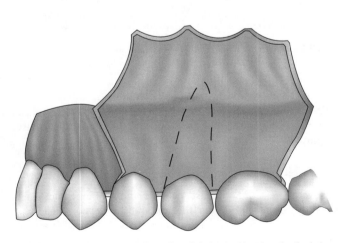

FIGURE 29.35 When outlining a flap, it is imperative that the flap's base be wider than its apex to ensure adequate blood supply. Peterson, Ellis, Hupp, Tucker. *Contemporary Oral and Maxillofacial Surgery*, 3rd ed. London: Elsevier, 1998.

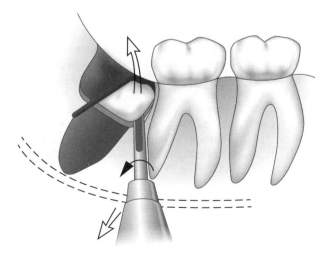

FIGURE 29. 38 Example showing necessary removal of alveolar bone, followed by sectioning of the tooth, in order to allow for a path of draw to extract the tooth. Peterson, Ellis, Hupp, Tucker. *Contemporary Oral and Maxillofacial Surgery*, 3rd ed. London: Elsevier, 1998. Figure 8-4c (p. 147).

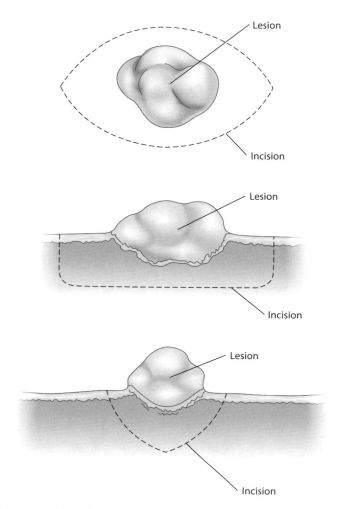

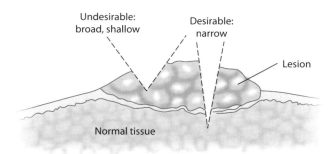

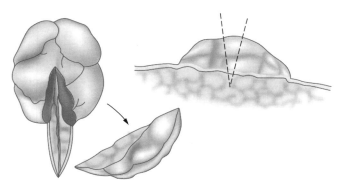

FIGURE 29. 40   Outline form for incisional biopsy. Peterson, Ellis, Hupp, Tucker. *Contemporary Oral and Maxillofacial Surgery*, 3rd ed. London: Elsevier, 1998. Figure 22-7 (p. 525).

FIGURE 29.39   Outline form for excisional biopsy. Peterson, Ellis, Hupp, Tucker. *Contemporary Oral and Maxillofacial Surgery*, 3rd ed. London: Elsevier, 1998. Figure 22-6 (p. 525).

Tuberculosis

Tuberculosis (TB) is a chronic infectious disease caused by *Mycobacterium tuberculosis* that remains present in areas without access to proper antimicrobials or healthcare infrastructure, high prevalence of human immunodeficiency virus/acquired immunodeficiency syndrome (HIV/AIDS), and unsanitary or crowded living conditions.

Head and neck manifestations of TB are not commonly reported; however, the oral cavity can be affected. Usually oral TB lesions appear as chronic, asymptomatic ulcerations that can be nodular, granular, or leukoplakic (Figures 29.41 and 29.42).

Kaposi's Sarcoma

Kaposi's sarcoma is a vascular neoplasm that was rarely reported prior to the AIDS epidemic. It has been linked to human herpesvirus 8. Oral manifestation of Kaposi's will appear as a bluish-purple macule or plaque, frequently on the palate (Figure 29.43).

Leishmaniasis

Leishmaniasis is a collective term that describes several types of infections transmitted by sandflies. Mucocutaneous

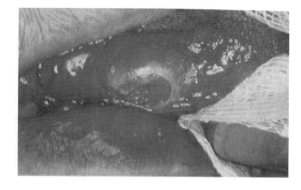

FIGURE 29.41   Oral manifestation of tuberculosis. Neville, et al. *Oral and Maxillofacial Pathology*, 3rd ed. Philadelphia: Saunders/Elsevier, 2008.

leishmaniasis is transmitted by the sandfly *Leishmania braziliensis* and can result in oral lesions. These oral lesions can be severely ulcerated, papillomatous, nodular, and destructive (Figure 29.44).

Areca Nut/Betel Leaves

In several areas of Southeast Asia, variations of areca nut chewing frequently occur. Often, the soft areca nut is combined with slaked lime and tobacco, and wrapped in betel leaves. This combination is chronically placed in the mouth, similar to chewing tobacco or snuff, often for its stimulating properties. Symptoms of chronic use can range from benign leukoplakia to severe conditions such as oral submucous fibrosis and squamous cell carcinoma (Figures 29.45 and 29.46).

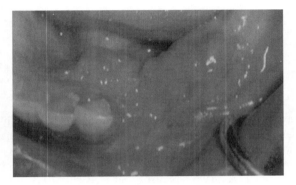

FIGURE 29.42   Oral manifestation of tuberculosis. Neville, et al. *Oral and Maxillofacial Pathology*, 3rd ed. Philadelphia: Saunders/Elsevier, 2008.

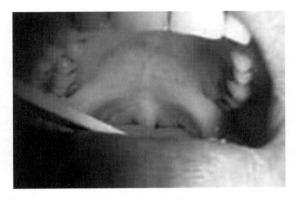

FIGURE 29.45   Oral submucosal fibrosis. Precancerous condition characterized by mucosal rigidity secondary to fibroelastic hyperplasia. Patients can present with severe trismus and mucosal pain. Unfortunately, these lesions do no regress with cessation of exposure. Squamous cell carcinoma has been found to develop at a rate of 8% over a 17-year period. Image by Ravi Mehrotra.

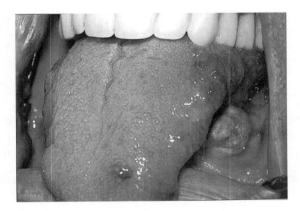

FIGURE 29.43   Typical oral presentation of Kaposi's Sarcoma. Marx, Stern. *Oral and Maxillofacial Pathology: A Rationale for Diagnosis and Treatment.* Chicago: Quintessence Publishing Co., 2003. Figure 2-95b (p. 109).

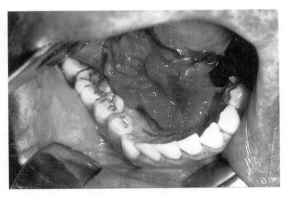

FIGURE 29.46   Squamous cell carcinoma of the oral cavity. Varied clinical presentations can include exophytic masses, endophytic lesions, leukoplakia, and or erythroplakia. Lesions can be completely asymptomatic or extremely painful. Marx, Stern. *Oral and Maxillofacial Pathology: A Rationale for Diagnosis and Treatment.* Chicago: Quintessence Publishing Co., 2003. Figure 7-59 (p. 338).

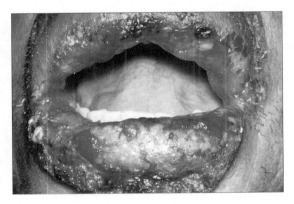

FIGURE   29.44   Tissue   destruction   common   with   Mucocutaneous Leishmaniasis. Marx, Stern. *Oral and Maxillofacial Pathology: A Rationale for Diagnosis and Treatment.* Chicago: Quintessence Publishing Co., 2003. Figure 2-95b (p. 109).

COMMENTARY

Rose Dina Premier, Haiti

Numbering Systems

Numbering systems are helpful for record keeping and inter-office communication (between dental staff), but not all practices use the same system. Haitian dentists use the Federation Dentaire Internationale (FDI). The FDI is a two-digit numbering system in which the first number represents the quadrant and the second number is the tooth number from 1–, beginning with the central incisors. Therefore, tooth numbering becomes 11 through 18 (maxillary right), 21 through 28 (maxillary left), 31 through 38 (mandibular left), and 41 through 48 (mandibular right). For deciduous teeth, we adopt the same system with quadrants, numbering the teeth 1 through 5 in each quadrant beginning with the central incisors.

When referring to the FDI verbally for deciduous teeth, we say five-three or six-two or seven-one or eight-five, and so forth. When writing, we represent the teeth as 51 through 55 (maxillary right), 61 through 65 (maxillary left), 71 through 75 (mandibular left), and 81 through 85 (mandibular right).

Odontogenic Infections

Odontogenic infections are treated similarly in Haiti and high-income countries (HICs). A dental diagnostic (palpation and percussion included) is often confirmed by a periapical dental radiograph. Depending on the severity of the infection, a panoramic radiograph is also sometimes necessary. Because a Panorex machine is not easily accessible, panoramic films are used most of the time to see the entire dentition, and a CT scan is the investigative tool of choice because it shows detailed anatomy of the joint and any pathology that may exist. The treatment is automatically the same.

Carcinoma

Carcinoma is a very dangerous oral lesion that is usually found on the lateral border of the tongue or on the floor of the mouth. Tobacco use, especially when connected with alcohol abuse, is thought to be a major culprit. The treatment of choice for most oral cancers is surgical excision.

Vesicular Lesions

Vesicular lesions start out as small, raised, fluid-filled areas on the mucous membrane. These vesicles soon rupture, forming a painful ulcer. These lesions are usually viral, although they may also be caused by allergies.

Recapping Needles

Preventing needlestick injuries is a priority. A recapping device can be used; it is a tool that holds the protective cap while protecting fingers from being stuck. Another approach is to place the protective cap on the work surface and scoop up the cap with the needle itself. Either way, a great deal of care is necessary in recapping syringes.

Dental Mirrors

A dental mirror is an important instrument that has many functions. Its primary use is to help the dentist see areas that cannot be seen directly. The term "indirect vision" refers to the situation in which a dentist looks into the mirror and sees a reflected image. Dental mirrors can also be used to reflect light into areas of the mouth that are difficult to see.

30

Orthopedic Surgery

George S.M. Dyer

Introduction

Epidemiology of Orthopedic Disease

In recent years, it has become increasingly clear that surgical illness—illness that can be treated by surgical means—is a major source of impairment in low- and middle-income countries (LMICs) around the world. This impairment translates into a huge burden of disability, lost productivity, and human misery. In turn, it has become clear that much of this impairment is musculoskeletal in nature. This connection should come as no surprise. In parts of the world where physical work is the principal or only means of making a living and the margin for economic survival is thin, even slight loss of strength, dexterity, or stamina can have grave consequences.[1]

It has been estimated by various aggregated statistical methods that approximately 11% of the total global burden of disease is surgically treatable.[2]

Of all musculoskeletal conditions causing impairment in the developing world, trauma is the single greatest contributing factor.[3] Trauma is a rising cause of death worldwide, particularly among young people aged 15–44 who are in the peak years of work productivity in the developing world.[3–6] However, treatable congenital conditions, infections, palsies, and other noninfectious acquired conditions also make a very large and probably underestimated contribution to overall suffering and lost productivity worldwide.

By conducting a house-to-house survey in Rwanda, Atijosan and colleagues created a compelling profile of the prevalence of various musculoskeletal impairments (MSI) and their impact. They screened a total of 6,757 individuals with a team of a trained physical therapists and medical assistants. They found an overall prevalence for MSI of 5.2%. Of these, 11.5% were congenital, 31.3% posttraumatic, 3.8% from musculoskeletal infection, 9.0% from neurological conditions such as palsies with skeletal impairment, and 44.4% were nontraumatic and noninfectious. The most common individual diagnoses were joint disease (13.3%), angular limb deformity (9.7%), and fracture mal- and nonunion (7.2%). They found that 96% of all cases required further treatment (Figure 30.1).[7]

Magnifying Effect

As impressive as these numbers are, this type of prevalence study does not fully explain the longitudinal and intergenerational effects of disabling injuries or other musculoskeletal events on a family unit. The effect is much worse when the ramifications of lost productivity are considered over time (Figure 30.2).

The primary and secondary effects of a head of household's loss of income dominate the WHO list of contributors to preventable global burden of disease: malnutrition, depressive disorders, intoxicant abuse, and family dysfunction.[8–10] Accordingly, the economic and social value of returning a productive person to full function is hard to overstate.

When the relatively low cost of many surgical interventions is considered, surgery looks like a real bargain.

Principles

Primum non nocere, first, do no harm, is the cornerstone of the Hippocratic Oath, and it is a good guiding principle for orthopedic surgery in the developing world as well. Orthopedic procedures are very appealing for visiting surgical teams. In this model, a group of specialists travels as a self-contained unit, bringing everything needed to do a highly specialized procedure, such as total joint replacement, with little or no reliance on the host country. The team and its equipment can be tailored efficiently to a single purpose. However, consider the immediate and long-term impact of the visiting surgical team's work.[11] Have the patients been adequately evaluated before surgery? What if there are serious medical complications during the procedures? Who will be qualified and available to evaluate and treat longer-term complications or conditions that arise? It is important to match the technology of a proposed intervention to the host environment.

Planning and Equipment

Perioperative Evaluation and Preparation

Cases should be carefully selected, and the entire preoperative and postoperative course planned to the greatest extent possible. This begins with being certain the patient understands the implications of the proposed operation and rehabilitation. Using a competent interpreter, if needed, explain how long the operation will take to perform and what the immediate risks are. Explain the entire course of recovery, including rehabilitation and pain management. Take nothing for granted in this regard. Will a Foley catheter be used in the operation? Will any part of the patient's body be shaved or otherwise altered? Include a truly comprehensive discussion.

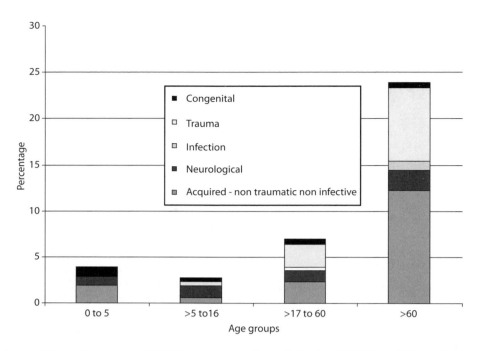

FIGURE 30.1. Prevalence and diagnostic categories of MSI, by age group. Atijosan O, Rischewski D, Simms V, Kuper H, Linganwa B, Nuhi A, et al. A national survey of musculoskeletal impairment in Rwanda: prevalence, causes and service implications. PloS one. 2008 Aug; 3(7): e2851.

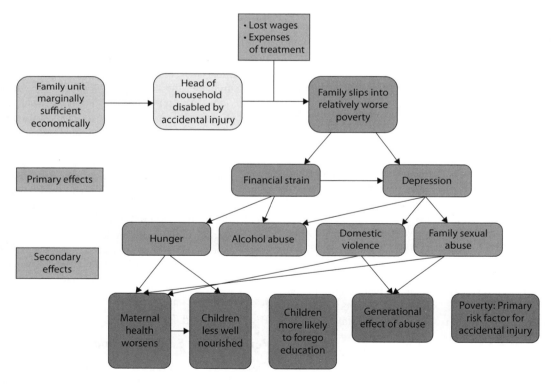

FIGURE 30.2. Implications for treatment and action. Image by George S.M. Dyer.

Comprehensively plan every step of the operation to be performed. What unexpected events are reasonable to predict? For example, if significant blood loss is a possibility, even an unlikely one, is banked blood available? If not, what will be the plan if significant bleeding is encountered? It is much better to cancel or alter a surgical agenda than to find yourself in a no-win situation far from home. It is reasonable to consider a dry run of particular

aspects of surgery in advance. This is especially true for complex operations involving a team whose members may not be used to working together or who are from different institutions.

Most important, what are the plans for after surgery? Who will see the patient in follow-up? If there are sutures or staples to be removed, who will do that? Will recovery require any supervised rehabilitation? If so, who will do that supervision? Will there be future visiting surgical teams or return visits by your team? When? All of these subjects should be discussed in detail before undertaking any operative procedures.

Fracture Nonunion

Chapters 49 and 51 are concerned with the acute presentation of fractures. However, so much of the musculoskeletal burden in the developing world relates to trauma that some chronic sequelae of fractures will be treated separately here.

Nonunion rates for nonoperatively treated fracture vary by part of the body, fracture-specific factors, and patient-related factors. It is likely that some chronically nonunited fractures will present. As with any evaluation and management of a fracture nonunion, begin by classifying the nonunion and attempting to determine why it occurred. Simple nonunions may be approached by improving immobilization, either surgically or by closed means. An infected nonunion or an atrophic nonunion is a greater challenge.

Some injuries, which are always treated promptly in high-income countries (HICs), are routinely treated late in the developing world. One example is femoral neck fractures in young adults. Although unfamiliar to many surgeons, there is good evidence to suggest that these should be treated even when they present late. Butt and colleagues reported satisfactory results following operative treatment of late presenting femoral neck fractures.[12,13] In this series, they used percutaneous cannulated screws with good results in 45 of 52 reported cases.

Nonunited tibia fractures are both common and particularly difficult to treat. The principles of nonunion surgeries are unchanging, but some aspects of the surgical tactic may be needed depending on resources. For example, circular frame or Ilizarov fixators may be difficult to maintain in LMICs. Intramedullary fixation, with or without grafting, may be preferable even if it results in leg length discrepancy.[13] Iliac crest bone grafting is the gold standard for atrophic nonunions, but the consideration of possible blood loss requiring transfusion must be factored in when operating in LMICs.[14,15]

Osteomyelitis

Infection of bone is a common chronic condition likely to be treated in a developing world setting. Other conditions such as degenerative arthritis may be more common, but osteomyelitis is likely to require operative treatment in any setting.

Although some of the resources available in such a setting may be different, the principles established for treating bone infections do not change. They include obtaining a good understanding of the patient's medical conditions that may affect ability to overcome infection (host factors), classifying the infection anatomically, and then treating it surgically. Surgical principles include debridement of necrotic bone and tissue with minimal trauma to healthy tissue and vascular supply, obtaining appropriate cultures, managing dead space, and stabilizing bone, if needed.

Figure 30.3 shows the classification of osteomyelitis proposed by Cierny and Mader.[16] Type I osteomyelitis confined to the medullary cavity is less common in LMICs, as it often results from

previous surgery. Deep soft tissue infection that extends to bone may produce type II osteomyelitis. Types III and IV are likely to be the dominant types seen, where a chronic bone abscess forms either with or without permeative destruction of the bone.

Surgical Principles

Debride thoroughly but not destructively. Avoid excessive stripping of periosteum from the bone. When dissecting, identify a plane outside the periosteum to maximize blood supply to the bone.[17] Within the infected bone, remove dead and devitalized bone tissue until there is punctate bleeding, which indicates that living, vascularized bone has been reached. If power equipment is available, this is done with a high-speed burr, but if not it can be done with curet, curved osteotome, rongeur, and Cobb elevator (Figure 30.5).

The determination of stable versus unstable bone loss is made after debridement. If the bone is unstable, then it must be stabilized, often by use of an external fixator. Some alternative solutions are possible for lower-cost external fixation as well. One described by Ismavel and colleagues involves using 2.5-mm

---

Anatomic type
Type I – Medullary osteomyelitis
Type II – Superficial osteomyelitis
Type III – Localized osteomyelitis
Type IV – Diffuse osteomyelitis

Physiologic class
A-Host – Good immune system and delivery
B-Host – Compromised locally (B^L) or systemically (B^S)
C-Host – Requires suppressive or no treatment; minimal disability; treatment worse than disease; not a surgical candidate

Clinical stage
Type + Class = Clinical stage

Example:
Stage IVB^S osteomyelitis = a diffuse lesion in a systemically compromised host

FIGURE 30.3. Cierny-Mader classification for osteomyelitis. Cierny G, 3rd, Mader JT, Penninck JJ. A clinical staging system for adult osteomyelitis. Clinical orthopaedics and related research. 2003 Sep; (414): 7–24.

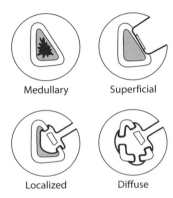

Medullary   Superficial

Localized   Diffuse

FIGURE 30.4. Graphical representation of the Cierny-Mader classification. Cierny G, 3rd, Mader JT, Penninck JJ. A clinical staging system for adult osteomyelitis. Clinical orthopaedics and related research. 2003 Sep; (414): 7–24.

K-wires to maintain the ankle plantigrade in two planes, at lost cost (Figure 30.6 and Figure 30.7).[18]

If there has been substantial bone loss or debridement but the bone is still mechanically intact, a useful way of predicting the need for fixation is that lesions that compromise more than 50% of bone cortex, over an area as large as the diameter of the bone, are at risk to fracture and should be protected by fixation.

Coverage

The last surgical principle of managing osteomyelitis is to bring blood supply to the devitalized tissue by maximizing the soft tissue envelope. If there is not sufficient good soft tissue after adequate debridement, then a flap may be needed. Free tissue or microvascular coverage may be beyond the capability of an LMIC, but many nonmicrovascular coverage options exist (Figure 30.8 and Figure 30.9).[19]

If none of these options is adequate and free tissue transfer with microvascular anastomosis is absolutely required, consider whether it is reasonable to perform microsurgery with loupes-only technique. Although extra time may be required, that drawback may be offset by the portability and reliability of loupes.[20]

Degenerative Conditions

In the Rwandan survey previously described, degenerative conditions were the second most common skeletal impairments found, after posttraumatic conditions. They are discussed last in this chapter, however, for several reasons. First, although painful and functionally limiting, degenerative conditions are unlikely to be life threatening. Because they generally come on gradually, the patient has the opportunity to become accustomed to the impairments and may tolerate them better than the sudden onset of impairment associated with trauma. Finally, surgery

for degenerative conditions, especially total joint replacement, is highly specialized and may be beyond the scope of many surgical settings in the developing world.

Globally, the amount of joint replacement surgery is on the rise. Some LMICs are building centers specifically geared

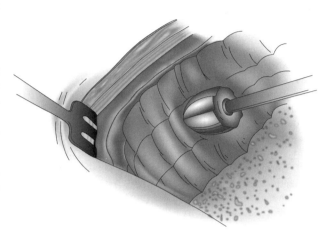

FIGURE 30.5. Bone is debrided until punctate bleeding is seen. A high-speed burr is shown here but hand instruments can be used instead.[16] Cierny G, 3rd, Mader JT, Penninck JJ. A clinical staging system for adult osteomyelitis. Clinical orthopaedics and related research. 2003 Sep; (414): 7–24.

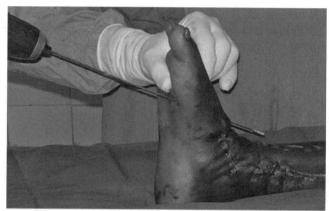

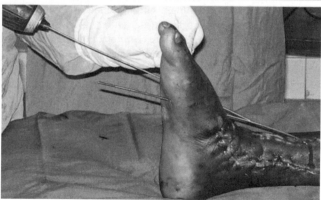

FIGURE 30.6. One K-wire is passed through the first metatarsal and the other through the fifth metatarsal. In this way the position of the foot can be controlled in both the coronal and sagittal planes.[18]

COMMON MICROORGANISMS IN ACUTE HEMATOGENOUS OSTEOMYELITIS

INFANTS:

Staphylococcus aureus
Group B streptococcus
Escherichia coli

CHILDREN UP TO 4 YEARS:

Staphylococcus aureus
Streptococcus pyogenes
Haemophilus influenzae

21 YEARS OR OLDER:

Staphylococcus aureus

ELDERLY:

Gram-negative rods
Septic Arthritis and Deep Infections of the Hands

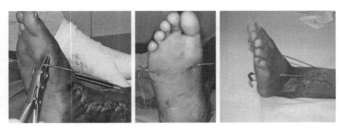

FIGURE 30.7. The wires are bent over to prevent injury to caregivers and damage to linens.[18]

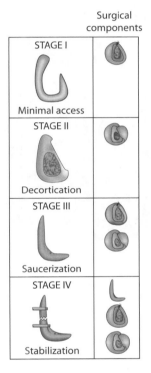

Surgical components

STAGE I Minimal access	
STAGE II Decortication	
STAGE III Saucerization	
STAGE IV Stabilization	

FIGURE 30.8. Surgical treatment according to Cierny-Mader stage.[16] Cierny G, 3rd, Mader JT, Penninck JJ. A clinical staging system for adult osteomyelitis. Clinical orthopaedics and related research. 2003 Sep; (414): 7–24.

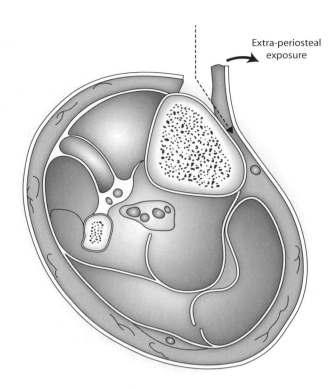

Extra-periosteal exposure

FIGURE 30.9. Avoid subperiosteal stripping in infection surgery.[17] Tetsworth K, Cierny G, 3rd. Osteomyelitis debridement techniques. Clinical orthopaedics and related research. 1999 Mar; (360): 87–96.

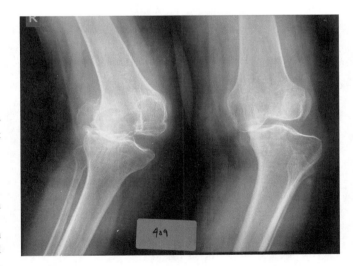

FIGURE 30.10. Preoperative radiograph of severe bilateral knee arthritis.[23] Image by Operation Walk Boston, Roya Ghazinouri and Thomas Thornhill.

toward these procedures, and at least one developing African country, Malawi, has established a total joint registry.[21]

Results are reported in rural settings that rival some Western referral centers. Stewart and colleagues reported a series of total knee and total hip replacements performed in rural Australia. There were no infections. In that group, 8.8% of knee patients had stiffness requiring manipulation, and 5.8% of hip patients had dislocations. Overall satisfaction was 97%.[22]

There is certainly a role for a visiting surgical team to do joint replacement surgery in an LMIC. The appeal of this is that joint replacement is a fairly discrete and predictable surgical event. The patients begin with an undeniably disabling and painful condition. After a few days of concentrated effort, they are left with a permanent improvement in health status. One orthopedic visiting surgical team dedicated to surgical

treatment of hip and knee arthritis is Operation Walk Boston.[23] This program, initiated in 2007 at Brigham and Women's Hospital in Boston, Massachusetts, USA, has partnered with a hospital in the Dominican Republic to provide joint replacement surgery once per year free of charge (Figures 30.10 through 30.16). More than 60 joint replacements are performed during each visiting surgical team's trip in a week's time. It must be emphasized, however, that it takes a whole year of preparation leading up to that week. Logistics planning for the visiting surgical team includes identifying all the patients well in advance, determining specific requirements for surgical implants and other expendable supplies as well as medications to be transported in advance. The total amount of material is enormous (Figures 30.10 through 30.16). The traveling team includes surgeons, anesthesiologists, operating room (OR) nurses, scrub techs, and recovery room and orthopedic staff nurses (Figures 30.10 through 30.16). A project of this scale would not be possible without the year-round partnership of the host physicians and nurses in the Dominican Republic. In addition to performing surgery, the team endeavors to include extensive hands-on and didactic training for the staff.

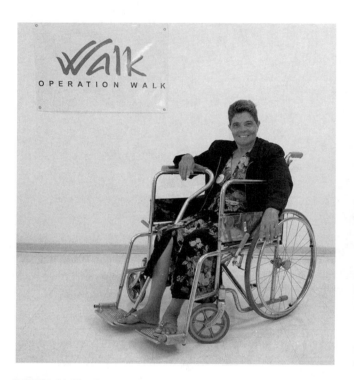

FIGURE 30.11. Preoperative photograph of patient bound to wheelchair by severe knee arthritis.[23] Image by Operation Walk Boston, Roya Ghazinouri and Thomas Thornhill.

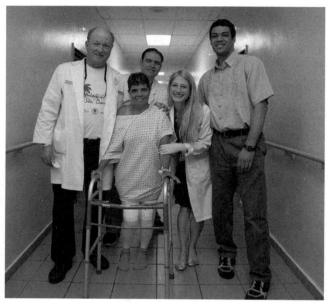

FIGURE 30.13. Postoperative photograph of patient standing after bilateral knee replacements.[23] Image by Operation Walk Boston, Roya Ghazinouri and Thomas Thornhill.

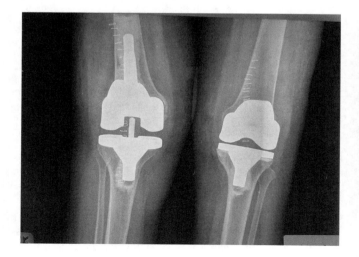

FIGURE 30.12. Postoperative radiographs of bilateral knee replacements.[23] Image by Operation Walk Boston, Roya Ghazinouri and Thomas Thornhill.

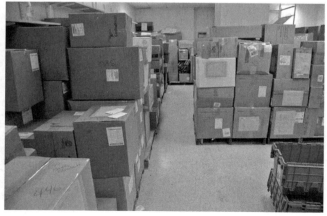

FIGURE 30.14. Orthopedic equipment stockpiled in advance of visiting surgical team's trip.[23] Image by Operation Walk Boston, Roya Ghazinouri and Thomas Thornhill.

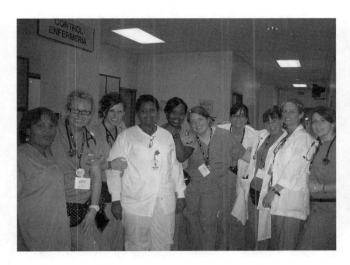

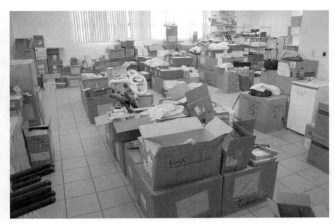

FIGURE 30.15. Anesthesia, medical, and other supplies.[23] Image by Operation Walk Boston, Roya Ghazinouri and Thomas Thornhill.

FIGURE 30.16. Orthopedic staff nurses and their Dominican counterparts.[23] Image by Operation Walk Boston, Roya Ghazinouri and Thomas Thornhill.

COMMENTARY

Ankur B. Bamne, Korea

The epidemiology of orthopedic disease focuses on the burden of impairment caused by various orthopedic ailments on societies. Musculoskeletal impairment is probably the most disabling condition, especially for people whose jobs involve manual labor. Nowhere is it more evident than in LMICs. In an estimate, half of the world's population lacks access to basic surgical care.[24] This is at a time when surgery is seen as a cost-effective public health measure.[25]

Trauma is an important cause of mortality and morbidity in young populations worldwide; these populations also happen to be the most economically productive. Losing the ability to earn a living can jeopardize a family's financial stability, especially in LMICs, which frequently lack disability insurance and other social benefits. There is also a significant burden of nontraumatic musculoskeletal disease. Considering these factors, the need for adequate treatment of these conditions and facilitating early return to work cannot be overemphasized.

The logistics and economics behind a visiting medical team can be enormous. However, there are many issues to be considered before embarking on these adventurous trips. Issues ranging from communication barriers to preoperative, intraoperative, and postoperative factors can jeopardize such an undertaking. Also, complex medical-legal issues can arise in the event of adverse outcomes. A better approach would probably be to train surgeons in LMICs to perform complex surgeries and help them to develop local healthcare infrastructure.

Principles behind managing fracture nonunions have been well described. Depending upon the type of fracture (infected vs. noninfected, hypertrophic vs. atrophic), specific management options have to be laid out. Surgeons in LMICs should have a lower threshold to accept certain complications like limb length discrepancy. Also, autogenous bone grafting may be the only option in the case of nonavailability of allograft bone or bone graft substitutes.

Osteomyelitis is one of the most common conditions encountered in LMICs. Lack of adequate treatment for acute osteomyelitis may lead to the development of chronic osteomyelitis (COM). Pathological fractures may develop when the bone is significantly weakened either by the disease process or by surgery itself. Soft tissue coverage is an important aspect in managing COM. Local flaps may be more feasible than microvascular free flaps in LMICs. Osteo-articular tuberculosis (TB) is still more highly prevalent in LMICs, including India, compared to many HICs. Acute TB and its sequelae is a significant source of morbidity in LMICs.

Congenital musculoskeletal ailments are a common occurrence in LMICs. India has the highest incidence of clubfoot in the world. Clubfoot cases are frequently undertreated either due to ignorance or lack of treatment facilities, especially in the rural areas. These individuals have little opportunity to become productive contributing adults in the society. Organizations like Cure Clubfoot are doing are a very important task of creating awareness and making treatment facilities available in the LMICs.

Life expectancy is increasing not only in HICs but also in LMICs.[26] This creates new challenges of facing degenerative ailments in aging populations. However, there are epidemiological differences between the Western world and many Asian and African countries with respect to degenerative arthritis. For example, primary hip arthritis is uncommon among Asian and African populations. Joint arthroplasty has revolutionized treatment of arthritic joints. Patients suffering from chronic pain because of arthritis seek dramatic improvement postarthroplasty. Also, many LMICs have made facilities for joint replacement available which are on par with their Western counterparts. More centers need to emerge to take care of the seniors in our societies whose activity is restricted because of arthritis. Also, because of cost constraints, newer advances like patient specific instrumentation may find limited utility in LMICs.

Orthopedic diseases can lead to severe impairment of function; however, their timely and adequate management can lead to good results and return to activity in both LMICs and HICs.

31

Pediatric Surgery

Doruk Ozgediz
Emmanuel A. Ameh

Epidemiology and Burden

Pediatric surgical conditions account for a significant portion of the burden of surgical disease in low- and middle-income countries (LMICs). This is partially due to regional demographics as more than half of the population is <18 years old in many countries and fertility rates remain as high as seven births per woman, even in countries with limited life expectancies. Prospective studies suggest that up to 85% of children in these settings will require surgical intervention by age 15.[1]

This chapter will discuss the care of selected common conditions encountered in a low-income setting; however, the reader is also referred to other subspecialty chapters in this book covering pediatric surgical conditions (e.g., urology [Chapter 43], otorhinolaryngology [Chapter 26], and orthopedics [Chapter 30]). In LMICs, all these conditions are likely to be managed by the same practitioner. Specifically, trauma comprises a large proportion of the burden of pediatric surgical conditions, and the reader is referred to Chapters 37 through 51 for the essentials of pediatric trauma care. In the North American environment, a significant portion (40% or more) of pediatric operations are for emergency conditions, and studies suggest this is comparable in LMICs.[2,3] A snapshot of selected inpatients on one day of the pediatric general surgery unit at Mulago Hospital (an LMIC national referral center) in Kampala, Uganda, reflects the broad spectrum of conditions treated there, ranging from trauma to congenital anomalies, oncology, and infectious diseases, and their attendant complications (Table 31.1).

In addition, the reader is referred to two other comprehensive recent textbooks covering this material in greater detail, one geared to the level of the district hospital and the other more to the tertiary center in Africa.[4,5]

Anesthesia Considerations, Vascular Access, and Critical Care

Frequently, the greatest perioperative morbidity and mortality in the care of pediatric surgical conditions is related to safe anesthesia and perioperative care. Some emergency conditions with high rates of effectiveness in the high-income countries (HICs) (such as airway or esophageal foreign bodies) may have a high complication rate in an LMIC due to anesthetic concerns.[6] Knowledge of the fundamentals of pediatric anesthesia and airway management and common pitfalls is essential before practicing in an LMIC.

The surgeon may be accompanied by an affiliated visiting anesthetic team but if not, should understand the availability of local resources: personnel, equipment, and expertise. In many settings, nonphysician clinicians may be the primary anesthesia providers and knowledge of the local practice is useful. There may be limited local experience with the postoperative recovery of patients. Particularly for elective cases, it may be useful to know the general volume of pediatric surgical cases (especially in neonates and infants). Even when focused on the surgical aspects of delivering care, perhaps the greatest contribution may be in assisting local personnel with overall readiness to perform operations on children. In some regions, especially outside of larger national referral hospitals, there may be no pediatric surgery performed other than by visiting teams.[7]

A general surgeon with primarily adult training must have a sense of the comfort level with a particular case if outside the scope of practice in their home environment. In uncertain cases, the surgeon may wish to consult with colleagues or local experts to determine the safety of specific elective cases. If there is a low volume of pediatric operations performed under general anesthesia, especially for neonates and infants, deferring the operation to an older age, perhaps >6 months old, may be considered, as the morbidity of general anesthesia is reduced. In the absence of anesthetic expertise, in neonates with an abdominal emergency it sometimes may be safer to perform the operation using abdominal field block with local anesthetic, if referral to a larger center is not feasible.

Sometimes the greatest challenge may be intravenous (IV) access, and the surgeon should be ready to establish IV access if routine peripheral sites fail for infants and small children. This is often exacerbated by delay in presentation, failure to thrive for chronic conditions, and acute dehydration with need for resuscitation. Vascular access may be performed by intraosseous route, cutdown (saphenous, external jugular, or umbilical in neonates), or percutaneous (external jugular vein). Many hospitals may not have a neonatal intensive care unit or capacity to ventilate pediatric patients. This should of course be considered for any elective case that may require postoperative respiratory support.

TABLE 31.1

Selected conditions present on pediatric surgery unit one day at Mulago Hospital, Kampala, Uganda 2010

Anorectal malformations

- 2-year-old with repaired vestibular fistula with re-fistula
- Neonate with cloaca
- Neonate with imperforate anus
- 3-year-old with fecal incontinence post-PSARP (posterior sagittal anorectoplasty)

Hirschsprung's disease

- 6-month-old status post Swenson with colostomy
- 3-year-old with enterocutaneous fistula post-stoma takedown
- 2-year-old post-Swenson operation with incontinence
- Infant with constipation and nondefinitive pathology for Hirschsprung's disease

Oncology

- 2-year-old with testicular rhabdomyosarcoma
- 4-month-old with sacrococcygeal teratoma
- 2-year-old with Wilms' tumor

Trauma

- 8-year-old with splenectomy post–blunt trauma
- 10-year-old with bilateral chest tubes s/p motorcycle crash

Infection

- 9-year-old boy with abdominal sepsis without source at laparotomy
- 5-year-old with postoperative enterocutaneous fistula after typhoid perforation
- 10-year-old s/p appendectomy
- 2-year-old with extremity gangrene after febrile illness
- 5-year-old with snakebite
- 1-year-old with wound tetanus

Miscellaneous

- 2-month-old with jaundice and possible biliary atresia

Electrolytes and Nutrition

Knowledge of the basic maintenance fluid requirements for infants and children is essential. For neonates, due to fluid overload in the first several days of life, maintenance fluids are limited to 60–80 cc/kg/day and D10 water is provided, with a gradual transition to ¼ normal saline solution if possible over the first week. During this time, healthy neonates gradually lose their innate excess sodium through a physiologic diuresis. Neonatal resuscitation skills and resources may not be available in the austere setting; currently a major World Health Organization (WHO) program, Helping Babies Breathe, is attempting to reduce neonatal deaths.[8] Generally, the "4/2/1" rule for maintenance IV fluids can be used for children (Table 31.2).

In other words, a 22 kg patient would require $(4 \times 10 = 40) + (2 \times 10 = 20) + (1 \times 2 = 2) = 62$ cc/hr. of IV fluid.

Potassium depletion is common, particularly in those with abdominal emergencies (e.g., intestinal obstruction or typhoid perforation) presenting late. This should be carefully corrected before surgery. Potassium replacement should also be considered postoperatively in patients who have had abdominal surgery and are NPO for more than 48 hours.

Especially for elective cases where blood transfusion may be necessary, local blood bank capacity should be evaluated. Blood volume per kilogram is highest in the neonatal period and decreases gradually at over 1 year old (Table 31.3).

Caloric requirements are also highest in the neonatal period and first year of life (100–150 kcal/kg/day) and gradually decrease to 25–35 kcal/kg/day in adulthood. Patients in many LMICs may not have access to parenteral nutrition or the diversity of enteral formulas available in an HIC. Even if available, enteral formulas or specific components of parenteral nutrition

TABLE 31.2

Maintenance fluid requirements for children

Weight	Fluid requirement
<10 kg	4 cc/kg/hr.
10–20 kg	+2 cc/kg/hr.
>20 kg	+1 cc/kg/hr.

TABLE 31.3

Blood replacement requirements for children

Age	Requirement
Preterm	90–100 cc/kg
Term	80–90 cc/kg
Infant	70–80 cc/kg
>1 year	70 cc/kg

may be available only in private pharmacies at an exorbitant cost to families. These factors should all be considered in operative planning and in any operation that may render a patient NPO for a prolonged period. Generally, parenteral feeding is indicated in children expected to be NPO for over 10 days. Enteral nutrition is always preferred if at all possible given the above factors. A higher proportion of children (20%–30%) in LMICs will be undernourished at presentation, contributing to higher rates of postoperative complications such as superficial and deep wound infections.[9] Though NPO guidelines vary by setting, in most settings a clear liquid diet can be taken up to 3 hours before surgery; breast milk for 4 hours.

Neonatal Bowel Obstruction

Perhaps the greatest difference between acute abdomen in the neonatal period in HICs and LMICs is that necrotizing enterocolitis, primarily a disease of prematurity, is rare in settings without a neonatal intensive care service and the capacity to care for the medical problems of prematurity. It will therefore not be discussed here. In the neonatal period, anorectal malformations (discussed below) are the most common source of bowel obstruction, followed by intestinal atresia-stenosis, Hirschsprung's disease (discussed below), and malrotation.

Malrotation

Malrotation generally presents (80%) with bilious vomiting in the term infant 1 month of age or younger. The infant with bilious vomiting should be presumed to have malrotation until proven otherwise. The disease is due to abnormal fixation of the bowel prenatally, leading to a shortened distance between the ligament of Treitz and the ileocecal junction and a narrow mesentery, resulting in heightened risk of twisting and a volvulus (Figure 31.1A and 31.1B). In the presence of abdominal distension and peritoneal signs, the patient may proceed to laparotomy without imaging, with IV access established and resuscitation underway while proceeding. A nasogastric tube should be placed to decompress the bowel.

Plain abdominal films may show a range of findings, from near normal-appearing bowel gas pattern, to a whiteout due to bowel edema and ascites, or pneumoperitoneum secondary to a perforated volvulus. An ultrasound may show swirling of the mesenteric vessels at the base of the mesentery with complete volvulus, though this may require an experienced pediatric radiologist to see. Though there is some controversy, the gold standard is an upper gastrointestinal contrast study, to identify the location of the ligament of Treitz (duodeno-jejunal junction) and to rule out other causes of proximal obstruction. The ligament of Treitz should be located to the left of midline and at the level of the duodenal bulb, at approximately the L1 pedicle. This study, however, may not be available in the LMIC, and laparotomy may be indicated based on clinical suspicion alone.[10]

A transverse laparotomy incision should be performed. Chylous ascites may be encountered in the presence of partial or intermittent obstruction. The bowel should be fully eviscerated. In the setting of midgut volvulus, the bowel is de-rotated in the counterclockwise direction and examined for improvement in perfusion. A pulse should be sought at the root of the superior mesenteric artery. This can also be evaluated by Doppler if available. The bowel can be covered with warm sponges, 100% oxygen administered by anesthetist, and a period of waiting of 10–15 minutes may be appropriate. In cases of questionable viability and demarcation, a second-look laparotomy may be planned for 12–24 hours if intensive care is available, and a temporary abdominal dressing may be devised. If the bowel is well perfused, a Ladd's procedure should be performed:

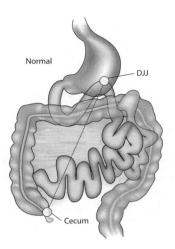

FIGURE 31.1A Normal rotation: The duodenal-jejunal junction (DJJ), or ligament of Treitz, and the ileocecal junction are fixed in a normal retroperitoneal location, maintaining a wide mesentery without a risk of volvulus. Illustration by Sani Yamout, MD.

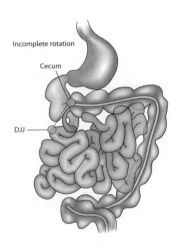

FIGURE 31.1B Incomplete rotation: The DJJ and the ileocecal junction are close, resulting in a narrow mesentery and an increased risk of volvulus. Illustration by Sani Yamout, MD.

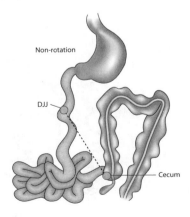

FIGURE 31.1C Nonrotation: The large bowel is on the left and the small bowel on the right side, without increased risk of volvulus. Illustration by Sani Yamout, MD.

1. The mesentery should be broadened at the base, which involves carefully freeing peritoneal adhesions in this area.

2. The ligament of Treitz should be taken down to straighten the duodenum and upper jejunum.

3. The small bowel should be placed on the right and the cecum in the left hypochondrium.

4. An appendectomy should be performed.

At the end of a Ladd's procedure, the intestine is left in a position of "nonrotation" (Figure 31.1C). This counterintuitive maneuver leaves the patient at the lowest risk of later adhesive bowel obstruction. After closure, feeds are commenced after evidence of return of bowel function as demonstrated by flatus.

Intestinal Atresia and Stenosis

Jejunoileal atresia and stenosis may have varied epidemiology, with an incidence ranging from 1 in 1,000 births in the African setting to 1 in 3,000 births in the United States.[11] Duodenal atresia may also be encountered but is thought to be less common.[12]

Neonates with atresia present in the early postnatal period with abdominal distension, vomiting, intolerance of feeds, and failure to pass meconium, while intestinal stenosis may not present until later in life. Plain abdominal X-rays may show the classic "double-bubble" in duodenal atresia or dilated intestinal loops in more distal atresias. Contrast enema may show a microcolon or may confirm meconium plugs or ileus, and for these conditions, the enema may be therapeutic and the patient may not require surgical intervention. Demonstration of colon continuity preoperatively also obviates the need to do this at laparotomy. Nasogastric decompression and IV resuscitation are necessary prior to laparotomy. Generally, nasogastric aspirate of >20–30 cc's in the newborn suggests obstruction.

Treatment at laparotomy depends on the type of atresia encountered (Figure 31.2).

Generally, the ends of the atresia must be resected before restoration of bowel continuity. At this time, the rest of the bowel distally can be flushed with normal saline to evaluate for the

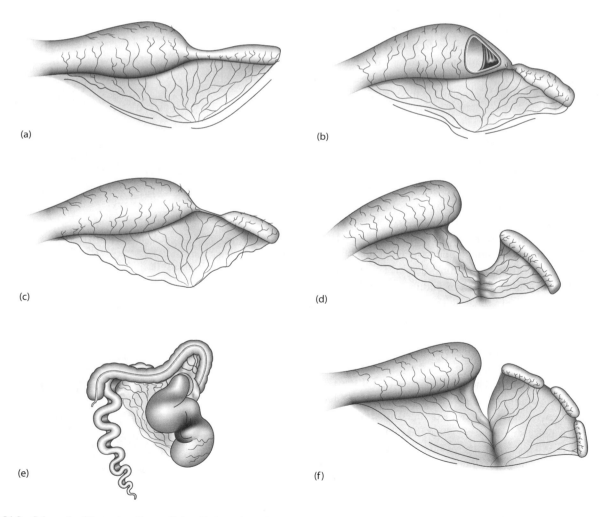

FIGURE 31.2 Schematic of the various forms of jejunoileal atresia. (a) Stenosis. (b) Type I: transluminal septum with intact bowel continuity. (c) Type II: 2 blind ending pouches with a fibrous cord in between, with intact mesentery. (d) Type IIIA: 2 blind ending pouches not in continuity with a mesenteric defect. (e) Type IIIB: "apple peel" or "Christmas tree" deformity with proximal jejunal atresia, large mesenteric defect, and varying length of distal small bowel with retrograde perfusion along a single vessel. (f) Type IV: Multiple intestinal atresias. Aguayo P, Ostile D. *Ashcraft's Pediatric Surgery.* 5th ed. Philadelphia: Elsevier, 2010.

presence of one or more additional atresias (4%). There may be a significant size discrepancy between dilated proximal bowel and decompressed bowel distal to the atresia. The approach may be dictated by the anatomy present. Sometimes resection of the bulbous end of dilated proximal bowel may facilitate anastomosis. An antimesenteric "slit" in the distal bowel may enlarge its diameter. Tapering enteroplasty or plication may also be performed on dilated proximal bowel to address the size discrepancy. Feeding is commenced after return of bowel function, and, if possible, total parenteral nutrition is maintained during this time. For more proximal atresias, a transanastomotic feeding tube and a gastrostomy tube may be particularly helpful in an environment without parenteral nutrition. While survival in HICs is >90%, it may be as low as 40%–50% in sub-Saharan Africa due to late presentation and the lack of parenteral nutrition.[13]

Other Abdominal Emergencies in Infants and Children

Pyloric Stenosis

While the incidence of pyloric stenosis is estimated to be 1 in 400 in some Caucasian populations, it is reported to be profoundly less in some other settings, for reasons that have yet to be elucidated. A recent audit from a tertiary center in Nigeria showed only 5 cases over 10 years, and 1 in the last 5 years.[14,15] Thus in some settings this will be exceedingly rare, and other conditions should be considered in the differential. The typical presentation is of projectile nonbilious vomiting at approximately 1 month of age. With a delay in presentation, infants may be profoundly dehydrated.[16]

On examination, the epigastrium is full, and active peristalsis of the dilated stomach may sometimes be seen moving from the left hypochondrium downward to the right side. The characteristic vomiting can be demonstrated by allowing the infant to suck on a pacifier, or the mother is asked to briefly breastfeed. A small mass (the "olive") can be palpated under the right hypochondrium with the index and long fingers of the left hand, drawing them downward as the infant suckles. The diagnosis is confirmed by abdominal ultrasound, with increased wall thickness and length (generally 4 mm × 17 mm). Upper gastrointestinal study is rarely necessary. The most common medical condition in the differential is reflux disease, and in cases of diagnostic uncertainty, feeds may continue to be attempted with the infant in the upright position, which should minimize vomiting if reflux disease is the cause.

The infant must be adequately resuscitated before proceeding to the operating room. Initial boluses should be with 20 cc/kg of normal saline, and urine output must be closely monitored. Inadequate resuscitation prior to general anesthesia may lead to postoperative ventilator dependence due to compensatory respiratory acidosis. Once the infant has begun to urinate, potassium may be added to the maintenance fluids. If electrolytes cannot be drawn, the clinician may have to rely on the urine output and clinical signs of hydration to assess readiness for surgery.

While there has been an increased trend to laparoscopy in HICs, in the HIC, this operation can be done through either a right upper abdominal incision or through a supraumbilical incision. The pylorus must be gently delivered into the wound and the serosa scored over its length. A blunt spreader can then be used to split the thickened muscle down to the level of the mucosa that will bulge through the myotomy, starting in the middle of the pylorus and extending in either direction. The pylorus extends from the duodenum, identified by the vein of Mayo (usually several small vein branches) to the gastric side, as identified by a change in direction of muscle fibers. Care should be taken at the edges of the myotomy as the muscles thin down to a normal size; these are the most common sites of perforation. If there is question of perforation, it may be confirmed by gentle gastric insufflation by the anesthesiologist and examination of the area in question. In case of perforation, the mucosa should be oversewn with a 5-0 absorbable suture on a round-bodied needle and a myotomy performed on the other side of the pylorus.

A nasogastric tube is not necessary postoperatively, and the infant can be fed with dextrose solution when he or she is vigorous and can progress to breast or formula feeding as tolerated. Vomiting of a lesser degree frequently occurs; the feed can be repeated and usually the vomiting does not occur more than once or twice. The infant is discharged home usually after 24 hours. Outcome is excellent if the pyloromyotomy is done well. Persistent vomiting after surgery may indicate an incomplete pyloromyotomy. An upper gastrointestinal contrast study should be done; if it shows gastric outlet obstruction, a repeat pyloromyotomy is necessary.

Intussusception

Intussusception occurs most frequently in the 3-month to 3-year age group and is most commonly idiopathic in origin, frequently due to a preexisting viral illness that may have produced intra-abdominal lymphadenopathy. The mesenteric lymph nodes, usually in the terminal ileum, are the most common lead point of the intussusception. In infants with gastroenteritis, vigorous peristalsis may also precipitate an intussusception. The intussusception is generally ileocolic (approximately 80%–90%) but can extend as far as the rectum or colon. In a minority of cases, the intussusception may be colo-colic, or small bowel to small bowel; the latter generally resolves spontaneously. There is no reliable population-level incidence data to evaluate whether intussusception is more common in the LMIC, but it is one of the most common causes of acute abdomen and bowel obstruction in children in LMICs.[17,18]

Classically, children present with fits of intermittent crampy abdominal pain (where the child draws his knees up to the chest) with intervening periods of normal behavior. It may or may not be possible to elicit a prior history of viral illness. There may be bilious or nonbilious vomiting, or red-purple "currant-jelly stools," an indicator of possible mucosal compromise. On physical examination, the abdomen is benign early, and later in the course becomes distended. The presence of peritoneal signs should raise concern for possible bowel compromise and mandates operative exploration. The child may have visible signs of dehydration and sepsis. Other causes of bowel obstruction, such as an incarcerated inguinal hernia, should be evaluated on physical examination. With early presentation, a mass in the right upper quadrant may be present. A rectal examination should be performed as well to evaluate for blood in the stool, and in the most extreme cases, the intussusception may protrude through the rectum (Figure 31.3), perhaps initially raising the question whether this may be rectal prolapse. Vital signs may reflect dehydration or septic response.

Plain abdominal films may show distended bowel loops consistent with intestinal obstruction or, in early cases, more normal appearing but for a paucity of gas in the right lower quadrant. In

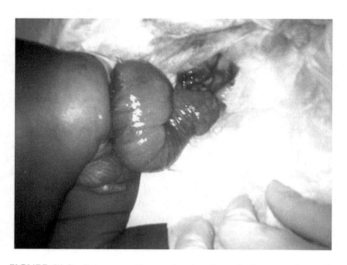

FIGURE 31.3 Intussusception prolapsing through the anus. Image by Emmanuel A. Ameh, MD.

the hands of an experienced radiologist, ultrasound may be confirmatory if the characteristic features of a target sign are present. With late presentation, pneumoperitoneum may be present. A contrast enema, in the hands of an experienced radiologist, may be therapeutic up to 80% of the time; however, this modality is frequently unavailable in a LMIC. The enema may be performed using air or water and is generally performed with the aid of fluoroscopy or ultrasound. In LMICs, surgeon-performed pneumatic reduction enema may also be performed safely in the operating room under general anesthesia.[19] If enema is available in the local environment, if the first attempt does not fully reduce the intussusception, it may be attempted again if some progress was made on the first attempt, in the absence of peritoneal signs or hemodynamic instability. Rarely, reduction by enema can result in perforation, and in extreme cases can result in abdominal compartment syndrome requiring emergency abdominal decompression with an 18-gauge needle at the bedside, prior to urgent laparotomy.

It should be stressed that the presence of peritoneal signs and clinical signs of sepsis mandate laparotomy. A nasogastric tube should be placed for decompression in the clinical setting consistent with a small bowel obstruction, the patient should be aggressively resuscitated with IV fluids, and the urine output monitored as closely as possible. As with other surgical conditions in the LMIC, patients often present with high-grade bowel obstruction and severe dehydration, and this compromises outcomes, with mortality rates of 8%–50% reported in these settings, compared to negligible mortality rate in HICs.[20]

In this age group, a primarily right-sided transverse or midline laparotomy may be performed. The bowel may be delivered, and the intussusception identified. The cecum may need to be mobilized. The intussusception should be reduced by milking the

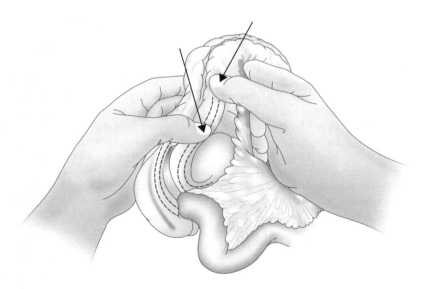

FIGURE 31.4 Depiction of intraoperative method to reduce intussusception. Aguayo P, Ostile D. *Ashcraft's Pediatric Surgery.* 5th ed. Philadelphia: Elsevier, 2010.

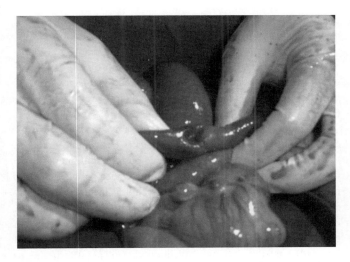

FFIGURE 31.5 Typical appearance of lead point of intussusceptions. Image by Doruk Ozgediz.

intussuscepted bowel from the distal end proximally (Figure 31.4 and 31.5) rather than trying to "pull it out" at the site of intussusception, as this may result in tearing of the bowel. Once reduced, the bowel should be evaluated for viability, and nonviable bowel should be resected and an anastomosis performed between ends of well-perfused bowel.

In cases where the intussusception is reduced nonoperatively, there is an approximately 10% risk of recurrence, and this should be stressed to the parents. In some cases, the intussusception may reduce on its own, without any intervention. Intussusception in the older child raises the question of a pathologic lead point, and this generally requires laparotomy for definitive diagnosis. The most common pathologic lead points are Meckel's diverticulum or polyps of the small and large bowel, malignant conditions such as small bowel lymphoma are also possible.

Appendicitis

Presentation of appendicitis in the child is quite similar to that in adults. Though in North America and Europe, the lifetime incidence of appendicitis is estimated to be 7%–8%, in Africa, it is estimated to be lower, closer to 1%–2%, perhaps due to variation in diet and the immune system. Peak incidence is in the 12–18 year age group; appendicitis is rare in neonates and infants.[21]

In most austere settings, the decision to operate for appendicitis will be based on history and physical examination alone, without the aid of any ancillary tests. However, imaging can be helpful. Plain films may be helpful in about 30% of cases, and may show a fecalith in the right lower quadrant, blurring of the psoas margin on the right, and scoliosis to the right on an upright film or an obstructive pattern. Ultrasound may be highly sensitive and specific, though this is mostly observer dependent. In an HIC, perforated appendicitis with abscess is generally diagnosed on computed tomography (CT) scan and imaging-assisted drainage may be performed with a plan for interval appendectomy several months later. This approach for perforated appendicitis is not possible in most LMICs without interventional radiology capacity, and nearly all such patients will require surgical intervention. Moreover, most patients with perforated appendicitis in these settings have general peritonitis at presentation, making an initial nonsurgical approach inappropriate.

In the child <4 years old, presentation with perforation is the rule, due to both the difficulty for young children to describe mild symptoms, and the fact that the omentum in young children is thinner and less able to contain infection. The patient with symptom duration >3 days who presents with a palpable right lower quadrant mass, but is pain-free and tolerating a diet, may be treated with antibiotics for 7–10 days and presumed to have appendicitis with contained perforation. This may be then followed up with interval examination. The need for later appendectomy in children treated nonoperatively is debated, as 19% of children with a fecalith and 9% without a fecalith go on to develop appendicitis again in the future.[22] A rectal examination should be performed in patients presumed to have perforation and abscess, and if initial nonoperative therapy is considered, transrectal drainage of a pelvic abscess can be performed under sedation.

An additional challenge is that fever, abdominal pain, and other symptoms similar to those of appendicitis are common in malaria endemic regions due to improper use of antimalarials. These medicines are readily available at pharmacies without a prescription. Parents may not seek medical attention until their child has not responded to a full course of therapy, and if they do so, may first see a traditional healer. These factors contribute to the frequent advanced presentation of diseases for acute abdominal conditions. In addition, the broader differential diagnosis for acute abdominal pain in children in the tropics must be considered, including, for example, intestinal perforation from infectious causes such as typhoid fever, infectious complications of malnutrition or immune suppression, and spontaneous bacterial peritonitis.

In the patient with diffuse peritonitis, a midline approach may be chosen to allow for adequate exploration and washout. In children the appendix may be ligated with a simple or pursestring suture, either antegrade or retrograde depending on the ease of dissection. Drains may be useful in localized abscess cavities. In the absence of formal Jackson-Pratt drains, other available rubber or soft plastic tubing or a corrugated rubber sheet may be used.

In extreme cases where the appendiceal stump is liquefied and the surgeon is concerned about the development of a cecal leak and subsequent colocutaneous fistula, a diverting loop ileostomy may be constructed, though this can have significant morbidity in an austere setting. A tube cecostomy, perhaps with a Foley catheter, may be more helpful and easier to manage in such a case. In other extreme cases, visceral edema from inflammation may be so extensive that primary fascial closure is not possible due to elevated intra-abdominal pressure. In these cases, a temporary abdominal closure may need to be devised, perhaps using a Bogota bag or a modified version (an opened-up urine bag can be used if a purpose-made bag is not available) for damage control laparotomy. Low-cost vacuum-assisted closure devices have also been described in these scenarios.[23] The care of these patients may be challenged by need for sedation for brief dressing changes, but this may be feasible through the use of short-acting but very effective and cheap anesthetic agents such as ketamine that are fairly available, may be given intramuscularly (IM), and have a good safety profile, even in austere settings.

Oncology

Lymphadenopathy and Lymphoma

The general surgeon is frequently called to evaluate "lumps and bumps" in children, often to establish the malignant potential of these lesions and to decide whether a biopsy is indicated. Most of the time, if there is a reasonable level of suspicion, a biopsy should be performed as this is a low-risk procedure that can give high-yield diagnostic information.

Lymphomas are generally classified as Hodgkin's (85% globally) and non-Hodgkin's (15%) type.[24] In sub-Saharan Africa, however, Burkitt's lymphoma is endemic and the most common type of lymphoma in children, often presenting with a mass about the jaw (Figure 31.6).

The high occurrence of Burkitt's may be partly due to an association and interaction between Epstein-Barr virus (EBV) and malaria that may also be affected by the influence of human immunodeficiency virus (HIV). In older children, other forms of lymphoma are more common.[25] Burkitt's lymphoma is one of the "small round blue cell" tumors of childhood, and one of the most rapidly dividing human tumors, with a doubling time of 24–48 hours. Its rapid growth leads urgency to its diagnosis and initiation of therapy, but fortunately also makes it very chemosensitive. Generally, the incidence of B-cell lymphomas has increased in high HIV-incidence areas, and HIV-related Burkitt's lymphoma has been shown to be less chemosensitive. Overall, it is estimated that the proportion of malignant to nonmalignant lesions in biopsied cervical nodes is similar between HICs and LMICs at approximately 12%.[26]

Initially, a careful history should be performed asking specifically about the size of the mass, other possible lymph nodes, and constitutional symptoms such as fever, weight loss, and lethargy. Risk factors for immune compromise should be evaluated and an HIV and purified protein derivative (PPD) tests should be obtained. Up to 18% of patients with HIV disease may present with adenopathy.[27]

Careful lymph node examination should be performed of all regions assessing whether nodes are fixed or mobile, matted, single or multiple, and whether there is associated abdominal organomegaly. Nodes persisting for more than 4 weeks, greater than 2 cm, nontender, hard or fixed, or those with rapid growth may be considered more suspicious for malignancy (Figure 31.7).

Any node in the supraclavicular fossa is considered suspicious and should be biopsied. In the cervical region, nodes in the posterior triangle are more suspicious for malignancy than those in the anterior neck. Concerning cervical or axillary (the most common locations) adenopathy should be investigated by chest X-ray (to rule out tuberculosis [TB] or a mediastinal mass). For patients with a mediastinal mass and cervical adenopathy, general anesthesia for biopsy should be avoided due to concern for cardiovascular collapse with induction of anesthesia due to potential airway compression by the mass.

With suspicion of infected nodes, a short course of empiric antibiotics may be administered. Without response or if nodes have persisted beyond 4 to 6 weeks, a biopsy should be obtained. Blood tests are unlikely to alter the need for a biopsy. A PPD may be placed as part of the workup for tuberculosis exposure; however, it should not be placed if Bacille Calmette-Guerin (BCG) vaccination is common in the local context. A single fluctuant tender node is more suggestive of acute suppurative lymphadenitis and can be treated with incision and drainage or needle aspiration with culture.

Tuberculous lymphadenitis is particularly common in high–HIV prevalence areas. Even in the absence of TB, lymphadenopathy may be the presenting symptom of HIV disease. This is in distinct contrast to the microbiology in North America, where infection with atypical mycobacteria is more common. BCG vaccination itself can also cause lymphadenitis in 36/1,000 vaccinations.[28]

As for biopsy technique, the reader is referred to Chapter 32 for a description of fine-needle aspiration biopsy (FNA) if one is to be performed. This procedure usually cannot be done in children without adequate sedation, and aspirate may not provide adequate tissue for flow cytometry required to diagnose lymphoma. An open incisional or excisional biopsy technique is preferred in most instances. In some cases, diagnosis may be obtained by bone marrow biopsy, or by aspirate of pleural fluid.

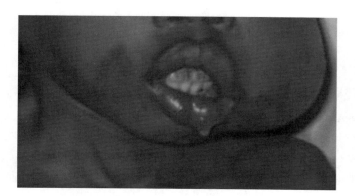

FIGURE 31.6 Burkitt's lymphoma. Image by Emmanuel A. Ameh.

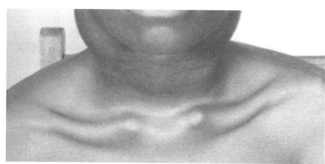

FIGURE 31.7 Cervical adenopathy concerning for lymphoma. Image by Emmanuel A. Ameh.

A wide spectrum of infectious and noninfectious diseases can also cause lymphadenopathy, and the reader is referred to other sources for a more complete discussion.[26]

Though lymphadenopathy may be the most common presentation of lymphoma in children, and the characteristic mandibular mass of Burkitt's lymphoma may be well recognized, other presentations include intussusception and/or bowel obstruction, abdominal mass, mediastinal mass, pleural effusion, or splenomegaly. In the rare cases of isolated bowel tumors with Burkitt's lymphoma, a complete resection, if possible, will be essentially curative, though postoperative chemotherapy will still be needed as the disease is multifocal. Most abdominal masses, however, will be unresectable, and only a biopsy needs to be performed in most cases with chemotherapy the mainstay of therapy. Staging laparotomy, once part of the management of lymphoma, is no longer indicated. Prognosis will depend on the local availability of chemotherapy programs as well as compliance with therapy.[30]

Wilms' Tumor

This is one of the most common embryonal childhood tumors, representing about 3%–20% of all malignant tumors in children in LMICs.[31,32] Patients may present with an abdominal mass, microscopic hematuria, hypertension, malaise, weight loss, or anemia. Pain with fever and a rapidly enlarging abdominal mass may indicate acute tumor rupture. In LMICs, due to often late presentation, a large abdominal mass is obvious at presentation. In these settings, anemia and malnutrition are present in more than 50% of the patients at presentation.[33,34] A minority of patients with Wilms' tumors have an associated named syndrome, and features associated with that syndrome may be present.

Abdominal ultrasound can identify the renal origin of the tumor and can assess the contralateral kidney, the ipsilateral renal vein, and the inferior vena cava for tumor extension. IV urography may show a distortion of the pelvicaliceal system of the affected kidney, and there may be non-excretion of contrast from that kidney. CT scan is most accurate in characterizing the extent of disease, but this is often unavailable or too expensive in LMICs. As a result, IV urography may be used more frequently. A soft-tissue needle biopsy of the tumor to confirm histological diagnosis can be done under ultrasound guidance (preferably using a Doppler ultrasound). Biopsy may be required also to exclude Burkitt's lymphoma. Open biopsy risks severe hemorrhage and tumor dissemination. A plain chest film should evaluate for pulmonary metastasis. The tumor should be staged and the National Wilms' Tumor Study (NWTS) or Société Internationale d'Oncologie Pédiatrique (SIOP) staging system can be used. In sub-Saharan Africa, >50% of patients present with stage III and IV disease.[35,36]

The treatment of Wilms' tumor involves surgery, chemotherapy, and radiotherapy. The NWTS and SIOP protocols can be used. The NWTS protocol advocates that resectable tumors are excised primarily. However, data suggest the SIOP protocol may be better suited for the LMIC setting.[37,38] This protocol consists of administration of preoperative chemotherapy for all patients, using vincristine and actinomycin D (given for 4 weeks and surgery in the 5th week) without histological diagnosis. This is aimed at reducing the tumor size to minimize the risk of intraoperative tumor rupture/spillage and increase the chance of complete resection. Following surgery, chemotherapy is continued based on risk stratification according to tumor histology (favorable or unfavorable) for a total of 18–24 weeks. Goals of surgery are abdominal exploration, complete tumor resection without spillage (in low-stage tumors), nephroureterectomy, lymph node biopsy at the renal hilum, and removal of the tumor from the renal vein or inferior vena cava in cases of tumor extension to these locations.

Wilms' tumor is presently considered a curable disease, and long-term survival can be expected for >80% of patients in HICs. In LMICs, however, the 5-year survival is below 50%, largely due to the late stage at diagnosis, comorbidities, and problems completing chemotherapy.

Congenital Anomalies

Anorectal Malformations

Anorectal malformations are one of the most common congenital anomalies encountered in neonates and children in LMICs, with an estimated incidence of 1 in 3,500 births. There is a wide spectrum of disease, ranging from limited perineal anomalies to complex cloacal anomalies requiring more complex reconstruction. Familiarity with the variations in presentation is essential (Figures 31.8A through 31.8E).[39] Most anomalies other than perineal fistulas can be approached in stages, with colostomy, followed by definitive repair (posterior sagittal anorectoplasty), and then colostomy takedown after several months.

Anomalies are generally classified as high or low. In male patients, the most common anomaly is high imperforate anus with recto-urethral fistula, while in female patients it is a low vestibular fistula. Only approximately 5% of male infants will have imperforate anus without fistula. Most babies with no anal opening at all will be referred for surgical evaluation within 24–48 hours of birth. Even if not diagnosed by trained birth personnel in a rural area, abdominal distension and failure to pass meconium will generally prompt parents to seek medical care. However, in LMICs, delay in presentation is common. The construction of a colostomy beyond this time period can be very challenging due to progressive abdominal distension, and perforation can occur in cases of further surgical delay. Other patients with an abnormally positioned anal opening who are able to stool with some difficulty may have a delayed presentation to later infancy or childhood. Sometimes these patients are treated unsuccessfully for chronic constipation due to presumed medical causes and suffer great morbidity. Girls with an uncorrected anteriorly displaced anal opening or rectovestibular fistula may live their whole lives with this anomaly. Some practitioners have raised concerns about future vaginal delivery in these patients; however, studies with sufficient long-term follow-up are lacking.

Delay in presentation and complications of anorectal malformations are the rule, either pre- or postoperatively.[40] A common scenario is one in which the surgeon is asked to "close a colostomy" that was created in the neonatal period, before the anoplasty has actually been done. In the acute neonatal setting, in the absence of an anal opening, a full physical examination should be performed. Anorectal malformations are part of the VACTERL association, which includes vertebral anomalies,

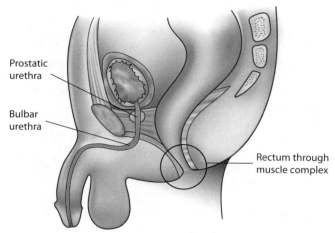

FIGURE 31.8A   Sagittal view of normal anorectal anatomy. Illustration by Sani Yamout, MD.

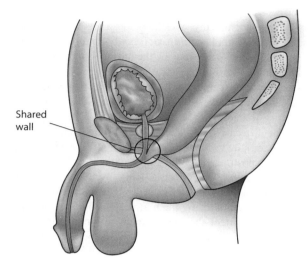

FIGURE 31.8B   Sagittal view of male with rectobulbar fistula. Illustration by Sani Yamout, MD.

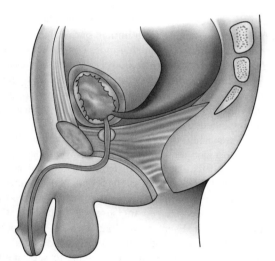

FIGURE 31.8C   Sagittal view of male with bladder fistula. Illustration by Sani Yamout, MD.

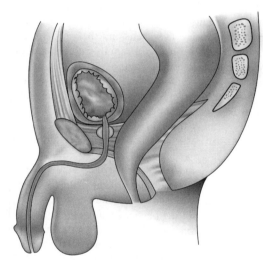

FIGURE 31.8D   Sagittal view of male with perineal fistula. Illustration by Sani Yamout, MD.

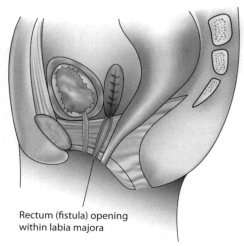

FIGURE 31.8E   Sagittal view of female with rectovestibular fistula. Illustration by Sani Yamout, MD.

cardiac defects, trachea-esophageal fistula, renal anomalies, limb anomalies, and distal spinal cord lesions. Cardiac auscultation may reveal a murmur; if available, an abdominal ultrasound should evaluate for renal structural anomalies. In the absence of hemodynamic instability, a formal echocardiogram may not be indicated. A careful perineal exam should be performed, noting the nature of perineum, the integrity of muscle formation, and palpable sacral defects. Generally, a "flat" bottom with poor muscle formation and sacral defects is associated with a high malformation, while a well-formed perineum is more suggestive of a low malformation. For an abnormally located anal opening in the perineum (i.e., perineal fistula), the size should be noted with the knowledge that most normal neonatal anal orifices accommodate a size 10–12 Hegar dilator. In girls, all orifices should be examined to ensure there is not a single orifice (cloacal anomaly, the rarest malformation).

An abdominal X-ray is likely to show distally dilated intestinal loops; a cross-table lateral X-ray (an invertogram should be done with caution as vomiting and respiratory complications may occur) may be used at 8–24 hours postnatally to estimate the distance from the rectum (should be visible with a column of air) to the perineal skin (marked with a radiopaque marker on the skin). If this distance is less than 1 cm, an experienced surgeon may choose to perform an anoplasty rather than a colostomy. If referred in the first day of life, one should wait 24 hours before the construction of a colostomy in case meconium passes in this time period to reveal a low malformation that can be primarily treated with a perineal procedure. The presence of a "bucket-handle" anomaly on the perineum suggests a low malformation that would be amenable to anoplasty, and sometimes a small previously undetected opening is revealed by gently using a small probe.

In cases of a large rectourethral fistula (as sometimes apparent by meconium staining of the urine), the baby may pass meconium in the urine and the bowel may rarely be decompressed with a Foley catheter passed through the urethral opening.

The creation of a colostomy for the newborn with acute abdominal distension with no anal opening may be a lifesaving procedure (Figure 31.9).

As recommended by Pena et al., this is done with a left lower quadrant incision.[39] The sigmoid colon is generally extremely distended on entry to the peritoneal cavity, and it may need to be decompressed prior to exteriorization. This can be done by placing a purse-string suture in the wall of the sigmoid and decompressing with a 25-gauge needle. The proximal and distal ends of the sigmoid colon should be clearly identified and the bowel should be divided. A divided colostomy is favored over a loop due to concern about partial diversion and spillover of stool. In addition, the colostomy should be constructed in the first mobile portion of the sigmoid colon to allow maximum bowel length for the later pull-through procedure. The distal colon-rectum should be washed out at the time of colostomy creation. The baby can then start feeding when the colostomy is functional and the abdomen decompressed. Most families in austere settings will not have access to stoma supplies, and providers and patients usually

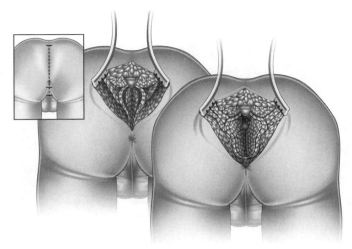

FIGURE 31.10A Basic depiction of a PSARP in a male with a recto-urethral fistula, posterior sagittal incision. Aguayo P, Ostile D. *Ashcraft's Pediatric Surgery*. 5th ed. Philadelphia: Elsevier, 2010.

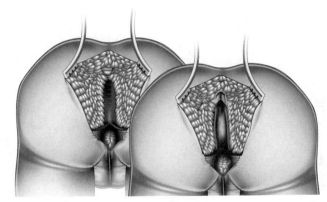

FIGURE 31.10B Basic depiction of a PSARP in a male with a recto-urethral fistula, exposure of the rectal wall after division of the midline parasagittal muscle fibers. Aguayo P, Ostile D. *Ashcraft's Pediatric Surgery*. 5th ed. Philadelphia: Elsevier, 2010.

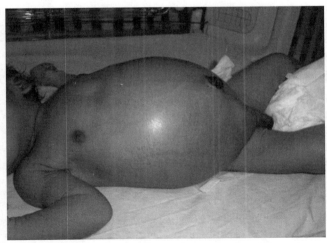

FIGURE 31.9 Newborn boy distended abdomen secondary to bowel obstruction from anorectal malformation. Image by Emmanuel A. Ameh.

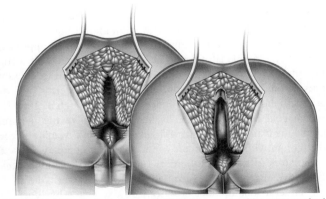

FIGURE 31.10C Basic depiction of a PSARP in a male with a recto-urethral fistula, depiction of the separation of the rectum from the urethra: 1) silk traction sutures placed on the rectum; 2) separation of the rectum from the urethra; 3) the rectum completely separated from the urethra. Aguayo P, Ostile D. *Ashcraft's Pediatric Surgery*. 5th ed. Philadelphia: Elsevier, 2010.

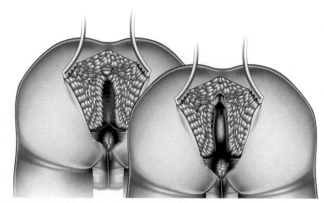

FIGURE 31.10D Basic depiction of a PSARP in a male with a recto-urethral fistula, passing of the rectum in front of the levator muscle complex. *Ashcraft's Pediatric Surgery*. 5th ed. Philadelphia: Elsevier, 2010.

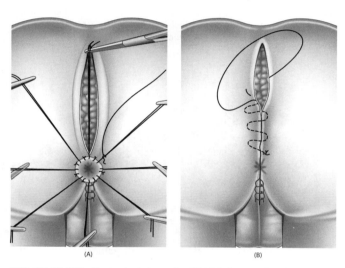

(A)   (B)

FIGURE 31.10E Basic depiction of a PSARP in a male with a recto-urethral fistula, anoplasty. Aguayo P, Ostile D. *Ashcraft's Pediatric Surgery*. 5th ed. Philadelphia: Elsevier, 2010.

improvise to care for the stoma with reusable materials such as napkins.

Approach to the definitive pull-through procedure depends on the type of malformation. In males, high malformations (prostatic or bladder neck fistula) will need an abdominal approach to ligate the fistula (if present) and mobilize the rectum, while low malformations can be approached through the perineum only through the standard approach of Pena (posterior sagittal anorectoplasty or PSARP) (Figures 31.10A through 31.10E).[39]

The goal of the operation is to fully mobilize the rectum, divide the fistula (if present) without urethral injury, and replace the rectum within the borders of the sphincter complex. Muscle stimulators to define the borders of the sphincter complex are expensive and may not be available locally; therefore, the visiting surgeon should either bring one or assemble a low-cost but effective alternative.[40,41] Use of diathermy set at low voltage may also be helpful in identifying the borders of the sphincter complex. Anesthesiologists in some settings may also have a nerve stimulator that can be used.

Prior to the PSARP, a distal colostogram should be done to identify the level of the malformation as well as the location of any fistula. Typically, no fistula may be identified as it might be plugged. In the absence of fluoroscopy, a series of X-ray images can be obtained using water soluble contrast flushed through the distal colon. If barium is used, it should be flushed out to prevent impaction in the distal colon.

In girls, for the most common malformation, a vestibular fistula, the surgeon must decide whether to perform a colostomy initially, with the repair (to "protect the repair"), or primary repair without diversion. There is also lack of consensus on the appropriate timing for surgery, whether in the neonatal period or delayed until the patient is several months old. This is dependent on the comfort of the surgeon in performing this procedure in the neonatal period and the condition of the patient. A newborn who breaks down her repair may need diversion and possible re-do surgery. Deep infection at the level of the repair also may result in incontinence; the best opportunity to achieve good results is at the first operation.

Postoperatively, rectal dilations should commence 10–14 days after surgery and can be continued at home by the child's caregivers. As Hegar dilators are generally unavailable, a smooth, appropriately sized candle covered by a glove with lube is a cheap suitable alternative for parents to continue dilations at home, as are other locally available soft supplies such as a rounded pen end and the caregiver's gloved little finger. For children beyond several months of age, dilations are poorly tolerated and most will put up quite a fight. As the anastomosis can scar down, follow-up is critical, and this must be stressed to families. Caregivers can also be taught digital dilation. These patients need to be followed through infancy and childhood as solid food is commenced and also through the period of toilet training. Children with low malformations have a tendency to constipation, and those with higher malformations tend more toward incontinence. Continued follow-up over these periods is critical as dietary modification and the introduction of laxatives or constipating agents may be necessary.

For the patient who has had a prior pull-through procedure who suffers from soiling, incontinence, and extensive perineal inflammation, in the absence of sophisticated investigations, the safest approach may be to once again create a sigmoid colostomy. The presence of anal stenosis may produce these symptoms, so stenosis should always be excluded before making a decision about treatment. In excluding stenosis, it should be noted that it may not always be at the anal verge and may be located slightly above.

Hirschsprung's Disease

Hirschsprung's disease is less common than anorectal malformations, at approximately 1 in 5,000 births, but the clinician should be aware of this entity. It is marked by a lack of ganglion cells (congenital aganglionosis) in the intestinal tract, generally (75%–80%) the rectosigmoid region. In LMICs, a delayed presentation of constipation, abdominal distension, and failure to thrive is the general rule for rectosigmoid disease (Figure 31.11).[40,42,43]

Patients with an absence of ganglion cells in longer segments of their bowel generally present in the neonatal period. Older patients have generally been treated for medical causes of distension such as parasitic infestations or tuberculosis. Historically,

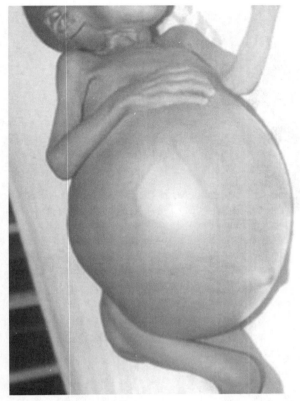

FIGURE 31.11 Delayed presentation of Hirschsprung's disease with bowel obstruction and failure to thrive. Image by Emmanuel A. Ameh and Doruk Ozgediz.

the disease was treated in three stages, with initial decompressing colostomy, a subsequent rectosigmoid resection and pull-through, and, finally, colostomy takedown. In most HICs, a one-stage procedure is now performed but frequently is not possible when a patient presents with long-standing constipation and neglected disease.

At initial evaluation, the patient should be examined for signs of peritonitis and enterocolitis. Enterocolitis is the primary cause of death in Hirschsprung's disease, and any patient presumed to have enterocolitis should be treated with broad spectrum antibiotics, rectal decompression, and irrigations, as well as bowel rest. A nasogastric tube may be necessary for temporary decompression, and laparotomy and fecal diversion may be necessary for inadequate decompression. At laparotomy, there may be a gross transition zone from dilated proximal ganglionated to contracted distal aganglionated bowel, and the colostomy should ideally be created just proximal to this gross transition zone. An ostomy created with aganglionated bowel is unlikely to function. Often the decision will need to be made without intraoperative pathology availability.

In the newborn period, the patient may present with signs of bowel obstruction and failure to pass meconium within 24 hours of birth, or may present with cecal perforation in the absence of atresia. A rectal examination may stimulate the passage of meconium. Plain X-rays are generally consistent with distal bowel obstruction. A contrast enema may not show a transition zone with dilated bowel proximal and decompressed distal

aganglionic segment within the first 2 weeks of life, and may appear normal if done prior to that time. Definitive diagnosis is provided by full-thickness rectal biopsy, usually done under general anesthesia or caudal block. While suction rectal biopsy is favored in many HICs, this is generally unavailable in an LMIC. The biopsy should be taken approximately 2–2.5 cm proximal to the dentate line and in the posterior midline. Biopsies taken too high risk intraperitoneal perforation, and too low risk the biopsy of the normal zone of hypoganglionated bowel just proximal to the dentate line. An anterior biopsy risks urethral (male) or vaginal (female) injury and should not be performed. Hallmarks of Hirschsprung's disease are absence of ganglion cells and hypertrophied nerve fibers in the submucosal and myenteric plexuses. One of the greatest challenges in the LMIC might be the absence of reliable pathology services to interpret biopsy results. In these cases the surgeon will have to use his or her best clinical judgment. However, definitive pull-through should ideally not be embarked upon without histologic diagnosis. Intraoperatively, a gross transition zone can be a guide. For the neonate with cecal perforation, the site may be resected and an ileostomy with a long Hartmann's pouch created, as this may represent a total colonic lack of ganglion cells.

The goal of definitive surgery is the removal of aganglionated bowel and the restoration of bowel continuity. The three common operations described are the Soave, the Swenson, and the Duhamel. A detailed description of each of these is beyond the scope of this chapter. No one procedure has proven superior to others, thus the surgeon should perform the procedure with which he or she is the most comfortable given the local environment. In the absence of safe neonatal anesthesia, the creation of a colostomy allowing the child to grow to an older age before definitive repair may be an acceptable alternative. For the patient presenting with massive fecal loading, on-table fecal washout will be necessary at the time of exploration and colostomy creation and a mucous fistula should ideally be created at this operation to facilitate continued postoperative washouts. If the proximal colon is markedly dilated and loaded with much feces, it may be safer to resect most of this segment to reach colon with manageable caliber. This will facilitate postoperative care and subsequent pull-through.

Even after a definitive pull-through procedure, patients with Hirschsprung's disease are at risk of enterocolitis, which may be lethal if not promptly addressed, and this should be stressed to caregivers. A regimen of dilations should be prescribed as described above for anorectal malformations. Most patients are followed at least to age 5, but many will go on to require stool management even after this period.

Abdominal Wall Defects

Surgeons are frequently involved in the management of abdominal wall defects in the neonatal period. Gastroschisis involves a full thickness defect in the abdominal wall to the right of midline, with exposed bowel outside the abdominal cavity, and in omphalocele, which is less common, the bowel is outside the abdominal cavity but is covered by a peritoneal lining.

In gastroschisis, immediate priority is resuscitation of the baby from third spacing, prevention of heat loss, and the administration

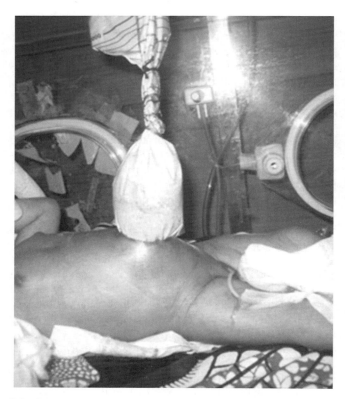

FIGURE 31.12 Gastroschisis covered with urine bag as temporary silo with bands noting serial reductions. Image by Emmanuel A. Ameh.

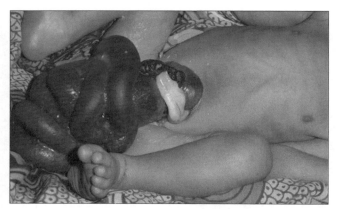

FIGURE 31.13 Gastroschisis with late presentation complicated by bowel ischemia. Image by Emmanuel A. Ameh.

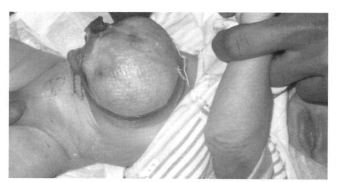

FIGURE 31.14 Omphalocele managed nonoperatively. Image by Emmanuel A. Ameh.

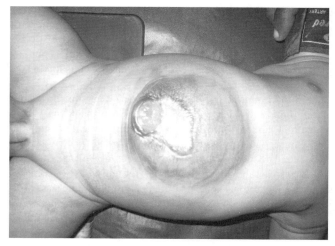

FIGURE 31.15 Same omphalocele 2 months after pressure dressing applied. Image by Emmanuel A. Ameh.

antibiotics to prevent infection in the exposed bowel. Over the last decade, there has been a trend to placement of a temporary silo, serial reductions, and delayed closure of the abdominal wall under general anesthesia. If primary reduction is not possible at initial evaluation in LMICs, a temporary abdominal wall covering should be devised. In the absence of a spring-loaded silo, a dressing using a plastic bag may be used that covers the abdomen and the lower extremities to retain heat and minimize fluid losses. A silo can be constructed by sewing together several pieces of urine bags (generally softer than IV fluid bags), sewing the edge of the bag to the fascia of the abdominal wall defect, then performing gradual bowel reductions once or twice a day (Figure 31.12).[44]

A Replogle tube should be placed for bowel decompression. In HICs, most babies have a 4–6 week hospital stay and a prolonged dependence on total parenteral nutrition (TPN) due to inflammation of the bowel and associated ileus that persists even after abdominal wall closure. This presents great difficulty in the absence of TPN. Even in the presence of a neonatal intensive care unit (NICU) and TPN, a recent South African series reported a mortality of 43%, primarily due to sepsis.[45] Volvulus and bowel ischemia may complicate gastroschisis (Figure 31.13).

If general anesthesia is unavailable to attempt primary reduction of the bowel, placement of the bowel into a silo and gentle reduction into the abdominal cavity can be accomplished without anesthesia over a period of a few days. Without excessive increase in intra-abdominal pressure, the abdominal defect can be temporary closed with the umbilicus or Wharton's jelly folded over, a temporary piece of mesh, or a suitable low-cost

local alternative. This may result in a delayed formation of a hernia at this site, but this may be acceptable in this setting. The resulting hernia can be repaired at a later date.

With omphalocele, associated defects are more common and these are more often the cause of mortality than the omphalocele itself. Blood glucose should be obtained, echocardiogram (if available) should be performed if there is an audible murmur, and

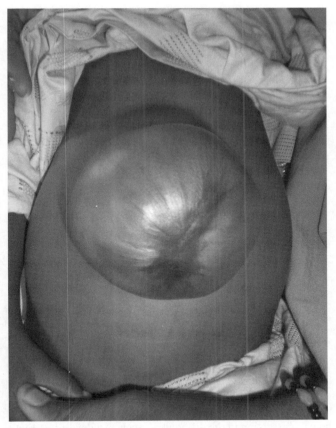

FIGURE 31.16 Same omphalocele healed after nonoperative management. Image by Emmanuel A. Ameh.

an abdominal ultrasound obtained. For smaller defects (<5 cm) primary closure is indicated. For larger defects, an escharizing agent such as 1% silver sulfadiazine (or native honey if the sac is infected) may be used to thicken the sac. The sac will progressively contract and the defect and associated hernia can be repaired when the child is older (Figures 31.14 through 31.16).

If the fascia cannot be closed, then skin only can be closed, leaving a hernia that can be repaired at a later date. With an intact peritoneal covering, there is usually no delay in gastrointestinal function and the baby can be started on feeds. Repairing the hernia at a later date may require the use of a mesh. If the sac is intact, serial gradual compression bandaging over a few weeks may help to facilitate earlier repair of the defect. If the sac ruptures and cannot be primarily repaired, a temporary silo can be devised in a similar manner described above, with serial reductions subsequently performed. In the infant with omphalocele, tetanus prophylaxis should be given if the mother did not receive this during the antenatal period or if the status is unknown.

Hernias and Hydroceles: Pediatric Aspects

Hernias and hydroceles are very common surgical conditions in children, regardless of context, affecting up to 1%–5% of term children and a higher percentage of premature babies. Hernias are more common on the right side, they more commonly affect males, and 99% are indirect hernias due to a patent processus vaginalis. Hernias in children are more commonly associated with some conditions such as abdominal wall defects and in children with ascites. Incarceration is more common in the neonatal period and poses not only risk to the bowel, but also risks of atrophy or frank necrosis of the ipsilateral testicle due to ischemia.

Generally, parents will report that the baby has had an intermittent bulge on either side. A careful physical exam should be performed. Both testicles should be examined to ensure they are descended, the genitalia should be examined, and the placement and size of the anal opening should be evaluated. If no hernia is initially palpated or seen, the examiner can induce increased abdominal pressure by gently holding the baby's arms and/or legs down. Trans-illumination may help to detect a hydrocele; if this is felt to be a noncommunicating hydrocele, which doesn't change in size, then operation can be deferred to age 1, as the majority of these self-resolve prior to that time (Figures 31.17A through 31.17D). An incarcerated hernia may be detected on rectal exam in infants.

Timing of repair is important. Ideally, infant hernias are repaired close to the time of diagnosis to minimize chance of incarceration; however, in an LMIC the availability and safety of neonatal general anesthesia should be considered as general anesthesia is preferred. Ketamine may also be used. Controversy remains over routine contralateral exploration, but most large retrospective series suggest that only a minority (7%) of children will develop a contralateral hernia.[46]

A standard high ligation of the hernia sac at the internal ring should be performed; this is the most important part of the procedure. Given the high preponderance of indirect hernias, a floor repair (i.e., Bassini or other) is generally unnecessary. In infant girls in particular, approximately 20% may contain the fallopian tube or ovary as part of a sliding hernia, and the surgeon should be prepared to invert the sac around a purse-string suture at the internal ring if necessary. In infants, the external ring and internal ring are nearly superimposed, and it may be unnecessary to open the external oblique to get adequate exposure of the internal ring. For large hernia sacs that extend into the scrotum, the scrotal portion of the sac does not need to be excised, as this may cause excessive bleeding and traumatize the cord structures for little gain. At the conclusion of the operation, if the testicle has been lifted out of the scrotum, it should be returned to its normal location to minimize the chance of iatrogenic cryptorchidism, a rare complication. In the case of transection of the vas deferens, it should be repaired with fine absorbable sutures.

If an incarcerated hernia is detected clinically, attempts should be made at reduction. Gentle pressure is usually able to reduce the hernia. If it cannot be readily reduced and the child is otherwise well, sedation may be given to increase the chance of success. If reduction was difficult, the patient should be observed at least for 4–8 hours to ensure that feeds are tolerated and that peritonitis does not develop. Ideally, the hernia repair should be performed in the next 2–3 days, allowing for some of the tissue edema in the cord to abate. Even several days later, the tissues and sac are likely to be more friable than normal.

In cases of suspected strangulation, and possible bowel compromise, reduction should not be attempted, and, as in adults, a groin exploration should be performed to evaluate the bowel. If this cannot be adequately performed through the groin, a laparotomy may be necessary.

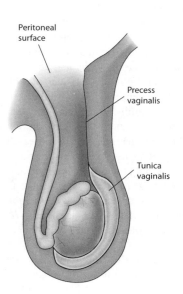

FIGURE 31.17A Schematic of differences between hernias and hydroceles, a normal groin. Illustration by Sani Yamout, MD.

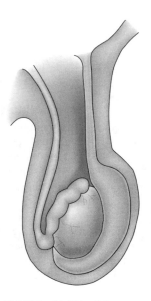

FIGURE 31.17B Schematic of differences between hernias and hydroceles, a communicating hydrocele. Illustration by Sani Yamout, MD.

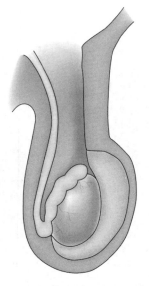

FIGURE 31.17C Schematic of differences between hernias and hydroceles, a non-communicating hydrocele. Illustration by Sani Yamout, MD.

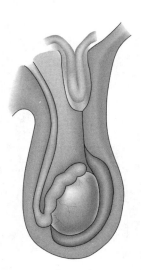

FIGURE 31.17D Schematic of differences between hernias and hydroceles, a hernia. Illustration by Sani Yamout, MD.

Surgical Infections

HIV and TB

In some regions, the prevalence of HIV in the pediatric population remains very high. Some high-prevalence countries have an adult prevalence of up to 26%; about 28% of adults who require treatments are on antiretroviral therapy.[47] Most children with HIV are infected through vertical transmission; the incidence of transmission can be reduced from 35% to approximately 10% with administration of nevirapine. As HIV-positive patients may initially present to the medical system with a surgical condition, surgeons should be familiar with the general criteria for diagnosis of HIV infection. An infant or child may present with adenopathy suggestive of HIV disease, of HIV-associated tuberculosis, or with a soft tissue infection secondary to immune compromise. HIV-infected children also have a higher incidence of lymphoma. Several HIV-defining surgical pathologies bear mention, such as spontaneous rectovaginal fistula or neonatal cytomegalovirus (CMV) enteritis. The symptomatic patient with HIV with an elective surgical condition should have surgery deferred until the medical status is optimized. Recent evidence suggests that circumcision may be effective prophylaxis as a component of HIV prevention programs, and some high-prevalence countries have adopted an official policy regarding circumcision and encouraged uptake of the procedure.

TB is more prevalent in high–HIV-prevalence countries, with an overall reported incidence of 0.7–2 per 1,000 children, and accounts for about 15% of bowel obstructions in children.[48] General workup may include skin test and sputum for acid-fast bacillus (AFB). For chronic abdominal symptoms, contrast studies (from above and below) may show thickened bowel wall or strictures, and in case of ascites, a paracentesis may be performed. A more chronic presentation may have other causes of bowel obstruction in the differential, such as a delayed presentation of Hirschsprung's disease. Rectal examination may detect fissures, fistula, or stenosis. Ultrasound may show bowel thickening or peritoneal nodules. Nodular disease may also suggest malignancy; ascites may also occur from other medical problems such as liver failure or malnutrition.

Tuberculosis of the abdomen may present as acute or chronic peritonitis or bowel obstruction. For chronic symptoms, if antitubercular therapy has not been started, this may be attempted for several weeks prior to surgery. Laparotomy may reveal thickened omentum, mesentery, or bowel wall. Copious ascites or adhesions may be present. Large or small bowel obstruction may occur due to thickening or strictures; presentation with frank bowel perforation is less common. High-grade strictures may require stricturoplasty in Heineke-Mikulicz fashion, and in cases of perforation, ostomy may be required due to peritoneal contamination. As TB cannot be "cleared" with surgery alone, the goals of operation are to treat the acute problem and to continue anti-tubercular chemotherapy postoperatively. Perforation is generally preferentially treated with resection and anastomosis rather than oversewing of the perforation alone, due to concern about tissue integrity around the site of perforation. Partial intestinal obstruction may be relieved with medical therapy over a period of months, and resection may be attempted in selected circumstances.

Typhoid Fever

Typhoid fever is a multisystem infection caused by *Salmonella*. The disease is transmitted by a fecal-oral route and is endemic in many LMICs, largely due to improper sewage disposal systems,

TABLE 31.4

Surgical complications of typhoid fever

Common	Less common
Intestinal perforation	Abscesses (hepatic, splenic, other)
Intestinal hemorrhage	Pancreatitis
Cholecystitis	Orchitis
Osteomyelitis	Pleural effusion

inadequate supply of clean water, and unhygienic environment. Twenty-one million cases occur annually, with children aged 5–15 primarily affected, though it does also occur in younger children.[49]

Children account for over 50% of patients with typhoid intestinal perforation, the most common and severe surgical complication, with a peak age incidence of 5–9 years. Boys and girls are equally affected.[49,51] In hospital-based reports, the overall intestinal perforation rate in children is 10%, increasing with age and reaching the highest rate of 30% by 12 years. The disease occurs year-round, but with a slightly higher incidence in the rainy season.[52] Untreated, several surgical complications can occur (Table 31.4).

Complications of typhoid fever frequently present late, and in LMICs, commonly after attempting treatment with over-the-counter antibiotics or local medications. Nearly 10% children with typhoid fever develop intestinal perforation while on medical treatment, which tends to mask the features.[50] Symptoms can include fever and headache. Abdominal pain sets in frequently after one week of onset of fever, and a sudden increase in abdominal pain suggests intestinal perforation or other intra-abdominal complication. Abdominal distension follows in patients with intestinal perforation but may also be present in those without perforation. Diarrhea or constipation may be present, and diarrhea may be bloody in those with intestinal hemorrhage. Jaundice suggests the development of cholecystitis or overwhelming infection. Chest pain and pain in the limbs are suggestive of complications in those areas.

The typical child who presents to the surgeon with typhoid is critically ill, particularly in cases of perforation. Signs of sepsis may be present, with dehydration and anemia, and many patients are malnourished due to delayed presentation. Respiratory examination is necessary to exclude complicating pneumonia or pleural effusion. The typical patient with intestinal perforation has abdominal distension and peritoneal signs, and frequently also has abdominal wall edema. These signs may not be as evident in patients who develop perforation while under medical treatment; in these patients, a high index of suspicion helps to make the diagnosis. In one report, abdominal rigidity was present in only one-third of children with intestinal perforation.[52] Rectal examination may identify a pelvic fluid collection (rectovesical or recto-uterine fullness) and the presence of blood in the feces. Any painful limb or superficial swelling may suggest osteomyelitis and abscess.

The diagnosis of intestinal perforation is mainly clinical, but laboratory tests and imaging may be necessary to guide treatment and also to exclude other conditions.[53] Serum electrolytes and creatinine should be drawn: in some patients, the electrolytes may be normal at presentation but a repeat analysis after resuscitation commonly reveals depletion. For this reason, the decision to operate should not be made until the electrolytes are analyzed after resuscitation. Hypokalemia and metabolic acidosis are common.

Complete blood count may identify anemia. The packed cell volume is often unreliable until after resuscitation, and hemogram should be the choice if it can be done quickly. Leukocytosis and neutrophilia are common in those with intestinal perforation. Blood should be grouped and cross-matched for pre-, intra-, and postoperative transfusion.

Radiograph of the chest and upper abdomen (erect film) should be obtained. Pneumoperitoneum is present in about 55%–66% of children with intestinal perforation but may be as high as 96% in those with typhoid colonic perforation.[54] The extent of pneumoperitoneum is important as it may be necessary to evacuate the air with an 18-gauge IV cannula preoperatively to improve respiration and reduce hypoxia. Evidence of pneumonia may be present on the chest radiograph. Abdominal ultrasonography can help to identify cholecystitis and also intraperitoneal abscesses. Other intra-abdominal conditions can be excluded. An X-ray should be performed on any limb suspicious for osteomyelitis.

Blood and urine, as well as an operative specimen of intraperitoneal fluid/pus, should be cultured to identify the *Salmonella* organism and any superimposed infections. In those in whom intraoperative diagnosis of cholecystitis (and its complication) is made, a sample of gallbladder contents should also be cultured. As a general guideline, in uncomplicated disease, blood culture is more likely to be positive in the first week of illness, urine culture in the second week, and stool culture in the third week, but these may overlap. Antibiotic sensitivity for all cultured material should be obtained.

Initial Treatment

Fluid and electrolyte deficits should be thoroughly replaced before surgical intervention. Inadequate resuscitation is a common cause of death in patients with intestinal perforation. Potassium repletion is particularly critical and should be commenced once the patient has an adequate urine output. The daily requirement of 1–2 mmol/kg can be started before receipt of electrolyte results after which the actual correction can be done.

A large bore (age appropriate) nasogastric tube should be placed for decompression and a urinary catheter placed to monitor urine output. Hemoglobin of <8 gm/dl should be corrected by whole blood transfusion before surgery to minimize hypoxia. In patients with evidence of coagulopathy, appropriate doses of intravenous vitamin K should be given for 5 days.

Frequently, the patients are hypoxic and require oxygen supplementation. If significant pneumoperitoneum was identified on chest/abdominal radiographs, the air should be vented by inserting an 18G cannula in the right hypochondrium, below the liver; this may help to improve respiration and oxygenation.

In uncomplicated typhoid fever, antibiotics are effective. However, once intestinal perforation and other surgical complications have developed, secondary infection by other bacteria requires broad-spectrum antibiotics. Commonly used antibiotic combinations in patients with intestinal perforation and other complications include:

1. Amoxicillin (or Ampicillin) + Gentamicin + Metronidazole
2. Third-generation Cephalosporin + Metronidazole
3. Ciprofloxacin + Metronidazole

The chosen antibiotic combination initially is given intravenously until temperature returns to normal, and can then be given orally (if oral form is available and the patient can achieve oral intake). The antibiotics should be given for 10–14 days.

Some patients are malnourished or nutritionally depleted. Parenteral nutrition, if available, should be given during the acute phase of the illness. When the patient is able to tolerate oral intake, a diet rich in proteins and carbohydrate should be given. Small frequent feedings are better tolerated than less frequent large-volume feedings.

Definitive Treatment of Surgical Complications

The definitive treatment for intestinal perforation is operative—to evacuate fecal contamination and prevent further contamination. Surgery should be done only when the child is adequately resuscitated. The choice of anesthesia is important. In patients who are very ill and considered poor anesthetic risks, use of muscle relaxants and anesthetic agents that may cause hypotension should be avoided. In such patients, use of ketamine is safe and effective, and recovery from anesthesia is not problematic. Once the peritoneal cavity is opened, any peritoneal fluid or pus should be cultured and all peritoneal collections evacuated. The intestines should be thoroughly examined; perforation(s) and near perforations are

usually located on the antimesenteric border. After identifying the perforation(s), the stomach, duodenum, large intestine, liver, and spleen should be inspected. Most perforations are located in the last 80 cm of the terminal ileum, but the jejunum and colon (cecum to sigmoid colon) may also be involved.[50,53,55] A surgical algorithm is illustrated in Figure 31.18.

The peritoneal cavity is irrigated with large volumes of warm normal saline. The abdominal fascia is closed according to the surgeon's preference. The skin can be closed primarily. However, in patients with anterior abdominal wall edema and those in whom the risk of surgical site infection is considered high (e.g., patients with severe peritoneal contamination with feces or pus), the skin is left open and dressed daily, and then a delayed primary closure can be done after 3–5 days if the wound remains clean.

The treatment of other surgical complications is summarized in Table 31.5.

Given the severity of infection and often delayed presentation in patients with typhoid intestinal perforation, complications following surgical treatment occur in 53%–79% of patients.[50,51,53,56] More than one complication can occur in the same patient. Each complication should be treated appropriately. The complication rate and mortality may be higher below 5 years of age. Mortality from intestinal perforation is high but varies widely from region to region (4.8%–41%).[51,53,56] Most mortality is from overwhelming infection, occurring usually after a mean of 4–5 days postoperatively. Abdominal pain of over 7 days is the primary important factor in predicting mortality. The number of perforations does not appear to affect mortality. Table 31.6 illustrates some of the perioperative complications of the disease in an LMIC.

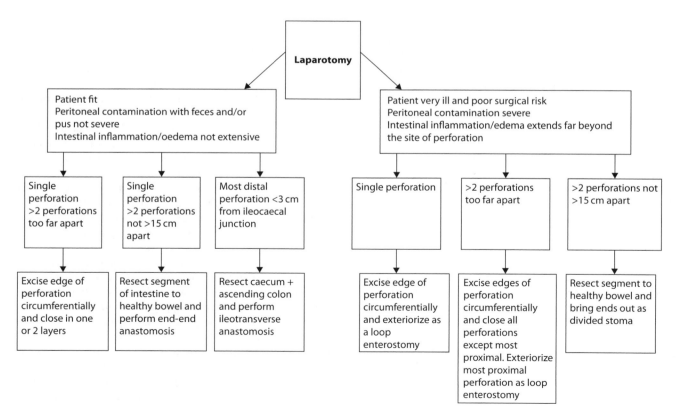

FIGURE 31.18 Surgical algorithm for complications of typhoid fever. Image by Emmanuel A. Ameh.

TABLE 31.5

Treatment of other complications of typhoid fever

Complication	Treatment
Intestinal hemorrhage	• Replace blood loss if severe. • Continue above antibiotics for 10–14 days. • If severe hemorrhage, keep patient in hospital for a few more days until bleeding has stopped (bleeding often recurs and may be more severe). • Most bleeding will stop on above treatment. • If bleeding persists, and coagulopathy is excluded, laparotomy and terminal ileal resection may be necessary (difficult to identify site of bleeding at surgery, and this should be last resort).

Cholecystitis	• If diagnosis certain and no general peritonitis, above antibiotics may suffice. Cholecystectomy may be necessary after 6–12 weeks to prevent recurrence and carrier state.
	• If above treatment fails or there's evidence of general peritonitis, do laparotomy + one of following:
	  – Tube cholecystostomy (especially if empyema or gangrene)
	  – Cholecystectomy (only if patient is not too ill and surgeon is experienced + appropriate surgical instruments)

Osteomyelitis	• Some of these patients may have sickle cell disease. • Give above antibiotics for 4–6 weeks (initially IV until acute phase over). • Drain associated abscess if present. • Give adequate analgesia. • Limb may need to be splinted and rested if pain is severe.
Abscesses	• May be located in various parts of the body, either superficial or deep. • Give antibiotics. • Drain as appropriate.

TABLE 31.6

Postoperative complications following treatment of typhoid intestinal perforation

Complication	Occurrence (%)
Early	
Malnutrition	61
Surgical site infection	49–59
Enterocutaneous fistula	6–25
Abdominal wound dehiscence	3–14
Intraperitoneal abscess	7–12
Perforation at new site	7–9
Anastomotic dehiscence	7
Prolonged ileus	
Late	
Adhesion intestinal obstruction	3
Incisional hernia	3

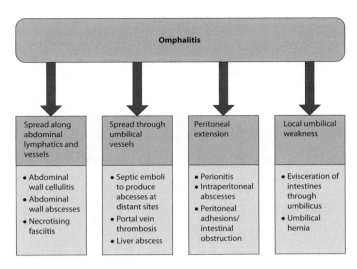

FIGURE 31.19 Pathogenesis of surgical complications of omphalitis. Image by Emmanuel A. Ameh.

Typhoid fever and its complications are preventable by simple public health measures. This disease condition is an area where the surgeon can play an important public health role in LMICs by participating in health education. Improvements in sanitation, proper waste and sewage disposal, and provision of clean drinking water are critical to the prevention. The Vi polysaccharide vaccine and the live attenuated oral Ty21a vaccine are currently the only vaccines considered safe and effective for the prevention and control of typhoid fever in individuals older than 2 years.[49,50]

Surgical Complications of Omphalitis

Omphalitis is an infection of the umbilicus and umbilical stump. It is predominantly a disease of newborns but can also affect infants. Although omphalitis is mainly a medical disease, surgical complications may develop. It is a significant cause of neonatal morbidity and mortality in LMICs, especially among infants delivered at home without skilled birth attendants and under unhygienic conditions. The incidence of this condition in LMICs has been reported as 2–7 per 100 live births.[57,58] In addition, the umbilicus is generally the portal of entry for cases of neonatal tetanus, still a problem in many LMICs.[59]

The pathogenesis of the surgical complications commonly encountered is shown in (Figure 31.19).

It is commonly caused by aerobic bacteria, including *Staphylococcus aureus* (most common pathogen), Group A streptococcus, *Escherichia coli, Klebsiella,* and *Proteus* species. In one-third of patients, anaerobic bacteria (*Bacteroides fragilis, Peptostreptococcus, Clostridium perfringens,* or *Clostridium tetani*) are involved.

The disease is usually noticed at 3–5 days of age in preterm infants and 5–9 days in term infants. The age at presentation for infants with complications has been reported as 5–75 days (median 33 days).[60]

The local signs of omphalitis include purulent or foul-smelling discharge from the umbilicus or umbilical stump, periumbilical erythema, edema, and tenderness. Pyrexia, hypothermia, and jaundice may be present. Other features will depend largely on the nature of presenting surgical complication. Omphalitis should be clinically differentiated from other conditions such as umbilical granuloma and the unusual vitelline duct and urachal anomalies.

TABLE 31.7

Treatment of surgical complications of omphalitis

Time scale	Complication	Clinical Notes	Treatment
Early	Necrotizing fasciitis	• Most common surgical complication • Starts initially as periumbilical cellulitis • Scrotum and abdominal wall commonly affected	• Antibiotics • Excision of all devitalized tissue • Local wound dressing until infection controlled • Cover defect by direct suturing, skin grafting, or flaps as appropriate
	Intestinal evisceration	• Usually small intestine, occasionally large intestine • Eviscerated intestine may be strangulated	• Cover intestine with moist gauze and place in transparent plastic bag (intestinal bag) • Umbilical defect may need extension • Cleanse intestine and return to peritoneal cavity • Nonviable intestine should be resected • If peritonitis present, do formal laparotomy and cleanse peritoneal cavity
	Peritonitis	• Could occur without abscess • Ultrasonography needed to exclude abscess	• If no abscess, antibiotics alone may suffice • If abscess present, do laparotomy and drain

	Distant abscesses	• May be retroperitoneal, hepatic, or elsewhere on the body
		• Abscesses need to be localized by appropriate imaging
			• Abscesses should be drained by:
			  – Percutaneous aspiration using wide bore needle under imaging (may need to be repeated)
			  – Open drainage

Late	Portal vein thrombosis	• Portal hypertension is the major consequence • Although early complication, the major consequence is late • A cavernoma may produce biliary obstruction	• Portosystemic shunt required if portal hypertension develops • Biliary obstruction should be treated appropriately
	Umbilical hernia	• A common problem • Usually asymptomatic but complications may develop	• Most would close spontaneously or significantly reduce in size by age of 2–4 years • If not closed by 4 years, or complication develops, surgical repair required
	Peritoneal adhesions	• A result of subclinical or treated peritonitis • Adhesions cause intestinal obstruction, which is usually not responsive to nonoperative measures	• Laparotomy and excision of adhesions required • Any gangrenous intestine to be resected

TABLE 31.8

Predisposing factors to necrotizing fasciitis in children

Predisposing factor	Examples
Chronic debilitating conditions	Malnutrition, anemia, vitamin B deficiencies
Specific infections and infestations	Specific bacterial infections (e.g., neonatal omphalitis, boils and abscesses, gingivitis, tuberculosis), HIV infection, measles, chicken pox, severe malaria
Trauma	Prick injuries, abrasions, cuts, etc.
Postoperative	Colostomy, appendectomy, dental procedures

A microbiological swab of the umbilicus should be sent for aerobic and anaerobic culture. In necrotizing fasciitis, tissue culture may give a better yield for anaerobes. A blood culture should be included when appropriate. An antibiotic sensitivity profile should be obtained to guide treatment. A blood count with differential for white cell counts may show a neutrophilia (or occasionally a neutropenia). Other investigations including plain abdominal radiography and ultrasonography may become necessary depending on complications suspected and to exclude differential diagnoses.

Prompt antibiotic administration normally controls uncomplicated omphalitis. Antibiotics specifically active against *Staphylococcus aureus* + an aminoglycoside + metronidazole to cover for gram-positive and gram-negative and anaerobic organisms are used. The duration of antibiotic treatment is usually 7–14 days, initially given parenterally. Tetanus prophylaxis needs to be given in most infants, to prevent development of tetanus. In addition to medical treatment for ongoing omphalitis, the surgical treatment depends on the presenting surgical complication (Table 31.7).

Uncomplicated omphalitis usually resolves if treated promptly. With delayed presentation and treatment, however, a mortality of 7%–15% has been reported.[60–62] Surgical complications result in mortalities as high as 38%–87%.[63–65]

Necrotizing Fasciitis

Necrotizing fasciitis (NF) is a rapidly progressive inflammation and necrosis of the skin, subcutaneous tissues, and the deep layer of superficial fascia and includes named infections.[62,63] NF may start spontaneously in apparently normal children, but it is most often preceded by other pathological conditions that

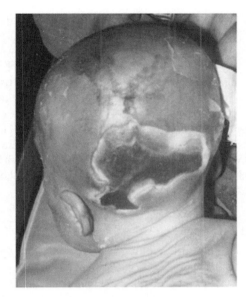

FIGURE 31.20 NF of the posterior scalp in a newborn. Image by Emmanuel A. Ameh.

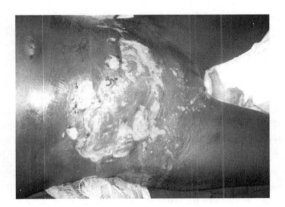

FIGURE 31.21 NF of the abdominal wall secondary to postoperative enterocutaneous fistula after appendectomy (Meleney's gangrene). Image by Emmanuel A. Ameh.

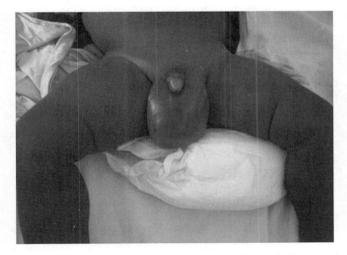

FIGURE 31.22 Fournier's gangrene in newborn. Image by Emmanuel A. Ameh.

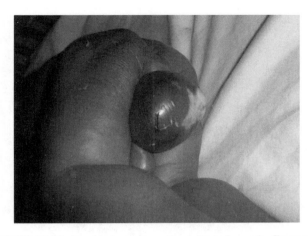

FIGURE 31.23 Fournier's gangrene in newborn. Image by Emmanuel A. Ameh.

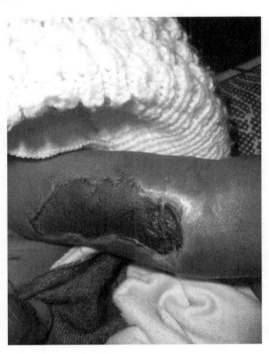

FIGURE 31.24 NF of the arm, Stage II. Image by Emmanuel A. Ameh.

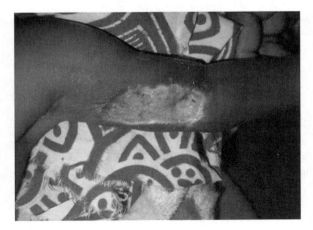

FIGURE 31.25 NF of the arm, Stage III, same patient. Image by Emmanuel A. Ameh.

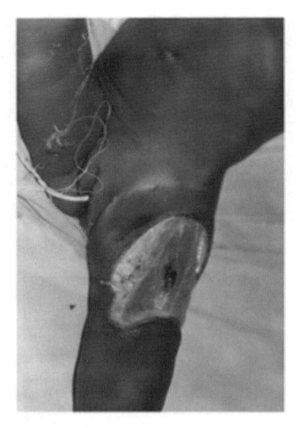

FIGURE 31.26 NF of the thigh (note exposed muscles). Image by Emmanuel A. Ameh.

lead to impaired host immunity, some of which are preferentially encountered in an LMIC (Table 31.8).

Aerobic pathogens are usually the primary tissue invaders. They destroy tissues and create an environment conducive for anaerobic or microaerophilic organisms, which are secondary invaders.[65,66] NF is polymicrobial in about 70%–80% of patients, and a wide spectrum of organisms are involved.[40,44–48]

NF can affect different parts of the body (Figures 31.20 through 31.26), and the clinical presentation is best categorized based on the various pathophysiological stages. The stages are mainly a progression from an earlier, less severe stage to a more severe stage if left untreated or poorly treated.[61,68,69]

Diagnosis of NF is mainly clinical, but a few investigations are necessary to help in the management of the patient:

1. Any discharge or swab from the wound is cultured (aerobic and anaerobic) to establish the bacteria involved in the process. Tissue culture may provide a better yield for anaerobic organisms. Blood cultures may be necessary in those with marked systemic features.
2. Leukocytosis is frequently present in the early stages of the disease.
3. Plain radiographs may show gas within the soft tissues at the early stages of the disease, but are rarely required to make the diagnosis.
4. Predisposing illnesses should be identified and guided by the degree of clinical suspicion. This may involve HIV testing, blood smear for malaria parasites, hemoglobin electrophoresis for sickle cell disease, and blood sugar to exclude diabetes mellitus.

General Treatment

As the bacteriology is usually polymicrobial, the initial choice of antibiotics should be broad to cover gram negatives, gram positives, and anaerobes. The antibiotic combination should take into consideration local sensitivity profiles. Combinations of cephalosporins + metronidazole, and penicillin + aminoglycosides + metronidazole have been found useful.[66,70,71] Tetanus prophylaxis (both active and passive) should be given to patients presenting with tissue necrosis.

Surgical Treatment

Even in the absence of obvious tissue necrosis, fasciotomy in the form of single or multiple linear incision(s) over the affected area may be necessary to achieve adequate compartment decompression. Thorough wound irrigation with antiseptics such as hydrogen peroxide or cetrimide and warm normal saline, then gentle packing with gauze in EUSOL® (hypochlorite solution) or natural honey helps to control local infection and halts progression of the disease. About 5–7 days after fasciotomy, when edema has subsided and infection reasonably controlled, skin closure can be achieved by suturing or skin grafting.

Prompt, adequate, and sequential debridement of all devitalized tissue is important to arrest progression of tissue necrosis. In very ill patients who may be poor anesthetic risks, debridement can be done at the bedside under analgesia and some sedation. Significant wound contraction could occur following adequate wound care, especially on the face, trunk, and perineum, but the final mode of wound closure also depends on the initial size. Any identified predisposing condition should be treated appropriately. This should be done simultaneously with treatment of the NF.

COMMENTARY

Milliard Derbew, Ethiopia

Pediatric surgery is a neglected specialty in sub-Saharan Africa. In this region, over half of the population is under the age of 18. The fertility rate is very high as well as the population growth, with proportionally high rate of congenital anomalies, trauma, and malignancies within this population. Despite the above facts, there are very few pediatric surgical facilities and pediatric surgeons in the region. In ten East and Southern African countries there are only 33 pediatric surgeons for over 300 million population (almost same population size as the United States). However, in the United States, there are over 1,000 pediatric surgeons, and the population is predominantly older unlike the sub-Saharan population. In 11 of the 47 sub-Saharan African countries, about 250 million people are 18 years old or younger, but there are only 130 practicing pediatric surgeons.

Without addressing the severe shortage of pediatric surgeons in sub-Saharan Africa, we will not be able to significantly reduce infant and child mortality.[72]

Another concern is most of the pediatric surgical patients present late in sub-Saharan Africa; as a result the disease is advanced and their outcome after treatment is not rewarding. Several factors contribute to the late presentation, including socioeconomic development, awareness, and barriers to transportation, shortage of pediatric surgeons, and shortage of facilities. The waiting list is very long for patients; it is a minimum of 1-year wait in Ethiopia, where I practice. Delays in intervention mean that the disease advances, where it ultimately results in higher rates of morbidity and mortality.

32

Oncology

T. Peter Kingham
Olusegun Alatise

Introduction

By 2050, the cancer burden could reach 24 million patients per year throughout the world, with 17 million cases occurring in low- and middle-income countries (LMICs).[1] Traditionally, in high-income countries (HICs), there are high rates of colorectal, lung, breast, and prostate cancer due to tobacco use, the Western diet, occupational carcinogens, and the Western lifestyle. These environmental and behavioral causes of cancer are often carcinogenic when combined with various genetic mutations. Up to 25% of cancers in LMICs, however, are caused by infections with hepatitis B virus (HBV), human papilloma virus (HPV), or *Helicobacter pylori* (*H. pylori*). In LMICs, the top five cancers among females from highest incidence to lowest are breast, cervical, stomach, lung, and colorectal. Cervical cancer accounts for a higher number of deaths, despite its lower incidence, when compared to breast cancer. The five most common cancers among males in LMICs are lung, stomach, liver, esophageal, and colorectal cancer. The total number of cancer deaths and disability-adjusted life years (DALYs) lost to cancer by World Bank region and country income level for 2001 showed that in LMICs there were 4,955,000 deaths with 74,752,000 DALYs lost compared to 2,068,000 deaths in HICs with 25,886,000 DALYs lost.

Cancer is already the second leading cause of death in the developed world, and its incidence in LMICs is rising, as 70% of predicted cases worldwide are now in LMICs. There are several reasons why cancer rates are rising in LMICs. Reasons include lifestyle choices such as sedentary lifestyle, tobacco, and obesity, combined with increased societal development causing longer life expectancy, as older age is a primary risk factor for cancer. For example, as infant mortality and maternal mortality rates have dropped, there is a higher proportion of older individuals in these populations.

The overall case fatality from cancer is determined by the ratio of incidence to mortality annually. It is estimated to be 75% in LMICs and 46% in HICs. Due to this high rate of case fatalities in LMICs, cancer accounts for more deaths than acquired immunodeficiency syndrome (AIDS), malaria, and tuberculosis combined worldwide. There are many reasons why cancer fatality rates are higher in LMICs when compared to HICs. These include poor oncology services, the advanced stage at presentation, lack of treatment choices, and poor compliance and follow-up. In the United States, there is 1 cancer center for every 5 million citizens, compared to 1 for every 48 million citizens in India. Cancer-oriented fellowships in surgery mean that there is 1 new trainee per 6 million citizens in United States compared to 72 million citizens in India.

There are several unique aspects to cancer care in LMICs:

- Surgeons are a vital component of public awareness efforts.
- Surgeons are often the primary caregiver responsible for all aspects of cancer treatments for solid tumors, including chemotherapy.
- Cancer prevention includes both environmental advocacy and screening.
- Coordinated cancer care with the development of cancer registries and cancer wards are emerging priorities.
- Palliative care is the most common role surgeons fill in LMICs to treat cancer patients.

Lack of public awareness is a major barrier to cancer care in LMICs. Given that many patients present to hospitals with late-stage cancers, the mortality rate of cancer patients seen at hospitals is high. The association of mortality from cancer with the hospital and medical establishment is one that leads many patients to avoid presenting to the hospital at any point if they fear they have a malignant process. For example, in a Philippines study of women who were taught to perform breast self-examinations, there were low follow-up rates with the medical establishment even in women with positive screening results.[2] The authors concluded that there was a lack of trust in the healthcare system and the available treatments. Given that surgeons are commonly the first and only physicians that deal with cancer patients in LMICs, their experience and knowledge can help dispel rumors and increase trust in the medical establishment. Palliative care also plays a role in lowering this barrier because if patients are made more comfortable during the process of dying, their families will at least be comforted in the knowledge that their loved one was well taken care of.

Cancer Prevention and Screening

Cancer prevention and screening are important facets of cancer care in LMICs. Tobacco use is one of the key factors responsible for the increasing cancer rates in LMICs. Poor diet, obesity, and lack of exercise are also factors. In the United States, obesity is associated with 20% of cancer deaths in women.[3] As the "Western lifestyle" becomes more common in LMICs, obesity rates are increasing.[4] Infectious diseases are also responsible for many cancers in LMICs. Infections cause a higher rate of cancer in LMICs than in other parts of the world, as high as 36% compared to 10% in HICs. Oncogenic viruses include HPV, Epstein-Barr virus (EBV), human immunodeficiency virus (HIV), and hepatitis B and C. These viruses can cause specific cancers, such as cervical cancer (HPV), liver cancer (HBV, HCV), and gastric cancer (*Helicobacter pylori* infection). Often these infectious causes can act in harmony with carcinogens. For example, aflatoxins found in contaminated grains are synergistic with hepatitis B in causing hepatocellular carcinoma (HCC). Viral causes also include AIDS. There are high rates of non-Hodgkin's lymphoma and Kaposi's sarcoma in African countries with high HIV/AIDS rates.[5] In addition, EBV-associated lymphoma and nasopharyngeal cancers in LMICs are 10- to 60-fold higher than in HICs (Table 32.1).[6]

There are primary prevention procedures that can reduce or end exposure to cancer-causing factors. These can include changes to lifestyle like nutrition or exercise, limiting exposure to environmental carcinogens, and tobacco control. Immunizations are an important part of primary prevention, given that HBV and HPV are responsible for a high percentage of cancers in LMICs. There is an HBV vaccine that can help reduce HCC mortality rates in vaccinated populations by up to 70%.[7] There is also an HPV vaccine against HPV strains 16 and 18. In studies that examined the efficacy of this vaccine, it was found that up to 95% of HPV 16 and 18 infections were prevented.[8] Multiple studies have shown that HPV vaccination of both men and women is important, as approximately one-third of HPV infections that can be prevented require male vaccination. Due to limited data about the prevalence of serotypes in LMICs, it is unclear if the HPV vaccine will be as successful in the LMIC setting as in HICs.

Industrialization has also caused an increase in air, water, and soil pollution. Construction materials, occupational exposures, and working conditions all play a role in increased cancer rates. Some studies have reported a link between chronic exposure to wood smoke, generated by burning wood in kitchens, and cervical intraepithelial neoplasms. Lead, often found in paint and water pipes, has also been associated with lung and stomach cancers. Radon exposure, generated by granite and limestone, has been associated with lung cancers. Awareness and advocacy programs to address these causes of cancer are an important public health component.

TABLE 32.1

Geographic associations with specific cancers

Cancer	Geographic region	Environmental factors
Stomach	East Asia, Chile	*H. pylori,* salt
Thyroid	India	Radiation
Cervical	South America, Africa, Asia	HPV
Liver	Africa, East Asia	Hepatitis B,C; aflatoxin
Oral	Southeast Asia	Tobacco chewing, areca nut
Lung	India, China	Indoor air pollution, tobacco smoking

Food safety is also an aspect of primary prevention. The dietary ingestion of aflatoxins, most specifically aflatoxin B1, is associated with HCC, due to synergism with HBV. The risk of liver cancer in patients with chronic HBV infection and exposure to aflatoxins can be as high as 30 times above baseline. There is also a link with increased risk and exposure to HCV, although this is not as well established. Strategies to reduce exposure to aflatoxins include improving post-harvest storage conditions, aflatoxin trapping agents, chlorophyllin, green tea polyphenols, and broccoli sprouts (that has shown in some rodent models to prevent cancer). Preventing contamination of grains is important. Chlorophyllin supplements can also reduce the carcinogenic properties of aflatoxins. Chlorophylls are found in green, leafy vegetables. Another treatment strategy to lower the risk of aflatoxin-induced HCC is to vaccinate patients against HBV.

Early detection and secondary prevention are another part of cancer control programs. For example, population-based screening programs can identify diseases at a stage that can still be treated with curative intention. Examples are breast self-examination, digital rectal exam for rectal cancer and prostate cancer, colonoscopy for colorectal cancer, or cervical surveillance. Resources are often limited for screening programs in LMICs. For cervical cancer screening, for example, cytology screening is difficult to establish and maintain given the requirement of cytotechnologists and laboratory infrastructure. A viable alternative for screening includes visual screening with acetic acid solution. With limited resources, cervical cancer screening conducted even once for women age 35 or older can have an effect on outcomes for large populations of women.

Serum tumor markers have little role in screening for cancers. They can, however, be useful in caring for patients with cancer. While they may assist in the diagnosis of a patient with a suspicious mass, their greatest utility is in following patients after surgical resection and/or chemotherapy treatments for a tumor recurrence. There are several useful tumor markers. In colorectal cancer, carcinoembryonic antigen (CEA) can be elevated. In prostate cancer, prostate specific antigen (PSA) can be elevated. In hepatocellular carcinoma, alpha-fetoprotein (AFP) can be elevated. Additionally, pathologic examinations for markers of tumor grade can assist in determining if the cancer is well differentiated and potentially slow growing or poorly differentiated and potentially more aggressive. In individual tumors like breast cancer, for example, there is a role for the pathologic analysis of hormone receptors to help classify the tumor as estrogen receptor (ER) positive/negative, progesterone receptor (PR) positive/negative, and HER-2 positive/negative. This distinction is important because it affects the treatment recommendations, especially using tamoxifen. It is also of prognostic significance as patients lacking all three receptors (triple negative) have worse outcomes. While the common presentation in patients in HICs is of an elderly woman with hormone receptor positive breast cancer, recent studies in LMICs have demonstrated that it is more common in that setting for patients to present at a younger age and with triple negative disease, compared to their counterparts in HICs.

Cancer Control Public Health Strategies

Coordinated cancer care is an emerging priority in LMICs. There are two aspects of this endeavor. The first is organizing cancer registries. This can be performed in collaboration with the World Health Organization (WHO) at a hospital, national, or regional level. The cancer registry relies on the pathologic diagnosis as the requirement for entry into the registry. This strong emphasis on basic pathologic analysis can be lacking in LMICs, but these services can be encouraged and expanded in the setting of a cancer registry. The data accumulated from a national cancer registry can assist in determining what cancers are public health priorities in that specific region. These data are also useful to assess cancer control projects over time. While cancer centers are common in HICs, this level of specialization is rarely necessary or afforded in LMICs. Developing a cancer ward within a large teaching hospital, however, is a way of coordinating cancer care.

Surgical procedures are also associated with cancer control. Circumcision, for example, is associated with a reduction in HIV transmission rates. Circumcision has been shown in two randomized controlled trials to lower transmission rates from females infected with HIV to males. This is of relevance to cancer control as HIV is associated with the development of cancers. In one of the initial randomized trials performed by Auvert et al. in 2005, the trial was halted at its interim analysis due to a relative risk of 0.40 (95% CI: 0.24%–0.68%; p<0.001). Thus, male circumcision is a surgical procedure that is an important part of public health initiatives in LMICs and can also assist in lowering rates of cancers that can be attributed to HIV.

Cancer Diagnosis

Surgery is one of the central treatments that can be offered to treat patients with cancers in LMICs. For solid tumors, it is generally considered the only way to obtain a cure. One challenge is how to adapt techniques that have been studied and reported in HICs and translate these data to practicing in LMICs. Breast cancer is a good example of this challenge (Figure 32.1). Breast cancer in LMICs often presents at a younger age and at more advanced stage. This is due to socioeconomic, cultural, and geographic differences when compared to HICs. Sentinel node biopsy has become an important diagnostic and staging tool in HICs. There are many obstacles to performing sentinel lymph node biopsies in LMICs, such as a lack of local expertise, multidisciplinary programs, training programs, quality assurance mechanisms, and supplies such as the gamma camera and radiotracers. Methylene blue dye is used in HICs in combination with radiotracers, so using this alone is one way to use this high-technology method in LMICs. This technique is of significant relevance in LMICs, where the majority of women present with advanced disease. Another aspect of caring for patients with breast cancer in LMICs is the lack of access to radiation therapy. Breast conservation is paramount in the treatment of many women with small breast cancers in HICs. Using this technique, however, is dependent on the availability of adjuvant radiation therapy. In locations without access to radiotherapy, a mastectomy is required to treat all breast cancers, regardless of size, in order to minimize local recurrences.

Clinical Assessment

Accurate diagnosis is very germane to the successful management of patients with cancer. It is the key to defining accurate causes of specific cancers, projecting the prognosis and course of the disease, and determining optimal therapy. While cancer diagnosis is confidently made following pathological or cytological examination of the tissue, some tumors do not afford themselves this opportunity before definitive treatments are planned due to the location of the tumor. Of note, among these diseases are gallbladder and pancreatic cancer. In these tumors and others like them, clinical judgment is vital in arriving at a diagnosis and planning for treatment. This becomes more important in LMIC settings because state-of-the-art, high-technology equipment is rarely available for diagnosis and treatment. In fact, in some remote parts of LMICs, accurate clinical diagnosis may be the only means of making the diagnosis (Figure 32.2).

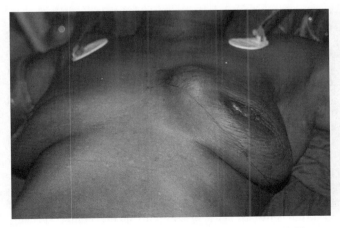

FIGURE 32.1 Breast cancer. Image by T. Peter Kingham and Olusegun Alatise.

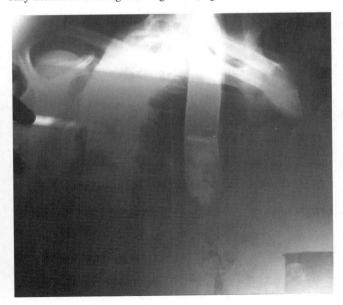

FIGURE 32.2 Advanced esophageal barium swallow. Image by T. Peter Kingham and Olusegun Alatise.

Late presentation is standard in most LMICs. Thus, patients usually present with large masses that may be neglected and ulcerated, especially in surface malignancies such as breast cancer. Most patients commonly present with features of anemia and malnutrition. When examining these patients, all systems must be reviewed to establish the presence of local and distant spread of the disease. For example, the presence of cough or backache in patients with colorectal or gastric cancer may give a clue to the occurrence of chest metastasis. Efforts should also be made to establish the presence of paraneoplastic syndromes when they can potentially be present. Examination of the patient must be methodical so as not to miss subtle clinical findings that can help diagnose and stage patients with cancer. Similar to trauma scenarios, patients should be examined from head to toe. A skull swelling, for example, may suggest skull metastasis, which will require further evaluation. Similarly, regional and other lymph node stations must be assessed to establish the presence of nodal involvement.

Cancer Diagnosis and Staging

The goal of investigating patients with cancer is to confirm the diagnosis and determine the sites of disease, extent of tumor burden, and any complications caused by the cancer. Local or locoregional treatments, such as surgery and radiation therapy, may be curative for localized disease. If the disease is widespread, although such local interventions may contribute to cure, they will be insufficient. Systemic treatment, for example with drugs or hormones, will be required. Unfortunately, the process of mapping out the extent of the disease in most LMICs is still crudely based on clinical examination, chest X-ray, and ultrasound. Within the limitations of these basic radiological investigations, a lot can be achieved when the investigation is done by experienced hands. All efforts should be made to maximize the use of abdominopelvic ultrasounds, especially in abdominal tumors, in locating the tumor, guiding percutaneous biopsies, and also detecting obvious signs of metastasis.

Computerized tomographic (CT) scans are now available in major cities in some LMICs. This facility is important in accurately staging cancers before a therapeutic treatment plan is instituted. Unfortunately, this procedure is quite expensive, and only a privileged few can afford it. This is due to a lack of health insurance schemes in most LMICs. In the absence of CT scan or other high-tech equipment like magnetic resonance imaging (MRI) and positron emission tomography (PET) CT scan, patients still require staging and treatment. Staging must often be performed with surgery (surgical staging) or solely on physical examination. Diagnostic laparoscopy with or without laparoscopic ultrasound is a good alternative for surgical staging with low morbidity, where it is available. Adequate surgical treatment can be offered to patients in the absence of all these facilities.

For most solid tumors, the first diagnostic question that must be answered is what type of tumor it is. To determine this answer, samples of a lesion can be obtained with a needle or with an open incisional or excisional biopsy. Fine-needle aspiration cytology is done to make cytological diagnosis before treatments are instituted. This is widely practiced in most LMICs because it is a fast, safe, and cheap procedure. In most centers, the results are available within hours of sampling. Unfortunately, the procedure has the disadvantage of not giving information on tissue architecture. For example, fine-needle aspiration biopsy of a breast mass can make the diagnosis of malignancy but cannot differentiate between an invasive and noninvasive tumor. Similarly, the occurrence of false negative could be as high as 15%, especially in small lesions. Hence, all cytological diagnosis must be supported by histological diagnosis using core biopsy. It is crucial to ensure that the histologic findings are consistent with the clinical scenario and to know the appropriate interpretation of each histologic finding. A needle biopsy for which the report is inconsistent with the clinical scenario should be either repeated or followed by an open biopsy. Fortunately, solid tumors in most LMICs are large, making it easy to obtain a biopsy and diagnose these tumors.

Core biopsy findings determine the tumor histology, grade, and type of the tumor using immunohistochemistry. These characteristics assist in definitive therapeutic planning. Biopsy specimens of mucosal lesions usually are obtained endoscopically (e.g., via colonoscope, bronchoscope, or cystoscope). Deep-seated lesions can be localized with ultrasound guidance and, where available, CT scan for biopsy. Open biopsies have the advantage of providing more tissue for histologic evaluation and the disadvantage of being an operative procedure. Incisional biopsies are reserved for very large lesions in which a definitive diagnosis cannot be made by needle biopsy. Excisional biopsies are performed for lesions for which either core biopsy is not possible or the results are nondiagnostic. Excisional biopsies should be performed with curative intent by obtaining adequate tissue around the lesion to ensure negative surgical margins. Marking of the orientation of the margins by sutures or clips by the surgeon and inking of the specimen margins by the pathologist will allow for determination of the surgical margins and will guide surgical re-excision if one or more of the margins are positive or are close for the presence of microscopic tumor. The biopsy incision should be oriented to allow for excision of the biopsy scar if repeat operation is necessary. Furthermore, the biopsy incision should directly overlie the area to be removed rather than tunneling from another site, which runs the risk of contaminating a larger field. Finally, meticulous hemostasis during a biopsy is essential, because a hematoma can lead to contamination of the tissue planes and can make subsequent follow-up with physical examinations much more challenging.

Cancer Treatment

In LMICs, surgery remains the definitive treatment and the only realistic hope of cure because even in conditions where other therapeutic measures may be equally effective, availability and affordability will be a constraining issue. Surgery has several roles in cancer treatment including diagnosis, removal of primary disease, removal of metastatic disease, palliation, prevention, and reconstruction.

Radical surgery for cancer involves removal of the primary tumor and as much of the surrounding tissue and lymph node drainage as possible not only to ensure local control but also to prevent spread of the tumor through the lymphatics. Removal of the primary disease can help to improve quality of life, especially in patients with large morbid tumors such as fungating breast cancers. Organ-sparing procedures such as quadrantectomy of the breast should be offered with care to cancer patients in these countries. One reason for this is due to poor follow-up and the culture in some LMICs. The affordability of surgery and availability of the operating theater in these countries cannot be guaranteed. It is important, however, to appreciate that high-quality, meticulous surgery taking care not to disrupt the primary tumor at the time of excision is of the utmost importance in obtaining a cure in localized disease and preventing local recurrence.

In certain circumstances, surgery for metastatic disease may be appropriate. This can help to improve quality of life and also to improve overall survival. This is particularly true for liver metastases arising from colorectal cancer, where successful resection of all detectable disease can lead to long-term survival in about one-third of patients. Though rarely available in most LMICs, with multiple liver metastases, it may still be possible to take a surgical approach by using *in situ* ablation with cryotherapy or radiofrequency energy. In many cases, surgery is not appropriate for cure but may be extremely valuable for palliation. A good example of this is the patient with a symptomatic primary tumor who also has distant metastases. In this case, removal of the primary tumor may increase the patient's quality of life but will have little effect on the ultimate outcome. Cases of fungating breast cancers are examples. Toilet mastectomy helps to remove the smell associated with this disease. Other examples include bypass procedures for obstructing jaundice from cancer of the head of pancreas. In inoperable cancer of the head of pancreas, cholecysto- or choledochojejunostomy may alleviate jaundice. Similarly, with inoperable cecal cancer, an ileotransverse anastomosis can help to relieve malignant bowel obstructions.

Other adjunctive therapies for cancer include chemotherapy and or radiotherapy. Radiotherapy machines are rare in most LMICs. When they exist, there is often a long waiting period. Frequent machine malfunctions due to the high volume of use and difficulty in maintaining these machines often worsen the situation. Unfortunately, some patients that manage to gain access to radiation therapy machines in LMICs end up with grave complications due to the outdated models of the machinery that are available. For example, most HICs have halted the use of cobalt radiation machines due to the difficulty in controlling doses and the scattering effect. This seems, however, to be the only type of machine available in most LMICs.

Chemotherapy is often prescribed by surgeons in LMICs for the treatment of solid tumors. This differs from the treatment paradigm in most HICs, where medical oncologists prescribe chemotherapy and treat chemotherapy side effects and nonsurgical complications. The use of chemotherapy can be problematic in LMICs. Generic drugs are difficult to obtain. Thus, the efficacy of available drugs may not be comparable to what is published in HICs. Agents commonly used include 5-fluorouracil, cyclophosphamide, methotrexate, Adriamycin, capecitabine, and oxaliplatin. Recently, some targeted therapies such as trastuzumab and bevacizumab have become available, although they are very expensive. Common indications and complications are listed in Table 32.2.

Palliative Care

Many patients with cancer in LMICs present to healthcare facilities with end-stage cancers. Palliative care is often the primary therapeutic option that is available given the late stage of disease (Figure 32.3). There are many symptoms that can be improved and sometimes alleviated. Antiemetics can be useful in treating patients with intractable nausea from their cancer or therapy.

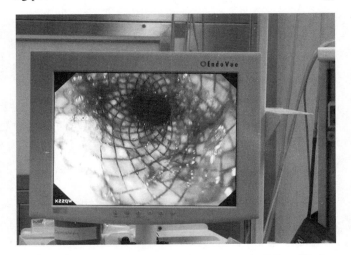

FIGURE 32.3 Palliative esophageal stenting. Image by T. Peter Kingham and Olusegun Alatise.

TABLE 32.2

Common chemotherapeutic agents

Agent	Mechanism	Route	Indication	Complications
5-Fluorouracil, Capecitabine	Antimetabolite–Pyrimidine analogue	IV, PO	Colon, breast, stomach, pancreas, ovary, head and neck, prostate, cervix, bladder	Myelosuppression, nausea, alopecia, diarrhea, hand-foot syndrome
Cyclophosphamide	Alkylating agent–nitrogen mustard class	IV, PO	Breast, ovary, lung, cervix, testicular, leukemia/lymphomas	Myelosuppression, alopecia, cardiac, renal, emesis
Methotrexate	Antimetabolite–folate antagonist	IV, PO	Breast, head and neck, lung, lymphomas, leukemias	Myelosuppression, renal failure, pneumonitis
Doxorubicin	Topoisomerase inhibitor–Anthracycline class	PO	Breast, lymphomas, bladder, thyroid, lung, gastric	Cardiomyopathy, myelosuppression, mucositis
Tamoxifen	Estrogen receptor modulator	PO	Breast	Amenorrhea, hot flashes, nausea, weight gain, venous thrombosis, endometrial cancer

Table created by T. Peter Kingham and Olusegun Alatise.

Medications, such as ondansetron, prochlorperazine, and dexamethasone, can help treat this symptom. Pain is one of the primary symptoms in patients with late-stage cancer. Sufficient supplies of opioids are often a problem due to government restrictions on opioid distribution. It is possible for surgeons to advocate for legal changes to allow for the compassionate use of opioids. Morphine delivered sublingual or subcutaneously is very effective at treating baseline pain. Concentrated morphine solutions and fentanyl are both useful for breakthrough pain. Symptoms of anxiety can be treated with lorazepam. Delirium can be treated with haloperidol.

One way to address the lack of availability of palliative care options is to use Community Volunteer Programs. This has been established in Uganda to treat patients with cancer and HIV/AIDS. The idea is to use the volunteers as bridges between the community and a facility that has some hospice capability.

The WHO has developed a Public Health Model with the aim of integrating palliative care into public health initiatives. This model includes training the healthcare workforce and the public, changing palliative care policies, and assuring an adequate supply of drugs. In many countries, palliative care is not recognized as a part of public health such that insurance companies won't pay for it. These include opioid availability workshops to identify barriers to opioid use, to inform regulators about the medical necessity for access to opioids, and to let regulators explain current and future regulations to physicians.

Cancer control strategies should focus on research, public health priorities, and implementation.[9,10] Research that is needed includes epidemiologic studies, risk factor assessment, cost effectiveness, and therapeutic trials. These data can help determine guidelines, priorities, and interventions that help create public health priorities. From these public health priorities, implementation strategies such as cancer screening, clinical training, cancer registries, and treatment access programs can be initiated. Surgeons play a vital role in all of these aspects of cancer care in LMICs, as they are frequently the sole physicians caring for patients with solid tumors.

Pediatric Neoplasms

For a discussion of pediatric malignancies in LMICs, including lymphomas and Wilms' tumor, please see Chapter 31.

COMMENTARY

Ruth Damuse, Haiti

In Haiti, like in other LMICs, there is a struggle to provide basic health care for the population. The healthcare system is unable to offer specialty services, including oncology, despite the growing evidence that the burden of oncological disease is increasing worldwide and in LMICs. Oncology is a field of medicine that is constantly evolving with continuous technological advances.

Oncologic surgery is limited in LMICs by several factors. The population has limited education about health care in general, and especially about prevention and early detection of cancer. There is a lack of strong national screening programs and a shortage of medical staff who specialize in oncology and oncology-related fields. There is also a limited supply of many cancer drugs. Targeted therapies are available, and they are shown to improve prognosis for several diagnoses, but they are often very expensive and therefore inaccessible in LMICs.

33

Infectious Diseases

Gita N. Mody
Sachita Shah
Robert Riviello

Introduction

Infectious diseases significantly impact the practice of surgery in low- and middle-income countries (LMICs). A surgeon operating in a tropical or remote setting requires a working knowledge of the locally endemic infectious diseases in order to care for these common conditions. Many of these diseases disproportionately affect people who are chronically undernourished or immunocompromised. Symptoms of infectious diseases can confound the presentation of even common surgical diagnoses and should be considered when evaluating a patient with abdominal pain, with lesions requiring biopsy, or undergoing evaluation for lymphadenopathy. The surgeon at the hospital or clinic must not only be able to surgically intervene on the manifestations of infectious diseases but must also be able to direct the perioperative monitoring and medical management.

This chapter both describes the presentation and treatment of infectious diseases treated primarily with surgery, particularly soft tissue infections, and reviews the most common communicable diseases that should be considered when evaluating a patient with surgical complaints. The surgical management of infections specific to defined anatomic regions will be covered in the relevant chapters of this book assigned to that anatomic region. A listing of cross-referencing infectious conditions covered in this book can be found at the end of this chapter (Table 33.1).

Soft Tissue Infections

Bacterial Soft Tissue Infections

A 10-year-old girl presented to the district hospital with a one-week history of increasing swelling over the anterior aspect of her upper left leg. She reported no fever or constitutional symptoms, and the swelling was warm, tender, nonmobile, and firm. The surrounding skin was intact with mild erythema. She initially reported no trauma, though on further questioning she reported having fallen while running about a year ago.

An X-ray shows no obvious bony changes or fracture. An ultrasound shows a 2 × 4-cm mass, deep to the fascial layer, with a hypoechoic center. The skin was cleansed

with iodine, a 16-gauge needle on a syringe was inserted, and a scant amount of purulent fluid was withdrawn. Incision and drainage was planned.

The above case is a typical presentation of pyomyositis, an intramuscular infection that typically becomes suppurative and is common in LMICs. Pyomyositis, subcutaneous abscesses, and intramuscular abscesses are among the most common indications for surgical interventions at the district hospital. For example, in one sub-Saharan hospital, pyomyositis accounted for up to 4% of hospital admissions.[1] Primary pyomyositis was originally described in and is typically seen in tropical settings, though the condition is being diagnosed more frequently worldwide, largely in immunocompromised patients.[2] The pathogenesis of pyomyositis is thought to be due to hematogenous spread of transient bacteremia from *Staphylococcus aureus* or group A *Streptococcus*.[3,4] However, patients in LMICs do not typically report a break in the skin or definite source of infection antecedent to presentation. Small wounds to the hands, feet, and nail cuticles caused by manual labor may serve as a common portal of pathogen entry. Trauma to the involved muscles (commonly the quadriceps, glutei, pectoralis major, serratus anterior, biceps, iliopsoas, gastrocnemius, abdominal, and spinal muscles) may be reported,[5] and multifocal infections are possible.[3]

Risk factors for pyomyositis include male gender, young adult age (20–45 years old), immune compromised status, and tropical climate.[3,5] Theoretically, the combination of poor nutrition, poor hygiene, endemic viral and parasitic infections, and lack of access to care predisposes patients to developing pyomyositis. High suspicion is warranted when a patient presents in an early stage with muscular pain and fever; however, patients typically present late, when a purulent collection has developed or when systemic sepsis has begun.[3] The differential diagnosis for pyomyositis includes other soft tissue infections, such as cellulitis, subcutaneous abscesses, clostridial infections, and necrotizing fasciitis; osteomyelitis; muscular trauma[5]; and soft tissue masses, including cancer. Vigilance in evaluating patients is necessary as pyomyositis can present anywhere in the body. Vague symptoms, including back pain, could be early evidence of disease, which when untreated, could become devastating.

The diagnosis of pyomyositis is confirmed by characteristic changes between muscle fibers on biopsy[3] or practically, when pus is evacuated from the muscle. Portable ultrasound (US) is an imaging modality that is increasingly available in developing and remote areas. The use of US can be extremely valuable in distinguishing cellulitis from an abscess, evaluating the presence and size of a fluid collection requiring drainage, and guiding needle placement for diagnostic aspiration of the fluid collection. Details on the use of ultrasound for diagnosing soft tissue infections are provided in Box 33.1 and Figures 33.1 and 33.2. More advanced imaging modalities such as computed tomography (CT) and magnetic resonance imaging (MRI), which can be helpful in

TABLE 33.1

Alphabetic listing of infectious disease conditions (synonyms in parenthesis) covered in this book.

- Abscess, bacterial
- Ameba
- Amoebiasis
- Appendicitis
- Ascariasis
- Aspergilloma (mycetoma, fungus ball)
- Buruli ulcer (tropical ulcer)
- Cellulitis
- Chagas disease (megacolon)
- Filariasis (onchocerciasis, elephantiasis)
- *Helicobacter*
- Hepatitis B
- HIV/AIDS
- Leischmaniasis
- Ludwig's angina
- Malaria
- Osteomyelitis
- Perirectal abscess
- Pott's disease
- Prostatitis
- Pyomyositis (tropical pyomyositis, myositis tropicans, tropical skeletal muscle abscess, tropical myositis, nontropical myositis, infectious myositis, or spontaneous bacterial myositis)
- Rabies
- Schistosomiasis
- Tetanus
- Trachoma
- Tuberculosis
- Typhoid
- Wound infections

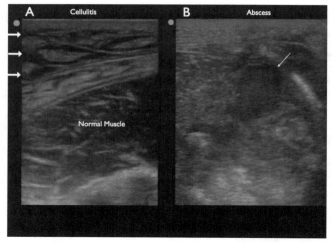

FIGURE 33.1 Ultrasound views of cellulitis (A) and abscess (B). A: Cellulitis. Arrows point to the area of cobblestoning. B: Abscess. Arrows point to the fluid collection. Image by Sachita Shah.

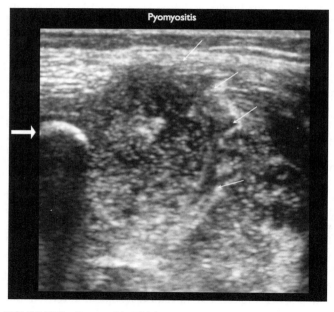

FIGURE 33.2 Pyomyositis. Thick arrow points to the fibula (hyperechoic bright bone). Thin arrows point to the muscle liquefied into pus adjacent to the bone. Image by Sachita Shah.

BOX 33.1   USE OF ULTRASOUND FOR DIAGNOSING SOFT TISSUE INFECTIONS

- Use a linear array ultrasound probe meant for superficial depths
- Consider a probe cover for purulent infections and use gel between the probe and skin
- Start with normal skin adjacent to the area of interest to visualize normal areas before moving on to the abnormal tissue
- Assess just below the skin for "cobblestoning" or fluid between subcutaneous tissue suggestive of cellulitis or edema
- Assess for hypoechoic or heterogeneous darker areas of fluid collections deep to the skin

    suggestive of abscess. Use calipers or the ruler on the side of the screen to assess size and depth of any fluid collections prior to drainage
- If purulent areas extend to disrupt normal muscle architecture or are in close proximity to bone, consider more serious infections such as pyomyositis or osteomyelitis
- Always clean the probe thoroughly after use to avoid transmission of infection to the next patient
- Potential pitfalls include thrombosed vessels appearing as an abscess and failure to identify a fluid collection if it exists

Exploring an abscess

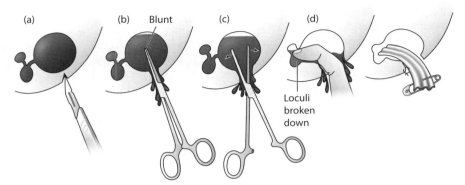

(a)   (b) Blunt   (c)   (d)

Loculi
broken
down

FIGURE 33.3 Use of latex glove finger as a drain to permit ongoing drainage of I&D site. Bewes P, Cairns J, Thorton J, King M. *Primary Surgery Volume 1: Non-trauma.* New York: Oxford University Press; 1990, p. 54, Figure 5.3.

BOX 33.2   COMMON PITFALLS

- The presentation of soft tissue infections in the developing world is often different than in the developed world. Deep infections involving the soft tissues, muscles, and bones, including in multifocal locations, are commonly seen in the developing world.
- Failure to completely access or irrigate abscess cavity is a common pitfall that can lead to ongoing illness for the patient.
- Local practice often involves aggressive, repeated wound toilet with hydrogen peroxide, providine iodine, or other caustic substances, which do not substitute from complete evacuation of the abscess cavity and can cause tissue trauma. Repeated use is discouraged.

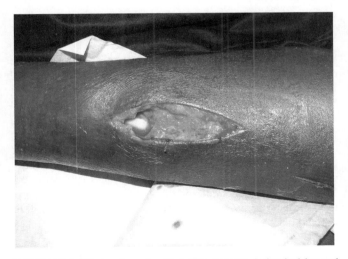

FIGURE 33.4 Photo of proximal left tibia exposed during incision and drainage of pyomyositis. Only the minimum amount of bone is exposed to adequately drain the purulent collection. Providing tissue coverage through approximated sutures or rotational flaps when needed should be considered to prevent bone dehiscence. Image by Gita Mody.

diagnosing soft tissue and bony infections, are typically not available or not cost-effective in LMICs. Attempting to obtain such studies will likely delay definitive care for these patients.

Treatment of a suppurative collection, either within or near muscle, always involves incision and drainage (I&D) and copious irrigation. Local anesthesia is less effective in areas of active infection. If a large I&D is planned or the patient is a child, consider using ketamine anesthesia and performing the procedure in the minor room or operating theater. If possible, send aspirated material obtained before I&D or at the time of the procedure for Gram stain and culture. If the material appears caseating, perform acid-fast stain. Start antibiotics (generally penicillin targeted toward *Staphylococcus* and *Streptococcus* organisms) in the nonseptic patient only after a sample for Gram stain has been obtained. If the patient is ill-appearing, consider broadly treating with ceftriaxone or other broad-spectrum antibiotic until the causative organism can be confirmed.

To drain the collection, make an adequately sized linear incision, oriented parallel to blood vessels and nerves and over the point of maximal tenderness and tenseness. Alternatively, a "finder" needle or ultrasound can be used to locate the fluid collection and plan the incision. To break up and evacuate all loculated collections, introduce and aggressively spread a blunt forcep or clamp, extending the incision if necessary. All necrotic muscle must be debrided. This may require a number of serial operations. Suturing in a drain or the finger of a latex glove (Figure 33.3) or making a cruciate incision can be considered to improve drainage.[6] If the depth of the purulence requires extension of the incision to the bone, care should be taken to avoid exposing large areas of bone (see Figure 33.4).

Serial examination of the patient and the wound is required even when I&D appears to have been adequate. In cases where purulent material was found to be adjacent to the bone, X-rays of the affected extremity should be reexamined to detect occult fracture as a possible source of the infection (as was the case in the child presented here). Serial images may be necessary to monitor for development of bony changes concerning for osteomyelitis. When bone is exposed in the wound, consideration should be given to treating the patient empirically for osteomyelitis with a 6-week course of intravenous antibiotics (for more details, see Chapter 30). A completely drained abscess should not require antibiotics. Foul-smelling bandages, purulent drainage, or failure of wound healing are signs of ongoing infection and should prompt repeat imaging, exploration, or referral as necessary.

In a patient with symptoms and signs of soft tissue infection but without a defined purulent collection, careful monitoring is still warranted. Cellulitis is a superficial skin infection, typically by *streptococci,* that affects minor skin trauma, lacerations, and surgical wounds and can be treated with penicillin antibiotics.[7] Lack of improvement of erythema should lead to further investigation, including cultures of tissues, imaging studies, and repeat exploration. Resistant organisms are likely less common in the developing world, but, at Mulago hospital in Uganda, roughly one-third of the *Staphylococcus aureus* isolated from surgical site infections were resistant to methicillin.[8] Necrotizing fasciitis, a rapidly evolving soft tissue infection caused by gas-producing organisms, leads to characteristic imaging findings and crepitance of the involved tissues on physical exam. Extensive debridement is often required, and referral to a facility that has a functioning intensive care unit (ICU) should be considered in a patient with confirmed necrotizing fasciitis as septic shock is the most common cause of death in such cases.

Other Causative Organisms

Organisms such as mycobacterium, fungus, and parasites also commonly cause soft tissue infections in tropical and subtropical climates. A careful history should be taken to identify exposures or occupations that may predispose to certain types of infections. Early directed therapy against the offending pathogen(s) is necessary to prevent chronic wounds. For example, the correct diagnosis and treatment of "tropical ulcers" may be elusive, as the epidemiology of these wounds is not well-known, and they affect poor and immunocompromised patients who may have limited access to healthcare.[9] These infections may have been treated by traditional healers before the patient seeks medical care, and typically present in delayed fashion with advanced infections or large, chronic, and nonhealing wounds.

Buruli Ulcer

Buruli ulcers are caused by infection of the skin and soft tissues, including muscle and bone, with toxin-producing *Mycobacterium ulcerans.* The mode of transmission is unknown, but it is thought to be due to contact with water or vectors that transmit the mycobacterium.[10] Buruli ulcers begin as a painless mobile nodules that progress to large, superficial painless ulcers, usually on the extremities.[11] For patients with suspected Buruli ulcers presenting to remote hospitals, the diagnosis can and should be confirmed with Ziehl-Neelsen (ZN) stains of wound material obtained by swabs[12] or fine-needle aspiration.[13] Patients with active disease should be treated with rifampicin, streptomycin, and amikacin for at least 8 weeks. Buruli ulcers can be quite morbid. Ulcers that do not heal despite 4 weeks of antibiotics may require excision, with a 4-cm margin often requiring extensive grafting.[14] Some authors have noted successful treatment with local hyperthermia to 40°C and with topical honey application.

Filariasis

Filariasis is a mosquito-borne helminthic parasite that causes destruction of infected lymphatic tissues. Surgically remediable conditions such as hydroceles can develop. Hydroceles form up to 40% of adult males in endemic areas.[15] Other common complications for filariasis are lymphedema and elephantiasis of the scrotum or limbs,[16] particularly in genetically susceptible individuals.[17] Bancroftian filariasis is one of three causative helminths (*Wuchereria bancrofti*) that can cause lymphatic filariasis. Ivermectin, diethylcarbamazine, and albendazole are among the chemotherapeutic regimens used to treat filariasis.[16]

A hydrocele is diagnosed by palpation of a nontender, nonreducible scrotal mass. Often, the testes cannot be felt when the hydrocele is large. While transillumination of the fluid-containing mass is a commonly described test, this may be difficult to accomplish in dark-skinned patients. Hydrocelectomy can reduce morbidity and improve quality of life in patients with lymphatic filariasis[18] and is safe and effectively performed in LMICs without sophisticated surgical equipment.[19,20] Complete excision of the hydrocele sac should be considered in patients with chronic bancroftian filariasis, in which the pathogenesis of hydrocele may be related to significant lymphatic damage by the adult filarial worms, as opposed to lymphatic obstruction by worm-induced granulomas.[21] More details on the operative technique for hydrocelectomy are found in Chapter 24.

Lymphatic filariasis can affect the genitalia in the form of acute or chronic hydrocele, acute scrotal pain, and breast or extremity swelling. Lower extremity lymphedema does not typically require surgical management and can be managed with compression, elevation, and anti-filarial drugs. Care should be taken to maintain skin integrity to avoid soft tissue infections.[22] In advanced, disabling cases of lymphedema or elephantiasis, amputation may be required. Wound healing is typically difficult in these cases, but with careful multidisciplinary care, successful outcomes can be achieved.[23]

Communicable Diseases: Management of Surgical Manifestations

The "big three" communicable diseases that affect patients in the developing world are human immunodeficiency virus/acquired immune deficiency syndrome (HIV/AIDS), tuberculosis (TB), and malaria. Evaluation of surgical patients with HIV/AIDS and the surgical management of common manifestations of AIDS, including Kaposi's sarcoma (KS), cytomegalovirus (CMV) colitis, gastrointestinal (GI) bleeding, and anorectal disease, are covered here. The drainage of tuberculosis empyema and surgical resection for complications of TB will be briefly reviewed. Management of typhoid perforation, gastrointestinal (GI) symptoms of malaria, and parasitic causes of abdominal pain will be covered in Chapter 42.

Human Immunodeficiency Virus/Acquired Immune Deficiency Syndrome

Roughly 33 million people live with HIV worldwide. While incidence of HIV is decreasing, deaths due to AIDS are also decreasing, and people with HIV are living longer.[24] Therefore, surgeons are increasingly involved in the care of patients with HIV/AIDS. The patient with HIV/AIDS may both be more susceptible to surgical disease due to general debilitation, multiple opportunistic infections, and malignancies, as well as be at increased risk of perioperative complications due to their immunocompromised[25,26] state. However, surgical morbidity and mortality are not increased in elective surgical care of patients with HIV or AIDS,[27] and surgery for trauma in HIV/AIDS patients has been shown to have good outcomes.[28] Emergent and urgent surgical procedures in AIDS patients should be approached with the patients' disease stage and goals of care in mind.[29]

For patients who are HIV positive, antiretroviral medications should be continued in the perioperative period. Universal precautions should be maintained while treating all patients, regardless of serostatus. The rate of HIV transmission from patient to healthcare workers after needle-stick injury is 0.3%,[30] and transmission from surgeon to patient has not been observed.[31]

KS is an angioproliferative soft tissue sarcoma associated with KS herpes virus and herpes virus 8 that is common in patients with immunodeficiency and is an AIDS-defining illness.[32] KS responds to highly active antiretroviral therapy and so is decreasing in incidence with more effective HIV treatment. Localized cutaneous and oral KS lesions may be observed, or treated with topical alitretinoin gel, radiotherapy, or intralesional chemotherapy, such as vinblastine. Generalized disease may be treated with doxorubicin-based systemic chemotherapy.[33] Lesions are often characteristic in appearance (purple or red nodules or papules) and do not require biopsy, but atypical lesions should be biopsied as bacillary angiomatosis is on the differential diagnosis.[34]

Resection of troublesome cutaneous lesions, even with margins, is not useful, as the surrounding skin will likely have pathological changes.[35] Electrocautery or topical silver nitrate application may be useful to treat slowly bleeding cutaneous lesions. Using nonadherent dressings, compression wraps, and extremity elevation may be useful as well. KS can cause lymphatic obstruction, leading to lymphedema. In severe or complicated cases of KS, including infection of KS lesions, amputation of the affected extremities may be required.[36,37] KS can also affect the GI tract and the lungs in as many as 50% of patients with cutaneous lesions,[38] occasionally leading to intussusception, obstruction, perforation, or hemorrhage with the need for surgery.[39–41]

GI tract perforation, obstruction, or bleeding can also occur in HIV patients due to CMV colitis, lymphoma, or fungal (candida) or mycobacterium infections.[42] The triage and management of patients with HIV/AIDS presenting with abdominal catastrophe follows standard principles. Emergent surgical intervention may be required. KS of the bowel should be resected or bypassed according to standard oncologic principles. CMV causes vasculitis, and so the affected bowel should be resected and consideration should be given to diversion. Non-Hodgkin's lymphoma, commonly occurring in HIV/AIDS patients, can cause massive intra-abdominal lymphadenopathy, leading to bowel obstruction.[42]

Other common surgical abdominal pathology, such as appendicitis or cholecystitis, may present unusually in HIV/AIDS patients, due to the lack of characteristic symptoms, leukocytosis, or fever, despite inflamed or perforated viscus. Thus, vigilance is required.

Anorectal surgery is the most common indication for an operation in the HIV-positive patient.[27] Notably, an immunocompromised patient with an anorectal abscess may not present with fever, skin induration, or erythema, nor with the typical amount of perianal pain as other patients. A course of postoperative antibiotics (ciprofloxacin, metronidazole) should be given in the immunocompromised patient despite adequate drainage. Other indications of anorectal surgery in HIV patients include anal fissure, fistula, anal condylomata (anogenital warts), and squamous cell cancer.[43] Excisional procedures for anal condylomata (as opposed to cryotherapy or laser therapy) are more likely to be carried out in developing settings. Excision with scissors may cause less tissue trauma than with electrocautery. Recurrence due to residual virus is common. Anal condylomata caused by human papillomavirus (HPV) may be associated with squamous intraepithelial neoplasia or squamous cell cancer due to co-infection with multiple HPV types.[44] Giant condyloma acuminatum (Buschke-Loewenstein tumor) is rare and difficult to manage, sometimes requiring abdominoperineal resection and/or complex reconstructions.[45] A low CD4 count is associated with postoperative complications, including poor wound healing, after anorectal surgery.[46]

Tuberculosis

TB affects 14 million patients worldwide and is the most common opportunistic infection in immunocompromised patients.[47] Tuberculosis requiring surgical management can affect most organ systems, including pulmonary (cavitary lesions, effusions, empyema, bronchopleural fistulas, pneumothorax, and bronchiectasis), gastrointestinal (bowel stricturing and obstruction and encasing peritonitis), and musculoskeletal system (Pott's disease of the spine and septic arthritis of the hip). Historically, thoracic surgery was developed to manage complications of TB.[48] TB should be considered in all patients in the developing world with effusions. In nearly 40% of empyema cases managed in the developing world hospital, TB is the causal agent.[49] Drainage of a tuberculous empyema requires a large-bore chest tube and at least a single-chamber chest tube drainage system (see Chapter 41 for details). Patients with tuberculous empyema more frequently require surgical procedures (drainage, decortication, closure of bronchopleural fistula, or thoracoplasty) and have poorer outcomes compared to patients with bacterial (*Staphylococcus aureus* or gram-negative bacilli) empyema[49,50]. Instilling fibrinolytic agents does not appear to improve outcomes or influence the need for surgery to aid drainage in empyema patients.[51] Antituberculosis treatment should be maintained for 6 months with a directly observed rifampin-containing regimen in new patients and according to drug subspecialty testing for previously treated patients.[52] Rarely, the purulent material involves the thoracic cavity and soft tissues, a condition called empyema necessitans, which requires surgery to drain the collection and obliterate the cavity.[53]

Multidrug-resistant tuberculosis (MDR-TB) is defined as TB resistant to isoniazid and rifampin.[54] There are 1–1.5 million existing and 440,000 new cases of MDR-TB worldwide,[54] with disproportionately more cases in LMICs, making MDR-TB a global health priority.[55,56] As exposure to MDR-TB regimens increases, extensively resistant strains of TB (XDRTB) are developing.[54] Surgical resection of affected pulmonary segments is increasingly used as a treatment adjunct to drug therapy in patients with highly drug-resistant or persistently positive sputum cultures.[57] Surgeons have reported postoperative mortality rates from 0%–6%, sputum culture conversion rates ranging from 60%–100%, and cure rates of 70%–90%.[58–63] A case series of 121 patients undergoing pulmonary resection in Peru was the first report of the use of pulmonary resection to treat MDR-TB in a low-income country.[64] The outcomes of patients treated with surgery for adjunctive treatment of MDR-TB compared to those not receiving surgery are still not known. Persistent cavitary lesions can also predispose to localized pulmonary aspergillomas (*Aspergillus fumigatus*) and may cause hemoptysis, requiring resection.[65]

Pediatric Considerations

For a discussion of surgically treatable infections pertinent to pediatric populations of LMICs, including HIV, tuberculosis, and typhoid, please see Chapter 31. Also not covered here is the surgical management of patients with tetanus, including neonatal tetanus. As these conditions are life-threatening, patients with tetanus or very high-risk wounds should be transferred to the highest level of care available after receiving immune globulin or antitetanus serum if available, and tetanus toxoid injection, penicillin, and airway support if needed.[66]

Conclusion

Surgeons working in LMICs and caring for the destitute ill will be called upon to intervene on a wide range of diseases. It is salient to point out that with infectious diseases, as with noncommunicable diseases, most of these conditions are a result

BOX 33.3   LMIC CONSIDERATIONS

- Unusual organisms can cause soft tissue infections, including Mycobacterium tuberculosis. Purulent material due to TB often appears caseating (cheese-like) infections and staining for acid-fast bacilli should be considered.
- Patients with immunodeficiency develop unique and common surgical diseases. These patients may present with variable symptoms and signs of surgical disease, including lack of leukocytosis or fever even with viscus perforation.
- Lack of resources does not permit lack of maintaining universal precautions. Protecting yourself, your colleagues, and your patients is of paramount importance. Wear eye goggles, double gloves, and protective aprons for all procedures.

of poverty more so than geography. The high incidence of pyomyositis, acute and chronic osteomyelitis, and Buruli ulcers is clearly related to poor nutrition and poor hygiene that result from poverty and lack of sufficient access to clean water. TB, thought to be a disappearing disease in the developed world prior to HIV/AIDS, never left the poor. TB will present in a multitude of fashions, in nearly every organ system. Surgeons will be called on to biopsy, drain, excise, resect, or bypass. In areas afflicted by high HIV prevalence, the surgeon may observe the HIV prevalence in hospitalized patients to be roughly double that in the baseline population. This will alter wound healing and complications seen at the hospital level. So many of the surgical interventions for infectious diseases bring an almost immediate benefit to the patient and to our colleagues in other disciplines, either by providing diagnosis, treatment, or palliation. In light of this, the surgeon working in LMICs is given a unique opportunity to significantly impact a disease burden that disproportionately affects the poor.

COMMENTARY

Samuel Abimerech Luboga, Uganda

This chapter has made a very important contribution to our understanding of the importance of surgery as a public health intervention, especially in a country like Uganda where infectious disease and its surgical prevalence is very high. It reminds us that many infectious diseases have concomitant surgical complications that must be taken into account and looked out for in evaluating patients presenting with infectious diseases. Surgical complications are sometimes the presenting complaint, as seen in, for example, swelling for

osteomyelitis (especially in patients with underlying immune compromise), or HIV/AIDS patients (especially children and elders). Surgery makes a major contribution to the prevention, diagnosis, care, and treatment of infectious diseases. Therefore, investment in prevention, care, and treatment (PCT) of infectious diseases should include adequate consideration for investment in building and maintaining capacity for surgical interventions that are often required for comprehensive management of patients with infectious diseases.

COMMENTARY

Peter M. Nthumba, Kenya

This chapter accurately presents some of the most common infections important to the surgeon working in LMICs. A few additional comments, including some unusual but important types of surgical infections that the surgeon working in this environment may see, are briefly introduced.

The HIV/AIDS scourge is such an important part of the surgical fraternity in Africa, and a few observations are necessary:

1. HIV/AIDS should now be considered a chronic illness that of necessity has its own peculiarities. This transformation in thinking is essential while offering care to patients with HIV/AIDS. Thus, with this consideration, selected patients who have AIDS are candidates for organ transplantation.

2. Patients with HIV/AIDS are at an increased risk for the development of malignancies. The duration of HIV infection, age greater than 40 years, and a history of opportunistic infection are the main determinants of the development of non-AIDS-defining cancers. Cutaneous malignancies are the most common non-AIDS-defining cancers among HIV-positive patients.

Part of the reason for insufficient debridement of wounds and infections—even when these are lifesaving—is the concern about the difficulties of covering vital structures that may be exposed during a debridement (i.e., neurovascular bundles, bone, and tendons). The "Principles of Reconstructive Surgery in Africa: A PAACS Publication", authored by surgeons who have worked or are working in Africa, is a useful free resource available at http://paacs.net/involved/paacs-resources/paacs-reconstructive-surgery-text/.

Cellulitis

The five cardinal signs of inflammation include:

1. Dolor—pain
2. Calor—warmth
3. Rubor—redness
4. Tumor—swelling
5. Functio laesa—loss of function

Of these classic signs, rubor, or redness, applies primarily to light-skinned races/individuals. It is difficult to discern in dark-skinned individuals. While pain, warmth, swelling, and loss of function are universal, failure to recognize the difficulties with redness in dark-skinned individuals has led to delays in the treatment of cellulitis. Additionally, cellulitis is a surgical infection and should be managed in collaboration with surgeons so that, should it fail to respond to antibiotic treatment, early surgical intervention is instituted. In my experience, reduction in edema (with skin wrinkling and desquamation) is the best sign of resolution, with the other signs resolving gradually.

Sadly, since there is no legislation in place, the extensive across-the-counter availability of antibiotics, including self-prescription, and poor antimicrobial stewardship across sub-Saharan Africa has led to the development of antibiotic resistance even with community-acquired infections. Worryingly, multidrug-resistant microbes are becoming increasingly common, even in rural hospitals.

Necrotizing Fasciitis

Necrotizing fasciitis that is peripheral, or in the extremities, should be treated aggressively; all involved fascia and skin should be excised, leaving normal/uninvolved skin at the edges. Central necrotizing fasciitis is fatal—once lower extremity necrotizing fasciitis involves the inguinal ligament, and/or extends into the retroperitoneum, the patient deteriorates rapidly to sepsis and death.

Fournier's Gangrene

Fournier's gangrene is an acute and rapidly progressive form of necrotizing fasciitis of the scrotum and perineum. Fournier's gangrene is a polymicrobial infection, including aerobic and anaerobic bacteria: *E. coli, Streptococcus* species, *Staphylococcus, Enterococcus,* and *Bacteroides.* It most frequently occurs in the background of immunosuppression, including diabetes mellitus and HIV/AIDS. Early recognition, aggressive debridement, and intravenous wide-spectrum antimicrobial administration is key to the management of Fournier's gangrene. In the elderly, sepsis may evolve early, leading to multi-organ failure and death. The resultant defects in survivors are a challenge to treat.

Tropical Diabetic Hand Syndrome

Tropical diabetic hand syndrome (TDHS) is an aggressive type of hand sepsis that results in significant morbidity and mortality among patients with diabetes in the tropics. Although akin to necrotizing fasciitis, TDHS affects all tissues down to bone. Glycemic control is easily achieved with debridement and insulin treatment. Hand, limb, or life salvage are more complex because clinical decisions are more difficult and compounded by the rarity of this condition; experience with the management of TDHS is limited across

Africa. Therefore, educating health workers, the patient (and other diabetics), and relatives is an important preventive measure.

Cancrum Oris

Cancrum oris or noma is aptly called "the face of poverty." It affects primarily children in sub-Saharan Africa, with 140,000 new cases reported each year. Ninety percent of these children die without any treatment, while survivors of the acute stage suffer extensive destruction of the midface, leading to progressive scarring, trismus, oral incontinence, and mandibulo-maxillary synostosis. The end result, in the survivor, may be severe facial disfigurement, speech difficulty, and progressive malnourishment. Surgical treatment is challenging.

SUGGESTED READING

1. Nthumba PM, Juma PI. HIV Infection: Implications on surgical practice. Chapter in HIV Infection - Impact, Awareness and Social Implications of living with HIV/AIDS, Pages 271–292. ISBN 978-953-307-343-9, edited by Eugenia Barros.
2. Sroczyński M, Sebastian M, Rudnicki J, Sebastian A, Agrawal AK. A complex approach to the treatment of Fournier's gangrene. *Adv Clin Exp Med.* 2013 Jan-Feb; 22(1):131–5.
3. Nthumba PM, Cavadas P, Landin L. The tropical diabetic hand syndrome: a surgical perspective. *Ann Plast Surg.* 2013; 70(1):42–46.
4. Nthumba PM, Carter LL. Visor flap for total upper and lower lip reconstruction: a case report. *Journal of Medical Case Reports* 2009, June 9, 3:7312.

34

Soft-Tissue Coverage and Flaps

Christopher D. Hughes
Nadine Semer

Introduction

Wounds and soft-tissue defects in low- and middle-income countries (LMICs) are often both more complex and more challenging to treat than the typical presentation in developed settings. A diverse spectrum of etiologies and an all-too-frequent delay in diagnosis and treatment demand an awareness of the basics of wound care and soft-tissue coverage, as well as of the reconstructive options available at the district level. This chapter will focus on the basics of soft-tissue coverage and will provide guidelines for both basic and advanced reconstruction.

The principles of wound management are covered in Chapter 36. Here we will begin by describing the principles of basic soft-tissue coverage, including a brief overview of the reconstructive ladder (Table 34.1) and key points about the nutritional requirements of patients with significant soft-tissue defects. We will then cover specific information about flap coverage, including a variety of local and distant flap choices.

Principles of Soft-Tissue Coverage and the Reconstructive Ladder

Wounds can be closed in a variety of ways, and the choice of treatment often depends on a variety of factors, including specific wound characteristics, available resources, functional outcome, surgeon experience, and the patient's overall clinical picture. The goals of any reconstructive effort should be aligned with the optimization of form and function and simultaneous minimization of morbidity. The final closure outcome depends on careful assessment of the wound and the subsequent selection of the most appropriate treatment.

All wounds and defects should be thoroughly cleansed and debrided (under local anesthesia if possible), evaluated for the presence of foreign bodies, and assessed for hemostasis prior to closure considerations. Once a defect has been cleaned and is appropriate for closure, tissue reconstruction can be accomplished in a variety of ways. The reconstructive ladder helps to organize these options into a simplified order to guide the surgeon's thought process and clinical management. Although there have been many variations on this reconstructive metaphorical model over the years, certain unifying themes are helpful in LMICs.[1]

A basic reconstructive ladder can be conceptualized as follows:

1. Closure by secondary intention
   - Useful for infected regions, wounds unable to be closed without tension
   - NOT appropriate for defects with exposed bone, tendon, or nerve
   - NOT appropriate for defects overlying joint creases
2. Primary closure
   - Need adequate skin to approximate wound edges
   - Best performed within 4–6 hours of injury if possible
3. Negative pressure wound therapy (NPWT)
   - May be especially useful in large defects
   - Several innovative technologies are making NPWT available at the district hospital level.
4. Skin graft
   - Full thickness or split thickness (see Chapter 40)
   - Required graftable bed to survive (grafts will have difficulty taking over tendon without paratenon, bone without periosteum, and cartilage without perichondrium)
5. Local flap (see below)
6. Distant flap (see below)
7. Free flap
   - Requires advanced surgical skill and resource availability. Generally not advised at the district level. Patients requiring free tissue coverage should be referred to a specialist facility.

A Few Words About Nutrition

Optimal nutritional status is important for proper immune function and wound healing and is, therefore, paramount to the success of any soft-tissue reconstruction. Especially in impoverished areas of LMICs, inadequate caloric, protein, vitamin, and mineral intake may be the cause for delayed/poor wound healing. Correction of nutritional deficiencies is an important component in wound care, and it may be wise to delay non-urgent

TABLE 34.1

The reconstructive ladder

1. Secondary intention
2. Primary closure
3. Negative pressure wound therapy
4. Skin graft
5. Local flap
6. Distant flap
7. Free flap

reconstructive surgery until the patient can be adequately supplemented.

Although nutritional adequacy depends on a variety of key ingredients, there are a few that deserve special attention because of their vital role in wound healing.[2]

Protein: Animal sources tend to be the most complete and balanced, but animal protein can be scarce in certain LMICs. Plant-based supplements including cereals and grains, rice and beans, milk, and noodles with cheese are therefore more common protein sources for many. If patients cannot get animal sources of protein, careful attention to a balanced plant-based diet should be considered.

Vitamin A: Vitamin A is a cofactor for collagen synthesis and is vital for wound healing. Good sources of vitamin A include dark green, leafy vegetables, liver, egg yolks, fortified dairy products, cereals.

Vitamin C: Vitamin C is another important cofactor in collagen synthesis. Good sources of vitamin C include citrus fruits, potatoes, tomatoes, broccoli, and peppers.

Vitamin E: Vitamin E helps to support proper immune function and overall health. It may be especially important in counteracting radiation-induced deficiencies in wound healing. Good sources of vitamin E include vegetable oils; whole grains; eggs; dark green, leafy vegetables; and seeds.

Zinc: Zinc plays a key role in wound epithelialization and helps to increase wound strength. Good sources of zinc include meat, fish, dairy, beans, and whole grains.

Flaps

For a thorough discussion of soft-tissue coverage via secondary intention, primary closure, and grafting, please see the chapters on skin grafts, wound care, and burns (Chapters 35, 36, and 40, respectively). The remainder of this chapter will deal only with flap-based soft-tissue coverage appropriate for practitioners in LMICs.

When faced with an open wound or significant scar contractures, the treatment goal is a healed wound with good functional outcome for the patient. A flap may be required for several reasons. The most common reasons to use flap coverage are when the wound cannot be closed primarily, when secondary closure would cause functional impairment, and when a skin graft will not take (poor vascularity, infection, etc.).

Potential wounds that may require flap coverage include:

- tissue loss in a flexion/extension crease (e.g., antecubital fossa);

- exposed tendons, bones, or other structures (dorsum of hand, open tibia/fibula fracture); and
- reconstruction of tight burn scar contractures.

A flap is a piece of tissue that maintains its own blood supply while being transferred from one area of the body to another[3]. It can be useful for soft-tissue coverage when the recipient bed has poor vascularity or even for infected wounds in some instances.[4,5] Flaps can also be used to cover vital structures and exposed bones. The tissue composition of the flap itself can be skin, muscle, bone, or fascia—alone or in combination.

Some flaps are based on named blood vessels, and as long as the vessel is not injured when raising the flap, the flap should survive. However, most of the flaps described below are those without a named blood supply; the circulation to the flap is from the dermal and subdermal plexi in the bridge of intact tissue. These flaps have more tenuous circulation than those with larger, dedicated vessels, and it is thus critical not to ask the flap to do more than it realistically can. To increase your chances of a successful flap, follow the 3:1 rule: the flap should be no longer than three times the base of the intact tissue bridge or flap pedicle.

If a skin marker is available, careful preprocedure outlining will help you plan appropriate and successful flap coverage. As noted above, ensure the flap base is as wide as possible to have more blood getting into *and out of* the flap. (Venous outflow problems are often the primary cause of flap death.) Regardless of the underlying vascular supply, the tip of the flap is the area most at risk of inadequate circulation. Unfortunately, the tip is usually the most critical part of the flap for wound coverage, and tension-free closure is therefore critical. Any tension in the repair can decrease blood flow and circulation and can result in partial flap loss. During flap elevation and insetting, watch capillary refill and watch for signs of venous congestion. In addition, it is critical to undermine widely around the wound and the flap in the appropriate plane to decrease tension on the closure.

There are many ways to classify flaps, but for practical purposes, it is simplest to classify them as *local* flaps or *distant* flaps with respect to the wound in need of coverage. Tissue for a local flap is located adjacent to the open wound, whereas a distant flap is created and taken from a part of the body away from the defect.

Local Versus Distant Flap

The distant flap is higher on the reconstructive ladder because, in general, this type of procedure is more technically challenging, and it creates two surgical sites that require postoperative care. However, distant flaps can still play an important role in reconstructive surgery in LMICs. The distant flaps highlighted below are technically appropriate even for nonspecialist trained surgical providers in LMICs. In general, deciding which flap to use depends on the local characteristics of the wound and requires thorough patient evaluation. Some important characteristics to consider include the following:

Location of wound: Begin by identifying spare/excess tissue that can be used for wound coverage. Pinch the skin of the cheek, trunk, or anterior calf for reference. On the face, back, abdomen, or inner arm, the skin is loose and the seemingly excess skin/tissue can be moved into a wound defect to facilitate closure. Thus, wounds in these areas are often amenable to local flap coverage.

These areas also represent potential donor sites for distant flaps. The lower leg and hand are examples of areas with tight skin and little tissue excess, so wounds in these areas often require distant flaps for coverage.

Nature of injury: The nature of injury can help guide your decision as well. A traumatic wound with significant surrounding soft-tissue injury and/or possible vascular injury would not be a good candidate for local flap coverage because the blood supply to the flap could be compromised. Therefore, a local flap would be selected when there is healthy, nontraumatized tissue adjacent to the wound which could be used for coverage. When there is no local tissue available, due to surrounding tissue trauma or no tissue excess, a distant flap may be the best coverage option.

In this chapter, we will cover the basics of local and distant flaps. More advanced methods of tissue transfer, including free flaps and synthetics (dermal matrices, tissue expanders, etc.), will not be covered; free tissue transfer is inappropriate for nonspecialist surgeons practicing in LMICs in most cases.

Specific Local Flaps

Local skin flaps are generally of two types: flaps that rotate on a pivot point (rotational, rhomboid/transposition) and those that don't (advancement flaps). Below are just a few examples of each type that may prove useful in LMICs.

Rotating Flaps

All rotating flaps rotate in an arc about a pivot point, and the radius of the arc represents the line of maximum tension in the flap (Figure 34.1).[4] Care should be maintained to avoid excessive tension along this line during flap closure, as too much tension can compromise the ultimate viability of the flap itself. Rotating flaps are useful in the coverage of sacral wounds and are applicable for a variety of wound sizes. They comprise a semicircular

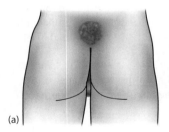
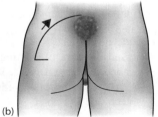
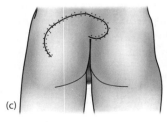

Rotation flap for closure of a sacral pressure sore. The donor site can be left open and allowed to heal secondarily, or a skin graft may be used if primary closure seems tight.

FIGURE 34.1 Rotational flap. Aston, et al. *Grabb and Smith's Plastic Surgery,* 6th ed. Philadelphia: Lippincott Williams and Wilkins, 2006, p. 154. Used with permission from the illustrator of the image, Nadine B Semer, MD, MPH.

flap of skin and subcutaneous tissue that can be rotated into an adjacent defect. Donor sites are usually able to be closed primarily or with a skin graft.

Procedure

1. Find the area of maximal skin laxity in the healthy adjacent tissue surrounding the wound or defect by pinching the skin.
2. Draw a line extending the wound edge in a curved fashion into this area until it seems that the flap can easily be rotated into the defect. Make sure you preserve a wide flap base. The curve is often an arc of 90–180 degrees.
3. Incise the flap along the drawn lines into the subcutaneous fat.
4. Undermine the flap widely in all directions to allow for adequate mobility.
5. If the flap is not rotating enough to fill the defect, you can make a small back cut at the flap base.
6. Rotate the flap into place and loosely suture (you can place a few Nylon tacking stitches to hold position if available). Use a few dermal polydioxanone (PDS) or equivalent sutures to secure the flap and take some tension off the skin. If the donor site cannot be closed primarily, you may need a skin graft to achieve complete closure, or additional undermining may help around the new defect.

Rhomboid (Limberg) Flaps

The Rhomboid flap is a type of transposition or rotational flap (Figure 34.2). Rhomboid flaps are useful for wounds or soft-tissue defects of the face, trunk, or extremity, especially in areas with limited adjacent tissue laxity. They typically provide an effective coverage area of about 5 cm in diameter.

Procedure

1. Find the area of maximal skin laxity in the healthy adjacent tissue surrounding the wound or defect by pinching the skin.
2. Draw a line approximately 75% of the total wound diameter into this area.
3. Draw another line of the same length at a 60-degree angle parallel to the wound edge. Take care not to make the angle too acute, so as not to narrow the pedicle.
4. Incise the flap along the drawn lines into the underlying subcutaneous fat. (Do not just take the skin.)
5. Undermine the flap and wound edges widely in all directions to allow for adequate mobility.
6. Rotate the flap into place and loosely suture. (You can place a few nylon tacking stitches to hold position if available.) Use a few dermal PDS or equivalent sutures to secure the flap and take some tension off the skin.

Advancement Flaps

Advancement flaps are moved (or "advanced") directly into the defect without pivot or rotation (Figure 34.3). As with rotational flaps, there are several modifications and types.

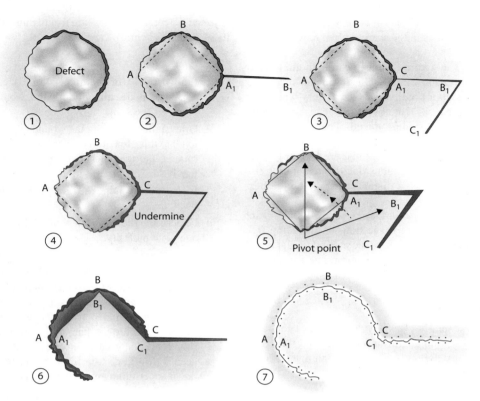

Rhomboid flap. *1:* Open wound in need of coverage. *2:* Draw a circle or rhomboid around the defect and, at the area of maximal skin laxity, a line 75% of the wound diameter. *3:* Draw another line of the same length at a 60° angle to the first line, taking care not to narrow the base of the flap. *4, 5, and 6:* Incise the lines. Undermine the area widely to allow transfer of the flap to the desired position and primary closure of the defect. *7:* Final appearance of closed wound.

FIGURE 34.2 Rhomboid flap. Aston, et al. *Grabb and Smith's Plastic Surgery,* 6th ed. Philadelphia: Lippincott Williams and Wilkins, 2006, p. 154. Used with permission from the illustrator of the image, Nadine B Semer, MD, MPH.

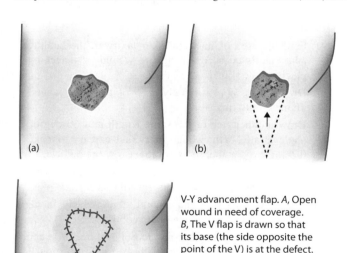

V-Y advancement flap. *A,* Open wound in need of coverage. *B,* The V flap is drawn so that its base (the side opposite the point of the V) is at the defect. Once the incisions are made, the tissue moves into the defect for coverage. *C,* The resulting wound is closed in a Y fashion.

FIGURE 34.3 V-Y advancement flap. Aston, et al. *Grabb and Smith's Plastic Surgery,* 6th ed. Philadelphia: Lippincott Williams and Wilkins, 2006, p. 154. Used with permission from the illustrator of the image, Nadine B Semer, MD, MPH.

V-Y Advancement Flaps

V-Y advancement flaps are particularly useful in regions with ample surrounding tissue laxity. They can be used for both large and small defects.

Procedure

1. Find the area of maximal skin laxity in the healthy adjacent tissue. Draw a V with the widest area of the V (base) at the wound edge and tapering gradually on each side to a point.
2. Incise the flap along the drawn lines down to but not including muscle. V-Y advancement flaps get their blood supply from deep underlying tissues (rather than from a bridge of surrounding skin), so it is important to transfer this tissue with the flap.
3. Primarily close the defect at the narrow point of the V to create the Y limb.
4. Use a few dermal PDS or equivalent sutures to secure the flap and take some tension off the skin.

Z-Plasty

The Z-plasty represents a critical resource in the armamentarium for reconstructive surgeons, perhaps especially in LMICs. The concept involves the transposition of two triangular flaps (or a "double transposition flap"), and it can serve several purposes. Primarily, the Z-plasty lengthens contracted linear scars and reduces longitudinal tension from scar contracture.[6] Additionally, the Z-plasty can reorient scars to improve functional and aesthetic outcomes, and it can reduce total scar width through the medialization of the lateral flaps (see Figure 34.4). When done correctly, Z-plasties further have the ability to restore elasticity in scar tissue by spurring collagen remodeling through tension release.[7] Z-plasties can be done singularly or in a series. Thus, these local flaps have particular use in LMICs in the release of burn scar contractures, especially when scars cross-flexion creases.[6]

Procedure

1. Inspect the wound or scar and determine the orientation needed for the Z-plasty. The original scar or defect will constitute the primary longitudinal axis.

2. Draw two limbs at each end of the axis line at an orientation between 30 and 90 degrees to the longitudinal axis. The classic angle for Z-plasty limbs is 60 degrees.

3. Each of these two limbs should ideally be the same length as the primary axis.

4. Plan, draw, measure, and measure again. It is always better to measure twice and cut once.

5. Infiltrate the area with local anesthesia.

6. Incise the Z-plasty along the drawn lines (excising the original scar if required), and carefully undermine each flap at the dermal-subcutaneous adipose junction. Take care to ensure that the flaps are appropriately thick. Flaps that are too thin may necrose due to a diminished blood supply, and flaps that are too thick will not rotate effectively.

7. Test the orientation of the flaps to the defects and assure that there is no significant tension on either of the flaps. If the closure seems "too tight," continue to sharply undermine each flap a bit more. If it is impossible to close the entire defect without tension, close what you can—a skin graft can subsequently be used to cover remaining bare areas.

8. Once the flap orientation is sufficient, use a temporary skin suture to hold the flaps in place at their tips. Take care not to manipulate the flap tips excessively, as these areas represent the regions most susceptible to necrosis and breakdown.

9. After securing the flaps with temporary sutures at the tip, begin to close the Z-plasty in two layers with dermal sutures followed by skin sutures. Suture choice is dictated by availability, surgeon preference, and reliability of patient follow-up. It may seem self-evident, but avoid nonabsorbable skin sutures in patients without prospects for follow-up.

Specific Distant Flaps

Since there are two distinct operative sites, distant flaps are often done under general anesthesia (Table 34.2). However, local anesthesia (or regional block when applicable) is sometimes preferable to prevent the patient from inadvertently pulling on the flap attachments when awakening from general anesthesia (see Chapter 6).

Chest/Abdomen Flap

These flaps would be appropriate for an open wound on the hand, wrist, or distal forearm with exposed tendons/bones.

Procedure

1. Ask the awake patient to position the injured hand over the chest/abdomen in the most comfortable position. Stay away from breast tissue.

2. Mark this area. The flap should be drawn in such a way that the hand can be comfortably attached to the chest, but you must make sure that the pedicle does not become kinked. Usually the flap is drawn so that the pedicle is based inferiorly, but it can be designed with almost any orientation. Be sure that no scars from previous injuries are located within the flap or pedicle.

3. Design the flap so that it is slightly larger than the defect.

4. Make the incision through skin and subcutaneous tissue and into the underlying fascia (the thin layer of connective tissue over the muscle). Do not incise the muscle. The fascia contributes to the blood supply of

TABLE 34.2

Techniques and critical points common to all local flaps:

1. If using local anesthetic, use dilute epinephrine (1:200,000 at most concentrated) or no epinephrine.

2. When undermining the flap, don't raise thin skin flaps. The incisions need to go into the subcutaneous layer, at depth of the wound.

3. Assess flap viability during the procedure. Most flap failures are either due to a lack of inflow or a lack of outflow. Keep the base of the flap wide and follow the 3:1 rule to ensure good inflow. During flap elevation, be gentle with the edges of the flap, and keep an eye on the bleeding from the flap edges or capillary refill of the flap, especially if you find you need to narrow the base of the flap to get it to rotate into the wound.

4. Sutures. Depending on suture availability and expected patient follow-up, you can use nylons on the skin (which will need to be removed later) or absorbable suture. It is always better to have small gaps in the skin edges compared to an over-tight approximation.

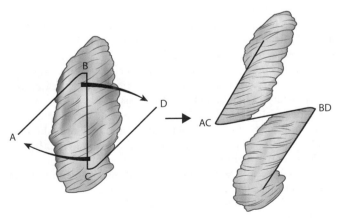

FIGURE 34.4 Z-plasty. Aston, et al. *Grabb and Smith's Plastic Surgery,* 6th ed. Philadelphia: Lippincott Williams and Wilkins, 2006, p. 154.

the flap; therefore, it is important to keep it attached to the flap whenever possible.

5. Elevate the flap off the deep underlying tissues.

6. Loosely stitch the three free sides of the flap in place. Use a few dermal sutures and then close the skin with interrupted, simple sutures. The closure does not have to be perfect. If the flap is stitched too tightly, it may compromise circulation and result in partial flap loss.

7. If possible, the donor site on the chest should be closed primarily, but usually a split-thickness skin graft is needed. Alternatively, if the wound is just a few centimeters in diameter, the donor site may be allowed to heal secondarily.

Inner Arm Flap

For smaller wounds of the thumb or fingers, the inner aspect of the upper arm has thinner skin with less subcutaneous tissue and thus is a good donor site for smaller hand wounds. The drawback is a more awkward patient position prior to flap division. The essentials to the procedure follow that described for the chest/abdomen flap above.

Cross-Leg Flap

These flaps are useful for an open wound/open fracture on the foot, ankle, or lower leg. Because the legs are immobilized and essentially sewn together for 3–4 weeks, this procedure can result in severe hip stiffness. Therefore, a cross-leg flap is best used in children or young adults.

Procedure

1. Determine the best position for the patient's legs prior to anesthesia. The orientation is such that a flap of tissue taken from the noninjured posteromedial calf must lie easily over the defect with the least patient discomfort.

2. Draw the flap on the posteromedial side of the calf, overlying the gastrocnemius muscle. The flap should be slightly larger than the wound defect.

3. The flap should be designed so that it is superiorly based.

4. Incise the skin, subcutaneous tissue, and fascia overlying the gastrocnemius muscle. Elevate the flap along the plane between the fascia and underlying muscle. The fascia must stay attached to the flap.

5. Move the flap over to the open wound.

6. Loosely stitch the three free sides of the flap in place. Place a few dermal sutures, and then close the skin with interrupted sutures. The closure does not have to be perfect.

7. The donor site should be covered with a split-thickness skin graft.

8. Place antibiotic ointment and saline-moistened gauze along the free undersurface of the flap. Apply antibiotic ointment around all suture lines.

9. The patient's legs must be immobilized together to prevent accidentally separating the legs and tearing the suture line. This is best achieved with plaster. Use a lot of padding under the plaster.

10. Cut out a window in the plaster and padding over the flap so that the flap can be observed and cleansed daily.

Dividing the Pedicle for Distant Flaps

Gradually, new vessels will grow into the flap from the recipient site. Usually the pedicle can start to be divided after 2 weeks. This can be done often with straight local anesthesia (*no* epinephrine). Cut across no more than a quarter of the width of the pedicle at a time, and suture the edges down loosely. Come back several days later to continue the process until completely divided. Alternatively, usually by 4 weeks the flap can be completely divided in one procedure.

To try to improve circulation/robustness of flap, you may consider performing a DELAY procedure. In the delay procedure, the flap edges are incised and the flap elevated off of its underlying tissue attachments. It is then sutured (loosely) back in place. This procedure places ischemic stress on the flap, and thereby makes the tissue dependent on the pedicle for circulation, without adding the additional stress of moving it to another location. Over the course of 10–14 days, the circulation within the flap and its pedicle becomes more robust. Subsequent tissue transfer can then be attempted after about 10–14 days.

Postoperative Care

Apply antibiotic ointment if available to the flap incisions and cover loosely with gauze dressings. The area can be cleansed daily with gentle soap and water or dilute saline 48 hours after the procedure. The flap should be checked daily to assess for viability and functionality.

The most common cause of initial flap failure is venous congestion, or an outflow problem. This can be caused by a number of different factors, including excessive flap compression, tension, or fluid accumulation under the flap. A helpful initial approach to a blue, swollen, and congested appearing flap is to first assure proper patient positioning and avoid any excess pressure on the region. Simply loosening or removing the bandage may also help to alleviate an outflow problem. Finally, if the flap appears to be under excessive tension, you can remove a few sutures. If it appears that fluid has accumulated under the flap, it should be drained: insert a clamp between sutures to open the space and promote fluid drainage.

After several postoperative days, inspection of the flap may indicate an area of purplish tissue, particularly at the tip, that may indicate ischemia and eventual tissue loss. If this area is not excessively large, a prudent management strategy may be to do nothing: as the tissue demarcates and dies over the next weeks, the underlying tissues will begin healing from below. As long as there are no signs of infection, this portion of the flap will serve as a biologic dressing, allowing the underlying tissue to heal from below. As with any postoperative wound in both the developed world and in LMICs, close follow-up and monitoring should be exercised for any concerning findings.

COMMENTARY

Jorge Palacios, Ecuador

The description of the principles and procedures in this chapter are very clear and accurate, especially for places in LMICs. The text is understandable to surgeons with expertise in general surgery who have to resolve injury requiring the use of flaps.

I must mark out the importance of using the appropriate instruments for preserving vascular and microvascular integrity; this is crucial in order to avoid manipulation of the flap directly with fingers. In LMICs, skin hooks are not always available for lifting and rotating transposition flaps. In our practice, we recommend the use of hypodermic needles with syringes sustained by bending the tip with a needle holder to also get the form of a skin hook.

COMMENTARY

Chona Thomas, Oman

In 1981, I began plastic surgery service in Oman with 10 beds and one assistant doctor. This was after I had completed my higher surgical training from the Oxford Group of Hospitals. I remained the only plastic surgeon in Oman until 1987. In the years following this, plastic surgery developed considerably in Oman. Our department of plastic surgery now has 90 beds with 25 doctors (12 of whom are trained plastic surgeons); it is currently the largest department of plastic surgery in all of the Middle Eastern countries.

I will focus my reflection on the years from 1981–1987, when I was the only plastic surgeon in Oman and had limited resources. After reviewing this chapter's text, I agree in principle but note that the application may differ in LMICs, depending on availability of facilities, manpower, and supportive services. The epidemiology of diseases that require plastic surgery may also vary. In Oman, road traffic accidents are the leading cause of death. For this reason, open wounds with or without fractures are very common, and these patients are usually referred to a plastic surgeon, or they have a plastic surgeon as part of their surgical team, which includes an orthopedic surgeon and a trauma surgeon.

My approach, especially when I was the only plastic surgeon, was try to do a primary closure or primary resurfacing with grafts or flaps after an aggressive surgical debridement, if not contraindicated due to lack beds in the hospital and supportive staff. Surgical debridement under general anesthesia is the key; a contaminated wound can be converted to a clean wound for the primary closure or resurfacing with split thickness skin graft, mostly meshed, or reliable flaps. For wounds in the head and neck region, preferably after the radical excision of malignant tumors, I used the safe delto-pectoral faciocutaneous flap and pectoralis major musculo-cutaneous flap. The forehead facio-cutaneous flap was selectively used for males since the forehead region is always covered by a turban or cap in the Middle East; this means that the cosmetic disfigurement is absent. My preferred flap for the hand was the groin flap. Of course, my approach differs for "problem wounds" (as titled in the chapter) secondarily due to vascular insufficiency, impaired cellular function, infection, nutritional imbalances, and malignancy. These problem wounds need an accurate clinical assessment followed by nonoperative management and later operative management, if indicated.

In short, my algorithm for soft tissue coverage in Oman is as follows:

1. Primary closure
2. Healing with secondary intention
3. Skin graft—split thickness, meshed, and full thickness
4. Local flaps
5. Distant flaps
6. Tissue expansion
7. NPWT
8. Free tissue transfer

COMMENTARY

Charles Furaha, Rwanda
Christian Paletta, Rwanda

We use flaps in Rwanda most commonly for the following conditions:

1. Open tibial wounds of the lower extremity
2. Soft-tissue wounds over joints such as the elbow, wrist, knee, and ankle
3. Severe burn or other traumatic scar contractures involving the neck, axilla, elbow, wrist, hand, anterior and posterior knee, ankle, and midfoot
4. Large soft-tissue defects following trauma; an infectious process such as empyema or necrotizing fasciitis; or extensive cancer resection of the scalp, face, chest, and abdomen
5. Pressure sores of the sacrum, coccyx, ischium, and greater trochanter

Based upon our resources, training, and experience, the following is our current thinking in terms of plastic surgery in LMICs or countries with too few or no plastic surgeons.

1. Free tissue transfer is technically possible. However, it requires a team approach and effort in addition to preoperative and postoperative skilled nursing and ICU care. Hence, we have found that it is not possible at this time to successfully embark on performing free flaps for wounds that would typically require such. Instead we use all possible and imaginable pedicle flaps whenever a skin graft is not the right thing to do, up to the point of using reverse sural cross-leg flaps when that is the only option (Figures 34.5, 34.6, and 34.7).

2. Oftentimes there are surgeons who can technically perform flap surgery who are not trained plastic surgeons. This type of surgical care must be done out of necessity but is not ideal or sustainable and may give a wrong perception of what plastic surgery can offer to patients and to other surgical disciplines. Poor preoperative judgments and inability to perform complex flap surgery may cause unnecessary morbidities while discouraging those surgeons to continue flap surgeries in the future. An example of this is seen when one starts a contracture release of a major joint like the axilla or the knee. It is not unusual to have exposed axillary or popliteal vessels. The operating surgeon must be prepared and have the knowledge, experience, and expertise to perform a latissimus dorsi, pectoralis major, or gastrocnemius flap in such cases.

3. For severe anterior burn scar contractures of the neck (Figure 34.8), we tend to favor the use of flaps as opposed to skin grafts. In addition, one of the key components to performing surgery on these patients is the availability of anesthesia staff trained in complex airway management such as rapid sequence induction and awake endoscopic intubation.

4. To avoid hematomas and seromas, and to facilitate flap adherence to the wound bed, suction drains are often an essential necessity for a period of time following flap surgery. Such drains are often unavailable, requiring the surgeon to improvise with the materials readily available (Figure 34.9). And whether one has a suction drain or must improvise, postoperative nursing care is critical for maintenance of continued wound suction.

5. When performing flap surgery, flap design is critical. It is helpful to have some type of marking device to aid in the design and orientation of a flap. Standard sterile skin markers may not be available. We have found that one can put a scratch on the skin with the backside of a surgical blade. Alternatively, we have used tongue blades sterilized in Cidex and fractured vertically as a marking device with methylene blue (Figure 34.10).

6. When I returned to Rwanda 2½ years ago as the first plastic surgeon to practice here, I observed that patients and healthcare providers in general had almost no awareness of what plastic surgery could offer. The need for plastic surgery services and backlog of patients was then and remains huge. In 2014 we now have an exponentially growing awareness of what plastic surgery can offer. As expected, this has resulted in an overwhelming demand which just one trained plastic surgeon cannot meet. The only sustainable long-term solution is to establish a training program for plastic surgery in Rwanda. We are initiating the steps necessary to make this happen.

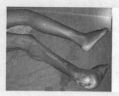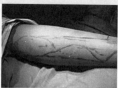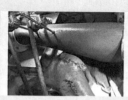

FIGURE 34.5 Fifteen-year-old with an unstable left heel wound following a grenade explosion with injury to his proximal ipsilateral posterior calf. He was successfully managed with a cross-leg reverse sural artery flap (RSAF) and temporary external fixator immobilization.

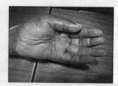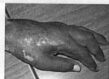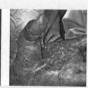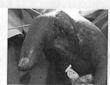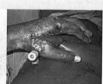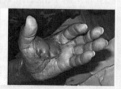

FIGURE 34.6 Young man 2 months following right upper extremity trauma including a proximal humerus fracture and soft-tissue loss of the left thumb web space from a motor vehicle accident, resulting in a severe thumb adduction contracture. An ipsilateral groin flap was used following release of the contracture and K-wire pinning of his carpometacarpal (CMC) joint.

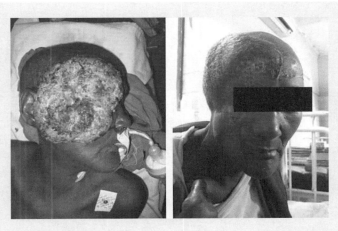

FIGURE 34.7 Sixty-year-old patient with extensive squamous cell carcinoma invading the zygomatic, orbital, auricular, and temporal regions. Following surgical resection including orbital exenteration, otecomy, and partial zygomatic and malar bone resection, closure was performed with a large rotational scalp flap and ipsilateral neck advancement flap and skin grafting to the flap donor sites.

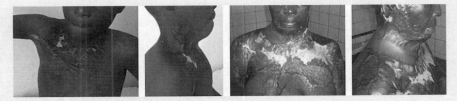

FIGURE 34.8 Young boy with severe neck and right axillary burn scar contracture (top left and top left center). Woman with extensive burn scar contractures following right posterior shoulder flap by visiting surgeons (top right and top right center). The distal 25% of the flap necrosed.

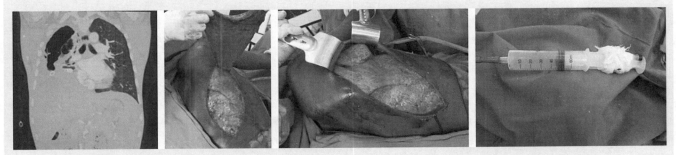

FIGURE 34.9 Young man with right chest empyema cavity. Latissimus dorsi muscle flap dissected and placed intrathoracically to obliterate the cavity. Suction drainage with improvised 60cc syringe.

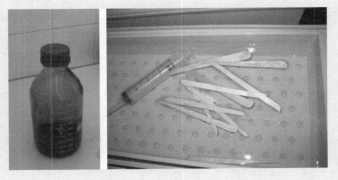

FIGURE 34.10 Methylene blue and vertically fractured tongue blades sterilized in Cidex for use as a surgical marker.

35

Skin Grafts

Ingrid Ganske
Jennifer Wall

Introduction

Competency in grafting is critical for an array of conditions, from coverage of freshly excised burns and reconstruction of burn contractures, to the closure of fasciotomy wounds, traumatic soft tissue avulsion, or superficial coverage of muscle flaps.

Lack of skin grafting expertise imposes a huge cost in low- to middle-income countries (LMICs) as patients consume valuable resources on the wards for weeks or months. Many patients with potentially graftable wounds that are instead allowed to heal by secondary intention ultimately suffer from wound colonization, infection, prolonged healing, and greater time out of work due to a lack of adequate dressing supplies and sterile conditions. Timely skin graft coverage of clean, granulating wounds can reduce individual patient morbidity and reduce the aggregate economic burden of disease.

Skin grafts comprise the intermediate rungs of the reconstructive ladder (see Chapter 34). Grafts are useful for closure of large superficial wounds that are too sizeable to be closed primarily and would take too long to heal by secondary intention, as well as wounds in delicate areas where contracture must be avoided (such as the eyelids, hands, and flexural surfaces). By definition, a graft is tissue that is completely removed from its blood supply on one area of the body and then replaced on another location in the body. Grafts develop nutrients and vascular in-growth from the wound beds in which they are placed in order to survive, or "take."

This chapter will describe the fundamental considerations and techniques for successful skin grafting.

Preoperative Considerations

Skin grafting can be an expeditious way to heal appropriately chosen wounds, but it is fundamentally a healing process that requires attention to all the factors discussed in Chapter 36, Wound Care. Systemic conditions must be optimized to ensure the graft heals; this includes nutritional repletion, avoiding tobacco, and tight glucose control.

Skin grafts require a vascular bed. Muscle and fascia accept grafts easily, as does the vascular fat of the face. Generally, grafts do not heal to exposed bone, cartilage, or tendon without their respective periosteum, perichondrium, or paratenon intact; however, if the surrounding tissue has adequate blood supply, grafts may bridge small defects.

Locally, the wound must be prepared prior to grafting. Acute wounds, such as freshly excised third-degree burns, are ready to graft when the wound has been debrided to a healthy vascular bed (Figure 35.1). Chronic wounds should demonstrate healthy-appearing, flat, red granulation tissue without surface film. Long-standing wounds can develop a fibrous covering and bacterial colonization that must be debrided prior to grafting. Common pathogens that colonize wounds include *Staphylococcus aureus, Escherichia coli, Proteus mirabilis,* and *Pseudomonas.* These can be treated appropriately with meticulous homemade Dakin's dressings (see Chapter 40 for further details) and typically do not require systemic antibiotics; nor is colonization with these flora a contraindication to grafting as long as the granulation tissue appears clinically healthy. The exception to this is *Streptococcus pyogenes,* which is a contraindication to grafting, as it routinely leads to graft failure. Wounds colonized with *S. pyogenes* tend to appear glazed and gelatinous, with friable granulations that bleed easily, and do not demonstrate evidence of marginal epithelialization at the wound edges. This specific colonization must be eradicated with antibiotics, local antiseptic (such as Hibiclens), and debridement.

Once there is evidence of a healthy vascular wound bed that is free of slough, grafting should be performed. Timely grafting decreases the risk of infection, wound contracture, and sustained metabolic demands and stress, which lead to cachexia, electrolyte imbalances, and nutritional deficits. If delay is necessary, then local dressings to reduce colonization and superinfection should be used, in addition to gentle compression and elevation to reduce edema, as well as nutritional optimization.

Wounds that do not demonstrate vascular tissue are most commonly the result of ischemia, from peripheral vascular disease, venous stasis, or irradiation. These wounds will not adequately support skin graft "take."

Types of Graft

Grafts are described as split-thickness or full-thickness based on the amount of dermis included. The thickness of the dermis determines how easily the graft takes, the degree of primary and secondary contracture, potential for reinnervation, as well as the resulting morbidity at the donor site. Split-thickness grafts are thinner and "take" more reliably, while full-thickness grafts have higher metabolic demands and greater tissue to revascularize,

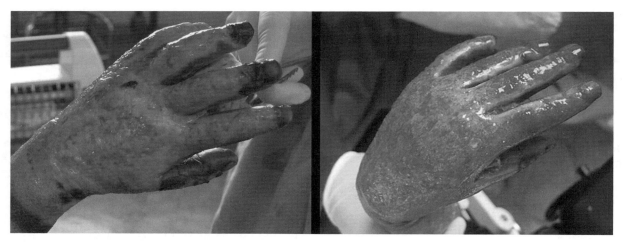

FIGURE 35.1   On the left, the patient's hand demonstrates significant fibrinous debris. On the right, the wound has been debrided to healthy bleeding tissue and is now ready to accept a skin graft. Images by Jennifer Wall.

and thus are more likely to fail. The thinner a graft, the less elastic and contractile it is at the time of harvest, but the more it contracts secondarily by scar in the long run, potentially leading to contracture, especially when placed across a flexure. Full-thickness grafts, with more dermal stability, are better able to tolerate trauma. Because they contain epidermal appendages, they are also able to grow hair and reinnervate by ingrowth of nerve fibers. However, the lack of remaining appendages at the donor site means that the donor site must be closed primarily or covered with a split-thickness graft. In practicality, this limits the amount of full-thickness skin that can be harvested and means these grafts are reserved for use on small defects in critical areas, such as across joints, on the hands, or on the face.

Full-Thickness Skin Grafts

Donor Sites

Common donor sites include postauricular skin, supraclavicular skin, the groin, the thigh, or the abdomen. Postauricular skin provides a good color match to the face, but the donor site is limited. The upper eyelid skin can be harvested and is an especially good match for the contralateral eye. Skin from the supraclavicular area is a relatively good match for the face, but inferior to postauricular skin (Figure 35.2). Larger full-thickness grafts can be harvested from the thigh or abdomen, in regions with skin laxity that can be closed primarily. Glabrous skin grafts to cover defects on the hands and fingers can be harvested from the hypothenar eminence or the instep of the foot.

Since full-thickness grafts remain relatively true to size after harvest, a template should be used to mark the area of skin that will be harvested. An elliptical pattern incision allows for closure without dog-ears.

Harvesting the Graft

Prior to excision, the marked region is injected with local anesthetic mixture containing epinephrine, to balloon the area. Incise along the outline of the graft. The graft can be retracted with a hook or pickups so that it is raised with visualization, in a subdermal plane, leaving fat on the donor side.

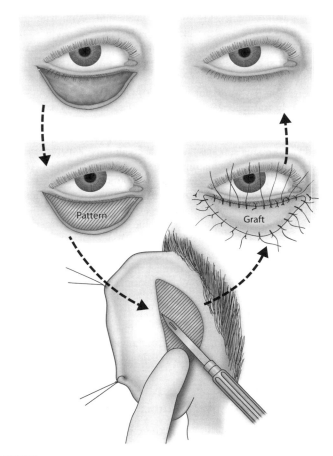

FIGURE 35.2   The lower eyelid is grafted with postauricular full-thickness skin graft, with the use of a template. McGregor AD and McGregor IA. *Fundamental Techniques of Plastic Surgery,* 10th ed. Philadelphia: Elsevier; 2000, p. 40.

Next, the fat is meticulously trimmed from the dermis of the graft. Residual fat will interfere with "take" of the graft. Place the skin graft under tension, draped over your finger. Use scissors to remove the fat. Although the goal is to preserve dermis, it is better to cut into dermis than to leave residual fat (Figure 35.3).

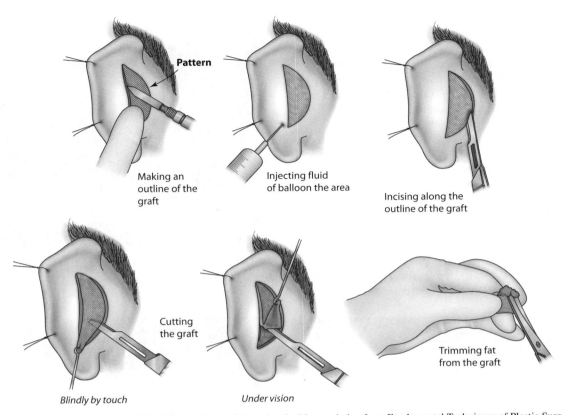

Pattern

Making an
outline of the
graft

Injecting fluid
of balloon the area

Incising along the
outline of the graft

Cutting
the graft

Trimming fat
from the graft

Blindly by touch

Under vision

FIGURE 35.3 Harvesting a postauricular full-thickness skin graft. Reprinted with permission from Fundamental Techniques of Plastic Surgery, 10th ed. McGregor AD and McGregor IA, "Free Skin Grafts", page 41, Copyright (2000), with permission from Elsevier. McGregor AD and McGregor IA. *Fundamental Techniques of Plastic Surgery,* 10th ed. Philadelphia: Elsevier; 2000, p. 41.

Applying the Graft

The wound bed should be clean and granulating as previously described. Meticulous hemostasis should be achieved to prevent hematoma from interposing between the graft and the bed. A few small slits can be made in the graft to prevent fluid accumulation under the graft. Do not mesh a full-thickness graft. Place the graft with the dermis side down. The premeasured graft fits the defect precisely. The graft is sutured in place with an adequate number of interrupted or running sutures to ensure good apposition of the edges. Care should be taken to achieve eversion of the edges. When placing the sutures, start on the graft side and drive the needle across to the recipient site—"ship to shore." This helps with both eversion and stabilizing the graft during suture placement.

Bolstering

"Take" of the skin graft relies on consistent, close apposition of the graft to the bed without shear or the development of underlying hematoma or seroma. This can be accomplished with a number of pressure dressings to bolster the graft to the recipient site.

Tie-over bolsters work well on the face and relatively flat surfaced wounds (Figure 35.4). When preparing a tie-over bolster, some of the sutures can be left long or additional sutures can be placed for the purpose of tying over a bolster. Lay a piece of nonstick material, such as Xeroform, antibiotic impregnated gauze, or tulle gras directly over the graft to prevent the dressing from adhering to the graft at the time of removal. Use a generous layer

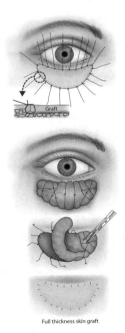

Full thickness skin graft

FIGURE 35.4 Tie-over bolster pressure dressing for a full-thickness graft to the lower eyelid. The full-thickness graft is sutured edge-to-edge to the surrounding recipient site. Sutures are left long to tie over the bolster. McGregor AD and McGregor IA. *Fundamental Techniques of Plastic Surgery,* 10th ed. Philadelphia: Elsevier; 2000, p. 42.

of antibiotic ointment over the graft along if there are no other nonstick dressing options. The bolus material is typically cotton wool or sterile gauze prepared in mineral oil, moistened with saline, or wrung with liquid paraffin. Apply sufficient padding with dry cotton or gauze to distribute the pressure evenly over the graft. Tie the sutures over the bolster, so that tension is also distributed evenly over the edges of the wound.

On the hands and fingers, tie-over bolsters may be too bulky or awkward, in which case a wrapped pressure dressing may be used, with the goal being complete immobilization of the graft. This can consist of a base layer of Xeroform or Vaseline gauze, covered by fluffed gauze, and bandages. For grafts placed over the hands, fingers, and flexural surfaces, apply a cast or splint. This is particularly true in children, in which case the joints proximal and distal to the graft site should be immobilized to prevent squirming out of the cast (Figures 35.5A through 35.5F).

A full-thickness skin graft typically heals in approximately 7–10 days. The bolster should remain in place approximately 7 days. If it develops malodor or drainage, remove the dressing

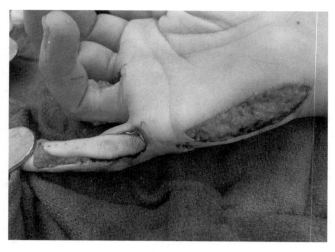

FIGURE 35.5C The graft is harvested, defatted, and placed dermis side down on the defect. Image by Peter Kim.

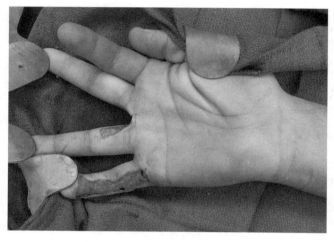

FIGURE 35.5A Full-thickness skin graft from the hypothenar eminence to cover a defect on the palmar aspect of a finger. Image by Peter Kim.

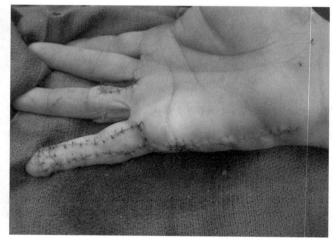

FIGURE 35.5D The graft is sutured in place with chromic sutures. Image by Peter Kim.

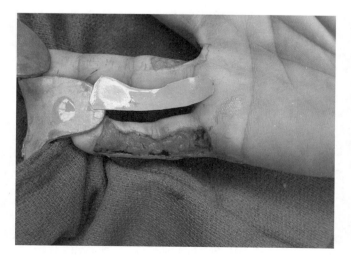

FIGURE 35.5B A template is used to measure the defect and mark a donor site. Image by Peter Kim.

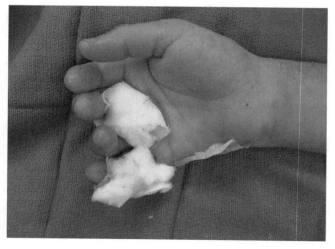

FIGURE 35.5E A pressure bolster of antibiotic ointment, xeroform, and cotton fluff is created. Image by Peter Kim.

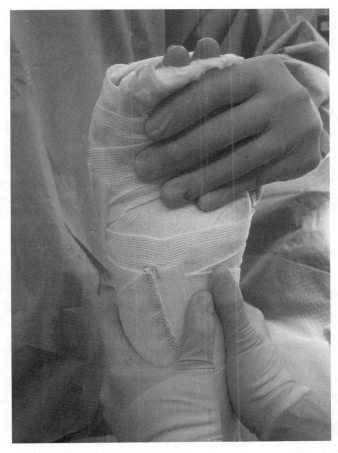

FIGURE 35.5F A splint is placed for graft stabilization. Image by Peter Kim.

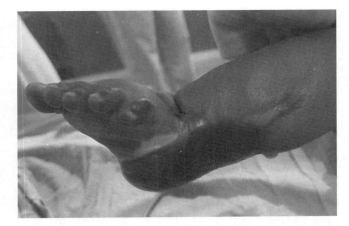

FIGURE 35.6A Burn contracture over lateral aspect of infant's ankle. Image by Jennifer Wall.

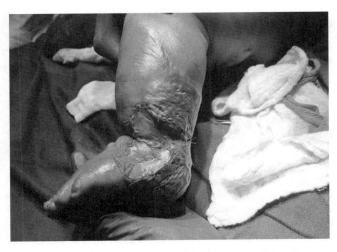

FIGURE 35.6B Full-thickness skin graft in place after excision of contracture. Image by Jennifer Wall.

sooner. When removing the bolster, use caution not to apply undue traction on the underlying graft. Moistening the dressing with saline will reduce sticking.

Aftercare

Apply antibiotic ointment to the graft once or twice daily for the next several days. Gently cleanse the area with saline at each dressing change. The graft can appear dusky for several days to weeks until it is fully revascularized. Sometimes the grafts will undergo epidermolysis, in which the epidermis will become black and peel off, revealing light-colored dermis below. This can look like graft failure. Be patient and continue the dressing changes. As long as the dermis is attached, the graft should heal. Once the graft is adherent and epithelialized, the dressings can be changed to a gentle moisturizer daily (Figure 35.6A, Figure 35.6B, Figure 35.6C, and Figure 35.6D). Care should be taken to avoid sun exposure and use sunscreen. The patient should not smoke during the healing period, or graft failure is likely.

Donor Site Closure

The donor site is closed primarily after undermining the skin edges sufficiently to achieve tensionless closure.

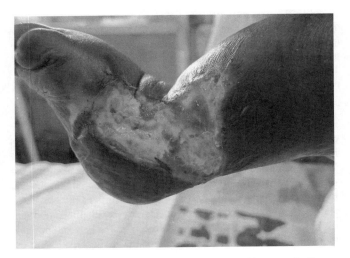

FIGURE 35.6C Epidermolysis of the skin graft, with exposed adherent dermis intact. Image by Jennifer Wall.

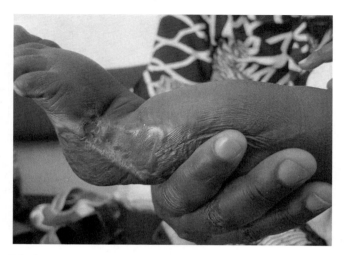

FIGURE 35.6D After reepithelialization of the graft. Image by Jennifer Wall.

Complications

Common reasons for full-thickness graft failure include hematoma or seroma between the flap and wound bed, infection, shear, insufficient wound bed vascularity, and residual fat on the graft that prevents ingrowth of vascularity from the wound bed. Hematoma can be avoided by meticulous hemostasis of the recipient site and avoiding shear trauma to the graft after it is in place. Seromas can develop when a graft is applied over a concave surface, particularly if the vascularized graft is lifted up from the underlying wound bed in the process of removing the bolster. Seromas will reaccumulate even when aspirated. When seromas occur, the overlying skin graft will continue to epithelialize on its deep surface from the cut ends of the pilosebaceous glands, and once this happens, it cannot re-adhere to the wound bed below. In this case, the affected portion of the graft must be incised and curetted on the deep surface so that it can re-adhere.

Split-Thickness Skin Grafts

A split-thickness skin graft (STSG) is indicated in most wounds that cannot be closed primarily, when closure by secondary intention is contraindicated (across joints), and for relatively large wounds (>5–6 cm diameter) that would take many weeks to heal secondarily.

Donor Sites

STSG donor sites are chosen based on a number of factors, including the size of graft needed, the importance of color match, and local convenience to incorporate both donor and recipient into the same prepped field or postoperative dressing. Common sites include the thighs and upper arms, flexor aspect of the arms, buttocks, back, abdomen, and scalp. The donor sites heal by epithelialization, but they always have some degree of discoloration at best and possible hypertrophic and keloid scarring at worst. The most readily accessible donor sites are often the most conspicuous sites for scars. Care should be taken to place the donor sites in discrete areas, yet ones that are easy to dress, give large surface areas, and will not cause positional discomfort for the patient in the recovery period. Do not harvest grafts over joint spaces, as this can cause contractures. Split-thickness grafts taken from the scalp will initially have hair, but since they do not contain the hair follicles, they will ultimately be hairless after grafting and hair will regrow at the donor site.

Anesthesia

Because of the large size of graft to be taken, the patient usually requires a regional block or general anesthesia for pain control. Locally, hemostasis-analgesia solution (HAS) is used, as described in Chapter 40. This consists of 1 liter NS 0.9% mixed with 50cc of 1% lidocaine and 2cc of epinephrine 1:1000. Epinephrine solution alone can be used if lidocaine is not available.

Instruments and Harvesting Techniques

A variety of instruments can be used to harvest the graft, including a Goulian/Weck knife, which is essentially a blade on a handle; variations of the Braithwaite knife such as the Cobbett, Watson, and Humby knives with a roller mechanism to control consistency of graft thickness; Silver's miniature knife for small grafts; or dermatomes, which are powered by electricity or air (Figure 35.7A through 35.7D). The Brown and Zimmer dermatomes are air-powered. The Model B Padgett is an electric dermatome that can be used with the proper electrical converter.

First, the skin should be cleaned and shaved of hair over the donor site. Any antibacterial solution used to prepare the surgical field should be washed off and the site dried. Inject the donor site subcutaneously with HAS to raise a rectangular area that is measured to match the wound. Apply a sterile mineral oil, K-Y jelly, paraffin, or soapy water to the area and to the knife that will be used.

The Humby knife and the dermatome have settings to adjust the thickness of the graft, ranging from approximately 0.011–0.015 inch (0.25–0.4 mm). But always check the opening of the blade, as these settings can be unreliable. One way to confirm a proper thickness setting is to run the beveled edge of a no. 10 blade along the opening of the Humby or dermatome–it should fit snuggly.

Position the patient so that the donor site area is as flat as can be, with surrounding muscle groups relaxed to avoid concavities and convexities that can increase the likelihood of inconsistent harvest depth. Have an assistant make the skin taught, with tongue depressors or manual retraction. The assistant applies pressure and spreads additional lubricant along the surface in a concerted forward motion a short distance in front of the knife.

Use the knife of choice in a back-and-forth pattern at a 45-degree angle to excise down to the surface of bright white healthy tissue. If fat is visible, the graft is too deep. As the knife moves back and forth over the skin surface, there should be little drag on the skin if proper lubrication has been applied. Assess the depth of the graft as it is harvested. A very thin graft will be translucent and will leave behind a high density of pinpoint bleeding on the donor site. A thicker graft will be more opaque and will leave a lower density of larger bleeding points. When you have taken a large enough graft, supinate the wrist, removing the knife from the skin. Use a scalpel to cut the skin graft from the donor site. It may be necessary to open the knife fully to remove the skin from the instrument (Figures 35.8A through 35.8C).

With power-driven dermatomes, large grafts of controlled width and thickness can be harvested easily without wasting skin between adjoining donor sites. When the donor site has healed evenly, it may be used again for repeat harvesting, although the dermis will be thinner on subsequent harvests. To harvest the graft, power the dermatome in the air prior to contact with the skin. Once the dermatome has landed on the skin, apply firm pressure downward and forward, holding the device at a 45-degree angle to the skin surface throughout the trajectory of the harvest. Slowly and steadily move down the donor site. When the dermatome reaches the end of the designated harvest site, gently lift it off the skin with the power on to completely free the graft from the donor site. Then turn off the device. The movement is commonly described as simulating an airplane landing and taking off right away. Carefully extricate the graft from the dermatome blade using forceps, with care not to tear or cut the graft.

Preparing and Applying the Graft

Place the skin graft on saline-moistened gauze until ready to inset the graft. "Meshing" involves making several small cuts in the

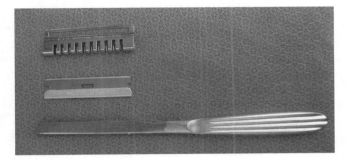

FIGURE 35.7A   Weck knife components. Image by Jennifer Wall.

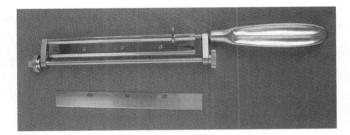

FIGURE 35.7B   Watson knife components. Image by Jennifer Wall.

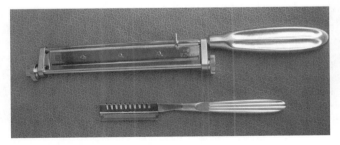

FIGURE 35.7C   Weck and Watson knives assembled. Image by Jennifer Wall.

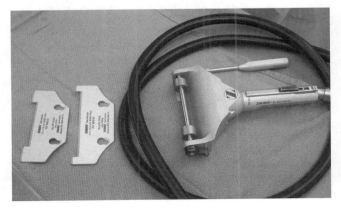

FIGURE 35.7D   Dermatome. Image by Jennifer Wall.

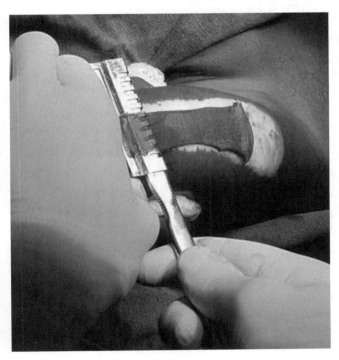

FIGURE 35.8A   Donor site harvesting using a Goulian knife. Image by Jennifer Wall.

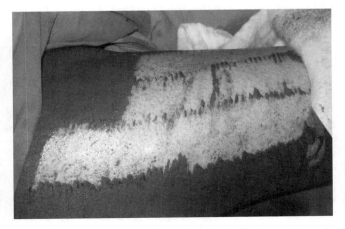

FIGURE 35.8B   Lateral thigh donor site after knife harvest. Image by Jennifer Wall.

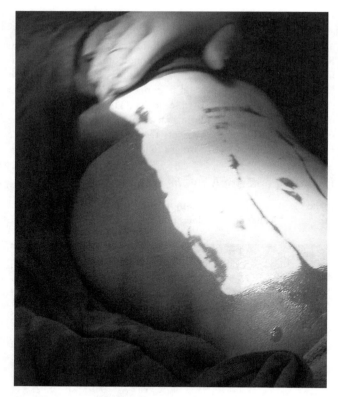

FIGURE 35.8C Back donor site after dermatome harvest. Image by Jennifer Wall.

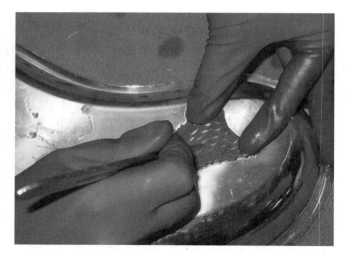

FIGURE 35.9 Hand meshing a split-thickness skin graft. Image by Jennifer Wall.

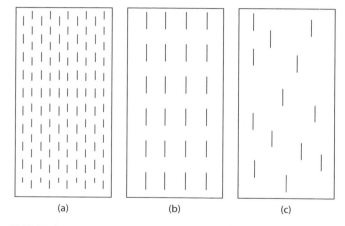

FIGURE 35.10 (a) Proper meshing pattern to provide optimal graft expansion. (b) Ineffective mesh pattern. (c) Ineffective mesh pattern. Image by Mellisa Stanislaw.

graft to prevent accumulation of blood and serum under the graft. It also expands the skin, creating a larger surface area and minimizing the amount of graft that must be harvested. Meshing can be done by hand or with a hand-cranked mechanical mesher. If meshing by hand, place the graft on a sterile cutting surface, such as an upside-down metal basin. With a scalpel, make a series of purposeful, staggered incisions to allow the graft to spread optimally (Figure 35.9 and Figure 35.10).

Mechanical meshers come in two varieties: those that require carriers and those that do not. The Brennan skin mesher has perforating rollers on the top and bottom which the skin is rolled through (Figure 35.11). The Zimmer mesher has a perforating roller on the top, and the skin graft is rolled under this on a ribbed carrier. A 1.5:1 carrier will create a graft that can spread an additional 50% in one direction. Spread the skin graft on the rough, corrugated side of the carrier. If it is placed on the smooth side, the graft will get cut to strands rather than be perforated. The graft may be placed either dermis or epidermis side up on the carrier. Slide the carrier through the mesher, carefully watching to ensure the graft does not roll up into the blades of the mesher after passing through.

If the graft has been placed dermis side up on the carrier, it is easy to take the carrier with meshed graft and place it face down on the wound to deliver the graft in the correct orientation. The graft will adhere only if the dermis side is placed face down. It is easy to maintain orientation if the patient has darker skin tone. Place the pigment side facing up and the white dermal side face down. In pale skin, this can be challenging to discern, but generally the dermis will have a shiny, moist appearance, while the epidermis will appear dry. If you are uncertain of the orientation, let the graft rest in your hand; the dermal side will curl inward at the edges (Figure 35.12).

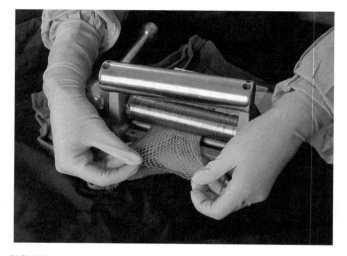

FIGURE 35.11 Brennan skin graft mesher. Image by Jennifer Wall.

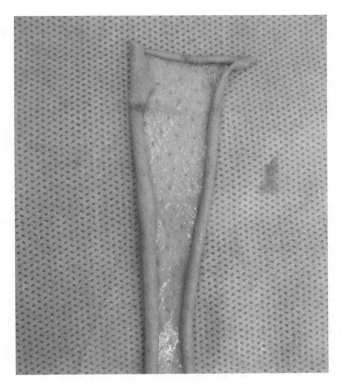

FIGURE 35.12 The dermis (up) appears shiny and curls inward. Image by Jennifer Wall.

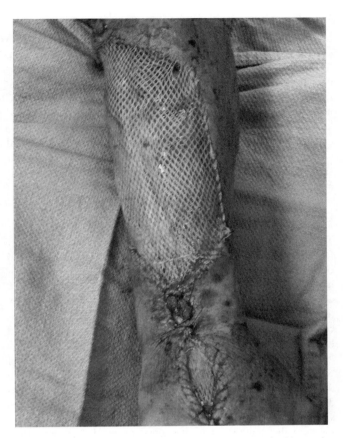

FIGURE 35.13 STSG sutured in place to forearm wound with running chromic suture. Image by Ingrid Ganske.

Place the skin graft on the recipient site and affix the graft around the perimeter with either sutures or staples. Rapidly absorbing sutures (chromic or catgut) work well, as this avoids the pain of suture or staple removal (Figure 35.13). Simple interrupted quilting sutures placed through the graft and the wound bed at regular intervals will help prevent shearing in the central portions of the graft. The surgeon's most common mistake is to assume that the graft will adhere with just a dressing. Be safe rather than sorry: secure the graft.

Bolstering

As with full-thickness grafts, STSGs must be carefully secured and bolstered to prevent shearing forces. Tie-over bolsters work well on flat surfaces, and compression wrap dressings work well on curvilinear surfaces. Place either a Vaseline gauze or generic petroleum gauze directly on top of the graft to prevent trauma at the time of removal. Gauze padding can be soaked in half-strength povidone-iodine solution, left damp, and applied over the top of the petroleum gauze in several layers. Then wrap over the gauze padding with several layers of dry gauze. Splint joints to prevent shear on the graft. Bolsters should be removed after approximately 5 days, or earlier in rainy, damp locations. For lower extremity grafts, the patient should remain on bed rest for 3–5 days, with extremity elevated, to reduce edema and prevent shearing, even if the graft is bolstered.

Aftercare

Apply antibiotic ointment to the graft once or twice daily for the next several days. If the graft has adhered, it is safe to gently cleanse the area with saline at each dressing change. After 10–14 days, the dressings can be changed to a gentle moisturizer daily. Care should be taken to avoid sun exposure and use sunscreen. The patient should not smoke during the healing period, or graft failure is likely.

Donor site treatment

Harvesting STSGs leaves variable degrees of dermal appendages behind, depending on the exact thickness of the graft in proportion to the dermis. The donor site can reepithelialize as soon as 7–10 days, but deeper grafts can take over 2 weeks. If the harvested graft is too thick, or if infection destroys the remaining appendageal remnants, then healing will take place from the wound margins unless the area is grafted with a STSG from elsewhere.

Donor sites can be quite painful for the first several days, followed by itching as the site heals. Pain can be reduced by the preoperative use of topical anesthetic.

At the time of surgery, the donor site can be dressed in a number of ways, generally categorized into moist and nonmoist dressings. Moist dressings include Tegaderm, OpSite, and other occlusive dressings. These are typically left in place until the wound has epithelialized, after 10–14 days. If fluid accumulates underneath the transparent dressing, this can be aspirated with a needle and the dressing patched with a small piece of additional dressing. Moist dressings have the advantage of being somewhat less painful but tend to be more expensive and often unavailable in LMICs.

Nonmoist dressings are inexpensive and have the added advantage of preventing donor site colonization with *Pseudomonas aeruginosa*, a common pathogen in humid, moist environments.

They can consist of solely a generous application of antibiotic ointment twice daily. Or, apply Vaseline gauze, covered with several layers of gauze moistened in povidone-iodine solution, followed by several layers of dry gauze and a wrap bandage. This dressing dries out over the next several days. After 7–10 days, remove the outer layers of gauze. The Vaseline gauze will gradually slough off as the underlying wound heals. Newly healed donor sites demonstrate a flaky, dry keratinized layer that is easily traumatized. Applying lotion and emollients for several weeks after the wound dries can help reduce irritation of this new skin. The donor site should be kept out of the sun. Sunscreen, if available, can be used once the wound has fully healed.

Complications

The primary reasons for STSG failure are similar to those for full-thickness graft failure, and include inadequately prepared or selected recipient sites, infection, hematomas from poor hemostasis, and seromas from poorly bolstered grafts. Smoking, edema, infection, ischemia, prior irradiation, foreign bodies, hypothermia, malnutrition, diabetes, and drugs such as corticosteroids and chemotherapy agents can all lead to poor wound healing and thus poor "take" of the skin graft.

Reduce donor site morbidity by taking the thinnest graft that will provide adequate coverage for the wound. Carefully check the dermatome thickness; harvesting a graft that is too thick can produce a new full-thickness injury at the donor site that then requires split-thickness grafting from elsewhere to heal. Also carefully measure the quantity of graft needed to avoid over-harvesting. Graft scars can contract and lead to additional deformity requiring Z-plasties or other local tissue rearrangement (see Chapter 34). If this happens, full-thickness grafts can be useful for contracture release defects, offering less scar contracture than STSGs.

If hematoma or seroma develops under a sheet graft or a full-thickness graft, the accumulated fluid can be rolled out or aspirated. However, remember there is a narrow window to appreciate and address fluid collections before the undersurface of the graft epithelializes and will no longer adhere to the underlying wound bed.

Special Graft Considerations

Meshing

Meshed STSGs are ideal for extremities and central body parts. The wider the mesh is made, the more total body surface area coverage provided (Figure 35.14). To minimize the scar and waffle appearance of a graft, use sheet grafts on the face and hands for a smoother and more aesthetic appearance. Sheet grafts also heal with less contracture than mesh grafts, ensuring a better functional result. On the digits, full-thickness grafts and unmeshed thick split-thickness grafts minimize the propensity for contraction.

Splinting

Along these lines, the importance of splinting grafted joints cannot be overstated, both for graft adherence in the initial healing stage as well for continuing use of nighttime splints and range of motion exercises to prevent long-term graft contracture.

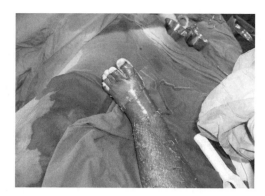

FIGURE 35.14 Meshed STSG to lower leg, with sheet STSG graft to foot. Image by Jennifer Wall.

Negative Pressure Wound Therapy

Negative pressure wound therapy (NPWT) has been used extensively in high-income countries (HICs) for STSG bolstering. Negative pressure dressings are created by placing non-adherent Vaseline gauze or Xeroform on top of the skin graft and then covering this with a porous sponge and a top layer of occlusive dressing. A hole is created in the occlusive dressing and suction tubing is connected to the sponge in the intermediate layer. Electric suction applies an evenly distributed compressive bolster to the underlying graft and a moist wound environment to facilitate wound healing. Limitations to widespread implementation of NPWT in LMICs include electrical requirements, high cost, and lack of technical knowledge, specific materials, and distribution channels locally. Mechanical, low-cost NPWT devices, composed of a bellows suction source and an occlusive dressing, are being developed for use in LMICs. These may soon provide another method of effective bolstering.

Suggested Reading

1. Angel MF, Giesswein P, Hawner P. Skin Grafting. In: McGregor AD, McGregor IA. *Evan's Operative Plastic Surgery: Fundamental Techniques of Plastic Surgery.* 10th ed. Churchill Livingstone: 2000.
2. Mody G, Zurovcik D, Kansayisa G, et al. Phase I Results of a Simplified Negative Pressure Wound Therapy Device for Use in Low Resource Settings [Internet]. 2011. Available from: http://clinicaltrials.gov/ct2/show/NCT01339429.
3. Thorne, C. Techniques and Principles in Plastic Surgery. In: *Grabb and Smith's Plastic Surgery.* 6th ed.
4. Schwarz RJ. Management of postburn contractures of the upper extremity. *Journal of Burn Care & Research.* 2007; 28: 212–9.
5. Voineskos SH, Ayeni OA, McKnight L, Thoma A. Systematic review of skin graft donor-site dressings. *Plastic and Reconstructive Surgery.* 2009; 124(1): 307–8.

COMMENTARY

Jorge Palacios, Ecuador

This chapter includes the best information and description about the utilization of skin grafts that I have read. The development of the exposition of the different procedures, method of application, assessment, and diagnosis allows a perfect understanding of the use of skin grafts.

I must reemphasize the author's section on common pathogens that colonize wounds. In our experience, we use a concentration of 20/1000 of chlorine Dakin's solution to treat the wounds contaminated with Pseudomonas, with incredible results in 72 hours, after three vigorous wound cleanings. Unfortunately, the abuse of antibiotics treatment will create the majority of infection problems and will result in drug-resistant microbes.

COMMENTARY

Charles Furaha, Rwanda
Christian Paletta, Rwanda

Based upon our experience in Rwanda, the surgeon's skill in improvising is essential. We have found the following to be not only helpful, but also often essential in managing an array of patients with a host of both acute and chronic wound and burn conditions:

1. Electrical power is not always consistently present during surgery and may terminate at any time for various lengths of time. Hence the use of a battery-operated headlight is an essential tool for the operating surgeon so that he or she can continue a procedure during a power outage (see Figure 35.15).

2. Dermatomes that require power (air-driven or electric) often fail due to poor maintenance and cleaning. In addition, they typically have expensive blades that patients or our facility cannot afford. Hence we often use the Cobbett, Watson, or Humby knifes, which have few movable parts, are easy to clean and resterilize (in Cidex for 15–20 minutes between procedures), and for which blades are less expensive and more readily available (see Figure 35.16). The graft thickness setting, skin tension, pressure applied while harvesting, the split graft, and knife angle at the donor site vary depending upon the experience and skill of the surgeon. We typically use a #10 or #15 blade to gauge the Humby dermatome blade setting and usually harvest our skin grafts at an angle between 5 and 15 degrees.

3. Sterile topical light mineral oil USP is ideal to lubricate a donor site. Often, this is not available. Hence the surgeon must be creative using another lubricant, such as the Vaseline obtained from the wrapping paper

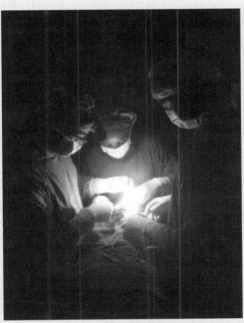

FIGURE 35.15 Dr. Charles Furaha continuing to operate during power outage.

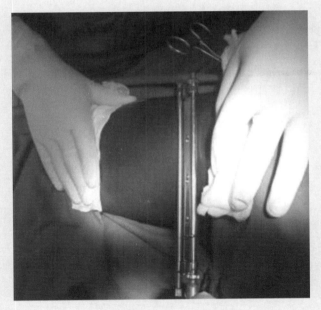

FIGURE 35.16 Freehand Braithwaite modified Humby knife placed at 5–15 degrees with assistant holding skin tense proximally and distally on the left anterior thigh of a patient.

sides of Vaseline gauze or another improvised lubricant, such as topical antibiotic ointments or K-Y Jelly.

4. The unavailability of routine postoperative splinting and physiotherapy following release and skin grafting for severe joint contractures, such as axilla, elbow, wrist, *metacarpophalangeal joints* (MPs), *interphalangeal* joints (IPs), and neck, increases contracture recurrence following grafting. Simple instructions to patients or parents explaining scar/graft massages and stretching and, whenever they can afford, silicone sheeting can be helpful. Due to lack of postoperative splinting, severe neck contractures may be best covered with flaps compared to skin grafting. Contracture recurrence is almost the rule when using skin grafts on the neck.

5. For very large skin grafts to the posterior trunk and perineum, improvised negative pressure therapy can be most useful to facilitate the development of granulation tissue in preparation for skin grafting. And in these areas where prevention of shearing can be difficult, NWPT can be beneficial and improve graft survival (Figure 35.17). We are still in the development stages of finding the best combination of NPWT dressing supplies that is economical, prevents fluid accumulation, can be easily applied by the nursing staff.

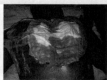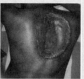

FIGURE 35.17 Back wound of a patient following resection of large sarcoma (top left). Negative pressure wound therapy applied (center). Back wound following a combination of NPWT and daily dressing changes prior to skin grafting (top right). Tumor resection by Orthopedic Oncology colleague Dr. Jennifer Kreshak.

6. Negative pressure therapy is a great technique to promote wound healing and at times as a substitute for flap coverage. It is especially useful with lower extremity wounds. Unfortunately, even improvised ones are still expensive and can be unreliable for district hospital settings. Currently, many individuals are working on NPWT technology that will hopefully result in less expensive applications both in referral and district hospital settings.

7. The use of extremity tourniquets is essential both to limit blood loss during debridement and in preparation for skin grafting. The surgeon must be careful to avoid overaggressive debridement under tourniquet and achieve complete hemostasis following tourniquet release.

36

Wound Care

Helena O.B. Taylor
Stephen R. Sullivan

Introduction

The goal of wound care is a healed wound with the best functional and aesthetic outcome. This chapter addresses the key considerations of wound preparation, closure, adjunctive treatments, postoperative wound care, and potential complications.

Wound Preparation

Examination

Wounds are the result of local trauma and can distract the healthcare provider from life-threatening injuries. Follow trauma protocols by assessing the ABCs (airway, breathing, and circulation) first and addressing life-threatening injuries before wound care. Wear gloves, eye protection, and a mask to protect against body fluids. Once a primary survey has been performed, obtain a complete history and perform a thorough physical examination, paying special attention to both the local wound environment and systemic factors that may affect wound healing. Evaluate the wound to determine the extent and complexity of injury, the tissues involved, the presence of foreign bodies contamination, and the degree of any previous injury. Note the wound size, location, bleeding, arterial or venous insufficiency, motor and sensory function, tissue temperature, and tissue viability. It may be necessary to probe ducts (e.g., the parotid duct or the lacrimal duct) to assess disruption. Radiographs may be required to rule out underlying bony injuries or retained foreign bodies.

Anesthesia

Anesthesia enables thorough irrigation, debridement, and optimal closure. Much can be accomplished under local anesthetic. While an anesthetic agent may be injected directly into the wound, it may be less reliable in inflamed or infected tissues and can distort anatomic landmarks used to align wound edges. Wherever possible, consider regional nerve blocks outside the zone of injury. Sedation or general anesthesia may be necessary if the patient is unable to tolerate local anesthesia (e.g., young children); the wound requires significant debridement, exploration, or repair; bleeding is difficult to control; or the required local anesthetic dose exceeds the maximum safe dose.

Local anesthetics are broadly divided into amides and esters. Amides (e.g., lidocaine, bupivacaine, and mepivacaine) rarely cause allergic reactions, whereas esters (e.g., tetracaine, procaine, and benzocaine) are metabolized to para-aminobenzoic acid, an allergen to some people. Lidocaine is the most commonly used local anesthetic because of its rapid onset of action (< 2 minutes), duration of action (60–120 minutes), relative safety in comparison to bupivacaine, and availability in multiple forms (e.g., liquid, gel, and ointment) and concentrations (e.g., 0.5%, 1.0%, and 2.0%). The addition of epinephrine to a local anesthetic (dilution of 1:100,000 or 1:200,000) produces vasoconstriction, aids in hemostasis, prolongs the anesthetic's duration of action, and allows a larger dose to be safely administered. Traditionally, local anesthetics with epinephrine have not been used in finger, toe, nose, ear, and genital wounds because of a theoretical risk of ischemia. Nevertheless, these adverse effects have not been documented by prospective studies and use is safe in these anatomical regions.[1]

Toxic levels of local anesthetics produce central nervous system effects such as vertigo, tinnitus, sedation, and seizures. These systemic toxicities may progress to cardiovascular effects such as hypotension, arrhythmias, and cardiovascular collapse. Treatment of an overdose is supportive, with oxygen, airway support, and, if necessary, cardiovascular bypass. The maximum safe dose of lidocaine without epinephrine is 3–5 mg/kg and 7 mg/kg with epinephrine. Aspirate before injecting to avoid intravascular injection. To minimize pain, buffer with sodium bicarbonate (1:10 ratio of sodium bicarbonate to local anesthetic), pretreat with a topical anesthetic (e.g., EMLA—a eutectic mixture of lidocaine and prilocaine), use a small-caliber needle (27- or 30-gauge), inject slowly, deliver subcutaneously rather than intradermally, and provide counterirritation.

Irrigation and Debridement

To promote healing and reduce the risk of infection, irrigate and debride necrotic tissue, foreign bodies, and contamination. First expose the wound and the surrounding local tissue. Trim hair with scissors or an electric clipper or retract with ointment. Avoid shaving with a razor because it potentiates wound infection. Avoid clipping eyebrows because they may not grow back and they aid in wound edge alignment. Prepare the surrounding skin with an antibacterial solution such as povidone iodine or chlorhexidine to help create a sterile field and limit contamination.

Irrigation methods include bulb syringe, gravity flow, and pulsatile lavage. These can be further divided into high-pressure (35–70 psi) and low-pressure (1–15 psi) systems. High-pressure pulsatile lavage reduces bacterial concentrations more effectively than low-pressure systems, but can cause more soft tissue disruption and penetration of bacteria into soft tissue. Merely running saline over a wound is of little value. To obtain continuous irrigation with effective pressures of 5–8 psi, wrap a saline bag in a blood pressure cuff, inflate to 400 mmHg, and connect the tubing to a 19-gauge angiocatheter.[2] Use nontoxic solutions (e.g., saline, lactated Ringer's solution, sterile water, or tap water). Irrigating with an antibiotic solution offers no advantages.

Sharply debride nonviable tissue and firmly embedded foreign bodies. If a significant quantity of questionably viable tissue precludes acute debridement and definitive wound closure, initiate dressing changes and delay wound closure. The wound can be closed when the tissue is declared to be either viable or necrotic and the necrotic tissue debrided.

Hemostasis

Hemostasis prevents hematoma formation, which increases the risk of infection and wound inflammation. Control hemorrhage with pressure, packing, wrapping, and elevating. Almost all bleeding can be controlled with prolonged directed pressure. If absolutely necessary, briefly apply a tourniquet to an injured extremity, but be aware that this is painful and may threaten the extremity. Stop hemorrhage with focused cauterization or vessel ligation. Do not blindly clamp or ligate vessels proximal to amputated parts, because an intact vessel is necessary for microsurgical replantation. Place drains if there is a risk of hematoma or fluid collection, but these are not a replacement for meticulous hemostasis.

Wound Closure

Materials

Following wound preparation, choose the appropriate materials for wound closure. Selection is based on tissue layer as well as wound type and location, potential for infection, the patient's ability to tolerate closure, and the degree of wound tension. Options for soft tissue closure include sutures, staples, tapes, and glues. Some wounds may require the consultation of a specialist surgeon, such as those with open bone fractures, or disrupted tendons or nerves.

Most soft tissues are closed with sutures. Sutures are categorized on the basis of material, tensile strength, filament, absorbability, and time to degradation (Table 36.1). Suture material may be either natural or synthetic. Natural fibers (e.g., catgut, cotton, and silk) cause more inflammatory reaction than synthetic fibers (e.g., polyglycolic acid, nylon, and polypropylene). Suture is a foreign body, which may generate an inflammatory response, interfere with wound healing, and increase infection risk. The number and diameter of sutures used to close a wound should be kept to the minimum necessary for wound edge coaptation.

Suture must support the wound until the tensile strength of the scar can withstand the wound tension. Tensile strength is defined as the amount of weight required to break a suture divided by the suture's cross-sectional area. It is typically expressed in an integer-hyphen-zero form. Larger integers correspond to smaller suture diameters. For example, a 3-0 suture is twice as heavy as a 4-0 suture. Suture material may be composed of either a monofilament (e.g., catgut, polydioxanone, and polyglyconate) or multifilaments (e.g., polyglycolic acid, polyglactic acid, and polyester). The interstices of multifilament suture may harbor organisms and increase the risk of infection. Nevertheless, multifilament suture is easier to handle, has less memory, and holds knots better than monofilament. Monofilament requires five knots for security, while multifilament may require only three or four knots. Knots must be square to be secure and must be only tight enough to coapt the wound edges but not strangulate the tissue. To minimize foreign body bulk and the risk of protuberance, cut buried suture ends near the knot.

Some suture materials are absorbable while others are permanent. Absorption of synthetic material (e.g., polyglycolic acid, polyglactic acid, and polydioxanone) occurs by hydrolysis and causes less tissue reaction than absorption of natural material (e.g., catgut), which occurs by proteolysis. Absorbable sutures are generally used to approximate dermis and superficial fascia.

Muscle lacerations should be repaired because muscle is capable of a significant restoration of strength. Approximate tendon lacerations to allow gliding and restore tensile strength. Either 3-0 or 4-0 multifilament polyester or monofilament polypropylene is a reasonable choice for muscle and tendon repair. Coapt the epineurium of severed nerves with tension-free primary repair using 8-0 to 10-0 monofilament nylon or repair with a nerve graft or nerve tube. Close deep fascial layers that contribute to the structural integrity of areas such as the abdomen, chest, and galea with 2-0 or 3-0 suture to prevent hernias, structural deformities, and hematomas.

The dermis is responsible for wound strength at the skin level and is usually closed with 4-0 suture. Sutures in the subcutaneous fat do little to aid in strength of the repair. Fat cannot hold sutures by itself, it has a poor blood supply, and suturing may lead to fat necrosis. If necessary for obliteration of dead space, place sutures at the fat-superficial fascia junction or the fat-dermis junction rather than in fat. Bury the dermal sutures and place 5–8 mm apart, with care taken to evert the skin edges. Nonabsorbable sutures (e.g., nylon, silk, or polyester) are most commonly used for the skin surface or deeper structures that require prolonged support (e.g., abdominal wall fascia, tendons, nerves, and blood vessels). For children, suture removal can be both emotionally and physically traumatic. Accordingly, consider using fast-absorbing suture material or a pullout continuous subcuticular suture in young children. At the skin surface, use fine sutures, staples, tapes, or adhesives to facilitate precise alignment. Evert skin edges with 4-0 to 6-0 nylon or polypropylene placed in the superficial dermis and the epidermis. The distance between the sutures and the distance between the wound edge and the suture insertion point should be equal to the thickness of the skin (epidermis and dermis combined).

Skin suturing technique varies depending on the nature of the wound. Simple interrupted sutures are useful for irregular wounds. Vertical and horizontal mattress sutures achieve good wound-edge eversion but can lead to ischemia and thus must not

TABLE 36.1

Suture materials and characteristics

Absorption	Material	Comment	Configuration	Tensile Strength at 2 Weeks (%)	Time to Degradation (days)
Absorbable	Plain catgut (bovine intestinal serosa)	Natural; high tissue reactivity	Monofilament	0	10–14
	Chromic catgut	Natural; treated with chromic acid, less reactive than plain	Monofilament	0	21
	Fast-absorbing catgut	Natural; heat treated	Monofilament	0	7–10
	Polyglytone 6211 (Caprosyn)	Synthetic	Monofilament	10	56
	Glycomer 631 (Biosyn)	Synthetic	Monofilament	75	90–110
	Polyglycolic acid (Dexon)	Synthetic	Mono/multifilament	20	90–120
	Polyglactic acid (Vicryl)	Synthetic	Multifilament	20	60–90
	Polyglyconate (Maxon)	Synthetic	Monofilament	81	180–210
	Polyglycolide (Polysorb)	Synthetic	Multifilament	80	56–70
	Polydioxanone (PDS)	Synthetic	Monofilament	74	180
	Polyglecaprone 25 (Monocryl)	Synthetic	Monofilament	25	90–120
	Polyglactin 910 (Vicryl RAPIDE)	Synthetic	Monofilament	0	7–14
Nonabsorbable	Polybutester (Novafil)	Synthetic; little tissue reactivity; elastic; good knot security	Monofilament	High	—
	Nylon (Monosof, Dermalon, Ethilon)	Synthetic; little tissue reactivity; memory necessitates more knots	Monofilament	High	—
	Nylon (Nurolon)	Synthetic; limited tissue reactivity	Multifilament	High	—
	Nylon (Surgilon)	Synthetic; silicon coated; limited tissue reactivity	Multifilament	High	—
	Polypropylene (Prolene, Surgilene, Surgipro)	Synthetic; limited tissue reactivity; slippery	Monofilament	High	—
	Polyethylene (Dermalene)	Synthetic	Monofilament	High	—
	Stainless steel	Least tissue reactivity; poor handling; artifact on CT scan; moves with MRI	Mono/multifilament	Highest	—
	Cotton	Natural	Multifilament	—	—
	Silk (Sofsilk)	Natural; extensive tissue reactivity; good knot security	Multifilament	Poor	—
	Polyester (Dacron, Mersilene, Surgidac)	Synthetic; high friction; limited tissue reactivity; poor knot security	Multifilament	High	—
	Polyester (Ticron)	Synthetic; silicon coated; limited tissue reactivity; good knot security	Multifilament	High	—
	Polyester (Ethibond)	Synthetic; polybutylate coated; limited tissue reactivity; good knot security	Multifilament	High	—
	Polyester (Ethiflex, Tevdek)	Synthetic; teflon coated; limited tissue reactivity; good knot security	Multifilament	High	—

Prucz R, Sullivan SR, Klein MB. ACS Surgery. Hamilton: Decker Intellectual Properties; 2012, p. 6.

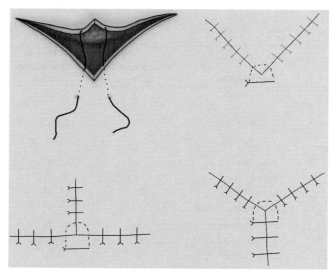

Method of insertion and application of the three-point suture

FIGURE 36.1   Three-point suture. Image by Bin Song.

be too tight. Half-buried horizontal and vertical mattress sutures are used for flap edges to minimize ischemia. For clean and linear wounds, a continuous intradermal or subcuticular suture is easy to remove and relatively inconspicuous without additional puncture wounds. Flap tips should be sutured with a three-point method to prevent strangulation (Figure 36.1).

Staple closure is less expensive and significantly faster than suture closure, and may provide a better aesthetic outcome for scalp wounds. Contaminated wounds closed with staples have a lower incidence of infection than those closed with sutures.[3] When used as the sole method of closure, staples eliminate the risk of a needlestick to the healthcare provider, which is an important consideration in caring for a patient with an unknown medical history. Staples do leave scars at their puncture sites, making them a poor choice for aesthetically sensitive areas such as the face.

Adhesive tapes (e.g., Steri-Strip) are hypoallergenic, have a long shelf life, and are porous. Superficial linear wounds in areas with little tension are easily approximated with tape alone. Tape spares discomfort associated with suture removal, prevents suture puncture scars, and avoids the emotional distress of suturing wounds on children. Advantages include wound edge immobilization, technical simplicity, comfort for the patient, minimal trauma, and lower infection rates in contaminated wounds than suture closure.[4] Disadvantages include the possibility of inadvertent removal and imprecise wound edge approximation. In addition, tape will not adhere to mobile areas under tension (e.g., the plantar aspects of the feet) or to moist areas (e.g., mucous membranes and groin creases). Wound edema can lead to blistering at the tape margins and to inversion of taped wound edges.

Tissue adhesives (e.g., octylcyanoacrylate) are a fast, strong, and flexible method of approximating wound edges. Compared with sutures, staples, and tapes, adhesive closure is faster and essentially equivalent in terms of aesthetic outcome, infection rate, and dehiscence rate for superficial lacerations.[5] Adhesives can be used on most parts of the body and on long wounds. Advantages include low cost, ease of application, and no need for needles or suture removal; their major disadvantage is lack of strength. Do not apply them to tissues within wounds but, rather, apply to intact skin at the wound edges, where they act to hold injured surfaces together. Tissue adhesives are not suitable for wounds in mucous membranes, contaminated wounds, deep wounds, or wounds under tension. Adhesives are particularly useful for superficial wounds or wounds in which the deep dermis has been closed with sutures.

Timing

The decision of when to close a wound may be critical in preventing infection while optimizing aesthetics. Choices include: 1) close the wound at the time of initial presentation (primary closure), 2) delay closure until after a period of healing or wound care (delayed primary closure), or 3) allow the wound to heal on its own (secondary closure). The decision depends on whether the patient is stable and able to undergo wound repair, whether nonviable tissue has been adequately debrided and foreign bodies removed, whether and to what degree bacterial contamination is present, and what the expected aesthetic outcome of immediate closure might be in comparison with that of delayed closure or secondary healing.

Primary closure provides optimal wound healing when two perpendicular, well-vascularized wound edges are approximated without tension. Scars are better tolerated than disruption of anatomic landmarks. Take care to identify the vermilion border of the lip, the eyebrow, or the hairline of the scalp and line up the wound edges appropriately. Handle tissue gently and use skin hooks or fine forceps to prevent wound edge trauma. Close from deep to superficial, placing sutures precisely, and with minimal tension.

Delay the primary closure if there is extensive bacterial contamination, a substantial amount of questionably viable tissue, or the patient is unable to undergo repair at the time of presentation. Delayed primary closure involves direct approximation of wound edges after a period (usually 4–5 days) of wound hygiene with good dressing changes. Delaying closure diminishes the incidence of infection in contaminated wounds if good wound care is provided in the interim.

Secondary closure is when the wound is left open and allowed to heal on its own. Healing depends on epithelization from the wound margins and contraction of the surrounding tissue. Frequent observation is essential as secondary healing can sometimes lead to contracture, a pathologic scar deformity. Secondary closure can yield acceptable results with specific wound types and anatomic sites. Puncture wounds, for example, heal well secondarily while diminishing the likelihood of infection. For both abrasions and puncture wounds, the functional and aesthetic results of secondary closure are generally as good as or better than those obtained by primary or delayed primary closure. Wounds on anatomically concave surfaces (e.g., medial canthal region, perineum) also heal with excellent results.[6] Secondary healing should also be considered for infected wounds, wounds with significant amounts of devitalized tissue, wounds with foreign bodies, and high-velocity wounds.

Closure by Wound Type

Abrasions

Abrasions are superficial wounds caused by scraping, which involve the epidermis and partial thickness dermis. They frequently heal secondarily within 1–2 weeks. Foreign body fragments can embed in and beneath the skin, and if the interval between injury and debridement exceeds 24–48 hours, the wounds will begin to epithelize and the embedded material will be trapped in the skin, resulting in traumatic tattooing. To avoid traumatic tattooing, sharply debride or scrub the abrasion with a brush. Once the wound is debrided, apply ointment or a semi-occlusive dressing to create a moist wound healing environment to speed epithelization. If needed, tape or glue may be used for epidermal approximation to prevent suture mark scars, which could be worse than the actual wound scar.

Puncture Wounds

Puncture wounds are typically left open, treated with wound care, and allowed to heal by secondary intention. Secondary closure reduces the risk of infection and yields a favorable aesthetic result. Grossly contaminated puncture wounds, such as cat bites, are at high risk for infection. These should be copiously irrigated at presentation, and systemic antibiotics are indicated.

Lacerations

The most common wound encountered by surgeons is generally a linear traumatic wound, known as a laceration. Primary closure within 6–8 hours of injury is desirable as it eliminates the need for extensive wound care, allows quick healing, minimizes the risk of infection, and minimizes patient discomfort. For sutured wounds, apply gauze to prevent bacterial contamination, protect the wound, and manage drainage. Dressings are required only for approximately 48 hours, by which time epithelial cells will have sealed the superficial layers of the wound and drainage ceases. Alternatively, apply an antibacterial ointment to minimally draining sutured wounds (see Topical Antimicrobials, below). Ointments maintain a clean and moist wound environment, which promotes healing. Clean wounds can be covered with a semi-occlusive dressing, which allows wound observation and optimizes epithelization, but has limited absorptive capacity.

Complex Wounds

Stellate, degloved, and mutilated tissues are known as complex wounds. Discuss with the patient the difficulties posed by these wounds. These wounds are often treated in the operating room (OR) under general anesthesia because of the extent of injury, need for tissue exploration, removal of foreign bodies, debridement of nonviable tissue, and repair of complex structures. Stellate wounds can be approximated with careful placement of interrupted and three-point sutures. Severely injured tissues may require excision as an ellipse, with closure of the resulting defect.

Degloving refers to circumferential elevation of skin and fat from muscle. The extent of tissue injury is often larger than appreciated. In the acute setting, debride devascularized tissues and observe questionably viable flaps of tissue. The degloved tissue segment may be primarily sewn back into its anatomic location, but avoid closure under tension as an injured but viable flap can quickly convert to ischemic and nonviable when pulled too tight. Consider delayed primary or secondary closure if primary closure leads to ischemia. With extensive degloving, the devitalized tissue may be thinned of subcutaneous fat and replaced as a graft.

Mutilating wounds (e.g., caused by machinery) are often severely contaminated and may involve injury to deeper structures. Prophylactic antibiotic therapy with an agent or combination of agents that offers broad-spectrum coverage is indicated. Repair of underlying bone, muscle, tendon, or nerve may require the operating room. For skin, loose closure should be performed. While tape or staples reduce the risk of infection, suture is often necessary. Avoid excessive amounts as well as multifilament suture, which is more prone to infection.

For complex wounds containing questionably necrotic tissue, foreign bodies, or other debris that cannot be removed sharply, wet-to-dry dressings are effective, simple, and inexpensive. Apply a single layer of coarse wet gauze, allow it to dry over a period of 6–12 hours, then remove. Necrotic tissue, debris, and exudate become incorporated within the gauze and are removed with the dressing. The disadvantages of wet-to-dry dressings are pain and damage to or removal of some viable tissue.

If tendons, arteries, nerves, or bone is exposed, use wet-to-wet dressings to prevent desiccation of these critical structures. Wet-to-wet dressings cause less tissue damage than wet-to-dry dressings but do not produce as much debridement. Most wet-to-wet dressings are kept moist with saline. Use an antibacterial solution (e.g., mafenide, silver sulfadiazine, silver nitrate, povidone iodine, or Dakin's solution containing sodium hypochlorite) on wounds with significant bacterial contamination.

Some wounds are difficult to dress and require special consideration. Do not use compression dressings on flaps or questionably viable tissue because they may cause ischemia. Temporarily immobilize wounds that traverse joints with a plaster splint. For large or irregular wounds, negative-pressure wound therapy (NPWT) is recommended as it conforms well to irregular shapes, removes excess wound fluid, stimulates granulation tissue, improves peripheral blood flow and tissue oxygenation, and reduces wound size.[7,8] Use caution with NPWT in wounds with exposed blood vessels or bowel. Although NPWT requires expensive dressings and equipment as well as electrical charging, less expensive devices are being tested and surgical providers in LMICs eagerly await disruptive technology with NPWT. NPWT has also been shown to decrease the need for more complex reconstructions, such as in exposed lower extremity fractures.[9]

Crush Injury

Crush injury can result in deep tissue damage leading to compartment syndrome, extremity loss, or death from rhabdomyolysis. Successful treatment depends on early diagnosis. Signs and symptoms include increasing pain that is out of proportion to stimulus, altered sensation, pain on passive stretching, weakness, tenseness of the compartment, pallor, poikilothermia, and pulselessness.[10] Compartment pressure can be measured, and compartment syndrome is diagnosed if the pressure exceeds 30 mmHg. Treat by restoring normal blood pressure if hypotensive, remove constrictive dressings or casts, and maintain the limb at heart level. If signs and symptoms persist, perform fasciotomies within 6 hours to prevent irreversible muscle necrosis. Check the serum creatine kinase and, if elevated, stabilize intravascular volume and confirm urine flow to prevent acute renal failure.[11] Renal dialysis may be necessary and life saving.

Extravasation Injury

Arterial or venous catheters may become dislodged or the vessel occluded, leading to extravasation of solutions into the interstitial space. Most extravasation injuries heal without complication. For extravasation of a small volume (<150 ml) of a nontoxic agent, manage conservatively with elevation of the limb and careful monitoring. Large-volume (>150 ml), high-osmolar contrast agents, cytotoxic agents, or chemotherapeutic drugs, however, can cause soft tissue necrosis and compartment syndrome. Treatment of these injuries is not standardized; it may include conservative management, hydrocortisone cream, incision and drainage, hyaluronidase injection, aspiration, irrigation, or fasciotomies in the case of elevated compartment pressures.

High-Velocity Wounds

Explosions or gunshots cause extensive tissue damage when the kinetic energy of high-velocity projectiles is released into the soft tissues. Although the entry wound can be small, the exit wound and interspace may contain large areas of ischemic and damaged tissue. Clothing and dirt may also be transmitted into the deep tissues. Radiographs may identify metallic foreign bodies. Identify and extensively debride injured tissue and foreign bodies. Not all fragments will be able to be removed. Leave wounds open to heal by delayed primary or secondary closure.

Bite Wounds

Human bite wounds are usually clenched fist wounds sustained while fighting. Puncture wounds in the metacarpophalangeal joint are at particularly high risk for infection. These "fight bites" are considered infected and must be treated with aggressive irrigation, usually in the operating room, and broad-spectrum antibiotic (e.g., amoxicillin-clavulanate). Obtain radiographs and explore wounds to evaluate for fractures or open joints. Delayed primary or secondary closure is advised due to the high risk of infection. Cat bites or scratches are at high (80%) risk of infection, while dog-bite wounds are at lower (16%) risk for infection, and prophylaxis with amoxicillin-clavulanate is appropriate.[12] Consideration should also be given to rabies treatment (see below). Puncture wounds should be left open and allowed to heal secondarily. Larger lacerations on cosmetically sensitive areas may be closed loosely with sutures, but patients must be advised regarding the possible risk of infection.

Adjunctive Wound Treatment

Prophylactic Systemic Antibiotics

For most wounds, prolonged antibiotic prophylaxis is not indicated. When it is called for, select an agent based on the bacterial species likely to be present. The anatomic location of a wound may also suggest whether oral flora, fecal flora, or skin flora is likely to be present. Gram staining can provide an early clue to the nature of the contamination. Ultimately, the choice of a prophylactic antibiotic regimen is based on the clinician's best judgment regarding which agent or combination of agents will cover the pathogens likely to be present. Wound categorization includes clean, clean-contaminated, contaminated, and dirty (Table 36.2).[13] Risk of infection correlates with wound category. Local factors, such as ischemia, radiation, and foreign body; and systemic factors, such as diabetes, acquired immunodeficiency syndrome (AIDS), and cancer, may increase the risk of wound infection. Prophylactic antibiotics can be considered in the presence of any of these factors. In addition, prophylactic antibiotics should be considered in patients with cardiac valvular disease or a prosthesis.

Topical Antimicrobials

Topical antimicrobials (e.g., antibiotic ointments, iodine preparations, sodium hypochlorite, and silver agents) significantly lower wound infection rates on open wounds and do not appear to impair epithelization in animal models.[14] Antibiotic ointments such as bacitracin, polymyxin, or triple antibiotic ointment (bacitracin, neomycin, and polymyxin B) are useful for abrasions, superficial burns, or along fresh suture lines. Patients may develop allergic dermatitis with prolonged use of these agents. Betadine (10% povidone with 1% free iodine) is an effective antiseptic,

TABLE 36.2

Classification and infection rates of operative wounds

Classification (class)	Infection Rate (%)	Wound Characteristics
Clean (I)	2–5	Atraumatic, uninfected; no entry of GU, GI, or respiratory tract
Clean-contaminated (II)	8–11	Minor breaks in sterile technique; entry of GU, GI, or respiratory tract without significant spillage
Contaminated (III)	15–16	Traumatic wounds <4 hours old; gross spillage from GI tract; entry into infected tissue, bone, urine, or bile
Dirty (IV)	28–40	Traumatic wounds >4 hours old; drainage of abscess; debridement of soft tissue infection

Cruse PJ, Foord R. The epidemiology of wound infection. A 10-year prospective study of 62,939 wounds. *Surgical Clinics of North America.* 1980 Feb;60(1):27–40.

often used for creation of a sterile field, which also promotes angiogenesis and fibroblast proliferation. Dakin's solution (half-strength 0.25% sodium hypochlorite) can be made inexpensively by diluting household bleach, and is useful for grossly infected wounds as well as promoting neodermal thickness and fibroblast proliferation. Silver has microbicidal effects on common wound contaminants and may also be effective against methicillin-resistant *Staphylococcus aureus*. Silver sulfadiazine (Silvadene) has broad antibacterial properties, maintains a moist wound, and has a relatively benign side effect profile (transient leukopenia is occasionally seen). It is useful for partial thickness burns.

Tetanus Prophylaxis

Tetanus is a nervous system disorder caused by *Clostridium tetani* and is characterized by muscle spasm. Wound severity is not correlated with tetanus susceptibility. Therefore, all penetrating wounds, regardless of etiology or severity, are tetanus prone, and a patient's tetanus immunization status must always be considered. Provide post-exposure prophylaxis per guidelines (Table 36.3).[15]

Rabies Prophylaxis

Rabies is an acute progressive viral encephalitis. Any mammal can transmit the virus, but carnivores and bats are the only viral reservoirs. Bite wounds in which the animal's saliva penetrates the dermis are the most common route of exposure. Consider vaccination prior to exposure if at high risk. Post-exposure treatment consists of wound care, infiltration of rabies immune globulin into the wound, and vaccine administration. Provide post-exposure prophylaxis per guidelines (Table 36.4).[16] Prior vaccination status determines the vaccination regimen (Table 36.5).[17]

TABLE 36.3

Recommendations for tetanus immunization

Tetanus Immunization History	Toxoid	Tetanus Immune Globulin (TIG)
Unknown	Yes	Yes
> 10 years since last booster	Yes	Yes
≥ 5 and ≤ 10 years since last booster	Yes	No
< 5 years since last booster	Yes	No

Note: Administer toxoid and TIG (250 units) with separate syringes at different anatomic sites. Toxoid is contraindicated if there is a history of a neurologic or severe hypersensitivity reaction after a previous dose. Local side effects alone do not preclude use. If a systemic reaction is suspected of representing allergic hypersensitivity, postpone immunization until appropriate skin testing is performed. If a contraindication to a toxoid containing preparation exists, use TIG alone.

*Pediatric diphtheria and tetanus toxoids and acellular pertussis vaccine (DTaP) for patients aged <7 years; tetanus and diphtheria toxoids (Td) if aged 7–10 years; reduced diphtheria toxoid and acellular pertussis vaccine (Tdap) (or Td if Tdap is unavailable) if aged ≥11 and <65 years; and Td for adults aged ≥65 years. Pregnant women should receive Td instead of Tdap, if possible.

Recommendations for Postexposure Interventions to Prevent Infection with Hepatitis B Virus, Hepatitis C Virus, or Human Immunodeficiency Virus, and Tetanus in Persons Wounded During Bombings and Other Mass-Casualty Events. [Image on Internet] 2008. [updated 2008 Aug 1; cited 2014 Jan 29]. Available from: http://www.cdc.gov/mmwr/preview/mmwrhtml/rr5706a1.htm#top [public domain]

TABLE 36.4

Rabies: Recommendations for post-exposure prophylaxis based on animal type

Animal Type	Animal Disposition and Evaluation	Patient Prophylaxis*
Dog, cat, ferret	Healthy and available for 10 day observation	Initiate prophylaxis immediately if animal exhibits rabies symptoms+
	Rabid or suspected rabid, no observation is indicated	Initiate prophylaxis immediately+
	Unknown	Consult public health official
Bat, skunk, raccoon, fox, and most other carnivores	Regarded as rabid unless brain laboratory tests are negative	Initiate prophylaxis immediately+
Livestock, horse, rodent, rabbit, hare, and other mammals	Consider each case individually	Consult public health official; rarely requires prophylaxis

*See Table 5 – Rabies: Recommendations for Post-exposure Prophylaxis
+If animal is euthanized for brain laboratory testing, stop prophylaxis if tests are negative for rabies.

Animal Type to Postexposure Prophylaxis. [Image on Internet] 2011. [updated 2011 Nov 15; cited 2014 Jan 29.] Availble from: http://www.cdc.gov/rabies/exposure/animals/domestic.html [public domain]

TABLE 36.5

Rabies: Recommendations for post-exposure prophylaxis

Treatment	Non-immunized Individuals	Previously Immunized Individuals
Wound care	Irrigate and debride the wound; apply a virucidal agent such as povidone-iodine solution.	Irrigate and debride the wound; apply a virucidal agent such as povidone-iodine solution.
Human rabies immune globulin	If possible, infiltrate the full volume (20 IU/kg) around wound(s). If necessary, administer remaining volume IM at another site. Do not use more than recommended dose. Use separate syringes and anatomic sites from vaccine.	Do not administer.
Human diploid cell vaccine or purified chick embryo cell vaccine	1.0 ml IM on days 0, 3, 7, and 14*	1.0 ml IM on days 0 and 3*

*Administer in deltoid for adults; anterolateral thigh may be used for children. To avoid sciatic nerve injury and reduce adipose depot delivery, the gluteus is not used.

Rabies Vaccines and Immunoglobulin Available in the United States. [Image on Internet]. 2011. [updated 2011 Apr 22; cited 2014 Jan 29]. Available from: http://www.cdc.gov/rabies/medical_care/index.html [publicdomain]

Postoperative Wound Care

Keep closed wounds clean and dressed for 24–48 hours after repair. Assess wounds at risk for infection within 48 hours of care. Teach the patient to look for signs of infection (e.g., spreading erythema, purulent drainage, and fever). After 48 hours, gentle cleansing with running water removes bacteria and crusting. Patients should not place tension on the wound or engage in strenuous activity in the first 6 weeks, while collagen deposition and tensile strength of the wound increases rapidly. After this period, tensile strength increases more slowly, eventually reaching a maximum of 80%–90% of normal skin strength.

The timing of suture or staple removal is a balance between optimal cosmesis and the need for wound support. On one hand, sutures should be removed early, before inflammation and epithelization of suture tracts occurs, usually by 7 days. But it takes a number of weeks for the wound to gain significant tensile strength, and early suture removal can result in dehiscence. Early suture removal is warranted for some wounds, particularly those in aesthetically sensitive areas under minimal tension. Facial sutures may be removed on day 4 or 5. Sutures in wounds subject to greater stress (e.g., wounds on the extremities or trunk) should remain in place longer (2–3 weeks), as should sutures in wounds sustained by patients who have impeded wound healing.

After suture removal, numerous methods are employed to minimize unsightly scar formation. The aesthetic outcome of a scar is largely determined by the nature and severity of the wound, which are outside the surgeon's control. The greatest impact a surgeon can have is by providing meticulous care when the acute wound is initially encountered. Postoperatively, massage, silicone bandages, pressure garments, and the application of lotion and sunblock may optimize outcomes. Nevertheless, the healing wound is fragile, and topical application of ointments to achieve an improved scar appearance may actually achieve the opposite result. Vitamin E, which is commonly applied to healing wounds, can induce contact dermatitis and cause scars to look worse.[18]

Chronic Wound Care and Impaired Wound Healing

A number of local and systemic factors can interfere with wound healing. Local factors include tension, infection, ischemia, hematoma, seroma, trauma, edema, and irradiation. Systemic factors include hypothermia, tobacco, malnutrition, diabetes mellitus, and drugs (corticosteroids or chemotherapy). Evaluate for these factors and take appropriate measures to improve the chances for optimal healing when possible.

Tension may lead to separation of wound edges. Causes of tension include absent tissues, inherent skin elasticity, poor surgical technique, movement of joints, or inadequate wound support. Minimize tension by undermining the wound edges during closure to allow easy coaptation. Limit surgical ellipses from wound edges to as narrow as possible and along relaxed skin tension lines. After suture removal, support the wound using tapes (e.g., Steri-Strips) for 3–6 weeks. Consider splinting wounds over joints. Tissues with dermal edges that do not bleed are ischemic. Monitor questionably viable tissue and debride when declared nonviable. Maintain intravascular volume and tissue perfusion with fluid or blood and provide supplemental oxygen if necessary. Rough handling of tissue edges with forceps causes additional iatrogenic injury. Avoid crushing the epidermis by handling wound edges gently at the dermal level with toothed forceps or fine skin hooks.

Hematomas and seromas increase the risk of wound dehiscence. Ensure hemostasis at the time of wound closure and correct bleeding diatheses. Close wounds over a drain if there is a large dead space, with significant risk for hematoma or seroma formation. Evacuate large hematomas or seromas before they solidify. Small hematomas or seromas can usually be observed as they often resorb. Edema results from the accumulation of fluid in the interstitial space. It may occur as an acute process due to inflammation or as a chronic process due to venous insufficiency, lymphatic insufficiency, or low plasma oncotic pressure. Edema inhibits healing. Clearing edema improves healing and may be accomplished by elevation, compression therapy, or NPWT.

Radiation irreversibly damages tissues and can cause wounds to heal slowly, or healed wounds to break down. Irradiated tissue is characterized by a thickened and fibrotic dermis, a thin epidermis, pigment changes, telangiectasia, decreased hair, and increased dryness. Wounds within irradiated beds may require tissue transfer for healing. Vitamin A supplementation can lessen the adverse effects of radiation on wound healing.[19]

Hypothermia impairs wound healing, increases the infection rate, and slows wound tensile strength. Prevent or correct hypothermia with systemic and local tissue warming to maximize wound healing potential. Supplemental oxygen benefits wound healing. Reduce the incidence of wound infection by improving the F_IO_2 with supplemental oxygen. Restore or improve the circulating volume by administering crystalloids or blood.

Tobacco smoking reduces tissue oxygen concentrations, impairs wound healing, and contributes to wound infection and dehiscence. Encourage acutely injured patients to stop smoking. Noninjured patients scheduled to undergo surgery should stop smoking at least 3–4 weeks before making an elective surgical wound.

Edema results from fluid accumulating in the interstitial space. It may occur as an acute process with trauma or as a chronic process due to venous insufficiency, lymphatic insufficiency, and a low plasma oncotic pressure. Edema raises tissue pressure, forms a fibrinous clot, and inhibits perfusion and healing. Clearing the edema is necessary and may be accomplished with compression or NPWT.[7,20]

Good nutritional balance and adequate caloric intake (including sufficient amounts of protein, carbohydrates, fatty acids, vitamins, and other nutrients) are necessary for normal wound healing. Protein is particularly important as it provides an essential supply of the amino acids used in collagen synthesis, and protein replacement and supplementation improves wound healing. Vitamin C deficiency causes scurvy, marked by failed healing of new wounds and dehiscence of old wounds. When low, supplement Vitamin C (100–1,000 g/day) to improve wound healing.[21] Vitamin K is necessary for blood clot formation and hemostasis, the first step in wound healing. Vitamin D is required for normal calcium metabolism and therefore plays a necessary role in bone healing. Dietary minerals (e.g., zinc and iron) are also essential for normal healing. Zinc replacement and supplementation can improve wound healing, but daily intake should not exceed 40 mg of elemental zinc.[21]

Diabetes mellitus is associated with poor wound healing and an increased risk of infection. Monitor and control blood sugar levels. Diabetic patients, with decreased acral sensation, must also closely monitor themselves for wounds and provide meticulous wound care. Many drugs impair wound healing. Corticosteroids, for example, inhibit all aspects of healing. In the setting of an acute wound that fails to heal, patients requiring corticosteroids may reduce the dose, administer topical or systemic vitamin A (25,000 IU/day orally),[22] and in extreme situations, supplement with anabolic steroids to restore steroid-retarded inflammation. Chemotherapeutic agents both hinder tumor growth and impair wound healing. Acutely wounded patients who have recently been treated with, are currently taking, or will soon begin to take chemotherapeutic agents, must be closely observed for poor healing and complications. Vitamin E (a-tocopherol) impairs collagen formation and causes inflammation. Despite its popularity, topical application can cause contact dermatitis and worsen the appearance of the scar.[18]

COMMENTARY

Ntakiyiruta Georges, Rwanda

This topic is excellently and comprehensively discussed in the chapter. I would like to add that one should consider performing an early diversion of stools for any perineal wound (from a gunshot wound (GSW), burn, or other cause), since persistent stool contamination will impair wound healing and any wound closure attempt (delayed primary closure or skin graft) will fail.

Another aspect of wound care is the management of wounds as a result of necrotizing fasciitis and Fournier's gangrene, both of which are highly prevalent in Rwanda. Both are life-threatening soft-tissue infections that are characterized by rapidly spreading inflammation and necrosis of the skin, subcutaneous fat, and fascia. The management of them involves good resuscitation measures, aggressive wound debridement, high doses of intravenous antibiotics, and regular relooks in the operating room. Delays in surgical treatment are associated with high mortality. Surgical debridement will result in an extensive wound. Wound healing takes a long period of time, and wound closure usually requires skin grafting.

Another aspect of chronic wound to highlight is chronic leg ulcers, also known as tropical ulcers. Tropical ulcers usually require antibiotics for up to 4 months and wound care. When there is good granulation tissue, the wound can be skin grafted. Tropical ulcers that have lasted for many years can undergo malignant changes.

Venous ulcers are also challenging, although leg elevation and leg compression with elastic bandages may help. Sclerotherapy of the varicose vein or varicose vein stripping are very useful in the management of nonhealing varicose veins.

The management of pressure sores in bedridden paraplegic patients is very difficult. The management principles for chronic wound are the same, but the most challenging in LMICs is the prevention of pressure sores in high-risk patients.

COMMENTARY

Sterman Toussaint, Haiti

Wound care is often one of the most challenging tasks for surgeons; it is critical for non-immediate life-threatening patients and sometimes for trauma patients. This chapter outlines a practical approach to wound care and pays particular attention to the initial aspects of wound management. This is very helpful for surgeons because, most of the time, the outcome of the healing process for any wound is tributary on the initial management.

It is also interesting in this chapter that the priority is not on the availability of unlimited resources and technology, but rather on the surgeon's basic and appropriate knowledge of wound management. However, it gives the surgeon the capacity to use the latest technological inventions, so any surgeon or surgery resident could use this as a good companion in the footpaths of daily wound management.

For coordinating ZL/PIH surgical activities in Haiti, where our network is concentrated in the countryside, the management of wounds is particularly more challenging because most of the time our patients have tried some empiric unadapted treatment before showing up to the hospital. We often have to deal with wounds that were initially dressed with a spider's web, horse or cow feces, or soil; in most of these cases, the patient was not vaccinated for tetanus.

It is also good to find that this chapter highlights the importance of the surgeon's experience in some cases, especially regarding the use of prophylactic antibiotics. However, some procedures, like skin graft and flaps, should be emphasized because neglected or complex wounds often need these procedures to heal.

Finally, since the sixteenth century when Ambroise Pare wrote *La Maniere de Traiter les Plaies* (The way to treat wounds), wound care has advanced, but initial wound management, especially cleaning the wound with soap and water, has remained the key to successful wound care.

COMMENTARY

Okao Patrick, Rwanda

Wound care is one of the pillars of surgical care. This chapter discusses the major aspects of wound care and clarifies many contentious topics. Good medical history and clinical examinations should be emphasized as part of the overall wound care. The cost of wound care can be markedly reduced if early and proper wound debridement and dressing is done because it will eventually allow early closure.

COMMENTARY

Okechukwu O. Onumaegbu, Nigeria

The goal of wound care remains a healed wound with the best outcomes in form and function. Adequate preparation of the wound without prejudice to the advanced trauma life support (ATLS) protocol is essential for this outcome. The use of regional anesthetic blocks outside the zone of injury is beneficial in freeing up the anesthetist (often in short supply) to attend to other pressing patient care. Where there is no anesthetist, this skill enables the surgeon to adequately, in dual role, attend to the surgical care of the traumatic wounds presenting.

Wound irrigation and debridement: Bulb syringes are not commonly available, but 20-ml syringes serve a similar purpose, albeit with less ease. With a number of patients presenting with wounds that have been treated with unconventional methods, assessment of these late presenting or chronic wounds may be preceded by serial dressing sessions using a "wet-and-dry" approach. An example of this approach is a wet/saline-wrung gauze inner layer overlaid with dry meshed gauze and cotton wool padding; this allows for moistening of the adherent agents on the wound floor and debridement of same. This allows for ambulatory initial management of these patients. The benefit is glaring in situations where bed space for inpatient care is a concern. Materials that have been found applied to wounds range from the identifiable and obliterating or desiccating like gentian violet, powdered contents of antibiotic capsules, and so on, to the unidentifiable and unimaginable. Wet-to-dry dressings changed every 6–12 hours are very effective but not usually feasible in our locality because of the manpower limitations for the required nursing care and the limited supplies from the central sterile supplies unit or, more often, its usually smaller equivalent.

Human bite wounds are more commonly on free-border facial structures like the lips, ala of the nose, and the pinna. They do not usually result from the incidental "fight bites" to the knuckles but from a deliberate attempt by a subdued opponent to inflict aesthetically relevant damage to his assailant. These structures usually present in such situations with full-thickness defects. Repair and reconstruction of these may be undertaken primarily by careful sharp excision of the often ragged edges. When contamination is deemed gross or indeterminable, a delayed primary approach is advised. Careful attention to the anatomic landmarks such as the white roll of the vermillion border of the lip may be enhanced by tattooing the relevant points with surgical ink using the tip of a small-caliber (23-gauge/25-gauge) hypodermic needle before local anesthetic infiltration and debridement. Additional excision of otherwise unaffected tissue may be necessary to obtain a better aesthetic result. For instance, crescentic excisions may be required lateral to the alae of the nose to facilitate apposition of a central upper lip defect without tension. In a not-so-related setting, a ray amputation may be required to improve the functional outcome in a low transproximal phalangeal traumatic amputation of the ring or middle finger, where replantation is precluded.

Brushing abrasions under saline or clean water irrigation, or with the added bubbling effect of dilute hydrogen peroxide solution irrigation on the wound, helps to prevent traumatic tattooing. Disposable brushes, however, are often a luxury, as are resterilizable brushes. The concept of resterilization is discouraged for fear of disease transmission. Sterile meshed gauze used as a brush will just as efficiently remove any ingrained dirt.

Degloving injuries are best laid back into position preferably over a wet single layer of gauze as they are often not clean wounds. Except for very lax elderly skin (which, however, has its own blood supply concerns) suturing the "flap" back into position is almost invariably going to be under tension.

Chronic wounds will almost always yield bacterial growth on culture of wound swabs. Antibiotic treatment should not be undertaken merely on account of a positive culture with demonstrated sensitivities. The clinical state of the wound and any associated systemic effects should guide the commencement of antibiotic therapy. The swab result may then guide the choice of antibiotic employed.

A word on leg ulcers in sickle-cell disease patients: Aggressive surgical skin cover either with local flaps or split skin grafts is often ill-advised, as these ulcers are notorious for recurrence. Adequate bed rest and judicious wound care with medication support (antimalarial prophylaxis, vitamin C in large doses of up to 1,000 mg daily, folic acid, and good hydration) are conservative approaches that yield remarkable healing in these ulcers.

Section IV

Trauma

37

Disaster Management

Susan Miller Briggs
Guy Lin

Introduction

The management of the medical and public health effects of contemporary disasters, whether natural or man-made, is one of the most significant challenges facing surgeons today. Disaster medical care is not the same as conventional medical care. Disaster medical care requires a fundamental change in the approach to the care of surgical patients to achieve the objective of providing the "greatest good for the greatest number of victims."

The demands of disaster medical relief have changed over the past decade, in the scope of medical care, the spectrum of threats, and the field of operations. Increasingly, civilian surgical teams are being asked to respond to complex disasters, with the spectrum of threats ranging from natural disasters to complex man-made disasters such war and terrorism. Many contemporary disasters occur in "austere" environments. An austere environment is a setting where access, transport, resources, or other aspects of the physical, social, or economic environments impose severe constraints on the adequacy of immediate care for the population in need (Figures 37.1 and 37.2).

Contemporary disasters follow no rules. No one can predict the time, location, or complexity of the next disaster. Similar to the ABCs of trauma care, disaster medical response includes basic elements that are similar in all disasters. The ABCs of the medical response to disasters include the following: 1) search and rescue, 2) triage and initial stabilization, 3) definitive care, and 4) evacuation. The difference in disasters is the degree to which certain capacities are needed in a specific disaster and the degree to which outside assistance (regional, national, or international) is needed. Rapid assessment by experienced teams of disaster responders will determine which of these elements are needed in the acute phase of the disaster to augment local capacities. Disaster management teams are based on "functional" capacities, not titles. Surgeons are uniquely qualified to participate in all four aspects of disaster medical response given their expertise in triage, emergency surgery, care of critical patients, and rapid decision making.[1,2]

Epidemiology of Disaster

Mass casualty incidents (MCIs) are events causing numbers of casualties large enough to disrupt the healthcare services of the affected communities (Figure 37.3). Demand for resources always exceeds the supply of resources in a mass casualty incident. Disasters may be natural or man-made, or a combination of the two. Natural disasters may be classified as sudden-impact (acute) disasters or chronic-onset (slow) disasters.

Sudden-impact disasters include:

- Earthquakes
- Tsunamis
- Tornados
- Floods
- Tropical cyclones, hurricanes, and typhoons
- Volcanic eruptions
- Landslides and avalanches
- Wildfires

Chronic-onset disasters include:

- Famine
- Drought
- Pest infestation
- Deforestation

Sudden-impact natural disasters generally cause significant morbidity and mortality immediately as a direct result of the primary event (e.g., traumatic injuries, crush injuries, or drowning), whereas chronic-onset disasters cause mortality and morbidity through prolonged secondary effects (e.g., infectious disease outbreaks, dehydration, or malnutrition).

Man-made disasters may be unintentional or intentional (terrorism). The spectrum of agents used by terrorists is limitless and includes conventional weapons; explosives; and biological, chemical, and radioactive agents. In addition to the possibility of a large number of victims, responders must be aware of the potential for secondary strikes directed at harming emergency personnel. More than 70% of terrorist attacks involve the use of explosive weapons and are a significant challenge for surgeons due to the complexity of injuries (primary, secondary, tertiary, and quaternary blast injuries).

Disasters involving weapons of mass destruction (biological, chemical, or radioactive agents), whether accidental or man-made

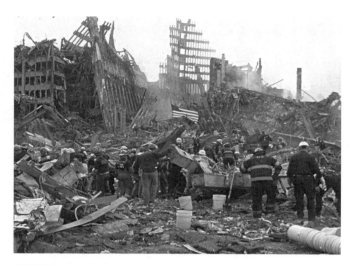

FIGURE 37.1   World Trade Center bombing, New York (2001). Image by Susan Miller Briggs.

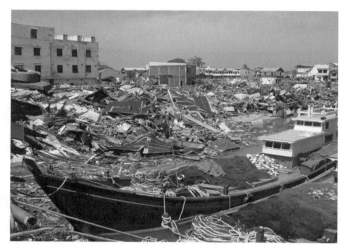

FIGURE 37.2   Tsunami, Banda Aceh, Indonesia (2004). Image by Susan Miller Briggs.

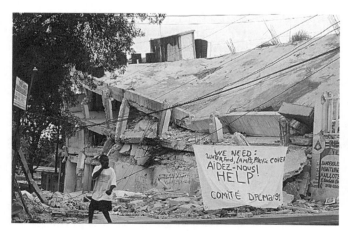

FIGURE 37.3   Haiti earthquake (2010). Image by Susan Miller Briggs.

mass casualty incidents, are a significant challenge for medical providers for three reasons[3]:

1. Weapons of mass destruction have the greatest potential to produce numbers of casualties large enough to overwhelm the medical and public health infrastructures. Such agents will also produce a category of victims known as "expectant" victims. This denotes a category of victims not expected to survive due the severity of injuries or underlying diseases and/or limited resources. This term was first used in conjunction with chemical warfare.

2. Weapons of mass destruction produce significant numbers of "psychogenic" casualties, greatly complicating medical providers' rescue efforts. Terrorists do not have to kill people to achieve their goals. Creating a climate of fear and panic to overwhelm the medical infrastructure achieves their goals. During the Sarin attack in Tokyo (1995), 5,000 casualties were referred to local hospitals. Fewer than 1,000 individuals were suffering from the effects of the gas.

3. Weapons of mass destruction will produce "contaminated" environments. Surgeons must be able to perform triage and initial stabilization and possibly operative care outside traditional hospital facilities. The necessity for decontamination prior to surgical care interventions further complicates rescue efforts.

Role of Surgeons in Disaster Medical Response

Search and Rescue

Many disasters, both natural and man-made, involve large numbers of victims trapped in collapsed structures (Figure 37.4). Many countries, including the United States, have developed specialized search-and-rescue teams as an integral part of their national disaster plans. Members of these teams, which receive

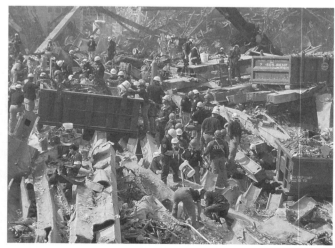

FIGURE 37.4   Search-and-rescue teams, Oklahoma City bombing (1995). Image by Susan Miller Briggs.

specialized training in confined space environments, generally include the following:

- A cadre of medical/surgical specialists
- Technical specialists knowledgeable in hazardous materials, structural engineering, heavy equipment operation, and technical search-and-rescue methodology
- Trained canines and their handlers

Triage and Initial Stabilization

Triage is the most important and psychologically challenging aspect of disaster medical response, both in the prehospital and hospital phases of disaster response. This is especially true in disasters occurring in austere environments where resources and evacuation assets are limited. Triage is the process of sorting casualties according to the level of care they require in a mass casualty incident. Patients' needs are matched with available resources.

Surgical disaster triage is significantly different from conventional triage. The objective of conventional surgical triage is to do the "greatest good for the individual patient." Severity of injury or disease is the major determinant of triage category as adequate resources are available for the care of the patient. The objective of disaster triage is to do the "greatest good for the greatest number of patients." In a mass casualty event, the critical patients having the greatest chance of survival with the least expenditure of time and resources (equipment, supplies, and personnel) are prioritized to be treated first. The major objective and challenge of surgical triage is to identify the small minority of critically injured patients who require urgent lifesaving treatments, including damage control surgery, from the larger majority of noncritical casualties. Review of the literature from major disasters estimates that 15%–25% of victims are critically injured, and the remainder of victims are noncritical casualties.

Triage errors, in the form of under-triage and over-triage, are always present in the chaos of mass casualty events. Under-triage is the assignment of critically injured casualties requiring immediate care to a "delayed" category. Under-triage leads to treatment delays with increased mortality and morbidity. Over-triage is the assignment of noncritical survivors with no life-threatening injuries to immediate urgent care. The higher the incidence of over-triage, the more the medical system is overwhelmed. In mass casualty incidents, especially explosions, triage errors more commonly involve over-triage than under-triage. Children are often over-triaged due to the emotional impact of injured children on medical responders. The level of acceptable over/under-triage in a mass casualty incident and the best method for evaluation of triage effectiveness in mass casualty incidents is still controversial. Various triage systems exist and, unfortunately, there is no universally accepted triage system for mass casualty incidents.

Triage is a dynamic decision-making process of matching patients' needs with available resources. Three levels of disaster medical triage have been defined. The level of disaster triage utilized at any phase of the disaster will depend on the ratio of casualties to capabilities. Many mass casualty incidents will have multiple levels of triage as surgical patients move from the disaster scene to definitive medical care.

Level 1: Field Triage

Field triage is the rapid categorization of victims who potentially need immediate medical care "where they are lying" or at a casualty collection center. Victims are designated as "acute" or "nonacute." Color-coding may be used. One effective way to begin Level 1 triage on a large number of victims is to instruct people to get up and move to a designated location. This will rapidly separate ambulatory (noncritical) individuals from nonambulatory (critical) victims.

Level 2: Medical Triage

Medical triage is the rapid categorization of victims by experienced medical providers at a casualty collection site or fixed or mobile medical facility. Medical personnel performing triage must have knowledge of various disaster injuries and illnesses. Victims are classified into the following categories:

- **Red (urgent):** Lifesaving interventions (airway, breathing, circulation) are required (Figure 37.5).
- **Yellow (delayed):** Immediate lifesaving interventions are not required (Figure 37.6).

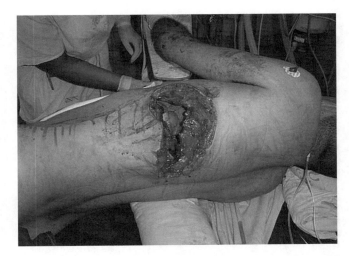

FIGURE 37.5   Severe crush injury to chest. Image by Susan Miller Briggs.

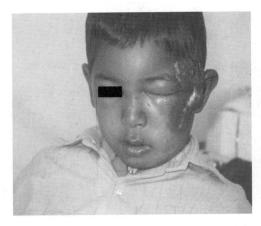

FIGURE 37.6   Crush injury to face. Image by Susan Miller Briggs.

- **Green (minor):** Minimal or no medical care is needed or psychogenic casualties (Figure 37.7).
- **Black:** Deceased victims (Figure 37.8).
- **Expectant category:** Classification of the expectant category of disaster victims is controversial. This triage category includes victims not expected to survive due to the severity of injuries (blast injuries; crush injuries; burns; or exposure to large quantities of chemical, biological, or radioactive agents) or underlying diseases and/or limited resources. Traditionally, this category of disaster casualties has been classified as "yellow or delayed" category. Currently, many triage systems classify expectant victims as a separate category with a different color designation. Some systems classify expectant victims in the black category.

Level 3: Evacuation Triage

Priorities for transfer to medical facilities are assigned to disaster victims using the same color classification as medical triage. Victims are matched to available receiving facilities. Often victims with minor injuries can be sent to more distant facilities, keeping closer facilities available for higher-priority victims. Rapid evacuation of critical casualties allows more time and resources for caring for the larger majority of non-critical victims.

Definitive Medical Care

Definitive medical care refers to care that will improve, rather than simply stabilize, a casualty's condition. Maximally acceptable care for all surgical patients is not possible in the early stages of the disaster given the large number of victims in a mass casualty incident. In the initial stage of the disaster, minimally acceptable surgical care (crisis management care or altered standards of care) to provide lifesaving interventions is necessary to provide the "greatest good for the greatest number of victims." Damage control surgery is an important component of crisis management care. In many disasters, local hospitals are destroyed, transportation to medical facilities may not be immediately feasible, or the environment may be contaminated. Mobile surgical facilities that can provide a graded, flexible response to the need for surgical care are the key to a successful surgical response (Figure 37.9).[4]

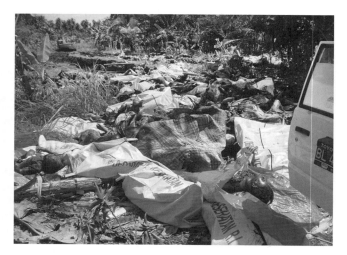

FIGURE 37.8 Fatality collection site. Image by Susan Miller Briggs.

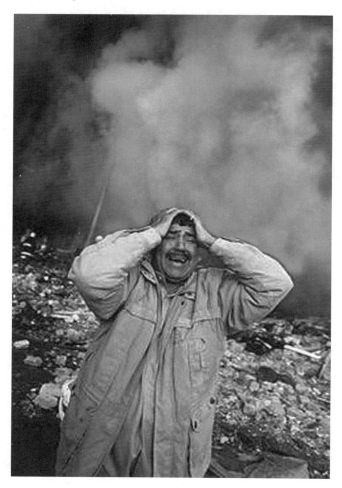

FIGURE 37.7 Psychogenic casualty following terrorist attack. Image by Susan Miller Briggs.

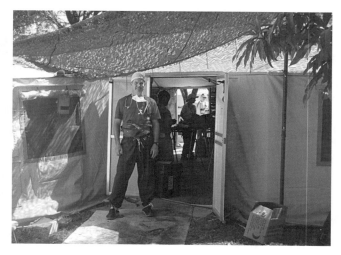

FIGURE 37.9 Mobile surgical field hospital. Image by Susan Miller Briggs.

Evacuation

Evacuation may be useful in a disaster to decompress the disaster area and provide specialized surgical care for specific casualties, such as those with burns and crush injuries. Surgeons with expertise in critical care are increasingly valuable resources in disasters. In most disasters, the large number of victims needing evacuation, especially in austere environments, will mandate the use of unconventional medical transport aircraft without medical crews (Figure 37.10).

Disaster Surgical Care at the Field Hospital

The "Minimally Acceptable Care" Concept

First of all, we need to find the appropriate balance between the complexity of the treatment needed and the number of patients being treated to save the most lives and prevent disability. The basic strategy is to direct limited resources toward treatment of those wounded that are expected to recover after surgical treatment with a short postoperative course.

As most victims sustaining severe torso or head injuries do not survive long enough to get medical treatment, surgical procedures are required primarily for the treatment of limb injuries. With a delay of several days many open fractures and severe soft tissue injuries become infected (Figure 37.11), and those wounded who survive the first 2–3 days may die later due to sepsis originating in their contaminated wounds. Timely surgical intervention can save lives. Amputation is sometimes the right solution for devastating limb injuries, but external fixation of fractures and aggressive debridement of soft tissues is feasible and can save many limbs (Figure 37.12). Most of these procedures can be performed under spinal anesthesia or a regional block, a particularly effective technique for a field hospital setting. The management of a mangled extremity usually requires prolonged hospitalization and repeated operations, sometimes with an uncertain functional result. Hence, such a treatment protocol will severely restrict the number of patients that can be treated and is not suitable for a mass disaster. To overcome these constraints, we recommend a short trial of limb saving—the "orthopedic minimally acceptable care"

limiting the number of surgical interventions to no more than two. This policy can save many limbs, without endangering the lives of those who eventually require amputation or are consuming precious resources on a nonsalvageable limb.[5-7]

The course of treatment is:

1. Intensive debridement of the infected extremity
2. External fixation of the fracture
3. Observation for 24–48 hours with administration of intravenous (IV) antibiotics and bedside debridement when needed

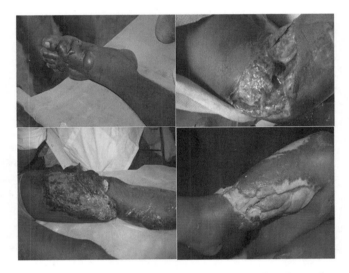

FIGURE 37.11 Injuries characteristic of disasters: neglected open fractures and severe soft tissue infections. Image by Guy Lin.

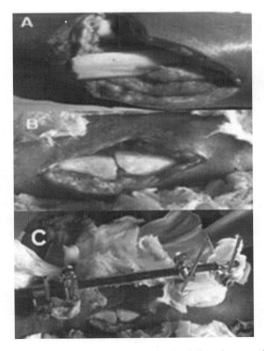

FIGURE 37.12 Treatment of a high-grade infected open fracture: Devascularized bone is excised (A), an acute shortening is performed bringing viable bone surfaces into contact (B), and external fixation (C).

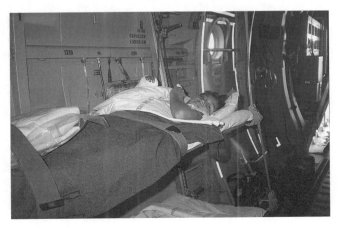

FIGURE 37.10 Air evacuation of crush injury victim. Image by Susan Miller Briggs.

4. Reevaluation and performing second surgical debridement or amputation

5. Discharge with oral (PO) antibiotics

6. Follow-up as "outpatients" and a "rescue" amputation for failures

Decisions may be influenced by the estimated availability of rehabilitation, prosthetic capabilities, wheelchair accessibility, and social services for disabled persons in the affected country. [8]

Although you can deal with some fractures without any imaging, effective treatment of limb injuries mandates X-ray imaging. Since hundreds of films are needed every day, a fluoroscopy machine is ideal. In the absence of a fluoroscopy machine, it is essential to minimize the number of X-ray images taken. Only one anteroposterior (AP) view is taken routinely. In most cases this view is adequate to understand the fracture configuration and treatment plan—either casting or pin placement in external fixation. Additional views are done selectively when deemed necessary. Postoperative radiographs are performed only in selected cases, mainly if there is any doubt regarding adequacy of fixation. Adhering to the "minimally acceptable care" concept, minor positional deviations are deemed irrelevant and would not be changed at this point.

With no conditions for internal fixation, closed femoral fractures in adults are also treated by external fixation (pediatric femoral fractures are managed with closed reduction and a spica cast) (Figure 37.13A and Figure 37.13B).[9,10] Femoral fractures carry a risk of life-threatening pulmonary complications as well as decubitus ulcers with prolonged immobilization. Moreover, this procedure may be lifesaving as immobilization by itself may be incompatible with life in an extreme disaster zone.

With the exception of femoral fractures in adults, all closed fractures are treated nonoperatively, sometimes with acceptance of residual deformity or joint incongruity. Having no other choice, femoral neck fractures are managed with external plaster boot to prevent rotation movements.

The "minimally acceptable care" can be extended to other anatomical regions such as mandibular fractures (Figure 37.14).

Acute trauma, surgical, and obstetrics emergencies are expected in any population. In many circumstances, patients in extremis cannot survive in an austere environment, and providing comfort measures only should be considered (see ethical dilemmas below). Decisions are supported by simple laboratory and imaging studies (i.e., ultrasound and plain X-rays). With limited resources, the rate of unnecessary laparotomy for trauma should be zero. As a rule, all stable patients sustaining any type of penetrating abdominal injury are managed expectantly until the development of signs of peritoneal irritation. Conservative management is also extended in chest trauma. For hemothorax, the decision to perform a thoracotomy is not based on "volume criteria" (e.g., chest drain output of 200 cc blood per hour). Autologous transfusion of blood draining out through the chest drains can help avoid thoracotomy in the stable patient.

"Simple" surgical emergencies, such as perforated peptic ulcer, have good prognosis with early surgical intervention and should receive priority. Also, basic obstetrics procedures may be lifesaving for both mother and fetus (Figure 37.15).

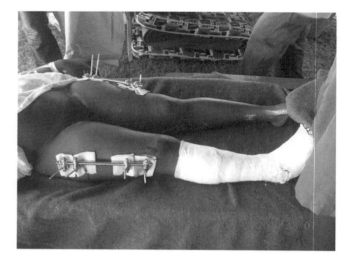

FIGURE 37.13A Multiple levels of closed fractures. Bilateral femoral fractures are treated by external fixations, and right tibial fracture is treated by closed reduction and a plaster of paris cast. Image by Guy Lin.

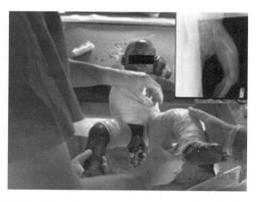

FIGURE 37.13B Closed reduction and a spica cast for a left femoral fracture in a 4-year-old boy. Image by Guy Lin.

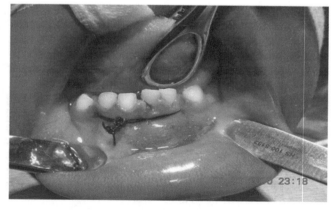

FIGURE 37.14 "Minimally acceptable care" for a mandibular fracture (arrow): minimal manipulation for reduction of the mandible and an external fixation, based on two teeth on each side of the fracture, with a prolene stitch. Eating ability is resumed. Image by Guy Lin.

The situation on the ground, the nature of patients' problems, and the availability of medical services change rapidly in a disaster. A daily revaluation of surgical strategies and priorities is needed. For instance, when a hospital capable of performing

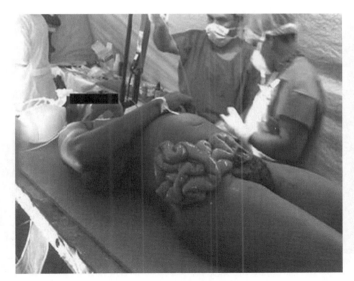

FIGURE 37.15 Haiti, January 2010. This woman underwent a "street" caesarean section and then brought with an open abdomen to the Israeli field hospital, sustaining tears of the uterus and the urinary bladder. Image by Guy Lin.

internal fixation is deployed in the area, external fixation of closed femoral fractures may not be needed.

Intensive care and dialysis services may be available at a later stage and influence our priorities, as referral to other facilities of patients for whom the capabilities of our hospital cannot offer any surgical or medical solution may become an option.

At any stage, collaboration between medical delegations, including exchange of patients, can greatly improve the operating efficiency and take advantage of the capabilities of each one. Central control can maximize the medical capabilities and allow the regulation of patients between different hospitals according to type of injury and occupancy.

Wound Care in Disasters

Debridement of wounds is the most common surgical procedure needed in disasters. Appropriate wound care requires dedication, as many wounded need a surgical debridement on a daily basis. There are no shortcuts. In general, these procedures are carried out under sedation. The sedation protocol is based on IV ketamine at a dose of 1 mg/kg with SaO_2 monitoring if available and O_2 supplementation if needed. Ketamine is a drug with a high hemodynamic and respiratory safety profile, with the advantages of a strong analgesic effect and the possibility for intramuscular admission. For mass treatment, a comfortable setup for bedside sedation should be prepared. Patients with infected wounds are hospitalized in the same area. Debridement kits including instrumentation, disinfectants, and disposal bags are prepared in advance. To save time and effort, 12 ampoules of 500 mg ketamine (10 cc each) are added to a half-liter saline bag to create a "family bag." Thus, a 620 cc of a 10 mg/cc ketamine solution is created. From this bag, we draw the appropriate dose for each patient. For less painful wounds and for those less infected, debridement can be done by the nursing staff and even by the patient himself (Figure 37.16). A surgical brush with hard fibers is particularly suitable for this purpose (Figure 37.17A and Figure 37.17B).

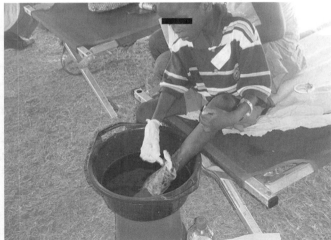

FIGURE 37.16 Haiti, January 2010. "Self-debridement" of an infected ankle wound. Image by Guy Lin.

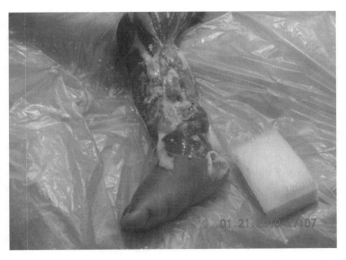

FIGURE 37.17A Before effective debridement of a major leg wound using a surgical brush. Image by Guy Lin.

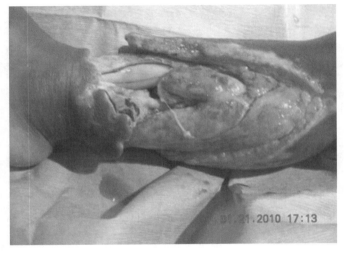

FIGURE 37.17B After effective debridement of a major leg wound using a surgical brush. Image by Guy Lin.

Management of infected trunk wounds is extremely difficult. Surgical debridement mandates general anesthesia, and obviously, amputation is not an option. If necrotizing fasciitis continues to spread despite repeated debridement, withdrawal of care should be considered (see ethical dilemmas below).

When a patient presents with a clean wound, coverage with an immediate skin graft is possible. Autologous skin, taken from an amputated limb, can be harvested and implanted on the wound (Figure 37.18).

In spite of significant delay, debridement and primary closure of facial and scalp wounds can be performed with slight risk of wound infection (Figure 37.19A, Figure 37.19B, and Figure 37.19C).

In most cases, soft-tissue coverage with skin grafts and flaps is performed at a later stage, about 10–15 days after the injury. At this point, the load of wounded decreases, and the operating room (OR) can schedule reconstructive operations. Also, at this time, the development of clean mature granulation tissue in the wounds enables successful "take" of the skin grafts.

The Disaster Zone Operating Room

Deploying an OR in a tent and supplying electricity through a small mobile generator enables surgical capability almost anywhere. Nowadays, the medical corps of many armed forces have lightweight, highly mobile, far-forward surgical teams. Such teams of the U.S. military performed many successful surgical procedures in Iraq and Afghanistan war zones.[11] These units can establish an OR and be prepared to operate within few hours and, therefore, are particularly suitable for disaster areas. Most of these units do not have a logistical backup. They have to join a larger force deployed in the field for logistic support.

However, military teams are designed to treat combat casualties. Hence, they need to be reinforced with the appropriate skills and equipment for a civilian population including children.

Despite careful planning, we may require items not prepared in advance. Therefore, with some creativity and improvisation talent, simple materials can be used to construct medical devices (Figure 37.20A, Figure 37.20B, Figure 37.20C, and Figure 37.20D).[12]

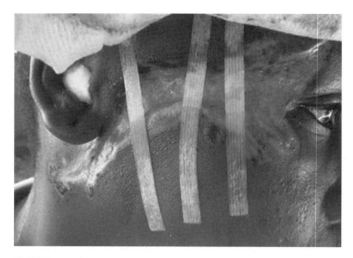

FIGURE 37.19A Neglected facial wound. Image by Guy Lin.

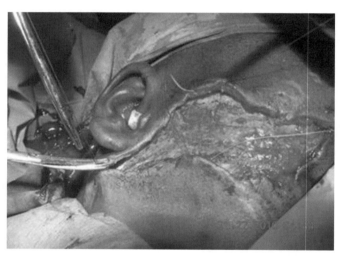

FIGURE 37.19B Surgical debridement. Image by Guy Lin.

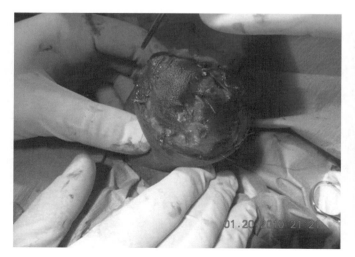

FIGURE 37.18 Immediate coverage of a clean stump: a full-thickness skin graft was taken from the amputated distal leg. Image by Guy Lin.

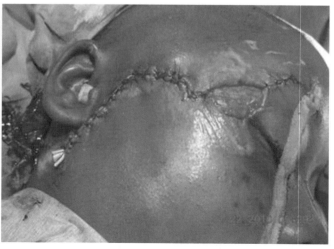

FIGURE 37.19C Primary closure. Image by Guy Lin.

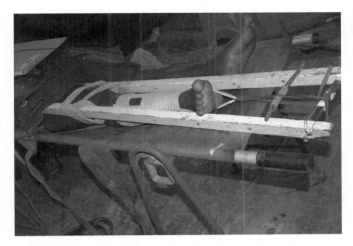

FIGURE 37.20A Improvised orthopedic device: traction device. Image by Guy Lin.

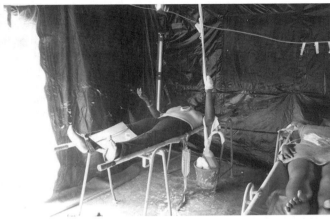

FIGURE 37.20B Improvised orthopedic device: traction device. Image by Guy Lin.

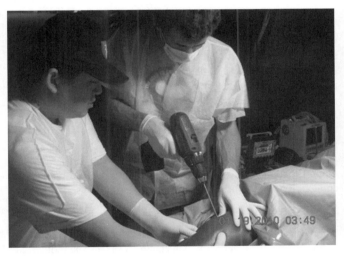

FIGURE 37.20C External fixation with an industrial drill. Image by Guy Lin.

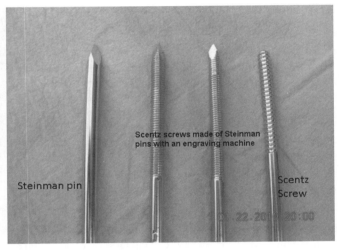

FIGURE 37.20D Self-made screws. Image by Guy Lin.

To perform many operations, an effective method for a "sterile supply" must be established. A method for cleaning, resterilization, and repacking of the surgical instruments should be developed. A heavy-duty autoclave is essential.

As general anesthesia is needed for some surgical procedures, a recovery "room" with ventilation and monitoring capabilities is required. These beds should be reserved for postoperative patients with good prognosis (see ethical dilemmas below).

The blood bank capability of a mobile OR is usually limited to refrigerated type O+ packed red blood cells, which are not ideal for children and women of childbearing age. Also, thrombocytes and coagulation factors may be desperately needed. A "walking blood bank" technique of fresh whole blood transfusion is feasible, and can be based on a preliminary screening of the medical personnel.[13]

Management of Crush Injuries/Crush Syndrome

Crush injuries are common after natural disasters (e.g., earthquakes, hurricanes, tornadoes, and landslides) as well as man-made catastrophes (e.g., wars, mining accidents, and terrorist attacks). Late mortality is occasionally attributable to rhabdomyolysis resulting in the crush syndrome.[14,15]

To prevent infections in tissues already lost, if the skin is closed, fasciotomies are not performed when medical care has been delayed for more than 24 hours. During debridement of open wounds, fasciotomy is performed when deemed necessary.

Crush-related acute renal failure (ARF) is a life-threatening complication of crush injuries that can be reversed. IV fluids infusion begins even before extrication of the injured from the ruins if possible. In the appropriate clinical settings, pink or cola-colored urine is diagnostic of rhabdomyolysis. Laboratory tests help to manage the patient but are not essential for making the diagnosis.

ARF caused by crush injury carries an 80% mortality rate, which can be reversed to an 80% survival rate with a good long-term prognosis, if hemodialysis is available. The leading cause of death is intractable hyperkalemia. The incidence of ARF related to crush syndrome depends on the amount of compressed tissues, the intensity of the compression, and the amount of time spent under rubble. More than half of those with renal failure will require renal replacement therapy (RRT). Conservative treatment for rhabdomyolysis includes a volume expansion phase with 5–7 L of 0.9% normal saline, together with a dose of 44.6 mEq of bicarbonate 3 times per day in the first day of treatment, followed by a high-dose phase of furosemide administration at a dose of 240 mg/d with monitoring of urine output by catheter. Treatment of hyperkalemia consists of calcium carbonate 10 ml, 4 times per day; insulin together with 10% glucose solution; and salbutamol (albuterol) inhalations 8 times per day.

The expected high prevalence of ARF due to crush syndrome should dictate solutions for the administration of RRT in the very early stages following disasters. In these early phases, hemodialysis availability is limited by the lack of necessary aseptic conditions, lack of running water, and the difficulty of coping with a very high patient load. Although less effective for clearance of potassium and other small molecules, peritoneal dialysis may be a short-term solution for patients with crush syndrome and ARF. The risk of peritonitis limits the use of the peritoneal catheter to a maximum of 4 days.

Peritoneal dialysis, although cumbersome, can be practiced in the field. RRT team, equipment, and protocols can be provided by the Renal Disaster Relief Task Force of the International Society of Nephrology. Besides treatment of various injuries and wounds, it is the surgeon's responsibility to create a peritoneal access. Although insertion of a peritoneal catheter can be done under local anesthesia, the procedure is better performed in the OR keeping strict sterile conditions. Priority should be given to this procedure in the time schedule of the OR. Continued care of these patients requires close cooperation between the surgeon and the nephrology team.

Ethical Dilemmas

The mission of the medical staff working in a disaster zone is to extend lifesaving medical help to as many people as possible. The need to manage limited resources that fall far short of the demands continuously presents the surgeon with complex ethical issues.[16] Every mass-casualty event raises ethical issues concerning the priorities of treatment, but a large-scale disaster with destruction of infrastructure can be exceptional in several ways. Under normal circumstances, triage involves setting priorities among patients with conditions of various degrees of clinical urgency to determine the order in which care will be delivered, presuming that it will ultimately be delivered to all. However, handling a situation in which it is impossible to treat everyone is unfamiliar to most of us, and contradicts our basic instincts as doctors.

The first triage decision we often had to make is which patients we would accept and which would be denied treatment. An admission policy of "first come, first served" is inconsistent with the mission of saving the largest possible number of patients.[17] In many cases, persons with the most urgent need for care are often the same ones who require the greatest expenditure of resources. Therefore, we first have to determine whether these patients' lives can be saved. The majority of the patients are going to present with limbs that are compromised by open, infected wounds. The natural history of untreated open fractures is infection, gas gangrene, and ultimately death. Clearly, the sooner after injury the patient received medical attention, the better his or her chances of survival. Late-arriving patients who already had sepsis have a poor chance of survival. But, there is no clear cutoff time beyond which patients cannot be saved. Patients presenting with septic shock and multi-organ failure or hemorrhagic shock with a need for massive blood transfusion can be assumed unsalvageable. Each case has to be evaluated individually, taking in consideration that resuscitating a patient with an extremely severe condition may mean rendering critical resources (e.g., a ventilator) unavailable to others for long periods. Also, admission of patients who need care far beyond the capabilities of the hospital (e.g., paraplegics) should be avoided. Resources should be saved for those who can benefit from appropriate medical treatment. Entrance to the medical facility should be restricted to prevent overcrowding and turning the medical facility into a refugee camp, a situation that will prevent the possibility of providing advanced medical care. These life-and-death decisions require reasonable conditions and should be taken by the most senior personnel. Admission principles should be determined in advance and then frequently updated by the team, based on the changing conditions, load at the hospital, available equipment, and options for cooperation with other medical forces. Serious mistakes can be made trying to evaluate who can benefit from advanced medical treatment among hundreds victims seeking medical care who come to the gate. We recommend preparing a designated triage area adjacent to the medical facility, which enables a slower and more accurate triage. Also, humanitarian aid and comfort measures for the dying can be provided in this area.

Withdrawal of care of patients who could possibly survive in modern hospital conditions is another unnatural course of action for physicians accustomed to treating all who have any chance of recovery. As medical options in a disaster zone can increase rapidly, withdrawal of care policy should be revaluated on a daily basis. Again, policy decisions must rely on a broad basis of team consensus, and then each case must be considered on its merits.[18]

COMMENTARY

Emmanuel Kayibanda, Rwanda

A disaster in the general context is an accidental or uncontrollable event in which a society undergoes severe danger. This may result in loss of people, loss of resources, and services disruption. In the hospital context, it is a large multiple patient incident (MPI) requiring mobilization of response capabilities beyond those locally available, and/or affecting infrastructure and medical capacity (e.g., earthquakes and infectious disease outbreaks). Disasters come in all shapes and sizes; they can be natural or man-made. They can come with days of prior warning or without any warning at all.

The situations of mass causalities are very sensitive, and the environment may negatively influence the management if not well supervised and scientifically conducted. The field triage at the scene of the accident is the most difficult because often no one is prepared. The patients are helped by the volunteers and first aid before the arrival of medical personnel; however, this is inefficient and may aggravate the patients' conditions. In low- to middle-income countries (LMICs), we usually do not have enough organized structures prepared to face such events. The army, police, and firefighter brigades usually play a big role in all disaster responses, but other services, especially many hospitals in suburban and rural areas, are not prepared for these impressive events.

The population is usually unfamiliar with the classic methods of triage and prioritization of patients to be treated at the scene of the incident and during transport. They cannot understand, for example, how the sickest patient is not the one who is assisted first, especially if the patient is their relative. And from there, everybody is seeking any influence that can help to care for their relatives, and this may interfere with the management plan.

We note here the important role of the incident commander (who must be a very senior person), his or her section commanders, and the security officers. The incident commander is often the hospital CEO, and he or she works under pressure because he or she is the one who receives a lot of calls from different places.

Another challenge in our settings is that a lot of people, especially those who have full medical coverage (with insurance or companies) are reluctant to be discharged from hospitals in these circumstances. This may create logistical problems, and the staff should be strong enough to refuse interferences, influences, and abnormal recommendations.

To address such emergencies, every organization (companies, national agencies, governmental or private services, hospitals, etc.) should establish a disaster preparedness plan, which provides guidelines for the management of the immediate actions and required operations.

These plans should be coordinated to provide an organized management system, the overall priorities during a disaster being the protection of lives, property, the community, and the environment. These preparedness plans should be designed to save the maximum number of patients in an organized and efficient manner. This means being continuously prepared with a proactive emergency management action plan for possible and eventual emerging incidents.

38

Initial Evaluation of the Trauma Patient

William P. Schecter

Introduction

The modern approach to the trauma patient is based on the Advanced Trauma Life Support (ATLS) program of the American College of Surgeons. The ATLS program was designed for high-income countries (HICs) and establishes both a protocol of care and a common language for all providers. The goal of care is transport of "the right patient to the right place at the right time." In other words, the patient should be transported as rapidly as possible to a hospital with clinical capabilities suitable to care for the patient's particular injuries. Unfortunately, most trauma patients in the developing world do not have access to hospitals with advanced trauma care capability, if they have access to a hospital at all. Transport may take hours to days. The relevance of ATLS to low- and middle-income countries (LMICs) has therefore recently been questioned.[1] Nevertheless, mastery of the principles of ATLS provides the individual with an organized approach, which can be modified based on the clinician's specific training, experience, and available resources.

Efficient care of the injured patient requires a fundamental change in mind-set. Two parallel processes, one therapeutic and one diagnostic, replace the traditional history and physical examination. We initiate treatment of physiologic abnormalities while pursuing the precise diagnosis. The goal is diagnosis and treatment of life-threatening conditions within 60 minutes of injury, the so-called golden hour. The ATLS program has four phases: the primary survey, the stage of resuscitation, the secondary survey, and definitive care.[2]

The Primary Survey

The primary survey has five components: airway, breathing, circulation, disability, and exposure (see Table 38.1). Although airway control is traditionally considered the first treatment priority, in an LMIC with limited or no access to blood, immediate control of active external bleeding is also of high priority. External hemorrhage should be controlled by direct pressure. Bleeding from the extremities can be temporarily controlled by application of a tourniquet proximal to the injury. A blood pressure cuff elevated to 250 mmHg secured with tape and placed over cast padding (if available) is a convenient tourniquet. Definitive control of massive hemorrhage requires urgent access to an operating room (OR).

Airway

There are three basic maneuvers in airway management: open the airway, give oxygen, and maintain cervical spine stability. If the patient is able to speak, the airway is intact. Oxygen, if available, should be given.

Cervical spine stabilization is unnecessary if the patient has an isolated penetrating injury. A neurologic injury caused by penetrating neck trauma is immediate. The cervical spine should be stabilized in all cases of blunt trauma. Stabilization is particularly important after blunt head or maxillofacial injury. The goal is prevention of delayed neurologic injury caused by instability. Although the utility of a cervical collar has recently been questioned,[3] cervical spine stabilization remains a sound principle following blunt injury.

If the patient is apneic, unconscious, or has signs of airway obstruction, the first step is a chin lift or jaw thrust. A chin lift is performed by placing the thumb underneath the chin and lifting forward, and a jaw thrust is performed by placing the long fingers behind the angle of the mandible and pushing anteriorly and superiorly (Figure 38.1). This maneuver lifts the tongue from the hypopharynx. If suction is available, it should be used to clear the airway. If not, clear the airway manually if necessary.

An oral airway, if tolerated, may keep the airway open, permitting spontaneous ventilation. If it is not tolerated, a nasopharyngeal airway may help (Figure 38.2).

The signs of upper airway obstruction are listed in Table 38.2. In general, an adult does not develop signs of upper airway obstruction unless the airway is 3 mm or less in diameter. Sweating is a sign of sympathetic discharge, an indication of hypercarbia. Patients with signs of upper airway obstruction unresponsive to a jaw thrust and oral airway require a definitive airway. The other indications for a definitive artificial airway are listed in Table 38.3.

There are two choices for establishing a definitive airway: endotracheal intubation and a surgical airway. A laryngeal mask is a good choice for temporarily controlling the airway if intubation is difficult or impossible. If the patient has satisfactory spontaneous ventilation, the surgical airway can be established under controlled conditions. If not, a rapid cricothyroidotomy is necessary. Endotracheal intubation is discussed in Chapter 6.

Cricothyroidotomy

The cricothyroid membrane is located between the thyroid and cricoid cartilage. I prefer a 2–3 cm transverse incision centered

TABLE 38.1

Primary survey

Airway
  Open airway
  Oxygen
  Stabilize cervical spine
Breathing
  Jugular venous distension
  Tracheal midline
  Symmetric chest wall expansion
  Chest wall pain and crepitus
  Bilateral breath sounds
Circulation
  External hemorrhage
  Pulse, peripheral perfusion
  Blood pressure
  2 large-bore IVs
  Blood for hematocrit, type and cross match
  2 L of warm crystalloid (in an adult)
Disability
  Glasgow Coma Scale
  Pupils
  Movement of extremities
Exposure
  Remove clothing
  Log roll the patient
  Keep the patient warm

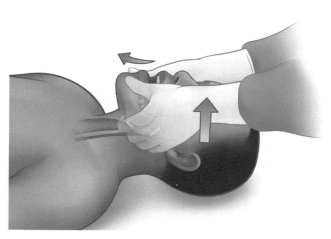

FIGURE 38.1 Jaw thrust. Image by Janet Fong, 2012 [updated 2013 Dec; cited 2014 Jan 27]. Available from: http://www.aic.cuhk.edu.hk/web8/ Hires/Modifiedjawthrustdhs2.jpg

over the membrane. Expect a lot of bleeding in the emergency situation. The patient is often struggling and the anterior jugular veins distended. Some surgeons use a vertical incision. If exposure is difficult, I make a vertical incision teeing off the transverse incision inferiorly in the midline. An assistant providing exposure with retractors is very helpful. The inferior portion of the thyroid cartilage is grasped with a tracheal hook stabilizing the airway and lifting it into the wound. Open the cricothyroid membrane with a knife, spread the incision with a clamp, and insert a small number 6 endotracheal tube or tracheostomy tube.

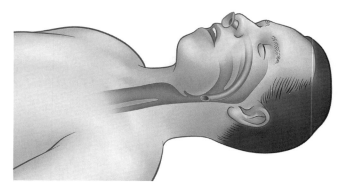

FIGURE 38.2 Nasopharyngeal airway. Image by Janet Fong, 2010 [updated 2013 Dec; cited 2014 Jan 27]. Available from: http://www.aic.cuhk .edu.hk/web8/Hi%20res/nasopharyngeal_CMYK.jpg

TABLE 38.2

Signs of upper airway obstruction

General signs of respiratory distress
  Tachypnea
  Tachycardia
  Flaring of the alae nasi
Specific signs of upper airway obstruction
  Inspiratory stridor
  Supraclavicular and intercostal retractions
  Inspiratory sternal retractions

TABLE 38.3

Indications for an artificial airway

1.	Hypoventilation
2.	Hypoxia
3.	Airway protection (unconscious patient)
4.	Pulmonary toilet

Once ventilation and oxygenation are restored, a formal tracheostomy can be performed in an OR if one is available. If not, the cricothyroidotomy tube can be left in place (Figure 38.3).

Commercial percutaneous cricothyroidotomy kits using the Seldinger technique are available. A needle is inserted into the trachea via the cricothyroid membrane and a wire passed through the needle. Make a small skin and subcutaneous incision. Pass the wire through the dilator over which sits a #6 cuffed tube. Then insert the dilator/tracheostomy tube unit into the trachea using the wire as a guide. Remove the wire and dilator, leaving the tube in place. Clinicians familiar with the technique, which requires some force, can place these tubes rapidly. However, in an emergency, use the most familiar technique. In any case, it is unlikely that you will have access to these kits in remote areas.

Breathing

There are five parts of the breathing assessment (see Table 38.1). The presence of jugular venous distension suggests a tension pneumothorax or cardiac tamponade. If symmetric breath sounds are present, jugular venous distension is most likely due to cardiac tamponade. A tracheal shift is a rare physical finding

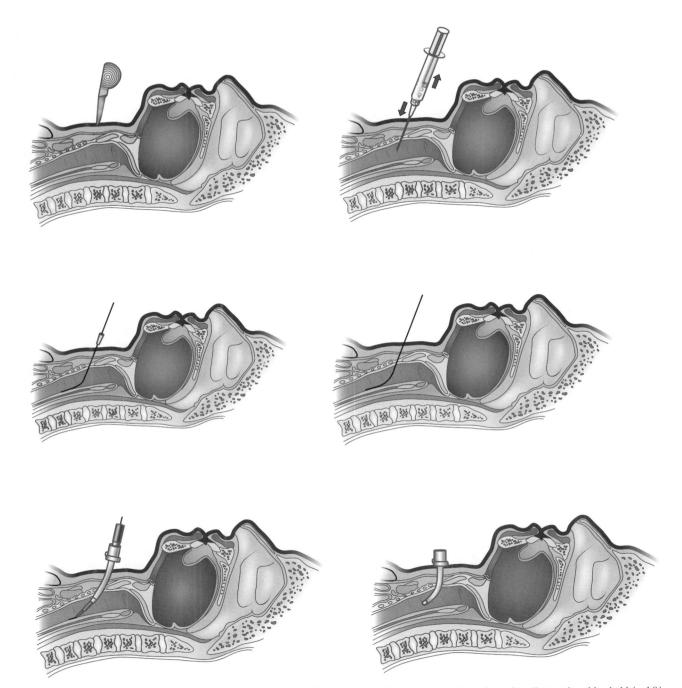

FIGURE 38.3 Cricothyroidotomy. Image by Janet Fong. 2010 [updated 2013 Dec; cited 2014 Jan 27]. Available from: http://www.aic.cuhk.edu.hk/web8/cricothyroidotomy.htm

associated with a contralateral pneumothorax. A tension pneumothorax more often is associated with asymmetric chest wall expansion and ipsilateral decreased breath sounds.

There are two life-threatening problems that must be immediately identified and treated in the "breathing" component of the primary survey: tension pneumothorax and hemothorax. Both of these problems are treated by tube thoracostomy and may occur simultaneously. A tension pneumothorax can be distinguished clinically from a simple pneumothorax by hypotension. Decreased breath sounds and hypotension require immediate pleural decompression without waiting for a chest X-ray.

Needle thoracostomy (Figure 38.4) will immediately decompress a tension pneumothorax. Insert the needle in the second or third intercostal space in the midclavicular line. Hit the rib with the needle and walk off the superior edge of the rib to avoid the possibility of injuring the intercostal artery which passes along the inferior portion of the rib. The needle thoracostomy will equalize the pressure between the pleural space and the atmosphere, resulting in a simple pneumothorax. Placement of a chest tube is therefore mandatory.

A chest tube should be placed under sterile conditions with sufficient local anesthesia. Use 30 cc of 1% Xylocaine in an adult

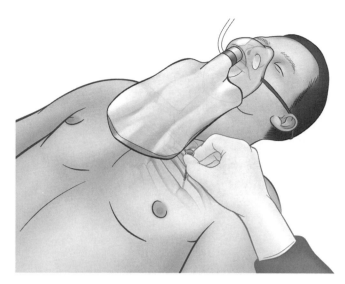

FIGURE 38.4 Needle thoacostomy. Image by Janet Fong, 2010 [updated 2013 Dec; cited 2014 Jan 27]. Available from: http://www.aic.cuhk.edu.hk /web8/Hi%20res/needle%20thoracostomy%20(janet).jpg

infiltrating the periosteum of the rib above and below the fifth intercostal space. Make the skin incision large enough to admit your index finger. A large clamp should be used to dissect the intercostal muscles. Then enter the pleural space. Insert your index finger into the pleural space to ensure that the lung is not stuck up to the chest wall. Then insert a #36 chest tube superomedially, making sure that all the holes in the tube are in the pleural space. Connect the tube to underwater seal and suture it in place. If you don't have commercial chest tubes, any sterile tube connected to underwater seal will serve the purpose.

Circulation

There are seven maneuvers included in the circulation component of the primary survey (see Table 38.1). Control of external hemorrhage is the first priority. In addition to extremity bleeding (previously discussed), bleeding from the scalp is a frequent problem. Dressing the scalp covers the wound but does not stop the bleeding. A running locking stitch will achieve a watertight closure allowing a clot to tamponade the bleeding. Skin staples are an alternative rapid closure if available. The patient can be taken to the OR for suture removal, wound toilet, and definitive hemostasis after stabilization.

A palpable radial pulse generally indicates a systolic pressure above 90 Torr. A weak, rapid pulse after trauma is a sign of hypovolemia. A blood pressure measurement will confirm hypotension. Two large-bore IVs (at least 16-gauge) are recommended for adults. Blood should be sent for type and crossmatch if you are fortunate enough to have a blood bank. Hypovolemia should be treated with a 2 L infusion of warm crystalloid solution. If the patient fails to respond, blood should be administered if available.

If there is a penetrating injury to the anterior chest and upper abdomen, consider the diagnosis of cardiac tamponade. Beck's triad (jugular venous distension, muffled heart sounds, and hypotension) is associated with cardiac tamponade. Pulses paradoxicus (a fall in systolic blood pressure > 10 mmHg on inspiration) is

associated with cardiac tamponade, tension pneumothorax, pulmonary hypertension, and obstructive lung disease. If an ultrasound machine is available, it will demonstrate the presence of pericardial fluid. It can also be used to guide pericardiocentesis.

Cardiac tamponade requires immediate treatment. If this diagnosis is suspected and you have access to an OR, transport the patient immediately. Maintain verbal contact with the patient. Mental status is an excellent sign of cerebral perfusion. Patients with tamponade frequently arrest on induction of anesthesia. The patient should be prepped and draped and the surgical team scrubbed before induction of anesthesia if possible. If the patient is stable and the diagnosis is in doubt, start with a pericardial window. This procedure involves making an upper midline abdominal incision through the fascia, elevating the xyphoid, grasping the pericardium with a hook to pull it inferiorly, and making a small incision in the pericardium. If there is clear fluid, hemopericardium is excluded. If blood is present, a left anterior thoracotomy or median sternotomy is required to expose and repair the heart injury.

If you don't have access to an OR, your only option is pericardiocentesis. This treatment is usually not effective unless the hole in the heart is small. I use an 18 spinal needle attached to a 12 cc syringe. If you have an intravenous (IV) extension tubing and a three-way stopcock, the operator can stabilize the needle while an assistant aspirates the blood. If ultrasound is available, it should be used to guide placement of the needle. If not, you will be unsure whether the blood you are aspirating is coming from the ventricle or the pericardium. If you have an electrocardiogram (EKG) machine and alligator clips, you can run a V-1 EKG strip and connect the V-1 lead to the needle as you insert it. Insert the needle in the subxiphoid position and aim toward the left shoulder. If you encounter an elevated ST segment (current of injury) during needle insertion, it means that the needle is in the wall of the ventricle. If you aspirate blood without a current of injury, the needle is most likely in the pericardium. There are commercial pericardiocentesis kits containing catheters which can be placed in the pericardium with the Seldinger technique. These catheters can be used for repeated aspiration but are most useful for serous collections.

Disability

The disability component of the primary survey is really a mini-neurologic exam. The word *disability* was used because it begins with the letter *D* (ABCDE). It has three components: examination of the pupils, mental status, and extremity motion (see Table 38.1). Symmetric pupils that respond to light indicate an intact reflex arc from the optic nerve to the third cranial nerve (carrying parasympathetic fibers from the Edinger-Westphal nucleus in the midbrain to the pupillary constrictor muscles). A unilateral dilated pupil after trauma is most often due to herniation of the uncus of the cerebellum over the tentorium cerebelli causing pressure on the ipsilateral 3rd cranial nerve. Direct ocular trauma or homatropine ophthalmic drops can also cause papillary dilation. Bilateral dilated pupils unresponsive to light with absent corneal reflexes are a poor prognostic sign associated with brain death.

Mental status should be assessed in all patients. A convenient universally accepted method is the Glasgow coma scale (see Table 38.4)[4]. Scores of 13–15 indicate mild disability. Scores of

TABLE 38.4

Glasgow coma scale

Eye opening	Spontaneously	4
	To speech	3
	To pain	2
	None	1
Verbal response	Orientated	5
	Confused	4
	Inappropriate	3
	Incomprehensible	2
	None	1
Motor response	Obeys commands	6
	Localizes to pain	5
	Withdraws from pain	4
	Flexion to pain	3
	Extension to pain	2
	None	1
Maximum score		15

TABLE 38.5

Life-threatening injuries requiring diagnosis and treatment during the primary survey

1.	Airway obstruction
2.	Tension pneumothorax
3.	Massive hemothorax
4.	Sucking chest wound
5.	Cardiac tamponade
6.	Shock

TABLE 38.6

Resuscitation stage

1.	Review ABCD
2.	Monitors (EKG, pulse oximetry, blood pressure, capnometer)
3.	Gastric tube
4.	Urinary catheter
5.	AP chest X-ray
6.	AP pelvic X-ray

8–13 indicate moderate disability. Severe disability, a Glasgow coma score ≤ 8, is an indication for intubation to prevent pulmonary aspiration of gastric contents.

If the patient moves all four extremities to command, paraplegia is excluded. If the patient is obtunded or unconscious, administer a noxious stimulus. Pinch the skin under the axilla. If the patient moves only the ipsilateral side, pinch the skin in the contralateral axilla. If the legs do not move, pinch the legs. If neither the upper nor lower extremities move, apply supraorbital pressure. A grimace or movement above the shoulders suggests quadriplegia. Be sure to record the findings. If the patient is later discovered to be paraplegic, the question always arises: "Was he paraplegic on arrival?"

Exposure/Environment

There are three parts of the exposure/environment section of ATLS: undress the patient, log roll the patient to examine the back, and then cover the patient to maintain warmth (see Table 38.1).

Complete exposure of the patient is important to exclude penetrating injuries. However, be aware of your surroundings. In an austere environment, you can affect outcome only by stopping external hemorrhage, opening the airway, decompressing a tension pneumothorax, and maintaining body heat. Exposing a patient in a cold environment without the possibility of treatment will adversely affect outcome.

Correct log rolling is a four-person job. One person maintains in-line traction on the head and one on the feet. Two people control the trunk. The patient is rotated 90 degrees. Look for signs of injury. Palpate the thoracic and lumbosacral spine looking for step-offs associated with a fractured spine.

Now is a good time to do a rectal exam when the patient is in the lateral position. Check for a high riding prostate, a sign of transection of the membranous urethra (almost always associated with a pelvic fracture), or gross blood (which could signify a bowel injury).

The life-threatening conditions which must be diagnosed and treated during the primary survey are listed in Table 38.5. It is important to carefully consider and either treat or exclude each of these diagnoses based on the clinical findings.

Stage of Resuscitation

After completion of the primary survey, proceed immediately to the stage of resuscitation (see Table 38.6). The first step is a review of A, B, C, and D. Is the airway still intact? If the patient was intubated in the primary survey, is the tube in the correct position? Does the patient have bilateral breath sounds? If a chest tube was inserted during the primary survey, is it still in the correct position? What is the chest tube output? Has there been a change in the hemodynamic status of the patient? If the patient was initially hypotensive during the primary survey, has he responded to the fluid challenge? If not, does the patient need blood? Has there been any change in the patient's mental status? The patient should be connected to a pulse oximeter, continuous blood pressure monitor, EKG, and capnometer, if available. If appropriate, arterial blood gases should be measured. In many hospitals in developing nations, these monitors are unavailable. If this is the case, the patient will have to be monitored by checking vital signs and mental status. The ATLS program prioritizes patient management. If there is a team of people available to manage the patient, monitors are usually connected to the patient during the primary survey. Nevertheless, they are listed in the stage of resuscitation because of their position in the hierarchy of priorities.

At this point, a urinary catheter and gastric tube should be inserted if indicated. All moderately and severely injured patients require a urinary catheter to monitor urine output. Inspect the perineum prior to insertion of the catheter. Perineal swelling and blood at the urethral meatus in addition to a high riding prostate are physical findings associated with urethral transaction. If an attempt to place a urinary catheter is unsuccessful, a suprapubic urinary catheter is usually required. In hospitals with specialist capability, a catheter can sometimes be passed with cystoscopic guidance after studying the injury with a retrograde urethrogram. Gastric intubation is indicated to treat gastric distension and prevent aspiration pneumonia. Pass the tube through the mouth instead of the nose in the presence of facial fractures to avoid inadvertent intubation of the cranial vault through a fractured cribriform plate.

The last component of the stage of resuscitation involves radiology. The most important film is the anteroposterior (AP) chest X-ray. Two liters of blood can hide in each pleural space in a supine injured patient with minimal physical findings on chest examination. Delay in obtaining a chest X-ray is a common cause of underestimation of severity of injury.

The next most important X-ray is an AP view of the pelvis. A major pelvic fracture can be an important cause of extraperitoneal pelvic hemorrhage. Early diagnosis is important to stabilize the fracture with a pelvic binder and arrange urgent angiographic embolization of the source of bleeding in the unlikely event that this technology is available.

Computerized tomographic (CT) scans of the neck have replaced crosstable lateral cervical spine films to exclude cervical spine injuries because of increased accuracy. If CT scans are unavailable, assume that the blunt trauma victim, particularly one with a head injury, has a cervical spine injury and maintain spine immobilization until the injury can be excluded clinically or radiographically.

The Secondary Survey

The secondary survey as envisioned by ATLS is a head-to-toe physical examination. As a concept, it has much broader application. In a real sense, images obtained in the CT scanner or angiography suite are part of "the secondary survey" since they identify injuries hidden to the clinician's natural senses. Similarly, an exploratory laparotomy or thoracotomy performed in an unstable patient facilitates precise diagnosis and treatment. The important point is initiation of effective treatment of all life-threatening injuries as soon as possible.

The head-to-toe physical examination should be a repetitive process. Each examination should be more detailed, focusing on subtle findings that may have been overlooked during the primary survey and initial examination. Life-threatening injuries should be treated immediately rather than delaying treatment until the end of the exam. In practice, treatment and examination proceed simultaneously. An abbreviated medical history is important. The mnemonic AMPLE is useful to emphasize the key points: allergy, medications, previous hospitalization and operations, last meal, events surrounding the injury (i.e., mechanism of injury). If the patient is responsive but requires intubation, take an AMPLE history if possible as preparations are being made for intubation. Now is a good time to get the name and phone number of a relative. Once the tube goes in, the opportunity is lost.

Head

Palpate the skull looking for scalp lacerations and depressed skull fractures. Actively bleeding scalp lacerations should be rapidly closed to control bleeding if this step was omitted in the primary survey. Examine the mastoid processes looking for a hematoma (Battle's sign), a finding associated with basal skull fracture.

Face

Palpate the supra and infraorbital rims, the zygomas, the nose, the maxilla, and the mandible. Examine the teeth. Do not put your fingers in the patient's mouth—you may be bitten! Search for periorbital hematomas (raccoon eyes) and cerebrospinal fluid (CSF) otorrhea and rhinorrhea. These signs are also associated with basal skull fractures.

Neck

Open the anterior portion of the cervical spine collar if the patient is wearing one. Reexamine the jugular veins and the trachea. Slip your hand behind the neck and feel for swelling or step-offs that may be a sign of cervical spine fracture. Reattach the anterior portion of the cervical spine collar.

Chest

Now take a moment and step back to observe the patient's respiratory pattern. It is easy to miss a subtle flail chest during the rush of the primary survey. Flail chest is a condition which occurs when there are two or more contiguous ribs fractured in multiple places in a segment of the chest wall. The injured segment is "free-floating." On inspiration, this segment will be paradoxically sucked into the chest while the rest of the chest wall expands. Fractures of the costochondral junctions on either side of the sternum can also result in a flail sternum. Some cases of flail chest can be treated by chest wall analgesia and pulmonary physiotherapy. However, if the work of breathing is too great or gas exchange deteriorates due to an underlying pulmonary contusion, intubation and positive pressure ventilation are essential.

Abdomen

Inspect the abdomen looking for bruises or evidence of penetrating injury. A "seat-belt sign," a bruise across the chest and abdomen caused by impact of the seat belt, is sometimes an indication of underlying small bowel and pancreatic injury. Look to see if the abdomen is scaphoid or distended. A distended abdomen may indicate free air from a ruptured viscus or intra-abdominal hemorrhage. If the patient is conscious, look for signs of peritoneal irritation. Your goal is to move the peritoneum with as little stimulus as possible. Ask the patient to cough. Abdominal tenderness after coughing is an important sign of peritoneal irritation. If the patient has an umbilical hernia, the peritoneum is just underneath the skin. Gently tap on the skin to elicit pain. Next, gently palpate the four abdominal quadrants looking for tenderness. Then percuss the four abdominal quadrants to give a graded stimulus to the abdomen. If no pain is elicited, deeply palpate the four abdominal quadrants. After deep palpation, release the pressure suddenly to search for "rebound tenderness."

Abdominal auscultation, while recommended by the ATLS, does not provide much useful information unless the patient has high pitched bowel sounds associated with a bowel obstruction (an unlikely presentation immediately after injury). Unfortunately, bowel sounds can be present after severe injury or "absent" in a perfectly normal patient. If a patient is unconscious or paralyzed, the abdominal physical examination is unreliable.

Pelvis

Although ATLS recommends gentle palpation of the pelvis to assess stability, I consider pelvic fracture to be a radiologic diagnosis. Vigorous movement of a fractured pelvis increases bleeding. If the patient has an "open book" pelvic fracture (i.e., a fracture of the pubic symphysis widening at the pelvic ring), reducing the fracture reduces the volume of the pelvis and probably limits bleeding due to the tamponade effect of the retroperitoneal hematoma. Immediate external fixation is unnecessary in the immediate postinjury period. Effective reduction can be temporarily achieved with a commercially available pelvic binder. Alternatively, a folded sheet placed under the patient and tightly secured anteriorly over the pelvis serves the same function.

Extremities

Inspect and palpate all four extremities looking for external rotation, malalignment, swelling, crepitus, or localized pain. Palpate and record the carotid, brachial radial, femoral, popliteal, dorsalis pedis, and posterior tibial pulses. Pay particular attention to pulses distal to a suspected fracture. Carefully examine and record sensory and motor function distal to a suspected fracture. Long bone fractures with a distal pulse deficit should be reduced by inline traction. All fractures should be immobilized and splinted. Avoid circumferential dressings or casts until you are sure that the patient has stabilized. Be alert to the development of a compartment syndrome (elevated pressure due to swelling in the subfascial compartments of the extremities), which may cause muscle and nerve death ultimately leading to loss of function and/or amputation. Pain and decreased sensation distal to the affected area are the first signs to appear. Swelling and firmness of the compartment and pain on passive motion are also associated findings. A pulse deficit is the last finding to appear. If you wait for a pulse deficit prior to fasciotomy, you have waited too long.

Neurological Examination

Now is the time to perform a more detailed neurological examination. Re-examine the patient's mental status. Examine cranial nerves II–XII. Do a detailed examination of the motor and sensory status of all four extremities. Examine the reflexes of the upper and lower extremities. A more detailed examination of the unconscious patient is beyond the scope of this chapter.

Potential injuries that should be diagnosed during the secondary survey are listed in Table 38.7. These injuries threaten the patient in a delayed fashion. The diagnosis and treatment of some of them may not be possible depending on the available resources.

TABLE 38.7

Potentially life-threatening injuries requiring diagnosis during the Secondary Survey

1. Simple pneumothorax
2. Pulmonary contusion
3. Flail chest
4. Blunt aortic injury
5. Esophageal perforation
6. Diaphragmatic injury
7. Intra-abdominal injury
   a. Intra-abdominal hemorrhage
   b. Hollow viscus injury
   c. Pelvic fracture

BOX 38.1   LMIC-SPECIFIC CONSIDERATIONS

Delayed transport means that many patients die before reaching hospital.

Inadequate or absent blood bank means that many patients will bleed to death after arrival to hospital.

Limited imaging capability means that many injuries will be missed.

Limited or absent surgical capability means that some patients with surgically correctable injuries will die.

Limited or absent ICU capability means that postoperative care will be rudimentary.

BOX 38.2   KEY POTENTIAL PITFALLS TO AVOID

Do not focus on the "obvious" injury. Focus on the primary survey.

Stop external hemorrhage!

Secure the airway early if required.

Don't miss a tension pneumothorax causing hypotension.

Synthesis

If you are in a facility lacking surgical or intensive care unit (ICU) resources, patients with life-threatening intrathoracic or intra-abdominal hemorrhage by this time will be dead due to uncontrolled hemorrhage. Patients with bowel injury and peritonitis will be dead in 24–72 hours of severe sepsis without surgical intervention.

Make a list of all known, suspected, and possible injuries. Do your best to exclude suspected and possible injuries given the available resources and the (im)possibility of transfer to another facility for definitive care.

If you have surgical capability, remember that hemostasis is the key factor in survival. Do not leave bleeding patients in the casualty ward expecting fluid resuscitation to improve the situation. Immediate transfer to the OR for control of hemorrhage, continuing resuscitation and completion of the diagnostic workup, is the key to success.

COMMENTARY

Sebastian O. Ekenze, Nigeria

Trauma is a major cause of preventable morbidity and mortality in LMICs. This is a growing health concern due mostly to the following factors: increasing sophistication and rapid growth of motorized transport without adequate safety precautions, increasing regional conflicts, and terrorism.

Significant challenges exist in the care of trauma patients in LMICs. These challenges are related to delayed presentation of trauma patients (due to lack of education, financial resources, and emergency vehicle services), capacity (lack of infrastructure and shortage of physical and human resources), and lack of proper emergency medical services. As a result, there is inadequate evaluation and management of trauma patients.

In the initial evaluation of trauma patients, it is important to emphasize that, while ATLS is the gold standard, its application in LMICs may need to be tailored to the capacity in this setting. Most health facilities in LMICs lack facilities for airway, breathing management, and vascular access. Facilities for focused resuscitation and investigations are also limited.

Understanding the principles of ATLS is thus indispensable in this setting to achieve an organized approach to the care of the injured patient. For the few patients who may present within the "golden hour" and those who present after a few hours with life-threatening conditions, the phases of ATLS (primary survey, resuscitation, secondary survey, and definitive care) may be applied as the facilities permit in order to achieve resuscitation, diagnosis, and treatment of the conditions. However, the cases that present late in poor clinical state (probably from inadequate or inappropriate treatment before presentation) may require a more thorough initial history and physical examination to determine the extent of the problem and the contributory factors.

In LMICs, the decision to operate during the initial evaluation of trauma patients with deteriorating clinical condition is critical especially in the event of inconclusive diagnosis due to lack of requisite diagnostic facilities. In such cases, it may be life-saving to undertake operative treatment based on clinical findings.

39

Amputation

Samuel C. Schecter
Nikolaj Wolfson

Introduction

Amputation is an important skill for physicians practicing in the developing world. Extremity injuries requiring amputation are caused by road-traffic accidents,[1] workplace injuries,[2] natural disasters, interpersonal violence, and warfare.[3] Neurovascular complications of diabetes compounded by poor nutrition are other leading causes of amputation.[4] When aggressive efforts at limb salvage fail, decisive and skillful amputation provides the best hope for survival and optimal functional outcome.

The goal of this chapter is to provide a practical guide for the evaluation and treatment of patients with devastating extremity injury requiring amputation.

General Principles

Approach to the Injured Patient

Triage of patients in both the rural and urban settings must be performed with consideration of the available resources. The approach to the patient with a limb-threatening injury is based on the principles of Advanced Trauma Life Support (http://www.facs.org/trauma/atls/). Once life-threatening injuries are identified and treated, attention is turned to the threatened limb.

Anesthesia

Major amputations may be performed with epidural, spinal, or general anesthesia. Immediate postoperative pain is decreased in patients receiving epidural or spinal anesthesia compared to general anesthesia.[5] However, there is no demonstrable difference in pain between the groups two years after amputation.[5] The type of anesthetic used for amputation must be appropriate to the available resources and the condition of the patient.

Wound Management

Management strategies depend on the type of extremity injury at presentation (Table 39.1). Proper assessment of the wound is essential.

Open vs. Closed Wounds

The most important factor dictating care of an extremity injury is the presence of an open or closed fracture or joint. An open injury is a skin laceration in communication with either the bone or joint space (Figure 39.1A). A closed fracture has no associated disruption in skin integrity (Figure 39.1B). Complete examination of the injured extremity is mandatory as small lacerations may be subtle but significant. Antibiotics active against *Staphylococcus* and *Clostridia* species and tetanus toxoid should be administered immediately upon identification of an open fracture. Open fractures or joint spaces require an exam under anesthesia, debridement of nonviable soft tissue, and copious irrigation. After induction of anesthesia, the extremity should first be washed with soap and water to remove gross contamination and then prepped and draped in a sterile fashion.

With an open fracture, the wound is explored and enlarged as needed to evaluate the fracture. Gross contamination must be removed. A scrub brush and a dilute solution of Betadine in sterile water or saline are used to scrub the exposed fracture. After scrubbing, the wound must be irrigated with copious amounts of normal saline, delivered under mild to moderate pressure. Some surgeons add bacitracin 50 units/ml to the irrigation solution, although there is only weak evidence to support this practice.[6] The wound is dressed open with a dilute Betadine-soaked gauze until the patient returns to the operating theater within 48 hours for reexamination.

An open joint requires special consideration because of the high risk of functional impairment should the space become infected. An open joint space is present if there is a tear in the joint capsule or evidence of a leak after injection of the joint space with methylene blue, or sterile saline. If there is a tear in the joint capsule, irrigation of the joint space with copious sterile saline is mandatory. If there is concern for compromise of the joint space without definitive evidence, inject a dilute methylene blue solution, or sterile saline, into the joint space in a clean, uncontaminated area and search for leak. When injecting methylene blue, intra-articular needle placement should be confirmed and a minimum of 50 ml injected into the joint space. If using sterile saline, an injection of between 155 ml and 194 ml will identify 95% of capsule injuries. If a leak is present the joint space will require irrigation.

TABLE 39.1

Wound management considerations

Open vs. closed wounds
Tidy vs. untidy wounds
Fracture classification
Crush injury
Neurovascular injury

Table created by Nikolaj Wolfson and Samuel C. Schecter.

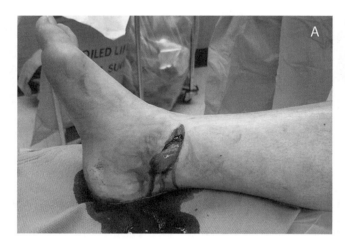

FIGURE 39.1A   Open ankle fracture. Image by Nikolaj Wolfson.

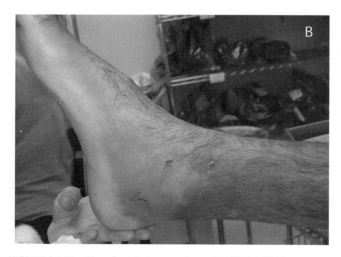

FIGURE 39.1B   Closed ankle fracture. Image by Nikolaj Wolfson.

Never perform a definitive repair of an open orthopedic injury on the first operative debridement. Patients will require multiple trips to the operative theater for wound evaluation and debridement prior to internal fixation of their injuries. Delayed primary closure of a clean wound is often possible following repeat assessment and offers the best chance of success.

Tidy vs. Untidy Wounds

Soft-tissue wounds are classified as tidy or untidy. A tidy wound is produced by a sharp object such as a knife or glass, and has minimal contamination and well-vascularized skin edges (Figure 39.2A).

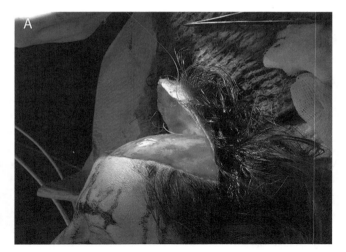

FIGURE 39.2A   Tidy wound to scalp with clean, well-defined edges. Image by Samuel C. Schecter.

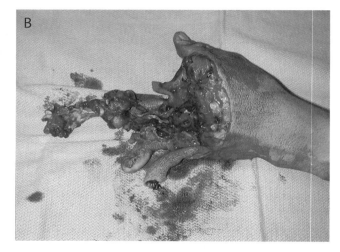

FIGURE 39.2B   Untidy wound of the hand with devascularized tissue and irregular borders. Image by Scott Hanson.

An untidy wound has irregular borders with areas of missing or devitalized soft tissue or bone (Figure 39.2B). The first step in the management of any wound is to cleanse and explore the wound. Tidy wounds require minimal debridement. Untidy wounds require debridement of all nonviable tissue. Both wounds will be left open, but patients with untidy wounds must return to the operating theater within 12–24 hours for further debridement as the initial assessment of soft-tissue viability is difficult.

Complex Fracture Management

Complex fractures, or fractures with extensive soft-tissue damage, may result in delayed union, non-union, or limb deformity (Figure 39.3A and Figure 39.3B). The risk of complications is greater in the presence of open, contaminated wounds. The Gustilo-Anderson classification of open fractures is a useful guide to risk stratification (Table 39.2).[7,8] Internal fixation is the optimal method of long bone fixation but should be delayed for

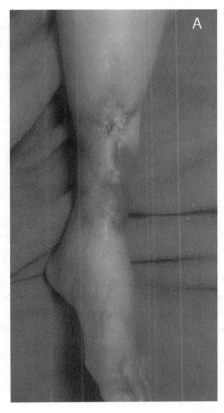

FIGURE 39.3A   Scarred soft tissue. Image by Nikolaj Wolfson.

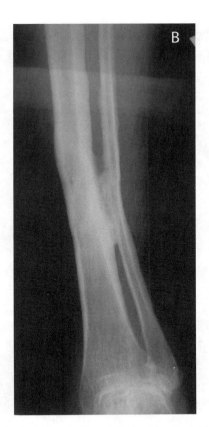

FIGURE 39.3B   Malunion of tibia and fibula with valgus deformity. Image by Nikolaj Wolfson.

TABLE 39.2

Gustilo-Anderson classification of open fractures[7,8]

Type	Soft-tissue injury	Other	Wound sepsis	Amputation rate
I	< 1cm	–	–	–
II	> 1 cm, < 10 cm	–	–	
IIIA	> 10 cm with available coverage	Segmental fractures, heavy contamination, high-velocity gunshot wounds	4%	0%
IIIB	> 10 cm without primary soft-tissue coverage	Periosteal stripping	52%	16%
IIIC		Vascular injury requiring repair	42%	42%

Table created by Nikolaj Wolfson and Samuel C. Schecter.

Gustilo IIIB or IIIC fractures due to the high risk of infection. These complex fractures, defined as open, multi-segment fractures with minimal native soft-tissue coverage, require cleansing, scrubbing, debridement, and placement of an external fixation device.

External fixation devices are either uniplanar or multi-planar. Multi-planar ringed external fixation devices maintain alignment and permit gradual increased weight-bearing while at the same time allowing for complex wound debridement and dressing changes (Figure 39.4). Patients may be required to have an external fixation device in place for many months if the fracture is not amenable to delayed internal fixation.

Crush Injury

Crush injury causes irreversible muscle injury with neurovascular compromise. The severity is difficult to determine immediately following injury. Crush injury should be suspected in the presence of limb swelling, erythema, skin pallor, pain with passive movement, paresthesias, and motor deficits. The clinical sequelae of crush injury are rhabdomyolysis, compartment syndrome, and renal failure due to myoglobinuria. Aggressive management, including external fracture fixation, wide fasciotomy, and fluid and electrolyte resuscitation, is essential to reduce the risk of renal failure, myonecrosis, and infection. Prompt amputation is indicated for severe soft-tissue injury associated with multi-organ failure.

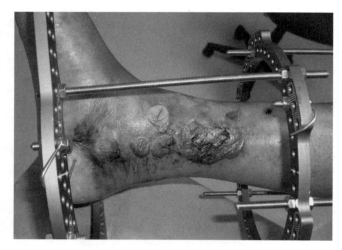

FIGURE 39.4 Multi-planar ringed external fixation device. Image by Nikolaj Wolfson.

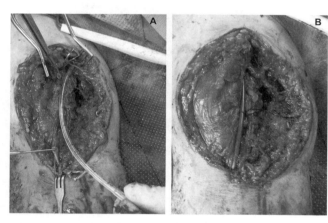

FIGURE 39.5 Vascular shunt placement for temporary limb perfusion. This patient suffered a transection of the brachial artery with a long gap defect. A) Sizing up a #4 pediatric feeding tube for placement into the arterial lumen. B) Shunt in place; notice the silk suture tied around the middle of the tube for identification. Images by William Schecter.

Neurovascular Injury

A major neurovascular injury directly threatens the viability and function of the limb. The first step is control of hemorrhage. Tourniquet placement above the level of an arterial injury can be life-saving and permit limb salvage if there is timely access to an operating theater.

Restoration of blood flow to an ischemic limb within 6 hours is essential. Rarely, if the warm ischemia time is very short, rapid fixation of a fracture is appropriate prior to revascularization. Almost always, revascularization should precede skeletal stabilization. Primary arterial repair is appropriate if a tension-free anastomosis is possible and minimal manipulation of the fracture is required.

Otherwise, a temporary vascular shunt (Figure 39.5) bridging the arterial defect permits rapid restoration of flow prior to skeletal stabilization. After stabilization is complete, an interposition graft of contralateral reversed saphenous vein or a synthetic graft can be used for definitive vascular repair. To reduce the risk of infection, autogenous vein is preferred. If the patient requires a damage-control operation because of hemodynamic instability, the arterial shunt may be left in place until definitive reconstruction can be safely performed.

When confronted with a combined arterial and venous injury, we recommend repair of the artery prior to the vein to rapidly restore blood flow to the extremity. Repair of the vein prior to the artery may sometimes be performed if warm ischemia time is short in an effort to prevent compartment syndrome. Attempts should be made to repair named veins above the popliteal fossa. Veins below the popliteal fossa need not be repaired.

Aggressive fasciotomies should be performed in all cases of prolonged warm ischemia time (greater than 2–3 hours) and crush injury.[9]

If the tibial nerve is disrupted, the patient loses sensation to the foot and plantar flexion. If the nerve injury occurs due to crush or high-velocity penetrating trauma, in conjunction with a complex or contaminated wound, primary amputation should be considered. If the nerve has been sharply transected (an unusual occurrence), it may be repaired with use of magnification.

Indications for Amputation

The decision to perform an amputation is based on a combination of patient, surgeon, and facility factors.

Patient Factors

The important patient factors include: the condition of the patient, the type of extremity injury, and the presence or absence of necrotizing soft-tissue or bony infection. Faced with a nonviable limb and the presence of hemodynamic and/or respiratory compromise, amputation of the extremity must be considered. Preservation of life over limb is paramount.

The type of injury sustained by the patient is a major determinant of the decision to perform an amputation and the method of amputation. The mangled extremity, involving neurovascular, skeletal, and soft-tissue structures with excessive tissue loss has a high potential for limb loss (Figure 39.6).[10] Attempts have been made to classify outcomes by the severity of damage to an extremity. Unfortunately, none of the scoring systems accurately predict the need for amputation.[11] Advancements in vascular and reconstructive surgery now permit salvage of severely mangled extremities in well-equipped centers. However, simplification of complex extremity wounds by amputation has merit in many austere settings.[12] All contaminated amputation wounds must be

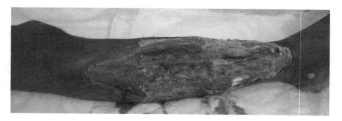

FIGURE 39.6 Mangled extremity with large soft-tissue and bone defect. Image by Nikolaj Wolfson.

left open to reduce the risk of extensive local infection and/or sepsis. A guillotine amputation, followed by definitive closure several days later, is recommended for contaminated and grossly infected wounds.

Surgeon and Facility Factors

The type of surgical intervention for the critical threatened limb depends on the skills and experience of the surgeon as well as the available resources for perioperative care. An attempt to salvage a mangled extremity is unwise in the absence of the necessary surgical skill set and facilities for long-term postoperative care and rehabilitation.

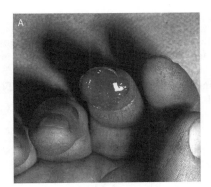

FIGURE 39.7A Amputated pulp of right third finger distal phalanx. Image by William Schecter.

Surgical Technique

Introduction

In an ideal setting, the care of amputation patients takes place in a multidisciplinary setting with skilled surgeons working in concert with nursing staff and physical therapists dedicated to orthopedic rehabilitation. In many low- and middle-income countries (LMICs) the workforce and equipment infrastructure is overwhelmed. Meticulous surgical technique and patient motivation must compensate for lacking services.

There are five steps to each amputation:

1. Planning and executing the skin incision
2. Dividing the bone
3. Transection of nerves and vessels
4. Soft-tissue flap closure
5. Dressing the wound

Each step is crucial to the patient's functional outcome.

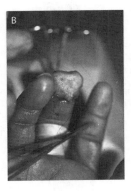

FIGURE 39.7B Full-thickness skin graft to amputation bed. Image by William Schecter.

Upper Extremity Amputations

Injuries requiring amputation of the upper extremity are usually the result of high-energy trauma. All attempts must be made to avoid amputation of the upper extremity because a poorly functioning arm is usually better than a good upper extremity prosthesis.[13] If amputation is required, preservation of maximum bony length is key.

Finger and Ray Amputation

Finger and ray amputation is a complex subject. The general surgeon must be familiar with basic finger amputation principles.

Fingertip soft-tissue avulsions should be left to heal by secondary intention, or covered with a skin graft (Figure 39.7A, Figure 39.7B, and Figure 39.7C).

Index finger amputations distal to the proximal interphalangeal (PIP) joint are treated with simple debriding of the bone surface followed by closure of the skin. To fashion the skin flaps for closure, the incisions should be made longitudinally on the medial and lateral aspects of the digit. If possible the dorsal flap should be shorter than the volar flap to allow the volar tissue

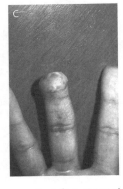

FIGURE 39.7C Three months after amputation. Image by William Schecter.

pad to cover the bony surface and be sutured to the dorsal flap without tension. The nerves must be identified and allowed to retract away from the wound edge. For amputations through or proximal to the PIP joint, the less experienced surgeon may elect for a simple debridement and closure as for distal injuries. The experienced surgeon may elect to perform a ray amputation of the index finger, transecting the second metacarpal bone in the mid hand. This amputation results in improved function, allowing the long finger to substitute for the index finger for maximal pinch strength.

Wrist Disarticulation

Wrist disarticulation is a better option than a transradial amputation if at all possible. If the radioulnar joint is intact, pronation and supination are preserved. The added length of the limb allows for improved power in the residual limb (Figure 39.8A, Figure 39.8B, Figure 39.8C, and Figure 39.8D).[14]

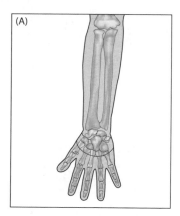

FIGURE 39.8A   Palmar view of planned flaps for wrist disarticulation. Illustration by Magdalene Brooke, MD.

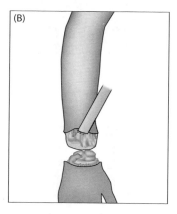

FIGURE 39.8B   Dorsal view of wrist and forearm demonstrating high ligation of arteries and nerves and transection of tendons. Illustration by Magdalene Brooke, MD.

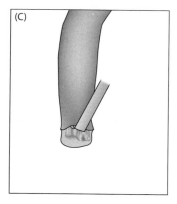

FIGURE 39.8C   Dorsal view of wrist after bones have been filed/rounded. Illustration by Magdalene Brooke, MD.

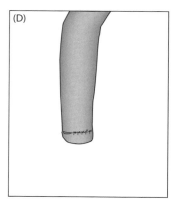

FIGURE 39.8D   Flap closure. Illustration by Magdalene Brooke, MD.

The steps of wrist disarticulation:

1. **Creation of skin flaps.** After prepping the arm from fingers to axilla, drape the arm allowing exposure of the entire upper extremity. A long palmar and short dorsal flap are outlined with a marking pen. The palmar flap should start 1.3 to 1.5 cm distal to the radial styloid process, move up to the palmar crease, and end 1.3 to 1.5 cm distal to the ulnar styloid process. Incision is made along the markings with a #10 blade scalpel to the bone. Care is taken to identify and doubly ligate the radial and ulnar arteries proximal to the level of wrist disarticulation. All tendons are transected at the wrist and allowed to retract into the forearm. The median, ulnar, and radial nerves are identified and transected well proximal to the level of bone transection. The nerves should be infiltrated with local anesthetic prior to transection. The joint capsule is divided and the hand removed from the field.

2. **Bone transection.** The radial and ulnar styloids are removed and the bones filed smooth.

3. **Debride soft tissue and hemostasis.** At this time, the soft-tissue edges are fashioned to allow clean closure of the wound. Hemostasis is achieved.

4. **Closure of flaps.** The palmar flap is placed across the exposed joint surface and the skin closed with 2.0 or 3.0 monofilament. A drain is left in place to evacuate hematoma.

5. **Dressing the wound.** Petroleum gauze or other non-stick dressing should be placed directly onto the suture-line followed by gauze and fluffs to protect the wound. An elastic bandage should be placed to hold the dressings in place and prevent swelling of the wound. The sutures will stay in place for 14–21 days prior to removal.

Forearm Amputation

1. **Creation of skin flaps.** After prepping the arm from fingers to axilla, drape the arm, allowing exposure of the entire upper extremity while wrapping the hand in a sterile towel. With a marking pen, outline anterior to posterior fish-mouth skin flaps. The length of

both anterior and posterior flaps should each be half the diameter of the arm at that level. Incision is made along the markings with a #10 blade scalpel to the bone. Care is taken to identify and doubly ligate the radial and ulnar arteries proximal to the level of bone transection. The median, ulnar, and radial nerves are identified and transected well proximal to the level of bone transection. The nerves should be infiltrated with local anesthetic prior to transection.

2. **Radius and ulna transection.** Bone length should be maximized. The ulna should be slightly longer than the radius for transections proximal to the mid-forearm. The radius should be 1–3 cm longer than the ulnar for transections distal to the mid-forearm. The periosteum is incised at the level of bone transection. The bone is transected with a Gigli saw, handheld bone saw, or cooled power saw and the edges filed smooth.

3. **Debride soft tissue and hemostasis.** The flexor digitorum sublimus is fashioned to a length to wrap around the cut radial and ulnar bones. The other muscles of the anterior compartment are transected at the level of the bone cut. The posterior compartment muscles are excised at the level of the bone cut. At this time, the soft-tissue edges are fashioned to allow clean closure of the wound. Hemostasis is achieved.

4. **Closure of flaps.** Myodesis is performed by sewing the flexor digitorum sublimus fascia to the fascia of the posterior compartment.[14] A closed suction drain is placed deep to the flap to evacuate blood. The subcutaneous tissue is closed in two layers of interrupted absorbable 3.0 sutures. The skin is closed with interrupted 3.0 monofilament sutures.

5. **Dressing the wound.** Petroleum gauze or other non-stick dressing should be placed directly onto the suture-line followed by gauze and fluffs to protect the wound. An elastic bandage should be placed to hold the dressings in place and prevent swelling of the wound. The initial dressing may stay intact for five days. The sutures will stay in place for 14–21 days prior to removal (Figure 39.9A, Figure 39.9B, Figure 39.9C, and Figure 39.9D).

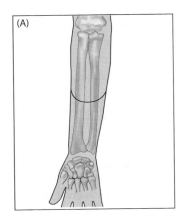

FIGURE 39.9A Planned flaps for forearm amputation. Illustration by Magdalene Brooke, MD.

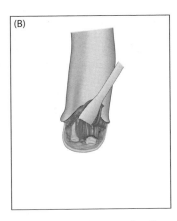

FIGURE 39.9B Post-transection demonstrating ligated arteries, nerves, and veins. Be sure to note that the ulna is longer than the radius. Illustration by Magdalene Brooke, MD.

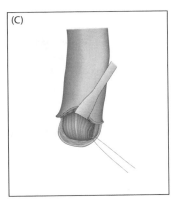

FIGURE 39.9C Myodesis. Illustration by Magdalene Brooke, MD.

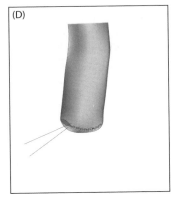

FIGURE 39.9D Flap closure. Illustration by Magdalene Brooke, MD.

Transhumeral Amputation

1. **Creation of skin flaps.** After prepping the arm from fingers to axilla, drape the arm, allowing exposure of the entire upper extremity while wrapping the hand in a sterile towel. With a marking pen, outline anterior to posterior fish-mouth skin flaps. The length of both anterior and posterior flaps should each be half

the diameter of the arm at that level. Incision is made along the markings with a #10 blade scalpel to the bone. Care is taken to identify and doubly ligate the brachial artery and vein proximal to the level of bone transection. The median, ulnar, and radial nerves are identified and transected well proximal to the level of bone transection. The nerves should be infiltrated with local anesthetic prior to transection. The anterior compartment musculature is transected 1.3 cm distal to the proposed bone transection site,[14] while the musculature of the posterior compartment is transected 4–5 cm distal to the bone transection site to allow adequate tissue for bone coverage.

2. **Humeral transection.** Humeral bone length should be maximized, but the bone cut must be made a minimum of 4 cm proximal to the elbow joint to allow proper prosthesis placement. The periosteum is incised at the level of bone transection. The bone is transected with a Gigli saw, handheld bone saw, or cooled power saw and the edges filed smooth.

3. **Debride soft tissue and hemostasis.** At this time, the soft-tissue edges are fashioned to allow clean closure of the wound. Hemostasis is achieved.

4. **Closure of flaps.** Myodesis is performed by bringing the longer triceps fascia forward to suture to the fascia of the anterior compartment musculature.[14] A closed suction drain is placed deep to the flap to evacuate blood. The subcutaneous tissue is closed in two layers of interrupted absorbable 3.0 sutures. The skin is closed with interrupted 3.0 monofilament sutures.

5. **Dressing the wound.** Petroleum gauze or other nonstick dressing should be placed directly onto the suture-line followed by gauze and fluffs to protect the wound. An elastic bandage should be placed to hold the dressings in place and prevent swelling of the wound. The initial dressing may stay intact for five days. The sutures will stay in place for 14–21 days prior to removal (Figure 39.10A, Figure 39.10B, Figure 39.10C, and Figure 39.10D).

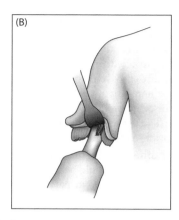

FIGURE 39.10B   Post-transection demonstrating ligated arteries, nerves, and veins. Illustration by Magdalene Brooke, MD.

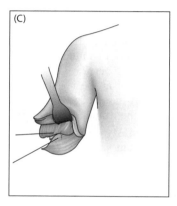

FIGURE 39.10C   Myodesis. Illustration by Magdalene Brooke, MD.

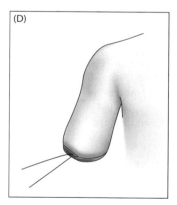

FIGURE 39.10D   Flap closure. Illustration by Magdalene Brooke, MD.

Lower Extremity Amputations

Toe Amputation

1. **Creation of skin flaps.** After prepping the foot and ankle with antiseptic scrub and paint, the foot is draped, allowing exposure of the foot. A sterile marking pen is used to outline fish-mouth flaps of skin allowing adequate, tension-free closure of the wound. The distal portions of the fish-mouth flaps are on the dorsal and

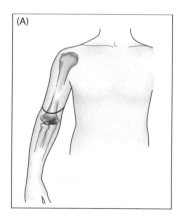

FIGURE 39.10A   Planned flaps for transhumeral amputation. Illustration by Magdalene Brooke, MD.

ventral sides of the toe. The proximal portions are on the medial and lateral aspects. Using a #15 blade scalpel, incision is made down to the bone along the markings. Using a periosteal elevator to raise the periosteum, flaps are created to the proximal third of the phalanx.

2. **Excising the bone.** Using bone shears or another sharp instrument, the proximal phalanx is transected. A rongeur is used to file down the sharp edges of the remaining bone.

3. **Debriding the soft tissue and tendons.** Excess soft tissue and tendon are sharply debrided with Metzenbaum scissors. Active bleeding is controlled with pressure and suture as needed.

4. **Closure of the flaps.** The skin flaps are brought together, without tension, with 2.0 nylon sutures placed in an interrupted fashion. Care should be taken not to crush the tissue edges with the forceps to allow a greater chance of healing.

5. **Dressing the wound.** Petroleum gauze or other non-stick dressing should be placed directly onto the wound followed by gauze and fluffs to protect the wound. An elastic bandage should be placed to hold the dressings in place. Important to note is that the dressing will be in place for at least 48 hours, and it is important to protect the patient's other digits by placing soft gauze or cotton between the toes prior to wrapping the foot.

Postoperative care should consist of non–weight bearing on the affected limb for a minimum of 48 hours, after which time the patient may begin to ambulate with careful unweighting of the incision by use of specialized orthotics. The stitches will remain in place for 14 days. Smokers are actively encouraged to quit smoking to facilitate blood flow to the extremity (Figure 39.11A and Figure 39.11B).

Below-Knee Amputation

The below-knee amputation is the critical amputation procedure for practice in LMICs because of the high prevalence of lower extremity injuries due to road traffic accidents. In certain areas, land mine injuries area also an important cause of major lower extremity injuries. A proper below-knee amputation will allow good prosthesis fit and restore function to a patient with an otherwise disabling injury (Figure 39.12A, Figure 39.12B, Figure 39.12C, and Figure 39.12D).

Steps to perform below-knee amputation:

1. **Creation of skin flaps.** After prepping the leg from foot to mid-thigh with antiseptic scrub and paint, the leg is draped, allowing exposure distal to the mid-thigh. A tourniquet may be applied to the upper thigh and used during the initial portion of the operation to minimize blood loss. A sterile marking pen is used to mark the site of planned bone transection and to outline the skin incision. The anterior skin incision should be a minimum of 2 cm distal to the tibial transection point. The anterior incision should be approximately two-thirds of the diameter of the lower leg. Using a #10 blade scalpel, incision is made down to the bone along the markings. The anterior tibial artery and vein as well as the deep peroneal nerve should be identified, and, under tension, individually doubly suture ligated and divided. The nerve may be injected with local anesthetic prior to transection to prevent excessive post-operative pain. To ensure a tension-free closure of the anterior and posterior skin edges, the length of the posterior flap should be approximately the diameter of the leg plus 3 cm. To prevent an unstable stump, only the skin, subcutaneous tissue, and gastrocnemius muscle are to be incorporated into the posterior flap. The soleus muscle and other soft tissue should be divided just proximal to the start of the posterior flap. The gastrocnemius muscle should be 5–8 cm in length to allow for proper padding of the tibia stump and myodesis. In the posterior aspect of the lower leg, the posterior tibial artery, peroneal artery, and tibial nerve must be identified and doubly suture ligated as previously described.

2. **Tibia and fibula transection.** When planning transection of the tibia, all efforts should be made to preserve

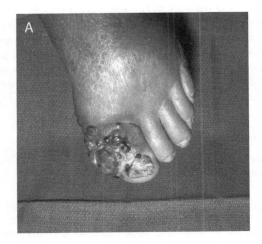

FIGURE 39.11A Squamous cell carcinoma of the left great toe. Image by William Schecter.

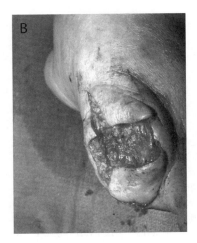

FIGURE 39.11B Amputation of left great toe and first ray. Image by William Schecter.

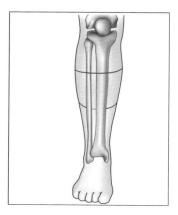

FIGURE 39.12A   Planned flaps for below-knee amputation. Illustration by Magdalene Brooke, MD.

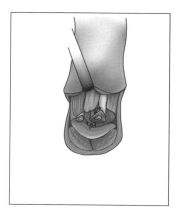

FIGURE 39.12B   Post-transection demonstrating ligated arteries, nerves, and veins. The fibula is transected proximal to the tibia. Illustration by Magdalene Brooke, MD.

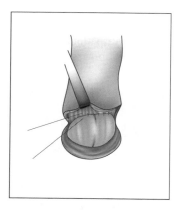

FIGURE 39.12C   Myodesis. Illustration by Magdalene Brooke, MD.

the tibial tuberosity. The tibial tuberosity is the insertion point for the patellar tendon, and its preservation will permit proper knee function postamputation. The ideal site of tibial transection typically preserves 50%–60% of the tibial length. Preservation of 60% of tibial length is the optimal length for prosthesis fitting. After dividing the soft tissue, the bone is circumferentially

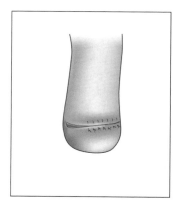

FIGURE 39.12D   Flap closure. Illustration by Magdalene Brooke, MD.

cleared of fascial attachments. Using a Gigli saw, handheld bone saw, or cooled power saw, the tibia is transected ensuring a 45-degree bevel in the anterior cortex. The cortical edges are then filed smooth. The fibula is transected with bone shears 1 cm proximal to the tibia cut.

3. **Debriding the soft tissue and tendons.** Excess tissue and tendon are sharply debrided with Metzenbaum scissors. If a tourniquet has been applied, it is released at this point. Active bleeding is controlled with pressure and suture ligation as needed.

4. **Closure of the flaps.** The wound is irrigated, and hemostasis achieved. The posterior flap is swung forward and the gastrocnemius fascia is sutured to the anterior periosteum or anterior cortex of the tibia. Myodesis, or the suturing of opposing muscle groups together, may be performed at this time. The soft tissue and skin should be closed in multiple layers of interrupted absorbable sutures. Skin should be closed with 3.0 or 4.0 monofilament vertical mattress sutures. Care is taken to avoid uneven closure, or "dog ears." A drain is left in place to prevent hematoma formation. The skin sutures will stay in place for a minimum of 14 days. Care should be taken not to crush the tissue edges with the forceps to allow a greater chance of healing.

5. **Dressing the wound.** Petroleum gauze or other nonstick dressing should be placed directly onto the suture-line followed by gauze and fluffs to protect the wound. An elastic bandage should be placed to hold the dressings in place and prevent swelling of the wound. Finally, the amputation stump, knee, and upper leg should be cast in extension to the mid-thigh to prevent joint contracture. A loss of 20 degrees of extension is a devastating complication as it will preclude the proper use of a prosthesis, making ambulation following amputation difficult at best. The plaster is changed between 2 and 10 days postamputation depending on the state of the wound at operation.

Above-Knee Amputation

An above-knee amputation carries a higher morbidity and mortality than below-knee amputations and, like the below-knee amputation, should be performed in a staged fashion if the wound conditions are unfavorable at first operation (Figure 39.13A, Figure 39.13B, Figure 39.13C, and Figure 39.13D). Preservation of femur length and myoplasty of adductor magnus to the lateral femoral cortex are the keys to good postoperative functional outcomes.

Positioning of the patient is the key to a successful operation. The patient should be supine with the hip flexed and a sterile roll placed under the thigh to maintain position.

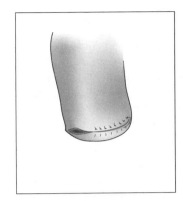

FIGURE 39.13D Flap closure. Illustration by Magdalene Brooke, MD.

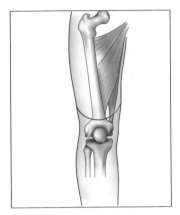

FIGURE 39.13A Planned flaps for above-knee amputation. Illustration by Magdalene Brooke, MD.

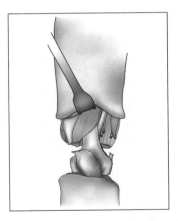

FIGURE 39.13B Post-transection demonstrating ligated arteries, nerves, and veins. Illustration by Magdalene Brooke, MD.

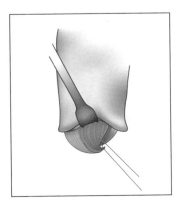

FIGURE 39.13C Myodesis. Illustration by Magdalene Brooke, MD.

1. **Creation of skin flaps.** After prepping the leg from foot to mid-abdomen with antiseptic scrub and paint, the leg is draped, allowing exposure distal to the groin. A tourniquet may be applied to the upper thigh and used during the initial portion of the operation to minimize blood loss. A sterile marking pen is used to mark the site of planned bone transection and to outline the fish-mouth skin incision allowing for anterior to posterior closure at the distal portion of the wound. Using a #10 blade scalpel, incision is made down to the bone along the markings. The quadriceps femoris is cut through its tendon above the patella. The adductor magnus is detached from its distal insertion for later transfer. The hamstrings and posterior muscles are divided just distal to the femur cut. The superficial femoral artery, deep femoral vein, and greater saphenous vein should be identified, divided, and doubly suture ligated. The sciatic nerve travels posteriorly and should be sharply divided well away from the edge of the wound to prevent nerve entrapment on closure. The nerve may be injected with local anesthetic prior to division to inhibit postoperative pain.

2. **Femur transection.** After dividing the soft tissue, the bone is circumferentially cleared of fascial attachments. Using a Gigli saw, handheld bone saw, or cooled power saw, the femur is transected 5 cm proximal to the most distal ventral skin edge incision. The cortical edges are then filed smooth.

3. **Debriding the soft tissue and tendons.** Excess soft tissue and tendon are sharply debrided with Metzenbaum scissors. If a tourniquet has been applied, it is released at this point. Active bleeding is controlled with pressure and suture ligation as needed.

4. **Closure of the flaps.** The wound is irrigated, and hemostasis achieved. With the femur in slight adduction, the adductor magnus is brought behind the femur and then attached to the lateral femoral cortex at the cut end under mild tension. Myodesis is performed by attaching the quadriceps tendon to the deep fascia of the posterior musculature. The soft tissue and skin should be closed in 2–3 layers of interrupted 2.0 absorbable sutures. Skin should be closed with 3.0 or 4.0 monofilament vertical mattress sutures. A drain is left in place

to prevent hematoma formation. The skin sutures will stay in place for a minimum of 14 days. Care should be taken not to crush the tissue edges with the forceps to allow a greater chance of healing.

5. **Dressing the wound.** Petroleum gauze or other nonstick dressing should be placed directly onto the suture-line followed by gauze and fluffs to protect the wound. An elastic bandage should be placed to hold the dressings in place and prevent swelling of the wound. Finally, the amputation stump should be cast in plaster to prevent major hip flexion and swelling in the healing phase. The plaster is changed between 2 and 10 days postamputation depending on the state of the wound at operation.

Other Lower Extremity Amputations

Transmetatarsal amputation, Syme's amputation, hip disarticulation, and forequarter amputation are beyond the scope of this chapter. Transmetatarsal and Syme's amputations are complex and usually require further training.

Complications of Amputation

Early complications of amputation are usually due to technical error or infection (Table 39.3). Postoperative bleeding is likely due to a missed vessel or a failure of suture ligation. Upon identification of hemorrhage, the surgical site should be uncovered an inspected. The patient may require a repeat trip to the operating room to halt surgical bleeding. Wound breakdown may occur from either closure of the wound under tension, or infection. Wound breakdown will delay fitting the amputation stump with a prosthesis, and may require a return trip to the operating room to revise the amputation. Infection in the immediate postoperative period is a risk in any contaminated field, and the reason why definitive closure of a grossly contaminated wound should be delayed. The effect of infection on postoperative recovery is the same as for wound breakdown with the added risk of osteomyelitis and sepsis.

Late complications of amputation include: stump instability, ulceration, contracture, phantom limb pain, neuroma, and heterotopic ossification. Stump instability is a complication of below-knee amputation caused by too bulky a muscular/soft-tissue envelope at the distal stump. The resultant soft-tissue

TABLE 39.3

Complications after amputation

Technical misadventure	Other	Rehabilitation + prosthesis
Delayed hemorrhage	Heterotopic bone formation	Ulceration
Skin flap breakdown	Infection	Contracture
Stump instability	Phantom limb pain	
	Neuroma	

Table created by Nikolaj Wolfson and Samuel C. Schecter.

mass does not provide a stable platform for weight bearing. Ulceration of the stump occurs from poor-fitting prostheses, adherence of skin to the bony surface, or from immobility. The key to avoiding ulceration is good stump and prosthesis care, ensuring soft-tissue coverage of the bone to prevent skin/scar tissue adherence, and relieving pressure points when sitting or lying for long periods of time. Contracture is a debilitating complication inhibiting proper limb function. Contracture is prevented by proper splinting in the immediate postoperative period and aggressive physical therapy following cast removal. Phantom limb pain is the sensation of feeling the amputated limb and occurs in up to 65% of patients at 1 year postamputation. The pain has been described as ranging from an itch to sharp and stabbing. A novel treatment approach is mirror visual feedback therapy which uses a mirror to modify the perception of pain in the affected limb.[15] Neuroma occurs from an overgrowth of neural and scar tissue and may prevent the patient from achieving maximal function. The risk of postoperative neuroma may be reduced by avoiding putting the nerves on stretch and avoiding electrocautery during surgery. Herterotopic ossification is the formation of bone in abnormal sites and occurs in up to 64% of stumps after amputation for high-energy trauma. Heterotopic ossification may lead to pressure point wound breakdown.[16] Treatment of heterotopic ossification consists of resizing the prosthesis or surgical excision of ossified lesions.

Conclusion

Amputation is a mandatory skill in the repertoire of a general surgeon practicing in LMICs. These operations, while simple in concept, are both life-saving and life-defining events. Proper operative judgment and surgical technique ensure the optimal outcome.

COMMENTARY

L.O.A. Thanni, Nigeria

Amputation is no doubt an important operation that results in alteration of the body image. The procedure is commonly performed in some high-income countries (HICs) with a prevalence of 17–30 amputations per 100,000 people in the population. In Nigeria, a low- to middle-income country (LMIC), the prevalence of amputation is about 1.6 amputations per 100,000 people in the population. The patient is most often a young male in the third or fourth decade of life in LMICs, whereas in HICs, he is more likely to be over the age of 70 years.

Knowledge and skill to perform minor and major extremity amputations should be possessed not just by the specialist orthopedic and trauma surgeon in the main city hospitals, but also by general surgeons and senior medical officers in general or district hospitals. This will reduce the need to transport patients over long distances to centers where the competence is available, thus helping to save limb and life.

Trauma resulting mostly from road crashes is the leading indication for amputation in LMICs. In some communities, ischemic gangrene complicating treatment by traditional bonesetters (TBS) is responsible for more than 20% of major amputations. While peripheral artery disease is very common in some HICs, it is an indication for about 2% of major amputations in LMICs. The most challenging clinical situation is when a major amputation is indicated but consent is withheld. An adult patient may withhold consent for the procedure simply because he cannot see his limb removed. Sometimes, an older adult, possible a family head, must consent to the amputation, even though he never visits the hospital. Sometimes, the family head will withhold consent and ask that the patient be brought home to him. When consent is finally given in many of these instances, the patient has developed sepsis and toxemia. It is little wonder that hospital mortality after major amputations is over 10%.

This book chapter will be very useful for doctors who are learning to perform amputations, and those who are already familiar with amputations; it is a good overview of the topic.

COMMENTARY

Michael O. Ogirima, Nigeria

Amputations in LMICs, like Nigeria, where I practice, are faced with lots of peculiarities and challenges. There are changing patterns of etiological factors for amputation due to changing lifestyles and increased violence in the society. There is gradual departure from infections and trauma to the extremities two decades ago to prevalence of noncommunicable diseases like diabetes mellitus, and peripheral vascular diseases. The traditional bonesetters are still preoccupied with obsolete methods of treating fractures and dislocations with attended risk of tight and wrongful splintage and ultimately gangrenous limbs. Gangrene is the ultimate reason why an extremity or part of extremity is accepted to be severed off readily in Zaria. It is therefore stressed that our patients should earn amputation rather than to succumb to the advice of the surgeon. Patients and their relations cope well psychologically with an amputee if the patient is allowed to accept the reality of a dead limb rather than anticipate a deadly or nuisance limb.

We are often faced with some difficulties in preoperative assessment of the viability of a limb with absence of current radiodiagnostic gadgets. Few centers are equipped with Doppler ultrasound machines. There is also competition for operation space with general surgical and gynecological emergencies. Many centers consider amputation as a minor procedure and would not readily accept it on their emergency list.

Postoperative care and rehabilitation of amputees also suffer some setbacks. There are very few centers for the production of artificial limbs and other orthotics for effectively rehabilitating our patients. Social rejection and denial of gainful employment are the worries and fears entertained by our patients when they are about to be discharged from the hospitals.

We need to train doctors on the techniques of good amputation, and there is need to continuously advocate for improved diagnostic gadgets in our health centers. Government should endeavor to train orthotists and prosthetists to keep up with ever-increasing demands.

40

Burns

Jennifer Wall
Gita N. Mody
Robert Riviello

Introduction

Encountering burn victims in a district or visiting hospital setting in a low- or middle-income country (LMIC) is an inevitable certainty for the visiting general or specialist surgeon. All too often, burn patients are found in the far corners of the hospital with little or no care. This unfortunate truth is not due to the staff's choice or intentional neglect of these patients, but is usually the consequence of their intimidation and lack of training to care for a burn patient with severe pain and specialized wound care needs. The majority of surgeons visiting LMICs likely do not specifically intend on treating burns. This chapter aims to guide the general surgeon through the fundamentals of acute burn care surgery and focuses on the resources (or lack thereof) that you will likely encounter.

The Burden of Burns in LMICs

The burden of burn injury, disfigurement, and death falls predominately on the world's poor. Ninety percent of all burn injuries occur in LMICs, accounting for the majority of the estimated 320,000 fire-related deaths per year.[1] With burn incidence as high as 6 million people annually in LMICs,[2] an unknown significant number survive their injuries with severe physical and emotional disabilities. In comparison, the United States encountered 45,000 burn-related hospitalizations and suffered 3,500 deaths in 2010.[3]

High-risk groups in LMICs include children <15 years old, and patients with comorbid diseases such as epilepsy and female gender. Fire-related burns are the only cause of injury in which global female rates of death outnumber those of men.[4] Females from Southeast Asia have the highest recorded burn death rate in the world at 16.9 deaths per 100,000 persons annually. Comparatively, total incidence in Africa is 6.1 deaths per 100,000 and 1.0 death per 100,000 in high-income countries (HICs).[1]

Risk factors differ greatly in HICs and LMICs. Interestingly, the combination of smoking and alcohol accounts for almost 50% of all fire-related deaths in HICs. Alternatively, low socioeconomic status heavily impacts the etiology of burns in LMICs, mainly due to the use of open pit fires needed to provide daily cooking, heat, and light to families living without electricity.

Other risk factors include loose-fitting clothing made of synthetic fibers, storage of a flammable substance in the home, ground-level stoves and fires, insufficient parental supervision, and parent illiteracy (Figure 40.1).[4]

Types of Burn and Clinical Presentation

The majority of all burns you will encounter will be flame and scald burns, seen disproportionately more in children less than 5 years old. Industrial burn injuries, including electrical injuries, will rarely be seen in the extreme rural setting, for obvious reasons. Flame, scald, steam, grease, contact, chemical, and electrical burns can present in any bodily location, with a spectrum from superficial to full-thickness wounds. Clinical presentation will dictate your care plan, but be mindful that the burn will evolve over the first 3–5 days after admission, with second-degree burns either converting to third-degree or beginning to heal (Figure 40.2A and Figure 40.2B).

Factors that may alter initial burn appearance include the use of home remedies, prehospital treatments provided by a local traditional healer, and delayed presentation. Common home remedies may include the application of flour, egg, toothpaste, gasoline, ashes, and herbs (Figure 40.3 and Figure 40.4).

Inscribed markings or tattoos in or around the wound are often a sign that the patient has been treated by a traditional healer before receiving hospital-based care (Figure 40.5).

First-Degree Burns

In first-degree burns, tissue damage is superficial, affecting the intact epidermis only, classified by hyperemia, pain, and lack of blisters. These burns are commonly known as sunburns and heal spontaneously within 7 days. First-degree burns are not included in the TBSA (total body surface area) calculation, as they do not cause physiologically significant fluid shifts.

Second-Degree Burns

Also referred to as partial-thickness burns, tissue involvement includes both the epidermis and varying depths into the dermal layer. Depending on the depth of the injury into the germinal layer

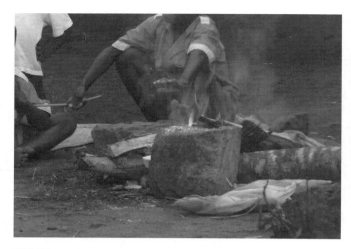

FIGURE 40.1 Malawian children light a ground-level fire unsupervised to cook a maize meal. Image by Jennifer Wall.

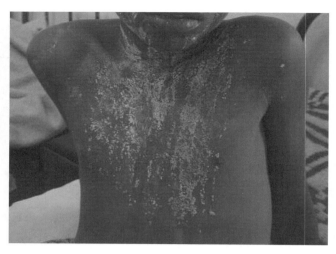

FIGURE 40.3 Flour home remedy for a second-degree burn. Image by Jennifer Wall.

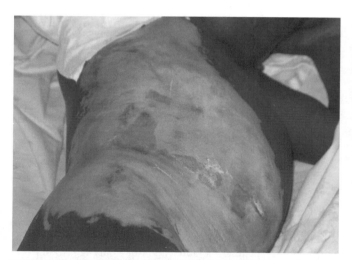

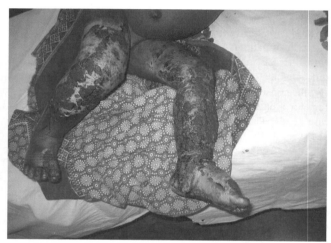

FIGURE 40.4 Fire ash home remedy for a second-degree burn. Image by Jennifer Wall.

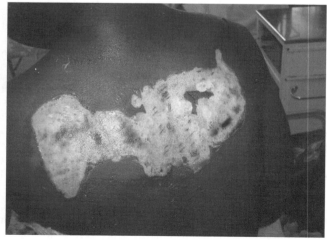

FIGURE 40.2A, B Conversion of second-degree burn on day 1 of burn to third-degree by day 5. Images by Jennifer Wall.

FIGURE 40.5 Hash marks are seared into a third-degree burn by a traditional healer in an effort to release evil spirits. Image by Jennifer Wall.

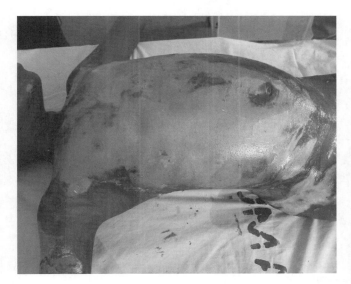

FIGURE 40.6 Superficial second degree-burn of the trunk. Image by Jennifer Wall.

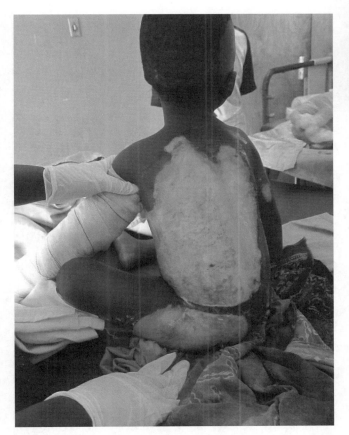

FIGURE 40.7 Deep second-degree burn, hospital day 4. Image by Jennifer Wall.

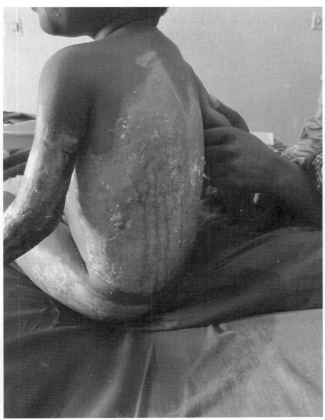

FIGURE 40.8 Same deep second-degree burn, with partial healing, hospital day 25. Image by Jennifer Wall.

Deep second-degree burns present with a range of appearances and can be difficult to classify at first glance (Figure 40.7). They may be blotchy red or white, a mix of moist or dry, demonstrate with decreased pain sensation, and be less likely to blanch.

It is often challenging to determine if these wounds require surgical excision and grafting. Classically, burn experts advocate for excision and grafting of any area not healed within 21 days to minimize the substantial risk of scarring and contracture formation. However, surgical risk needs to be weighed and the total open TBSA needs to be considered. The spontaneous healing of some burn wounds will surprise you when treated with expectant, nonoperative management (Figure 40.8).

This is especially true of burns over large, flat surfaces, rather than over mobile joints. Factors that are favorable to healing in this depth of burn appear to be young age, proper wound care, good nutritional support, and breast-feeding. Practitioners should have a lower threshold to debride and graft these burns if they involve a joint surface or if the wound clearly is not showing any signs of healing progression.

Third-Degree Burns

Also referred to as full-thickness burns, these destroy both epidermal and dermal layers and commonly penetrate into the fatty tissue. In contrast to second-degree burns, these wounds usually have a yellow, waxy, or leathery appearance (Figure 40.9). This is termed eschar, formed by coagulated protein.

of the dermis, the burn may be regarded as superficial, deep, or indeterminate and will reflect in the healing time of these injuries.

Superficial second-degree injuries should heal the epidermal layer with topical treatment within 14 days (Figure 40.6). The classic appearance is marked by the presence of blisters and bright pink, moist tissue underneath. These burns blanch to touch and are extremely painful.

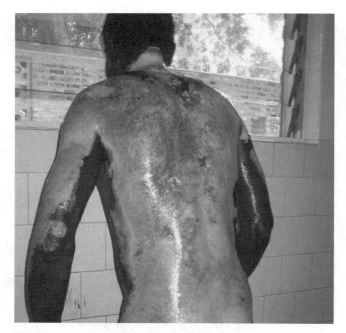

FIGURE 40.9 Third-degree burn. Etiology: Flame burn during a seizure. Image by Jennifer Wall.

Most notably, third-degree burns have a lack of pain to touch initially (due to the destruction of the superficial nerve endings and lack of circulation to the area) and do not blanch. It should not be misconstrued that third-degree burns are completely painless. The contraction and diffuse inflammatory process that sets in by postburn day 2 or 3 can be severely uncomfortable. The patient's experience of pain is heightened by the lack of narcotic pain control that is all too common in LMICs. Full-thickness burns should be excised and skin grafted in the early postburn period to optimize survival and reduce scarring and contracture.

Fourth-Degree Burns

Burns can be further categorized into fourth-degree; these are full-thickness burns that also destroy muscle, tendon, or bone. These burns are typically seen in victims who have had long-standing contact with the burn source or electrical injuries. Because skin grafts will not adhere to the avascular surface of a tendon or bone, treatment options can be challenging in the LMIC setting. Dead structures must be debrided, and kept moist and infection-free, until a healthy granulation bed can form over these structures to ultimately accept a skin graft (Figure 40.10A, Figure 40.10B, Figure 40.10C, Figure 40.10D, and Figure 40.10E). Occasionally, drilling into the marrow of an exposed bone is necessary to promote coverage with granulation. However, fourth-degree burns of the extremities commonly require amputations.

Chronic Hypergranulation

Patients with third-degree, long-standing open burn wounds will classically develop red, raised, and painful granulation tissue (Figure 40.11).

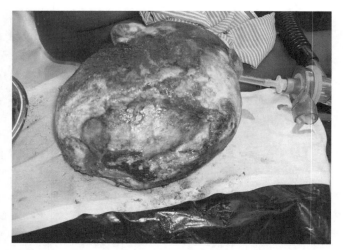

FIGURE 40.10A Fourth-degree burn of scalp, hospital day 7. Image by Jennifer Wall.

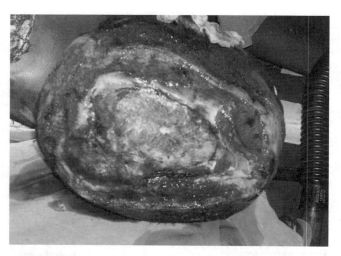

FIGURE 40.10B Status, postdebridement, hospital day 14. Image by Jennifer Wall.

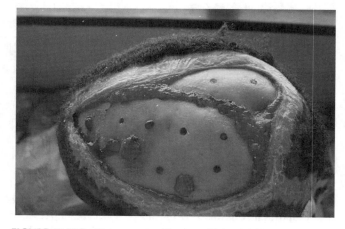

FIGURE 40.10C Status, posttrephination with hand drill. Granulation tissue coalescing slowly. Hospital day 180. Image by Jennifer Wall.

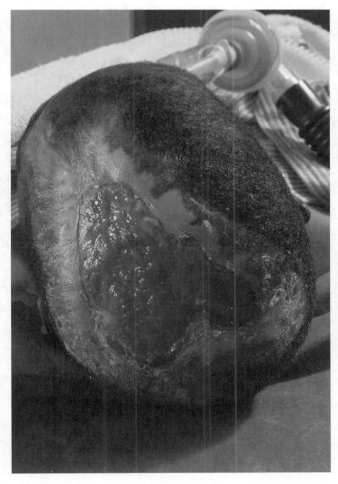

FIGURE 40.10D Complete granulation bed, fit for grafting. Hospital day 300. Image by Jennifer Wall.

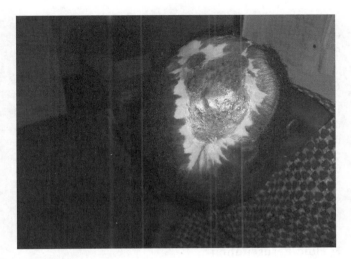

FIGURE 40.10E Fourth-degree burn healed. Hospital day 370. Image by Jennifer Wall.

This tissue often makes very poor healing progression, and patients will do better with aggressive debridement of the granulation tissue and concurrent skin graft closure. It is of utmost importance to assume these wounds are bacteria-colonized. First

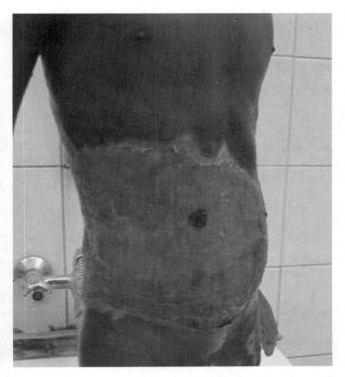

FIGURE 40.11 Granulation tissue. Image by Jennifer Wall.

treat topically (see Dressings) and consider systemic antibiotics, if there are signs of associated infection, before attempting to place a skin graft.

Primary Survey

Remember that burn patients are trauma patients. As such, you should approach them with a standard advanced trauma life support (ATLS) approach. Specialized considerations in the primary and secondary survey for burn patients follow.

A: Airway

Inhalation injury must be suspected when mechanisms of injury include closed-space fires (i.e., poorly ventilated homes), facial burns, unconscious patients, and hoarse or stridorous patients (Figure 40.12). You will lack the convenience of an arterial blood gas or a carboxyhemoglobin test and need to rely completely on your clinical judgment. Do not rely on a pulse oximetry reading to help you to determine the diagnosis, as it will usually be normal in the early postinjury period. Hypoxia is a late sign of inhalation injury.

Signs and symptoms of inhalation injury include swollen airway, singed facial/nasal hairs, carbonaceous sputum, and soot in the mouth or nose.

If you have a high suspicion for an inhalation component and your hospital has the capability to maintain a ventilated patient, the patient should be intubated before upper airway edema makes it impossible to do so.

If there is no capacity to intubate or transfer the patient to a higher level of care, conservative measures should be taken.

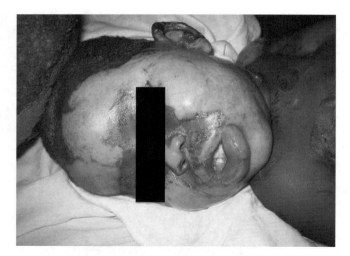

FIGURE 40.12   Burn pattern with high risk of inhalational injury. Image by Jennifer Wall.

Elevate the head of the bed, provide supplemental oxygen, and consider low-dose anxiolytics and analgesics to keep the patient calm, increasing doses gradually as tolerated.

B: Breathing and Ventilation

Ensure that the patient is achieving full chest expansion with breathing. If a patient is tachypneic (>20 breaths/min), determine if the cause is pain or anxiety, or if the patient attempting to compensate for a restrictive or central cause. If the patient is found to have full-thickness restrictive wounds of the chest, escharotomy should be performed immediately to restore chest expansion and adequate ventilation (Figure 40.13).[5] Supplemental oxygen should be given to all patients with suspected inhalation injury.[6]

C: Circulation

Check the patient's pulse. It is important to check on limbs affected by burns and especially those that are circumferentially burned. Burns that are circumferential pose the highest risk of compartment syndrome. Signs and symptoms of compartment syndrome include pain (on passive range of motion), pallor, pulselessness, paraesthesia, poikilothermia (cold), and paralysis. Immediate treatment with escharotomy is indicated to restore blood supply to the affected body part; at times a fasciotomy is required. Incision lines medial and lateral on a limb are ideal to avoid major blood vessels and nerves. If decompression is accomplished via incising the eschar, this is called an escharotomy. If perfusion is inadequate after an escharotomy, you can easily convert your incision deeper to incise through the fascia layer, termed fasciotomy.[5] Late presentation or delay in this procedure can result in the need for amputation, sepsis, or death.

D: Disability

Determine neurological status. Keep in mind that patients with comorbid neurological diseases—including persons with epilepsy, developmental delays, and history of cerebral malaria—are

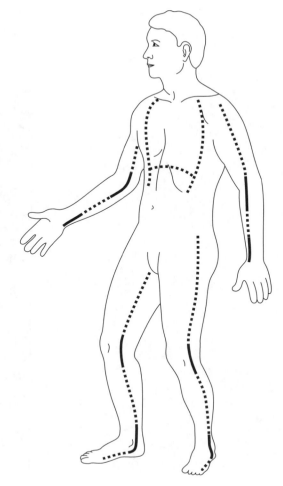

FIGURE 40.13   Locations of burn escharotomies.[5] Mozingo D. Surgical Management. In: Carrougher G (ed). *Burn Care and Therapy,* 1998. Figure 10-1, p. 234.

often at high risk for burn injuries. These conditions need to be taken into account when determining baseline neurologic status.

E: Exposure

Fully exposing the patient is necessary on initial examination to determine the extent of injury. However, burn injuries place the patient at high risk for hypothermia due to the rapid evaporation and heat loss that occurs with open burns, particularly those with large TBSA. It is important to cover the patient with warm blankets during initial work-up and keep the room warm if possible. Work expeditiously to get the patient in a proper dressing to avoid detrimental hypothermia.

F: Fluid Resuscitation

1. Obtain weight (kg).
2. Estimate TBSA of second- and third-degree burns using the Lund–Browder chart (Figure 40.14).[7] A quick estimate can be obtained by using the patient's hand surface area (palm and fingers) as a rough estimate to equate 1% TBSA.

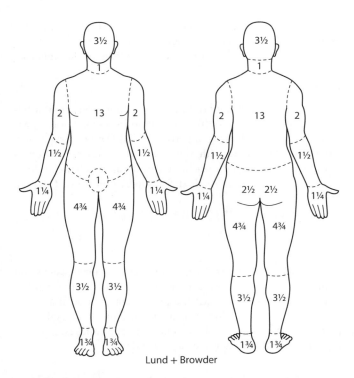

FIGURE 40.14 Lund–Browder burn map.[7] Mlcak RD, Buffalo MC. Prehospital management, transportation, and emergency care. In: Herndon DN (ed). *Total burn care,* 2nd ed. London: Saunders Elsevier, 2001: 67–77.

3. If the patient has a TBSA of 15%–19%, place a peripheral intravenous (IV) and start maintenance intravenous fluids (IVF) (0.9% NS or LR).

4. If the patient has a TBSA of 20% or greater, place 1–2 large–bore peripheral PIVs (or a central venous line if this is available at your hospital).

5. For 20% burns or greater, initiate IVF resuscitation with 0.9% normal saline (NS) or lactated Ringer's (LR) according to the Parkland formula:

   • 4cc x wt (kg) x % TBSA = X ml
   • Give ½ X ml divided by 8, per hour for the first 8 hours.
   • Give the next ½ X ml divided by 16, per hour for the next 16 hours.
   • After the first 24 hours, give a maintenance IVF rate.
   • Children require additional maintenance IVF rate with D5 ½ NS in addition to the Parkland formula due to loss of glucose stores. However, this can be challenging if two PIVs cannot be obtained. You can help compensate for this glucose loss if enteral feeds can be started in the early period.

6. To monitor resuscitation, place a urinary catheter to monitor urine output with a goal of 0.5cc/kg/hr in adults and 1.0cc/kg/hr in children. If a Foley catheter is unavailable, consider weighing cloth diapers or towels.

7. If urine output does not reach this goal, provide IVF bolus with the same fluid type at 5–10cc/kg until the goal is reached.

8. Check electrolytes if possible.

9. Elevate head of bed 30 degrees.

10. Place supplemental O_2.

Resuscitation Physiology

Large burn injuries, >20% TBSA, are complicated by massive fluid and vascular shifts unique to thermal trauma. Fluids are shunted from the intravascular to the extravascular space, causing extremes of edema. Responsive mediators are believed to be the cause of this capillary permeability, including histamine and bradykinin. The ultimate goal of fluid resuscitation is to support the patient during the critical first 24–48 hours of fluid shifts and hypovolemia. Although resuscitation formulas are used as a guideline for fluid management, individual clinical response to the therapy needs to be strictly monitored and resuscitation should be adjusted appropriately.[8]

Signs of hypovolemia may include restlessness, confusion, anxiety, oliguria, or anuria. Peripheral edema is inevitable with IVF resuscitation and should not be mistaken as fluid overload.

Secondary Survey

Obtain details regarding who, what, when, and why, and an A-M-P-L-E history (allergies, medications, past illnesses, last meal, events related to the injury). Keep in mind that it is essential to use a knowledgeable translator for all interactions with the patient, assuming you do not share a common first language.

• Determine depth and TBSA percentage of the burn if not performed previously.
• Provide pain control (see the Pain Control section).
• Emergency procedures should be performed at this time if necessary (escharotomy, fasciotomy, or sloughectomy).
• If there are suspected corneal burns, treat them (see the Eye Burns section).
• Select the best dressing for the observed wound (see the Dressings section).
• IV antibiotics are not indicated in the initial burn period unless a patient presents late with an overtly septic wound. Be inquisitive regarding the patient's living conditions and daily work duties to assess his or her infection risk.
• Tetanus toxoid should be provided to all child and adult burn patients.
• Perform laboratory testing (depending on your available testing resources).

Pain Control

Providing pain control is absolutely essential. Although the normal selection of narcotics you are accustomed to may be lacking in the LMIC setting, good options will likely exist. Disregard the hearsay that your patients in LMICs will have a higher pain tolerance; this is an unacceptable and unethical assumption.

Always consider the combination of the following;

- IV or intramuscular (IM) narcotic as needed for breakthrough pain and dressing changes (i.e., morphine or hydromorphone), plus
- Around-the-clock anti-inflammatory (i.e., ibuprofen) every 6 hours, plus
- Around-the-clock analgesic/antipyretic (i.e., acetaminophen/paracetamol) every 4 hours, plus
- Ketamine IM/IV as needed for dressings that are large, for burns that require debridement, in children, and/or for poorly tolerated dressings due to pain or anxiety.

Good practice dictates that all patients receive analgesic premedication 30 minutes prior to starting a dressing change.

Debridement

To debride or not to debride has been a long-standing point of contention among burn providers for superficial second-degree burns. Keep it simple. If a blister is <2 cm it is acceptable to leave the blister intact to serve as a biological dressing. If blisters are large, cross a joint surface, or are painful due to fluid pressure, then debride and place an appropriate dressing. Eschar that can be easily removed (pseudo eschar) should be removed either at the bedside or in a pain-controlled environment such as the operating room.

Dressing Options

HICs conventionally use closed dressings as opposed to open dressings (meaning no dressing) for a multitude of reasons. Open dressings are commonly seen in LMIC facilities that have poor funding, lack of resources, and staff shortages. If at all possible, antibiotic-impregnated closed dressings are the option of choice as they provide pain relief, reduce infection, and allow for better extremity movement and mobilization out of bed. The downside is they tend to be costly and a skilled staff member needs to change them.

All burn wounds should be washed with a common household soap and clean water prior to placing a dressing. Some hospitals prefer using a dilute Savlon (chlorhexidine) or povidine iodine solution for cleansing depending on their protocols. Household soap is just as good and usually the cheaper option.

Silver Sulfadiazine 1% (AgSD)

This can be applied to dry gauze and applied directly to the burn. Wrap over with dry gauze to keep in place. Its chemical activity lasts 12 hours after applied; however, in an LMIC it is reasonable to change just once a day. Silver sulfadiazine is ideal

for superficial and deep second-degree burns. It also penetrates eschar of a third-degree burn well.

Clinical activity: Effective against *Pseudomonas aeruginosa*.

Honey

Honey's wound healing properties including promotion of tissue growth and epithelialization due to its weak acidity, proteolytic enzymes, hydrogen peroxide, and osmotic properties. Honey can be mixed with vegetable oil or water, applied to dry gauze, and placed over the burn. It can be changed daily or every other day. It is ideal for superficial second-degree burns.

Clinical activity: Effective against *Staphylococcus aureus*.

Papaya

The pulp of the papaya fruit can be mashed, applied to gauze, and used on deep second-degree burns. This common fruit is helpful to promote slough of eschar and provide antimicrobial activity. Proteolytic enzymes, chymopapain and papain, contained in the pulp are thought to provide the chemical debriding action. The dressing should be changed every other day.

Eusol (Edinburgh University Solution of Lime)

Eusol is used primary to de-slough deep second-degree burns. It is mixed with liquid paraffin. This is a chemical debriding agent that should be changed daily. Although it has some antibacterial action, it does not have antimicrobial activity against *Pseudomonas*.[6]

Gentian Violet (GV) Paint 0.5%

This bright violet liquid has antifungal and disinfectant properties. It is used best on scattered small areas of granulation tissue <0.5 cm. Dab it on the surface, allow it to dry, and leave it open to air. Reapply daily. It helps to reduce dressings when the patient is near healed.[6]

Options for Septic Burns

Acetic Acid 0.5%

Common vinegar (5%) can be diluted to 0.5% by mixing 1 part vinegar to 9 parts water.[6] Apply it to dry gauze and change the dressing twice daily if possible. Dilute vinegar is used for infected wounds and burns.

Clinical activity: Effective against *Pseudomonas*.

Dilute Chlorine 0.25%

Common bleach (3.5%) can be diluted with 13 parts water and 1 part chlorine (70 ml of 3.5% bleach mixed with 930 ml clean water to make a 1-liter supply). Apply it to dry gauze, place the gauze over the wound, and change it twice daily if possible. This preparation is also ideal for granulation tissue that is being prepared for surgery in the future days to ensure the wound is clear of bacteria before skin graft application.

Clinical activity: Broad-spectrum antimicrobial.

TABLE 40.1

LMIC burn dressing options

Wound Type	Appearance	Treatment options	Frequency
Superficial second-degree	Pink, +blanch, moist, +pain	1-Petroleum gauze with or without triple antibiotic 2-AgSD 3-Honey, with or w/o mixture in vegetable oil	Daily
Deep second-degree	Red or pale, +/- eschar, decreased blanch	1-AgSD 2-Eusol 3-Papayal	Daily
Third-degree	Pale, yellow, leathery, decreased pain, + thick eschar, - blanch	Options pregrafting: 1-AgSD 2-Dilute chlorine 0.25% 3-Papaya 4-Eusol	Daily
Hypergranulation	Bright red, painful, bleeds	1-Dilute chlorine 0.25% 2-Papaya 3-Zinc oxide crm 5%–15%	Daily
Septic	Purulent, foul-smelling, +/- cellulitis	1-Dilute chlorine 0.25% 2-Acetic acid 0.5%	Twice daily
Skin graft	Mesh or sheet	1-Petroluem gauze with or w/o triple antibiotic ointment 2-Petroleum gauze, then ½ strength Betadine soaks, then dry gauze	Unocclude POD# 3–5, then q 2–3 days
Donor site	White, moist dermis tissue, +/- bleeding	1-Petroleum gauze, then ½ strength Betadine soaks, then dry gauze	Unocclude POD# 10–14, then q 2 days
Escharotomy/fasciotomy site	Incision through eschar to fat tissue or fascia	1-Petroleum gauze, keep moist	Daily
Spotty granulation	Small areas of granulation <0.5 cm	1-GV paint 2-Petroleum gauze	Apply daily until healed

Splinting

All joints in the acute burn and the postoperative grafted burn should have a splint placed during the hospitalization period, as well as several weeks postoperatively if possible. Wound contracture risk exists up to an entire year after the injury or graft has been placed.

The cheapest and most cost-effective way to prevent a life-long disability is to place a simple splint over the joint surface. There are multiple ways to make a cheap splint, including with cardboard, wood, or tongue depressors. Ensure the splint is padded well and changed when it becomes saturated. The best option is to use plaster of paris (POP) if available. Use it as a custom-fit, dorsal or ventral slab over the joint. Remove it daily and replace the gauze wrap. If the effort is put forth to keep the inner layer clean, you should be able to use the same splint for the entire course of the hospitalization (costing less than $2).

Most large joint contractures can be avoided with one splint. However, contractures of the very young in the distal digits (fingers/toes) can be unavoidable, as bone growth may be faster than what their new healed skin (or graft) can accommodate (Figure 40.15). Contracture releases are ultimately needed for a victim who suffers functional impairment. Sadly, only 3% of disabled children attend school in LMICs.[2]

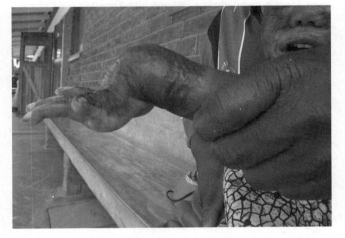

FIGURE 40.15 Severe contracture of child's hand despite skin grafting. Image by Jennifer Wall.

Referral Criteria

Depending on the resources of your hospital or clinic, you may be in a better position to treat a burn than the next level of referral. First determine if the site you intend to refer to knows how to treat burn patients and is indeed a higher level of care. For example, you may have a patient with a suspected inhalation injury and would opt to transfer to a facility with a ventilator and intensive care unit (ICU); however, this option doesn't exist in many countries.

If a higher level of care exists, then almost every burn except for the smallest and most benign ones should be transferred as a general rule.

Before any transfer takes place, ensure that primary and secondary surveys are accomplished, necessary emergency procedures are performed, and pain control is provided. Apply a loose, dry dressing for transfer to avoid heat loss.

Excision and Skin Grafting

Early excision and grafting is the standard of care and among the most effective treatments for third-degree burns to decrease morbidity and mortality, particularly among high-TBSA burn victims. Studies have consistently demonstrated decreased hospital stay, less hypertrophic scarring, and improved function and return to work rates with early excision and wound closure technique.[9]

Hemostasis-Analgesia Solution (HAS)

- Mix 1 liter NS 0.9% with 50cc of 1% lidocaine and 2cc of epinephrine 1:1000. If this quantity of lidocaine is not readily available, you can use the epinephrine dilution solely.

Tangential Excision Technique

- Place a tourniquet or inflated blood pressure (BP) cuff if excising an extremity.
- Excise the area of the burn with your knife of choice in a back-and-forth pattern until healthy bleeding tissue is achieved. The angle with which you hold your knife and the amount of downward force you apply to the tissue with the knife will affect the depth of your cut, in addition to the depth of the guard setting on the knife.
- Achieve hemostasis either with electrocautery or gauze soaked in hemostasis-analgesia solution (HAS) applied to the area, with pressure if necessary.
- Wrap circumferentially with a mild pressure dressing and release the tourniquet.
- Revisit the excised site after 10 minutes and work on further hemostasis if necessary.
- Harvest the donor site.

Fascial Excision Technique

- If the burn is >15%, fascial excision should be considered to minimize blood loss if you have an available electrocautery.
- Start by incising the wound edges with electrocautery and excising sections at a time. Excise down to the fascia, ensuring strict hemostasis at each myocutaneous perforating vessel during the entire procedure.
- HAS can be applied to the fascia surface if bleeding is excessive with saturating 4x4 gauzes.
- Harvest the donor site.

Donor Harvest and Graft Placement

See Chapter 35 for more detail on skin grafts.

- Inject the donor site subcutaneously with HAS superficially to raise a rectangular area.
- Smear mineral oil, K-Y jelly, or soapy water to the intended donor area. Anterior and lateral thighs are ideal donors because they are easy to dress and give a large surface area.
- Have an assistant make the skin taught, either with penetrating towel clamps or tongue depressors.
- Use your knife of choice in a back-and-forth pattern at a 45-degree angle to excise down to the surface of bright white healthy tissue (Figure 40.16). If you are into the fat layer, you are too deep!
- Dip the graft in saline and place it on a sterile wood cutting board (assuming no skin mesher). Mesh the skin with an 11 blade scalpel in a purposeful, staggered pattern to allow it to spread optimally (Figure 40.17).
- Place the skin graft on the recipient site dermis side down.
- Affix the graft with either sutures or staples. Rapidly absorbing suture (chromic, catgut) is particularly useful in children, as this avoids the pain of suture removal (Figure 40.18).

Be safe rather than sorry—secure the graft.

Surgical Dressing Options

See Chapter 35 for more detail on skin grafts.

- Place either a Vaseline gauze or generic petroleum gauze directly to the graft.
- Soak sterile gauzes in half-strength povidine-iodine solution, leave them damp, and dress over top of the petroleum gauze with several layers.

TABLE 40.2

Comparison of procedural resources

Procedure	HIC Resource	LMIC Resource
Desloughing	Norsen debrider	Tongue depressor/washcloth
Escharotomy/fasciotomy	Electrocautery	Scalpel/forceps
Escharectomy	Watson/Goulian knife	Scissor/forceps/scalpel/Goulian
Skin harvest	Powered dermatome	Goulian/Watson blade
Skin mesh	Brennan skin mesher	Scalpel/wood cutting board

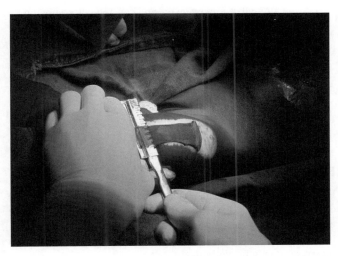

FIGURE 40.16 Donor harvesting with the Weck (Goulian) blade. Burn surgery knives: Goulian blade, Goulian guard, Goulian assembled handle set, Watson blade, Watson handle set. Image by Jennifer Wall.

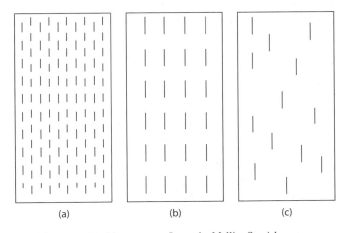

(a)   (b)   (c)

FIGURE 40.17 Meshing patterns. Image by Mellisa Stanislaw.

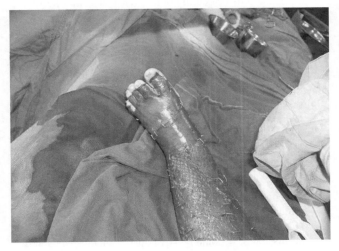

FIGURE 40.18 Sheet graft of foot, mesh graft of leg. Secured with donated skin staples. Image by Jennifer Wall.

- Wrap over with several layers of dry gauze. If over a joint space, splint appropriately with POP.
- Unocclude on postoperative day (POD) 5, or earlier if you are in a rainy, damp season.
- Consider bed rest for the patient for 3–5 days depending on the site of the graft if you are worried about shearing.
- Donor site dressing: Use the same procedure as for the graft site; unocclude POD 10–14, and expect it to be healed by POD 14.

Postoperative Pearl

- Postoperative fever in the LMIC burn patient is not necessarily indicative of atelectasis as assumed in a HIC. First rule out malaria, if your patient is from a malarial area. If you cannot get an immediate result, treat empirically.

Watch-and-Wait Theory

There can be benefits to waiting to excise on a subset of patients with deep second-degree or indeterminate depth burns. Patients of young age, with <15% TBSA burns, with good nutrition, and/or who have been breast-fed have a high potential to heal. An assumed third-degree burn at first glance can ultimately heal in 3–5 weeks. The appearance is marked by thick, white, damp tissue in the early stages. Week-by-week progression is seen in the thinning of this white to a lighter pink color, exposing dermal components. Healing is noticed from the bottom up as well as from the peripheral edges.

Nutrition

Burn patients suffer from a hypermetabolic state after a severe injury, increasing their energy expenditure by 60%–100% above normal. If energy needs cannot be met, the consequence is rapid loss of lean body mass, impaired immunity and wound healing, organ dysfunction, and possible death.[10]

Providing an adequate high-protein and carbohydrate diet will be a substantial challenge in the LMIC setting. If a patient is deemed greater than 20% and feeding tubes are available, place a tube. If a feeding tube is not an option, be resourceful in utilizing local produce and market foods.

Focus on a high-protein and high-carbohydrate diet. The carbohydrate recommendation for adults is 7 g/kg weight and protein is 2 g/kg weight daily. High-protein examples per portion include:

- ½ cup dried beans = 8 grams
- 1 egg = 7 grams
- 8 ounces cow's milk = 8 grams
- 1 ounce chicken, fish, or meat = 7 grams
- 2 tablespoons peanut butter (or Ready-to-Use Therapeutic Food [RUTF]) = 9 grams

Homemade Tube Feed

This high-energy milk formula can be provided enterally either orally or via feeding tube to provide 440 kcals, 8 g fat, 10.5 g protein, and 42 g carbohydrates per feed.[6] Mix the following:

- 1 cup vitamin fortified skim milk powder
- 60 cc oil
- ½ cup sugar
- 300 cc water

Troublesome Burn Injuries

Eye Burns

Burns of the face require a high suspicion of corneal injury. As a Wood's lamp and staining capacity is unlikely to be available, it is best to empirically treat all suspected eye burns to avoid the devastating complications of a missed injury. Not all patients will be able to relay that they have eye pain or blurriness; this is especially true in young children. Corneal abrasions and ulcerations are the most commonly found eye injuries associated with burns (Figure 40.19).

- Treat empirically.
- Consult ophthalmology if available.
- Treat topically with chloramphenicol or tetracycline drops.

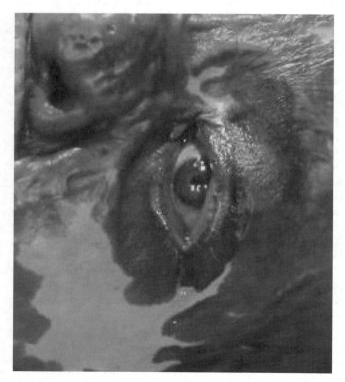

FIGURE 40.19 Severe facial scarring and ectropion in a patient who received no treatment for her full-thickness burns. Burn etiology: Fall into fire during a seizure episode. Image by Jennifer Wall.

- If eyelid burns are extensive and causing ectropion and lagophthalmos, consider tarsorrhaphy to protect the cornea from exposure.
- If chemical burn is suspected, irrigate with water for one hour then treat with topical antibiotics.
- Do not patch the eye.[11]

Risks of not treating a corneal abrasion are progression to corneal ulceration, infection, and ultimately blindness.

Electrical Burns

Because electrical current seeks the path of least resistance, the current travels quickly through the soft tissues along the interface of muscle and bone. Burns are deep, usually all third-degree, and often cause deep muscle injury similar to a traumatic crush injury, requiring fasciotomy.

The principles of debridement for electrical burns remain the same as for other burns: All dead tissue must be removed and the patient may even require an amputation. Myoglobulinuria may be present, revealing dark red or tea-colored urine due to rhabdomyolysis occurring as a compounding complication in association with the electrical injury. Treatment of rhabdomyolysis requires adequate perfusion of the kidneys via fluid resuscitation. Pay careful attention to urine output with a goal of 75–100 cc/hr in adults and 1.5 cc/kg/hr in children[6] until the dark color urine has cleared.

Chemical Burns

Both alkali and acid burns must be neutralized by dilution with copious water irrigation for an hour after the injury (including eye burns). The depth of these burns may be hard to classify in the early stages but will declare themselves within a few days. Treat as a thermal burn injury after dilution, choosing the appropriate topical dressing according to the depth.

LMIC Specific Considerations

- Epilepsy will be found commonly as a comorbid disease in burn victims. Seizure-related burns usually carry a high mortality as epileptics will fall into a cooking fire face first with sustained contact with the flames. Traditional beliefs may create a barrier to treating persons with epilepsy with standard medications. Persons with epilepsy are at times viewed as "possessed" or contagious, and thus ostracized from their families and social networks.
- Malaria claims the lives of nearly 800,000 persons per year in LMICs. Ninety percent of malaria deaths occur in Africa alone.[12] Signs and symptoms of malaria will be masked by the burn picture. Although fevers are common in burn patients simply due to the burns, malaria must always be ruled out in endemic areas (Figure 40.20). Many patients are positive before admission or become positive during a lengthy hospital stay. Consider testing all patients upon admission and again when a fever mounts.

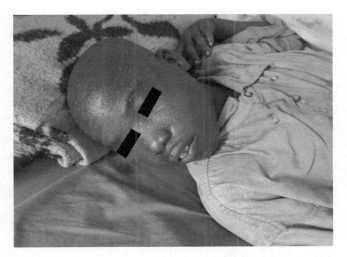

FIGURE 40.20 A burn patient mounts an extreme fever, hospital day 2, secondary to malaria infection. Image by Jennifer Wall.

- Traditional healers are culturally and historically respected community members who treat common ailments, chronic disease, and acute injuries, including burns and epilepsy. Their treatment plans often differ from those recommended by Western medicine standards. Discretion and sensitivity are of importance when changing modalities or recommending a new care plan. Patient education regarding a new treatment is often accepted well by patients.

Prevention

HICs are succeeding in burn prevention strategies in large part due to technological advances. Smoke detectors alone have accounted for a 61% decrease in all house fires.[1] Reliable plumbing with thermostat regulation and electrical wiring is not even a remote possibility for the foreseeable future for most households LMICs, much less so for those living in urban or rural poverty. However, the lack of technological and financial resources is only a part of the problem. Burn causation in LMICs is significantly tied to cultural norms and behavior patterns. Prevention programs targeting social determinants of injury and behavior patterns require persistence, educational programs, and precise execution.[13] Generations of families have survived by allowing young children to care for even younger siblings. A child will know how to gather wood, light a cooking fire, and prepare a simple meal by the age of 6.

Complicating matters, unforeseen burn mechanisms have arisen from foreign aid organizations despite their best intentions. The distribution of mass mosquito nets has led to more hut fires as candles lit bedside ignite the nets while children lay helpless and caught inside. School feeding programs have led to an increase in scald injuries, as large vats of boiling porridge are cooked on the ground level with young children nearby. Most known burn prevention programming is carried out at the small nongovernmental organization (NGO) and missionary level rather than at the agency, corporation, or government level. Injury prevention is given a much lower priority than disease prevention because of the relative lack of funding and advocacy.[13]

Current LMIC burn prevention strategies include solar cooking, solar electricity, educational school programming, drama programming, targeted epilepsy treatment, parent education, and children's literature, including culturally appropriate coloring and comic books. To learn more about burn prevention strategies used in rural Africa, visit http://africaburnrelief.com/About_Us.html.

Helpful Items to Bring

- Goulian or Watson knife with replacement blades
- Portable pulse ox (including batteries)
- Dressing supplies (Do not bring highly specialized, expensive dressings that are not sustainable at your host site.)
- Sterile operating room (OR) instrument pack (toothed forceps, fine scissors, and heavy tissue scissors)
- Sterile staplers (This will decrease the length of a large burn case significantly and the local staff will likely be eager use them.)
- Staple removers
- Battery-powered head lamp
- Educational handouts, slide shows

COMMENTARY

Nivaldo Alonso, Brazil

The authors provide a comprehensive explanation about the diagnosis and treatment of burns, although the incidence of burns is significantly different in LMICs compared to HICs. In Africa, there are 8.7 burns per 100,000 people every year (OMS data from 2004), compared to 0.2 burns per 100,000 people every year in Europe and 0.7 burns per 100,000 people every year in North America. In Brazil, where I practice, the resources disbursed for public health are high (BRL$63 million/year) and high incidence is worrisome, especially since it is preventable.

Two major causes of burn in children are scald burns and domestic accidents with fire. Domestic accidents sometimes occur in LMICs when children are left at home with only supervision from older siblings; this is very difficult to address because it is related to financial constraints.

It is critical that LMICs offer education about how to treat a burn initially. It is important for people to know that traditional practices of treating burns with sugar, butter, or other basic goods should be avoided. Instead, the wound should be washed and covered with wet cloths.

It is also important that LMICs prioritize prevention of burns. The implementation of several laws has helped to reduce burn incidence; one example is seen in the prohibition of domestic use of liquid alcohol, which encourages a switch to rubbing alcohol. In some parts of Brazil, advertising campaigns using local newspapers and comic books have also helped to reduce the incidence of burns caused by domestic accidents. Furthermore, media advertising to stimulate medical education is also important because doctors are not always well prepared to deal with burn treatment. Additionally, on an individual level, burns can be prevented by smoke detectors (which need to be installed in homes), and controlled water temperature.

Suggested Reading

Gawryszewski, Vilma Pinheiro et al. Public Hospital Emergency department visits due to burns in Brazil, 2009. *Cad. Saúde Pública* [online]. 2012, vol.28, n.4 [cited 2014-01-11], pp. 629-640.

Child injuries and violence. World Health Organization. http://www.who.int/violence_injury_prevention/child/en/

Cartilha para tratamento de emergência das queimaduras/ Ministério da Saúde, Secretaria de Atenção à Saúde, Departamento de Atenção Especializada. – Brasília : Editora do Ministério da Saúde, 2012. 20.

COMMENTARY

Daniel Chimutu, Mongolia

When a small American NGO first offered assistance to Nkhoma Hospital, a rural hospital in Malawi, I was one of the people who was initially trained to manage burns. I was also taught some surgical skills, and I learned debridement, skin grafts, fluid resuscitation, pain management, and wound dressing techniques. When these volunteers first entered our site, we thought our program might fail because of our limited resources, staff shortages, struggling infrastructure, and lack of skill. But the volunteers offered hope for our program.

With the return of teams to train counterpart professionals, our relationships strengthened and the hospital staff could see the transformation in the management of burn cases and epilepsy cases at Nkhoma Hospital, and in Malawi overall. Previously, we had been treating burn cases as normal wounds, and many people lost their lives or suffered unfortunate complications. But with our improved program, we have reduced the number of deaths and complications, including contractures and amputations, from burns. We now have a survival rate that is close to 85%. We are also able to identify, treat, and follow all the epileptic patients in our catchment area, and even those beyond our catchment area, with the introduction of a burn prevention program.

Additionally, visiting specialty surgeons help manage highly complicated cases and impart knowledge in the local clinicians. My surgical skills have greatly improved as a result. It is my hope that visiting staff will continue to assist programs like ours, and consider staff exchange visits from Malawi to the United States. We also hope for additional funding opportunities for burn conferences, which provide exceptional learning opportunities for health professionals in LMICs.

COMMENTARY

David Morton, Malawi

Nkhoma Hospital is a rural visiting surgical team hospital in Malawi, Africa. Like most rural African church hospitals, it requires a number of sources of funding to meet its operational budget. Historically, the church health units were set up to provide health care to the indigenous people. During colonial times, the initial health care and facilities provided by the colonial administrations were set up for the colonial officials. As colonial governments developed health care for the local people, health care became part of the government responsibility; this continued after independence. However, due to lack of resources, most sub-Saharan African (SSA) governments depend upon the church-run health units to provide a significant percentage of health care for their populations, and these units are often in the more rural and therefore poorer areas of the country. In Malawi, the Ministry of Health estimates that up to 40% of health care is provided by church units. Because the church units are serving a poorer percentage of the population and because they exist specifically to care for the poor and needy, church units do not charge what services actually cost since that would make their services unaffordable for the very people they exist to serve. This is especially true for more expensive or sophisticated services such as burn care and treatment of chronic diseases such as epilepsy. Our particular hospital has three sources for funding to cover its operational expenses: patient fees (usually significantly subsidized), Malawi government grants for basic salaries of an established staff and for reimbursement of care under service level agreements, and donations (usually from churches, individuals, or organizations from outside Malawi). Over the past four years, the average percentages of income provided are 50% from the Malawi government, 30% from donations, and 20% from patient reimbursement of fees. Some conditions, however, result in significant disability, carry significant public health risks, or are too heavy a burden for the local population to carry even at the subsidized rates charged.

These conditions, including burn care, epilepsy, tuberculosis (TB), human immunodeficiency virus (HIV), obstetric fistulas, and, to some extent, malaria, are treated for free, are more heavily subsidized, or are assisted through Ministry of Health vertical programs funded by large external donors such as the Global Fund or Pepfar.

Although the Malawi government is committed to providing health care to its population, it does not have the resources currently to provide even what the Ministry of Health calls the "Essential Health Package," which is basically free under-fives care for the most common illness, antenatal and obstetrical care, and care for the most common chronic noncommunicable diseases. Often government hospitals and health centers will not have a consistent supply of medications or supplies to consistently provide good health care, especially for more specialized conditions, such as burns or epilepsy. Nkhoma has experienced receiving patients who have been minimally treated in government health centers and have come to Nkhoma to get some care, but often in a worse condition because of the delays. Also, with chronic diseases such as epilepsy, we have seen patients who have been treated with a variety of anti-epileptic medications simply because the government unit gives the patient the drug it happens to have at the time, rather than having a consistent supply of a number of drugs which would allow more rational dispensing. It is not always easy to understand why the Ministry of Health units are not better supplied and equipped, though often it is a combination of lack of resources, planning difficulties centrally, frequent stock outs, and inadequate supervision.

Church health units tend to focus on some of these more specialized conditions (burns, epilepsy, obstetrical fistulas, cervical cancer, and diabetes) because successful appeals can be made to outside donors to enable the hospital to care for patients who would otherwise have limited options for their, at times, very distressing conditions.

41

Thoracic Trauma

Abraham Lebenthal
Alexi Matousek

Introduction

In high-income countries (HICs), death in trauma patients has a trimodal distribution death at the scene or in the first hour (50%), death in the next 1–4 hours (30%), and late death (20%). Thoracic trauma is a significant cause of immediate and delayed patient mortality. In contrast, in the developing world, with limited emergency medical services and prolonged transport times from injury to care, significant thoracic injuries may lead to even more early deaths with late deaths becoming more unusual. Life-threatening thoracic injuries that must be recognized and addressed immediately include airway loss or obstruction, tension pneumothorax, hemopneumothorax, pericardial tamponade, and great vessel injury. The goal of this chapter is to teach the nonthoracic surgeon "pattern recognition" and "simple procedures" to convert urgent, life-threatening situations into salvageable and stable conditions with minimal resources and training.

Chest trauma typically leads to lung injury (contusion, consolidation, or atelectasis) and disruption of chest wall mechanics (rib fractures, diaphragmatic injuries, muscle contusions, and pain). The overall decrease in chest wall compliance is additive to the decrease in lung compliance seen because of contusion or consolidation. Together, over time, this can lead to a vicious cycle of hypoxia, hypercarbia, and acidosis. The majority of patients who suffer from thoracic trauma and reach a medical facility alive can be managed with small lifesaving interventions. Examples include: a surgical airway, tube thoracostomy, and pericardial window. Only a minority of patients with thoracic trauma will require thoracotomy (<10% blunt, 15%–30% penetrating). These simple interventions are relatively easy to master and may convert an unstable patient with a life-threatening injury into a stable patient. Late sequelae of chest trauma include adult respiratory distress syndrome and pneumonia, especially in patients with rib fractures and large pulmonary contusions, which can lead to preventable deaths if not managed properly.

Initial Management

The management of thoracic trauma includes establishing and maintaining a patent airway, ensuring adequate respiration (relief of pneumothorax, tension pneumothorax, and hemothorax) by external ventilatory support as needed, and aiding circulation (hemorrhage control, volume resuscitation, relief of tamponade, etc.). Hypoxia is the most serious result of chest injury. It can be due to loss of airway or altered breathing and must be treated immediately.

On examination, the patient's vital signs (pulse, blood pressure, and respiratory rate) and mental status will give an indication of the severity of injury. The trachea should be central in the neck. If the trachea is deviated, pneumothorax should be suspected in the hemithorax that is contralateral to the direction of tracheal deviation (the pressure of the pneumothorax pushes the trachea away). The rib cage is examined by pressing along the ribs bilaterally. If a step, instability, or tenderness is found, fractures are suspected. Subcutaneous emphysema, rib fractures, and hemodynamic instability suggest significant injury to the lung (contusion), possible pneumothorax, and possible significant hemothorax. If lung sounds are distant or nonexistent in one hemithorax, a pneumothorax or hemothorax should be suspected. If the patient has distant heart sounds, a narrow pulse pressure, and distended neck veins, cardiac tamponade should be suspected. It is important to remember that anoxia (and shock) will lead to anxiety, combative behavior, and confusion. Additionally, it is important to remember that one can exsanguinate into the chest cavity. For all injuries, the need for antibiotic coverage and tetanus vaccination should be addressed. A quick neurological assessment as well as full exposure is essential for accurate assessment of patient's injuries, enabling the proper diagnosis of injuries dictating the correct sequence of therapy. Please see Chapter 38 for a discussion of airway management.

Tension Pneumothorax

Prompt diagnosis and therapy are essential for surviving significant thoracic injuries. The surgeon must have a high index of suspicion for conditions in patients with a patent airway who are unstable with impaired breathing. The most serious of these conditions is tension pneumothorax. When identified, immediate treatment converts a life-threatening injury to a non-life-threatening condition.

Diagnosis

Clinical signs of tension pneumothorax include: air hunger, dyspnea, cyanosis, distention of neck veins, tracheal deviation, diminished breath sounds on the side the trachea is deviating away from, tachycardia or bradycardia, hypotension, severe anxiety, confusion, and combative behavior.

Surgical Management

Upon identification, the physician should immediately perform needle decompression. A strong gush of air should immediately exit, with the patient immediately improving from a cardiovascular standpoint; if this does not happen completely, an additional needle can be inserted. If the patient stabilizes, the physician continues the primary survey according to advanced trauma life support (ATLS) protocol and then places a chest tube during the resuscitation phase. Alternatively, if air is obtained and the patient does not stabilize, a chest tube is immediately placed.

Needle Decompression

This is the quickest, safest, and least technically demanding procedure for converting a tension pneumothorax, which is life-threatening, to a simple pneumothorax. It should be done expediently and immediately upon diagnosis.

Equipment: A 14- or 16-French intravenous (IV) cannula, and an alcohol swab.
Positioning: Supine.
Procedure: The area just under the second rib on the midclavicular line of the affected side is cleaned with an alcohol swab. A 14- or 16-French IV cannula is then is inserted into the chest immediately superior to the third rib (avoiding the neurovascular bundle that runs inferior to each rib). A gush of air should be heard. In the event that the patient does not stabilize, an additional catheter is placed. If this fails to achieve results, a chest tube is in placed.
Caution: Needle decompression of a tension pneumothorax is a temporizing measure facilitating temporary stabilization of the patient. This should never be used as the only treatment. Once carried out, a chest tube should be placed as soon as possible.

Tube Thoracostomy

The indication for placing a chest tube as well as urgency must factor into the speed at which the tube is placed. The procedure can be performed anywhere with the proper equipment and training.

A patient suffering from a symptomatic tension pneumothorax which has not been relieved by needle decompression needs an urgent tube placed with only vital steps quickly taken (alcohol swab, a larger incision, relief of tension, placement of tube, and tube anchoring with heavy suture). This is in contrast to a tube placed to drain a chronic effusion or empyema where all steps to maintain sterility must be taken.

A chest tube is typically a long plastic tube with multiple holes at its end, but any at least mildly stiff sterile tube of the right diameter would suffice. Chest tubes can be straight or right angle. Straight tubes are primarily used to drain air and blood, while right-angle tubes are primarily used to drain pus. The size of a chest tube depends on its diameter and is listed in French. Straight chest tubes may contain an inner needle or trocar. Typically a 28-French chest tube will evacuate air, while a 32-36-French chest tube is needed for evacuation of blood in adult patients. Chest tubes have numbers in centimeters written along their side. It is important to note that the zero marks the distal end of the last hole and not the end of the tube. Typically, a straight chest tube should be inserted to 20 cm (from the skin) for an adult female and 24 cm for an adult male, to assure that it reaches the apex of the hemithorax. Remember; one can always pull it back, but space contamination can occur if the tube is advanced inwardly sometime after its insertion.

Equipment: A scalpel, Metzenbaum scissors, strong surgical sutures (#1 or 2 silk), needle driver, 2 Kelly clamps, sterile drapes, antiseptic wash, 10–20 cc of 1% lidocaine, 10 cc syringe, and a 21-gauge long needle.
Anesthesia: Local injected subcutaneous (SQ) by the surgeon, as well as rib blocks. If available, patient can receive small amount of intravenous sedation, such as ketamine.
Antibiotics: 2 g Ancef for coverage of skin flora may be given if available.
Positioning: The patient lays supine, a folded sheet placed under the affected side in order to obtain a 20- to 30-degree elevation. The arm on the affected side is either a flexed over the head and taped, or strapped straight next to the body in the way that will insure non-interference during the procedure.
Procedure: A fully gowned, gloved, and masked surgeon preps the chest widely with an alcohol-based solution. The chest is then draped in the area of the fifth intercostal space anterior axillary line. The edge of the nipple is left in view. Three towels are placed to form a triangle. The fifth rib is palpated just posterior to the anterior axillary line, lidocaine is injected under the skin in this area, and then into the deep tissue. Then 2–3 cc of lidocaine is then injected just inferior to the lower border of the posterior fourth and fifth ribs. Care is taken to avoid injury to the long thoracic nerve.

A horizontal incision at least 2½ times the diameter of the chest tube is made through the skin. If the patient is unstable, muscular, or obese, or placement is difficult, the skin incision should be widened (a prudent surgeon would make a larger incision from the start for these patients). Using scissors, the subcutaneous tissue is spread vertically to avoid the thoracodorsal and long thoracic vessels. The apical portion of the fifth rib is palpated and the intercostal muscles anchoring into this are divided using scissors. The dissection should be bloodless, all sources of bleeding including inadvertent intercostal injury must be controlled. It is much easier for a novice to place a chest tube at a 90-degree angle with the skin and ribs—do not attempt to tunnel the tube. Using a clamp, the intercostal muscles are split along the upper edge of lower rib. A rush of air should be heard upon entering the chest cavity if a simple or tension pneumothorax is present.

In the event of a hemothorax, blood and clot will evacuate. Empyema pus will discharge, if culture or Gram stain are possible, then exudate should be collected sterilely using a syringe. Empyema and effusions may be loculated. A gloved-finger inserted into the thoracotomy opening can feel the pleura, lung, and chest wall and rule out significant adhesions. If found, loculations can be gently broken up using a suction tip; however, care must be taken to avoid causing bleeding while doing so (by pushing into the lung or hilar structures). Complete evacuation of blood or pus from the cavity is important to decrease future morbidity.

Choose a straight chest tube to evacuate air and blood. Place it into the chest through the incision guided by mini-thoracotomy guided by a clamp or a trocar inside the chest tube that has been pulled back 1 cm. Insert it with a twisting corkscrew motion pointing toward the posterior chest and then directed apically. It is *not* advisable to place a chest tube with a trochar fully in place due to the danger of injury to additional viscera. However, when the trochar is withdrawn by 1 cm, it makes chest tube insertion simpler since the trochar gives the chest tube firm strength, enabling passage through a small thoracotomy, while preventing insertion injuries caused by its sharp point. If resistance is encountered, the tube should be partially withdrawn and then corkscrewed in. For an apical tube, insert the tube to 20 cm for an adult female and 24 cm for an adult male. For empyema, a right angle tube, if available, is placed toward the costophrenic angle. The area around the chest tube is closed in multiple layers. The chest tube is secured with a heavy 2.0 silk suture, and an omega stay suture is placed around the tube to enable additional anchoring as well as future closure if desired.

Pitfalls

Extrathoracic tube: The tube is not inside the pleural space, but is in the chest wall. One can decrease the chance of this happening by using a larger incision and good analgesia.

Injury to the spleen or liver: The chest tube was placed too low or the hemidiaphragm is elevated; this is unrecognized and the chest tube is forced into a visceral organ, causing damage and bleeding. This may be prevented by first inserting a finger into the thoracotomy opening to confirm pleural position, and then placing the tube.

Laceration of lung or heart: Multiple adhesions, unrecognized, may be preventable by placing a finger into chest and palpating. Blunt, gentle division of adhesions and a limit on the amount of force utilized will decrease the chance for this possibly lethal complication.

Incomplete drainage of infection: Chest tube inserted; however, due to positioning as well as to loculations, it does not completely drain the cavity. Division of adhesions may decrease the chance of this complication.

Incomplete drainage of air: The chest tube may be too small, plugged with blood or fibrin, or may not be in an adequate position. Replacement with a larger tube or the placement of a second tube may manage this. Also, "stripping" of fibrinous material from the chest tubing may help remove fibrin and blood plugs.

After insertion, it is preferable to connect the chest tube to a collecting system with at least a water seal to prevent contamination. Suction enables active evacuation and drainage of the pleural cavity. Initial simple systems utilized suction but had no control over suction strength, and lacked the advantage of water-seal systems. However, they are easy to make with reusable jars and tubing (Figure 41.1).

A more complex, "closed system" separates the patient from the suction by utilizing a water seal (See Figure 41.1a, b or c), can have adjustable suction control (Figure 41.1b and c) and can have separate drainage and water seal bottles making removal of the drainage bottle easier (Figure 41.1c). The addition of a water column enables calibration of the suction by increasing or decreasing

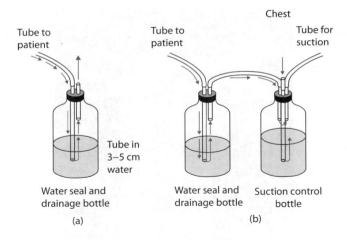

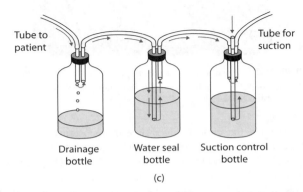

FIGURE 41.1 Closed system drainage. Miller-Keane M. *Encyclopedia and Dictionary of Medicine Nursing and Allied Health.* 7th ed. Philadelphia: Elsevier, 2005.

the water column. Industrially produced systems are available and are typically used in HICs (Figure 41.2).

When suction and a collection system are not available, then drainage through a Heimlich valve to a bag is the best option. The Heimlich valve is a one-way flutter valve, invented by Henry Heimlich in 1963, that enables air and liquids to evacuate the pleural cavity and then collect in a bag, preventing suctioning of external contents into the pleural cavity.

An improvised valve can be made if neither a suction device nor a Heimlich valve is available. This is fashioned as follows: The middle finger can be cut off a surgical glove and then tied with a heavy silk tie to the end of the chest tube, cutting off the distal tip. The chest tube is then inserted into the middle of a drainage bag. This is then secured to the chest tube achieving an improvised "closed" one-way system.

Chest Tube Management

Although there is general agreement among surgeons on the indications and techniques for chest tube insertion, there is no consensus on the subsequent management of these tubes following placement. Management practices are often institution based and physician specific according to training and preferences developed from anecdotal experience. Subsequent management of the chest tube must be individualized to the patient, taking into

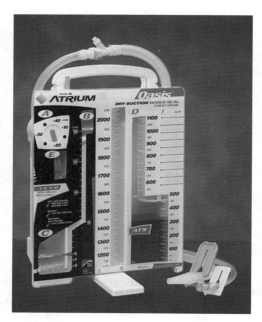

FIGURE 41.2 Industrially produced chest drain system. Model 3650 ATS Chamber. [Internet]: Atrium. Available from http://www.atriummed.com/en/chest_drainage/oasis.asp

consideration the indication for tube thoracostomy, whether or not the patient has had pulmonary resection, mechanical ventilatory dependence, and presence or absence of bronchopulmonary fistula. Premature chest tube removal, as well as unnecessary delays in removal, can lead to longer hospital stays and unjustified costs.

The timing of chest tube removal in regard to drainage volume has been investigated by Younes and colleagues in a prospective randomized trial.[1] There was no major difference in the rate of fluid accumulation and need for thoracocentesis between groups of drainage amounts of ≤100 ml/day, ≤150-ml/day, or ≤ 200 ml/day, respectively. Using the threshold of daily drainage of less than 200 ml could lead to quicker removal of the chest tube, reducing hospitalization time.

When removing a chest tube, some surgeons recommend pulling the tube when the patient is in maximal inspiration and others in maximal expiration. A prospective, randomized trial by Bell and colleagues to evaluate whether a recurrent pneumothorax (PTX) was more likely with chest tube removal at end-inspiration or end-expiration concluded that the risk of recurrent PTX was similar between both groups and that either method of chest tube removal was safe.[2]

Another area of controversy is the use of suction or water seal in patients with a continuous air leak. Many surgeons will place a small leak on higher levels of suction (up to –40 mmHg) in an attempt to pull the lung tighter into the pleura and seal the leak. Other surgeons feel that high levels of suction stent open leaks, and will place the chest tube to water seal. Many surgeons feel a daily chest X-ray is indicated for every patient who has a chest tube in place. In LMICs, such a strategy may not be practical, and X-rays may be obtained only with changes in suction parameters or changes in clinical status.

One practice that should be avoided is clamping a chest tube for several hours prior to removal to ascertain whether

a pneumothorax accumulates. While this is an acceptable strategy if monitoring is excellent, it is a dangerous choice in almost all realistic scenarios due to the risk of tension pneumothorax.

The ideal chest tube management algorithm has yet to be determined. Specifically, wide variation in management practices exists in regard to the timing and parameters under which chest tubes should be removed, the best method of removal, and the need for chest X-rays to monitor patients pre- and postremoval. Specific strategies should be tailored to individual patients and settings.

Lung and Airway Injury

The vast majority of traumatic injuries of the lung are self-limited. These include: contusion, intraparenchymal hemorrhage, laceration, and air leak due to parenchymal injury. They can usually be managed with simple supportive measures (oxygen supplementation, adequate pain control, and early ambulation) or procedures such as tube thoracostomy as necessary.

Diagnosis and Initial Management

A massive air leak after chest tube insertion may be due to an injury to a major bronchus, typically the proximal mainstem bronchus near its insertion to the carina. These patients present with massive subcutaneous emphysema and tension pneumothorax. Chest tube insertion results in a high-volume continuous air leak and on chest X-ray the lung does not reinflate. Additional chest tubes are placed and, if despite placement of these tubes the lung does not reinflate, an airway injury is suspected. This may be confirmed with a chest X-ray demonstrating a "dropped lung" despite multiple functioning tubes.

Surgical Management

If the patient is able to ventilate adequately, a small bronchial tear may heal without operation, but a larger tear requires a posterolateral thoracotomy, repair, and likely postoperative ventilatory support. In the operating room, the tear is typically found on the posterior wall of the mainstem bronchus within an inch of the carina. The edges of the tear are debrided and repaired with interrupted sutures. The repair may be buttressed with a flap of nearby pericardium if possible. This would obviously require advanced capabilities.

Deep Lung Lacerations

Lung lacerations are usually self-limited and can be treated with tube thoracostomy and supportive measures. The lung receives its blood through a low-pressure system. The normal pulmonary arterial pressure is around 30 mmHg, thus evacuation of clot and resuscitation will usually lead to hemostasis. Rarely, surgical intervention is warranted. If the pulmonary hilum is found to be the source of major hemorrhage on exploration, the left anterior incision should be extended posteriorly. The inferior pulmonary ligament is found heading inferiorly away from the hilum in the mediastinum. It can be released and the lung can be torsed 180 degrees to achieve immediate hemostasis. Additionally, one-lung ventilation (of the noninjured lung) will lead to shunting of blood away from the collapsed lung, thus decreasing blood loss. Depending on the surgeon's skill set, the injured vessels can be repaired directly with fine simple sutures. The injured vessel can be approached from the hilum or through exploration into the laceration in the lung parenchyma via tractotomy. Alternatively, the involved segment or lobe can be resected. The patient's overall condition and available postoperative resources need to be considered before embarking on a large exploration and complex pulmonary procedure.

Chest Wall Injuries

Rib Fractures

Rib fractures are often diagnosed with tenderness on physical examination, or as a result of a chest X-ray finding. Typically, ribs are not "fixed" mechanically or splinted like other bony fractures. Thus, as the broken ribs rub on the exposed periosteum >17,000 times a day, a pain cycle gradually increases over time, leading to decreased lung volumes and splinting of the chest wall. Atelectasis can lead to lung consolidation, which over time can become infected, and the patient develops pneumonia. This cycle can be anticipated and treated with an aggressive cocktail of pain medications with diagnosis (do not wait for pain to develop). This cocktail typically includes "leap-frogging" scheduled alternating doses of acetaminophen and a nonsteroidal analgesic every 3 hours so that the patient receives each medication every 6 hours, plus an opiate for breakthrough pain. These patients should be ambulated aggressively.

Flail Chest

A subset of patients with rib fractures have instability of the chest wall, and an even smaller number have paradoxical motion of the chest wall on breathing known as "flail chest." This is typically found on physical examination by indentation of the involved segment of chest wall on inspiration and protrusion of expiration. This paradoxical chest wall motion can impair ventilation, and these patients will need very aggressive pain control to prevent pneumonia. If available, an epidural catheter should be placed and the patient should receive bolus or patient-controlled analgesia through this for a number of days. Alternatively, multiple rib blocks can be performed in the involved segments. If successful, the blocks can be repeated as they wear off. A subset of these patients will require intubation and positive pressure ventilation until their rib cage has become stable enough to support their own ventilation.

Circulation

The mechanism of injury is very important in understanding the likely culprit of hypovolemic shock that originates in the thorax. A number of intrathoracic injuries can cause hypovolemic shock,

including: injuries to the great vessels, heart, lungs, and chest wall. Typically, injury to the great vessels leads to immediate death at the scene. Their repair is complex and beyond the scope of this chapter.

Diagnosis and Initial Management

The "cardiac box" is the area between the nipples from the clavicles to the costal margins, and penetrating injuries in this area are at high risk for causing an injury to major vascular structures or the heart. A stab wound in "box" in a hypotensive patient warrants immediate exploration if possible. If not possible, intervention should be directed by physical exam and available resources. If breath sounds are absent or muffled, a needle decompression should be done as above. If breath sounds are clear and equal, and pericardial tamponade is suspected by muffled heart sounds and/or jugular venous distension in the face of hypotension, a needle pericardiocentesis may be attempted as a temporizing maneuver. The lungs work under a low hemodynamic pressure system, and thus bleeding from lung lacerations is generally more survivable. Chest wall injuries, including rib fractures, can also lead to significant intrathoracic bleeding as well as ongoing parenchymal injury to the lung. Undrained blood in the thorax can lead to chronic fibrothorax, and may serve as a medium to encourage space infection.

Resuscitation Phase

Two wide-bore intravenous catheters, if available, are placed peripherally, and fluid resuscitation is begun as indicated with saline or Ringer's lactate solution. If available, a portable chest X-ray is taken in the trauma bay. The chest X-ray is reviewed systematically, the lungs are examined for aeration and contusion; a white-out of the hemithorax may signify a massive hemothorax. The pleural cavities are examined for pneumothoraces and hemothoraces. Small blood collections may be found in the costophrenic angles. The heart and pericardium are assessed for contour. A large or "Mateus bottle" contour can be a sign of hemopericardium. The diaphragm position is evaluated as well as aeration of the visible abdominal contents. The bony structures are examined for fracture. The mediastinum is assessed for width, the presence of the aortic knob on the left and the superior vena cava shadow on the right, and any air.

Adjuncts

Chest X-Ray

Table 41.1 shows possible findings on CXR and the corresponding differential diagnoses to consider.

FAST

When ultrasound is present, a focused assessment with sonography for trauma (FAST) exam can be used to assess the pericardium for effusion. A skilled examiner can also find air or blood in the costophrenic angle.

TABLE 41.1

Summary of radiographic findings and associated injuries

CXR Finding	Diagnoses to Consider
Respiratory distress without X-ray findings	CNS injury, aspiration, traumatic asphyxia
Any rib fracture	Pneumothorax, pulmonary contusion
Fracture first 3 ribs or sternoclavicular fracture-dislocation	Airway or great vessel injury
Fractured lower ribs (9 to 12)	Abdominal injury
Two or more rib fractures in two or more places	Flail chest, pulmonary contusion
Scapular fracture	Great vessel injury, pulmonary contusion, brachial plexus injury
Sternal fracture	Blunt cardiac injury
Mediastinal widening	Great vessel injury, sternal fracture, thoracic spine injury
Persistent large pneumothorax or air leak after chest tube insertion	Bronchial tear
Mediastinal air	Esophageal disruption, tracheal injury, pneumoperitoneum
Gastrointestinal (GI) gas pattern in the chest (loculated air)	Diaphragmatic rupture
Nasogastric (NG) tube in the chest	Diaphragmatic rupture or ruptured esophagus
Air fluid level in the chest	Hemopneumothorax or diaphragmatic rupture
Disrupted diaphragm	Abdominal visceral injury
Free air under the diaphragm	Ruptured hollow abdominal viscus

ACS Committee. *The ATLS Student Manual.* 6th ed. Chicago: American College of Surgeons; 2008.

Tube Thoracostomy

If clinical suspicion exists for hemorrhage into a pleural cavity, with or without imaging, a thoracostomy tube should be expediently placed as previously described. Output on insertion should be recorded as well as hourly output.

Thoracotomy

Indications

Thoracotomy should not be attempted unless a trained surgeon is present and the patient has lost vital signs within the last several minutes. In an environment where thoracotomy may be performed with appropriate personnel present, indications for immediate exploration of the chest include:

- Stable patient with >1500 cc upon initial chest tube insertion or more than one third the patient's calculated blood volume
- Persistent blood requirements despite receiving blood products and output greater than 250 cc an hour for a few hours
- Penetrating injury to the "cardiac box": medial to the nipple line or scapular tip line
- Unstable patient with significant hemothorax
- Cardiac tamponade: Beck's triad: muffled heart sounds, elevated venous pressure, decreased arterial pressure

Procedure

In penetrating trauma to the left of the sternum, a left anterior thoracotomy would be the incision of choice. In right-sided penetrating trauma, a midline sternotomy would be preferred.

A cardiac laceration injury from an anterior penetrating injury typically involves the right ventricle. It can be approached through an anterior lateral thoracotomy or midline sternotomy. The pericardium is opened, and double-armed monofilament pledgeted 2.0 mattress sutures are placed. Care is taken when sewing a beating heart to time the placement of the suture with diastole. It is essential to slide the needle smoothly through the tissue in order not to enlarge the hole. In the event that additional stitches are needed, they are placed until complete hemostasis is obtained. Great care must be taken to avoid injury to named coronary vessels, which can typically be seen pulsing in the ventricular wall muscle.

Emergency Room Thoracotomy

Procedure: Anterior lateral thoracotomy (Figure 41.3).

Indication: Penetrating trauma to the "box" leading to severe shock or witnessed recent loss of signs of life.

Aim: Urgent identification of bleeding source or cross-clamping of the aorta if the source is not readily visible, with volume resuscitation and rapid control of bleeding source.

Equipment: Alcohol or Betadine, sterile drapes, a large scalpel, long scissors, long blunt forceps, long needle drivers, aortic clamps (straight and curved), a large chest wall retractor, large malleable retractor, large sponges, a strong working suction device, 2.0 silk sutures and ties, teflon pledgets if available (if not, pericardium can be used), large chest tubes, and a chest tube collecting system (preferably with suction).

Optional but beneficial: Linear staplers with reloads (preferably Endo GIA), vascular as well as heavy tissue loads.

Technique: The surgeon stands to the patient's left, using a large blade (22), rapidly cutting down to intercostal muscle. In a female patient, cut along inferior mammary fold and elevate the breast off the inferior aspect of the pectoralis muscle. Divide the intercostal muscle along the upper edge of the sixth rib, enter the chest, and place the chest wall retractor between the ribs, using suction to remove any blood encountered. Pack the chest and then systematically assess for the source of hemorrhage. The next steps are directed as necessitated by the injury encountered. Incise the pericardium vertically with scissors parallel and anterior to the phrenic nerve, taking into account the beating heart and timing incisions appropriately. The patient's volume status

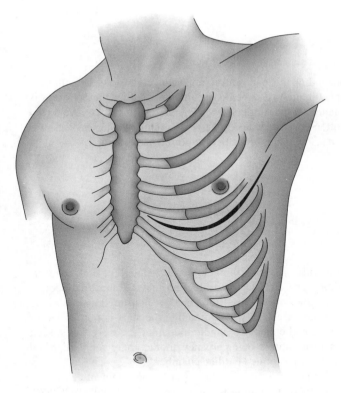

FIGURE 41.3 Anterolateral thoracotomy. Henning R. *Critical Care Cardiology*. Philadelphia: Elsevier, 1989.

can be assessed by observing the heart for distention or collapse. Cardiac activity may also provide some sense of whether the patient will survive or not. Vigorous cardiac contraction implies a greater chance of success. A sluggish or still heart is less likely to respond to volume resuscitation. If faced with the evacuation of a large or ongoing volume of hemorrhage from within the pericardium, a cardiac laceration may need to be controlled and repaired as above. This may require extending the incision medially (horizontally) into or beyond the sternum using heavy scissors to obtain adequate exposure.

If the patient is in extremis, the descending aorta can be dissected circumferentially. The surgeon bluntly dissects around the aorta with his index finger, taking care not to inadvertently injure the esophagus or avulse direct intercostal perforators. A straight aortic clamp can then be placed temporarily, enabling rapid resuscitation. Clamping the aorta can provide a short window of opportunity in which surgical bleeding that led to hypovolemic shock can be controlled. If this maneuver is necessary, survival is unlikely unless a bleeding source can be promptly identified and addressed.

Pitfalls

- Transection of chest wall arteries leading to unnecessary bleeding and possible long-term disability (internal mammary, thoracodorsal, long thoracic, and intercostal)
- Lung injury, upon rapid entrance to the chest
- Phrenic nerve injury upon opening of the pericardium (runs from anterior-lateral to the thoracic inlet sloping along the pericardium posterior to the hilar structures
- Cardiac injury when opening the pericardium (remember timing of surgical actions when operating in and around a beating structure)
- Esophageal injury when getting around the aorta in order to clamp

Diaphragmatic Laceration/Rupture

Surgical Management

Surgical repair of the diaphragm is possible through a thoracotomy or a laparotomy. For the general surgeon a midline laparotomy may be the most comfortable approach. Abdominal contents are reduced back into the abdomen and then the diaphragm is repaired by placing multiple interrupted pledgeted (if available) mattress stitches (2.0). Williams et al. describe a mortality rate of 23% in a large series of traumatic diaphragmatic ruptures in an urban level 1 trauma center in the United States.[3] This mortality rate is reflective of the fact that associated injuries are usually present. In LMICs where there is a lack of blood banking capability, attention to prompt hemorrhage control must be the surgical strategy. The diaphragm can be repaired in a delayed procedure. The left phrenic nerve originates in the 3 o'clock position in the center of the diaphragm, in the midaxillary line just lateral to the crura. The nerve branches then fan out circumferentially toward the periphery. The diaphragmatic vessels originate as direct branches off of the aorta and superior vena cava and follow the nerves. A similar pattern occurs on the right with the origin of the nerve at 9 o'clock in the inferior lateral region of the inferior vena cava. The neurovascular bundles must be avoided during the repair to prevent a postoperative paralyzed diaphragm.

COMMENTARY

Koffi Herve Yangni-Angate, Cote d'Ivoire

The incidence of thoracic trauma cases is increasing in low- and middle-income countries (LMICs) in Africa. Thoracic trauma is the result of accidental injury, as seen in automobile collisions (sometimes from unsafe roads), and intentional injury, as seen in stabbings or gunshot wounds. We often see lesions, including those in rib fractures, lung contusions, hemothorax, pneumothorax, or hemo-pneumothorax. Tube thoracostomy is generally the surgical procedure used with success. We do not often see cardiac and great vessels injuries, injuries of the trachea and major bronchi, or ruptured diaphragms.[4-6]

COMMENTARY

Ikechukwu A. Nwafor, Nigeria

In LMICs like Nigeria, where I practice, thoracic trauma continues to be one of the leading causes of morbidity and mortality among the young and old, with an estimated mortality rate of 40%. The unique challenges in the management of thoracic trauma can be divided into trauma that occurs in the field, in accidents and emergency situations, in the operating room, and in the intensive care units or wards.

In the field, trained paramedics are few to nonexistent. Ambulance services are poor. Patients often present late to accident centers. Once patients get to the accident center, it may be very difficult to diagnose them because the technology may not be available; this includes a chest X-ray, computed tomography (CT) angiography, or magnetic resonance angiogram (MRA). For this reason, the doctor must rely mainly on his or her clinical skills to diagnose the patient.

In the operating room, the requisite equipment is usually inadequate or absent. For example, we may not have a facility for video-assisted thoracic surgery (VATS), and echocardiography and electrocardiogram may be unavailable or, if available, may be malfunctional or nonfunctional if we do not have electricity. Additionally, the staff is not skilled or motivated enough to handle moderate to severe cases, such as resuscitative or emergency thoracotomy for a ruptured aorta or perforated cardiac chamber.

In intensive care units and wards, management of patients with thoracic trauma in these areas faces many challenges, ranging from infrastructure to equipment to personnel. Ventilators, pulse oximeters, portable chest X-ray machines, transducers for central lines, and portable echocardiography machines including the consumables are either lacking or inadequate when available.

In conclusion, management of chest trauma cases, especially high-profile ones, is grossly inadequate in LMICs like Nigeria.

42

Abdominal Trauma

Alexi C. Matousek
Thomas G. Weiser
Selwyn O. Rogers

Introduction

This chapter provides an overview for treating patients in low- and middle-income countries (LMICs) who present with abdominal trauma. Management of specific organs is discussed.

Specific Considerations for LMICs

History and physical exam are keys in the diagnosis and management of abdominal trauma. Attention to cultural context and language will facilitate an accurate history and physical examination. While a proper history and physical examination are needed, there are a number of important pitfalls to avoid when working in an LMIC.

Inadequate, inappropriate, or poorly executed operations will cause excess harm, morbidity, and mortality, and end up stressing an already under-resourced system. In addition, they will add significant financial and social burdens on a family. The best chance for a good outcome is during the first operation. Due to geographic constraints, patients often present much later in the time course of their injury. Long distances and significant delays in care render patients dehydrated, metabolically deranged, and physically compromised. Appropriate resuscitation prior to surgery is essential to prevent cardiovascular collapse in these patients. Finally, surgical outcomes are frequently linked to the reputation of the health center, and intraoperative or postoperative deaths, even if unavoidable, can reflect poorly on the facility. As such, the response may be later presentation and a vicious cycle of moribund patients whose likelihood of survival is negligible and resultant decline in hospital reputation.

General Principles

Mechanism of Injury

Abdominal trauma may be divided by mechanism of injury. Blunt trauma usually results from falls or motor vehicle crashes that may lead to multiple injuries. Blunt trauma may present a difficult diagnostic scenario, for often the external exam reveals few physical abnormalities. In such instance, a high index of clinical suspicion is essential. Any abrasion or evidence of abdominal wall trauma should alert the clinician to the possibility of occult intra-abdominal injury. Such patients should be treated with extreme caution and care, as their initial history and presentation can be deceivingly benign.

Penetrating abdominal trauma usually results from the piercing of the abdominal cavity by a sharp object such as a knife, lance, or even a tree branch, or by violation of the cavity by a projectile such as bullet or shrapnel. Ballistic injuries can be disarmingly small, and can also be located at a distance from the abdominal cavity, such as the leg, arm, chest, back, or buttock. Depending on the trajectory of the missile and the position of the patient when struck, a missile can exit the patient or come to rest at a very peculiar distance from its original point of entry. Any and all structures in between the point of entry and exit (or final position) of a missile are at risk of injury, and a careful and methodical examination must be undertaken should the patient require an operation. One note of caution regarding the external exam should be mentioned: penetration of the rectum and vagina can cause internal damage with little external visible injury and should not be overlooked during the initial assessment of a traumatized patient, particularly one who is unresponsive.

As a general rule, patients who have a penetrating injury with violation of their peritoneum should be taken to the operating room for exploration. However, such an undertaking should not be without consideration. Good evidence has accumulated demonstrating that even patients with a penetrating mechanism can be managed nonoperatively if they remain hemodynamically normal and stable, are closely monitored by a trained clinician, and remain free from peritonitis and increasing abdominal rigidity. Any patient who presents with hemodynamic compromise or peritonitis should be immediately explored in the operating room.

No matter what the mechanism, the two most immediate life-threatening concerns are bleeding and bowel leakage. Any patient who presents with hemodynamic instability, or becomes unstable within the first 12–24 hours of injury, should be taken urgently to the operating room.

Initial Evaluation

Evaluation of an injured patient begins with a rapid but thorough history and physical exam. Important information includes the time and mechanism of injury, whether others were injured or killed at the same time or from the same mechanism,

BOX 42.1 LMIC-SPECIFIC CONSIDERATIONS

In the management of the multiply injured patient or a traumatized patient:

1. Attention to the available resources (e.g., blood products, intensive care unit capacity, nursing care) is essential.
2. Attention to airway, breathing, and circulation is paramount.
3. Adequate IV access is mandatory to ensure fluid resuscitation.
4. Suspect a diaphragmatic injury in a patient with a significant traumatic mechanism and many associated injuries.
5. Serial chest X-rays in intubated patients can confirm the diagnosis days to weeks after injury.
6. Nasogastric tube decompression can alleviate dyspnea with a herniated stomach.
7. A chest tube is usually required for associated rib fractures and hemopneumothorax.

and the amount of blood lost at the scene. An initial physical exam should rapidly identify airway or respiratory compromise, hemodynamic instability in the form of tachycardia or hypotension, obvious sources of bleeding, new weaknesses and disabilities, the level of consciousness, and any obvious anatomic deformities or injuries. After identifying and correcting any life-threatening airway, breathing, or circulatory issues, a complete secondary exam is essential. This includes careful inspection, auscultation, palpation, and percussion of the abdomen and a digital rectal exam to look for bleeding. In women, a careful manual vaginal exam is also important as fullness in the rectovaginal pouch may indicate hemoperitoneum. Abrasions or bruising on the abdominal wall should raise concerns about possible internal injury, as should any tenderness to palpation, rigidity, or guarding. Equivocal exams should be repeated every 30–60 minutes, ideally by the same clinician so progression of peritonitis can be identified and operative management undertaken without undo delay.

Ancillary Tests

Laboratory tests should be obtained if possible to establish a baseline hemoglobin level. However, hemoglobin levels will not drop until the patient receives intravenous (IV) resuscitation, and the white blood count may not rise until infection and peritonitis set in, or may rise from the stress response alone.

Plain chest and pelvis X-rays can be a useful adjunct to the physical exam. If a portable X-ray machine is available, these can be obtained after the initial physical examination without moving the patient. A chest X-ray may reveal a widened mediastinum, pneumothorax, or rib fractures. Abdominal films should be taken with the patient upright if possible. Features to look for are disruptions to the curve of the diaphragm, pleural effusions, fractures to the lower ribs, air under the diaphragm, and foreign bodies.

If available, ultrasound examination can help make a diagnosis, but knowledge of its use and the ability to interpret the images are fundamental. With an experienced ultrasonographer, the space between the liver and kidney, the space between the spleen and kidney, around the bladder, and within the pericardium should reveal no fluid collections in normal patients. Fluid around any of these structures should raise suspicion of an intra-abdominal injury and prompt operative exploration in the hemodynamically unstable patient.

In locations without ultrasound, a diagnostic peritoneal lavage or aspirate (DPL/A) can be useful if internal hemorrhage is included in the initial differential diagnosis. In locations with more resources, computed tomography (CT) scanning or diagnostic laparoscopy can be extremely helpful.

Management Strategies

Depending upon the mechanism and clinical status of the patient, operative management versus observation of patients who suffer abdominal trauma is indicated. Prior to initiation of a plan, attention to airway, breathing, and circulation; adequate IV access; and fluid resuscitation are paramount.

In the hemodynamically unstable patient, the presence of gross blood from a DPL/A or free fluid in the abdomen on ultrasound is an indication for emergent laparotomy.

In the hemodynamically stable patient, free fluid on ultrasound is not an absolute indication for urgent surgery, as it cannot differentiate solid organ injury from hollow viscus injury. In such cases, diagnostic peritoneal lavage can help reveal the nature of the injury. If the sample reveals gross blood, succus, or food particles, or is so murky as to render the fluid opaque (some use the criterion of being unable to read newspaper print through the fluid sample), then exploratory laparotomy should be performed. If negative, it should be kept in mind that DPL may be falsely negative in the early period after trauma. The decision to operate should be based on the clinical judgment of the individual surgeon.

Penetrating wounds to the abdomen and lower chest should raise suspicion of abdominal injury. In the absence of peritonitis, abdominal wounds can be locally explored to investigate if the peritoneum has been violated. If there is any doubt that the peritoneum may have been entered (i.e., penetration of the anterior abdominal fascia), the patient may undergo a laparotomy to evaluate for intra-abdominal injury or be carefully observed for development of peritonitis over a 24- to 48-hour time period. Laparoscopy may also be employed, if available, to inspect the abdomen. If penetration of the peritoneum is noted on laparoscopy, an exploratory laparotomy must be performed. If CT is available, it can be very useful in the management of hemodynamically stable trauma patients.

When preparing for an operation, the extent of injury is rarely clear. Positioning and wide scrub preparation are essential (Figure 42.1). Patients should be laid supine on the table and prepped from chin to knees with the groins exposed and genitalia covered. This allows access to the chest, abdomen, neck, and groins. For isolated extremity or neck injuries, prep the groins as well as the chest to facilitate exposure and vascular control, and to allow for vein harvesting should this be necessary. During positioning and preparation, communication with the anesthetic and nursing teams is essential: prepare the entire operating room (OR)

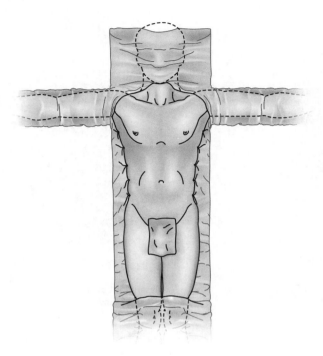

FIGURE 42.1 Patient positioning and preparation for a trauma exploratory operation. Hirshberg A, Mattox K. *Top Knife: The Art and Craft of Trauma Surgery.* Castle Hill Barns: TFM Publishing, 2008, p. 7.

BOX 42.2 POTENTIAL PITFALLS TO AVOID

1. Operating outside of your comfort zone could lead to a patient's death.
2. Preemptive maneuvers to address acidosis, avoid hypothermia, and correct coagulopathy can save lives.
3. Inadequate exposure leads to prolonged operative times and potential morbidity and mortality.
4. Leaving a missed injury:
   a. GE junction
   b. Ligament of Treitz
   c. Mesenteric border
   d. Posterior wall of transverse colon
   e. Extraperitoneal rectum
5. Placing excess tension on the greater curve of the stomach during inspection, causing avulsion injury to the short gastrics and/or spleen.
6. Decide on a damage control approach early if the patient has a large physiologic insult.
7. Consider leaving the skin open in cases with gross gastric spillage, especially with intraperitoneal bleeding to prevent skin infections.

---

team for what to anticipate. Making use of this time to gather appropriate instruments, place lines, and verbalize an operative plan will help prevent delays once the operation gets underway.

Damage control surgery refers to a strategy of controlling bleeding and contamination in a severely injured and metabolically compromised patient without attempting to provide definitive repair of all injuries. It has been described and is used in HICs where intensive care units provide support and resuscitation to these patients. It has only a limited role in LMICs. However, in select patients with survivable injuries, there may be a role for delayed repair of intra-abdominal injuries if this allows appropriate resuscitation and to limit the initial surgical insult.

Injury to Stomach, Bowel, and Mesentery

Definition and Clinical Presentation

Hollow viscus injuries are unusual in blunt trauma but significantly more common in penetrating trauma. The patient may have diffuse peritonitis with a rigid, distended abdomen on presentation.

Surgical Management of Hollow Viscus Injury

If hollow viscus injury is suspected, broad-spectrum antibiotics should be administered prior to incision. If injury is confirmed, antibiotics should be continued for 24 hours; however, they should be discontinued after this as there is no evidence for continuing antibiotics after 24 hours, even in cases of gross peritoneal contamination. If free intraperitoneal blood and succus are encountered upon entering the abdomen, hemostasis

takes priority. The abdomen should be packed in all four quadrants with absorbent pads and the bleeding controlled prior to any repair of a hollow viscous injury. If spillage from a bowel injury is obscuring the operative field, temporary control can be achieved by placing clamps on the injured bowel to prevent ongoing spillage.

Once hemostasis is achieved and adequate resuscitation has been performed, the entire length of the bowel should be systematically evaluated from the ligament of Treitz to the ileocecal valve, and the entire colon inspected to the level of the peritoneal reflection deep in the pelvis. Special care should be taken to inspect both sides of the bowel, especially the mesenteric border as a perforation may occur into the mesentery without spillage into the abdomen (Figure 42.2). Any enterotomies should be controlled as they are encountered to prevent excess spillage. If there are an odd number of holes in the gastrointestinal (GI) tract after penetrating trauma, three possibilities exist: one injury is tangential, the missile is in the lumen of the bowel, or there is another injury which is not yet identified. Be sure to compulsively examine the entire GI tract to ensure no injury has been missed.

Specific Injuries

Stomach

Be sure to examine both surfaces of the stomach by entering the lesser sac and reflecting the stomach superiorly to examine the posterior surface. An intramural hematoma should be unroofed and evacuated. If there is no penetration of the mucosa, simple silk interrupted seromuscular sutures will sufficiently repair the injury. Larger lacerations can also be repaired primarily using

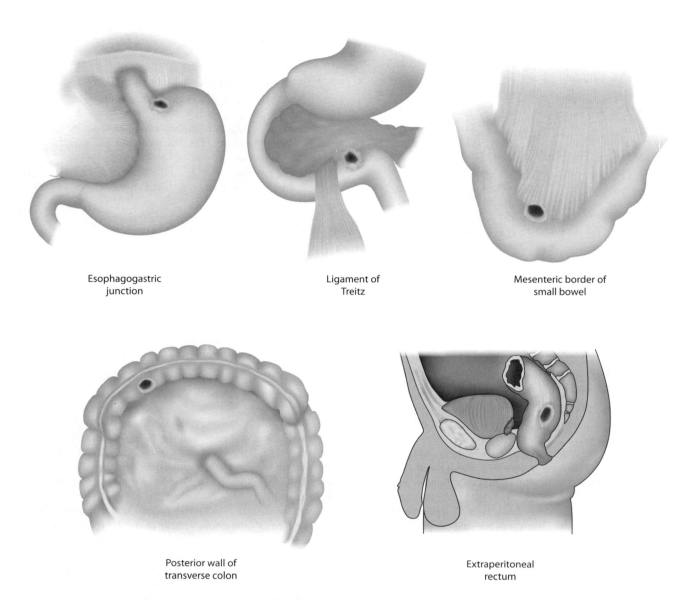

Esophagogastric
junction

Ligament of
Treitz

Mesenteric border of
small bowel

Posterior wall of
transverse colon

Extraperitoneal
rectum

FIGURE 42.2   Commonly missed bowel injuries. Hirshberg A, Mattox K. *Top Knife: The Art and Craft of Trauma Surgery.* Castle Hill Barns: TFM Publishing, 2008, p. 73.

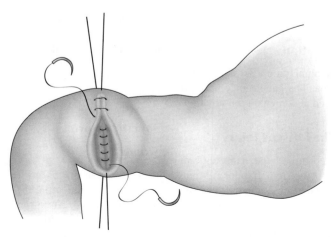

FIGURE 42.3   Pyloroplasty. Souba W, Fink M. *ACS Surgery,* 6th ed. Hamilton: Decker Publishing, 2007.

slow absorbable sutures, taking care to close both the mucosa and serosal layers as the gastric mucosa is well vascularized and has a propensity to bleed. Use the gastric cardia to reinforce the repair if the injury is near the gastroesophageal junction. If the wound involves the pylorus, conversion to a pyloroplasty (Figure 42.3) can help prevent future stenosis. More severe injury to the stomach is rare, as most patients die before laparotomy, but in the case of significant tissue loss with partial devascularization, a partial gastrectomy should be performed and either a gastroduodenostomy or gastrojejunostomy (Figure 42.4A and Figure 42.4B) created based on the presence of other injuries.[1] A complete gastrectomy with Roux-en-Y reconstruction may be necessary for an injury that involves a large amount of tissue loss and devascularization. If the patient is severely injured with a large physiologic insult, a damage control operation may be a wise choice before the lethal triad of hypothermia, acidemia, and coagulopathy ensues. Leaving the abdominal incision open in the case of spillage is wise.

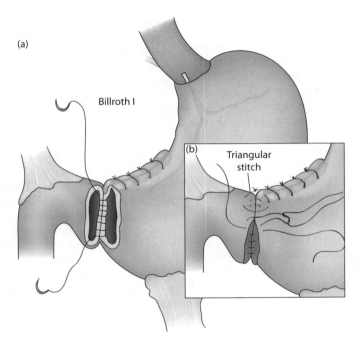

FIGURE 42.4A Gastroduodenostomy reconstruction (Billroth I) for injuries to the stomach that require a partial gastrectomy. Souba W, Fink M. *ACS Surgery,* 6th ed. Hamilton: Decker Publishing, 2007.

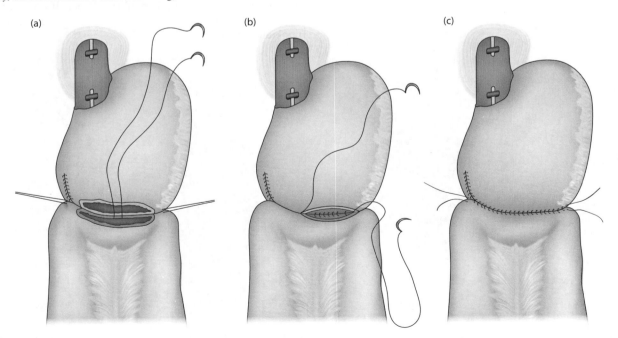

FIGURE 42.4B Gastrojejunostomy reconstruction (Billroth II) for injuries to the stomach that require a partial gastrectomy. Souba W, Fink M. *ACS Surgery,* 6th ed. Hamilton: Decker Publishing, 2007.

Duodenum

A simple duodenal injury can be repaired primarily in transverse fashion using absorbable sutures to avoid narrowing the lumen. Consider opening the duodenum anteriorly to either inspect the mucosal surface for a posterior injury, or to repair a posterior injury from inside the lumen. If the injury requires more than just a short suture line, or the repair appears tenuous in any way, perform a pyloric exclusion (Figure 42.5). Place closed suction drains near all but the most pristine, short suture lines.

A pyloric exclusion is performed by making a longitudinal incision just proximal to the pylorus and extending a few centimeters proximally along the antrum of the stomach. Pull the pylorus proximally with clamps and oversew the pylorus with heavy suture in big bites (0 Vicryl or equivalent). Then bring up a loop of jejunum and create a gastrojejunostomy, and finish with a feeding jejunostomy tube. Vagotomy is not required.

A large duodenal injury comprising more than 50% of the circumference can potentially be debrided and anastomosed end-to-end, but many times there is not enough length. If the patient is stable with no other active injuries, a Roux-en-Y reconstruction is possible. However, in most cases, it is most prudent to attempt reconstruction in delayed fashion, and not during the initial operation.

Small Bowel

Enterotomies discovered upon laparotomy should be temporarily controlled at the time of their discovery to prevent excess spillage. Clamps may be used to seal an enterotomy during the initial phases of the trauma laparotomy. Once hemorrhage is controlled, the entire small bowel should be inspected in systematic fashion from the ligament of Treitz to the ileocecal valve, taking care to investigate the mesenteric border for bleeding.

Once all enterotomies have been identified, the decision must be made to do a damage-control operation or proceed with definitive repair. This decision should be based on the total physiologic insult the patient has endured, and not the presence of hypothermia, acidosis, and coagulopathy, as once any of these ominous signs have developed, it is often too late.

If the decision has been made to perform a damage-control operation, the bowel may be left in discontinuity. Cotton tape can be used to ligate the bowel on either side of an enterotomy to prevent spillage (Figure 42.6).[1] The abdomen should then be temporarily closed. The simplest way to temporarily close the abdomen is to use several penetrating towel clips to close the skin without any closure of the fascia or subcutaneous tissue. This method is quick, but still leaves the patient vulnerable to abdominal compartment syndrome. Alternatively, a sterile IV fluid bag can be opened and the plastic sewn to the edges of the wound. A vacuum-pack can be fashioned by placing a sterile plastic drape over the bowels and into the paracolic gutters. Closed suction drains are placed on top of the plastic sheet and covered with sterile towels. The entire abdomen is then covered in a plastic adhesive sheet, and the drains placed to suction. The patient can then be stabilized in an intensive setting. Definitive repair may be undertaken when the patient is stable enough to allow abdominal closure without tension.

If the patient is stable, definitive repair may be considered at the time of the initial surgery. Hematomas in the bowel wall should be unroofed to inspect for penetration through the mucosa. Serosal tears in the bowel wall can be oversewn with interrupted sutures. Small enterotomies less than 50% of the diameter of the bowel can be repaired in one or two layers in a transverse orientation to avoid luminal narrowing. Injuries that are greater than 50% of the diameter of the bowel should be resected and an anastomosis performed.[2] Small bowel anastomoses can be sewn in one or two layers, depending on surgeon preference (Figure 42.7).

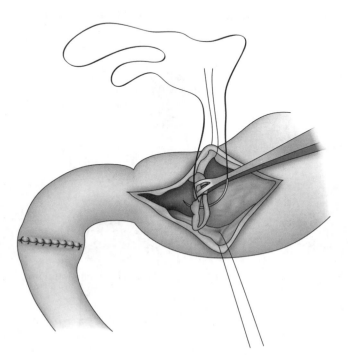

FIGURE 42.5 Pyloric exclusion. Hirshberg A, Mattox K. *Top Knife: The Art and Craft of Trauma Surgery.* Castle Hill Barns: TFM Publishing, 2008, p. 126.

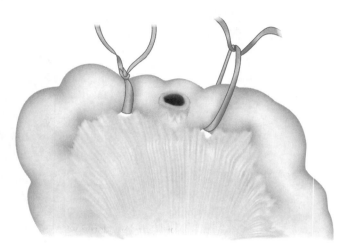

FIGURE 42.6 Cotton tape ligation. Hirshberg A, Mattox K. *Top Knife: The Art and Craft of Trauma Surgery.* Castle Hill Barns: TFM Publishing, 2008, p. 75.

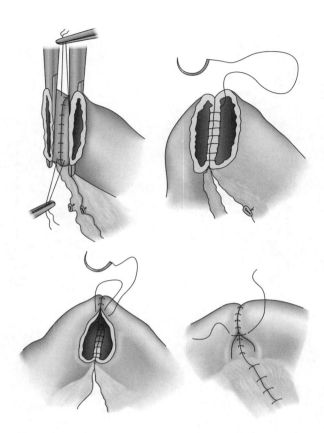

FIGURE 42.7 Two-layer hand-sewn small bowel anastomosis. Souba W, Fink M. *ACS Surgery,* 6th ed. Hamilton: Decker Publishing, 2007.

Colon

Colonic injuries can be particularly devastating if they are missed, and one must be especially vigilant when inspecting the colon for injury during the laparotomy for trauma. If there is any question, the colon should be mobilized to inspect the posterior surface. Do not leave any hematoma on the colon, no matter how small, without unroofing it and inspecting for perforation.[1]

Injuries to the colon that comprise less than 50% of the diameter of the colon should be repaired primarily if there is no peritonitis and the patient is stable during the operation. Partial-thickness defects can be closed in a single layer of inverting seromuscular sutures. Full-thickness lacerations should be closed in one or two layers. Injuries that destroy more than 50% of the diameter of the colon, or have extensive tissue loss or a devascularized segment, should be managed with resection and anastomosis.

Historically, traumatic injury to the colon was managed by colostomy in nearly all cases. Today, more than 90% of colonic injuries can be managed with primary repair or resection and anastomosis. Delayed skin closure may be wise in cases with significant spillage. Foreign bodies should be removed when possible to prevent abscess formation. Diversion with a transverse loop colostomy (Figure 42.8) should be considered when there is peritonitis, the operation is delayed from initial injury, or when the patient has sustained a significant injury.

The location of the injury is a major determinant in the decision to perform an anastomosis. Injuries to the right colon should be managed with primary repair or a right hemicolectomy with anastomosis between the terminal ileum and transverse colon. Injuries to the left colon are more difficult. If the patient is young, and has not sustained a large physiological insult, resection and anastomosis may be considered. However, for any patient who is slightly unstable, is elderly, or has significant comorbidities, closing the distal colon as a Hartmann's pouch and performing a proximal diverting colostomy is the more prudent option.

Rectum

A missed rectal injury can have devastating consequences. Therefore, any trauma patient with penetrating wounds to the abdomen, thigh, buttock, perineum, or groin should be carefully examined to rule out rectal injury. Every patient should receive a rectal examination followed by rigid proctoscopy if any injury is suspected.

Injuries to the rectum above the peritoneal reflection should be treated in the same manner as left-sided colon injuries. Injuries to the rectum below the peritoneal reflection can usually be explored and repaired, with fecal diversion via end or loop colostomy. If the injury is difficult to access, or exploration would risk damage to the surrounding nerves and genitourinary organs, then presacral drainage with diversion via end or loop colostomy should be considered. Presacral drainage is performed with the patient in lithotomy position. A curvilinear incision is made between the coccyx and the anus. The presacral space is

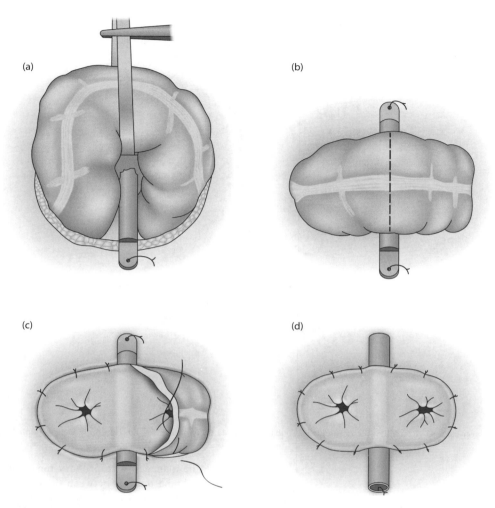

FIGURE 42.8   Transverse loop colostomy. Souba W, Fink M. *ACS Surgery,* 6th ed. Hamilton: Decker Publishing, 2007.

entered using blunt dissection, and penrose drains are placed in the space and sutured to the skin (Figure 42.9). They are then gradually withdrawn several days after the initial operation.

Mesentery

In contrast to the bowel, the mesentery will bleed profusely when injured. An expanding mesenteric hematoma should be controlled with manual pressure or gentle handling in between clamps. Mesenteric bleeding should be controlled as close to the source of bleeding as possible to preserve the maximum vascular supply to the remaining bowel. If the hematoma is at the root of the mesentery, do not immediately open the hematoma as it may conceal a lacerated superior mesenteric vein, which would be further injured with blind clamping. Instead, pinch off the root of the mesentery with your hand and then carefully explore the hematoma. Optimize your exposure, light, and position, and then make a careful repair. Blind stitching can result in ligation of major vessels such as the superior mesenteric artery, causing bowel ischemia.[1]

Injuries to Diaphragm

Definition and Clinical Presentation

The diaphragm may be injured in either blunt or penetrating trauma. In either scenario, the injury usually occurs on the left as the right hemi-diaphragm is protected by the liver. The diagnosis can be especially difficult as the initial chest X-ray can be normal and the patient may not be symptomatic until weeks later.

Differential Diagnosis

The initial chest X-ray may show elevation of the diaphragm, hemothorax, gas shadow overlying the hemidiaphragm, or a nasogastric tube positioned in the chest, which is classic for the condition.[3] The injury may produce severe dyspnea or may be asymptomatic for weeks. If the patient is on ventilatory support with more than 5 cm H_2O of positive end-expiratory pressure (PEEP), the abdominal contents may not herniate, and the injury may only become apparent as the PEEP is weaned and the

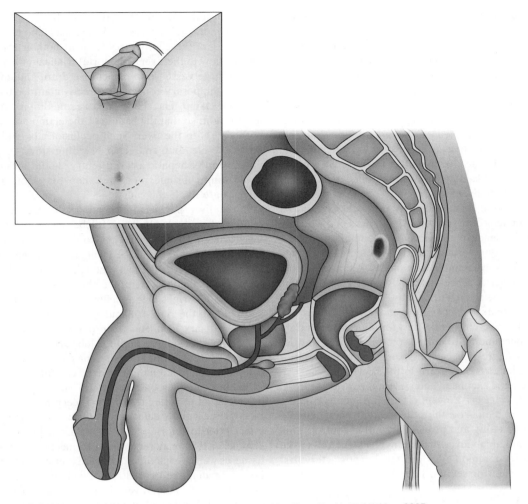

FIGURE 42.9   Presacral drainage. Souba W, Fink M. *ACS Surgery,* 6th ed. Hamilton: Decker Publishing, 2007.

abdominal contents start to rise into the chest. Therefore, serial chest X-rays should be obtained to avoid a missed diaphragmatic injury.[4]

CT scanning has become commonplace in the evaluation of trauma patients in HICs but may not be available in many LMICs. If laparoscopy is available, it may be reasonable to explore a hemodynamically normal patient with a penetrating injury with a laparoscope.

Procedure Highlights

Diaphragm injuries are most easily approached via laparotomy. A chest tube usually should be inserted first, taking special care to avoid injuring herniated abdominal organs that are displaced into the chest. Repair is facilitated by decompressing the stomach with a nasogastric tube, mobilizing the left lobe of the liver to the patient's right, and gently retracting the abdominal contents out of the chest. The edges of the torn diaphragm should be grasped with long clamps to gently bring them into view. Use large No. 1 monofilament nonabsorbable sutures in running fashion to close the defect. Some advantage may be gained by using gentle traction on one suture while taking the next bite.

Interrupted sutures may be placed first to take tension off the continuous repair. Occasionally, the defect is too large to enable primary closure, and a polypropylene mesh must be inserted. Alternatively, if there is loss of chest wall integrity with multiple rib fractures, the diaphragm may be resuspended from higher ribs to allow closure.[2]

Solid Organ Injury

Liver Injuries

The liver is the most commonly injured solid organ following blunt trauma, and given its size and position, is also frequently injured in penetrating injuries as well. Blunt injuries typically affect the liver substance and hepatic veins, while penetrating injuries are more frequently associated with hepatic arterial injury. Controlling bleeding is the main concern with hepatic trauma. As the liver is difficult to expose and repair, areas that are not bleeding are best left alone. The feared retrohepatic injury to the vena cava is happily a fairly rare occurrence, but when present is difficult to control even in the most experienced of hands.

Exposure is usually through a midline laparotomy; however, this can be extended by T-ing the incision laterally to the right to obtain adequate visualization in extreme cases. In addition, should suprahepatic vena cava control become necessary while performing total hepatic vascular isolation, extension to the chest with a partial or full sternotomy or right thoracotomy is also an option.

Initial management of bleeding liver injuries requires prompt packing of the right upper quadrant (Figure 42.10). If this controls bleeding, attention can be turned to other areas of the abdomen, and once enteral contamination and other sources of bleeding are identified and controlled, reexamination of the liver can proceed more systematically. If bleeding appears controlled, palpation of the entire surface of the liver is warranted to evaluate the extent of injury. Medial mobilization of the liver to look at its posterior aspect and inferior vena cava is not worth the risks of dislodging clot if there is no evidence of uncontrolled bleeding.

Packing should be done systematically by placing laparotomy sponges over obvious tears and lacerations as well as along the right lateral and posterior aspects of the liver between it and the diaphragm to compress the liver medially. This will often reapproximate edges of tears and lacerations and provide hemostasis in the majority of cases. This works best for injuries to the right lobe; the left is much more difficult to compress in this way. Be aware that overly aggressive packing can occlude the inferior vena cava and reduce venous return to the heart, and can also impede diaphragmatic excursion and elevate airway pressures.

If bleeding remains brisk despite packing, control of the vascular inflow can temporize the situation long enough to aid identification of bleeding and provide definitive control. This is done by a Pringle maneuver, which involves encircling the triad of portal vein, common bile duct, and hepatic artery first with a finger by blunt dissection lateral to medial sweeping

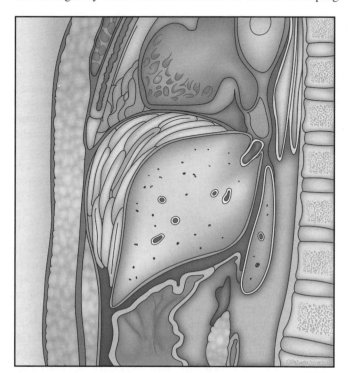

FIGURE 42.10 Hepatic packing. Souba W, Fink M. *ACS Surgery,* 6th ed. Hamilton: Decker Publishing, 2007.

underneath the portal structures and then bluntly penetrating the lesser omentum between the stomach and left liver. Gentle squeezing of these structures restricts both arterial and portal venous flow to the liver. The portal triad can then be encircled with a large vessel loop or penrose drain and compressed to provide temporary control, or directly clamped using a curved vascular clamp. The clamp is passed medial to lateral (patient left to right) so that the handle of the clamp does not interfere with access to the liver. Such occlusion also aids in diagnosis of the bleeding source: if bleeding slows or ceases, then portal vein or hepatic arterial injury should be suspected, but if bleeding continues unabated, hepatic venous or vena cava injuries are likely the source.

If the liver parenchyma continues to bleed, mobilize the injured lobe completely. The left lobe can be mobilized by incising the falciform ligament close to the body of the liver all the way to the diaphragm. The triangular ligament is divided by sweeping a finger underneath the lateral edge and retracting the lobe caudad, being aware of the phrenic vein just superior to the ligament. The right lobe is mobilized by retracting it medially and incising the right triangular ligament lateral to medial up to the coronary ligaments, then freeing the anterior and posterior coronary ligaments until the lobe is completely mobile. The hepatic veins enter the inferior vena cava (IVC) in this area, so complete mobilization must be done carefully.

Small lacerations on the surface can be packed with gauze or omentum, or sutured with wide, deep bites using absorbable monofilament and a blunt needle. Gauze can also be packed into a tear prior to suturing if reexploration is planned. Larger lacerations or tears may require debridement to remove devitalized tissue, as well as exploration to identify torn vessels that need ligation. Extending the laceration is fraught with risks, but can help identify specific injured vessels that can subsequently be ligated or repaired. While undertaking this, individual vessels encountered on the way to the depth of the laceration should be ligated.

If a through-and-through injury is encountered, particularly one crossing both lobes of the liver, tamponade of the tract can be achieved using a red rubber catheter threaded through a penrose drain. The penrose is tied at the distal end, the catheter then introduced, and the drain tied tightly at its base around the drain. Once this makeshift balloon is tested for leaks by infusing the red rubber catheter with saline, it can be maneuvered through the hole in the liver and the balloon inflated with saline to fill the tract and tamponade the injury. By bringing the catheter out of the abdominal wall through a separate stab incision, it can be retrieved after removing the saline without requiring reexploration.

Drainage of liver injuries is controversial; however, if bile is clearly noted, wide drainage will help prevent bile peritonitis and may control bilomas.

Portal Triad Injuries

Injuries to the portal structures are usually due to penetrating mechanisms. If they are localized between the pancreas and the liver, control of bleeding with pressure, wide mobilization, and direct repair is possible. If both the hepatic artery and portal vein are injured, at least one needs to be reconstructed. If, however, just one is injured and the patient is unstable, it can be ligated.

The common bile duct should be repaired over a T-tube to allow biliary drainage.

Splenic Injuries

The spleen is the second most commonly injured solid organ in blunt trauma. While nonoperative management has been the mainstay of conservative treatment, splenectomy of an injured spleen plays an important role in control of hemorrhage during trauma laparotomy. Delayed splenic rupture and bleeding can occur up to several weeks following injury, and careful evaluation and management plans should be undertaken for patients treated conservatively.

At the time of operation for hemodynamic instability or peritonitis and following abdominal packing, if the packs in the left upper quadrant are blood soaked and bleeding continues from this area, the spleen needs to be evaluated. However, if no evidence of bleeding is present, the spleen can be palpated and left in place if no injury is noted. The most important maneuver for evaluating an injured spleen is complete mobilization. From the patient's right side, the spleen should be retracted toward the midline with the left hand. Attachments between the spleen and the diaphragm are incised starting at the lower pole of the spleen and moving cephalad along the curve of the spleen toward the esophagogastric junction. Careful traction avoids unnecessary injury to the capsule or extension of lacerations. Once this plane has been divided, the spleen is lifted anteriorly and medially and a plane created between the spleen and the left kidney. This lifts the spleen and distal pancreas as a unit, bringing the hilum into the incision. Clamping of the hilum should proceed as close to the spleen as possible; clamping of the proximal portion only is required, as the spleen will be removed after division of the hilar vessels. These should be suture ligated with absorbable suture. If the tail of the pancreas has been divided, suction drainage should be placed in the splenic bed.

If the patient is not unstable and can tolerate splenorrhaphy, simple lacerations can be repaired with absorbable monofilament mattress sutures with a buttress of pledgets to prevent tearing of the capsule and to provide hemostasis. Splenic preservation is most important in young patients, in whom the risk of overwhelming postsplenectomy sepsis is greatest.

Pancreatic Injuries

Injuries to the distal body and tail of the pancreas can be approached in similar fashion to the spleen. In fact, in emergencies the spleen should be mobilized as previously described and the pancreas with it, and they should both be resected. The first step is to evaluate the surface of the pancreas by entering the lesser sac. This is done by retracting the stomach superiorly, the transverse colon inferiorly, and dividing the bloodless plane of the gastrocolic ligament slightly to the left of midline. This provides access to the lesser sac, and if injury is evident, wider exposure is required. Continue dissection of the gastrocolic ligament until the stomach is freely mobile and the entire surface of the pancreas is exposed. If a hematoma is present, it can be evaluated by incising the peritoneal surface overlying the pancreas. Benign-appearing injuries can be more complex than anticipated, and should prompt the removal of the distal pancreas.

Similar to splenic mobilization, once a plane is developed between the spleen and left kidney, this plane can be continued medially beneath the tail and body of the pancreas all the way to the aorta and superior mesenteric artery. If a laceration is present but does not appear likely to interrupt the duct, or if the patient is doing poorly, wide closed suction drainage is appropriate. Place drains around the area of the injury and abort further attempts at pancreatic exploration. If a deep injury to the pancreatic parenchyma is evident and ductal injury likely, pancreatic resection is warranted. The spleen and pancreatic body and tail are lifted into the wound and the base of the pancreatic body is clamped with a noncrushing clamp. The distal edge is then divided, and the cut edge oversewn with a running nonabsorbable monofilament, being careful not to pull though the fragile pancreatic parenchyma. If the duct can be seen, it can be oversewn with a figure-eight stitch, but as this is frequently too small to be found, time should not be wasted looking for it. A closed suction drain should be placed in the pancreatic bed to control leakage.

Injuries to the head of the pancreas should be controlled with drainage and packing. A "trauma whipple" in austere circumstances is ill advised and highly lethal.

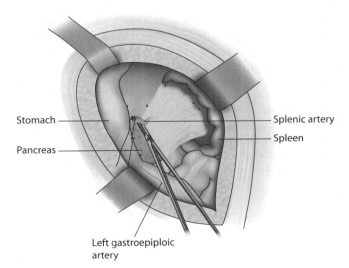

Stomach

Pancreas

Splenic artery

Spleen

Left gastroepiploic artery

FIGURE 42.11 Control of the splenic artery during splenectomy. Souba W, Fink M. *ACS Surgery,* 6th ed. Hamilton: Decker Publishing, 2007.

Conclusion

Managing patients with abdominal trauma in LMICs can be challenging. With limited diagnostic and therapeutic options, often no clear understanding of the underlying condition can be definitely ascertained before going to the OR for an exploratory laparotomy. Good preoperative resuscitation is mandatory for success, and close cooperation with staff and colleagues is vital. Strong history taking and physical diagnosis skills, along with flexibility and a firm understanding of general surgical principles, are needed to care for these patients.

COMMENTARY

Rodolphe R. Eisenhower Jean-Louis, Haiti

The management of suspected or proven major vascular injury in LMICs may differ significantly from common practice in HICs in several respects. In rural Haiti, where I practice, there is no efficiently organized prehospital care system; most severe vascular injuries never reach a hospital. For those patients who do survive long enough to reach a hospital, it is not uncommon to receive them 12 hours after injury occurred; sometimes, it is even longer than 12 hours. Many hospitals also do not have sufficient quantities of blood available to attempt a major vascular repair, even if someone on staff is trained to do so and has the other necessary materials.

At my hospital in rural Haiti, we generally apply the following decision paradigm given our resource limitations. In hemodynamically stable patients who present more than 6 hours after injury and who are found to have nonexpanding retroperitoneal (RP) hemorrhage at the time of laparotomy, we will generally not attempt an exploration regardless of the location of the bleeding. We usually have no more than two units of blood available in our blood bank, so we rely on the compressive nature of the RP hematoma to staunch the bleeding. Exploring the retroperitoneum carries a high risk of exsanguination "under the eyes of the surgeon."

If the patient presents less than 6 hours after injury, all Zone 1 hematomas will be explored. If the patient has been stabbed, we are likely to attempt an exploration as the probability of a successful primary repair is higher for stabbing victims than for gunshot victims. Management of Zones 2 and 3 hematomas is similar to management in HICs in patients who present soon after injury.

In cases of expanding retroperitoneal hemorrhage or hemodynamic instability, an attempt can be made to expeditiously perform a primary repair. First, manual pressure is used to attempt to occlude the vena cava and iliac vessels to slow bleeding. A medial visceral rotation is performed, and an attempt to locate the bleeding source is made. We will attempt a primary repair if possible. Most great vessel injuries that cannot be repaired primarily are not survivable in our setting.

If the retroperitoneum was opened by trauma or by the surgeon, and no discrete source of bleeding is found, then the installation of packing can be useful, taking care not to compress the renal veins. Arteriography or other endovascular interventions are not available in Haiti.

In summary, the management of major abdominal vascular injuries in LMICs varies considerably with the available resources and the usual time course of presentation. Additionally, in our cultural context, a surgeon may be held more responsible for the death of a patient who undergoes a desperate operation and dies in the operating room or after the procedure than in a case where a patient dies of his or her injuries without undergoing an operation. Therefore, more caution must be taken than in HICs before commencing an operation that is unlikely to succeed.

COMMENTARY

Emmanuel Kayibanda, Rwanda

Trauma is a leading cause of mortality and morbidity all over the world, particularly in LMICs. This is due to the fact that many cases in district hospitals are handled by medical officers who do not have enough expertise to handle trauma cases. Other patients are referred to provincial or teaching hospitals and are also handled by junior postgraduates who may not have the expertise or, if they are more senior, are not familiar with trauma concepts.

Knowing that the best chance for a good outcome for trauma patients is during the first operation, everything should be done to get a correct diagnosis, appropriate treatment, and adequate follow-up.

The most common causes of blunt abdominal trauma include motor vehicle crashes, assaults, falls, automobile–pedestrian accidents, work-related injuries, intimate partner violence, and child abuse. Gunshot wounds are particularly frequent in LMICs, especially within the last decade, and are a source of many abdominal traumas.

Blunt abdominal traumas are more frequent than penetrating abdominal traumas. All the intraperitoneal organs can be injured. The injury of retroperitoneal organs can lead to a retroperitoneal hematoma that can leak in the peritoneal cavity if it is extensive. In case of associated pelvic trauma, always have in mind an intraperitoneal rupture of the bladder.

The Airway, Breathing, Circulation, Disability, Exposure (ABCDE) concepts are the guiding principles of the patient examination. Remember that a patient with an abdominal trauma may have extra-abdominal injuries.

The investigation tools of full blood count (FBC) and diagnostic peritoneal aspirate (DPA) can be done everywhere. DPL and ultrasonography are very useful and may be available in many centers. A CT scan and diagnostic laparoscopy that may be available in some teaching hospitals are helpful and save many patients.

Appropriate resuscitation prior to surgery is one of the most important factors in preventing morbidity and mortality. It allows facing efficiently intraperitoneal bleeding, performing safe bowel anastomosis, and minimizing stomas that are very harmful in LMICs.

Training medical personnel to manage trauma patients is crucial. Refresher courses are very useful for those who have been trained.

43

Urologic Trauma

Kristen R. Scarpato
Hiep T. Nguyen
Richard N. Yu

Introduction

Trauma is a leading cause of morbidity and mortality worldwide. Motor vehicle collisions and violence account for the vast majority of these injuries. After the initial resuscitation, successful treatment of traumatic injuries requires a multidisciplinary approach. Injury of the genitourinary (GU) tract occurs not uncommonly, accounting for approximately 10% of all traumatic injuries.[1] The kidney is the most frequently injured GU organ, with the bladder, the urethra, the ureters, and the external genitalia in decreasing order of frequency.

Renal Trauma

Etiology

The kidney is the most frequently injured urologic organ despite being well protected in the retroperitoneum. Injuries can range from minor disruptions in the renal capsule to complete fracturing of the kidneys. Obtaining the full details of the accident is an essential part of the workup for any traumatic injury, especially when it comes to the recognition of renal injury. Renal damage often results from blunt trauma, including motor vehicle collisions, falls, and assault. The importance of obtaining information regarding the extent of the impact cannot be understated, as it may correlate with the degree of damage. Penetrating injuries such as stab and gunshot wounds can also violate the retroperitoneum and injure the kidney. It is necessary to note the characteristics of the weapons used because knowledge of the mechanism of injury will aid in prompt diagnosis.

Diagnosis

Prompt diagnosis begins with a complete history and physical exam, including the details surrounding the trauma and subsequent signs and symptoms of renal injury. Hematuria, gross or microscopic, is the best indicator of traumatic GU injury.[2] Although not specific to renal trauma, blood in the urine should raise the index of suspicion that the kidneys may be involved. It is important that the first urine specimen be analyzed. It is essential to recognize that the degree of hematuria does not correlate with severity of injury. Patients who present in shock, or quickly become unstable, may have sustained a traumatic renal injury and diagnosis should be prompt. Hemorrhagic shock is often seen with severe renal injury and, in conjunction with hematuria, may indicate significant renal injury.

Renal traumatic injury is often diagnosed by imaging studies performed shortly after a traumatic event. The genitourinary tract should be imaged after trauma in all pediatric patients and in adults with penetrating trauma with gross hematuria, blunt trauma associated with gross hematuria, or blunt trauma associated with microscopic hematuria and shock.[3,4] In the developed world, computed tomography (CT) scan with contrast is the preferred imaging modality because the parenchyma, vascular structures, and collecting system can be visualized (Figure 43.1A, Figure 43.1B, and Figure 43.1C).[5]

Findings suggestive of renal injury include medial hematoma, urinary extravasation, and delayed or absent nephrogram. Alternatively, renal sonogram can be beneficial as it allows the parenchyma and associated fluid collections to be visualized. However, it is not definitive in diagnosing vascular or collecting system injuries, nor can it clearly define lacerations of the renal parenchyma. However, it is fast, affordable, and easy to perform, often being done in the trauma bay as part of the focused assessment with sonography for trauma (FAST) exam. There may be a limited role for other forms of renal imaging, such as intravenous pyelography (IVP) and arteriography. Single-shot IVP (a single abdominal X-ray obtained 10 minutes after IV injection of 2 ml/kg of contrast material) intraoperatively may be helpful in the evaluation of a retroperitoneal hematoma discovered during exploration.[6] Arteriography lends itself to the diagnosis of vascular injuries not clearly seen by other imaging modalities.

The classification of renal injury is dependent upon imaging studies. The most widely used system is the American Association for the Surgery of Trauma Organ Injury Severity Scale, which grades injuries from I–V (Table 43.1).[7]

Management

Management ranges from observation to surgical intervention based primarily upon the patient's clinical condition. It is often the associated nonurologic injuries that determine the

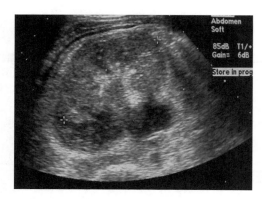

FIGURE 43.1A Radiological evaluation of Grade IV renal injury following a motor vehicle accident. US demonstrates a hematoma and disruption of the renal parenchyma. Image by Kristen Scarpato, Hiep T. Nguyen, and Richard N. Yu.

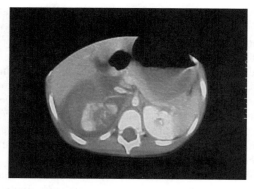

FIGURE 43.1B Radiological evaluation of Grade IV renal injury following a motor vehicle accident. CT demonstrates fracturing of the kidney with significant perirenal hematoma. Image by Kristen Scarpato, Hiep T. Nguyen, and Richard N. Yu.

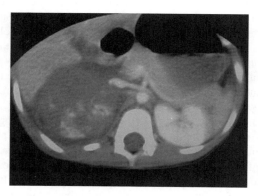

FIGURE 43.1C A magnified version of the CT image in Figure 43.1B. Radiological evaluation of Grade IV renal injury following a motor vehicle accident. CT demonstrates fracturing of the kidney with significant perirenal hematoma. Image by Kristen Scarpato, Hiep T. Nguyen, and Richard N. Yu.

course of management in these patients. In hemodynamically stable patients with any grade of renal injury based upon definite imaging studies, observation is preferred. Indeed, the vast majority of blunt renal trauma can be managed conservatively.[4] Patients who are clinically stable with high-grade injuries can be managed with bed rest, serial hematocrits evaluation, frequent monitoring of vital signs, and serial imaging. If vitals and labs remain stable, patients may ambulate once gross hematuria

resolves and ultimately be discharged from the hospital with close follow-up.

Renal exploration, reconstruction, or nephrectomy for renal trauma is not commonly indicated. However, there are certain scenarios that require operative management, including persistent renal bleeding and expanding or pulsatile perinephric hematoma. Relative indications for surgical intervention include urinary extravasation or arterial injury. For open exploration, a transabdominal approach with early control of the renal vessels is preferred.[8] During renal reconstruction, adequate exposure should be achieved and all nonviable tissue should be debrided. If reconstruction is not possible, partial nephrectomy may be indicated. In cases of extensive renal damage or hemodynamic instability, nephrectomy may be warranted.

Complications

There are several immediate and long-term complications associated with renal trauma. When the collecting system has been injured, there may be ongoing urinary extravasation leading to urinoma and perirenal infections. These patients require close monitoring in a hospital setting and occasionally will require a placement of a ureteral stent. However, the majority resolves spontaneously. In the weeks following injury, patients may experience delayed rebleeding requiring bed rest. There is limited data regarding the development of hypertension as a long-term complication.

Alternatives in an LMIC

Limitations in the diagnosis and management of renal trauma in developing areas are often related to imaging capability. While plain films and ultrasounds are usually available, the more advanced technologies of magnetic resonance imaging (MRI), CT scan, and angiography are frequently unavailable, limiting definitive diagnosis. Clinicians are forced to rely heavily upon history and physical exam, in conjunction with ultrasound or IVP when available. Often surgical exploration is performed as a substitute for imaging. Again, it should be emphasized that most renal injury can be managed nonoperatively; surgical exploration can lead to worsening of the renal injury, renal loss, and increased blood loss. If surgical exploration is contemplated, it is essential to achieve renal vascular control (through a retroperitoneal incision over the aorta medial to the inferior mesenteric vein) prior to opening up the retroperitoneal hematoma and exposing the injured kidney (Figure 43.2).

Ureteral Injuries

Etiology

Diagnosing ureteral injury requires a high index of suspicion, as they may not be immediately apparent. More often than not the injury goes unrecognized, until the patients develop subsequent fever, leukocytosis, and pain. Traumatic ureteral injury can be the result of external trauma but frequently occurs iatrogenically during abdominal surgery or ureteroscopy. External trauma is a rare cause of ureteral injury and will typically occur in the

TABLE 43.1

American Association for the Surgery of Trauma Organ Injury Severity Scale

Grade	Type	Description
I	Contusion Hematoma	Microscopic or gross hematuria, normal imaging Subcapsular, nonexpanding, no parenchymal laceration
II	Hematoma Laceration	Nonexpanding perirenal hematoma confined to renal retroperitoneum <1cm parenchymal depth of renal cortex without urinary extravasation
III	Laceration	>1 cm parenchymal depth of renal cortex without urinary extravasation or collecting system damage
IV	Laceration Vascular	Parenchymal laceration extending through renal cortex, medulla and collecting system Main renal artery or vein injury with contained hemorrhage
V	Laceration Vascular	Completely shattered kidney Avulsion of renal hilum, devascularized kidney

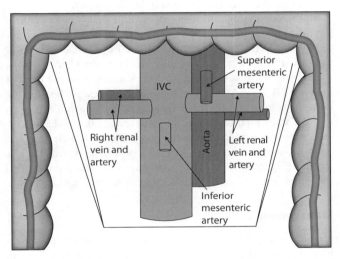

FIGURE 43.2 During renal exploration for trauma, vascular control should first be performed by incising through the retroperitoneum over the aorta medial to the inferior mesenteric vein. Image by Hiep T. Nguyen.

setting of a catastrophic event with high mortality.[9] Significant blunt trauma has been associated with ureteral injury, more commonly resulting in ureteropelvic junction (UPJ) disruption. More commonly, ureteral injury from the external trauma will result from a penetrating insult such as with a knife or a bullet, which may directly transect the ureter or injure its blood supply, leading to ischemia and resultant necrosis.

Iatrogenic ureteral injury can be seen following a variety of surgical procedures but is more frequently observed after gynecologic, colorectal, and vascular surgeries.[10] Injury has been reported following open, laparoscopic, and robotically assisted procedures. A clear understanding of anatomic relationships is crucial to prevent ureteral damage. Manipulation of the ureter alone can cause transient edema and obstruction with resultant hydronephrosis. Endoscopic surgery, such as for stone disease, is another potential source of injury. Risk factors for these injuries include the length of procedure, the surgeon's experience, previous abdominal or pelvic radiation, the method of stone treatment, and the stone burden.

Diagnosis

Awareness of the risk of potential ureteral injury is a key part of the diagnosis. Intraoperative recognition, especially during laparoscopy, requires a high index of suspicion and a thorough understanding of anatomy, while postoperative diagnosis requires knowledge of the typical signs of delayed presentation. Hematuria may be an indication that ureteral injury has occurred, although it is not consistently present. Ureteral injury is difficult to diagnose radiographically since findings such as urinary extravasation are frequently nonspecific or subtle. Retrograde ureterography, if available, is often the most diagnostic and is helpful for picking up missed injuries.

Management and Complications

Options for management and the potential associated complications are dependent upon the nature and location of the injury. The success in the management of ureteral injuries is dependent upon the maintenance of well-vascularized tissue. Injuries of the ureters from external trauma often require surgical intervention. Contusion of the ureter at any location may require internal stenting; less often, ureteroureterostomy is required.[9] In the case of partial ureteral transaction, a spatulated, watertight primary repair is frequently employed. Injuries of the upper ureter may be repaired by excision and primary re-anastomosis, autotransplantation, or bowel interposition, while mid-ureteral injuries may require transureteroureterostomy. Distal ureteral injury may be repaired by ureteroneocystotomy with or without the use of a psoas hitch or Boari flap.

In cases of iatrogenic ureteral injuries, a primary ureteroureterostomy may be performed if the injury is noted immediately. When the diagnosis is delayed, management options include immediate stenting or open repair. If the ureter is ligated surgically, it may be possible to remove the ligature and simply place a stent. If the ligation results in ischemic, nonviable tissue, a ureteroureterostomy or reimplant may be required. Ureteroscopic perforation may be stented, while ureteral avulsion should be treated in the same manner as in cases of open or laparoscopic ureteral trauma. In certain cases, percutaneous nephrostomy may be desirable to divert urine from the site of injury. However, subsequent management of the ureteral injury is still required.

Alternatives in an LMIC

In LMICs, there is reliance upon the history and physical exam for diagnosis. If IVP is available, it may aid in diagnosis. Lack of more advanced imaging modalities does limit the ability to diagnose ureteral injury in some instances, although radiography is frequently nonspecific and unhelpful in the majority of cases of ureteral injury. Percutaneous nephrostomy placement may be helpful in the diagnosis and temporary management of ureteral injury, but this option may also be unavailable or be associated with greater complication rates in LMICs.

Surgical repair of ureteral injury frequently requires advanced surgical technique, and therefore it is essential that surgeons in these locations have adequate education and tools, such as fine sutures and stents for the management of ureteral injuries. The distal ends of the injured ureter should be mobilized but in a limited fashion to preserve the blood supply to the ureter. Devascularized or necrotic tissue on the ends of the ureter should be resected back until healthy bleed is encountered. Next, the ends of the ureter should be spatulated to allow for a wide anastomosis. Fine absorbable sutures (such as 6.0 chromic or Vicryl) should be used for the anastomosis. A double J-stent should be placed to ensure proper healing. When primary anastomosis is not possible, a nephrostomy tube should be placed and delayed repair should be performed at a later time.

Bladder Injuries

Etiology

Bladder injuries are rarely seen in isolation and are frequently associated with pelvic fractures.[11] Though well protected in the pelvis, bladder injury may occur following blunt trauma involving rapid decelerations (such as in motor vehicle collisions), crush injuries, or assault. Penetrating injury to the bladder is often the result of surgery, especially during gynecologic procedures, but may also occur from gunshot wounds to the pelvis or abdomen.

Diagnosis

Patients with bladder injury may complain of suprapubic pain, inability to void, or bloody urine. However, symptoms may be subtle or masked by other injuries. Bladder injury should be considered when there are penetrating injuries to the pelvis or lower abdomen; not uncommonly, findings on physical examination may not be obvious (Figure 43.3).

Gross hematuria, although seen in other forms of urologic trauma, is the most consistent sign of bladder injury. When bladder

injury is suspected, a catheterized specimen should be obtained; however, if concomitant urethral injury is suspected, then radiographic evaluation (retrograde urethrogram) should be performed prior to instrumentation.[12] Imaging studies are essential in the diagnosis of bladder injury. Blunt trauma combined with hematuria, gross or microscopic, often warrants radiographic studies especially when pelvic fractures are suspected. Absolute indications for cystography include gross or microscopic hematuria in the setting of penetrating injury to the pelvis or lower abdomen, as well as gross hematuria associated with pelvic fracture. There is a high likelihood that bony fragments may lacerate the bladder or that the bladder may tear when shear forces disrupt the pelvis. In this setting, cystography should be performed immediately to confirm the presence and location of bladder injury.

Retrograde cystogram, using plain film or CT will confirm the diagnosis in most cases. A plain film should be taken prior to the administration of contrast, followed by an anteroposterior film when the bladder is adequately filled (Figure 43.4A). Finally, a drainage film should be taken to evaluate for posterior bladder injury. If CT is used, drainage films are not necessary because the posterior bladder can be clearly visualized. In the case of extraperitoneal bladder rupture, radiography will reveal a flame-shaped collection of contrast material in the pelvis (Figure 43.4B). Contrast outlining loops of bowel is indicative of intraperitoneal bladder rupture (Figure 43.4C). Pelvic sonogram may also be used and may show a decompressed bladder and intraperitoneal free fluid.

Management

Simple extraperitoneal bladder rupture may be managed conservatively with large diameter Foley catheter drainage; a follow-up cystogram is recommended approximately 14–21 days after the injury.[13] In the absence of residual bladder injury, the catheter may be removed. Extraperitoneal bladder rupture may also be closed if the patient is undergoing surgery for other abdominal or pelvic injuries. For complicated bladder injuries such as intraperitoneal rupture, bladder neck injury, penetrating bladder trauma, concurrent vaginal or rectal damage, or in the setting of pelvic fracture, immediate open repair is warranted. These injuries are unlikely to heal with conservative management alone.[13] Repair of the bladder should be with an absorbable suture in one or two layers. It is important to achieve a watertight closure, especially

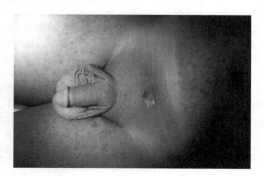

FIGURE 43.3   Gunshot wound to the suprapubic area. Note the minimally physical findings. The entrance wound may not be obvious prior to shaving the suprapubic area. Image by Kristen Scarpato, Hiep T. Nguyen, and Richard N. Yu.

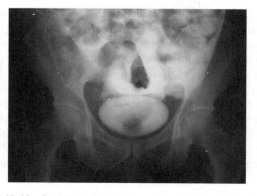

FIGURE 43.4A   Radiological evaluation of bladder injury following blunt pelvic trauma. Plain X-ray cystogram demonstrates an intraperitoneal bladder rupture with contrast outlining the bowels within the peritoneum. Image by Kristen Scarpato, Hiep T. Nguyen, and Richard N. Yu.

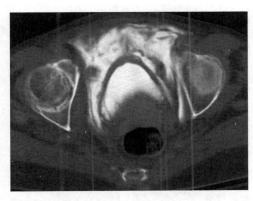

FIGURE 43.4B Radiological evaluation of bladder injury following blunt pelvic trauma. CT demonstrates extraperitoneal bladder rupture. Image by Kristen Scarpato, Hiep T. Nguyen, and Richard N. Yu.

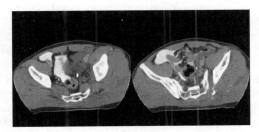

FIGURE 43.4C Radiological evaluation of bladder injury following blunt pelvic trauma. CT demonstrates intraperitoneal bladder rupture. Image by Kristen Scarpato, Hiep T. Nguyen, and Richard N. Yu.

when orthopedic hardware has been placed, to prevent subsequent infection. When injury occurs in the area of the trigone, the ureteral anatomy should be defined; administration of indigo carmine or methylene blue intravenously will help identify the ureteral orifices. The ureters should be reimplanted if injury has occurred. The bladder should be drained with a large-caliber catheter following repair, and repeat imaging should be obtained 2–3 weeks following surgery. Patients should be maintained on perioperative antibiotics to minimize the chance of infection.

Complications

Patients often do well with timely diagnosis and proper management. It is when injury is unrecognized that complications occur. They include fistula, stricture, and urinary incontinence. Patients with missed diagnosis of bladder injury may initially present with fever, acidosis, azotemia, or sepsis.

Alternatives in an LMIC

Diagnosis and treatment of bladder trauma in an LMIC is not unlike workup and management of these injuries in a more developed setting. Although CT cystograms may be unavailable, diagnosis may be made with plain film cystogram. The same surgical indications and principles apply and are unlikely to be deviated from, as repair requires basic materials and skills. If radiological evaluation is not available at the time of evaluation, a Foley should be placed and left to drainage. Subsequent follow-up

evaluation with a cystogram will be needed to ensure that there is no intraperitoneal bladder rupture.

Urethral Injuries

Etiology

Injury may occur at the level of the posterior or anterior urethra, each with different mechanisms of injury and manifestations.[14] Anterior urethral damage is usually isolated and occurs in the setting of straddle injuries, and less often from penetrating trauma. Posterior urethral injury frequently occurs following blunt trauma, especially in cases in which the bony pelvis has been disrupted. The fixed location of the posterior urethra between the urogenital diaphragm and puboprostatic ligament make it more susceptible to damage from shear forces.

Diagnosis

There are several important signs of urethral injury, including blood at the meatus, inability to void, palpable bladder, perineal hematoma, vulvar edema, and a high-riding prostate.[15] Exam of the external genitalia is a key component in the diagnosis of these injuries that should not be overlooked during the initial trauma assessment. Inability to pass a urethral catheter is indicative of urethral disruption; the procedure should be aborted until further imaging can be performed. Retrograde urethrography (RUG) should be performed with urethral injury is suspected, especially in cases in which blood is seen at the meatus. The severity of urethral injury can be graded based on the findings seen on RUG:

1. Grade I: urethral contusion with a normal RUG but blood at the meatus (Figure 43.5A)
2. Grade II: stretch injury (Figure 43.5B)
3. Grade III: partial disruption (Figure 43.5C)
4. Grade IV: complete disruption <2 cm (Figure 43.5D)
5. Grade V: complete disruption > 2 cm or with prostate/vaginal laceration (Figure 43.5E)[16]

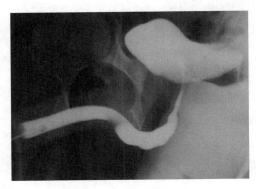

FIGURE 43.5A Grading of urethral injury. Grade I: urethral contusion with a normal RUG but blood at the meatus. Image by Kristen Scarpato, Hiep T. Nguyen, and Richard N. Yu.

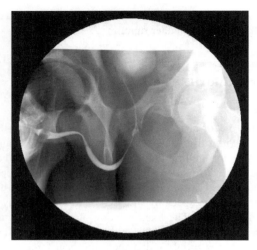

FIGURE 43.5B Grading of urethral injury. Grade II: stretch injury. Image by Kristen Scarpato, Hiep T. Nguyen, and Richard N. Yu.

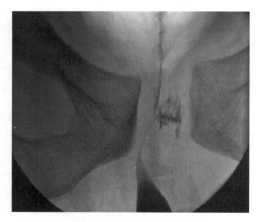

FIGURE 43.5C Grading of urethral injury. Grade III: partial disruption. Image by Kristen Scarpato, Hiep T. Nguyen, and Richard N. Yu.

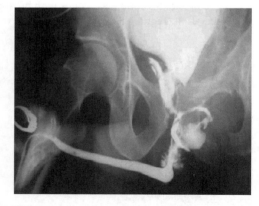

FIGURE 43.5D Grading of urethral injury. Grade IV: complete disruption < 2cm. Image by Kristen Scarpato, Hiep T. Nguyen, and Richard N. Yu.

Management

Initial management of urethral trauma remains controversial.[16] Traditionally, drainage with a suprapubic tube (SPT) has been the standard of care. Open placement of an SPT is commonly

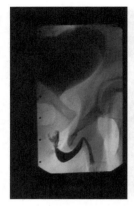
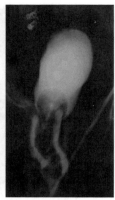

FIGURE 43.5E Grading of urethral injury. Grade V: complete disruption > 2 cm. or with prostate or vaginal laceration. Image by Kristen Scarpato, Hiep T. Nguyen, and Richard N. Yu.

used, and a large-bore catheter is placed. This effectively drains the bladder and helps divert urine from the area of injury. When open repair for concurrent injuries is not indicated, an SPT can be placed percutaneously using a small trocar or dilator. More recently, primary realignment has been advocated, especially in the setting of incomplete urethral tears. A single gentle attempt at passage of a Foley is unlikely to convert a partial urethral tear into a complete tear. This can be attempted in an antegrade or retrograde fashion, commonly over a wire, which has been placed into the bladder under cystoscopic guidance.

Immediate repair of posterior urethral disruption inevitably leads to increased complications requiring reoperation. Therefore, delayed reconstruction after placement of an SPT or primary realignment is recommended. Urethroplasty is indicated when the urethral scar tissue is well developed and other traumatic injuries have been stabilized, usually several months after initial insult. Patients should undergo preoperative imaging to clearly define anatomy and surgery is ideally performed through a perineal approach.

Female urethral disruption presents a unique problem due to the short length of the female urethra.[17] Open repair is preferred in this situation to prevent subsequent urethral stenosis and may aid with recognition of other injuries, such as vaginal or rectal lacerations. Placement of a catheter alone has yielded poor long-term results.

Complications

Complications following urethral disruption are not uncommon and include incontinence, impotence, recurrent stenosis, and anejaculation. It is often difficult to distinguish surgical complications from those of the original traumatic injury. Nevertheless, it is essential to have a thorough understanding of surgical management options and techniques in order to minimize the chance of these complications.

Alternatives in an LMIC

The initial management of urethral injury is similar in LMICs, including SPT placement and catheter drainage. Diagnosis can be made based upon clinical findings and simple radiographic imaging. However, when delayed reconstruction is indicated, the availability of advanced surgical technique may be the limiting factor in definitive management.

Penile Injuries

Etiology

The penis is most commonly injured in the erect state when the tunica albuginea is more susceptible to fracture. Forceful sexual intercourse may result in a buckling injury. The penis may also be subject to penetrating trauma (from stabbing or gunshot wounds, or animal and human bites) or in severe cases even amputation.

Diagnosis

History and physical exam alone are often sufficient to diagnosis penile traumatic injury.[18] A cracking and popping sound associated with pain, rapid detumescence, and classic "eggplant" sign is diagnostic of penile fracture (Figure 43.6). Additional studies are not required in most cases. External trauma will be easily

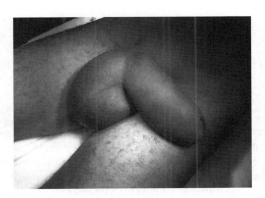

FIGURE 43.6 Appearance of penile fracture. Image by Kristen Scarpato, Hiep T. Nguyen, and Richard N. Yu.

identified and should fit with the history provided. If there is concern for urethral injury, a urethrogram should be performed immediately.

Management

Management depends upon the mechanism of injury.[19] When the penis has been fractured, it should be immediately explored and repaired with absorbable sutures. The patient should have a one-month course of antibiotics. Gunshot wounds to the penis should also prompt immediate surgical exploration with removal of the bullet, debridement of nonviable tissue, and copious irrigation with a postoperative prolonged course of antibiotics. Animal and human bites both require immediate exploration, debridement, and antibiotics. However, animal bites should be closed immediately while human bites are usually contaminated and should not be closed primarily. A traumatically amputated penis requires microsurgical repair ideally with postoperative suprapubic catheter drainage. When microsurgical techniques are not available, realignment of the urethra and corporal bodies macroscopically has acceptable results.

Complications

Penile trauma and repair can ultimately lead to undesirable cosmesis and plaque formation, infection and abscess, penile curvature, and erectile dysfunction. Prompt surgical intervention can decrease the likelihood of long-term complications, especially in the case of penile fracture.

Alternatives in an LMIC

Management of penile trauma depends upon prompt recognition and intervention regardless of the setting. In areas with limited resources, management may be hindered by the availability of microsurgical supplies and technique. In general however, there is unlikely to be discrepancy in the diagnosis and treatment of these injuries.

COMMENTARY

Demberelnyambuu Batsukh, Mongolia

In children, 94% of renal injuries are caused by blunt trauma. In Mongolia, where I practice, 34%–68% of all genitourinary tract injuries result mainly from falls (especially during horseback riding) and motor vehicle accidents. The small size of children increases their vulnerability to more severe kidney damage. Children's kidneys are more vulnerable to severe kidney damage than adults' kidneys because their kidneys are relatively smaller in proportion to their abdominal size, and are less protected because of poor development of Gerota's fascia and perirenal fat; the lower two ribs are not completely ossified until 25 years of age; and the persistence of fetal lobulations allows easier parenchymal disruption.

Modern management of trauma in children has evolved around a multidisciplinary approach involving pediatricians, surgeons, urologists, emergency physicians and other appropriate healthcare providers. In children, blunt renal trauma should be managed conservatively. If initial radiography studies are abnormal, follow-up studies are recommended in 6–8 weeks, and a final check—including urine analysis; blood pressure, and IVP—should be performed 1 year after injury. About 5%–10% of injuries can be categorized as critical and immediate operative intervention is necessary. The indications for surgical intervention are renal bleeding, urinary extravasation, shattered kidney/grade V injury/and vascular injury. The injured kidney should be explored transperitoneally through an upper transverse incision depending on the age of the child and the degree of trauma. If the renal vessels on the injured side are isolated before exploration of the kidney, they can be clamped should heavy bleeding be encountered when Gerota's fascia is entered. Total renal exposure is important, because multiple injuries might present. It is important to place vessel loops on the renal vasculature before exploring the hematoma and kidney. Clamping of the renal artery is not necessary. Bleeding often can be controlled with finger compression. All clot and nonviable tissue should be removed and hemostasis obtained. When faced with a significant vascular injury, I would undertake partial or total nephrectomy. When the collecting system has been opened, a drain should be placed only until urine is not draining. This will help avoid infecting the retroperitoneum and hematoma. Postoperatively, you need to watch for delayed bleeding, infection with abscess formation, formation of a urinoma, and open or closed urinary leakage. Long-term follow-up is required after renal trauma because of the possible late complications such as arteriovenous fistula, hypertension

(40%), renal atrophy (15%), renal calculi (5%), and secondary hydronephrosis (25%).

Ureteral and bladder injuries are uncommon and account for only 4% of all genitourinary traumas in children. In most cases they are iatrogenic. Iatrogenic ureteral trauma could happen during operations of bowel abnormality and gynecological surgeries. Lower ureteral injury may occur in conjunction with pelvic fractures. The bladder in children occupies more abdominal position than in adults and is more vulnerable to rupture at the time of blunt trauma, especially when it is full. Blunt trauma is the cause of 80%–95% of all bladder injuries; more than 70% of them are due to pelvic fractures. Iatrogenic bladder injury can occur during cystoscopy or open operative procedures such as umbilical artery catheterization in newborns and inguinal herniatomy.

Injuries to the anterior urethra are caused by blunt or penetrating trauma, placement of penile constriction bands, and iatrogenic injuries from procedures. Injuries to the posterior urethra occur after pelvic fractures, mostly as a result of motor vehicle accidents. Injuries vary from simple stretching (25%) to partial rupture (25%) and complete disruption (50%).

COMMENTARY

E. Oluwabunmi Olapade-Olaopa, Nigeria

Urologic trauma is common in sub-Saharan Africa (SSA). In Nigeria, where I practice, urologic trauma is responsible for approximately 10% of admissions in our unit, 50% of which are due to urethral injury. The sections on alternatives for management of trauma to the individual organ in an LMIC included in this chapter present a generally comprehensive guide for the trained surgeon.

Interestingly, despite the oft-described general insufficiency of infrastructural and equipment resources in SSA, perhaps the most important challenges to the management of diseases or injury in the subcontinent are the delay in presentation of the patients (due to the lack of an ambulance system both for patient retrieval from the accident site and for transfer between hospitals) and the variability of surgical expertise and equipment (and thus standard of care) available at individual medical centers. Indeed, the majority of the mortality and morbidity from trauma in SSA is due to attempts at care in insufficiently equipped and staffed centers, with belated transfer to better-resourced centers in the region. There may also be a delay in the recognition of urologic trauma at the hospital of first presentation, as these injuries often accompany other major injury. Thus, current guidelines on trauma care in SSA now emphasize immediate transfer of trauma cases as quickly as possible to the nearest hospital where trauma services are available, delaying only to resuscitate patients with immediately life-threatening conditions. In addition, the training of surgeons (and other healthcare workers) is being ramped up by local surgical colleges and associations (e.g., West African

College of Surgeons; College of Surgeons of East, Central, and Southern Africa; and the Pan-African Urological Surgeons Association) often in collaboration with foreign experts/nongovernmental agencies (NGOs) (e.g., Tropical Health Education Trust and IVUMed) to increase the quantity and quality of expertise available in the subcontinent.

Also important, though, is the need to appreciate that the determination to offer best practice care in the face of scarce resources in SSA has resulted in many innovations (devices, surgical techniques, and healthcare strategy), some of which are applicable to the rest of the world. Prominent among these is the EAT-SET (Emergency Auto-Transfusion Set; www.eat-set.com), which sieves blood lost into the peritoneum that can then be auto-transfused safely. This device reduces mortality from blood loss due to scarcity of blood and its products. EAT-SET has won many awards worldwide and has now been patented in 9 countries. Also noteworthy is the modification to the technique of early realignment of traumatic urethral disruption using rigid retrograde endoscopy only. This enables successful repair of this injury (a major proportion of the workload in our unit) in the outpatient clinic with satisfactory medium-term results.[20,21] This innovation has reduced the cost and morbidity of the injury. This innovation has also impacted the management of the injury, especially with regard to income lost while awaiting definitive surgery, the reduction in demand for operating room time, and the cost of admissions and the operation. Finally, the strategy of deploying medium-level surgeons and other healthcare professionals as first-responders during mass gatherings minimizes the effect of the scarcity of highly trained trauma teams in the region. This reduces the morbidity of injuries occurring at the events, and the transfer rate to the secondary and tertiary centers.

SUGGESTED READING

EO Olapade-Olaopa et al. On-site physicians at a major sporting event in Nigeria. Prehospital and Disaster Medicine, 21: (1), 40–44, 2006.

COMMENTARY

Emile Rwamasirabo, Rwanda

In LMICs, renal injuries are less prevalent than intraperitoneal injuries. Blunt traumas are most common; penetrating injuries are rare. When there is evidence of gross hematuria, patients are transferred to referral centers relatively quickly. Diagnosis is based on an ultrasound, and symptoms of gross hematuria and lumbar tenderness; medical officers in district hospitals will usually diagnose. Contrast CT-abdomen is only available in referral centers in which the grading is established. Grades IV and V are rarely seen, likely either because patients do not survive long enough to make it to the referral center, or because speed limits for motorcycles on our roads prevent serious accidents. Management is mostly conservative, but it is not uncommon to see late presentation with misdiagnosed, infected urinomas that require surgical drainage and sometimes nephrectomy due to secondary bleeding.

Iatrogenic causes lead to most of the ureteral injuries in our setting; this is especially true following caesarian section or caesarian-hysterectomy performed by medical officers in district hospitals. Ureteral injuries are usually diagnosed late, except in case of ureterovaginal fistula or rarely ureterouterine fistula (3 days). Cases of obstructive renal failure due to bilateral ureteric ligation are not rare; we have also handled cases of massive urine ascites with renal failure several weeks after caesarian-hysterectomy due to bilateral ureteric injury and fistulization of the urine into the peritoneal cavity. Diagnosis is based on sonography, intravenous urography (IVU) or CT-abdomen, or MRI, where possible. Ureteroneocystostomy with temporary stenting is generally the main treatment modality.

Both blunt and penetrating bladder injuries are routine occurrence in accidents and emergency units. Extraperitoneal bladder rupture, especially when associated with pelvic fracture, is diagnosed relatively early as all patients are immediately transferred by ambulances to referral centers. Retrograde urethrocystogram rules out associated urethral injuries and confirms the nature of the bladder injury. However, it is not rare to see associated urethral injuries that have been mismanaged by overzealous health workers who hurriedly insert urethral catheter without any indication to do so; this further complicates the grade of the urethral injury.

Noncomplicated and moderate rupture is generally managed conservatively.

Intraperitoneal injuries are generally seen late, especially when caused by blunt trauma; it is not rare to receive patients several days after they have been transferred with infected urine ascites. We have also seen cases of repeat laparotomy because of ascites recurrence that resulted because the first laparotomy had missed the small hole in the bladder dome. Attention has to be drawn to the quality of the retrograde cystogram to make sure the bladder filling is adequate; a partial filling of the bladder misses the small hole in the dome indeed. Repair of the bladder whole is the norm.

Both anterior and posterior urethral injuries are common in Rwanda. The diagnosis (or the suspicion) of urethral injuries in district hospitals is made on the basis of urethral bleeding or pelvic crash. The localization and the grading of the injury are done in referral centers where all patients are taken by ambulances. The diagnosis is confirmed by the retrograde urethrogram. The management follows the traditional guideline, meaning suprapubic cystostomy and no urethral catheterization unless there is evidence of ability to pass some urine through the urethra, in which case a gentle catheterization is done under endoscopic control. However, cases of inopportune catheterization and deflation of the balloon in the pelvic hematoma outside the ascended bladder/prostate are not uncommon. The definitive urethra rupture repair is generally performed in 3 months through a perineal approach; it is sometimes useful to use the transpubic approach in the cases in which the initial management has been late or inappropriate, resulting in severe sepsis and therefore extensive fibrosis with the prostate still high in the pelvis.

Patients with penile injuries (rupture of the tunica albuginea or penile amputation) are normally sent to the referral centers, although the appropriate conservation of the amputated part is not widely known to health workers. The number of cases of penile glans amputation following blunt circumcision techniques has considerably decreases following a nationwide circumcision training campaign. Repair of the tunica albuginea, urethral realignment, and corporeal bodies' approximation are the main treatment modalities.

44

Neurosurgical Trauma

Benjamin C. Warf

Introduction

The assumptions for this chapter are the same as that for its companion, Chapter 25, Neurosurgery: that the reader has basic surgical skills but is not a neurosurgeon; he or she is practicing in a hospital with limited resources; neuroimaging such as computed tomography (CT) or magnetic resonance imaging (MRI) are not readily available; and emergency transport to a neurosurgical facility is not an option. We will focus on the acute management of patients with cranial or spinal trauma, concentrating on those interventions that both can and must be done, and are likely to alter the patient's outcome.

Cranial and spinal trauma is responsible for an enormous burden of disease in the developing world. A major factor contributing to the prevalence of such trauma is motor vehicle accidents, potentiated by unsafe roads, unsafe vehicles, unsafe drivers, non-use of passenger restraints and motorcycle helmets, and inadequate enforcement of road safety laws. Areas of insecurity or conflict are also commonplace. Furthermore, low- and middle-income countries (LMICs) typically have no system for emergency medical transport or on-site intervention and, if such existed, there is typically no receiving facility able to provide the basic interventions that constitute trauma life support. The physician providing surgical care in this context may be called upon to provide emergency care to patients suffering from trauma to the head or spine who have been brought in by family members without the benefit of initial care, such as airway management or cervical spine immobilization. These situations can be very challenging and sometimes overwhelming.

Pathophysiology of Head Injury

There are two components to a head injury: 1) the primary injury directly resulting from the energy delivered to the head, and 2) the secondary injury that can develop in response to the initial event. The basic mechanisms of primary head injury include: acceleration, impact, and penetration. Such injuries can occur alone or concurrently.

Primary Injury

When the head is accelerated (or decelerated) severely, movement of the brain within the skull can cause compression, expansion, and shearing of the brain parenchyma as well as movement of the brain relative to the skull. Mechanisms include high-speed impact motor vehicle accidents and falls (sudden deceleration) as well as cranial impacts that suddenly accelerate the stationary skull (like a blow to the head with a blunt object). These mechanisms typically include an impact, which will be considered below. Acceleration forces can cause direct mechanical trauma to the brain tissue, intraparenchymal contusion or frank hematoma from torn blood vessels, cortical contusion from impact of the brain against the inner table of the skull, and subdural hematoma from shearing of cortical veins coursing from the brain to the dura. Generally speaking, acceleration forces are associated with some of the poorest outcomes.

In addition to some component of acceleration, impact delivers energy locally to the point of contact. This can lead to scalp laceration, linear skull fractures, and depressed skull fractures sometimes associated with cortical contusions or hematomas, or laceration of the dura or cortex. Breech of the dura and cerebrospinal fluid (CSF) leakage through the laceration present the risk of subsequent central nervous system (CNS) infection. Bleeding from fractured bone, or worse, a torn penetrating artery (classically, the middle meningeal artery that penetrates the temporal bone), can result in an expanding epidural hematoma (Figure 44.1).

Penetrating injuries to the skull can be of low or high energy. The classic example of the latter is a gunshot wound, in which the high-speed projectile transfers tremendous destructive energy to the surrounding brain as it decelerates along its path. Damage from lower energy penetrations (such as knives, machetes, arrows, shards of wood or metal, or low-velocity projectiles) is more confined to the actual tract. Both types of penetration can cause bleeding inside or outside the brain, dural laceration with CSF leakage, and transit of bone, skin, or debris intracranially.

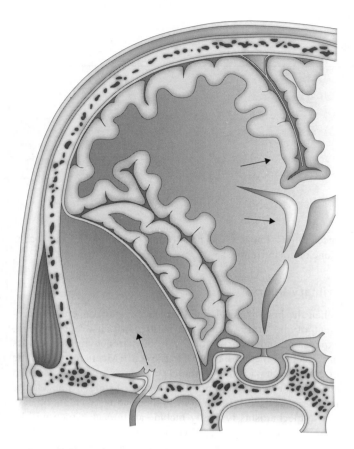

FIGURE 44.1   Epidural Hematoma. Coronal section through the brain and skull [image on the Internet]. 2013 [cited 2014 January 27]. Available from: www.5minuteconsult.com/viewImage/7051664/

Secondary Injury

The worst enemies of the brain-injured patient are hypoxia and hypotension. Brain and spine injuries often occur in the context of accompanying injuries that may contribute to these sequelae by way of blood loss or injury to the chest or airway. In addition, patients with isolated brain injury can suffer apnea or airway compromise as a direct result of CNS dysfunction. These can contribute to early and sustained ischemic injury in the brain beginning soon after the initial injury.

The brain's response to parenchymal injury and ischemia can include vasogenic and cytotoxic edema as well as dysregulation of cerebral blood flow. These all lead to increased extracellular and intracellular water or increased blood volume, respectively, within the limited, fixed volume of the cranial cavity. Since water is incompressible, the result is a rise in the intracranial pressure, which causes a further decrease in brain tissue perfusion and worsening ischemia.

Regional areas of brain tissue swelling as well as evolving hematomas either within (intracerebral hematoma) or outside (subdural or epidural hematoma) the brain can cause shifts of the affected areas beyond their normal boundaries and compression of neighboring brain regions. A classic example of this is herniation of the medial temporal lobe across the tentorial edge with subsequent compression of the midbrain, resulting in coma and death (Figure 44.2).

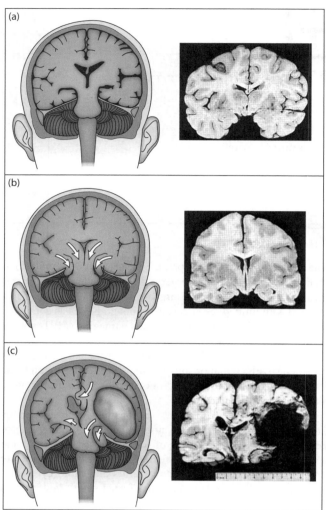

FIGURE 44.2   Intracerebral hematoma with transtentorial and subfalcine herniation. Plum F. *The Diagnosis of Stupor and Coma*, 3rd ed. London: Oxford Press, 1980, p. 92.

Management of the Head-Injured Patient

Initial Evaluation

Upon presentation of any injured patient, the initial response is attention to the ABCs of airway, breathing, and circulation. These principles are covered elsewhere in this book, but it is worth reiterating here. Once again, the worst enemies of the brain-injured patient are hypoxia and hypotension. One must also add hypoventilation, since hypercarbia exacerbates vasodilatation of the cerebral vasculature and subsequent aggravation of elevated intracranial pressure (ICP). Since cervical spine injury is a common accompaniment of a significant head injury, the neck should be immobilized in the neutral position until a fracture or subluxation can be ruled out by X-ray. If the patient requires endotracheal intubation, this should be done in neutral position with an assistant holding the head and applying modest axial traction.

The neurologic examination is important and, in this context, straightforward. An excellent place to begin is assessment of the patient's level of consciousness, and this is facilitated by use of the standard Glasgow Coma Score (GCS) (Figure 44.3). This establishes a baseline against which improvement or deterioration can be measured in an objective way. Such objective measures can help assess the severity of the injury and aid in the communication with other caregivers. Posturing, whether "decerebrate" (extensor) or "decorticate" (flexor), indicates severe injury with release of the normal cerebral-level controls on these primitive brainstem level reflexes (Figure 44.4). The pupillary examination is also important. Nonreactive and dilated pupils connote a severe brainstem injury. Asymmetric pupils can be an early warning sign of transtentorial herniation (described above) as the 3rd cranial nerve, lying between the tentorial edge and the midbrain, typically becomes compressed prior to significant compression of the midbrain itself. An initially normal pupillary examination is important to document as well, since a change may prompt life-saving intervention. In addition, one should determine whether the movements of arms and legs are symmetric or asymmetric. Development of lateralized weakness

Feature	Scale	Score
	Responses	*Notation*
Eye opening	Spontaneous	4
	To speech	3
	To pain	2
	None	1
Verbal response	Orientated	5
	Confused conversation	4
	Words (inappropriate)	3
	Sounds (incomprehensible)	2
	None	1
Best motor response	Obey commands	6
	Localize pain	5
	Flexion–Normal	4
	Flexion–Abnormal	3
	Extend	2
	None	1
Total Coma 'Score'		3/15–15/15

FIGURE 44.3 Glasgow Coma Score. Plum F. *The Diagnosis of Stupor and Coma*, 3rd ed. London: Oxford Press, 1980, p. 66.

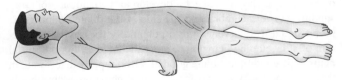

(a) Extension posturing (decerebrate rigidity)

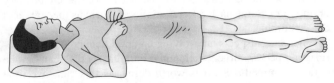

(b) Abnormal flexion (decorticate rigidity)

FIGURE 44.4 Posturing. *Winn R. Youmans Neurological Surgery Volume 4*, 6th ed. Oxford: Elsevier Saunders, 2011, p. 3434.

or posturing suggest an evolving intracerebral or extracerebral (epidural or subdural) hematoma involving the contralateral hemisphere (on the side opposite the weakness), which may be important in determining the side of operative intervention if such is to be undertaken. However, it is important to know that herniation of the medial temporal lobe can push the contralateral cerebral peduncle of the midbrain against the contralateral tentorial edge causing weakness on the same side as the hematoma and dilated pupil. Thus, a progressively dilating pupil is a more reliable lateralizing sign, typically indicating the side of the expanding mass.

Patients who present with fixed and dilated pupils and a low GCS have a very poor prognosis for survival under the best of circumstances, and there is typically little that can be done with limited resources. The patient for whom one can make a difference in the context of limited resources is the one who doesn't look "too bad" on initial presentation (for instance, GCS >7, symmetric and reactive pupils, and a symmetric motor examination), giving evidence that the primary brain injury was not severe, and who subsequently deteriorates over the course of care (e.g., declining GCS, a changing pupillary or motor examination), suggesting that a secondary process (such as a developing hematoma or increasing ICP with decreasing cerebral perfusion) is evolving.

Of course, if brain imaging by CT is available, this is an invaluable tool especially in regard to delineating a hematoma that should be evacuated. If not available, skull X-rays, though of limited usefulness, can be of benefit in identifying the presence and location of a skull fracture. Although not the case for the majority, a fracture should elevate one's suspicion for an epidural hematoma, and if clinically indicated, can help guide the initial site chosen for burr hole placement.

Management

In the stable patient, it is critical to monitor and maintain airway, oxygenation, and blood pressure with whatever monitoring is available (e.g., electrocardiogram [EKG], O$_2$ saturation, frequent assessment of blood pressure, and pulse). In the patient with a significantly reduced level of consciousness, endotracheal intubation is typically warranted. Furthermore, as explained above, frequent, directed neurological assessments are paramount. Close monitoring by informed nursing personnel around the clock is mandatory. Significant changes need to be dealt with swiftly. Neurologic assessments should include assessment of level of consciousness (as guided and objectively documented by the GCS), pupillary examination (size and reactivity), and an assessment of motor function to look for lateralizing signs.

Management of Elevated Intracranial Pressure

As noted above, brain edema and shifts in blood volume from dysregulation of cerebral blood flow can lead to elevations of pressure within the closed compartment of the skull. This leads to decreased tissue perfusion and oxygenation and further brain injury. Diagnosing increased ICP is best done by invasive monitoring, but, with limited resources, the only method at hand will likely be placement of an external ventricular drain (EVD). This can be used with excellent results to both measure and treat elevated ICP.

After clipping hair and appropriately prepping and draping the scalp in the area, local anesthesia (such as 0.25% Marcaine with 1:200,000 epinephrine) is used to infiltrate the incision site. A 1–2 cm incision is made centered at the intersection of a sagittal plane through the right mid-pupillary line and a coronal plane just anterior to the tragus (or just anterior to the coronal suture, which can be palpated). It is important to avoid making the opening near the midline, which is the location of the superior sagittal sinus. A burr hole is created with a hand drill, such as a Hudson brace and bit as detailed in the following section, centering the hole according to the landmarks just described. The dura at the base of the burr hole can be penetrated by touching it with the tip of a hemostat while applying monopolar electrocautery (e.g., a Bovie) to the hemostat. This will create a small dural opening with cautery that is unlikely to bleed. The catheter, with the stylette in place, is directed at an angle perpendicular to the plane that is tangent to the point of entry. The ventricle should be entered with spontaneous egress of CSF at a depth of around 5 cm, and the stylette removed while holding the catheter in position. The catheter should not be passed deeper than 6 cm, and if no CSF is encountered it is withdrawn fully, redirected slightly, and passed again. While maintaining the position of the catheter in the ventricle, pinching it off at the point of its exit from the skull, the other end should be tunneled to a separate exit site a few centimeters away, brought out through a stab incision, and anchored to the scalp with a series of tacking stitches that are snug, but do not occlude the catheter. An EVD must be connected to a sterile closed drainage system. EVD drainage systems are available. If this is not an option, then drainage into a vented empty glass intravenous (IV) fluid bottle can be constructed with IV tubing. The point at which the droplet of CSF forms at the end of the tubing prior to dropping into the chamber should be raised above the level of the ear just to the point at which the droplets stop forming. The vertical height in centimeters from the tragus of the ear to the droplet is a good approximation of the intracranial pressure in centimeters of water. Pressures above 20 cm are elevated. If the drainage height is fixed at 20 cm, then pressures above that level will cause CSF drainage, and help maintain ICP in the normal range.

If the patient is sufficiently brain-injured to warrant placement of an EVD (generally, a GCS <7), endotracheal intubation should be performed first. Not only are patients with altered levels of consciousness at risk for airway obstruction, but also hypoventilation and hypercarbia can greatly exacerbate intracranial hypertension (elevated ICP). Furthermore, in the face of elevated ICP, moderate hyperventilation of the patient can acutely decrease the ICP through induced hypocarbia with resultant constriction of the cerebral arterioles, thus decreasing the total blood volume in the intracranial compartment. This is a first-line treatment for acutely elevated ICP, although prolonged, extreme hyperventilation can be detrimental and should not be maintained.

Unfortunately, diffuse cerebral edema will squeeze CSF out of the cranial cavity, and the ventricles may become very small. This can make the initial catheter placement difficult, and CSF drainage may subsequently become very slow. Furthermore, in the face of collapsed ventricles, ICP measurement can become inaccurate. If the patient has a declining level of consciousness (GCS) and CSF drainage with hyperventilation are unable to improve the patient's condition, particularly if persistent ICP elevation is documented, pharmacologic means may be necessary.

Pharmacologic Management

Mannitol can be given in bolus injections of 0.25 g/kg body weight up to 1 g/kg. This can be repeated as needed, but there is a danger of inducing dangerous hypernatremia from the diuretic effect, and the patient's serum sodium levels will need to be monitored with prolonged mannitol use. In general, it should be given in the smallest effective dose, and not exceeding 1 g/kg body weight over 4–6 hours. If the serum sodium level reaches 160 or greater, mannitol must be discontinued. This agent may act by decreasing the viscosity of blood, which in turn increases the cerebral blood flow and induces vasoconstriction in those areas of the brain where autoregulation is intact. It should also be noted that IV fluids given to the patient should be either normal saline or lactated Ringer's solution or its equivalent. Hypo-osmolar fluids are to be avoided.

Elevated ICP can be exacerbated by the normal vasodilatory response to ischemia, which causes a further rise in ICP, which worsens the ischemia, and thus induces a vicious cycle. This can sometimes be broken by the use of pressor agents to elevate the blood pressure, which increases cerebral perfusion and induces a reflexive vasoconstriction that can lower the ICP. Patients should be kept euvolemic and normotensive as a baseline, but if ICP is spiraling out of control, the induction of hypertension can arrest the process. The cerebral perfusion pressure (CPP) is defined as the difference between mean arterial pressure (MAP) and the ICP (CPP = MAP – ICP). This should ideally be maintained above 50 mm Hg. (When measuring ICP in cm of water, the pressure is converted to mm of Hg when dividing by 1.3). If the ICP is, for instance, sustained at 40 mm Hg, then the mean arterial pressure would need to be raised to above 90 mm Hg to achieve a minimum CPP of 50 mmHg.

Exploratory Burr Holes and Craniectomy for Hematoma Evacuation

If a patient presents with, or develops, an asymmetric pupillary examination, particularly if accompanied by a change in consciousness or lateralizing motor signs (weakness or posturing on one side), one should suspect a developing hematoma (epidural, subdural, or intracerebral) on the side of the dilated pupil. This is the signal to intervene with a potentially life-saving evacuation of a developing hematoma. For patients in whom the initial neurologic condition is quite good and who rapidly deteriorate in this way, the likely diagnosis is epidural hematoma (commonly associated with a skull fracture), since patients with subdural and intracerebral hematomas tend to have had a more severe primary brain injury. Some have referred to this scenario as the "talk and die" syndrome.

When one suspects an evolving epidural hematoma in a deteriorating patient, urgent action is required. If a CT scan can be obtained immediately, it is worth doing, as this can save time in the operating room. In the absence of imaging, it takes courage to proceed on clinical grounds alone. One must remember that a negative exploration is completely forgivable and the risks involved are nominal, while failure to act risks an unnecessary death. If there are clues as to the location of intervention, such as a skull fracture noted by X-ray or a prominent scalp hematoma, begin there. If there are no guiding signs, begin in the temporal squamosa on the side ipsilateral to the dilated pupil. Motor signs, as explained above, can be on either side. The method for making the burr hole is described in Chapter 25.

Hair is clipped and the side of the head is prepped. A vertical linear incision is made through the skin, then the temporalis fascia and muscle, beginning at the zygoma 1 cm anterior to the tragus and extending upward for about 3 cm. A periosteal elevator and monopolar electrocautery are used to dissect the muscle from the underlying bone and a self-retaining retractor is placed. The skull is penetrated with a hand drill, such as a Hudson brace and bit. Care must be taken to prevent "plunging" of the drill as it penetrates the inner table of the skull. The force applied must be primarily that of twisting the drill bit, and not of pushing downward. The bit should be allowed to "carry itself" through the bone. The inner table is reached after the diploic space has been fully penetrated and the marrow elements give way to pure white bone. Penetration of the inner table as the bit turns through it can be felt distinctly. Assessing the depth of the hole periodically can aid in this process. Additional edges of bone may be removed with a small curette, and bleeding from the bone edges can be controlled by pressing bone wax into the bleeding spaces. If there is no epidural hematoma, the dura will be seen deep to the inner table. If either liquid blood or a solid clot is encountered, the burr hole is enlarged by biting away the edges of bone circumferentially using a Kerrison, Leksell, or other available rongeur. The clot can be decompressed with suction and irrigation, and occasionally with the help of a cup forceps in the case of solid hematoma. The bone opening is enlarged, lengthening the incision as necessary, until the majority of clot has been removed and the dura expands outward. The source of bleeding is identified; in this case, the source is typically arterial and associated with a skull fracture. Bleeding is controlled with bipolar electrocautery where the artery is accessible and with bone wax where it penetrates the skull. If available, Gelfoam soaked in thrombin or Surgicel can be laid over the dural surface and tucked just under the margins of the craniectomy prior to closure of the muscle, fascia and skin.

If no epidural clot is found, a small opening can be made in the dura to disclose underlying subdural hematoma. If none is present, then close the incision (the dura can be left open) and move to the next site. If subdural hematoma is encountered, the incision is enlarged and bone opening performed as described above in order to open the dura sufficiently to evacuate the clot and reveal the decompressed cortical surface beneath. A ventricular catheter or red rubber catheter can be gently passed circumferentially to irrigate in all directions in an attempt to remove as much hematoma as possible. With a limited exposure, the source of bleeding might not be determined, but is typically venous and may have already abated. The culprit is commonly one or more torn veins that bridge the cortical surface and the dura. When found, these can be controlled with bipolar electrocautery or tamponade.

If exploration in the temporal location is unrevealing, the posterior parietal and frontal regions are explored. If a very large hematoma is encountered, the burr holes can be connected with a Gigli saw to elevate the entire bone flap as shown in Figure 44.5.

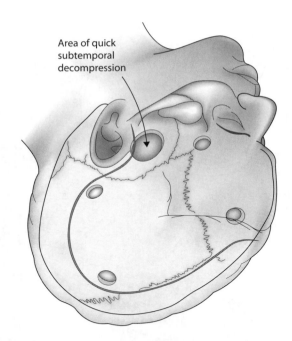

Area of quick subtemporal decompression

FIGURE 44.5 Exploratory burr holes and small temporal craniectomy. *Winn R. Youmans Neurological Surgery Volume 4*, 6th ed. Oxford: Elsevier Saunders, 2011, p. 3434.

If all areas are negative, one must consider whether to proceed with the same routine on the other side of the skull.

It should be borne in mind that these are extreme measures taken in the face of grave circumstances when imaging studies for diagnosis are not available. Clinical indications of an expanding epidural or subdural hematoma may confound an actual focal cerebral edema or an intracerebral hematoma. Thus, a negative exploration is entirely possible, and should be expected on occasion. However, the results of decompressing an expanding epidural hematoma in a deteriorating patient who did not have a significant primary brain injury are dramatic. It can mean the difference between death and having a normal patient walk out of the hospital in a few days. On the other hand, there is little to lose from a negative exploration in a patient that is deteriorating from other less treatable causes.

Depressed Skull Fractures

A closed depressed skull fracture with no overlying scalp laceration in a neurologically intact patient is primarily a cosmetic issue and does not require emergency management. This patient, if stable and alert, can be transferred non-emergently to a neurosurgical facility if possible. A patient presenting with an open depressed skull fracture is at risk of meningitis or intracerebral abscess if this is not washed out, debrided, and closed. This does constitute an urgent problem that can and should be dealt with unless transfer for treatment by a neurosurgeon can be done right away.

The patient is taken to the operating theater and placed under general anesthesia. A large area of scalp surrounding the lesion is clipped free of hair, prepped, and draped. The existing scalp laceration (which is typically irregular or stellate) is lengthened as needed to expose the full perimeter of the depressed bone (Figure 44.6). Scalp bleeders are dealt with first to secure a dry

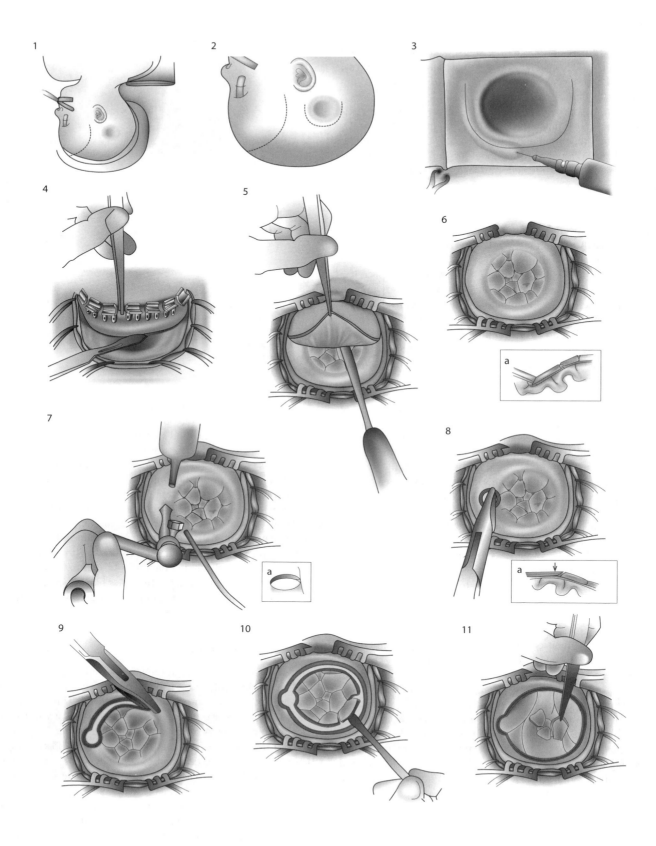

FIGURE 44.6 Steps for elevation of depressed skull fracture. Shillito J, Matson D. *An Atlas of Pediatric Neurosurgical Operations.* Oxford: Elsevier, 1982, p. 103.

operative field. Self-retaining retractors are placed to maintain the exposure. Sometimes purchase can be obtained on an edge of fractured bone in order to leverage this up to be grasped and removed. Once the first piece is removed, the others typically follow much more easily. However, if this proves infeasible, a burr hole (using the technique described above) can be made in the intact skull just at the edge of the fracture, and an instrument (preferably a Penfield dissector or a Freer elevator, but one can also use as a small periosteal elevator or an osteotome) can be gently manipulated into the epidural space beneath the depressed bone and pry it up. Alternatively, the burr hole can be used as the starting point for removing the depressed bone piecemeal with a Leksell or Kerrison rongeur, or for performing a craniotomy around the periphery of the depressed fracture by rongeuring bone circumferentially (Figure 44.6). As much as possible, it is desirable to remove larger pieces of bone intact so they can be washed and replaced to minimize the resulting cranial defect. As bone is removed, the underlying dura is inspected for tears, which should be repaired by primary closure if possible. If a significant dural defect cannot be closed primarily, a locally harvested graft of pericranium taken from the exposed undersurface of the adjacent scalp should be used to complete the closure. Prior to dural repair, the defect should be inspected for the presence of any bone fragments that have penetrated the cortical surface. These must be carefully removed, and bleeding controlled with bipolar electrocautery. Prior to any closure, the area must be copiously irrigated with antibiotic solution of bacitracin or gentamycin. Large bone pieces that could be used to repair the cranial defect should be inspected for debris or frank contamination. If the wound was not severely "dirty" (as in the case of an animal bite) bone can be thoroughly scrubbed and soaked in antibiotic solution and replaced. Bone can be loosely secured to the intact skull by sutures passed through small holes made with a twist drill or a towel clip. Rigorous hemostasis must be insured prior to proceeding with repair of the scalp defect.

Penetrating Cranial Injuries

Low-velocity penetrating injuries, such as from knives, machetes, arrows, spears, or other implements, will present either after the offending instrument has been removed or with it still in place. If it has been removed, one should proceed as described above with repair of an open depressed skull fracture. In this case, there may be intracerebral, subdural, or epidural hematoma that also requires evacuation. Furthermore, the tract must be visually inspected—but not physically explored—for retained foreign bodies or debris that can be readily and safely extracted. Copious irrigation with antibiotic solution and repair as described above must follow. In the case of a retained implement, no attempt should be made to remove this at the bedside. The patient must be taken to the operating theater, placed under general anesthesia, and the entire area thoroughly prepped. A long object protruding and interfering with the operation can be cut short if possible while avoiding any manipulation that would disturb the buried portion. A scalp incision is fashioned so as to incorporate the penetrated skin in the incision, and thus raise a flap while leaving the weapon in place. A burr hole is placed (as described above) adjacent to the bone defect and used as the starting point for rongeuring away bone to form a craniectomy

that extends circumferentially around the weapon that provides sufficient exposure to deal with bleeding and dural repair. The dural defect from the penetration is carefully lengthened on either side of the offending object, being careful to avoid injury to underlying cortex. This is facilitated by passage of a grooved director or dental instrument beneath the dura to protect the brain and having an assistant cut on top of it. Similarly, a second linear dural incision is created perpendicular to the first to form a "+", and the four corners of the resulting cruciate incision are reflected back to expose the brain around the tract. Accessible brain tissue around the margin of the tract is coagulated with the bipolar, and then the object is gently and smoothly withdrawn in the direction along its axis to avoid any lateral movement of the object's distal tip within the brain. Upon completion of its removal, the tract is inspected for bleeding, which can be controlled by placement of Surgicel strips or thrombin-soaked Gelfoam. In the event of significant bleeding, cotton balls saturated with half-strength hydrogen peroxide can be placed into the tract and left for several minutes to tamponade the bleeding prior to their removal. Irrigation with bacitracin or gentamycin solution should precede dural closure with simple running 4-0 stitches (neurolon, prolene, or Vicryl). The scalp is then closed in layers. Treatment with broad-spectrum IV antibiotics for 2 weeks is advisable.

The effects of low- and high-velocity missile injuries were described above. The main treatment goals for treating gunshot wounds to the brain are: 1) debridement and closure of the entrance wound (described above for penetrating injuries); and 2) management of elevated intracranial pressure from brain swelling as already described. Generally speaking, "through-and-through" gunshot wounds through the middle of the brain are eventually fatal under the best of circumstances.

Management of the Patient with a Spinal Injury

Initial Evaluation

Spinal injury should be anticipated as a possibility in any victim of significant trauma, such as a road traffic accident or a significant fall. The secondary survey of the patient, after addressing airway, breathing, and circulation, should include inspection of the neck and back for overt signs of trauma as well as palpation to look for areas of tenderness. Until spinal injury is ruled out, the neck should be immobilized in a rigid collar. If such is not available, immobilization can be achieved by positioning sandbags, linen rolls, or liter IV bags placed on either side of the head (with the patient supine and the neck in neutral position) and strapping tape across the forehead and the sand bags from one side of the stretcher to the other. Also, when turning the patient, he should be log rolled without extending or flexing the thoracic and lumbar spine.

Anteroposterior (AP) and lateral X-rays of the cervical, thoracic, and lumbosacral spine, as well as an open-mouth odontoid view (if possible) should identify most significant fractures or dislocations. The pertinent neurologic examination assesses for sensation along the dermatomes, strength in the individual muscle groups of the upper and lower extremities, and an assessment of anal sphincter tone.

Management

In an LMIC, operative intervention for acute spinal cord decompression or spinal stabilization is typically not an option. Patients who are identified as having a spinal column fracture should be immobilized and placed on bed rest until arrangements for evaluation by a neurosurgeon or orthopedic surgeon can be made. Such an expert assessment will be necessary to determine whether or not a fracture is unstable, and whether and what type of immobilization should be maintained. Guidelines for this are outside the scope of this text.

Patients having "complete" cord injuries as defined by flaccid paralysis, loss of sphincter tone, and absence of sensation below a defined spinal dermatomal level have a very poor prognosis for recovery of any function. Patients with incomplete injuries may see gradual recovery of some function. The efficacy of steroids in the acute treatment of spinal cord injury remains controversial. Given the expenditure of resources necessary and the need for early initiation of treatment, such measures are likely infeasible in these contexts.

Spinal Cord Injury Without Radiographic Abnormality in Children

Young children can present with spinal cord injury in the absence of any fracture or subluxation seen on X-ray. This has been termed SCIWORA (spinal cord injury without radiographic abnormality). Young children can more easily have a reversible spinal subluxation without fracture because of their immature anatomy, which results in a brief spinal cord compression or impact. The child presents with motor and sensory loss commensurate with the injury level, but spine X-rays look normal. In these situations, one should assume there has been ligamentous injury and ongoing spinal instability. In the case of a cervical neurological level the neck should be immobilized in a rigid collar. In the case of a thoracic neurological level, bed rest should be maintained until some sort of immobilization can be arranged. If nothing else can be obtained, a plaster cast can be fitted that will prevent flexion and extension of the thoracic spine. These precautions are intended to avoid additional spinal cord injury from abnormal motion at the injured segment until the ligamentous injury has healed. At the end of 12 weeks, flexion and extension lateral spine X-rays can be obtained to look for abnormal motion indicating ongoing instability. If this is the case, the patient will need to be referred for a spinal stabilization procedure.

Conclusion

The patient with a severe brain or spinal cord injury has a poor prognosis for recovery in the best of circumstances. However, in the context of an LMIC, there are a few circumstances in which intervention can be of significant benefit and is at times life-saving.

Suggested Reading

Winn HR (ed.). *Youmans Neurological Surgery*. 6th ed. Philadelphia: Elsevier and Saunders, 2011: Ch. 333–335.

Plum F, Posner JB. *The Diagnosis of Stupor and Coma*. 3rd ed. Philadelphia: F.A. Davis Co., 1980.

COMMENTARY

John Mugamba, Uganda

Given the increasing number of vehicles on our roads, especially motorcycle "taxis," and the inadequately trained and inexperienced riders (highway code), we are seeing a rapid increase in the number of patients with multiple injuries. Head and spinal cord injuries are not uncommon. There are very few neurosurgeons in sub-Saharan Africa (SSA); they cannot provide services for the increasing population. This shortage is unlikely to be addressed in SSA in the very near future. Dr. Benjamin Warf touches on this crucial subject in the chapter, and outlines the need to reduce the morbidity and mortality from secondary events or insults after road traffic accidents. I do agree that a general surgeon or physician is capable of doing this. The chapter addresses all the practical aspects and, in a way, demystifies the fear we all carry in dealing with neurosurgical emergencies.

45

Maxillofacial Trauma

Daniel J. Meara

Introduction

In low- to middle-income countries (LMICs), regional trauma centers often do not yet exist, and with increasing industrialization and urbanization, maxillofacial trauma is increasing, resulting in a significant burden to emergency rooms. Limited access to care, inappropriate triage protocols, delay in definitive care, and limited resources, including surgeons, often are obstacles to optimal patient care. Fortunately, facial trauma alone is rarely a threat to life unless uncontrolled hemorrhage or airway compromise is present or anticipated. However, a systematic approach to maxillofacial trauma is essential to avoid occult injuries and provide comprehensive care to the injured patient. For a detailed review of advanced trauma life support (ATLS) principles and the initial evaluation of the trauma patient, please see Chapter 38.

The Physics of Facial Injuries

Speed, shape, density, and mass of the striking object directly affect the type and severity of facial injury.

High Impact	Low Impact
←Supraorbital rim/Frontal Sinus----------- Zygoma/Nasal Bones→	

Thus, the type of facial fracture should intimate the forces involved in the injury and may provide a suggestion of associated underlying injuries.

Physical Examination Keys

Inspect facial structures for asymmetry. Critical, "can't miss" elements include the following:

- Inspection of scalp for lacerations, as significant blood volume can be lost quickly
- Inspection for an orbital hyphema to minimize long-term visual changes
- Gross visual acuity assessment for baseline comparisons
- Extraocular movement evaluation to rule out muscle entrapment
- Finger tonometry for intraocular pressure assessment and need for lateral canthotomy and cantholysis
- Inspection of nasal septum for septal hematoma formation and need for incision and drainage to prevent a saddle-nose deformity
- Inspection of nasal passages for clear drainage, suggestive of cerebrospinal fluid (CSF) leakage and underlying injuries
- Evaluation for associated soft tissue injuries to vital structures such as the lacrimal apparatus, parotid duct, and facial nerve
- Check of facial motion—temporal bone fracture can lead to facial paralysis
- Check of ears for otorrhea and mastoid bruising

Concomitant Injuries

Head injuries are commonly associated with maxillofacial trauma. Mulligan et al. report in a 2010 retrospective review of more than a million trauma patients that 28.7%–79.9% sustained head injuries, 4.9%–8.0% cervical spine injuries, and 2.8%–5.8% concomitant head and cervical spine injuries.[1]

Frontal Sinus

The frontal sinus is a pyramidal, air-filled cavity that lies between the lamina of the frontal bone. The size and shape of this sinus varies among individuals and between the two sides. Nonetheless, frontal sinus fractures require a significant force, between 363 kg and 727 kg, to fracture and are usually the result of high-velocity impacts.[2] Anatomically, the frontal sinus floor forms two-thirds of the medial orbital roof and has both anterior and posterior tables. Management of frontal sinus fractures is dependent upon the involved tables, cosmetic deformity, involvement of the nasofrontal duct, and the presence of a CSF leak.

Anterior Table

Isolated anterior table fractures are typically repaired only to correct cosmetic deformities. Displacement of the anterior table greater than the width of the bony table itself is a guide to the possible need for correction, but definitive need is often undetermined until facial edema has resolved.

Posterior Table

Correction of frontal sinus fractures with posterior table involvement is often predicated on CSF leakage as a result of a dural

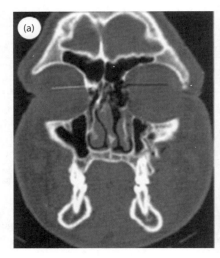 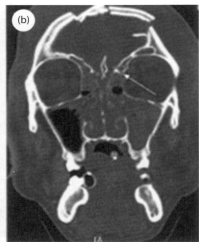 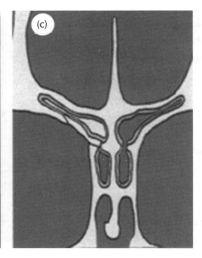

FIGURE 45.1 Coronal CT images demonstrating sinus outflow obstruction. Stanwix, et al. Frontal Sinus Fracture Diagnosis. *Journal of Oral and Maxillofacial Surgery.* 2010.

tear. Neurosurgical consultation as to the need for dural repair and cranialization is often required.

Nasofrontal Duct

The nasofrontal duct (NFD) is located posteromedial in the frontal sinus and drains into the middle meatus. Computed tomography (CT) imaging, if available, can facilitate determination of patency of the NFD (Figure 45.1).

Surgical Correction

If warranted, the first decision based on the goals of treatment is access to the fractures. If an associated laceration is present, this may often be used to address the underlying bony injuries and may be extended with a 15 blade as needed. If no lacerations exist, then two main surgical techniques can be employed. A W-plasty type of incision hidden in the eyebrows and across the glabellar region can be created with an 11 blade. Ideally, however, a well-positioned coronal incision allows excellent access for reconstruction, including pericranial flap creation, cranial bone graft harvesting, and any associated neurosurgical procedures. Further, bony fracture segments can be stabilized with wire or plate fixation. Obliteration of the sinus, if required, demands removal of all sinus mucosa and obliteration of the sinus cavity itself, such as with fat or bone. The nasofrontal duct must also be addressed via obliteration or reconstruction. Reconstruction can be achieved with placement of an 18 French red Robinson catheter or a number 26 chest tube. Once secured from the frontal sinus ostium to the middle meatus, the tract is allowed to heal and remucosalize and then the stent may be removed intranasally after approximately 3 weeks (Figure 45.2).

Complications

Mucopyoceles can develop up to 20 years after the traumatic event. Thus, long-term follow-up is recommended.

Naso-orbital-ethmoid

The naso-orbital-ethmoid (NOE) complex consists of the medial orbital walls, the nasal bones, and the nasal projection of the frontal bone. Physical examination often demonstrates telecanthus and instability of the medial canthal ligament and central bony fragment. Further, clinical examination includes the bowstring and Furness tests as well as direct intercanthal measurements.[5] Intercanthal distance in adults is approximately 35 mm. An acute nasofrontal angle may be noted as well as ophthalmic nerve hypoesthesia. Three fracture types are typically delineated (Figure 45.3).

Surgical Correction

Surgical management is complex and often requires secondary reconstruction. Initial emphasis is placed on restoration of orbital volumes, recreation of nasal contours, over-correction of the intercanthal distance, and restoration of midface projection. Access is optimized via a coronal incision, unless a significant laceration preexists in the area. Paranasal Lynch incisions are an alternative for access but often are less esthetic (Figure 45.4). Transnasal fixation with nonabsorbable sutures is a critical step in surgical reconstruction if the medial canthal tendon insertion is disrupted. Over-correction is suggested and semi-rigid external bolsters are essential to prevent pseudotelecanthus (Figure 45.5A, Figure 45.5B, Figure 45.5C, Figure 45.5D, and Figure 45.5E).[6]

Complications

Complications include persistent soft-tissue thickness due to inadequate bolstering, nasal dorsal defects, and lacrimal apparatus disruption presenting as epiphora, which will likely require definitive repair (Figure 45.6).

Nasofrontal duct reconstruction

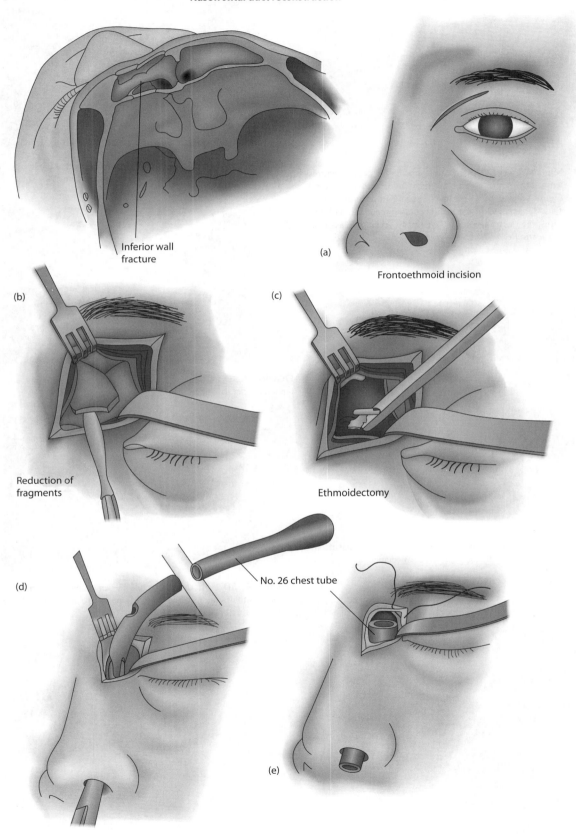

Inferior wall fracture

(a)

Frontoethmoid incision

(b) Reduction of fragments

(c) Ethmoidectomy

(d)

No. 26 chest tube

(e)

FIGURE 45.2　Nasofrontal duct reconstruction. Mathog, et al. *Atlas of Craniofacial Trauma*. Philadelphia: W.B. Saunders Company, 1991.

Nasoethmoid orbital fracture classification

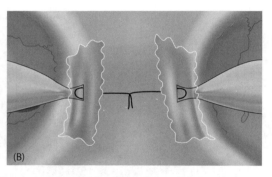

Type I   Type II   Type III

FIGURE 45.3 Markowitz et al. Classification scheme for NOE fractures based on the relationship of the medial canthal tendon and the central bony fragment. Figure created by Gino Inverso using information from: Markowitz BL, et al. Management of the medial canthal tendon in nasoethmoid orbital fractures: the importance of the central fragment in classification and treatment. *Plastic Reconstructive Surgery.* 1991; 87(5):843–53.

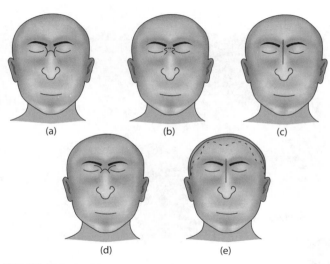

(a)   (b)   (c)

(d)   (e)

FIGURE 45.4 Variable surgical incision types for access to the nasofrontal region: a) H-shaped, b) bilateral z, c) midline, d) W-shaped, and e) coronal. Image by Gino Inverso.

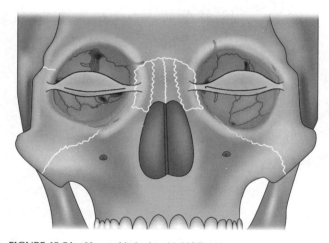

FIGURE 45.5A Naso-orbital-ethmoid (NOE) anatomy. Image by Bin Song.

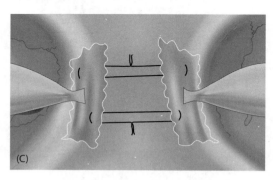

FIGURE 45.5B Trans-nasal wiring of medial canthal tendons to bony segments, with narrowing of the NOE complex. Image by Bin Song.

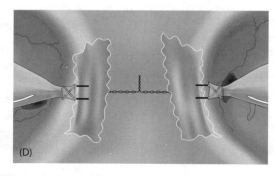

FIGURE 45.5C Trans-nasal wire fixation of bony segments, with canthal tendons intact. Image by Bin Song.

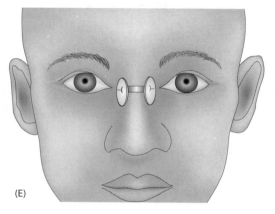

FIGURE 45.5D Alternative technique for trans-nasal wire fixation of medial canthal tendon to the bony segment, to narrow the NOE complex. Image by Bin Song.

FIGURE 45.5E Trans-nasal fixation to limit pseudo-telecanthus. Image by Bin Song.

CANALICULI REPAIR

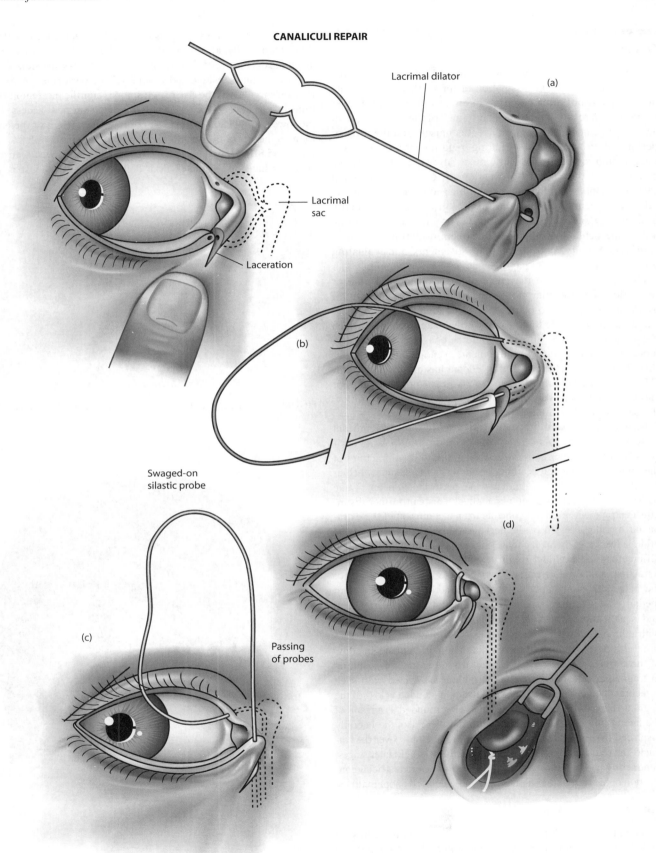

Lacrimal dilator

(a)

Lacrimal sac

Laceration

(b)

Swaged-on
silastic probe

(c)

Passing
of probes

(d)

FIGURE 45.6 Steps for canalicular repair. Mathog R, Loechel W. *Atlas of Craniofacial Trauma*. Philadelphia: W.B. Saunders Company, 1991.

Orbital

The orbital floor bone is extremely thin, and a direct blow to the globe usually results in dissipation of forces that fractures the floor of the orbit, often resulting in a blowout fracture. Lesser fractures can result in rotational "hinging" of the bony fragment and impingement of the inferior rectus muscle and the inferior periorbital tissues. Such a finding requires prompt surgical intervention to relieve the entrapment, allowing for free range of motion of the eye and prevention of long-term functional sequelae. Ophthalmologic consultation should be part of the initial treatment algorithm to assess the globe itself, especially prior to any surgical intervention. Goals include establishing a baseline ocular examination; documenting intraocular pressure, visual acuity, and extra-ocular movements; and evaluating for globe injury, afferent papillary defect, and hyphema.

Physical examination may note diplopia on upward gaze or restriction of extraocular movements. Thin-slice CT imaging, if available, is superior to plain films as an adjunct to the clinical examination, as subtle findings may only be appreciated on such high-resolution scans. Surgery should be considered for: 1) diplopia secondary to physical entrapment; 2) enophthalmos greater than 2 mm, best determined after edema has dissipated; and 3) CT scan measured orbital floor defects greater than 1 cm.[7] For cases that do not clearly require surgery, the surgeon must follow the patient closely to monitor for any delayed changes.

Medial orbital wall fractures can also result in significant increases in orbital volume that must be addressed to avoid horizontal diplopia, and progressive enophthalmos.[8] For all fractures of the orbit, forced duction is an important test to determine whether muscle entrapment exists and can be performed on an awake patient after topical anesthetic is applied. This can further distinguish entrapment of orbital contents from a contusion of the extraocular muscle, a lesion of the nerve, or simple congestion of the orbit. However, early on, if a muscle is swollen, it may be difficult to differentiate the swelling from true entrapment. A pseudo–Duane retraction syndrome or retraction of the globe and narrowing of the palpebral fissure upon attempted abduction may occur with medial wall fracture associated with medial rectus entrapment, and is pathognomonic for this complication.[9] Medial wall fractures with ethmoid-orbital fractures can cause damage to the nasolacrimal drainage system and the medial canthal ligament. In some of these fractures, the medial canthal tendon is injured, resulting in traumatic telecanthus. A clinical finding associated with such detachment or severance of the medial canthal tendon is loss of the angular shape of the canthus, thus appearing rounded as a result of the lateral pull of the orbicularis oculi muscle. Also, the laterally displaced tissues of the upper and lower eyelids may cover the caruncle, the semilunar fold, and a portion of the sclera. In later stages, contracting necrotic muscles, orbital fat atrophy, or cicatricial contraction of the retrobulbar tissues may cause delayed enophthalmos.

Surgical Correction

Emergent issues such as a retrobulbar hematoma are addressed first. In an attempt to preserve vision, a lateral canthotomy and inferior cantholysis are performed immediately if orbital compartment syndrome is present (Figure 45.7). Surgical access to the orbital floor can be achieved via a transconjunctival, subciliary, subtarsal/mid-lid, or lower lid incision. Transconjunctival

incisions result in no skin incisions and less incidence of ectropion. Technically, all sutures should be below the conjunctiva to avoid iatrogenic corneal abrasions. The subciliary incision is the most technique sensitive and should only be performed by experienced surgeons as the risk of ectropion is significant.[10] Subtarsal (mid-lid) or lower lid incisions also provide surgical access, but the lower lid incision is the least cosmetic as a result of the anatomical merger of eyelid and malar skin types (Figure 45.8A and Figure 45.8B). Medial access is often best achieved via a transcaruncular incision.[11] Isolated floor defects are best reconstructed

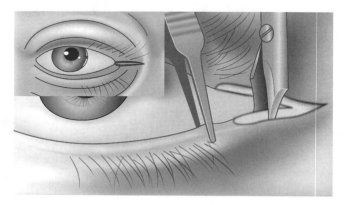

FIGURE 45.7 Lateral canthotomy and inferior cantholysis. Image by Karen Goodall.

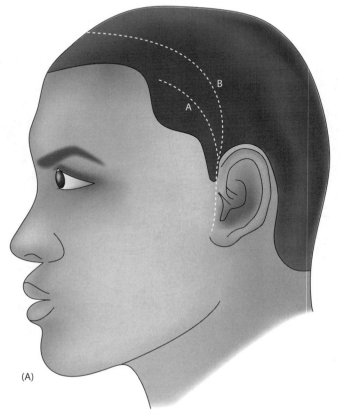

(A)

FIGURE 45.8A Incision designs for orbital-related surgical access. Image by Bin Song.

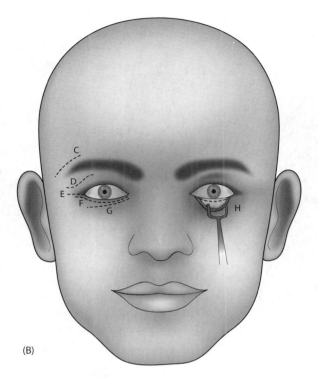

FIGURE 45.8B Incision designs for orbital-related surgical access. Image by Bin Song.

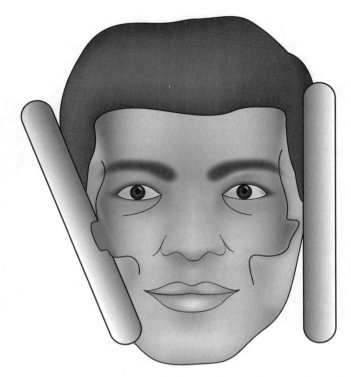

FIGURE 45.9 Simple tongue blade analysis of malar projection and symmetry. Gustav OK. *Textbook of Oral Surgery*, 4th ed. Philadelphia: Mosby, July 1974.

with autogenous bone (split calvarium), nasoseptal cartilage, or alloplast implants such titanium-reinforced polyethylene implants. Alternatively, for orbital floor reconstruction, the maxillary antrum can be packed with ribbon gauze to buoy the orbital floor back into position until scarring has occurred below the globe to stabilize its position.[12] Dissection distances within the orbit must be monitored to avoid the optic nerve, approximately 40–45 mm from the orbital rim.[13]

Complications

Prolonged V2 paraesthesia, scleral show, ectropion, entropion, and diplopia can be long-term sequelae even with surgical intervention.

Zygomaticomaxillary Complex and Arch

The zygomaticomaxillary complex (ZMC) fracture or tetrapod fracture incidence increases with the development of the paranasal sinuses, as well as the increased prominence of the zygoma with growth.[14] The zygoma is a confluence of four main articulations: 1) zygomaticofrontal, 2) zygomaticosphenoid, 3) zygomaticotemporal, and 4) zygomaticomaxillary. Clinical findings include maxillary nerve hypoesthesia, malocclusion, trismus, subconjunctival hemorrhage, increased transverse dimension, and loss of malar projection (Figure 45.9). Significant displacement results in increased orbital volume and enophthalmos that may initially be camouflaged by edema. Ophthalmologic assessment is critical to establish a baseline ocular examination, and, as with isolated orbital fractures, the etiology of visual acuity abnormalities must be determined before facial fracture repair and positive findings require prompt attention.

Surgical Correction

Nondisplaced fractures or minimally displaced fractures can be managed conservatively, but cases with coronoid impingement, enophthalmos, or significant fracture displacement require intervention. Typically, two points of fixation are usually adequate to stabilize the fractures and restore the facial projection. The zygomaticosphenoid suture is critical to visualize postreduction so as to evaluate for any residual rotational deformities that would result in orbital volume and esthetic changes.[15] Approaches include an intraoral Keen incision in the maxillary vestibule and an upper eyelid, blepharoplasty-like, crease incision. Use of the brow incision should be minimized, especially in females, due to the potential for postoperative alopecia. A limited transconjunctival approach for concomitant orbital rim and floor repair is well tolerated. Alternative access to the zygomatic arch can be achieved via a Gillies approach through the scalp and medial to the superficial layer of the deep temporal fascia overlying the temporalis muscle (Figure 45.10).

Noncomminuted fractures, especially of the zygomatic arch, can be reduced with a towel clamp (Figure 45.11). For zygomaticomaxillary complex fixation, wire or plate fixation is preferred via intraoral and/or facial incisions with an external splint secured with permanent suture passed under the arch for stabilization of the zygomatic arch component. If no rigid forms of fixation are available, the zygomaticomaxillary complex, like orbital floor reduction, can be ideally positioned and stabilized with robust packing of the maxillary antrum by a Caldwell-Luc approach, which prevents sagging and allows for healing prior to complete removal (Figure 45.12A, Figure 45.12B, Figure 45.12C, and Figure 45.12D).[12]

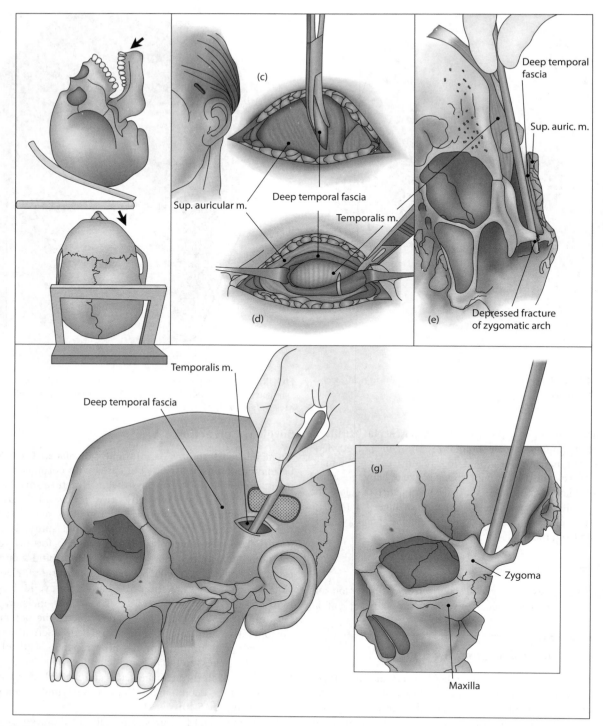

FIGURE 45.10   Zygomatic arch reduction vial scalp or Gillie's approach in contrast to the oral, Keen approach. Lore and Medina. *An Atlas of Head and Neck Surgery*, 4th ed. Philadelphia: W.B. Saunders Company, 2004. Figure 13–23, p. 621.

Complications

Failure to address displaced fractures typically results in a lack of anterior-posterior projection and an increased transverse widening of the face, both of which result in a loss of symmetry and lack of cosmesis.

Nasal

Nasal fractures are the most common facial fracture in adults due to the nose's prominence and thin, bony skeleton. The mechanism of injury is useful in focusing the clinical examination as a glancing

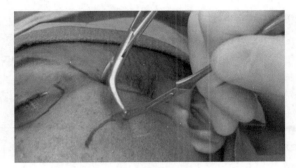

FIGURE 45.11 Simple towel clamp technique for isolated zygomatic arch treatment. Carter T, Bagheri S, Dierks E. Towel Clip Reduction of the Depressed Zygomatic Arch Fracture. *Journal of Oral and Maxillofacial Surgery.* 2005; 63:1244–1246.

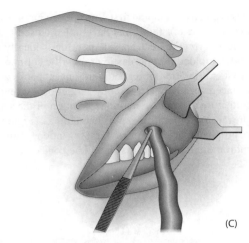

FIGURE 45.12C Ribbon gauze packing of the maxillary sinus for zygoma stabilization or orbital floor reduction. Image by Bin Song.

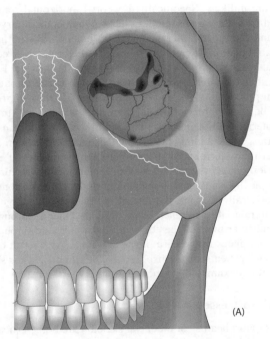

FIGURE 45.12A Ribbon gauze packing of the maxillary sinus for zygoma stabilization or orbital floor reduction. Image by Bin Song.

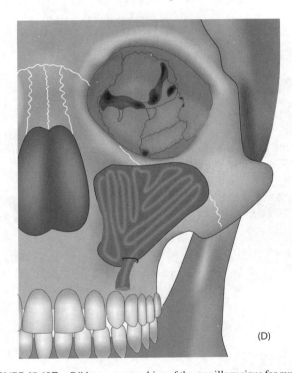

FIGURE 45.12D Ribbon gauze packing of the maxillary sinus for zygoma stabilization or orbital floor reduction. Image by Bin Song.

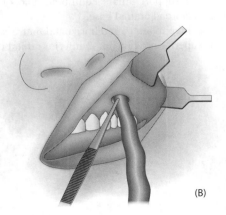

FIGURE 45.12B Ribbon gauze packing of the maxillary sinus for zygoma stabilization or orbital floor reduction. Image by Bin Song.

or tangential blow will often result in different injuries than a direct frontal force. Patients will often present with considerable nasal bleeding that should be addressed immediately with posterior and anterior packing as needed (Figure 45.13). For instance, Foley catheter can be used to tamponade posterior nasal bleeds not amenable to simple packing. Clinical examination is often all that is necessary for diagnosis; treatment planning and additional imaging are warranted only if other maxillofacial injuries are suspected.

Surgical Correction

Surgical intervention is required for 1) uncontrolled hemorrhage, 2) drainage of a septal hematoma, 3) cosmetic deformity, and 4) functional impairment of airflow through the nares. Closed reduction is typically attempted first with open reduction reserved for complex fractures or those that have failed closed reduction. After surgical correction, extranasal splinting is ideally accomplished with a molded thermoplastic or metallic splint or a plaster nasal cast. Antibiotic-impregnated intranasal packs or ribbon gauze is placed to augment the bony reduction by tenting the bony architecture and also to maintain position of the septum as well as prevent postoperative septal hematomas (Figure 45.14). Systemic prophylactic antibiotics for prevention against toxic shock syndrome and endocarditis should be considered.[16,17]

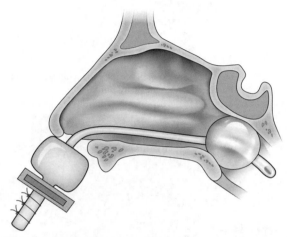

FIGURE 45.13 Anterior and posterior nasal packing for significant nasal hemorrhage. Image by David Randall.

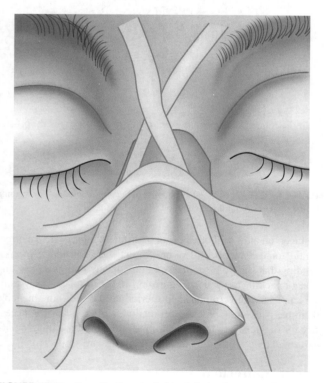

FIGURE 45.14 Complications include a left, hard extranasal splint/cast to protect the bony reduction and right, silastic intranasal stents. Lore and Medina. *An Atlas of Head and Neck Surgery*, 4th ed. Philadelphia: W.B. Saunders Company, 2004. Figure 13-2, p. 599.

Complications

- Persistent deformity or nasal airflow obstruction.
- "Saddle-nose" deformity if nasoseptal hematomas are not addressed.
- Major morbidity and even mortality if hemorrhage is not aggressively treated.

Maxillary

Midface patterns of fracture, as delineated by Rene Le Fort in 1901, are rare until aeration of the paranasal sinuses (Figure 45.15). In what is an oversimplification, Le Fort fracture patterns are typically presented in three classical and pure forms, despite the reality that in facial trauma such pure fracture patterns are unlikely. Specifically, Le Fort I, horizontal fractures, extend from the nasal septum to the zygomaticomaxillary junction and then to the pterygomaxillary junction, disrupting the pterygoid plates. The maxilla represents the bridge between the cranial base superiorly and the dental arch inferiorly. Le Fort II, pyramidal fractures, extend from the nasal bridge through the frontal processes of the maxilla, inferolaterally through the lacrimal bones and inferior orbital floor/rim and inferiorly through the anterior wall of the maxillary sinus. Le Fort III, transverse fractures, create a total craniofacial dysjunction. These fractures start at the nasofrontal and frontomaxillary sutures and extend posteriorly along the medial wall of the orbit. The fracture pattern typically continues along the floor of the orbit and continues superolaterally through the lateral orbital wall and zygomatic arch. Intranasally, a branch of the fracture extends through the perpendicular plate of the ethmoid, the vomer, and through the pterygoid plates to the base of the sphenoid. As a result of this path, such patients are predisposed to CSF rhinorrhea and should be carefully examined for such findings.[18]

Facial Buttresses

The "support beams" of the facial skeleton are both vertical and horizontal buttresses (Figure 45.16).[19] The three main, paired vertical buttresses are: 1) nasomaxillary, 2) zygomaticomaxillary, and 3) pterygomaxillary. Additional bolstering exists in the form of an unpaired midline frontoethmoid-vomerine buttress. These vertical support pillars equilibrate and diffuse vertical forces over the broad cranial base.

Similarly, three main, paired horizontal buttresses exist in the form of: 1) superior orbital rim, 2) inferior orbital rim extending

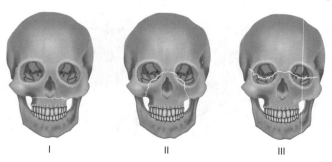

I   II   III

FIGURE 45.15 Le Fort I, II, and IIIF pure fracture patterns. Image by Gino Inverso.

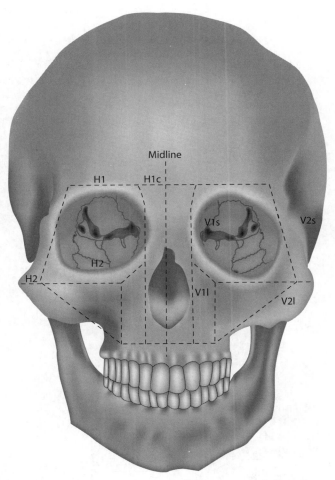

Midline

H1 H1c

V1s V2s

H2

H2 V1l

V2l

FIGURE 45.16 Schematic of the horizontal and vertical facial support buttresses. Image by Gino Inverso.

into the zygomatic arch, and 3) maxillary alveolus and palate. However, in comparison to the vertical buttresses, the horizontal support beams are less stout and less force resistant, resulting in fractures with vertical injury propagation.[20] Surgical correction, regardless of the technique, requires restoration of all facial buttresses to restore facial form and function.

Surgical Correction

Maxillomandibular fixation in conjunction with semi-rigid or rigid fixation is typically required. As an alternative to miniplates, interosseous wiring to stabilize the fractures at key points of fixation is viable. For instance, at the nasofrontal suture or the zygomaticomaxillary buttress, 24-gauge stainless-steel wire is passed through a hole on each side of the fracture line and tightened, securing the segments. Circumzygomatic and other suspension wiring techniques can be employed for Le Fort I, Le Fort II, and Le Fort III fractures (Figure 45.17A, Figure 45.17B, and Figure 45.17C). Extraskeletal fixation is a viable treatment modality often reserved for extensive fracture comminution and/or panfacial injuries as the "ex-fix" may be the only means of stabilization. However, this method may apply excessive or misdirected forces onto the fracture segments and therefore cause shortening or further deformity of the midface.[21]

Complications

Significant craniofacial deformity is likely if all fractures are not accurately addressed or if misdirected forces or vectors are applied with fixation during the healing period. For midface fractures, resuspension of the soft tissue envelope is critical to avoid unsightly scars and loss of soft-tissue support.

Mandible

Mandible fractures are quite common and unique due to the shape of the mandible, the functional requirements (deglutition, phonation, and mastication), occlusion with the maxillary dentition, and articulation with the cranial base. Fractures are typically categorized by anatomical location: 1) symphysis, 2) parasymphysis, 3) body, 4) angle, 5) ramus, 6) coronoid, 7) subcondyle, 8) condyle, and 9) dentoalveolar. Further, condylar fractures are categorized into three main types: 1) intracapsular/condylar head fractures, 2) condylar neck fractures above the sigmoid notch, and 3) subcondylar fractures through the sigmoid notch. Physical examination is often adequate to make an accurate diagnosis, but radiographs can be of great assistance, especially with condylar-associated fractures. Restoration of form and function is uniquely challenging in mandibular fractures.

Patterns of Injury

Symphyseal fractures tend to occur in conjunction with subcondylar fractures and angle fractures with a fracture of the contralateral body or condyle.

Occlusion

Unlike long bone fractures or most isolated midface fractures, the foundation for a successful reconstruction of a fracture of the mandible is predicated upon either restoration of the patient's occlusion or contact of the teeth. Failure to address the fracture-related occlusal discrepancy will certainly result in a suboptimal clinical outcome.

Surgical Correction

As with other facial fractures, emergent issues can arise when bilateral parasymphyseal or body fractures are noted secondary to muscle pull posteriorly, often creating airway compromise. The ABC's (airway, breathing, and circulation) of critical care management must be performed to stabilize the patient prior to any definitive fracture repair. Once the patient is stable, the goals of intervention are to restore facial form (esthetics) and function (occlusion and range of motion). As is understood, bony reduction and immobilization is necessary for ideal bony healing in most cases. Thus, only clinically stable, incomplete, and nondisplaced mandibular fractures without malocclusion or other sequelae are amenable to conservative (nonoperative) treatment. Specifically, limitation of jaw motion and a strict, nonchew diet are essential. All other fractures must be immobilized for a period of time to allow for healing of the bony segments while maintaining an ideal occlusal scheme. Closed reduction via maxillomandibular

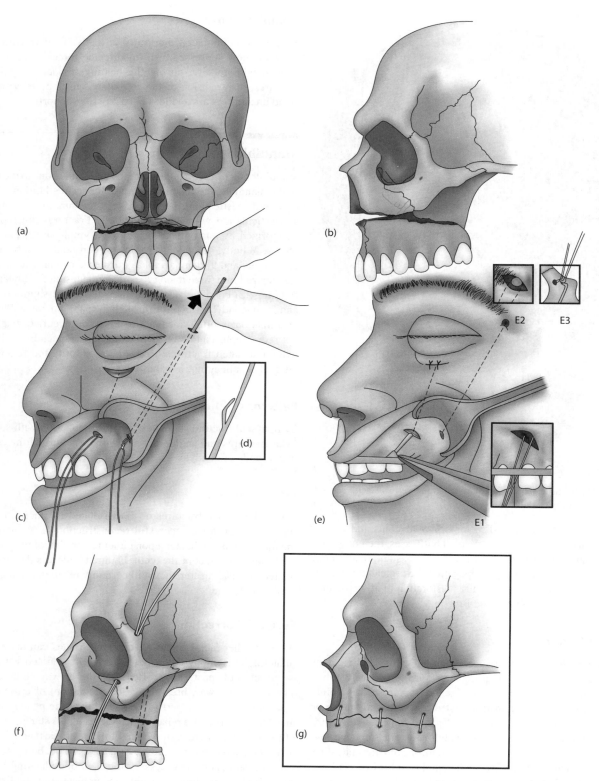

FIGURE 45.17A Circumzygomatic wires and maxillomandibular fixation for Le Fort I fractures. Lore and Medina. *An Atlas of Head and Neck Surgery*, 4th ed. Philadelphia: W.B. Saunders Company, 2004. Figure 13-28, p. 631.

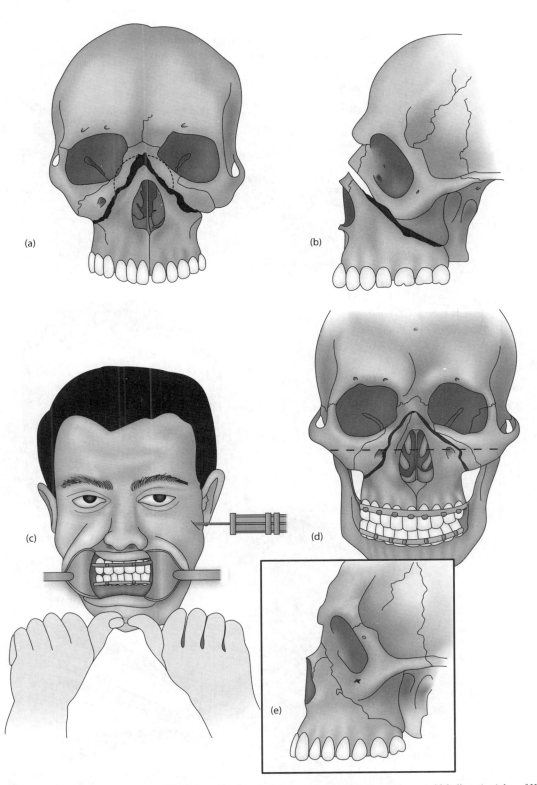

FIGURE 45.17B   K-wire fixation through the malar eminences and wire suspension for Le Fort II fractures. Lore and Medina. *An Atlas of Head and Neck Surgery*, 4th ed. Philadelphia: W.B. Saunders Company, 2004. Figure 13-29, p. 633.

Repair of Le Fort III/malar fractures (*Continued*)

Suspension technique (*Continued*)

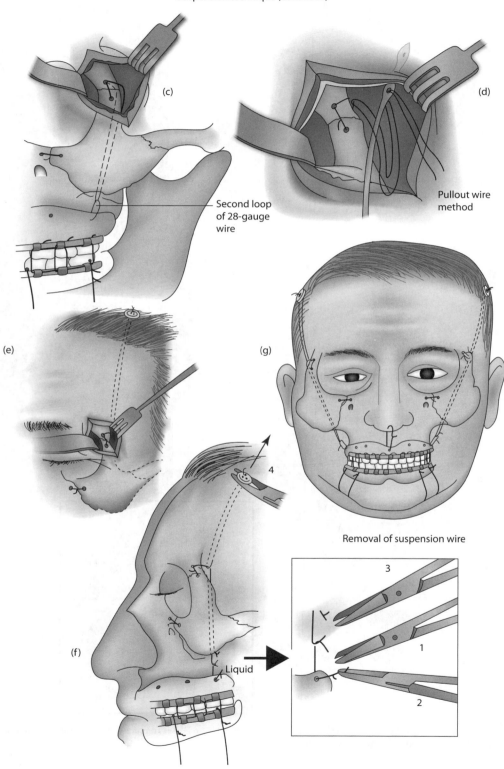

FIGURE 45.17C Wire suspension for Le Fort III fractures. Mathog, et al. *Atlas of Craniofacial Trauma*. Philadelphia: W.B. Saunders Company, 1991.

fixation can be easily achieved and in a timely manner with Erich arch bars, Ivey loops, or intermaxillary fixation screws. Also, stone models can be idealized and a lingual acrylic splint can then be designed to stabilize the mandible in the correct position during healing (Figure 45.18A, Figure 45.18B, Figure 45.18C, and Figure 45.18D).

Alternative technique of IVY loops

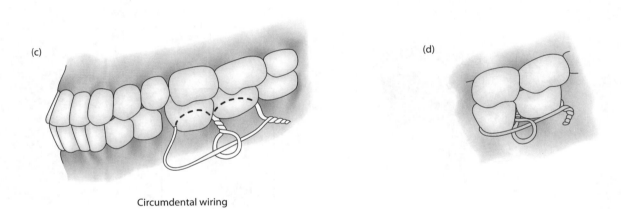

(a)

(b)

(c)

Circumdental wiring

(d)

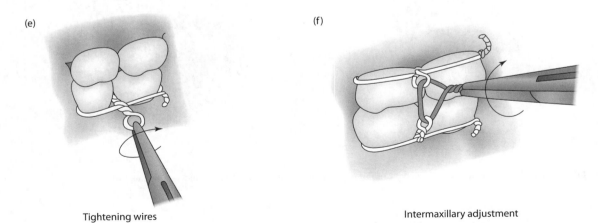

(e)

Tightening wires

(f)

Intermaxillary adjustment

FIGURE 45.18A Ivey loops. Mathog, et al. *Atlas of Craniofacial Trauma*. Philadelphia: W.B. Saunders Company, 1991.

Intermaxillary fixation for condylar fracture

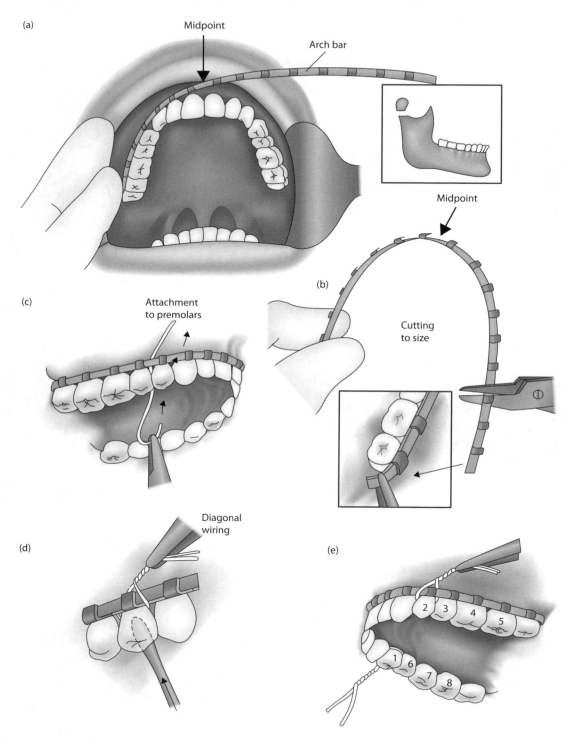

FIGURE 45.18B   Erich arch bars. Mathog, et al. *Atlas of Craniofacial Trauma*. Philadelphia: W.B. Saunders Company, 1991.

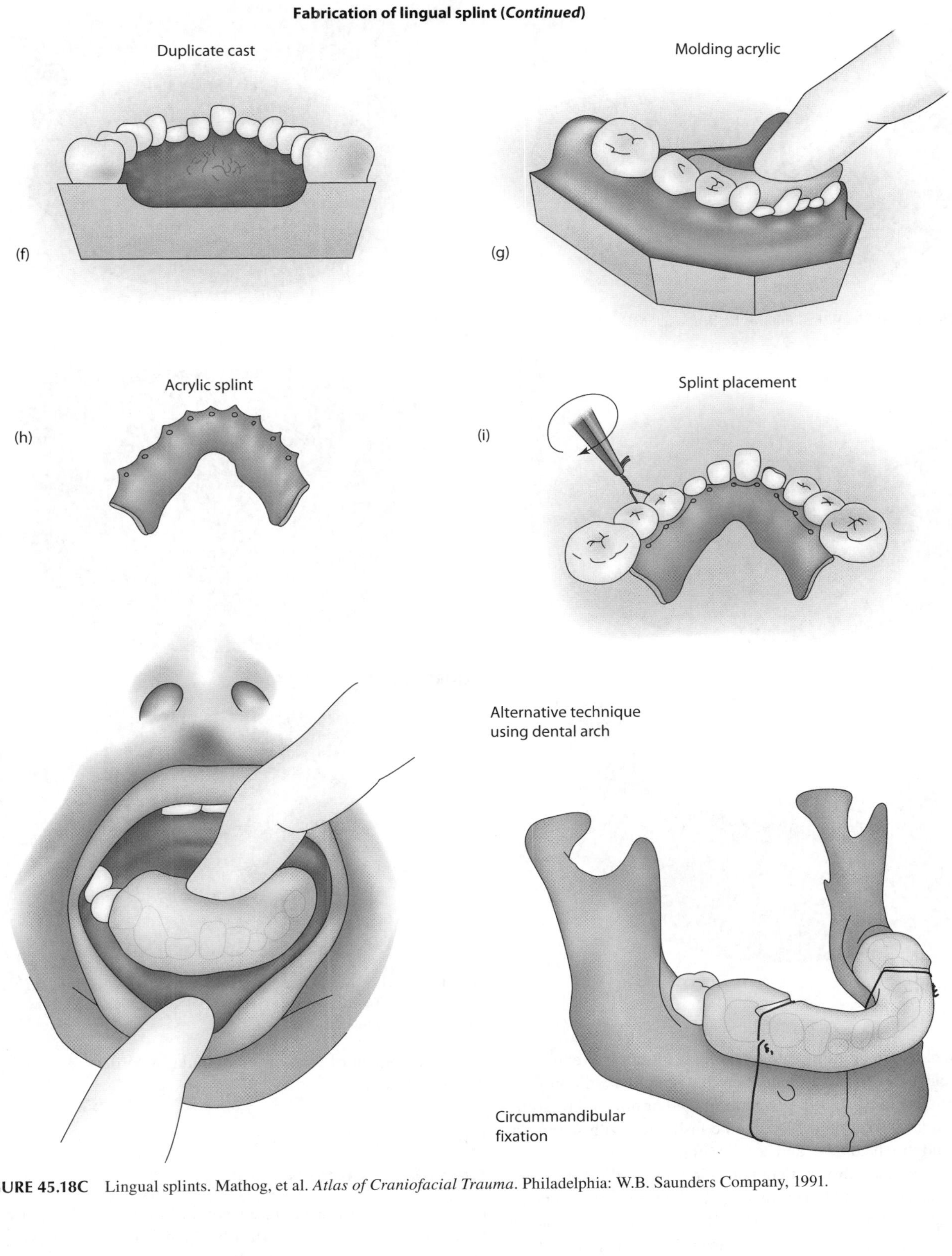

Fabrication of lingual splint (*Continued*)

Duplicate cast

(f)

Molding acrylic

(g)

Acrylic splint

(h)

Splint placement

(i)

Alternative technique
using dental arch

Circummandibular
fixation

FIGURE 45.18C Lingual splints. Mathog, et al. *Atlas of Craniofacial Trauma*. Philadelphia: W.B. Saunders Company, 1991.

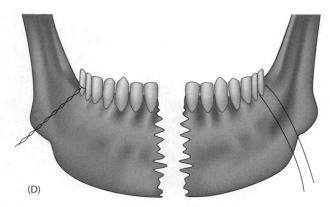

FIGURE 45.18D   Rison Wires. Figures by Bin Song, MD, PhD.

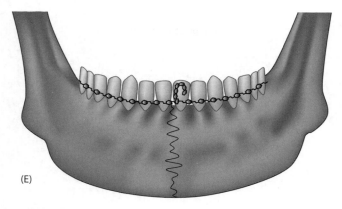

FIGURE 45.18E

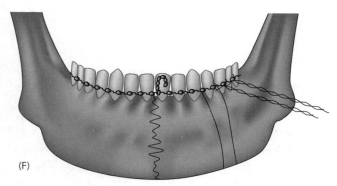

FIGURE 45.18F

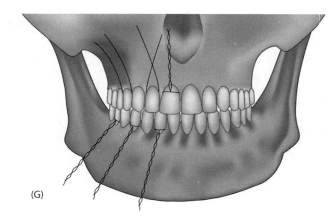

FIGURE 45.18G

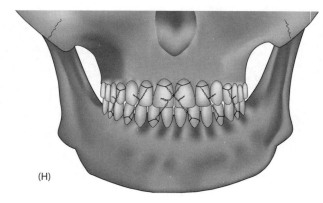

FIGURE 45.18H

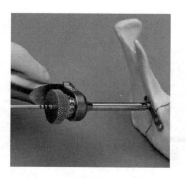

FIGURE 45.19 Mini-plate fixation. Used with permission from: MatrixMANDIBLE Technique Guide. ©DePuy Synthes CMF, a division of DOI 2013. All rights reserved.

If available, wire or mini-plate fixation via intraoral or extraoral incisions enhances the bony reduction and simplifies the postoperative period (Figure 45.19). For comminuted or infected fracture sites, an external fixation device can be fashioned with screws, a modified endotracheal tube, and acrylic (Figure 45.20). Regardless of the treatment modality, patient education and participation are most critical with mandibular fractures and success may depend on compliance. Further, when maxillomandibular fixation is employed, airway management and preparation are paramount.

Complications

Complications include malocclusion, lower facial transverse widening when a symphyseal fracture is not appropriately repaired, and development of temporomandibular disorders, especially in condylar fractures.

Special Considerations

Edentulous Fractures

In the setting of associated mandibular atrophy, wire or mini-plate fixation will often be inadequate. External fixation is required unless stable bony reduction can be achieved, which would then allow a period of intermaxillary fixation utilizing the patient's dental prosthesis or gunning-type splints and circummandibular wiring (Figure 45.21A and Figure 45.21B).

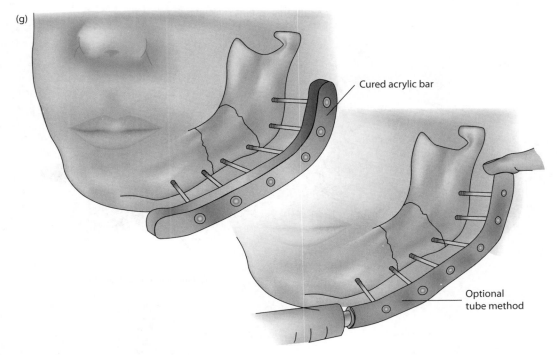

FIGURE 45.20 External fixation technique. Mathog, et al. *Atlas of Craniofacial Trauma*. Philadelphia: W.B. Saunders Company, 1991.

Comminuted Fractures

Maxillomandibular fixation or external fixation is instrumental in achieving bony union in areas of comminution. Wire or mini-plate fixation is difficult and often counterproductive.

Intracapsular Condylar Fractures

Contrary to most subcondylar treatment algorithms, intracapsular fractures are actually best treated by maintaining jaw function and range of motion, so as to minimize any chance of ankylosis.[22]

Dentoalveolar

Dentoalveolar trauma is a common occurrence at all ages. Concomitant alveolar segment bony fractures may coexist with soft-tissue lacerations of the tongue and lips. Comprehensive evaluation should attempt to account for missing and possibly swallowed or aspirated teeth or foreign-bodies, especially in obtunded patients. Plain films are often most useful to evaluate for the presence of foreign bodies the soft tissues. A nonchew diet is critical, and avoidance of contact activities is mandatory.

Surgical Correction

Luxated adult teeth should be repositioned and avulsed teeth reimplanted ideally within 60 minutes.[23] Stabilization should then be instituted with bonded braided wires or arch bars, with care taken to avoid extrusion of the unstable teeth. Dentoalveolar segment fractures can usually be reduced and stabilized with arch bars or rigid wire fixation.

Complications

Tooth loss and malocclusion can occur despite appropriate treatments.

Pediatric Pearls

- Estimates suggest that 1%–15% of facial fractures occur in the pediatric age group.[24]
- Only approximately 1% of facial fractures occur in patients less than 5 years of age.
- No "golden hour" exists in pediatric trauma as for adults.
- In pediatric trauma, only a "platinum half-hour" exists in resuscitation.[25]
- Three main growth centers may be affected by injuries during growth:[23]

  1) the nasomaxillary complex
  2) the orbits
  3) the condylar-ramal elements

- In addition, surgical intervention may contribute to any growth disturbance; thus thoughtful perioperative planning is of vital importance.
- Pediatric patients are more prone to cranial vault and superior orbital roof fractures due to the prominence of the forehead and the lack of a cushioning effect from the frontal sinus that is absent or underdeveloped in younger children.[24]

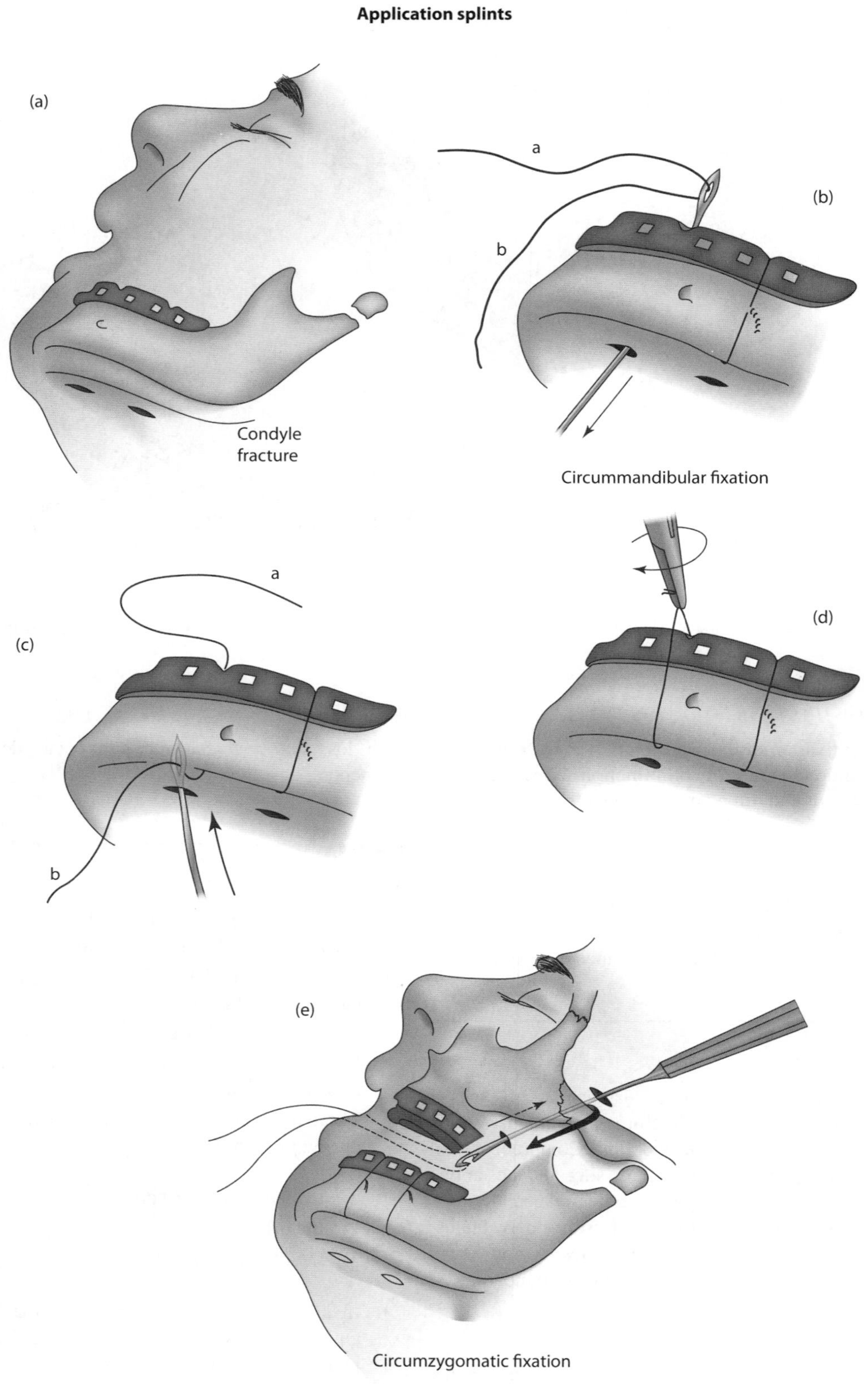

Application splints

FIGURE 45.21A Circumzygomatic fixation of gunning splints or existing dental prosthesis. Mathog, et al. *Atlas of Craniofacial Trauma*. Philadelphia: W.B. Saunders Company, 1991.

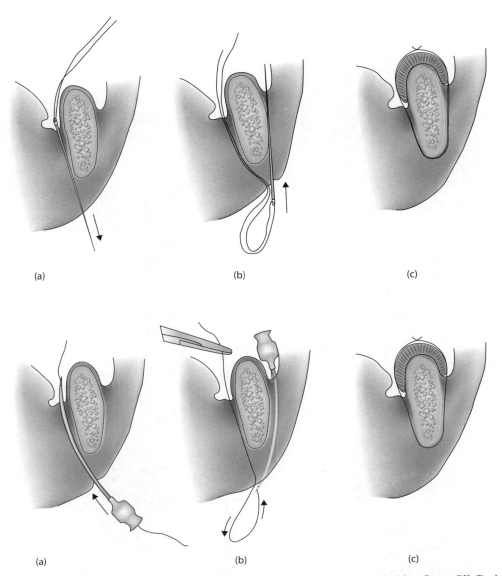

(a)　　　　　　　　(b)　　　　　　　　(c)

(a)　　　　　　　　(b)　　　　　　　　(c)

FIGURE 45.21B　Alternate method, using a simple hypodermic needle or angiocatheter for circumferential wiring. Gustav OK. *Textbook of Oral Surgery*, 4th ed. Philadelphia: Mosby, July 1974.

- Midface fractures become more prevalent with development of the paranasal sinuses.[14]
- In contrast to "blow-out" orbital floor fractures in adults, in children orbital floor "blow-in" fractures are likely to occur as a result of orbital trauma. Due to the pliable nature of bone in children, the orbital floor bone often recoils, resulting in a "trap door" phenomenon involving the inferior rectus muscle and the inferior periorbital tissues.[24]
- Maxillomandibular fixation for midface or mandible fractures should be no more than 1–2 weeks' duration, especially with condylar fractures so as to prevent ankylosis (Figure 45.22).[22]

- Ivy loops and Risdon wires are often needed for maxillomandibular fixation (MMF) due to the shape of the deciduous dentition and inability to fashion arch bars.
- The mixed dentition must be considered when plating jaw fractures.
- Deciduous teeth that are avulsed should not be reimplanted as damage to the underlying adult teeth may occur.[23]

Facial trauma management requires a systematic approach that is patient specific and restores function and esthetic form.

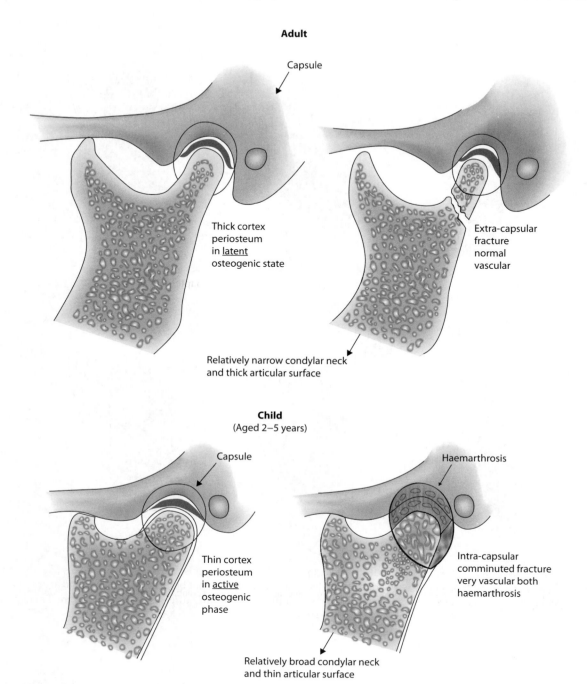

Adult

Capsule

Thick cortex
periosteum
in <u>latent</u>
osteogenic state

Extra-capsular
fracture
normal
vascular

Relatively narrow condylar neck
and thick articular surface

Child
(Aged 2–5 years)

Capsule

Haemarthrosis

Thin cortex
periosteum
in <u>active</u>
osteogenic
phase

Intra-capsular
comminuted fracture
very vascular both
haemarthrosis

Relatively broad condylar neck
and thin articular surface

FIGURE 45.22   Pediatric anatomic and physiologic mandibular condyle. Hall RK. *Pediatric Orofacial Medicine and Pathology.* London: Chapman & Hall, 1994.

COMMENTARY

Bin Song, China

This chapter has provided straightforward and valuable information on various maxillofacial surgery topics, and it concisely covered the general principles that one needs to know for managing patients. The techniques described in the chapter are quite simple, and feasible in LMICs.

I would like to highlight the importance of preoperative and postoperative physical examinations, which are critical and "can't miss." In China, we had a case of blindness after surgical repair of orbital fracture. A patient who had a blowout orbital floor facture came to us for correcting his morphological deformity. We managed to insert additional implants to restore the volume of orbit and "overcorrect" the enophthalmos, so that when the edema dissipated, the eye could be restored to normal. The patient did not have any complaints on the first postoperative day, although he did have some visual problems, which he thought was common after an ophthalmic operation. On the second postoperative day, the patient found that his eyesight was rapidly declining; he complained to us only at that time. Upon physical examination, we learned that the patient had completely lost his vision in that eye. Urgent CT scan showed that his optic nerve was stretching due to excessive implants as well as edema in the orbital. We rushed to the operating room to decompress the optic nerve; unfortunately, the patient did not have his vision recovered in spite of the rescue managements. I believe the optic nerve could be saved in the earlier postoperative time upon revealing the visual issue with a gross visual acuity assessment, as listed in the "Physical Examination Keys" in this chapter.

All in all, this chapter is a valuable, essential reference for surgeons, especially those in LMICs, to manage patients with maxillofacial injuries.

COMMENTARY

C.C. Uguru, Nigeria

The incidence of maxillofacial trauma is very high in Africa, with most cases being consequences of RTAs and numerous armed conflicts. This has resulted in many skilled practitioners in the management of such skeletal injuries.

Maxillofacial surgeons are often called to see the patient after the accident and after emergency physicians have stabilized the patient. In many cases, before the patient is seen by a maxillofacial surgeon, the primary suturing for soft-tissue injuries has been done, or the patient has traveled many miles to see the specialist. We do not have regional trauma centers in Nigeria, but a majority of maxillofacial injured patients will ultimately end up in the teaching hospitals, as these centers are often the only places where skilled surgeons are available. This inadvertently delays treatment and may lead to complications that could have been avoided if skilled manpower was more widely available.

Plain film radiotherapy is widely available, but advanced imaging like CT scans is not always available for diagnosis of fractures. The use of bone plates for treating fractures is gradually coming into the mainstream, but most surgeons are more at ease using archbars and wires to achieve reduction and immobilization of most jaw fractures.

Although a multidisciplinary approach is advocated for treatment of many maxillofacial injuries, in my experience this is not always easy. It is difficult for a multitude of reasons, ranging from lack of a required specialist like a neurosurgeon in many centers, to inability to coordinate theater time for required surgeons and the jack-of-all-trade mentality of many doctors.

Follow-up care and rehabilitation are not always possible because either such programs do not exist in many hospitals, or the patients do not bother to come back and accept any disability or deformity after initial care is given. This unfortunately is almost always due to their inability to pay for further treatment, as most treatment is paid for out-of-pocket, or the distance they have to travel to get specialist treatment, which is very long and costly.

Health insurance in many African countries is more theory than a reality, and any policies that are available do not cover dental and maxillofacial treatment.

Even with the myriad of problems that exist, maxillofacial trauma management has improved in the last decade and will continue to improve as more specialists are trained both at home and in HICs, and as more resources are devoted to healthcare in Africa.

46

Ophthalmic Trauma

Matthew C. Bujak
Geoffrey C. Tabin
Benjamin J. Thomas

Introduction

An estimated 1.6 million people worldwide are bilaterally blind, and an additional 19 million are blind in one eye, as a result of ocular trauma; many more suffer from significant vision loss due to trauma.[1,7] Populations of low- and middle-income countries (LMICs) are at increased risk for ocular trauma due to an increased incidence of traumatic workplace incidents (especially in the agricultural setting), road accidents, and domestic accidents.[4-6] Additionally, war and civil strife impose a high risk of trauma on select populations.[2] However, the morbidity of ocular trauma can be mediated through timely implementation of medical care. With proper tools and training, the global surgeon can treat injuries in a primary care setting and thereby reduce the severity of lifelong impairment brought on by vision loss.

Physical Examination Techniques

Equipment

Although a slit lamp is the ideal tool for providing a thorough ophthalmic exam, a comprehensive examination can still be performed with minimal equipment. The following tools are recommended: a bright penlight or other adjustable light source, a cobalt blue filter for the torch or ophthalmoscope, a near vision card, a handheld magnifier, cotton-tipped swabs, fluorescein dye strips, topical anesthetic (e.g., proparacaine hydrochloride 0.5% ophthalmic drops), and dilating drops (e.g., cyclopentolate 1%) (Figure 46.1A and Figure 46.1B).

Examination

Physical examination should begin with a general inspection of the traumatized area, with attention to the forehead, cheeks, eyelids, and—finally—the eye itself. Identification of anatomic landmarks and tissue planes helps to determine how best to proceed with the ocular exam.

If the patient is able, baseline ocular function tests, such as checking visual acuity and ocular motility, should be done as soon as possible. These can be facilitated by placing a drop of topical anesthetic agent in the eyes. To administer the drop, the lower lid should be gently pulled away from the globe and 1 to 2 drops administered. Care should be taken at all times to avoid undue pressure on the globe, both during administration of the drop and when opening the eyelids for ocular examination. If needed, as in cases of severe lid swelling or ecchymosis, two smooth curved retractors (Desmarres retractors) can be gently slid underneath the upper and lower eyelids when the eye is sufficiently anesthetized to allow for inspection and functional testing (Figure 46.2).

Visual acuity measurements range from no light perception (NLP), light perception (LP), hand motion (HM), and counting fingers (CF), to identification of common optotypes on a near card or distance target. Vision should be tested both at distance and at near with the patient wearing his or her spectacles. A pinhole occluder (easily produced by making a few <0.5 mm holes in an index card) can be used to grossly estimate the patient's best corrected visual acuity (BCVA). At times, eyelid swelling or ecchymoses can make it difficult to open the eye, but preserved visual acuity even through a small opening of the eyelids is reassuring that the globe has not been severely damaged. Pupillary testing, specifically looking for a relative afferent pupillary defect (RAPD), provides a gross functional measure of the retina and optic nerve. Extraocular muscle motility testing and confrontational visual field assessment both provide useful information about the integrity of the eye and surrounding orbit. Finally, in cases of unilateral trauma, the status of the uninjured eye provides a somewhat reliable baseline of normal ocular function for the patient.

Moving forward from baseline functional testing, the globe should be examined with a bright light source and magnification, if possible. A systematic "outside-to-inside" method helps the examiner avoid missing important diagnostic clues. First, begin by assessing the position of the eye relative to surrounding bony structures, looking especially for proptosis (eye bulging forward) or enophthalmos (eye sunken in). These observations help corroborate the findings of motility testing, as mentioned above. Extraocular motility is assessed by having the patient direct his or her attention to the examiner's finger as it moves between the six cardinal positions of gaze, with attention for limitation that may signify entrapment of extraocular muscle, mass effect in the orbit (e.g., from tissue edema or hematoma), cranial nerve paresis, or rupture of the globe.

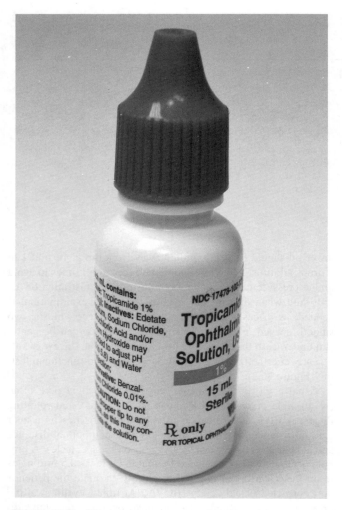

FIGURE 46.1A   Dilating drops are conventionally packaged with a red top. After instillation, 15 to 30 minutes are required to achieve full pupillary dilation. (Accredited to Benjamin Thomas, John A. Moran Eye Center / University of Utah.) Image by James Gilman, Moran Eye Center, Salt Lake City, UT.

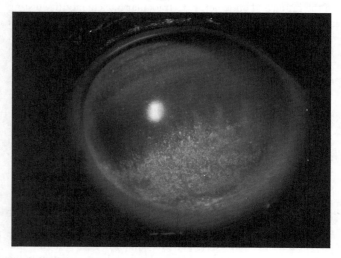

FIGURE 46.1B   Dense, central corneal staining in the area of a traumatic corneal abrasion, made evident with application of fluorescein day and cobalt blue filter. Image by James Gilman, Moran Eye Center, Salt Lake City, UT.

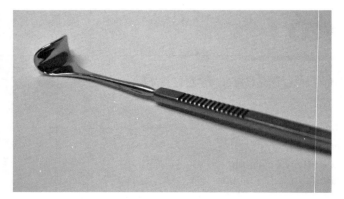

FIGURE 46.2   Desmarres retractor. Image by Benjamin Thomas, John A. Moran Eye Center/University of Utah.

Then, the eyelids are examined closely, noting any lacerations of the eyelid margin and/or canalicular system. Small external lacerations should be carefully explored, as these may lead to the discovery of foreign bodies within the lids, globe, or orbit.

Next, the examiner should conduct a thorough assessment of the conjunctiva and sclera for tears, hemorrhage, or abnormal pigmentation that could help to identify an open globe or foreign body entrance wound. Even small subconjunctival hemorrhages may obscure a full thickness defect in the globe. Any brown, grey, or dusky tissue protruding from the globe, or associated with a wound, is highly suspicious for open globe injury. Other signs of globe rupture include a soft eye (hypotony), 360-degree subconjunctival hemorrhage, and unusual shallowing or deepening of the anterior chamber. Additionally, corneal lacerations, unless small and self-sealing, can be associated with a "peaked" or "tear-drop" pupil, as iris tissue is drawn forward to the wound.

After thorough anterior segment evaluation, dilating drops should be instilled and inspection of the lens and posterior segment carried out. In cases of ocular trauma, the lens may be mobile, subluxed, or completely dislocated, depending on the degree to which the suspensory zonules are ruptured. Examination of the optic nerve, vessels, macula, and periphery with an ophthalmoscope provides additional information on the extent of trauma. In the absence of an ophthalmoscope, red reflex testing can help identify vitreous hemorrhage, which may obscure posterior ruptures, retinal tears or detachments, or subretinal hemorrhages.

If referral to a specialist is required, or if an open globe injury is suspected, a hard protective shield should be taped in place over the injured eye. Administration of oral fluoroquinolone or chloramphenicol, along with broad-spectrum topical antibiotic drops, should be considered, especially if time to evaluation by a specialist may be delayed.

Anatomy of the Eye

Before beginning any procedure, the surgeon should have a thorough understanding of ocular and periocular anatomy. The following is a basic introduction to ocular anatomy (Figure 46.3) that will help guide the procedures outlined in the next two sections.

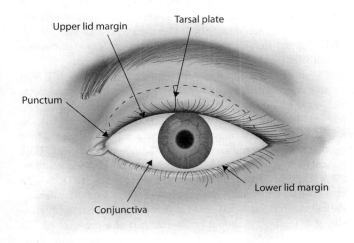

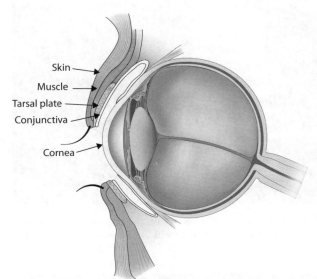

FIGURE 46.3 Basic anatomy of globe and eyelids. Image adapted from the World Health Organization (WHO). Reacher M, Foster A, Huber J. *Trichiasis surgery for trachoma: the bilamellar tarsal rotation procedure.* Switzerland: WHO; 1998, p. 3.

The Eyelid

Eyelid skin is thin, loosely adherent to underlying tissue, and supplied by a highly vascular network of vessels. The orbicularis muscle lies just underneath the eyelid skin and acts to close the eyelid. Below the orbicularis lies a firm collagenous plate—termed the tarsus—that gives the eyelids their structural integrity. Within the tarsus lie the Meibomian glands—sebaceous glands that open up onto the lid margin just posterior to the eyelashes. The tarsal plate is 10 mm high in the upper lid and only 5 mm high in the lower lid. A shiny and transparent layer of conjunctiva lines the back of the tarsal plate. This conjunctiva covers the entire backside of the eyelid (palpebral conjunctiva), folds over itself to form the conjunctival fornices (forniceal conjunctiva), and then extends over the surface of the globe to cover the sclera (bulbar conjunctiva). It attaches firmly near the corneoscleral limbus, where it fuses to the underlying Tenon's capsule.

Medially, two puncta, located in the upper and lower eyelids, provide the outflow of tears into the lacrimal canaliculi, the nasolacrimal sac, and eventually the nasolacrimal duct, which drains into the inferior meatus of the nose.

The Eye

The cornea is an avascular, collagenous structure—on average, approximately 540 μm in thickness—that provides a transparent refractive surface to the eye. The corneal stroma is covered by corneal epithelium that is continually replenished by proliferating stem cells residing in the corneoscleral limbus, at the junction where the cornea meets the opaque sclera. As mentioned above, the conjunctiva fuses with underlying Tenon's capsule to the sclera just peripheral to the corneoscleral limbus. The eye can be subdivided into three compartments: the anterior chamber, the posterior chamber, and the vitreous cavity. Aqueous fluid fills the anterior chamber, anterior to the iris plane. It is produced by the ciliary body, in the posterior chamber (posterior to the iris plane, anterior to the zonules) and then flows through the pupil into the anterior chamber to eventually drain in the angle formed by the cornea and the iris. The vitreous is a gelatinous substance that fills the cavity posterior to the intraocular lens. The lens itself is a crystalline structure supported by 360 degrees of zonules that hold it firmly in place behind the iris.

At the posterior aspect of the vitreous cavity, internal to the scleral wall of the eye, lies the neural structure of the retina and the substantive vascular choroid. The nerve fibers of the retina course posteriorly to the optic nerve, which then passes posteriorly through the orbit toward the optic nerve chiasm.

Blunt Trauma

The eyelids have an extraordinary blood supply, with only loose attachment of tissue to underlying bony structures. Thus, large hematomas may result even when little damage has occurred to the eye. Conversely, blunt injury may produce very few external signs of trauma despite significant damage to the globe.

Hyphema

Diagnosis

Any direct blow to the eye may damage intraocular structures. The eye distorts under pressure, springs back into shape, and tearing and bleeding of the tissues may result. Intraocular blood tends to either fill the vitreous, as vitreous hemorrhage, or layer out in the anterior chamber in the form of a hyphema. (Figure 46.4A and Figure 46.4B) The presence of intraocular blood signals an increased likelihood of damage to the iris, subluxation of the lens, cataract formation, retinal damage (tear or detachment), globe rupture, and subsequent traumatic glaucoma.

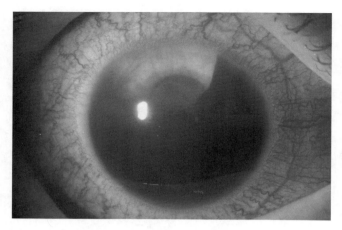

FIGURE 46.4A Hyphema. As blood fills the anterior chamber, note the horizontal line formed as it begins to settle. Image by Matthew C. Bujak.

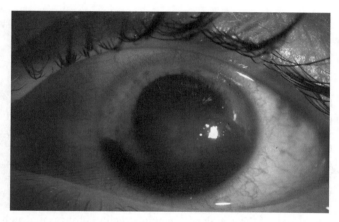

FIGURE 46.4B Hyphema. With time, blood will turn darker and begin to clear from the anterior chamber, clearing the visual axis. Image by Matthew C. Bujak.

Thus, a comprehensive ocular exam is necessary in every case of ocular trauma.

In the setting of hyphema, black and Mediterranean patients should be screened for sickle cell disease (or trait), as problems with resorption of intraocular blood can be compounded in these patients. A high risk of complications necessitates close follow-up in these patients. Other factors requiring closer observation include: hyphema greater than one-third of the anterior chamber depth, visual acuity worse than 20/200, elevated intraocular pressure (IOP), or recent nonsteroidal anti-inflammatory drug (NSAID) or aspirin use.

Management

In straightforward cases, hyphemas should be managed conservatively with bed rest, with the head of the bed elevated 30 degrees to facilitate inferior displacement and layering of blood. A potent cycloplegic agent, such as atropine 1%, improves comfort and minimizes the chance of re-bleeding from iris movement. Mild analgesics such as acetaminophen may be administered, but NSAIDs and aspirin are to be avoided. Topical steroids such

as prednisolone acetate 1% are administered 4 times daily and tapered over the course of several weeks. If a corneal abrasion is present, topical antibiotics should be used in the absence of steroids. Topical steroids may be started once the corneal abrasion re-epithelializes.

IOP should be monitored daily in higher-risk cases. If IOP is greater than 30 mmHg, it should be treated with a topical beta-blocker (e.g., timolol maleate 0.5% ophthalmic drops), administered to the affected eye twice daily. If this is unsuccessful, the following treatments may be added sequentially: topical alpha agonist (e.g., brimonidine tartrate 0.2% three times a day [TID]), topical carbonic anhydrase inhibitor (dorzolamide hydrochloride 2% TID), oral acetazolamide 500 mg twice a day [BID], or—in rare cases—intravenous mannitol (1–2 g/kg) over 45 minutes. Patients with sickle cell disease or trait should have more aggressive IOP control; it should be maintained at a pressure of less than 24 mmHg. Management of the sickle cell population, however, is more problematic. Although topical alpha agonists may be used, they can reduce anterior chamber pH and potentially induce sickling. Systemic diuretics should also be avoided, as they may induce a sickle cell crisis. If a systemic carbonic anhydrase inhibitor is necessary, oral methazolamide (50 mg PO q8h) is preferable to acetazolamide. Finally, if pressure cannot be controlled, referral should be made to an ophthalmologist for further surgical management.

Orbital Fracture with Extraocular Muscle Entrapment

Blunt ocular trauma can damage the surrounding bony orbit by two proposed mechanisms (see Chapter 45). In brief, one theory postulates that direct trauma to the globe pushes the eye back into the orbit, thereby greatly increasing orbital pressure. With a sudden increase in orbital pressure, the weakest bony portion—the orbital floor—may buckle inferiorly ("blow out") into the maxillary sinus. Also, the thin lamina papyracea of the medial wall may fracture into the ethmoid sinuses. An alternate theory proposes that forces transmitted to the orbital rim cause fracturing of the thin orbital floor.

Diagnosis

Regardless of the exact mechanism of fracture, the examination and management are the same. When examining a patient with blunt ocular trauma, particular attention has to be paid to the position of the globe. A large fracture of the orbital floor can cause the eye to appear sunken in. In the acute phase, this may not be readily apparent, and the eye may, in fact, appear proptotic due to retrobulbar hemorrhage and/or tissue edema. The patient should be evaluated for numbness of the cheek and upper teeth, as orbital floor fractures may be accompanied by hypesthesia in the distribution of the infraorbital nerve. The bony orbital rim should be palpated for point tenderness and "step-off" deformity. Extraocular motility should be assessed in the six cardinal positions of gaze, and the patient should be asked about diplopia or pain with eye movement.

If an orbital floor fracture is present, entrapment of the inferior rectus muscle may occur. This entrapment usually limits upgaze of the affected eye, and the patient will report vertical diplopia and/or sharp pain behind the eye when attempting to look up.

These fractures can be particularly worrisome in young patients under 20 years of age, as increased bone pliability in this age group predisposes them to "trapdoor" fractures of the floor. A "trapdoor" fracture occurs as the fractured orbital floor springs back to its original position and entraps the belly of the inferior rectus muscle or its associated tissues. The resultant muscle ischemia causes significant pain and can lead to necrosis of the muscle if not dealt with urgently. Remarkably, these serious injuries may present with few external signs aside from severe pain and limitation of upgaze and, thus, have been termed "white-eyed blowout fractures."

Management

The young patient with painful entrapment must be referred urgently to an ophthalmologist for emergent repair and release of the entrapped muscle. All other floor fractures can be referred to an ophthalmologist for repair 7–14 days after injury.

It should also be noted that many orbital floor fractures do not require surgical repair. Patients are often asymptomatic, without any disruption of ocular motility or position, upon resolution of posttraumatic edema. Indications for delayed repair of an orbital floor fracture include: diplopia in primary gaze (when looking straight ahead), notable enophthalmos, or a greater-than-50% defect of the orbital floor upon CT scan imaging.

Conservative management of orbital floor fractures immediately after the inciting trauma consists of the following: noseblowing precautions, nasal decongestants (e.g., pseudoephedrine spray for 14 days), broad-spectrum oral antibiotics (e.g., cephalexin 250 to 500 mg PO four times a day [QID] for 14 days), and ice packs to the periorbita for the first 48 hours. Isolated medial wall fractures are rarely repaired and are treated in a similar conservative manner. Although rare, orbital roof fractures necessitate immediate neurosurgical consultation.

Traumatic Retrobulbar Hemorrhage

Diagnosis and Initial Management

The orbit has a rich vascular supply and is, thus, predisposed to hemorrhage with ocular trauma. In most cases, retrobulbar hemorrhage is tamponaded by the bony confines of the orbit and causes few problems aside from mild proptosis and ecchymosis, which resolve spontaneously with time. Occasionally, a retrobulbar hemorrhage can continue to build, causing three distinct problems: proptosis with subsequent inability to close the eye and exposure, elevated IOP, and pressure on the optic nerve causing a compressive optic neuropathy.

Inability to close the eye can cause serious problems to the cornea from exposure. It should be treated with copious lubrication and prophylactic topical antibiotics.

If IOP is elevated above 30 mmHg, it can be treated with topical and oral IOP-lowering medications as outlined previously in the hyphema section. However, if IOP elevation is refractory to medical management, it may require treatment through surgical release of the eyelids with a lateral canthotomy and inferior cantholysis. This procedure also needs to be performed urgently if there is suspicion of optic nerve compromise from the elevated orbital pressure. Decrease in visual acuity, diminution in color

vision, particularly red colors, and a relative afferent pupillary defect (RAPD) are all signs of optic nerve compromise. These should be checked immediately upon presentation, and—if positive—surgery is required to relieve orbital pressure.

Surgical Management

Lateral canthotomy and inferior cantholysis is a powerful, low-risk, and relatively easy procedure that can be sight-saving during an emergent retrobulbar hemorrhage. It can be performed under conscious sedation in a minor procedures room and does not require general anesthesia in an operating room. The goal of the procedure is to perform a soft-tissue decompression of the orbit by disinserting the lower eyelid from its periosteal attachments.

After cleaning the procedure site, topical anesthesia (e.g., lidocaine 2% with epinephrine) is injected subcutaneously around the lateral canthus. A hemostat is clamped horizontally on the lateral canthus for a full minute to compress the tissue and reduce bleeding. Blunt Westcott or Stevens scissors are used to make a full-thickness horizontal cut in the lateral canthus. This step, though providing little soft-tissue decompression, gives access to the inferior crux of the lateral canthal tendon.

The next step involves releasing the periosteal attachment of the eyelid by cutting the inferior canthal tendon. The lower eyelid is grasped with toothed forceps (e.g., Adson or Bishop Harmon forceps) and tractioned away from the globe. Closed scissors are placed into the wound, oriented vertically, pointing downward. The scissors are "strummed" in an anterior-posterior direction over the inferior attachment of the lateral canthal tendon until the resistance of the tendon is felt against the closed scissors. Once the tendon has been identified, it is cut with the scissors pointing down toward the nose. If it is fully cut, the lower eyelid should fall away from the globe easily. After successfully dividing the inferior attachment of the lateral canthal tendon, pressure is maintained over the incision to control bleeding. Antibiotic ointment is placed on the incision and an eye pad is folded over the skin wound.

Postoperative Management

If successful, a cantholysis should relieve orbital pressure within approximately 15 minutes (Figure 46.5). There should be a corresponding decrease in IOP and an improvement in optic nerve function. The patient should be monitored closely for the first 8–12 postoperative hours as hemorrhage can recur, even if the pressure seems resolved initially.

Interestingly, a large percentage of lateral canthotomies and inferior cantholyses will heal spontaneously with good cosmesis, and most do not require any further surgery to repair the eyelid. In some cases, the inferior canthal tendon may be re-sutured to the inner aspect of the lateral orbital rim within 1–2 weeks after resolution of the retrobulbar hemorrhage.

Pitfalls

Inadequate soft tissue release: If the inferior crux of the lateral canthal tendon is not fully transected, the orbital pressure may not be adequately released. The surgeon must ensure that the tendon is fully cut and the lower eyelid and its attachments can be displaced easily from the orbit.

Bleeding: The eyelid is highly vascular, and the initial cut of the canthotomy can cause significant bleeding, which can obscure the surgical field. Pressure is usually sufficient to stop bleeding and cautery is rarely required.

Trauma to globe: Inadvertent damage to the eye can be caused by the surgical instruments employed in a canthotomy and cantholysis. The surgeon should use blunt scissors, such as Westcott or Stevens scissors, to minimize the chance of iatrogenic injury to the globe.

Postoperative follow-up: Patients must be monitored closely for re-bleeding in the first 12 hours, and optic nerve function and IOP should be checked regularly during this period. If complete eyelid closure is still not possible, the patient should be maintained on copious lubrication with ointments and prophylactic topical antibiotics.

Lacerations

Lacerations may result from forceful blunt trauma or from injury with sharp objects. A detailed comprehensive exam must be performed, as a small laceration to the eyelid may be accompanied by a sight-threatening laceration to the globe.

Eyelid Laceration

Diagnosis and Initial Management

When an eyelid laceration is present, blunt eyelid retractors (Desmarres retractors) should be used to complete a full ocular exam, with particular attention to signs of globe laceration

or rupture (see the section on open globe injuries later in this chapter). Superficial lacerations not affecting the lid margin can be closed easily with interrupted 6-0 plain gut sutures or, alternatively, silk. If fat is noted to prolapse through the eyelid, there should be significant concern for deeper injury. This signifies that the orbital septum has been violated; repair should ideally be performed by an ophthalmologist to minimize postoperative ptosis and other complications. If available, a computed tomography (CT) scan should also be ordered to look for deeper injury.

If the lid margin has been lacerated, special attention should be paid to the technique of closure, as permanent lid deformity may result from improper closure, causing subsequent epiphora and poor cosmesis (Figure 46.6). If the medial aspect of the eyelids is violated, the lacrimal puncta should be identified and probed to ensure that they are intact. Lacerations involving the lacrimal puncta or other elements of the canalicular system should ideally be repaired by an ophthalmologist within 3 days to prevent scarring and closure of the tear drainage system.

Eyelid Margin Laceration Repair

To prepare for repair of a marginal eyelid laceration (Figure 46.7), the eyelid and periorbital skin are cleaned with 5% povidone-iodine solution, after instilling topical anesthesia into the eye. Topical anesthesia (e.g., lidocaine 2% with epinephrine) is injected subcutaneously into the surrounding eyelid. The wound should be irrigated aggressively with saline and explored further to delineate length and depth.

As with other periorbital lacerations, the skin closure is performed with absorbable sutures (e.g., 6-0 Vicryl). However, the most important step is approximation of the tarsus with 1–2 silk sutures. This silk suture is placed in the eyelid margin to span the wound, using the "grey line" made by the external margin of the muscle of Riolan, entering and exiting 2 mm from the laceration edge. This suture is not tied but instead is put on traction with a

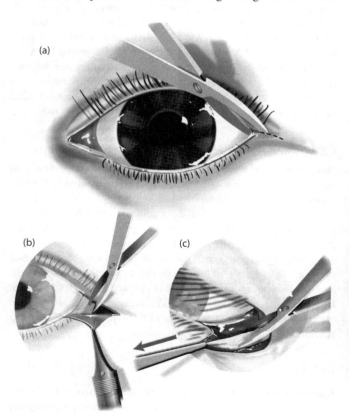

FIGURE 46.5   Lateral canthotomy and inferior cantholysis. Image adapted from Gertensblith A, Rabinowitz M. *Wills Eye Manual*, 4th ed. Philadelphia: Lippincott Williams & Wilkins, 2008. Figure 3.10.2.

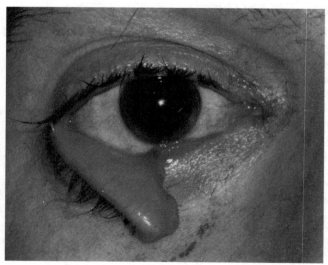

FIGURE 46.6   Marginal eyelid laceration. Involvement of the eyelid margin near the medial canthus should cause concern for canalicular involvement. Image adapted from Gertensblith A, Rabinowitz M. *Wills Eye Manual*, 4th ed. Philadelphia: Lippincott Williams & Wilkins, 2008. Figure 3.8.2.

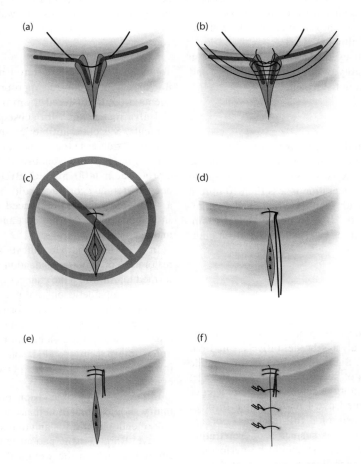

FIGURE 46.7 Repair of a marginal eyelid laceration. Image adapted from Gertensblith A, Rabinowitz M. *Wills Eye Manual,* 4th ed. Philadelphia: Lippincott Williams & Wilkins, 2008. Figure 3.8.4.

hemostat. This suture should provide good anatomical approximation of the eyelid margins without any notching of the lid contour. Several absorbable sutures (usually 3–4 in the upper lid, 2–3 in the lower lid) are then used to approximate the anterior aspect of the cut tarsus, depending on the length of the wound. These sutures should be placed in a partial-thickness fashion through the tarsus; if they go full-thickness, passing through the posterior conjunctiva, they will abrade the cornea. The tarsal sutures are tied down and cut short. The marginal suture is then tied down, leaving a long tail. If necessary, a second marginal suture may be tied just anterior to the initial suture, also leaving a long tail. Absorbable (Vicryl or plain gut) sutures are then used to close the length of the skin laceration in an interrupted manner. Finally, the long tail(s) of the marginal sutures are imbricated in the knot of the absorbable skin suture closest to the margin. This will ensure that the marginal suture ends do not evert and abrade the cornea. Antibiotic ointment is placed on the wound and the eye is patched closed.

Postoperative Management

The tarsal sutures provide the integrity of the closure and do not need to be removed. The silk lid margin sutures should be removed in 5–10 days. If plain gut suture was used to close the skin, it can be left to resorb on its own. If a quickly absorbable suture was not used, the skin sutures should be removed in 4–7 days. Antibiotic ointment should be applied to the wound 3–4 times daily for 2 weeks.

Pitfalls

Lid notching: If the tarsus is not approximated well, it may splay open, or heal unevenly and result in significant lid notching. The surgeon must ensure proper alignment of the eyelid when placing the marginal sutures. To minimize postoperative notching, the incision should have a slightly "pouty" appearance at the conclusion of the case (see Figure 46.7), as this will flatten during wound healing to yield a smooth eyelid contour.

Corneal abrasion: Iatrogenic corneal abrasion may occur if sutures are passed in a full-thickness manner through the palpebral conjunctiva. To avoid this complication, the surgeon must evert the eyelid after suturing the tarsus to ensure that the sutures have not passed full-thickness. The eye may be checked postoperatively with fluorescein dye to ensure that there is no irritation from sutures.

Lacrimal duct laceration: If there is any question of disruption of the canaliculi, the surgeon must thoroughly assess the integrity of the tear drainage system. Lacrimal duct lacerations should be repaired by an ophthalmologist.

Deeper injury: As with all eyelid lacerations, the surgeon must be attentive to the possibility of deeper orbital injury, particularly if prolapsed fat is seen in the wound.

Conjunctival Lacerations

A conjunctival laceration should induce high suspicion for an underlying scleral laceration, and a thorough exam should be undertaken (Figure 46.8). If there is no evidence of damage to the globe, and the conjunctival laceration is less than 10 mm, it can be treated conservatively with prophylactic topical antibiotics administered four times daily. If it is greater than 10 mm, then closure with absorbable sutures (e.g., 8-0 Vicryl) in an interrupted fashion is indicated.

Open Globe Injuries

Diagnosis

Open globe injuries are defined as compromised integrity of the sclera or cornea; they should always be definitively ruled out in patients with ocular injury. Signs of globe rupture include decreased vision, 360 degrees of subconjunctival hemorrhage, soft globe, shallowing or deepening of anterior chamber, irregular "peaked" pupil, or pigmented uveal tissue visible through a scleral wound. If the diagnosis of a full-thickness corneal laceration is not certain but there is suspicion of penetration into the anterior chamber, a Seidel test should be performed. To perform this test, a cobalt blue light is directed at the eye while a moistened fluorescein strip is brushed over the wound. A wound leak can be visualized as the stream of aqueous fluid turns the fluorescein from dark to bright green. If the Seidel test is initially negative and suspicion is high for open globe injury, very gentle digital pressure can be applied in select cases to facilitate a positive Seidel test and ensure that a self-sealing, full-thickness wound is not missed. If available, a CT scan can be used to assess the scleral wall, look for intraocular or orbital foreign bodies, and assess the walls of the orbits.

Management

Tonometry should be deferred in the setting of obvious full-thickness globe rupture. Appropriate analgesic and anti-emetic agents are administered to minimize the chance of increased Valsalva maneuver, with subsequent expulsion of intraocular contents. Systemic antibiotics should be administered immediately to decrease the chance of endophthalmitis. Intravenous cefazolin (1 g intravenously [IV] every 8 hours) and oral ciprofloxacin (400 mg PO BID) is an effective regimen. If needed, tetanus toxoid should be administered. In all cases, a rigid shield should be placed over the eye, and the patient should be confined to bed rest and fasting until further surgical management.

In a severely traumatized eye in which there is no chance for restoration of vision, enucleation or evisceration should be performed to minimize the chances of a rare autoimmune response, termed sympathetic ophthalmia, in the fellow uninjured eye. This procedure should be performed within 14 days of the initial injury, or can be done at presentation or 7–14 days after primary repair of the ruptured globe. Immediate enucleation or evisceration is rarely recommended; some physicians believe that delaying the procedure allows the person to better cope with the loss of an eye.

If there is salvageable vision, primary repair of the open globe injury should be instituted as soon as possible to minimize the risk of endophthalmitis and to restore the structural integrity of the eye. Rarely, if the patient is reliable and there is no incarceration of iris in the wound (for wounds less than 3 mm in length), then the full-thickness incision can be observed closely without surgical repair. In this case, topical antibiotics should be administered 6 times daily along with a daily cycloplegic drop (e.g., atropine 1% ophthalmic drops). A rigid protective shield is a requirement. Partial-thickness corneoscleral wounds can be managed in a similar conservative manner but require definitive surgical repair if there is significant wound gape or override.

Corneoscleral Lacerations and Open Globe Repair

Many cases can be repaired using peribulbar anesthesia and a Van Lint eyelid block. (Retrobulbar anesthesia is not advised, as posterior orbital pressure can lead to expulsion of intraocular contents.) If available, repair under general anesthesia may be easier. Depolarizing anesthetics should be avoided as the resultant muscle contraction may also cause extrusion of intraocular contents. The surgeon should gently sterilize the periorbital skin, drape the surgical site, and insert the lid speculum without applying pressure to the globe. Additionally, the surgeon should prepare to intra-operatively culture the wound edges, any excised tissue, or any foreign body on plates of blood agar and chocolate agar, thioglycolate broth, and/or Sabouraud agar (if fungal inoculation is suspected).

The approach to repair depends on the extent and location of the injury, and whether or not the laceration crosses the corneoscleral limbus. If the injury crosses the limbus, or is situated

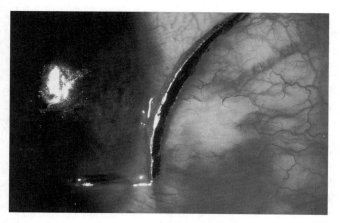

FIGURE 46.8 Conjunctival laceration. Black pigment deep within the scleral wound or the corneal wound indicates full-thickness laceration that must be repaired emergently. Image by Matthew C. Bujak.

on the sclera, a 360-degree peritomy should be performed to allow adequate visualization of the entire wound. To perform the peritomy, the conjunctiva is grasped adjacent to the limbus with fine-toothed forceps (e.g., 0.12 Castro-Viejo forceps). As the conjunctival tissue is pulled away from the globe, blunt Westcott scissors are used to vertically incise both the conjunctiva and the underlying Tenon's capsule. The incision is extended 360 degrees around the limbus, alternately using blunt dissection to separate the conjunctiva from the underlying sclera, then sharply dividing the freed conjunctival tissue at the limbus.

Once the peritomy is complete, the full extent of the wound must be identified. Care should be exercised if gelatinous vitreous is noted in the wound, as undue traction may lead to retinal tears. If uveal tissue is prolapsing through the wound, an attempt should be made to reposit it back through the wound with either a spatula or a viscoelastic ophthalmic product. If it cannot be repositioned, it may be carefully excised; however, this should be done with care as cutting uveal tissue may cause bleeding (and the potential complication of sympathetic ophthalmia—see above—should always be in consideration). If iris tissue has been exposed out of the wound for more than 72 hours, it should be excised rather than repositioned, as it is likely necrotic and could lead to postoperative inflammation.

The wound should be closed with nonabsorbable nylon sutures (e.g., 8-0 nylon). The wound edges should be gently lifted with forceps while passing the needle in a partial-thickness manner (approximately 75-percent thickness), so as not to incorporate uveal tissue into the wound. The typical suture should be approximately 1.5 mm in length with spacing of about 1 mm between sutures. These interrupted sutures should be continued posteriorly in a zipper-like fashion to close the full extent of the corneal wound. In a large scleral rupture that extends posterior to the equator of the globe, the posterior wound may be difficult to reach. The posterior extents of a wound may be best left unsutured, as attempting to close them surgically is difficult and may cause further undue damage to the globe.

Once the sclera is repaired, the cornea should be sutured (Figure 46.9) with a smaller nylon suture, using a spatulated needle. Whereas the sclera is closed in a zipper-like manner, the cornea should be closed by sequentially bisecting the wound. Corneal sutures should be placed at 90-percent depth, entering the cornea at a 90-degree angle and following the natural curve of the needle through the stromal tissue. Full-thickness bites should be avoided as the suture may act as a conduit for microorganisms. The optimal length of corneal sutures is also approximately 1.5 mm with a similar 1 mm spacing between individual sutures. Longer sutures are used if the tissue is macerated, while shorter sutures are used in the central visual axis to minimize scarring and postoperative astigmatism. The suture ends are cut short, and the sutures are rotated until they are buried in the cornea or sclera. If the corneal sutures are not buried, the patient will complain of exquisite discomfort postoperatively due to exposed suture edges (Figure 46.10A, Figure 46.10B, Figure 46.10C, and Figure 46.10D).

When the corneal wound is being sutured, balanced salt solution (BSS) or viscoelastic is periodically injected through the wound into the anterior chamber with a fine blunt cannula. This ensures that the anterior chamber does not collapse and allows for more precise closure of the corneal wound. At the conclusion of the case, the anterior chamber should be formed and stable. A Seidel test with a fluorescein strip can be done to ensure that there is no leakage from the wound. Although minimal leakage through an inadvertent full-thickness suture bite can be left alone, as it will self-seal over few days, cyanoacrylate glue may be applied to a leaking wound in conjunction with a bandage contact lens for closure. A contact lens alone may help by providing resistance to outflow, if a leak persists. At the conclusion of surgery, a broad-spectrum antibiotic (e.g., cefazolin 100 mg) is injected subconjunctivally and an eye patch is placed over the eye. In the developing world, subconjunctival steroid injections should be avoided due to increased risk of infection.

Postoperative management

If possible, IV antibiotics should be continued for 3 days and oral antibiotics for a full 10 days. The patch and shield are removed on postoperative day 1 and the eye is reexamined to ensure proper closure of the wound and stability of the anterior chamber. Topical fortified antibiotics are administered hourly (e.g., vancomycin 50 mg/ml and ceftazidime 50 mg/ml). If not available, they can be substituted with a topical fluoroquinolone (e.g., moxifloxacin 0.5% ophthalmic drops). A cycloplegic drop (e.g., cyclopentolate 1%) is given 3 times daily for patient comfort, to reduce intraocular scarring, and to help maintain a deep anterior chamber. A topical steroid (e.g., prednisolone acetate 1% ophthalmic drops) is administered 4–6 times daily and tapered over 4–6 weeks as inflammation subsides. The injured eye should be shielded at all times (even during sleep) for 6–8 weeks while healing occurs. The corneal sutures can be slowly removed beginning 3 months postoperatively. The scleral sutures can be left indefinitely but need to be removed should they become exposed.

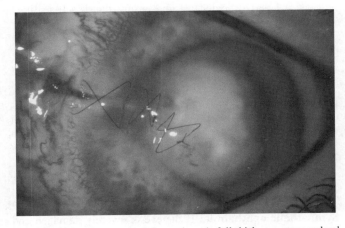

FIGURE 46.9 Corneoscleral laceration. A full-thickness corneoscleral laceration that has been repaired with 10-0 nylon on the cornea and 8-0 Vicryl on the sclera. Typically, single interrupted sutures are used to close the wound; however, "X" sutures knotted in a 3-1-1 manner can also be used to approximate the wound as was done in this case. Nylon should be used on the cornea, however. Vicryl can be substituted for nylon on the sclera. Image by Matthew C. Bujak.

Simple full-thickness corneal lacerations

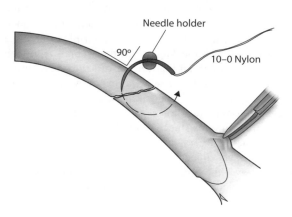

FIGURE 46.10A Repair of a full-thickness corneoscleral laceration. Technique for placing stitches through the cornea (cross-section). Image adapted from Hersh PS, Zagelbaum BM, Cremers SL. *Ophthalmic Surgical Procedures*. New York: Thieme Publishing, 2009. Fig. 28.2.

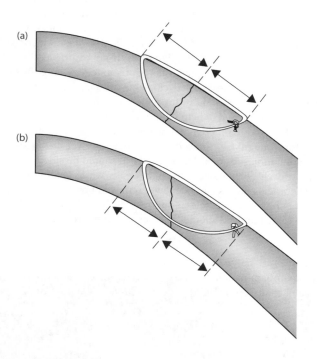

FIGURE 46.10B Repair of a full-thickness corneoscleral laceration. The cornea should be approximated evenly, without overriding of either wound edge, to promote the best possible postoperative result. Image adapted from Hersh PS, Zagelbaum BM, Cremers SL. *Ophthalmic Surgical Procedures*. New York: Thieme Publishing, 2009. Fig. 28.3.

Pitfalls

Sympathetic ophthalmia: If the eye is severely damaged and visual potential is negligible, it should be enucleated or eviscerated within 2 weeks to minimize the development of sympathetic ophthalmia. Sympathetic ophthalmia is a very rare autoimmune condition wherein exposure of damaged uveal antigens leads to an intense autoimmune reaction in the fellow uninjured eye.

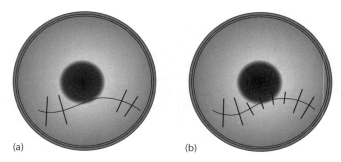

FIGURE 46.10C Corneal wounds should be closed by sequentially bisecting the wound, with the longest sutures at the ends of the wound and shorter sutures at the middle. Image adapted from Hersh PS, Zagelbaum BM, Cremers SL. *Ophthalmic Surgical Procedures*. New York: Thieme Publishing, 2009. Fig. 28.4.

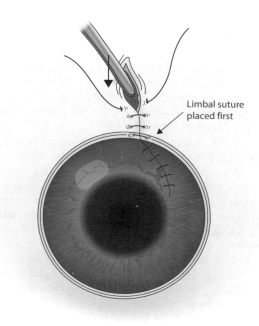

FIGURE 46.10D Repair of a full-thickness corneoscleral laceration. Technique for repairing lacerations that cross the corneoscleral limbus. Image adapted from Hersh PS, Zagelbaum BM, Cremers SL. *Ophthalmic Surgical Procedures*. New York: Thieme Publishing, 2009. Fig. 28.10.

Posterior scleral rupture: Posterior ruptures should be left to heal alone as attempted surgical repair is difficult and may cause further damage to the eye.

Postoperative infection: Endophthalmitis is the most devastating complication of open globe injuries. The eye should be monitored closely for infection and a rigid regimen of antibiotics should be maintained. Topical and oral anti-fungals should be considered in the setting of injury with vegetable matter (e.g., injury in an agricultural setting).

Intraocular foreign body: If a retained intraocular foreign body is suspected, closure of the wound should be delayed and the patient should be referred to an ophthalmologist. Iron, steel, copper, and vegetable matter are particularly toxic to the eye. Other metals such as nickel, aluminum, and zinc are mildly inflammatory. Glass, lead, stone, and coal are relatively inert. Still, even inert substances can be toxic to the eye due to a coating or chemical additive and should, therefore, be removed.

Chemical and Thermal Injuries

Diagnosis and Initial Management

Chemical injuries of the eye require immediate treatment, before transport to a medical facility and, upon arrival to triage, even before vision testing (Figure 46.11A, Figure 46.11B, and Figure 46.11C). Copious irrigation should be instituted immediately with saline or Ringer's lactate solution and continued for at least 30 minutes. If sterile fluids are not readily available, tap water (or even milk) can be used. One should not attempt to use acidic solutions to neutralize alkaline injury, or vice versa. A drop of topical anesthetic and a wire lid speculum can facilitate irrigation. Additionally, IV tubing can be connected to an irrigation solution and used to irrigate the ocular surface and the conjunctival fornices for a full 30 minutes.

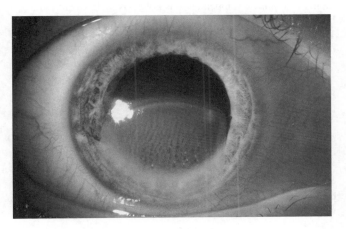

FIGURE 46.11A Chemical or thermal corneal injuries. Moderate injury with partial corneal opacification and associated conjunctival injection and chemosis. Image by Matthew C. Bujak and Geoffrey C. Tabin.

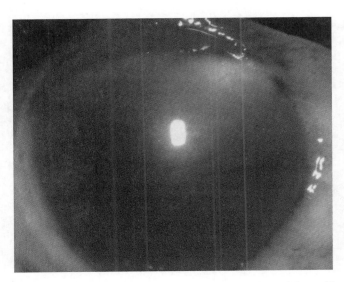

FIGURE 46.11B Chemical or thermal corneal injuries. Severe injury, with full corneal opacification and complete limbal blanching. Image adapted from Gertensblith A, Rabinowitz M. *Wills Eye Manual,* 4th ed. Philadelphia: Lippincott Williams & Wilkins, 2008. Figure 3.1.1.

Ten minutes after finishing irrigation, the pH of the ocular surface must be checked using a pH strip. Irrigation should continue until a neutral pH of 7.0 is achieved, which may require multiple liters of irrigating solution. The fornices should be swept with a moistened cotton swab to remove any chemical debris or particulate matter.

The extent of ocular injury depends on the concentration of the chemical, the exposure time prior to irrigation, and the acidity or alkalinity of the inciting substance. Alkaline injuries tend to be more destructive, as these substances saponify tissue proteins and penetrate more easily than acidic substances, which induce a barrier of coagulative necrosis.

Referral to an ophthalmologist is a matter of severity: mild corneal burns may cause little more than punctate epithelial erosions or small epithelial defects. In these cases, the eye typically appears injected, but no areas of limbal ischemia or "blanching" are noted. After thorough irrigation, these may be treated similar to a corneal abrasion (see the section on lacerations).

Moderate cases exhibit greater degrees of chemosis and injection, increased corneal edema, and may have segments of limbal "blanching." These cases will need long-term monitoring by an ophthalmologist, and urgent referral for guided therapy is likely beneficial in most cases.

Severe burns, however, should be referred immediately for management by an ophthalmologist. These cases are marked by ominous blanching of the perilimbal conjunctiva, severe chemosis, corneal edema and opacification. A burn of the periocular skin often accompanies severe corneal burns. These patients should ideally be managed by an ophthalmologist and may require hospital admission for close monitoring. As in the case of mild injuries, prophylactic antibiotics, cycloplegia, and analgesia should be administered. Additional treatment should include debridement of necrotic tissue and a topical steroid (e.g., prednisolone acetate 1%) applied 4–9 times daily. The topical steroid should be gradually tapered at 7–10 days as its prolonged use can potentiate melting of the cornea—again, close management by an ophthalmologist is necessary in these cases.

IOP must be monitored daily because the secondary intraocular inflammation can cause elevated pressure. If the IOP is greater than 30 mmHg, oral acetazolamide at a dose of 500 mg

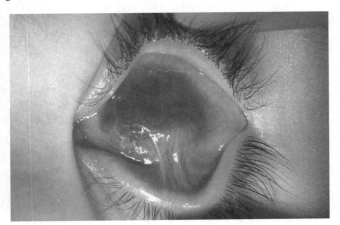

FIGURE 46.11C Chemical or thermal corneal injuries. In the absence of appropriate therapy, long-term complications include formation of ocular surface scars and symblepharon, with corneal scarring and neovascularization. Image by Matthew C. Bujak and Geoffrey C. Tabin.

twice daily can be given. If this is insufficient, a topical beta-blocker (timolol 0.5% BID) may be added. A pressure patch may be applied between drops to improve comfort and facilitate epithelial healing, as long as infection is not suspected.

During follow-up evaluations, a glass rod (or even the sterilized end of a thermometer) may be used to sweep the fornices and lyse any adhesions between the eyelid and the eye itself. If adhesions are present, lysis of adhesions should be done every day or every other day. Severe burn patients must be monitored closely. Patients with uncontrollable glaucoma, or progressive thinning or full melting of the cornea should be urgently referred for more definitive care by an ophthalmologist.

COMMENTARY

Ifeoma Ezegwui, Nigeria

The concept of a global surgeon managing some types of ocular trauma in a primary care setting is desirable. The challenge is defining who the global surgeon is—a medical doctor in general practice (general practitioner), the ophthalmic nurse, or the optometrist.

In Nigeria, where I practice, most general practitioners, apart from managing lid lacerations, refer any other eye trauma to the ophthalmologist. To function effectively as a global surgeon for primary eye care, the general practitioner will need some training. The optometrist is not trained to carry out any surgical procedures on the eye. Although ophthalmic nurses by legislation are permitted to carry out limited operative procedures on the eye, they do not function independently. They are posted to facilities that have ophthalmologists (full-time or visiting).

Most health facilities where primary eye care can be sought (e.g., general (district) hospitals or primary health centers) do not have any basic equipment for eye care (not even a vision chart), but there is an optometrist or a visiting ophthalmologist attached to the facility. Materials such as fluorescein strips, 8-0 Vicryl sutures, 9-0 nylon sutures, and appropriate surgical instruments will generally not be provided in such facilities.

Some of the recommended topical medications are not commonly available. Cyclopentolate is not as available as atropine, homatropine, and tropicamide. Similarly, prednisolone acetate 1% is not as available as dexamethasome, betametasome, or fluorometholone. Hard protective eye shields are also not widely available.

Late presentation after eye injury is a challenge in LMICs. Patients first seek help from patent medicine dealers or even traditional eye medications before resorting to a health facility. A patient with traumatic hyphema, for example, may not present to the hospital until corneal blood staining has set in.

In conclusion, the cadre of health workers to function as a global surgeon should be defined. The personnel should then be appropriately trained and equipped, and this manual will be very valuable.

COMMENTARY

John Nkurikiye, Rwanda

This chapter is well designed with a systematic flow of data.

On ocular motility examination, where it is said that the patient follows the examiner's finger, there is a process I use when the patient's visual acuity is reduced. I hold the patient's finger and move it in the cardinal positions. Proprioception will make it possible even for the blind.

The common ocular injuries are well covered with clear definition of which lesions should be sent to the ophthalmologists for proper management and clear details on how to do the repair for the less complicated cases.

47

Soft-Tissue Injuries of the Face

Christopher D. Hughes
Julian J. Pribaz

Introduction

Soft-tissue injuries of the face can be common in resource-poor settings in resource poor settings of low- and middle-income countries (LMICs) where trauma constitutes a significant source of surgically treatable morbidity and mortality. Injuries can range from superficial abrasions to deep lacerations that may or may not involve the craniofacial skeleton. For any traumatic facial injury, a thorough examination of the wound is necessary to completely define the extent of the trauma and to assess for proximity to specialized structures.

The goal of this chapter is to describe the common soft-tissue injuries of the face that may typically be encountered at the district level in areas with limited resources. Injuries to the maxillofacial skeleton will not be covered here (see Chapter 45 for information on maxillofacial trauma).

We will begin by highlighting the core principles associated with nonbony facial trauma, including care for abrasions, lacerations, avulsions, and bites. We will then cover specialized regions, including the scalp, forehead/cheek, lips/tongue, nose, and ear.

General Principles

Thorough evaluation of facial wounds is important but should only be conducted after the initial primary and secondary trauma surveys are complete. Once the patient is clinically optimized and stable, all facial wounds need to be thoroughly evaluated, under local anesthesia if available. Consideration should be given to both extent and mechanism of injury, as crush injuries can often result in significantly greater adjacent tissue damage than laceration.[1]

The face is an extremely vascular region. This rich vascularity does provide a certain level of resistance to infection, but it can also result in a significant risk of hemorrhage associated with traumatic injuries. Tamponade and control of hemorrhage should also be paramount prior to wound treatment.

Once the patient is stabilized, all wounds need to be thoroughly irrigated and debrided to remove dirt and foreign bodies, and to reduce the overall risk of infection. Retained foreign debris can also result in permanent tattooing, and care should be taken to clean the wound as much as possible. If available, tetanus prophylaxis should be administered. Dead or devitalized tissue can be sharply debrided, and ragged or beveled wound edges can be sharpened, but tissue conservation should be the goal for all injuries involving the face and specialized facial structures.[2]

Abrasions

In general, all abrasions should be thoroughly cleaned and kept moist as much as possible. Treatment with a topical antibiotic ointment can help combat infection and can result in more rapid epithelialization of the wound. Patients should be cautioned to avoid excessive sun exposure to the area for up to 1 year to protect against ultraviolet (UV) damage to the healing area. Unprotected sun exposure can result in persistent erythema and pigment changes to the affected area.

Lacerations

The repair of facial lacerations demands careful handling and attention to both functional and cosmetic outcomes. As with all injuries, hemostasis should be assured. Layered closure is typically preferred in most regions of the face, and obliteration of any potential dead space should be an important consideration to prevent hematoma, seroma, or infection. Use 4-0 or 5-0 absorbable suture for the approximation of deeper tissues and a 5-0 or 6-0 monofilament for the epidermal layer. Try to evert the skin edges as much as possible. When planning skin closure, traditional teaching suggests the use of relaxed skin tension lines as a guide for orientation. However, the nature of the traumatic injury often dictates the orientation of the defect and its subsequent closure. As long as the deeper layers are well approximated, it is usually better to loosely approximate the skin rather than risk edge necrosis with over-tightened sutures. Facial sutures can be placed closer together than normal; usually 1–2 mm from the skin edge and 3 mm apart is recommended.[3] Sutures may be removed in 5–7 days.

Avulsions

Avulsive injuries to the face require careful planning in repair. Depending on the region of injury (see the following sections), avulsions may require undermining, local flap coverage, or skin grafting for complete closure. Again, as with any trauma, patient stabilization should be a priority over complex wound closure. Use

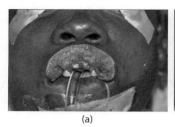
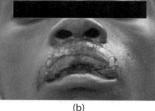

(a)   (b)

FIGURE 47.1   Use of avulsed tissue as a graft or biologic dressing. Images by John G. Meara.

of the avulsed tissue itself as a graft should always be an important consideration in LMICs where more complex closure options are often not available. In the best-case scenario, the amputated or avulsed tissue will heal to the defect like a skin graft and will provide adequate coverage. Even if the temporary graft ultimately fails, it provides a useful biologic dressing for immediate wound coverage (Figure 47.1).

Bites

Bite wounds can present fairly commonly in LMICs. These wounds are most commonly associated with dog bites, but bites from any animal (and human) are frequent as well.[4] Bites often require close attention to prevent increasing infection and worsening soft-tissue loss, and thorough irrigation and washout is necessary for all bite injuries. Antibiotic coverage should be broad spectrum; amoxicillin/clavulanic acid (or equivalent) is the recommended agent for polymicrobial coverage. In facial bite injuries *only,* consideration may be given to primary closure of the wound after thorough irrigation and antibiotic prophylaxis (Figure 47.2). Close follow-up is necessary.

As with any complex injury in LMICs, primary consideration should be given to stabilization and repair of form and function. Complex injuries requiring advanced reconstruction in these settings are probably best treated with stabilization and primary repair initially, followed by transfer to a more specialized center if available.

Anatomic Regions

Scalp

Evaluation

Scalp injuries can be masked by hair and dried blood, so a thorough examination of the patient's head is important in any trauma situation. Hair should be shaved if necessary. The extensive vascularity of the scalp offers some level of defense against infection, but also confers an additional risk of hemorrhage. Aggressive hemostasis with both pressure dressings and epinephrine-containing anesthetic (if possible) should be attempted with all injuries to the scalp region.

Management

Anatomically, the scalp is composed of five distinct layers: skin, subcutaneous tissue, galea aponeurosis, loose connective tissue, and periosteum (simplified by the mnemonic, SCALP [Figure 47.3]). Stop any major bleeding identified with suture

Summary of Optimal Suture Material for Specific Facial Wounds

Site of Injury	Optimal Suture Size*	Optimal Suture Material (Good Alternate Choice)
Cheek, forehead, or nose skin	5–0, 6–0	Nylon, Prolene† (chromic for children or patients who cannot return for suture removal)
Ear skin	4–0	Nylon (chromic)
External tongue mass	4–0	Chromic (Vicryl/Dexon)‡
Eyelid skin	5–0, 6–0	Nylon (chromic)
Frontalis (forehead) muscle	3–0, 4–0	Polydioxanone (Vicryl/Dexon, chromic)
Galea (scalp)	3–0, 4–0	Polydioxanone (Vicryl/Dexon, chromic)
Lip or intraoral mucosa	4–0	Chromic (Vicryl/Dexon)
Lip muscle	4–0	Vicryl/Dexon (chromic, polydioxanone)
Lip skin	5–0, 6–0	Nylon (chromic)
Nasal Mucosa	5–0	Chromic
Scalp skin	3–0, 4–0	Nylon (staples, chromic)
Subcutaneous tissue	4–0, 5–0	Vicryl/Dexon (chromic)
Tongue muscle	3–0	Vicryl/Dexon (chromic, polydioxanone)

*It you have a choice, these sizes are recommended.
†Prolene can be substituted whenever nylon is recommended.
‡Vicryl is a polyglactic acid; Dexon is a polyglycolic acid. They are essentially interchangeable.

FIGURE 47.2   Suture choices. Semer NB. *Practical Plastic Surgery for Non-Surgeons.* Philadelphia: Hanley and Belfus, Inc., 2001, pp. 145–159.

ligation if need be. Because of the extensive vascular supply to the region, prolonged venous oozing is common with traumatic injuries, so expedited closure is the best way to ultimately mitigate blood loss. With full-thickness injuries to this region, the galea should be closed with interrupted 4-0 absorbable suture to ensure adequate tissue approximation and to protect against deeper infection. The skin can then be reapproximated with monofilament or with a skin stapler if available.

Forehead

Evaluation and Management

Soft-tissue injury to the forehead should be treated as any other laceration of the face: thorough irrigation and debridement with appropriate tissue closure as described above. One important thing to remember with soft-tissue injuries to this region is the anatomical proximity of the frontal sinus (see Chapter 45).

Cheek

Evaluation

Lacerations to the cheek can involve multiple layers, including skin, underlying subcutaneous tissue and/or muscle, and the intraoral mucosa. Injuries to this region should be thoroughly evaluated to determine the depth and extent of the traumatic insult.

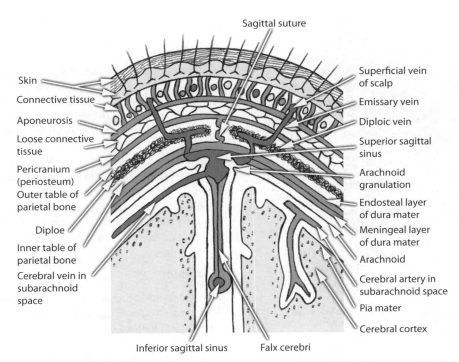

FIGURE 47.3 SCALP: skin, subcutaneous tissue, galea aponeurosis, loose connective tissue, and periosteum. Snell RS. *Clinical Anatomy for Medical Students,* 5th ed. Philadelphia: Lippincott Williams & Wilkins, 1995.

Lacerations of the cheek require a careful examination and knowledge of the anatomical location of both the patient's facial nerve and parotid gland and duct in relation to the traumatic injury.

Treatment

Full-thickness lacerations to the cheek should be repaired in layers after thorough evaluation and washout. The intraoral mucosa should be closed first, taking care *not* to include the opening of Stenson's duct in the suture line of your repair.

1. Use absorbable 4-0 or 5-0 suture.
2. Take care not to include too much tissue in each bite (mucosa only).
3. Take bites near the wound edge and evert the edges.
4. Mucosa only needs to be approximated.

Once the intraoral mucosa is closed, the wound should be irrigated again to decontaminate the oral flora as much as possible. Next, close the remaining defect in layers with a few 4-0 absorbable sutures, including the muscle layers if possible. Failure to approximate the muscle layers can result in a subsequent unilateral facial weakness that may be misdiagnosed as a nerve injury. The remaining traumatic defect can often simply be closed by closing the skin with interrupted 4-0 Nylon/monofilament sutures. To prevent hematoma/seroma formation, take care to obliterate as much dead space as possible. As with all repairs involving the cheek, take care not to include too much tissue or take too big bites to avoid including important structures in your repair.

Special Considerations: Facial Nerve Injury

New onset facial asymmetry can provide a quick diagnostic clue to the extent of a potential facial nerve injury. Be sure to assess facial symmetry prior to the administration of local anesthesia. If the injury is medial to a line dropped vertically from the patient's lateral canthus to the corner of the mouth, only peripheral branches of the facial nerve could have been injured, and you should not spend time trying to identify and repair them.

If the injury is lateral to this line and there are signs and symptoms concerning for a facial nerve injury, it is possible to attempt a facial nerve repair. Consideration should be given to surgeon expertise and resource availability prior to attempting the procedure. While facial nerve repair should be done within 72 hours of injury to stimulate the distal branches, initial wound closure and referral might be a more appropriate treatment option in certain situations.

To properly identify the region of the injured nerve, the wound needs to be thoroughly evaluated with careful inspection of the anatomy (Figure 47.4). Good lighting and proper magnification (e.g., loupes, if available) will be keys to success. Begin the dissection of the cheek through the anterior base of the parotid. The branches of the facial nerve are deep to the deep fascia (superficial muscular aponeurotic system [SMAS]) and the facial musculature. The parotid duct is a good anatomic landmark as the facial nerve lies in the same plane as the duct. The buccal branches usually lie in close proximity.

If the nerve itself has been transected without an appreciable gap, the ends of the nerve may be approximated with one or two single 7-0 nylon sutures. If there is a significant gap between the ends of the transected nerve, do not attempt to repair the nerve primarily. Mark each end with one suture and refer the patient for nerve grafting if possible. Again, adequate lighting

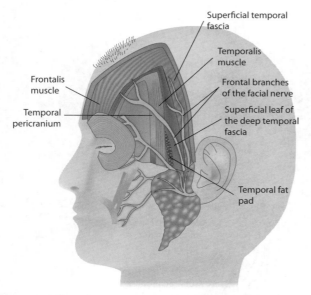

FIGURE 47.4   Facial nerve diagram. Thorne C. *Grabb and Smith's Plastic Surgery.* 6th ed. Philadelphia: Lippincott Williams & Wilkins, 2006, p. 359.

and magnification are extremely important for success in facial nerve repair.

Special Considerations: Parotid Duct Injury

The parotid duct (or Stenson's duct) runs just inferior to the middle third of a line drawn from the patient's tragus to his ipsilateral oral commissure. The intraoral opening of the duct is usually located behind the second maxillary molar. Patients can develop a sialocele or a fistula if an injury to the parotid duct is missed or not repaired. Therefore, if the traumatic injury to the cheek transects the duct and it is identifiable, repair may be attempted after thorough wound evaluation and irrigation.

To evaluate for a ductal injury:

1. Cannulate Stenson's duct intraorally with an angiocatheter if available.
2. Flush the duct with saline to observe for extravasation in the wound.
3. Fluid extravasation indicates the presence and location of the ductal injury.

To repair a ductal injury:

1. Appropriate magnification with loupes or a microscope (if available) will be essential for success.
2. Stent the duct with an appropriate gauge angiocatheter exiting through the oral duct opening.
3. Use 7-0 or smaller suture to primarily repair the duct over the stent and secure the loose end of the angiocatheter to the oral mucosa with a single suture.
4. Leave the stent in place for 1–2 weeks, although it may work its way out on its own.

Lip

Evaluation

Lip lacerations require can involve mucosa only, the vermillion border, or can be full-thickness injuries that involve skin, muscle, and mucosa. Careful planning is required in the reapproximation of the orbicularis oris and alignment of the vermillion border. Irrigate the wound as with all other facial soft-tissue injuries.

Important landmarks with respect to lip injuries include the vermillion border, wet mucosa, and dry mucosa. When repairing defects in this region, it is important to align these regions as closely as possible to prevent obvious deformity. Some authors suggest that a mismatch in the vermillion of even 1 mm can be obvious at a normal conversational distance.[5]

Treatment

The area should be anesthetized with local anesthetic if possible. Alternatively, a local block can be used.
For mucosal injuries only:

1. Align the wet mucosa with wet and the dry mucosa with dry.
2. Use 4-0 absorbable suture to reapproximate the mucosa, taking care to evert the edges.
3. Tie at least 5 knots in all lip sutures.

For injuries that cross the vermillion border but are not full-thickness:

1. Use a tacking stitch in the white border just above the vermillion to align the borders.
2. Remove and realign as necessary.
3. Once the borders are aligned, the skin can be closed with 5-0 or 6-0 suture and the mucosa closed with 4-0 or 5-0.

For full-thickness injuries:

1. Repair the inner mucosa first. Use 4-0 absorbable suture and evert the edges.
2. Irrigate the wound with saline once the inner mucosa is closed.
3. Assure hemostasis, especially in the region of transected orbicularis oris.
4. Use absorbable 4-0 or 5-0 suture to reapproximate the muscle layer with interrupted figure of eight stitches. Take care not to include mucosa in this layer of the repair.
5. Repair the skin and vermillion border as described above.

Tongue

Evaluation and Treatment

Because the musculature of the tongue retracts when transected, the extent of tongue injuries often appears larger than it really is. After thorough irrigation, tongue lacerations can often be repaired rather simply. Administer lidocaine with epinephrine prior to repair. If possible, use a 3-0 long lasting absorbable sutures in figure of eights in the deep muscle layer to bring the wound together. The tongue edge can then be closed with 3-0 chromics. If layered repair is not practically possible, you may repair the tongue edges with 3-0 or 4-0 absorbable suture with larger bites to encompass more of the deeper layer.

Nose

Evaluation

The nose is composed of three layers: skin and soft tissue, cartilaginous framework, and the mucosal lining. Injuries and lacerations to the nasal region can encompass any or all of these layers; therefore, knowledge of the anatomy and a thorough evaluation of the wound are necessary to properly restore both form and function. As with most regions of the face, all injuries should be examined and irrigated prior to closure. Prior to repair, inject the region with local anesthesia. This will not only help with pain control, but the epinephrine will also increase visibility during repair. The overriding goal with nasal reconstruction is to restore the anatomy to its pretraumatic state as much as possible.

Treatment

For injuries to the skin only:

1. Reapproximate the wound edges with 5-0 nonabsorbable sutures, placed a few millimeters from the wound edge. Be sure to evert the wound edges, using mattress sutures if needed.
2. Be sure to align the alar rim as closely as possible in your repair to avoid notching and deformity.

For injuries involving the nasal cartilage:

1. Transected cartilage can be repaired primarily with 5-0 monofilament suture. Avoid excessive suturing in the cartilage.
2. Close the skin as above.

For injuries involving nasal mucosa:

1. If there is excessive bleeding of the injured mucosa, local anesthetic injection with epinephrine can be helpful.
2. Small, 4-0 or 5-0 chromic sutures can be used to reapproximate mucosal edges.
3. Irrigate the wound following mucosal closure. Repair remaining lamellae as above.
4. Pack the affected nare with gauze, coated in antibiotic ointment if possible. Leave the packing in place for a few days to promote wound healing.
5. Patients with full-thickness nasal injuries involving the mucosa should be prophylactically treated with an oral antibiotic (cephalosporin) while the packing remains in place.

Ear

Evaluation

Traumatic injuries to the ear can be challenging, and can be classified as either partial-thickness or full-thickness. Soft-tissue loss in multidimensional planes often results in exposed cartilage, which can lead to deformity and infection. Care should be exercised to conduct a thorough evaluation of the extent of ear injuries, and, in general, conservative debridement of both skin and devitalized cartilage is prudent to prevent significant deformity. Postoperative follow-up is especially important to identify and treat hematomas.

Treatment

Explore the wound thoroughly to evaluate for cartilaginous involvement. Cartilage that has been stripped of perichondrium should be conservatively debrided. If there is no cartilaginous injury and the skin over the cartilage can be primarily closed, suture the edges together with interrupted 4-0 or 5-0 absorbable suture. If cartilage is exposed, be sure to irrigate the wound thoroughly and remove any dirt or debris. Close the skin as before, and try to include perichondrium in the suture to reapproximate the cartilage in the same repair as the skin. In general, it is not advised to place sutures directly into the cartilaginous framework itself.

If a significant portion of the patient's pinna is removed or destroyed from the injury, primary repair becomes even more challenging. Large defects can be managed in several potential ways, depending on surgeon expertise and referral availability. In general in LMICs, it is likely preferable to close the skin of any significant ear injury and refer to advanced reconstructive care if possible.

If the defect cannot be closed, however, and referral for advanced reconstruction is possible, the wound can be packed with antibiotic impregnated gauze and kept moist. Frequent dressing changes are essential to protect against infection and prevent desiccation. This should only be done as a temporizing method prior to definitive treatment.

Partial avulsion or amputation may be able to be primarily repaired if an attached segment remains intact. If possible, loosely reapproximate the avulsed or amputated segment with a few sutures. Loose approximation is key to avoid strangulating the remaining regional blood supply. Injuries involving significant structural loss without any attached segments can be treated with skin grafting from the contralateral postauricular region or with advancement or rotational skin flaps from the ipsilateral pre- or postauricular region. Again, these advanced closures should only be performed if necessary in a stable patient and in the hands of an experienced reconstructive surgeon.

Postoperative Care

Postoperative care of ear injuries requires special mention because of the risk of hematoma formation. Undetected and untreated, hematomas of the ear can lead to significant deformity (cauliflower ear), and therefore need to be evaluated and addressed. Following repair of an ear injury, properly placed dressings can help prevent this hematoma formation. Use antibiotic ointment coated gauze directly on the repair site. Use several pieces of gauze as "fluffs" and pack circumferentially around the ear. Use another piece of gauze to then wrap around the head to keep the ear dressing in place and to keep an appropriate amount of pressure on the repair site. Keep the dressing in place for 24–48 hours. Particularly with ear injuries, it is important to closely monitor the repair site.

If a hematoma does develop, the patient may present several days postoperatively with pain, swelling, and/or discoloration of the affected area. To evacuate the hematoma, remove the sutures and drain the collection. Thoroughly irrigate the wound again, and loosely repair as before. Redress the wound as previously done. Oral antibiotic prophylaxis may confer an additional level of protection against postoperative infection in these cases as well.

LMIC-Specific Considerations

Keep the following in mind when treating soft-tissue injuries in LMICs.

1. Control of bleeding should be a paramount consideration with facial injuries. Expedited closure of defects is the best way to control hemorrhage.
2. Consider using avulsed or amputated tissue as a graft or biologic dressing.
3. Partial avulsions or amputations may be primarily repaired by loosely reapproximating the tissue with a few sutures, taking care to avoid strangulating the remaining blood supply.

Key Pitfalls to Avoid

Do not attempt to do too much. Advanced reconstruction in the setting of facial trauma in LMICs is usually not appropriate. Priority should be given to bleeding control and the restoration of the anatomy.

COMMENTARY

Nivaldo Alonso, Brazil

This compilation of basic principles for treating facial soft-tissue injuries is a helpful guide for practitioners in areas with limited financial and medical resources. It is important to note, however, that larger countries frequently have areas that are without widespread medical resources. For this reason, first responders and emergency transportation are especially important. In addition, local nurses are essential, and they need to be trained to control bleeding, clear airway obstructions, and prevent infection. Aside from essential basic emergency care, there are also areas that require specialized knowledge from first responders. One example is seen in areas where the patient has suffered a large animal bite and the first responder needs to know what to do with the avulsed body part. Another example is seen in Brazil, where providers need to know how to respond to patients who have been scalped in boating accidents. High-quality surgical treatment has been proven to be essential for the patient's quality of life, and also for the community's economic stability. We continue to search for the key to providing consistent, specialized, high-quality care in these areas with unique needs. Providers who lack expertise in specialized emergency care could possibly benefit from educational videos. Telemedicine is another powerful educational tool to consider.[6,7]

48

Spinal Trauma

Andrew K. Simpson
Mitchel B. Harris

Introduction

Spinal trauma can be devastating for patients and their families, even with the technology of the most advanced medical and surgical care. Spinal trauma in the developing world can affect entire communities and local economies, especially if the injuries are associated with a neurological deficit. In high-income countries (HICs) the standard of care for such injuries necessitates rapid prehospital care, stabilization, advanced imaging techniques, spine subspecialty care, and often early surgical intervention. In the developing world, however, there is no comparable infrastructure to support these pillars of modern spine care. Though the lack of resources is not unique to spinal trauma care, the consequences of spinal trauma in association with neurologic deficit are particularly challenging and can quickly consume the limited available resources. The goal of this chapter is to identify the challenges to managing spinal trauma acutely and during rehabilitation in the developing world.

Epidemiology

The annual incidence of spinal cord injury (SCI) is estimated to be approximately 40 cases per million population.[1] Chiu et al. recently reviewed the literature on spinal cord injury and compared epidemiologic data from low- and middle-income countries (LMICs) and HICs and brought to light several systematic differences that may aid us in determining what changes we can make to improve the quality of spine care in the third world.[2] First, the mortality rate with SCI in LMICs was twice that in the majority of HICs. This is likely due to the high cost of rehabilitative care and resources needed to maintain health in cord-injured patients that are simply not available in LMICs. The most common ertiology of SCI in the LMICs is falls, while motor vehicle accidents are the predominant cause of SCI in developed nations. SCI most commonly affects males between the ages of 30 and 50 universally, regardless of national resources.

A well-done prospective epidemiologic study on SCIs, performed in Nepal, demonstrated similar population data.[3] Of all patients with cervical spine injuries presenting to the hospital, 79% had neural deficits, greater than half of these with tetraparesis. From a prehospital care perspective, more than 80% of patients were transported without any neck immobilization in a vehicle unsuitable for a spine-injured patient. The average time from injury to hospital presentation was 2 days. Though data on spinal trauma in developing nations is limited, certain themes are pervasive. Specifically, spinal trauma and spinal cord injury occur with a similar incidence to HICs and in a similarly young population, there are high rates of neurologic injury associated with spinal trauma, and there is inadequate prehospital care to prevent progression of neurologic injury in the setting of unstable injuries.

Prehospital Care

The field care of the patient from the time of injury to the time of hospital presentation is vitally important and ideally should follow strict protocols (i.e., advanced trauma life support, or ATLS). One of the principal difficulties in managing spinal trauma and spinal cord injury in the developing world is that the vast majority of patients with SCI have complete neurologic injuries at the time of initial presentation, obviating the potential for any neurologic recovery.[4-6] This is in stark contrast to HICs, where patients more often present with incomplete injuries.[7]

In HICs this process is managed by experienced emergency medical service (EMS) workers who often arrive on the injury scene within 20–30 minutes. These individuals are trained to recognize and presume spinal injury and specifically and methodically immobilize the cervical spine and initiate log roll precautions. Patients are then taken to designated trauma centers, generally arriving within hours. After initial assessment and diagnosis, patients either receive definitive care or are transferred to a tertiary center. This entire process, even if requiring transfer, often occurs on the temporal order of hours.

In direct contradistinction to this expedient prehospital regimen described, LMICs often do not have the infrastructure to support organized prehospital trauma care and first aid at the scene of an injury. Solagberu et al. evaluated prehospital care in Nigeria by identifying how patients in road traffic accidents arrived at a hospital.[8] The study found that 50% of patients were brought in by family members or relatives, 40% were brought in by police or federal road safety corps, and the remaining few percent by bystanders. Regardless of the mode of prehospital transport, in the vast majority of cases no medical interventions were performed prior to hospital arrival. Based on these data and what we know about the importance of prehospital care in HICs, the necessity for training first responders in basic trauma life support must be emphasized and deemed to be the first step toward improved care. Even with unlimited resources, we can do little to affect the neurologic outcome of patients who present with complete neurologic injury; therefore, the first step toward improving spine care in LMICs is to address prehospital care from a systems perspective to improve the outcome of patients with incomplete neurologic injury.

Initial Management and Diagnostic Techniques

Harris et al. recently reviewed the initial assessment of the multiple-trauma patient with an associated spine injury and emphasized the importance of ATLS principles and identifying life- and limb-threatening injuries.[9] Once these injuries are addressed, spinal column assessment and neurologic protection should be the highest priority. In the spinal cord–injured patient, the simple administration of oxygen and maintenance of systolic blood pressure (BP) >90 has proved beneficial.[10] Data from Canada found that approximately 40% of spinal injuries occurred in the context of the multiply injured patient with other nonspinal injuries.[11] Given the significant number of spinal injuries that occur in multiply injured patients, significant attention should be paid to spinal immobilization and clinical detection of potential cervical or thoracolumbar spine injury.

In LMICs, plain radiography is a limited resource and advanced imaging is rarely available. Though the most sensitive and specific studies for both cervical and thoracolumbar injuries are computed tomography (CT) scans and magnetic resonance imaging (MRI), these modalities cannot be relied upon in the developing world and practitioners should become adept at clinical evaluation and interpretation of plain radiographic imaging.[12] In patients with suspected spinal trauma, plain radiographic evaluation should be performed when available. Radiographs of the cervical spine, if adequately performed, can detect the majority of clinically significant injuries. A single adequate lateral radiograph of the cervical spine has been shown to detect 74%–93% of clinically significant injuries. Further, complete radiographic series of three views with anteroposterior, lateral, and open-mouth views has been shown to have as high as 99% sensitivity.[13–15] Plain radiographic evaluation of the thoracolumbar spine should include anteroposterior and lateral views, with great attention paid to the junction where the immobile thoracic spine meets the mobile lumbar segments, as this area incurs the greatest proportion of injuries. Moreover, injuries to the upper and mid-thoracic spine are more inherently stable and are less likely to require any operative intervention or bracing.

Occult spine injuries can be easily overlooked, especially in cases of polytrauma. Sengupta et al. demonstrated that cervical spine injuries are almost five times more likely to be missed than thoracolumbar injuries and that missed injuries are most often the result of failure to obtain the appropriate or technically adequate radiographs.[16] In LMICs, where imaging capabilities are limited, the rate of missed injuries in the initial evaluation of patients will be inherently greater.

From a practical standpoint, polytrauma patients should be immobilized by whatever means possible in the field or upon evaluation and undergo standard cervical spine clearance protocols. Patients with significant cervical or thoracolumbar pain should be evaluated with corresponding plain radiographic evaluation. Advanced imaging, if available, may be utilized further down the care algorithm in instances of suspected spinal injury (i.e., localized axial or radicular pain and/or neurologic deficit) where radiographs have failed to reveal a clear etiology.

Treatment

The primary goals in the evaluation of patients with spinal injury in the developing world are identifying the injuries requiring treatment and having access to facilities that have the capacity to treat such injuries. Patients with incomplete spinal cord injury have the greatest potential for functional long-term neurologic recovery[7]. Patients with complete spinal cord injury, however, especially those with injuries more than 24 hours old, are far less likely to make significant functional improvements despite surgical intervention. Unfortunately, while most patients in the developed world present with incomplete spinal cord injuries, those in LMICs most commonly present with complete paraplegia.[4–6,17] This disparity in presenting neurologic status is presumed secondary to inadequate prehospital care and evacuation protocols in LMICs.

Which patients should have spine surgery? In an environment where surgical resources are limited, this question can only be answered on an individual case basis where many factors are considered. Some generalizations, however, can be made in regard to priority of operative intervention. Spinal surgery can provide essentially two things: (1) decompression of the neural elements and (2) restoration of biomechanical stability simultaneous to optimal spinal column realignment. Surgery in LMICs is in itself a limited resource. For example, a young healthy patient with an acute isolated thoracic spine fracture-dislocation with incomplete neurologic deficit would be a high-priority surgical candidate as he has great potential for recovery with decompression and immobilization of this region where bracing is relatively ineffective. On the other hand, a patient with a mid-cervical spine fracture with complete cord injury that is in adequate alignment presenting days out from injury is less likely to have as much incremental benefit from surgery rather than immobilization in a hard cervical orthosis.

Over the past decade, there has been an increased trend toward nonoperative management of many traumatic spine injuries. In neurologically intact patients, the vast majority of traumatic subaxial cervical spine injuries and thoracolumbar injuries can be treated successfully with nonoperative management. In cases of complete cord injury, there is a substantial risk of acute wound infection with surgery.[18] Further, patients with complete cord injuries frequently incur urinary and pulmonary infections, which often lead to transient bacteremia and ultimately can result in seeding of the spinal instrumentation. If this results in late infections, it can be difficult and costly to treat. All told, there is significant evidence to support the nonoperative management of the majority of patients with spinal trauma who are neurologically intact or have complete cord injuries. In regard to managing patients in LMICs, this is certainly encouraging as surgery is a very limited resource. Nonetheless, there are patients with significant instability requiring instrumentation and incomplete cord injuries that would benefit from surgical treatment.

Practically speaking, the two predominant principles dictating spinal trauma care are neurologic status and injury stability. For simplicity's sake, patients can be neurologically classified as intact, complete cord injury, or incomplete cord injury, meaning some degree of neurologic deficiency. Injury patterns are either stable or otherwise. Although neurologic status and injury pattern stability obviously exist on a spectrum and have multiple complex classification schema, they are beyond the scope of this chapter and spinal trauma management can most easily be understood in these broad terms.

In LMICs, acute surgical intervention is likely not feasible, leaving those delivering care with options for immobilization, such as bracing with a cervical or thoracolumbar orthosis, or maintaining a patient on bed rest with log roll precautions. If available, the application of cervical traction may be utilized in unstable cervical injuries such as fracture-dislocations.

Cervical spine fractures without dislocations in either intact patients or those with complete cord injuries should be initially placed in a collar and, if possible, seen in a regional center by providers with spine care training. Patients with incomplete cord injuries have far more potential to either improve or deteriorate neurologically and, as such, should be carefully immobilized as effectively as possible with utmost importance placed on their timely transfer to regional facilities where they can be managed by a spine surgeon. Patients with cervical fracture dislocations and partial neurologic injury should undergo cervical traction as soon as possible to restore alignment, decrease cord compression, and maximize the potential for neurologic recovery. Cervical traction will require an experienced practitioner placing cervical tongs and the addition of incremental weight to restore cervical alignment, which is confirmed by repeat radiographic evaluation and must be maintained by halo placement, continuation of traction, or hard cervical orthosis, depending on the injury pattern.

Thoracolumbar injuries are less effectively immobilized with external orthoses than their cervical counterparts. As such, bracing can help to some extent when mobilizing patients with more inherently stable injuries, such as compression or burst fractures, but is certainly not ideal in cases of more unstable flexion-distraction injuries where the anterior, middle, and posterior spinal columns are compromised. Here again, even with modern medicine and unlimited resources, there is little potential to effect significant neurologic recovery in patients with complete cord injuries. However, patients with unstable thoracolumbar injuries who are neurologically incomplete or intact should be maintained on bed rest with log roll precautions and transferred to regional facilities where spine specialty care is available for definitive management.

Rehabilitation

The vast majority of care of the spinal trauma patient with neurologic compromise takes place beyond the hospital, as these patients require long-term support for problems with skin breakdown, urinary dysfunction, and infections. In the modern healthcare system, these patients are placed in dedicated SCI centers and managed by multidisciplinary teams. These teams are rarely available in the developing world. Rathore et al. looked at rehabilitation for SCI and found that there are only a handful of organized SCI wards in the developing world, and even in such centers there is a lack of many of the members of standard multidiscipinary rehabilitation teams.[19] Many SCI patients are cared for on general surgical, orthopedic, or neurosurgical wards and often managed by providers not trained in the conservative or operative management of such injuries. Perhaps improved training of physicians and staff on such wards with regard to skin care, ulcer prevention, mobility and transfer assistance, and so on, may provide improved daily care to such patients in periods of hospitalization.

Complications

Complications after spinal trauma with neurologic injury in the developing world are the same complications we see with the most modern health care, though they occur with greater frequency.[20] Jain et al. looked at SCI patients in a tertiary center and found that most patients were arriving approximately one week after their injury, already frought with complications of pressure sores, urinary tract infections, and deep vein thromboses.[21] Some of the factors contributing to this increased complication rate are inadequate pressure ulcer risk assessment and preventative technologies, and little access to disposable catheters for clean intermittent cateterization. Later complications, such as pulmonary infections and sepsis, contribute to a large percentage of the mortality in SCI patients. Long-term mortality and life expectancy data on SCI patients in LMICs, however, do not exist as many patients are lost to follow-up and systems for tracking patients are not in place.

Future Goals

To improve clinical outcomes for spinal trama patients in LMICs, we need to improve the organization of spinal trauma care services beginning with prehospital care delivery and extending to multidisciplinary rehabilitation centers. The first goal should be to define the magnitude and nature of the problem. National registries are difficult in the most modern of countries, yet to define the scope of the problem in an LMIC, a national or regional registry of spinal trauma with epidemiological data focusing on the mechanisms of injury, patient demographics, and treatment is required. Perhaps the most realistic and cost-effective intervention would be to deliver education to potential first responders, as there is currently no centralized effort in effective immobilization and safe transportation. Current knowledge suggests that the majority of SCI patients in LMICs are brought from the injury scene to the district hospital by government workers, which is essentially a captive population of individuals that could be trained in more effective prehospital care. Without attention to prehospital care improvement and spine precautions in the field, patients will continue to present initially with complete injury for which little can be done at this point to affect their overall neurologic outcome.

A second and perhaps equally important focus would be to create regional centers where "all" spinal injuries are sent for evaluation and treatment. In the United States, the creation of regional SCI centers greatly improved the understanding of spinal injuries and facilitated the advent of treatment protocols and outcomes studies.[22] By creating centers that pool resources for spine care, more standardized and thoughtful programs can be implemented for both acute and long-term care of these patients.

Standardized management protocols for spine evaluation in both isolated injuries and the multiply injured patient should be developed based on the resources available at a particular site. Such algorithms would define the necessary studies or examinations used for spine evaluation as well as when further imaging or intervention is needed that may necessitate transfer to a tertiary center. Further, these algorithms should be designed by regional spine surgeons in conjunction with district hospitals such that they may account for local resources and provide a standard that improves outcomes but is also achievable. Though the specific protocols would be dependent on regional resources, priority should be given to young patients with incomplete neurologic injuries who present early after injury and have evidence of unstable fracture patterns such as fracture dislocations. These patients should be mobilized carefully and in a timely fashion to tertiary centers where advanced diagnostic imaging and surgical care are available.

COMMENTARY

Ankur B. Bamne, Korea

Spinal trauma is a relatively common occurrence around the world. However, limited resources available in LMICs make it difficult to manage these challenging injuries in a timely and effective manner. Poor infrastructure makes adequate prehospital care and stabilization a difficult undertaking. Contrary to HICs, many LMICs do not have paramedical staff in place to respond to patients at the site of injury and transport them safely to a treatment facility.

Falls remain the leading cause of spinal injuries in LMICs. Poor working conditions among the unskilled manual workers, coupled with lack of adequate safety measures, make them vulnerable. However, motor vehicle accidents are a close second as the mode of injury. Patients are transported to the hospitals by untrained individuals, and they usually do not get any prehospital care. These injuries commonly have associated injuries like pelvic, proximal tibia, and calcaneal fractures, making early care during the "golden hour" extremely important.

The principles of early management of patients with suspected spine injuries are well described. Plain radiographs may be the only available means of investigation in many hospitals in LMICs. Plain radiographs, if acquired properly, are very helpful for subsequent management. However, often it is difficult to get good-quality radiographs from multiply injured patients, which is the leading cause of missing serious cervical spine injuries.

The density of the initial neuro-deficit (complete/incomplete) is the most important prognostic factor for these injuries, with incomplete injuries commonly having better prognosis for recovery. However, in the absence of adequate prehospital care, many patients in LMICs present with complete paresis.

Surgery for spinal injuries should be considered taking into account numerous factors: the site, the level of injury, the extent of neurologic injury, the instability of the spinal column, and the duration since injury. The limited available surgical resources in LMICs should be reserved for patients who might derive the most benefit from such an intervention.

The need for proper rehabilitation of SCI patients cannot be overemphasized. However, LMICs commonly lack centers for dedicated rehabilitation units. SCI patients are cared for by untrained individuals in poorly equipped facilities. In the light of these factors, many SCI patients develop complications like pressure ulcers, pulmonary infections, and urinary tract infections, and their mortality during the first year posttrauma is very high.

Many factors need to be considered to improve outcomes of SCI patients. Prevention of falls and implementing adequate safety measures can go a long way in preventing these injuries in the first place. Development of adequate infrastructure and prehospital care, training of first responders, and development of dedicated spine care centers and rehabilitation units are needed. Taking into account factors like local terrain and resources, specific protocols need to be designed considering regional variations. Adequate research to identify epidemiological trends, patterns of injury, and outcomes also can help.

49

Upper Extremity Trauma

Paul T. Appleton
Joseph P. DeAngelis

Injuries to the Shoulder Girdle

Acute trauma to the shoulder girdle commonly results in shoulder pain and dysfunction. When fractures, dislocation, and separations occur as a consequence of blunt injury, accurate diagnosis and appropriate treatment produce good results in the majority of patients with little long-term disability. In most cases, falls and collisions result in direct trauma to the shoulder. In young patients, high-energy accidents (e.g., car accidents) increase the severity of the injury, while lower energy trauma (e.g., falls from standing height) may lead to substantial injury in the elderly.

All evaluations should begin with a detailed history, as the mechanism of injury provides considerable insight into the extent of the injury, concurrent problems, and the most appropriate treatment.

The physical examination of a person with an injured shoulder must include a comprehensive examination of the cervical spine, the neurologic status of the involved limb, and a careful vascular exam. Comparison with the unaffected limb is essential to an accurate diagnosis.

Though rare, there are a few injuries to the shoulder girdle that warrant urgent treatment—open fractures, limb ischemia, and dislocations. Open fractures (fractures in which the skin has been compromised) should be treated with prompt, appropriate antibiotic therapy followed by a formal irrigation and debridement of the open fracture whenever possible. In most cases, surgical treatment of the fracture often follows irrigation and debridement.

Vascular injuries to the shoulder require particular attention. While there is good collateral circulation in the upper arm, trauma to the brachial artery can result in an ischemic limb and the need for emergent exploration and possible revascularization. Immobilization of the fracture will minimize trauma to the supporting soft tissue and limit any concomitant injury, while appropriate consultation or transfer of care can be arranged.

Shoulder dislocations are relatively common and should be promptly reduced. A dislocated glenohumeral joint should never be left untreated. Delays in treatment can result in serious neurologic and vascular injury as well as irreversible damage to the articular cartilage. Appropriate radiographic examination is essential to confirm the reduction of the humeral head in the glenoid.

A complete radiographic assessment of the shoulder requires a minimum of two projections taken in orthogonal planes (perpendicular to each other). In this way, any anterior-posterior (AP) view (Figure 49.1) may be paired with an axillary lateral view

(Figure 49.2). However, in a patient with an injured shoulder, positioning for the axillary view may prove too painful or challenging. For this reason, a scapular-Y view (supraspinatus outlet view) can be used if, and only if, it is paired with a true AP projection. The scapular-Y view is by convention a view of the glenoid en fosse. In this way the resulting two images are orthogonal to each other and allow for accurate assessment of the shoulder.

A scapular-Y view should never be used in isolation, and must never be used in the absence of a true AP (Grashey) projection. Failure to obtain a complete set of shoulder radiographs, or a pair of images orthogonal to one another, may result in a missed diagnosis and compromise patient care.

Fractures

Clavicle Fractures

Clavicle fractures commonly result from a direct blow to the shoulder, and in majority of cases these injuries are successfully treated without surgery. As the only bony strut connecting the arm to the trunk, the weight of the upper extremity generates a considerable deforming force. For this reason, sling immobilization can be used to support the arm, thereby decreasing the stress on the clavicle and improving patient comfort.

Midshaft, diaphyseal fractures represent more than 80% of clavicle fractures (Figure 49.3). With or without comminution, 4 weeks of sling immobilization produces good outcomes with fewer skin-related complications than figure-of-eight bandages. Range of motion is permitted to tolerance, while weight bearing should be delayed until the fracture callus has matured. Early return to contact sports or repetitive lifting may lead to complications and prolonged disability. For this reason, 12 weeks of recuperation have been recommended prior to participation in collision-prone activity and weighted overhead movements.

Distal (or lateral) clavicle fractures should be treated based on their degree of displacement, as disruption of the coracoclavicular ligament complex results in significant deformity at the fracture. When widely displaced, these injuries combine a clavicle fracture with disruption of the ligamentous complex that couples the clavicle with the scapula. The position of the fracture relative to the origin of the conoid and trapezoid ligaments determines which structures are at risk, while the amount of displacement illustrates the extent of the injury. Widely displaced, fractures within 2 or 3 cm of the acromioclavicular joint constitute a

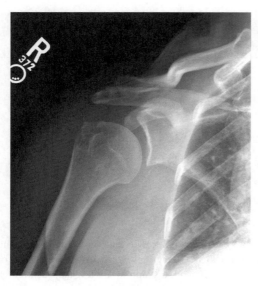

FIGURE 49.1   AP view of shoulder. Image by Paul T. Appleton and Joseph P. DeAngelis.

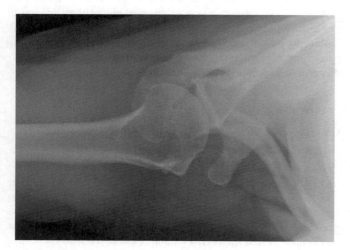

FIGURE 49.2   Axillary lateral view of shoulder. Image by Paul T. Appleton and Joseph P. DeAngelis.

complete disruption of the coracoclavicular ligaments. This pattern of injury represents a higher level of trauma and may warrant surgical intervention to restore normal function of the upper extremity.

Fractures of the Scapula

Scapular fractures are uncommon injuries and most can be treated successfully with conservative care. Careful evaluation should determine if there is extension of the fracture into the articular surface of the glenoid as intra-articular fractures with significant displacement (greater than 2 cm) may benefit from open reduction and internal fixation. Injuries that involve a significant portion of the articular surface (greater than 25%) should be followed for signs of glenohumeral instability. These cases often result from impaction of the humeral head into the glenoid in a fall onto the shoulder or on an outstretched arm,

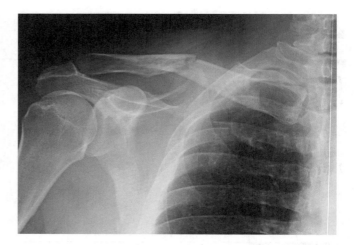

FIGURE 49.3   Clavicle fracture. Image by Paul T. Appleton and Joseph P. DeAngelis.

and represent a pattern of trauma comparable to a shoulder dislocation.

When appropriate for closed treatment, patients with scapular fractures benefit from sling immobilization to decrease the downward pull that results from the hanging arm. Early motion will improve shoulder function in the long term but should be limited to tolerance. Rehabilitation of the injured shoulder girdle should emphasize postural training, periscapular stabilization, and range of motion.

Fractures of the Proximal Humerus

In patients with osteoporotic bone, falls from standing height often result in proximal humerus fractures. The management of these injuries should be informed by the patient's premorbid level of function, his or her handedness, the degree of displacement, and the number of fragments present. In response to blunt trauma, the proximal humerus fractures in relatively consistent patterns. The primary fracture lines involve the greater tuberosity, the lesser tuberosity, the surgical neck of the humerus, and the anatomic neck of the humerus. Because the rotator cuff inserts on the greater and lesser tuberosities, the resulting pull of the rotator cuff musculature is responsible for the deforming force on these fracture fragments and can lead to migration of the fracture fragments if left unchecked. To this end, the greater the number of fracture fragments and the wider the fracture displacement, the more severe the injury and correspondingly the more likely the patient is to benefit from surgical reconstruction of the proximal humerus.

Nondisplaced fractures, regardless of the number of parts, are best treated with sling immobilization followed by gentle range of motion based on the patient's level of comfort. This same approach can be used to address minimally displaced and impacted fracture of the surgical neck (Figure 49.4). However, in circumstances where the tuberosities are displaced or the surgical neck is fractured, surgical intervention may offer a better functional outcome by restoring a normal anatomic relationship to the muscular forces about the shoulder girdle. Similarly, surgical neck fractures with significant displacement and varus angulation benefit from open reduction and internal fixation. As with all intra-articular injures, a fracture line extending into the articular dislocations are best treated with sling immobilization. Posterior dislocations require careful attention. In the absence of airway or vascular compromise, prompt reduction should be performed under general anesthesia with thoracic surgical support available. Emergent intervention is warranted in patients presenting with a posterior sternoclavicular dislocation in extremis.

The glenohumeral joint has the greatest degree of freedom of any joint in the body. As a consequence, it is susceptible to dislocation. Commonly, the humeral head dislocates anteriorly in response to trauma to the shoulder. Posterior and inferior dislocations occur less frequently. The classic teaching suggests that patients who have been electrocuted or have sustained a seizure should be closely examined for a posterior dislocation due to violent contracture of the posterior shoulder musculature.

Patients with anterior shoulder dislocations will hold their arm slightly abducted and externally rotated. Because the humeral head is anterior to the glenoid, internal rotation will be limited and the shoulder will appear squared-off due to the prominence of the acromion overlying an empty glenoid fossa. Conversely, patients with posterior shoulder dislocations have limited external rotation because the humeral head is posterior to the glenoid and attempts at external rotation lead to further bony contact. In an inferior dislocation, the head of the humerus sits below the glenoid resulting in obligatory abduction of the arm. Referred to as a luxatio erecta, this rare pattern of injury has a characteristic pattern of presentation and the head of the humerus can be palpated in the axilla as it rests on the chest wall.

In all cases, a complete set of accurate radiographs will confirm the diagnosis (Figure 49.5). As discussed earlier, a complete set of radiographs must include two views taken orthogonal (perpendicular) to one another and may include either a true AP projection (Grashey) with a scapular-Y view or any AP view with an axillary lateral. Use of these images allows for accurate diagnosis and ensures the quality of care.

All dislocated joints should be reduced as soon as possible to restore normal tissue alignment, decrease tension on vital structures, and minimize secondary sequalae of the dislocation. The principle holds true of glenohumeral dislocations. A variety of techniques have been described, and familiarity with these different methods allows for flexibility in administering care.

The traction-countertraction relies on two people to provide opposing lines of pull. With a sheet around the patient's torso, one provider pulls countertraction while the other applies axial traction to the affected limb.

In the Hippocratic technique, a single practitioner applies pressure to the patient's dislocated humerus using his foot in the axilla. Simultaneous longitudinal traction is applied with his hands to the affected arm.

The Stimson, Milch, and scapular manipulation methods require the patient to be prone with his or her arm hanging off the bed or table. In the Stimson technique, weights are hung from the affected extremity to fatigue the muscles as the arm hangs down, leading to a reduction. With the Milch technique, manual traction is applied to the arm to aid in the reduction. With one hand in the patient's axilla, the opposite hand is used to manipulate the arm, gently abducting while pressure is applied to the humeral head. Once fully abducted, the arm is externally rotated to complete the reduction. The scapular manipulation technique combines the traction method of the Stimson method with gentle

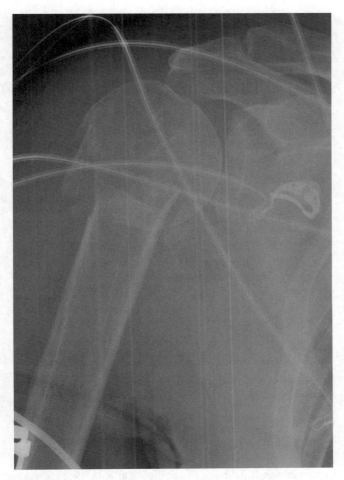

FIGURE 49.4 Minimally displaced proximal humerus fracture. Image by Paul T. Appleton and Joseph P. DeAngelis.

surface of the humeral head should be scrutinized closely for irregularities in the subchondral bone. These "head-split" patterns are rare, but when they are displaced, they can result in significant long-term disability if not appropriately treated.

Dislocations

In the shoulder girdle, there are three joints that are at risk for injury. Dislocations can occur at the glenohumeral joint as well as at the sternoclavicular joint, while an injury to the acromioclavicular joint is regarded as a shoulder separation. These injuries can occur in isolation, often following a direct blow to the shoulder, or in combination with other forequarter injuries.

Dislocations of the sternoclavicular joint are rare. However, if unrecognized, a posterior sternoclavicular dislocation can compress the trachea, esophagus, or the great vessels at grave risk to the patient. For this reason, careful examination of the clavicle should include evaluation of the medial clavicle and its relationship to the sternum. If an irregular contour is identified, raising concern for a sternoclavicular dislocation, a serendipity view of the chest should be obtained. This additional radiograph is centered at the manubrium with a 40-degree cephalic tilt. In an anterior dislocation, the clavicle will be anterior to the interclavicular line, while a posterior dislocation will reveal the clavicle below this line. Anterior

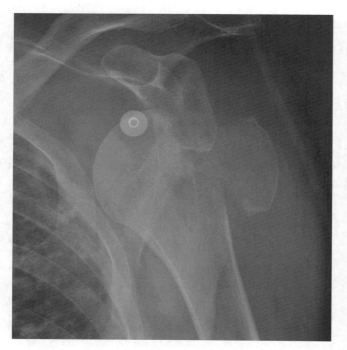

FIGURE 49.5   Anterior shoulder dislocation. Image by Paul T. Appleton and Joseph P. DeAngelis.

manipulation of the scapula. Weights are affixed to the prone patient's arm. Once the muscles are fatigued, the practitioner lifts the inferior angle of the scapula medially, allowing the humeral head to reduce into the glenoid.

Acromioclavicular Injuries (Shoulder Separations)

The acromioclavicular (AC) joint is an articulation between the hyaline cartilage articular surfaces of the acromial process and the clavicle. The joint is stabilized by a combination of dynamic muscular and static ligamentous structures, which allow a normal anatomic range of motion. Direct downward forces can disrupt this joint, usually causing the clavicle to be malpositioned superior to the acromion. The severity of the injury depends on the magnitude of damage to the ligaments between the acromion and clavicle. As more force is applied during trauma, more ligamentous structures are disrupted, causing the clavicle to become more superiorly displaced and often causing prominence under the skin. The majority of AC separations can be treated with a sling for comfort, allowing the patient to begin gentle pendulum exercises as pain permits. The sling is usually worn for 2–3 weeks depending on the patient's level of comfort. Rarely is surgery indicated for these injuries.

Humerus Shaft Fractures

Fractures of the humeral shaft can occur in any age group and are usually due to a rotational injury or direct blow. Fortunately, most of these fractures heal uneventfully without the need for operative intervention. One must be certain to examine for neurovascular injuries.

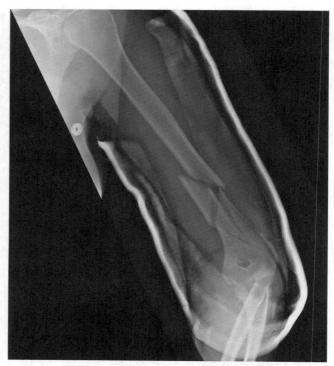

FIGURE 49.6   Humerus shaft fracture. Image by Paul T. Appleton and Joseph P. DeAngelis.

Evaluation

There is significant muscle covering the humerus, and open fractures are less common. Often there is an obvious deformity of the upper arm in addition to swelling and pain. One should be certain to evaluate the entire upper extremity to ensure that an elbow dislocation or forearm injury is not missed as these can be associated with higher energy injuries. A thorough neurovascular exam should be performed as well assessing a radial pulse at the wrist and hand function including radial, median, and ulnar nerve function. The radial nerve (due to its close proximity to the humeral shaft) is the most commonly injured neurovascular structure. If injured, patients may present with a wrist drop or the inability to extend their thumb. There may be associated paresthesias in the dorsum of the hand near the thumb web space.

Diagnosis

X-rays of the humeral shaft are diagnostic and no further imaging is required (Figure 49.6). If there is any question about associated injuries in the arm, a thorough physical examination including range of motion of the joints should be assessed. If the diagnosis is uncertain, further X-rays of the elbow and forearm can be obtained.

Treatment

Fortunately, most humeral shaft fractures can be treated very effectively with nonoperative management. In general, it is not necessary to manipulate the humerus shaft into better alignment as there is risk of injuring the radial nerve during manipulation. A U-type splint can be placed around the elbow extending up to

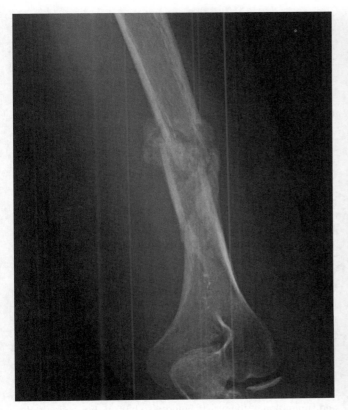

FIGURE 49.7 A healed humerus shaft fracture at 4 months. Image by Paul T. Appleton and Joseph P. DeAngelis.

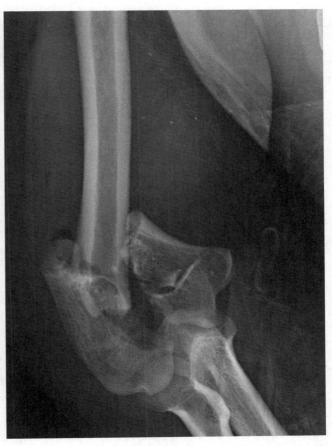

FIGURE 49.8 A distal humerus fracture. Image by Paul T. Appleton and Joseph P. DeAngelis.

the shoulder initially, and after pain is improved and swelling has decreased, a fracture brace can be fabricated to allow motion at the elbow and shoulder. Braces should be worn for 8–12 weeks and can be removed as healing has progressed and there is no motion at the fracture site, and pain has decreased. Malalignment of the humerus shaft can be well tolerated with minimal loss of function or obvious deformity. In general, it is acceptable to have up to 30 degrees of angular deformity (Figure 49.7). Open fractures should be irrigated and closed, and then a fracture brace can still be utilized. Indications for operative treatment (usually with a plate and screws) include an associated vascular injury requiring repair, and a floating elbow (where an operation of the forearm will be required). An open injury with a radial nerve palsy is worth exploring to assess for a laceration of the nerve. All other radial nerve palsies can by followed and will most likely recover. Patients should be warned that it can take up to a year for full nerve recovery, and they should be encouraged to wear a wrist splint as possible to prevent any contractures caused by the associated wrist drop. They should also be encouraged to continue range of motion of the wrist.

Supracondylar Humerus Fractures

Fractures that occur at the distal third of the humerus and can extend into the joint surface are called supracondylar fractures. They are usually due to higher energy mechanisms of injury than humeral shaft fractures. Given the involvement of the joint, these can be difficult fractures to manage.

Evaluation

Patients will present with pain, swelling, and deformity around the elbow. Given the smaller amount of soft tissue around the elbow, these injuries are more likely to be open, and thorough examination for any skin lacerations or punctures should be performed. The appearance can be similar to elbow dislocations; one should make certain that the injury is a fracture rather than a dislocation as it is important to reduce the dislocations to avoid long-term loss of function that is easily preventable.

Diagnosis

X-rays of the distal humerus or elbow are usually diagnostic (Figure 49.8).

Treatment

Fractures that do not involve the joint surface can usually be treated nonoperatively with either a long arm cast or a fracture brace similar to that used for a humeral shaft fracture. Those that involve the joint are ideally treated with open reduction internal fixation if resources are available. These can be complex injuries to fix, and a referral to a tertiary center should be considered if possible (Figure 49.9). If resources are not readily available, an attempt at closed reduction can be made with longitudinal

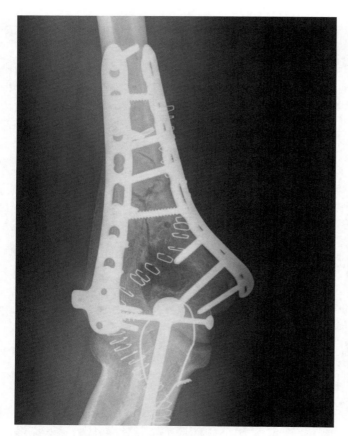

FIGURE 49.9 Following surgical repair of a distal humerus fracture. Image by Paul T. Appleton and Joseph P. DeAngelis.

traction on the arm and manual manipulation of the bone at the elbow to adjust the malalignment. The bone can usually be easily palpated at the distal humerus. Following reduction, the arm should be placed in a long posterior splint. The reduction should be assessed by X-ray following the manipulation. If tools are available, one can try placing the arm in gentle traction, placing a Steinman pin in the ulna, and attempting to reduce the fracture. Patients can be placed in traction for about a month, but should then start motion of the elbow once healing has begun.

One must keep in mind that when treating these injuries in a long arm cast that immobilizes the elbow, loss of motion will frequently occur. It is best to try immobilization of a manipulated supracondylar fracture for a couple of weeks followed by a fracture brace that allows some motion at the elbow to prevent stiffness.

Elbow Dislocation

Elbow dislocations usually occur as a result of a direct fall on an outstretched upper extremity. The majority of dislocations occur in the posterior or posterolateral direction (meaning the olecranon has moved posterior to the distal humerus).

Evaluation

There is usually an obvious deformity at the elbow and significant pain. Patients are unable to flex or extend at the elbow and cannot rotate their forearm. Open injuries should also be assessed as any laceration/puncture wound likely directly communicates with the joint and diligent exploration and washout is essential to avoid a septic arthritis. A thorough neurovascular examination should be performed.

Diagnosis

X-rays are diagnostic and, if possible, both an AP and lateral view should be obtained to assess the position of the dislocation (Figure 49.10A and Figure 49.10B).

Treatment

Elbow dislocations should be reduced as soon as possible. Adequate sedation is usually required. If general anesthesia is not available, one can consider an intra-articular injection of lidocaine to help reduce pain prior to reduction. Traction should be applied to the extremity in slight flexion. Direct posterior pressure should be placed on the olecranon, pushing it anteriorly. If the dislocation is posterolateral, some pressure should be placed on the olecranon, directing it medially. Following reduction (which is usually accompanied by an audible or palpable "clunk"), the elbow stability should be assessed in addition to the reduction. If successfully reduced, one should be able to flex and extend the elbow without any blocks to motion. Pronation and supination at the wrist should also be full. Following reduction, the elbow can be placed in a posterior splint for 2 weeks. Ideally, postreduction X-rays can be obtained to ensure that there is no remaining subluxation of the joint. The splint should be left on no longer than 2 weeks, at which point the splint should be removed and motion begun. Immobilizing the elbow for longer than 2 weeks can lead to significant loss of motion. If it is impossible to keep the elbow reduced due to instability, one should consider urgent referral to a tertiary care–type facility if possible. Alternatively, an external fixator can be placed around the elbow to hold it reduced but should not remain on much longer than 2–3 weeks to keep the elbow joint from becoming very stiff.

Olecranon Fractures

Fractures of the olecranon usually occur as a result of a direct fall on the elbow. The triceps insert broadly over the olecranon, and displaced fractures can result in the inability to extend the arm. In addition, displaced fractures can result in some degree of instability of the elbow joint and dislocations can be associated with this injury.

Evaluation

Patients usually present with pain, swelling, and a deformity at the elbow. It is often possible to palpate a gap in the olecranon as it is usually easily palpable given the small amount of muscle covering the bone. Patients usually cannot extend the arm. If small avulsions or minimally displaced fractures are present, one should carefully assess the patient's ability to extend his or her arm at the elbow.

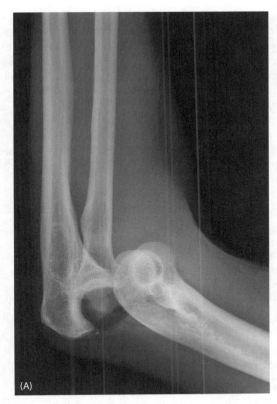

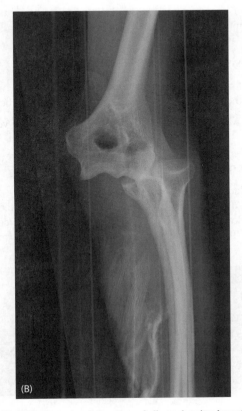

FIGURE 49.10A Posterior elbow dislocation. Image by Paul T. Appleton and Joseph P. DeAngelis.

FIGURE 49.10B Posterior dislocation of elbow showing lateral displacement. Image by Paul T. Appleton and Joseph P. DeAngelis.

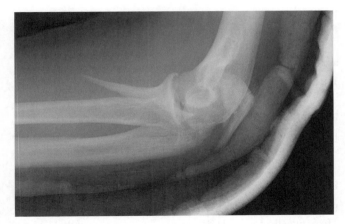

FIGURE 49.11 Displaced olecranon fracture. Image by Paul T. Appleton and Joseph P. DeAngelis.

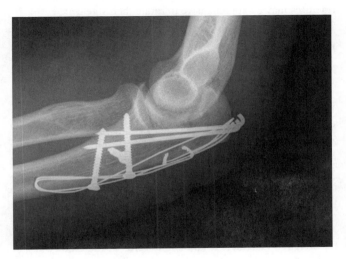

FIGURE 49.12 Olecranon fracture repaired with tension band. Image by Paul T. Appleton and Joseph P. DeAngelis.

Diagnosis

X-rays of the elbow are usually diagnostic and should be scrutinized for associated injuries such as a dislocation or fracture of the radial head (Figure 49.11).

Treatment

Nondisplaced fractures can be immobilized in a long arm cast. Placing the arm in extension rather than at 90 degrees may place less stress on the olecranon by relaxing the triceps and minimizing the chances of displacement. Patients may begin mobilization after 2–3 weeks, allowing passive motion only at first to prevent displacement of the fracture by the pull of the triceps muscle.

Displaced fractures are best treated operatively. If resources are not available, one could try a closed reduction by manipulating the displaced olecranon fracture in extension and placing a cast. Simple operative treatment includes excising the olecranon fracture fragment if small and advancing the triceps mechanism, suturing it to the ulna. Alternatively, a tension band construct is a simple and effective means of treating these without complex equipment needed other than a couple of Kirschner wires and a strand of wire (Figure 49.12).

If operative fixation is performed, the elbow should be immobilized for no longer than a couple of weeks to prevent the loss of motion.

Radial Head and Neck Fractures

The radial head is the proximal part of the radius that articulates with the distal humerus along with the olecranon. The elbow joint is complex in nature, and subtle fractures or subluxations can cause significant disability and loss of motion (Figure 49.13).

Evaluation

Patients usually present with pain at the elbow and an effusion. There may be no visible deformity. The pain is usually localized to the lateral side of the elbow. Given the function of the radial head with pronation and supination of the forearm, patients with fractures may be apprehensive to rotate their forearm.

Diagnosis

X-rays of the elbow are diagnostic.

Treatment

Most radial head and neck fractures are either non- or minimally displaced. Patients can be placed in a posterior splint of a sling for 7–10 days for comfort. They should gradually begin motion at the elbow as soon as pain is tolerated. Displaced fractures can often be reduced in a closed manner. The radial head can usually be palpated on the lateral side of the elbow just anterior to a line drawn between the tip of the olecranon and the lateral humeral condyle. Pressure right over the radial head while applying longitudinal traction and slight varus at the elbow may be sufficient. Gently rotate the forearm while pressure is applied. A postreduction X-ray should be performed, and the elbow can be immobilized in a posterior splint for 2 weeks before starting gentle motion to prevent significant loss of motion at the elbow. Fractures that are comminuted or remain displaced and cause a block to motion should be treated operatively if resources are

available. The fracture can be fixed internally with screws or excised if motion is blocked and resources to repair the fracture are not available. If considering excision, it is imperative to rule out an injury to the ligamentous complex between the radius and ulna in the forearm. If there has been an injury and the radial head is excised, significant shortening of the radius can occur, causing disability and pain at the wrist in addition to possible elbow dislocation. Always palpate the wrist in a patient with a radial head fracture to ensure there is no injury or dislocation of the distal radial/ulna joint. If the fracture is not reconstructable and the elbow remains unstable, one should consider a radial head replacement if resources are available.

Forearm Fractures

The forearm is made up of two long bones: the radius and ulna. The two bones articulate with each other both proximally at the elbow and distally at the wrist. Their relationship can be complex, and even minor injuries can cause a dramatic loss of motion in the upper extremity. Most fractures are the result of a direct fall on the upper extremity.

Evaluation

Fractures can occur in either the radius or ulna alone or in both bones. There is usually an obvious deformity and pain if the fracture is displaced. Patients usually cannot rotate the arm after these injuries due to pain or disruption of the complex anatomy of the forearm. A thorough neurovascular exam is critical as compartment syndrome can occur with higher energy injuries.

Diagnosis

X-rays of the forearm are diagnostic. It is imperative to include films of the elbow and wrist as well to make certain there is not an associated injury such as a radial head dislocation or distal radio-ulnar dislocation (Figure 49.14).

Treatment

Nondisplaced fractures can be treated nonoperatively. Initially, they should be placed in a splint that crosses the elbow and extends down to the wrist. After 2 weeks, this can be converted to a cast. To prevent displacement, there should be no rotation of

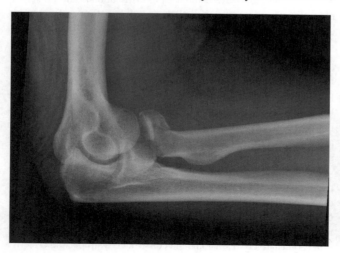

FIGURE 49.13 Displaced radial head fracture. Image by Paul T. Appleton and Joseph P. DeAngelis.

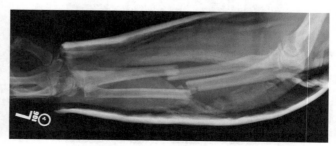

FIGURE 49.14 Both bone forearm fracture. Image by Paul T. Appleton and Joseph P. DeAngelis.

the forearm; to accomplish this, a Munster cast can be applied. The cast should have flares around the elbow to prevent rotation, but allow flexion and extension at the elbow joint.

Displaced fractures should be treated operatively with plates and screws if resources are available (Figure 49.15). If operative fixation is not an option, a closed reduction of the fracture can be attempted. Skeletal traction can be placed to help realign the fracture. After a couple of weeks of traction, a cast can be applied. When using skeletal traction, one must very cautious that ischemia of the upper extremity does not occur with prolonged traction. Frequent neurovascular exams are imperative.

Distal Radius Fractures

Fractures of the distal radius are one of the most common injuries seen by orthopedic doctors. Most injuries are the result of a direct fall on an outstretched upper extremity. Distal radius fractures can be associated with low-energy falls in the elderly population or higher energy accidents in younger patients. Many of these fractures can be treated nonoperatively in a cast, but occasionally the fracture pattern is unstable enough that surgical intervention is required.

Evaluation

Patients can have an obvious deformity to the wrist with swelling and pain. A thorough neurovascular examination should be performed focusing on both pulses and capillary refill in the fingertips in addition to sensation in the median, ulnar, and radial nerve distributions. The most common sensory defect is in the median nerve with resultant decreased sensation in the index and middle fingers. The median nerve traverses the wrist through the narrow carpal tunnel, and any deformity of the distal radius can put significant stress on the median nerve.

Diagnosis

X-rays, including an AP and lateral of the wrist, are usually diagnostic. It is important to differentiate between a distal radius fracture and a dislocation of the carpus, which can look similar on physical examination. The most important imaging to review is the lateral view of the wrist as the most important predictor of functional outcome is the degree of dorsal tilt of the wrist on the lateral view (Figure 49.16A and Figure 49.16B).

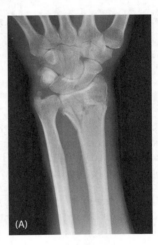

FIGURE 49.16A   AP view of a distal radius fracture. Image by Paul T. Appleton and Joseph P. DeAngelis.

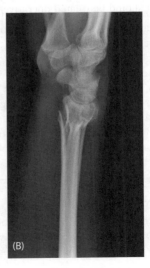

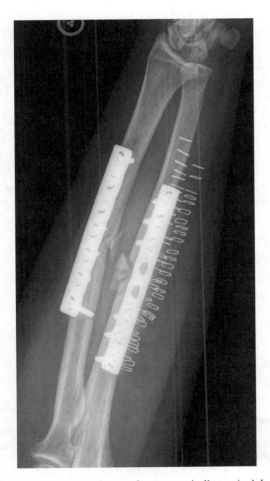

FIGURE 49.15   Both bone forearm fracture surgically repaired. Image by Paul T. Appleton and Joseph P. DeAngelis.

FIGURE 49.16B   Lateral view of a distal radius fracture with some dorsal displacement. Image by Paul T. Appleton and Joseph P. DeAngelis.

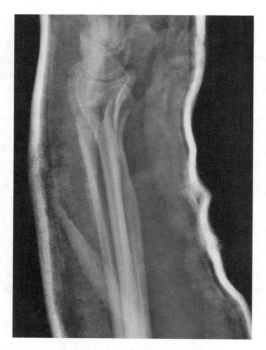

FIGURE 49.17   Postreduction views of a distal radius fracture. Image by Paul T. Appleton and Joseph P. DeAngelis.

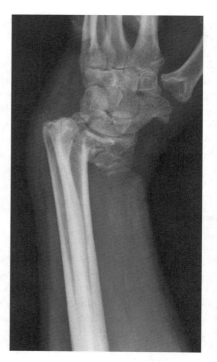

FIGURE 49.18   Volarly displaced distal radius fracture. Image by Paul T. Appleton and Joseph P. DeAngelis.

Treatment

Nondisplaced distal radius fractures can be treated in a short arm splint or cast for 6 weeks. It is important that casts leave the fingers free so that patients do not get stiff and are allowed unlimited motion of the fingers during the casting period. Fractures that are dorsally displaced can be reduced with a hematoma block and placed in a well-padded splint with some pressure against the back of the wrist to prevent repeat displacement (Figure 49.17).

Occasionally, it is very difficult to hold more complex fractures in position in a cast. If there is difficulty maintaining alignment, an external fixator can be used with two pins in the radius proximal to the fracture and two pins in the index finger metacarpal. K-wires can also be used to augment the external fixator if holding the fracture in position with the external fixator does not provide enough support.

Fractures of the distal radius that occur with volar (palmar) displacement can be very difficult to hold in position in either a cast or external fixator as the entire wrist can sublux off the front of the distal radius (Figure 49.18). If resources are available, placing a volar plate can be very effective for treating these (Figure 49.19).

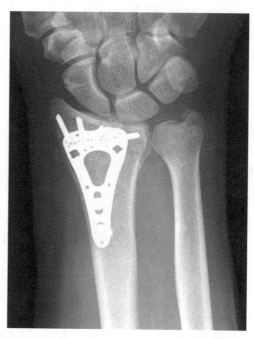

FIGURE 49.19   Distal radius fracture treated with a volar plate. Image by Paul T. Appleton and Joseph P. DeAngelis.

Suggested Reading

Bucholz RW, Heckman JD, Court-Brown CM, et al. (eds.). *Rockwood and Green's Fractures in Adults*. 7th ed. Philadelphia: Lippincott Williams & Wilkins, 2010.

Browner BD, Green NE, Jupiter JB, et al. (eds.). *Skeletal Trauma: Basic Science, Management, and Reconstruction*. 4th ed. Philadelphia: WB Saunders, 1997.

COMMENTARY

Ankur B. Bamne, Korea

There is a higher prevalence in low- to middle-income countries (LMICs) than in high-income countries of low-cost motorcycles as a primary mode of transportation. Even a low-energy trauma in such a scenario makes people vulnerable to serious injuries, especially to the upper extremity. Many patients in LMICs seek medical attention from untrained, inexperienced laypeople. These bonesetters have no medical training and commonly splint injured parts with wooden sticks and a tight wrapping. This leads not only to outcomes like nonunion and malunion, but also to serious complications like compartment syndrome, or even gangrene. The compartment syndrome is frequently untreated and develops into a Volkmann's ischemic contracture. It is at this stage that the patient presents to a tertiary hospital. Although it an exception rather than the rule, such outcomes for trivial injuries are not acceptable in today's environment.

In India, pediatric injuries of the upper extremity are often left untreated when they are mistaken for sprains. This leads to complications like malunion. Cubitus varus following malunited supracondylar humerus fracture in the pediatric age group is very commonly seen in India.

Certain treatment modalities may be more commonly used in LMICs. For example, fixation of both bone fracture of forearm is commonly done with nails rather than plates in many centers with inadequate facilities. Also, distal radius fractures are more likely to be treated conservatively. These lead to a higher incidence of malunion with its functional consequences.

Thus, the trauma to the upper extremity and the subsequent morbidity in the form of loss of dexterity and strength has a profound effect on individuals involved in manual labor. It is imperative that these should be adequately treated and the patients returned to their pre-injury status as much as possible.

The mechanism of injury in shoulder trauma may be direct (impact on the shoulder) or indirect (fall on the outstretched hand). The severity of injury may be low-energy or high-energy depending on the mode of injury. The usual scheme of evaluation of patients with shoulder injuries begins with a history, physical examination, and subsequent investigations. Shoulder injuries that require "emergency" management are open fractures, associated vascular injuries, and dislocations. It is important to image the shoulder in two orthogonal views on plain radiographs.

Midshaft clavicle fractures are common. A majority of the fractures can be treated nonoperatively with sling immobilization. The skin over the fracture may break down if one of the fragments is tenting the skin. Distal third clavicle fractures sometimes need operative treatment.

Scapular fractures are uncommon. Most of the scapular fractures heal well because of the extensive muscular coverage of the scapula and good vascularity. Intra-articular displaced fractures may need operative fixation.

Fractures of the proximal humerus are seen in elderly osteoporotic patients with low-energy trauma. Fractures may be displaced or nondisplaced. Three-dimensional computed tomography (CT) scans can be helpful in delineating the fracture anatomy, especially intra-articular fractures. Nondisplaced fractures can be treated nonoperatively. Proximal humerus locked plates have revolutionized fixation of multi-fragmentary fractures.

Dislocations of the sterno-clavicular joint are extremely rare injuries. Posterior dislocations can compress the trachea, esophagus, or the great vessels. They need prompt reduction. The glenohumeral joint, being the most mobile joint in the body, is also the most commonly dislocated joint. The most common type of dislocation is the anterior dislocation. Posterior dislocations are seen postseizure or postelectrocution due to the powerful contraction of the shoulder internal rotators. Inferior dislocation is extremely uncommon. Different types of dislocations have classic deformities. After adequate plain radiographs, emergent reduction should be undertaken. Many different maneuvers have been described for reduction of the glenohumeral joint. Postreduction, the shoulder should be immobilized for a duration depending upon the age of the patient to prevent the possibility of recurrent dislocation.

In acromioclavicular (AC) joint injuries, the clavicle is commonly displaced superiorly due to injury to the acromio-clavicular and/or coraco-clavicular ligaments. These injuries are classified according to the grade and direction of clavicular displacement. Higher grade injuries need operative intervention.

Humerus shaft fractures occur across all age groups. The mechanism of injury can be varying. A careful assessment of neurovascular status of the extremity must be made. Radial nerve palsy (RNP) is present in 10% of the cases. Pain radiographs usually are sufficient to diagnose humerus fractures. It is important to include the shoulder and elbow joint in the images to avoid missing associated injuries. After initial splinting, most of the humerus fractures in adults can be managed nonoperatively by a functional brace. A closed fracture associated with RNP does not need operative intervention. However, exploration of the radial nerve should be done if it is associated with open humeral fractures.

Supracondylar fractures occur at the distal metaphyseal flare of the humerus. They may or may not be intra-articular. Careful distinction from elbow dislocation should be done. Extra-articular fractures may be treated nonoperatively. Intra-articular fractures need open reduction and internal fixation in an attempt to restore articular congruity.

Elbow dislocation occurs due to a fall on the outstretched hand. Posterior and posterolateral displacements are common. The three-point bony relationship of the elbow will be disturbed. Emergency closed reduction should be performed and the elbow immobilized for no more than 2–3 weeks.

Olecranon fractures occur due to direct injury. A gap at the fracture is commonly palpable. Active extension at the elbow is not possible due to discontinuity in the extensor mechanism. Nondisplaced fractures may be treated with immobilization in extension, whereas displaced fractures need open reduction internal fixation (ORIF).

Radial head fractures are relatively uncommon injuries. Physical examination will delineate tenderness directly over the radial head. Closed reduction of displaced fractures may be done and subsequently treated with immobilization. Range of motion may be resumed when pain decreases. Displaced fractures may be fixed with screws. Comminuted fractures may need radial head excision.

Fractures of the forearm are common injuries. Physical examination and radiographs are diagnostic. Careful assessment has to be done to rule out compartment syndrome. Because of the interosseous membrane between the two bones and the movements of pronation and supination, fractures of the forearm are now considered intra-articular and need ORIF. Dynamic compression plating gives good results.

Fractures of the distal radius are extremely common. The mode of injury may be high-energy (in the young) or low-energy (in the elderly). Patients with Colle's fracture have a typical deformity called "dinner fork" deformity, due to the dorsal displacement. Radiographs are diagnostic and define the fracture pattern. Nondisplaced fractures do well with a cast immobilization. Displaced fractures need reduction and fixation. A residual deformity at the level of the wrist may remain after fracture healing due to collapse in the cancellous bone.

50

Hand Trauma

Simon G. Talbot
Amir H. Taghinia

Introduction

This chapter on hand trauma will focus on infectious, traumatic, and posttraumatic conditions that one may encounter in underserved populations. Although patients in high-income countries (HICs) often present acutely, it is not uncommon for patients in low- and middle-income countries to present late and, most often, with other complicating factors. Thus, it is critical for the clinician to consider advanced cases of common scenarios as an explanation for a condition that he or she has never seen. Furthermore, follow-up care of traumatic or infectious conditions can be problematic as distance, education, and financial hardship often prevent return visits. Therefore, it is also important that the clinician consider the likelihood of continued care. For example, in certain circumstances, it may be more prudent to perform an amputation and immediate closure of a fingertip injury as opposed to several weeks of dressing changes to allow secondary healing. Although the latter approach would preserve length, the need for frequent dressing changes and follow-up, and the possibility of infection due to poor sanitation, may increase the risk of complications. Similar reasoning should apply to placement of drains, which may end up staying in place for months.

This chapter will discuss the diagnosis and treatment of acute traumatic injuries (including sharp lacerations and crush injuries), burns, and infections. Special attention will be given to emergent conditions including bleeding, pyogenic infections, and compartment syndrome. The delayed presentation of acute trauma or burns can be complicated by acute or chronic infections. The same principles of treating infections apply in these conditions. We will also discuss the diagnosis and treatment of late sequelae of trauma and burns. These include scar contractures, joint stiffness and malalignment, malunions, nonunions, and chronic wounds. The diagnosis and treatment of these conditions will be considered in the setting of underserved populations.

Basic Hand Anatomy

A basic knowledge of hand anatomy is critical for diagnosis and treatment. This point cannot be overemphasized. With adequate knowledge of anatomy, the practitioner needs very few additional diagnostic studies to arrive at an accurate diagnosis. Indeed, there are few circumstances in which the examination distal to

an injury does not provide a convincing and definitive diagnosis of the injured structures. Probing the wound to assess the nature and extent of injury is simply wrong.

Topographical Anatomy

Knowledge of the topographical anatomy of the hand is important for communication between practitioners. Typically, one refers to the dorsal or palmar aspect of the hand. The terms *distal* and *proximal* provide relative measures of position. *Radial* and *ulnar* are preferred to *medial* and *lateral* because the latter two terms can be confused based on pronation or supination of the hand (Figure 50.1).

Skeleton

The wrist, or carpus, sits on the distal radius and distal ulna and is made by eight carpal bones. Distal to the wrist are five metacarpals, and these create the basic hand unit. Each finger has three additional bones, the proximal, middle, and distal phalanges (Figure 50.2). The thumb has two phalanges, the proximal and distal phalanges. The joint upon which the proximal phalanx articulates with the metacarpal head is the metacarpophalangeal (MP) joint. In the fingers, there are two interphalangeal joints—proximal (PIP) and distal (DIP). Each joint is surrounded by a set of ligamentous structures that protect it against mechanical stresses. The volar plate is a strong ligamentous structure that protects against dorsal translation. On each side of the joint lie the collateral ligaments. The proper collateral ligament spans from the middle portion of the condyle proximally to the volar aspect of the phalanx distally. The accessory collateral ligament spans from the middle portion of the condyle to the volar plate and provides additional stability to the joint. Dislocation of a joint usually indicates a tear in at least two of these structures.

Tendons

The flexor tendons are located on the palmar surface of the hand and forearm. The origins of these flexors lie in the forearm and the insertion in the hand and digits. There are two flexor tendons for each finger; they enter the hand through the carpal tunnel. The superficial flexors (flexor digitorum superficialis, FDS) flex the PIP joints, whereas the deep flexors (flexor digitorum profundus, FDP) flex the DIP joints. There

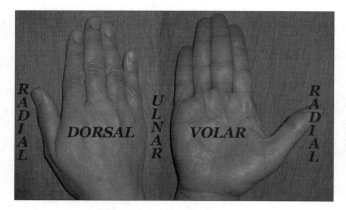

FIGURE 50.1 Topographical anatomy of the hand. Image by Amir Taghinia.

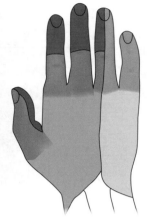
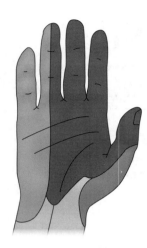

FIGURE 50.3 Sensory nerve distribution of the hand. The medium-gray area is median nerve innervated, the dark-gray area is radial nerve innervated, and the light-gray area is ulnar nerve innervated. Image by Amir Taghinia.

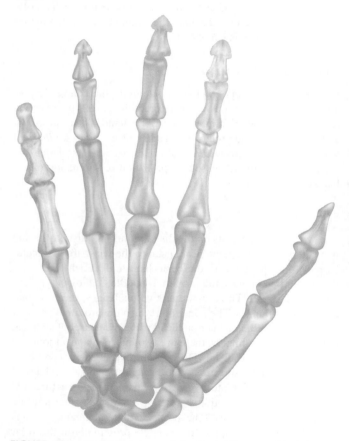

FIGURE 50.2 Skeletal anatomy of the hand. There are 14 phalanges, 5 metacarpals, and 8 wrist bones. Image by Amir Taghinia.

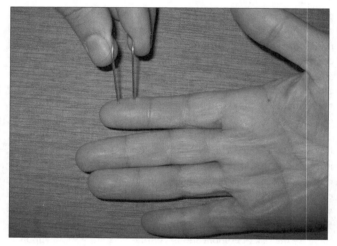

FIGURE 50.4 Testing 2-point discrimination is easily done using a paper clip. Image by Amir Taghinia.

is only one flexor tendon to the thumb (flexor pollicis longus). Extension in the digits is complicated and is mediated by a harmonious interplay of intrinsic and extrinsic muscle-tendon units. Each digit has a single extrinsic extensor tendon—except for the index and small fingers, which have an additional, independent extensor.

Nerves

The palmar surface of the hand is innervated by the median and ulnar nerves. The median nerve enters the hand in the carpal tunnel radially, just below the transverse carpal ligament. It then provides motor function for the intrinsic muscles of the thumb and sensation to the palmar surface of the thumb, index finger, middle finger, and radial aspect of the ring finger. The ulnar nerve enters the hand in Guyon's canal and divides into sensory and motor branches. The sensory branch provides sensation to the small finger and ulnar aspect of the ring finger. The motor branch innervates the hypothenar muscles, the volar and dorsal interossei, and the adductor of the thumb. Sensation to the dorsum of the hand is provided by the dorsal sensory branch of the ulnar nerve (ulnar dorsum) and the sensory branch of the radial nerve (radial dorsum) (Figure 50.3).

The ideal way to examine for a sensory nerve deficit is using two-point discrimination. For nerve injuries, it is best to test moving two-point discrimination. This can be easily done with a paper clip (Figure 50.4). The examiner asks the patient to shut his or her eyes and gently runs the tips of the paper clip on the ulnar or radial side of the finger. Normal moving two-point discrimination is about 3 mm; anything above 8–9 mm should be considered abnormal.

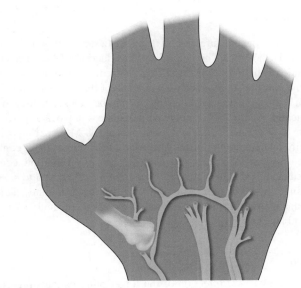

FIGURE 50.5   The radial artery (RA) and ulnar artery (UA) communicate via the superficial palmar arch (shown) and deep palmar arch (not shown). MN is the median nerve and UN is the ulnar nerve. Note the ulnar artery is radial to the ulnar nerve. Image by Amir Taghinia.

Vessels

The arteries of the hand are palmar and the veins are dorsal. The arterial blood supply is provided by the radial and ulnar arteries. These two arteries meet in the palm, forming a deep and superficial palmar arch (Figure 50.5). In most patients, the ulnar artery is the dominant supplier of the hand. It provides the major contribution to the superficial arch, whereas the radial artery provides the major contribution to the deep arch. Common digital arteries to each web space originate from the superficial arch. Once they reach the MP joint level, each common web space vessel gives off an ulnar and radial digital artery to its neighboring digit. These arteries then travel with their associated nerves—the neurovascular bundle—palmarly on each side of the digit. In the digits, the arteries are dorsal to the nerves.

Basic Tenets of Hand Surgery

In treating hand conditions, several basic principles should be followed. These principles apply to the hand and complement the basic principles of surgery. The first principle was mentioned in the introduction—examine distal to the injured area. The examination distal to the area of injury is more revealing about the nature of the injury than inspection of the injured site. Probing the wound is rarely the correct maneuver.

When considering an operation, the other two principles are securing adequate anesthesia and use of an operating tourniquet. Because of the consistent anatomy of the sensory nerves in the hand, and because of their proximity to the skin, obtaining pain-free conditions is relatively easy in the hand. With four injections, the surgeon can render the entire hand anesthetic. These sites are the median and ulnar nerves in the palmar wrist and the radial and ulnar nerves on the dorsum wrist. Obtaining adequate

anesthesia is critical because a patient who has pain is likely to move and compromise the repair of small structures. Also, the patient is less likely to come back for follow-up care.

Technique

Using 5 ml of local anesthesia (50/50 mix of long-lasting bupivicaine and short-acting lidocaine is ideal) for 4 sites (20 ml total), the wrist is prepped with alcohol. The median nerve is anesthetized by using a short 25-gauge needle that enters at the distal wrist flexion crease ulnar to the palmaris longus tendon and is directed radially 45 degrees and palmarly 45 degrees. The ulnar nerve is anesthetized by entering just dorsal to the flexor carpi ulnaris tendon with the needle directed radially. The ulnar nerve is ulnar to the ulnar artery (Figure 50.6). The sensory branch of the ulnar nerve can be anesthetized on the dorsum of the wrist by making a skin wheal just distal to the ulnar styloid. Finally, the radial nerve is anesthetized by injecting down to the radius 3 fingerbreadths proximal to the radial styloid and withdrawing the needle while instilling the 5 ml of local anesthesia. The ulnar nerve and median nerve blocks take about 10 minutes to work.

Use of a tourniquet is also critical. The hand has a rich blood supply, and bleeding can severely limit visibility. When properly administered, a tourniquet minimizes blood loss and provides a clean operative field with minimal morbidity. A well-padded upper-arm pneumatic tourniquet should be placed, the limb exsanguinated with an esmarch bandage, and the tourniquet inflated to 250 mmHg for most patients. If only an esmarch is available, this can be used to exsanguinate the arm, and is then wrapped over itself several times at the proximal extent to function as a tourniquet, while unwrapping the distal end to allow surgery. If none of this equipment is available, elevation of the arm with digital pressure over the brachial artery followed by

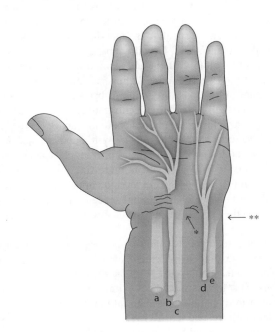

FIGURE 50.6   Injection sites to anesthetize the median (*) and ulnar (**) nerves. The ulnar artery (not shown) is radial to the ulnar nerve. a = flexor carpi radialis tendon, b = median nerve, c = palmaris longus tendon, d = ulnar nerve, e = flexor carpi ulnaris tendon. Image by Amir Taghinia.

inflation of a blood pressure cuff may be an alternative, but the cuff requires frequent observation to ensure that it remains inflated. If a prolonged tourniquet run is anticipated, the limb should be allowed to perfuse 30 minutes for each 2 hours of tourniquet time. In an awake patient, the tourniquet should not be used for more than 30 minutes as it can be quite uncomfortable.

There is a theoretical risk of spreading an infection or malignancy proximally if the limb is exsanguinated prior to tourniquet inflation. In these cases, the esmarch can simply be started more proximally, or the limb elevated with 1 minute of compression on the brachial artery prior to inflation of the tourniquet.

Infections

It is common to see infections in underserved communities and LMICs. The practitioner should be aware of local common infections that may be rare in the developed world. Furthermore, the practitioner should be aware of advanced presentations of common infections.

Basic Principles

When diagnosing and treating an infection, the clinician should consider three potential factors: host factors, inoculum, and organism(s). Host factors include those that may predispose the host to infection. These may include comorbidities such as diabetes or immunosuppression or wound beds with necrotic tissue. Necrotic tissue does not have blood flow, so the host cannot mount an immune response and antibiotic medications cannot penetrate these tissues to kill the microorganisms. Inoculum speaks of the amount of contamination. For example, a wound that was created by a clean knife is far less likely to get infected than a bite wound that contains a large number of microorganisms. The last factor, the organism(s), speak to the fact that some organisms are more virulent than others. Certain subspecies of streptococcus pyogenes can be quite virulent and a small inoculum can cause severe infections, whereas other strains are innocuous.

Most hand infections are caused by skin flora such as *Staphylococcus aureus* and are due to trauma. As there are multiple moving structures and multiple potential spaces in the hand, the initial bacterial inoculums may move to another adjacent site where the local defenses are weaker. For example, a small inoculum in the flexor tendon sheath is more likely to develop into a pyogenic infection because of the potential space within the sheath; this is an avascular potential space rich in nutrients. The infection can then spread all across the finger along this potential space.

In treating infections, the stand-alone surgical tenets are drainage of abscesses and debridement of nonviable tissues. These principles alone should cure a great majority of problematic infections. Host factors should be optimized, including control of blood sugar in diabetics. The material that is drained is sent for Gram stain, culture, and sensitivity, if available. Once cultures are back, antibiotics should be tailored to the offending organism(s). After drainage and adequate debridement, the wound should be allowed to stay open. If a small opening is created, a wick or drain should be placed to keep the wound well drained.

Specific Hand Infections

Paronychia

This is a pyogenic infection of the soft tissue surrounding the nail. It is thought to be caused by introduction of bacteria via the side of the nail. Pain, swelling, and redness around the nail are the cardinal signs. If left alone, most of these spontaneously drain, but improvement in symptoms can be quicker if they are surgically drained. Although some authors advocate partial removal of the nail, this is seldom necessary. Most paronychia require a small stab incision at the site of the abscess and complete drainage. A small wick may then be placed to allow continued drainage. Alternatively, the patient may be asked to soak the finger in warm water 4–6 times per day for 20 minutes. This amount of soaking is necessary to keep the skin moist so the wound heals slowly.

Felon

This is a pyogenic infection of the finger pulp. Patients present with severe, throbbing pain on the volar surface of the finger. A small transverse mid-lateral incision should be placed to drain the abscess. The septae that span the palmar skin and the distal phalanx should be bluntly divided to make sure the entire abscess has been drained. It is common for patients to experience mild to moderate anesthesia/dysesthesia in the pulp for many months thereafter. If allowed to fester, the pyogenic pressure can build up in the pulp and necessitate in the bone, causing osteomyelitis.

Collar-Button Abscess

This pyogenic infection involves the dorsal and volar soft tissue of the hand in the webspace. Initially, it may start as a dorsal or volar infection that spreads to the other side through a small opening, thus forming two simultaneous abscesses that communicate. The key objective is to drain both dorsal and volar components; this can be done through small incisions. Care should be taken to avoid injury to the neurovascular bundles in the webspace.

Flexor Tenosynovitis

This is an infection of the flexor tendon sheath. The diagnosis can be made by assessing for Kanavel's signs: 1) finger is held in flexion, 2) finger is swollen like a sausage, 3) there is tenderness at the A1 pulley area (between the distal palmar flexion crease and the metacarpophalangeal flexion crease), and 4) there is pain with passive extension of the finger (Figure 50.7). When caught early with mild signs and symptoms, the condition can be treated with intravenous antibiotics. However, if more advanced, surgical drainage is required. Our preferred method is to make two incisions, one palmar incision at the A1 pulley and another midlateral incision at the A3 or A5 pulley. The finger is drained and cultures are sent. A small, perforated pediatric feeding tube is then threaded from proximal to distal within the sheath. The wounds are left open and the tube is irrigated with normal saline for 24–48 hours. If the infection has infiltrated the subcutaneous tissues, a larger midlateral incision may be necessary. The

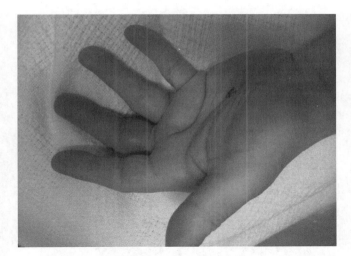

FIGURE 50.7 Early flexor tenosynovitis. The finger is held in flexion and passive extension is painful. There is swelling and redness distal to the A1 pulley. Image by Amir Taghinia.

mid lateral incision can be allowed to remain open and heal secondarily. Avoid making zigzag palmar incisions on the finger as these increase the risk of an open wound with exposure of the flexor tendon.

Other Space Abscesses in the Hand

The fascial investments over the intrinsic muscles of the hand help to create additional potential spaces in the hand. These include the midpalmar space and the thenar space. The flexor tendon sheath of the small finger can extend proximally and communicate to the flexor tendon sheath of the thumb via a potential space (termed Parona's space) in the distal forearm. Abscesses within these locations should be drained. Because of the proximity of multiple important structures, drainage in the operating room under tourniquet is advised. For a detailed anatomical description of these spaces, the reader is referred to other sources.

Burns

Burns in the hand are more common on the dorsal surface. Palmar burns are less common, but more prone to functional problems. In diagnosing and treating a burn, the clinician must first focus on the basics of resuscitation, including the airway and breathing. Inhalation injury, as evidenced by singed nasal hairs and soot in the sputum, can cause significant morbidity and needs to be assessed carefully. The degree and extent of burns on the body should be assessed and carefully documented. Herein, the pathophysiology and overall management of the burn patient will not be covered; instead, we will discuss management of burn injuries in the hand alone.

Depth of Burn

It is important to estimate the depth of a burn because it determines management. Burns injure the skin at various levels. Superficial burns that affect only the epidermis are first-degree. Examples include burns caused by sun exposure. The rete ridges

of the skin are maintained and visible. Those that involve a portion of the dermis are termed second-degree. Sensation is maintained but the rete ridges may not be visible. Blistering, which usually occurs 1–2 days after injury, often indicates a second-degree burn. Third-degree burns involve the entire thickness of the dermis. The skin usually has a pale, white appearance and is insensate. Fourth-degree burns extend into the subcutaneous tissues. Despite these guidelines, diagnosing the depth of an acute burn can be difficult, even with experienced eyes. Waiting a few days may be necessary to allow the injury to "declare."

Acute Treatment

The acute treatment of the burned patient involves basic life resuscitation measures. Once the patient is stable, attention can be directed to the hand. Management is tailored to the depth of injury. First- and second-degree burns are usually observed and treated with topical antibiotics such as bacitracin. We usually avoid silver sulfadiazine in the hand because the rich blood supply of the hand can allow systemic absorption and potential complications. Most burns of the dorsal hand can be allowed to heal secondarily—this includes small third-degree burns that do not compromise the paratenon (the thin fascial covering of the tendon). In contrast, even small third-degree burns on the palm and palmar digits can cause severe flexion contractures, especially if they occur on a flexion crease. These should be excised and resurfaced with full-thickness skin grafts (Figure 50.8). Large, third-degree dorsal wounds should also be excised and grafted. Split-thickness sheet grafts are usually adequate and provide an aesthetically acceptable treatment in most cases.

Late Treatment

The late treatment of burns in the hand usually addresses scar contractures. Deep second-degree and third-degree wounds that are allowed to heal secondarily—especially those on the palmar surface—can lead to scar contractures that compromise function. In these cases, treatment usually involves some sort of release procedure with resurfacing. It is critical to assess the status of the neighboring joints. If the scar contracture is long-standing, it is possible that the joints are stiff and may benefit from release. The surgeon who plans for a joint and scar release simultaneously should be prepared to do a flap reconstruction. Often after joint release, the flexor tendon and other vital structures become exposed in the wound and these will not take a skin graft. Furthermore, with a flap reconstruction, the patient can start immediate range of motion exercises (as opposed to skin graft, which requires a period of immobilization).

Small contractures across flexion creases or in webspaces can usually be treated with local tissue rearrangement such as Z-plasty. This is a simple but powerful technique of releasing a tight scar by recruiting tissue in a direction perpendicular to the scar (Figure 50.9; see also Chapter 34). For larger contractures, release and skin graft or flap reconstruction is required. A good example of this is for reconstruction of the first webspace. Multiple Z-plasties rarely improve a first webspace contracture because the contracture is usually extensive and there is little tissue laxity on either side of

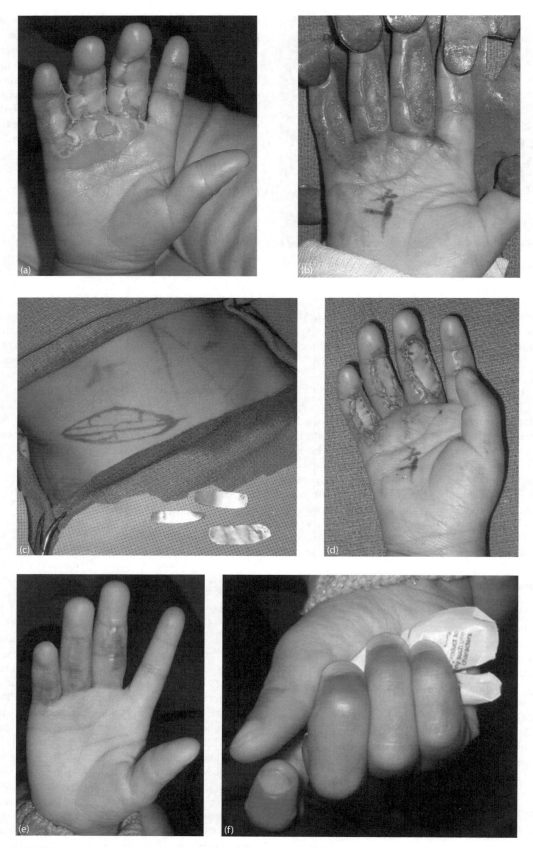

FIGURE 50.8 Treadmill burn in the young child. The white areas in (a) indicate full thickness injury; these areas should be excised (b) and exact-template full-thickness skin grafts using suture pack templates (c) should be applied (d). Long-term outcome is shown in (e) and (f). Images by Amir Taghinia.

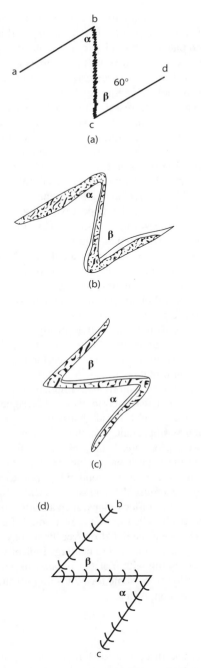

FIGURE 50.9 (a) The scar contracture spans from point b to c. The central limb is oriented on the scar. (b) The incisions are made and flaps are created. (c) Usually the flaps will then auto-rotate into their desired configuration. (d) Final appearance shows that the distance from b to c is lengthened. Images by Amir Taghinia.

the web. A semicurved, transverse incision to release the webspace followed by skin grafting or flap resurfacing is usually necessary.

In the case of skin grafting, several key technical maneuvers can assure success. If the procedure is done under tourniquet, the tourniquet should be deflated and careful hemostasis obtained prior to placing a skin graft. Hematoma is a major reason for skin graft loss. For dorsal releases, a split-thickness sheet graft works well. For palmar releases, full-thickness skin grafts work better. A great place to harvest full-thickness grafts is the lower abdomen

and upper inguinal area. If a large full-thickness graft is anticipated, one should consider tissue expansion in the lower abdomen.

Once the skin graft is harvested and hemostasis obtained, it should be carefully sutured to the edges of the defect under a small bit of tension. The next consideration is avoidance of shear. A cotton bolster may be used to secure the skin graft in the palm and dorsum; however, bolsters on the fingers are cumbersome. Here, we have found that simple compression gauze followed by immobilization in a cast is sufficient. The cast is left on for 2–3 weeks. After removal, the patient may start range of motion exercises.

Trauma

Hand trauma is common in the developing world. Frequent manual labor and a lack of safety equipment and regulations are significant contributing factors. A thorough understanding of hand anatomy and performance of a good physical examination are of key importance in determining what structures are injured, which need repair, and how extensive surgical repair will be. Timing of presentation may also alter available management options. While delayed presentation will rarely preclude surgical management, it may require more extensive dissection, grafting, or use of other structures to accommodate tissues that have shortened with time, such as tendons.

Sharp Injuries

When presented with a sharp injury, adequate examination to determine which structures are injured is critical. If necessary, local anesthesia and/or the use of an esmarch as a tourniquet can aid in accurate diagnosis by removing a patient's apprehension due to pain and allowing visualization of structures in a bloodless field.

After completing an examination, the necessary equipment must be gathered. All possible equipment, including sutures that may be required, should be obtained prior to proceeding. Loupe magnification should be used if possible. Typically, a simple Littler scissor, small needle holder, toothed Adson forceps, and several small-sized sutures are all that is absolutely necessary. More complex injuries may require more specialized equipment such as tendon passers, clamps, K-wires, and drills. Where patient follow-up is limited, absorbable 5-0 plain gut in the skin is often a good choice. More specific sutures may be necessary if specific structures, such as tendons, require specialized repair. Next, the hand should be adequately anesthetized (see earlier discussion). A basic principle of all acute hand trauma is debridement and irrigation to reduce bacterial load. The hand should be cleaned of all gross debris and then prepped, typically with povidone-iodine or chlorhexidine. Next, all nonviable tissue is debrided to ensure optimal healing. This is particularly important on the palm of the hand where the thick skin must be sutured with excellent eversion to ensure dermis-to-dermis apposition. A very thorough irrigation is next used to wash away any microscopic foreign material and reduce bacterial load. At this stage, each specific injury should be managed in turn.

Nail-bed injuries are very common. They typically occur with lacerations or crush injuries of the distal digit. Due to the nail's intimate association with the distal phalanx, a tuft fracture almost always includes an injury to the overlying nail matrix. A subungual hematoma is also often a sign of an underlying injury. To repair these nail-bed injuries, the nail should be removed by sliding the tines of a blunt scissor under the nail from the hyponychium to just proximal to the eponychial fold. By spreading the scissors, the nail plate can be freed from its attachments and removed. The matrix itself should then be repaired using 6-0 or smaller plain gut suture. The nail is then trimmed into a "guitar pick" shape, replaced, and held temporarily in place with an absorbable suture at its base. A new nail will grow out over months and the old nail "splint" can be removed in due course.

Extensor tendon injuries are also common and generally can be easily repaired. In the forearm and dorsal hand, the traumatic laceration can be extended to gain access, usually in a Z shape to allow proximal and distal extension. In the digits, incisions may be extended in the mid-lateral lines to gain better exposure. Key considerations in the digits include preservation of the central slip and terminal extensor. Conversely, loss of one of the two lateral bands is acceptable. Tendon ends should be debrided to ensure that good-quality tendon is incorporated in the repair. A 3-0 or 4-0 permanent suture such as nylon, polypropylene, or polyester should be used. Numerous techniques have been described, but a simple four-stranded repair using a modified Kessler suture and/or mattress suture is usually sufficient. Immobilization in an extended position for 1–2 weeks with gentle passive followed by active motion until full healing has occurred at 6–8 weeks is usually adequate.

Flexor tendon injuries can be significantly more complex than their extensor counterparts due to the interplay of both superficial and deep tendons and the presence of the digital pulleys. Several key principles should be considered. First, when both tendons to any digit are injured, ideally both would be repaired. However, if suboptimal surgical conditions exist or where repair of both will limit the excursion of either, a digit can function adequately with only the deep tendon. Second, incisions on the palmar aspect of the hand should not cross flexion creases perpendicularly. Instead, Brunner (zigzag) incisions or mid-lateral incisions should be used. Third, tendon gliding of the flexor tendons is of paramount importance. Keeping the repair to a minimal bulk and removing pulleys when they inhibit gliding may be necessary. Only the A4 and half of the A2 pulleys are considered essential for normal digit function. The pulleys keep the tendons close to the bone so there's no bow-stringing during flexion. Fourth, early protected motion is critical to prevent adhesions of a freshly repaired tendon. Flexor tendons are typically repaired with a four-stranded technique such as a cruciate repair or a modified Kessler augmented with a box suture. As with extensor tendons, 3-0 or 4-0 permanent sutures are appropriate. Additionally, an epitendinous running 5-0 or smaller suture is used to improve tendon gliding and increase strength of the repair. Postoperatively, the hand is splinted with an extension-blocking splint, and then started on an early motion protocol at around 1 week.

Vascular injuries are likely irreparable without significant surgical training and specialized equipment. Suffice it to say, injuries to both the radial and ulnar arteries will require emergent revascularization if the hand is to survive. Similarly, injuries to both vascular bundles of a digit will require emergent repair or amputation. An injury to only one artery will not usually cause a major deficit due to redundancy in the arterial tree. However, keep in mind that an arterial injury is frequently associated with a nerve injury due to their proximity in most areas of the hand. One key point is that if revascularization will be attempted or a patient sent to another facility for formal repair, it is important *not* to clamp a bleeding vessel. This can damage the vessel irreparably and risks inadvertent injury to an adjacent nerve. Local pressure is preferred. If an artery is injured and the decision is made not to repair it, careful suture ligation is most reliable. Note that pressure will often stop even arterial bleeding unless only a partial vessel wall laceration has occurred, in which case vasospasm will hold the vessel laceration open.

Injuries to nerves in the upper extremity may range from simple (a digital nerve) to devastating (any of the three major nerves in the forearm). Repair is not emergent, but should occur within days to weeks for optimal outcome. Ideally, nerves should be repaired with microscopic magnification or high-powered loupes. The epineurium is repaired with meticulous interrupted nylon sutures of 8-0 or smaller size. A repair should be tension-free, and a nerve graft from the sural nerve or a nerve branch in the forearm may be required. Alternatively, a conduit, such as a section of native vein or those commercially available, may be used. The hand is typically immobilized for 1–2 weeks to allow the repair to consolidate.

Injury to the skin and soft tissue is implicit in any sharp trauma. As mentioned previously, debridement and irrigation are of primary importance. Careful and thorough closure of skin with good eversion is important, and the use of absorbable sutures is often most appropriate. Where closure is not possible, skin grafting from the hypothenar eminence or distant sites may be performed. But where bone or tendon is exposed, more complex methods will be required for closure. Local tissue rearrangement with Z-plasties or local flaps, such as cross-finger flaps, can be used effectively when options are limited, but when larger areas need coverage, pedicled or free flaps may be necessary. Good dressings are important to healing. Typically, a petroleum-impregnated dressing with moistened gauze to wick blood from the closure, followed by some form of immobilization to prevent shearing and tension, is ideal.

Fractures

A comprehensive discussion of forearm, wrist, and hand fractures is beyond the scope of this chapter (see Chapter 49 for more on upper extremity trauma). However, some basic principles can make management much easier. First, determining the stability of a fracture is essential in determining optimal treatment. Fractures that are nondisplaced, remain reduced after reduction, or are simple transverse or short oblique fractures are usually (but not always) stable and can be treated with simple immobilization. Long oblique, spiral, or very comminuted fractures are typically unstable. To accommodate swelling, a splint is usually placed first followed by a cast, if necessary, at approximately 1 week. In the developing world, this is typically a short forearm cast for forearm and wrist fractures and either a thumb spica, volar resting splint, or ulnar gutter for hand fractures. In the digits, aluminum splints or buddy taping may be most appropriate. For unstable fractures, fixation with percutaneous K-wires or internal plates and screws is usually required. For grossly contaminated open fractures, external fixation is preferred until the wound is controlled.

Second, fracture reduction is a key part of managing any displaced fracture. This can be done with either a hematoma block (local anesthetic directly injected into the location of the fracture) or a regional block (such as a wrist or digital block). Numerous reduction maneuvers are described, but the principle involves traction, recreation of a deformity, and manipulation into an anatomic position. Note that reduction may be limited by tissue interposition or ongoing deforming forces such as tendon pull, both of which constitute unstable configurations. Following reduction, the fracture must then be immobilized. Fractures should be immobilized until pain-free and/or radiologic signs of bridging bone are seen. This will usually be around 4 weeks in the digits, 6 weeks in the hand, and up to 8 weeks in the wrist and forearm. Third, several specific fractures warrant special consideration. These include scaphoid fractures and fractures of the base of the thumb metacarpal, which require more extensive fixation as these may be inherently unstable and prone to long-term complications.

Dislocations

Dislocations in the hand are common. In the digits these usually require simple traction and reduction (after a digital block) followed by splinting. Early reduction is critical as delayed presentation may preclude reduction without surgical release of the joint capsule and collateral ligaments. Where joint instability or fractures exist or where tissue interposition (such as the volar plate) limits reduction, operative management may be required. Concurrent injury to various structures such as the central slip or volar plate may cause boutonniere or swan-neck deformities, respectively, and will usually require surgical repair. Dislocation of the carpal bones is a significantly more serious injury. Rapid reduction with anesthesia, muscle relaxation, and traction should be performed as soon as possible. Injury to the carpal ligaments is common, and compression of the median nerve is possible. Operative decompression of the carpal tunnel and/or operative fixation of the wrist with closed or open techniques may be required.

Crush Injuries

Crush injuries are very common in industrial settings. Many of the principles of repair of individual structures from the prior section apply. It is always important to recognize that injuries from crushing will often create internal damage that is not immediately apparent. Again, a thorough examination is the most effective way to determine what is injured. Another important consideration is the propensity for development of a compartment syndrome. This occurs when pressure within a fixed space in the hand or forearm exceeds end capillary pressure, causing ischemia of the contained structures. Diagnosis and management will be discussed in the following sections.

Bites

Numerous types of bites can occur, and the specifics of each will be unique to the area of the world in which they occur. Cat, dog, and human bites remain the most common. Cat bites typically cause deep-tissue inoculation after which the tract closes over. Infection often progresses rapidly, requiring early drainage and intravenous antibiotics, typically with ampicillin-sulbactam or its equivalent. Dog bites tend to be more open, reducing the risk of deep infection, but more often injure various structures. Human bites are usually the result of a fight. Where a tooth enters a joint (termed a "fight bite" when this occurs to the fifth metacarpophalangeal joint), the joint is susceptible to septic arthritis and requires arthrotomy and wash-out. More exotic bites may occur in the developing world. Again, several principles apply. An initially unremarkable injury can progress to a large area of tissue necrosis due to various toxins in many insect, spider, or reptile bites. Thus, observation of a bite wound over several days is important. A thorough debridement of necrotic tissue may be necessary. Incomplete debridement will ultimately delay ultimate wound closure. Skin grafting or local flaps may be necessary. For all bites and resulting hand infections, management of edema by splinting and elevation is almost always necessary and effective.

Compartment Syndrome

Recognition of a compartment syndrome of the hand or upper extremity is of unparalleled benefit to a patient. Treatment is relatively simple, but if this goes undetected, the sequelae can be devastating, such as a Volkmann's ischemic contracture. Compartment syndromes occur when the pressure in a closed compartment exceeds end capillary pressure. This may occur from a fracture, hematoma, crushing injury, infiltrate, bites, burns, tight dressings, or any number of other causes.

Diagnosis

The diagnosis of a compartment syndrome is primarily clinical. Pain on passive extension of the muscles in the compartment is the sine qua non in an awake patient. The other cardinal signs of pallor, paresthesias, pulselessness, paralysis, and poikilothermia typically occur later. In an obtunded patient or where there is doubt as to the diagnosis, the use of a Stryker side-port needle or a simple arterial line connected to a pressure transducer will allow adequate measurement of the pressure within a compartment. A typical cutoff for diagnosis is a compartment pressure of greater than 30 mmHg or less than a 30 mmHg difference between the compartment pressure and the diastolic blood pressure.

Treatment

The treatment of compartment syndrome is emergent fasciotomy of the involved compartments. In the forearm this is usually performed with a volar lazy-S incision extending from the mobile wad to the wrist in the supinated arm. The muscle fascia must be incised, and typically the pressurized muscle will protrude into the incision. The carpal tunnel should be released distally, taking care to only incise the transverse carpal ligament and preserve all neurovascular structures and tendons. Particular care must be taken not to injure the median nerve or palmar cutaneous branch of the median nerve at the wrist, which will lie ulnar and superficial to the main nerve. A dorsal forearm incision is not often required.

Compartment syndrome in the hand is less common, but release should be done through two dorsal incisions over the second and fourth metacarpals to release each of the interosseous compartments, hypothenar and thenar incisions, and a carpal tunnel incision if not already done (Figure 50.10). Digits can be released from mid-lateral approaches, avoiding the ulnar border of the thumb and small finger and the radial border of the index finger, as these surfaces are important in sensation. Minimally invasive incisions with subcutaneous fasciotomies are generally not adequate for acute compartment releases, especially where equipment and monitoring are limited.

Amputations

In addition to the discussion that follows, see Chapter 39.

Principles of Amputation in the Upper Extremity

Patients may *present* with partial or complete amputations or, particularly in the developing world, amputation may be the preferred method of treating a complex injury or infection. Remember that a well-performed digital amputation may give a patient a rapid, functional result far sooner and with far less risk of complication than a complex repair or revascularization.

When patients present with a complete amputation, a decision must be made whether to attempt replant of the part, requiring microvascular surgery, or whether a completion amputation will be more appropriate. Where facilities are limited, the indications for digital amputation are significantly expanded. They include, at least, any irreparable digit, an isolated devascularized, unmanageable infection, or malignancy. Whenever possible, the thumb, hand, and forearm should be preserved.

The term *partial amputation* is used to describe a wide number of presentations. In these situations, the key decision is whether the part is vascularized. If it is vascularized, attempting soft-tissue and bony repair is usually preferable unless the part is severely mangled.

A further common scenario is injury to a digital tip. When bone is not exposed, many people advocate dressing changes to allow healing by secondary intention, while maintaining length and sensibility. A decision must be made as to whether this is feasible in the developing world where frequent dressing changes may be impractical and/or risk infection. Similarly, a skin graft (such as a hypothenar graft) may require more care and follow-up than is available. In these situations, a rapid and very functional completion amputation of a tip with primary or local flap closure may be the best option. Where necessary, a volar-based V-Y flap can be used to ensure pulp coverage of the distal tip. Where a significant portion of nail matrix is present, residual nail, or a splint made from a foil suture wrapper, should be placed to prevent synechiae between the eponychium and nail matrix (Figure 50.11). If only a remnant of the nail matrix is present, this will

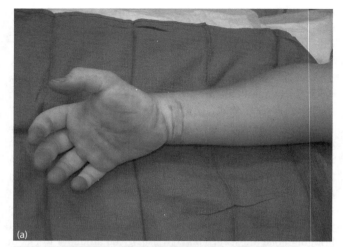
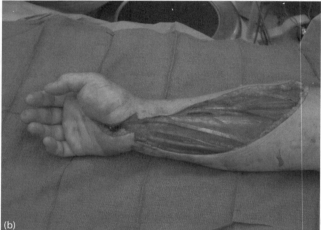
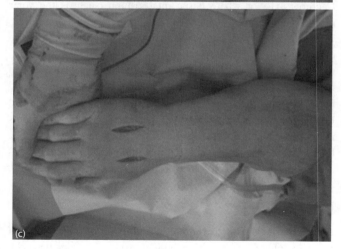

FIGURE 50.10 A severe compartment syndrome is shown in (a). This should be treated with a wide fasciotomy of the forearm (b) and possibly hand (c).

often need to be ablated (both the matrix and the volar aspect of the eponychium) to prevent troublesome partial and malformed nail growth in the future.

Tip amputations are also a special case in which two fundamental deformities must be avoided. First, the flexor digitorum profundus should be left attached to the distal phalanx where

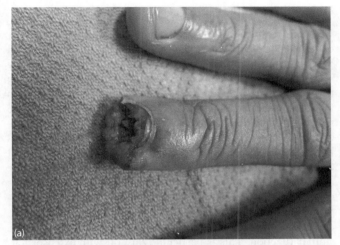

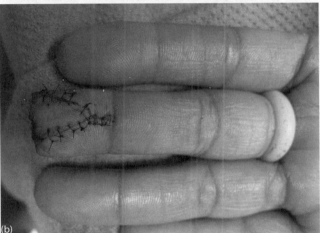

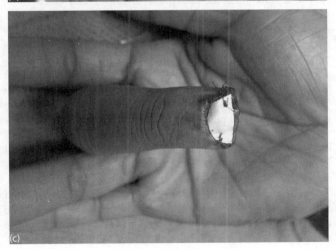

FIGURE 50.11 A traumatic digit tip amputation shown in (a) can be easily treated with a V-Y flap closure (b) and stenting of the eponychial fold (c). Images by Amir Taghinia.

A key parameter for a usable digit is length. An amputation (or completion amputation) must shorten the bony skeleton enough to allow appropriate coverage with primary closure or local flaps. However, maintaining length of the skeletal framework will maximize function. Keeping tendon insertions in the remaining phalangeal bones is also important to maintain flexion and extension. For example, a distal tip amputation should strive to maintain the terminal extensor and flexor digitorum profundus to allow motion through the distal interphalangeal joint and retain power grip. The same is true of an amputation through the middle phalanx in which the tendon insertions to the base of the phalanx should be maintained. In the proximal phalanx, the tendons may be attached to bone or periosteum to maintain movement of this bone, which otherwise does not receive tendon insertions. A further consideration is whether to perform a ray amputation versus amputation at the metacarpophalangeal joint when an entire digit requires amputation. While a ray amputation is generally cosmetically more acceptable and avoids the problem of small objects falling through an interdigital space, in manual workers, maintenance of palmar width by amputating at the metacarpophalangeal joint is usually preferable to help with power grip.

Sensation in the digit is usually maintained unless a more proximal injury is present. More problematic is the development of neuromas from digital nerve endings. These can often be prevented by dissecting out the nerves, placing these on slight stretch, and either burying the ends in muscle or allowing them to retract, thus preventing a nerve end from direct apposition with the new pulp.

Where an amputation occurs through a joint, the cartilage should be removed from the distal end of the proximal bone. This will allow better adherence of the new pulp tissue to the underlying corticocancellous bone and a more stable digital tip.

Gangrene

Gangrene refers to two distinct entities: wet and dry gangrene. Dry gangrene refers to tissue necrosis from avascular necrosis. This may occur when a vascular injury to a digit is left untreated or when underlying disease (such as diabetes) impairs small vessel circulation. In these situations, auto-amputation is usually preferable, whereby the underlying tissues are allowed to heal by secondary intention and the nonviable part is "pushed" off. Minor local flap procedures or trimming of bone may be necessary to ensure adequate bony coverage. This method maximizes length and sensibility of the affected digit. Wet gangrene implies infection and may be primary or secondary to tissue necrosis from any cause. In contrast to dry gangrene, wet gangrene requires urgent surgical management to debride all nonviable tissue. Infected wounds should be left open and treated with simple but frequent dressing changes and ongoing debridement until a healing and granulating wound bed is present, which may then be closed or grafted.

Late Sequelae of Trauma and Burns

In the developing world, it is very common for patients to present with delayed sequelae of untreated or suboptimally treated injuries. These may be difficult or impossible to correct. However, several principles can be followed to minimize

possible, to avoid a lumbrical plus deformity in which migration of the tendon proximally may cause paradoxical extension of the digit when attempting to flex it. Second, the flexor and extensor tendons should *not* be sutured together on the tip to avoid a quadriga deformity, whereby extension of uninjured digits is checked by inability to extend an injured digit.

the development of these late complications. In addition, several simple techniques can be used to treat a large number of functional complications.

Prevention of Skin and Joint Contractures

Prevention of contractures is an important consideration. When treating burns, early excision and grafting of deep second- and all third-degree burns has been shown to reduce contractures from secondary healing. Circumferential burns may need urgent escharotomy and/or fasciotomy to prevent ischemia of the deeper tissues, which can also contract. Full-thickness grafts on the digits and unmeshed (sheet) *thick* split-thickness grafts minimize the propensity for contraction. Avoidance of incisions that cross flexion creases perpendicularly is also a critical preventive measure. The use of Brunner incisions, mid-lateral incisions, or incisions that cross flexion creases at less than 90 degrees is almost always preferred.

Also very important is the use of splinting and therapy. Joints that are immobilized while soft tissues, burns, tendons, or fractures heal should be splinted in an intrinsic plus position with the wrist extended, metacarpophalangeal joints flexed, and interphalangeal joints extended. This position maximizes stretch on the collateral ligaments of each joint, thereby minimizing the development of joint contractures. Where a contracture has been present for some time, progressive splinting to increase the flexion or extension of a joint by passive stretching may be effective.

Early motion and therapy after any hand injury or surgery is a good rule of thumb. Aggressive and active motion is typically delayed for several weeks until full healing has occurred. But passive motion of all joints in the hand is important to prevent the development of joint contractures and tendon–soft-tissue adhesions, which may limit an otherwise perfect repair.

Treatment of Skin and Joint Contractures

For contractures that present late, the use of release and grafting or Z-plasties may be very effective, and easily performed in an outpatient setting. Where joint contractures have been long-standing, joint capsulotomy may also be necessary with release of the accessory collateral ligaments. Release and grafting is preferred for more severe soft tissue contractures. An incision is made transversely across the contracture, and the soft tissue freed either side. A graft is then sewn into the resulting defect and an extension splint placed. The same principles apply for this grafting in this technique as for burn resurfacing to minimize recontracture. Where a more minor contracture is present, this may be treated with a Z-plasty or a series of Z-plasties. In this technique, a longitudinal incision is made along the line of maximal tension, and Z-plasty flaps are created (usually with an angle around 60 degrees) and then transposed. This alters the line of maximal tension to a direction perpendicular to it.

Delayed Treatment of Nerve and Tendon Injuries

Delayed treatment of nerve and tendon injuries is typically complicated and beyond what can be accomplished without good hospital facilities. These structures will retract, leaving significant deficits that prevent primary apposition. Nerves may be grafted using the sural nerve or smaller nerve branches in the forearm. Tendons may be treated by grafting, but due to the nature of the pulley system over the flexors of the hand, this often confers the need for a two-stage repair in which a tunnel is made with a silastic spacer and a full-length tendon graft using the palmaris or plantaris is performed later. To avoid the need for multiple procedures in the developing world, tenodesis or tendon transfers may be a better option. Tenodesis is performed by joining a distal tendon stump to an adjacent tendon, and allows function of a tendon to be paired to another with a similar function. This is particularly useful with extensor tendons where isolated motion is less critical. Tendon transfers may also be used, by using redundant or less critical tendons to perform a new function. For example, the extensor indicis proprius tendon may be transferred to a distal extensor pollicis longus tendon for thumb extension. A variety of tendon transfers have also been described to compensate for loss of function of any of the major nerves of the forearm, utilizing various semi-redundant tendons, including the flexor carpi ulnaris, palmaris longus, and the flexor digitorum superficialis to the long and ring fingers.

Malunion and Nonunion

Treatment of malunions and nonunions in the forearm and hand can also be complex and difficult. The primary sequelae of these outcomes include pain, arthritis, and poor function (due to suboptimal positioning and tendon imbalances). Appropriate correction typically requires X-ray and/or fluoroscopy with methods for good bony fixation, such as K-wires or internal fixation. Correction of malunions can often be achieved using a wedge osteotomy with fixation. Correction of a nonunion must first address the reason for the nonunion (such as infection, poor vascularity, excessive motion, or tissue interposition), secondarily remove all callous and fibrous tissue, and finally ensure a repair with good fixation. Malunions or nonunions in the developing world that involve the small joints of the hand may be best treated with arthrodesis depending on the situation.

Treatment of hand injuries in LMICs can be challenging. Armed with a basic understanding of hand anatomy and applying the basic tenets of upper-extremity surgery, physicians can treat a variety of common pathologies that affect the hand. These include infections, burns, trauma, and the chronic conditions associated with untreated or poorly treated patients. It is important to consider amputation as a reconstructive procedure, not necessarily a failure. In situations of limited resources, a simple tourniquet and local anesthesia block of the hand can allow the surgeon to undertake substantial procedures with minimal discomfort.

Suggested Reading

Wolfe SW, Hotchkiss RN, Pedersen WC, et al. *Green's Operative Hand Surgery*. 6th ed. New York: Churchill Livingstone, 2010.

Mathes SJ (ed.). *Plastic surgery, Vol. 7: The Hand and Upper Limb, Part 2*. 2nd ed. Philadelphia: Saunders Elsevier, 2005.

Beasley RW. *Beasley's Surgery of the Hand*. New York: Thieme, 2003.

American Society of Surgery of the Hand. *The Hand: Primary Care of Common Problems*. 2nd ed. London: Churchill Livingstone, 1990.

Medical Council of Malawi data, January 2014.

Fielder S, Mpezeni S, Benjamin L, Cary I. Physiotherapy in Malawi—a step in the right direction. http://www.medcol.mw/mmj/?p=1545.

I Kakande, N. Mkandawire, MIW Thompson. A review of surgical capacity and surgical education programmes in the COSECSA region. A collaboration between the Royal College of Surgeons in Ireland (RCSI) and the College of Surgeons of East Central and Southern Africa (COSECSA). *East and Central Africa*.

COMMENTARY

Nyengo Mkandawire, Malawi

Hand injuries pose a major management challenge, particularly in LMICs where economies are predominantly agrarian based and most citizens rely on manual work for economic activities. In most LMICs nonphysician clinicians or nonsurgeons are the primary, or sometimes the only, providers of trauma care and thus need to be well versed in the basic care of hand injuries. All cadres of healthcare workers must therefore receive training and education, tailored to their level of clinical practice, to be able to understand anatomy of the hand, do a physical examination, be aware of conditions or injury mechanisms with potentially devastating outcomes, initiate management appropriate to level of training, appreciate the need of working with rehabilitation professionals to maximize outcome, and be advocates for measures to prevent hand injuries and adverse outcomes.

For instance, in a country like Malawi with a population of 14 million people against 32 general surgeons, 9 orthopedic surgeons, and 2 plastic surgeons, nonsurgeons treat the majority of hand injuries. Even after receiving initial treatment, aftercare and rehabilitation are seriously compromised due to the severe shortage of rehabilitation services with only 38 physiotherapists, 10 occupational therapists, and 76 diploma-level rehabilitation technicians for the entire population. With increasing industrialization, the incidence of hand injuries is increasing. A significant proportion of such industrial injuries would be prevented if working conditions and occupational health and safety regulations were enforced strictly.

Limited microbiology services and narrow choice of available antibiotics seriously affect the management and prevention of hand infections. Without microbiological assessment, the best management of infection is to do thorough and aggressive debridement and "blind and judicious" use of antibiotics using local knowledge of drug availability and sensitivities.

In LMICs, delayed presentation worsens outcomes and affects definitive treatment of hand conditions that would otherwise have a good outcome. Factors contributing to delayed presentation include: poor education and lack of knowledge on the part of both patients and healthcare providers, distance to healthcare facilities, lack of transport, traditional beliefs on disease causation and health-seeking behavior, and delays within the health system even if a patient presents early at the first point of contact. These same factors also affect patient follow-up and aftercare, thus compromising the outcome.

It is unlikely that high-end surgery such as revascularization of amputated digits, open reduction and internal fixation of fractures, or complex nerve and tendon reconstruction would be readily available outside a few specialist centers. It is therefore imperative to be able to offer definitive treatment that would minimize adverse outcomes—to provide the shortest possible treatment time while maximizing functional outcome. For example, amputation of a severely damaged digit may offer superior functional outcome compared to salvaging such a digit.

This chapter gives a broad overview of the challenges in the management of hand injuries in LMICs. It reviews basic anatomy of the hand and outlines clinical presentation and management of common hand conditions.

51

Lower Extremity Trauma

Paul T. Appleton
J. Kent Ellington
John Y. Kwon

Pelvic Fractures

Pelvic fractures occur as a result of high-energy trauma and often have associated injuries such as abdominal trauma and injuries to the genitourinary system. Pelvic fractures can be life-threatening due to significant trauma and associated blood loss. This is especially true with high-energy unstable pelvic fractures. These injuries are very complex, and in low- and middle-income countries (LMICs), limited resources may make it quite difficult to treat these injuries.

Anatomy

The pelvis is made up of three bones—the sacrum and two innominate bones, created by the fusion of the ilium, ischium, and pubis. The bony pelvis is held together by intricate ligamentous structures that contribute to the bony stability of the pelvis. Vascular, neurologic, and genitourinary structures sit within the pelvis and can be at high risk of injury during pelvic trauma.

History

Pelvic fractures can be as simple as an isolated pubic ramus fracture in an elderly person following a fall from standing to as complex as life-threatening injuries from a high-speed motorcycle accident.

Evaluation

Physical examination findings include:

1. Labral or scrotal swelling and ecchymosis
2. External rotation or shortening of one of the extremities
3. Pain with palpation or compression over the iliac wings

A thorough genitourinary exam is critical to rule out any fracture that may have penetrated the vaginal mucosa in females.

Diagnosis

An anterior-posterior (AP) S-ray of the pelvis is the most important initial image to obtain and can give an overview of the injury.

The initial AP view of the pelvis can quickly tell the magnitude of the injury and whether or not the fractured pelvis is inherently unstable. Initial findings on the AP pelvic view can guide the treating physician toward immediate steps such as placing a sheet or pelvic binder around the patient to help decrease pelvic volume and subsequently tamponade and slow acute blood loss. If X-rays are available, an inlet and outlet view may be helpful for understanding the pattern of injury. Computed tomography (CT) scan is also very helpful for operative planning but unlikely to be available in remote settings.

If X-ray is not available, one can suspect a displaced pelvic fracture if the patient has significant pain with palpation and pressure over the iliac crests, and on examination one or both of the legs are held in external rotation as the entire pelvis may have been forced open.

Classification

Pelvic injuries can be one of three main patterns: anterior/posterior compression (APC), lateral compression (LC), and vertical shear (VS) injuries.

APC injuries are comprised of three subgroups depending on the amount of anterior displacement of the pubic symphysis anteriorly and associated disruption of the posterior pelvic ring. Stable APC I injuries have little widening of the anterior pubic symphysis (less than 2 cm). APC II injuries have widening greater than 2cm, but the posterior sacroiliac ligaments are intact. APC III injuries are more significant in that both the anterior and posterior ligamentous or bony structures are disrupted and the pelvis is unstable (Figure 51.1). This is the most common severe injury seen in pedestrians. The so-called open-book pelvis injury can cause a significant amount of blood loss.

LC injuries are most commonly caused by a fall landing on one side. They can also be the result of a motor vehicle collision where the pedestrian is struck from the side. LC I injuries have a pubic ramus fracture and usually an associated impaction of the posterior sacroiliac (SI) joint (small buckle fracture). LC II injuries usually have a pubic ramus fracture anteriorly and an associated "crescent fracture" posteriorly. This is described as a fracture of the iliac wing just lateral to the SI joint. LC III fractures are usually the result of a crush injury where there is a compressive type of injury at one SI joint and an open-book

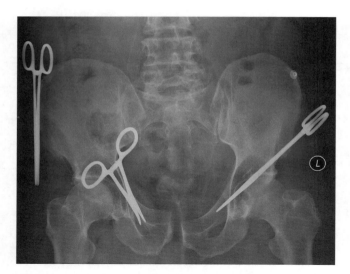

FIGURE 51.1 A typical APC III (open-book pelvic fracture). Image by Paul T. Appleton, J. Kent Ellington, and John T. Kwon.

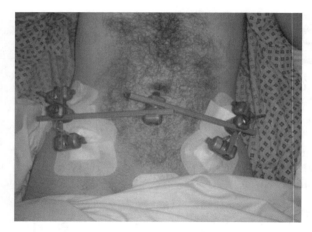

FIGURE 51.2 Clinical photograph of a two-pin external fixation construct. Image by Paul T. Appleton, J. Kent Ellington, and John T. Kwon.

injury pattern on the other with some widening and opening of the contralateral SI joint. The pelvic ring fracture is internally rotated on one side and externally rotated on the other.

VS injuries are usually the result of a fall and are severe injuries causing increased blood loss and concomitant vascular/neurologic injury. X-rays show vertical displacement of the hemipelvis, often with complete dislocation of the SI joint.

Treatment

Initial treatment depends on the injury pattern. APC II or III injuries, once diagnosed, can be treated with a sheet wrapped around the patient's sacrum and pelvis. This can help decrease pelvic volume and subsequently blood loss. If equipment is available for placing an external fixator on the pelvis, following sheet stabilization, this can be considered for APC II and III type injuries. External fixator pins should be placed into the iliac wings and then an anterior bar connected over the abdomen once the iliac wings have been compressed (Figure 51.2). An external fixator can be placed without radiography in the operating room. If resources are available, these patients should be referred into a tertiary care facility where they can undergo definitive treatment of their injuries. If this is not an option, they should remain non–weight-bearing on the injured side for 12 weeks. Patients can use crutches allowing weight bearing on the unaffected side. An external fixator should remain in place for 3 months.

If no surgical equipment is available, treatment options include keeping the patient on bed rest with a sheet or pelvic binder around the pelvis. One must be very cautious if a sheet is to remain in place for more than a couple of hours and be diligent to inspect the skin under the sheet or binder for any signs of pressure ulcers.

Simple LC I fractures can be treated with early mobilization where weight bearing is permitted. More severe type II and III injuries will need their weight bearing limited on the side of the injury. If the affected hemipelvis is significantly displaced, an external fixator can be placed into the iliac wings and manipulation attempted.

VS injuries can be treated with traction to try to reduce the pelvic dislocation. A traction pin can be placed in the femur on the affected side, and this may help to reduce the dislocation. If

no further resources are available, patients should be left in traction for 8–12 weeks. Weekly X-rays should be obtained during the first month to assess the position of the pelvis under traction. If able to reduce the pelvis with traction, an external fixator can be placed in the iliac crests to allow stabilization to let the patient get out of bed and off traction.

Fractures of the Acetabulum

Fractures of the acetabulum (hip socket) generally occur in younger patients as the result of motor vehicle collisions. Hip dislocations can often occur with acetabulum fractures, and it is important to make this diagnosis early as early hip reduction can be critical for long-term outcomes/function. Fractures of the acetabulum are some of the most difficult fractures to treat operatively, and only specialists familiar with this surgery and the anatomy of the pelvis should attempt any surgical repair.

Evaluation

Physical exam will likely show increased pain with any motion of the hip. If there is an associated dislocation, the extremity is usually shortened and internally rotated. Physical examination should include careful inspection of the remainder of the extremity as there can be a high association of knee and foot and ankle injuries. A neurovascular examination is also important with injuries to the sciatic nerve, which is the most common associated neurologic injury due to the proximity of the sciatic nerve to the posterior wall of the acetabulum. Patients with injuries to the nerve will likely lack the ability to extend their great toe or dorsiflex the ankle.

Diagnosis

X-rays are critical for this diagnosis and can often be made on a simple AP view of the pelvis. It is imperative to rule out a posterior hip dislocation associated with the fracture, and a lateral view of the hip may be essential. The fracture classification of acetabular fractures is complex and beyond the scope of this book. The most important determinate of outcome is the concentric reduction of the hip in the acetabulum to prevent debilitating arthritis.

Treatment

Fractures of the acetabulum that are stable and minimally or non-displaced can be treated with protective weight bearing for 12 weeks. If the fracture is associated with a dislocation and the hip and is unstable, it is best treated at a specialist facility for definitive care. If definitive operative treatment is not available, patients should be placed in traction for 12 weeks and then begin gradual weight bearing. If the hip is not dislocated but the fracture is displaced, disrupting the acetabular surface, the ideal treatment would again be a referral to someone experienced in managing these injuries. In reality, if limited resources are available, traction for 8–12 weeks will help unload the pressure on the acetabulum, allowing it to heal without further displacement. It may be possible to reduce some fractures with traction, and weekly X-rays should be obtained to assess the position of the fracture during traction.

Hip Dislocations

Hip dislocations are usually the result of high-energy trauma and were discussed in the acetabular fracture section. However, occasionally a patient can have a hip dislocation without an associated acetabular fracture. It is important to recognize these injuries quickly as interventions can prevent lifelong disability. The vast majority of hip dislocations are posterior; however, anterior dislocations can occur as well.

Evaluation

The affected leg is usually shortened, flexed slightly at the hip, and internally rotated if a posterior dislocation. For anterior dislocation the hip is more likely to be slightly extended with the leg shortened and externally rotated. A thorough neurologic exam is imperative. It is also important to be aware of associated injuries on the same limb.

Diagnosis

On examination the affected extremity is usually shortened and externally rotated. X-rays of the hip will usually show the dislocation; however, it can be as subtle as a nonconcentric hip seen on the plain films. Always compare the contra-lateral hip on the AP of the pelvis for reference.

Treatment

Hip dislocations should be reduced as soon as possible with conscious sedation. Posterior dislocations can be reduced by flexing the hip to 90 degrees and pulling upward, while internally rotating the hip. Anterior dislocations are reduced by gently abducting the hip, pulling traction and internally rotating the leg. Once reduction is confirmed by X-rays, patients should observe protected weight bearing (partial weight bearing—about 30–40 pounds of pressure maximum) for 3–4 weeks until their pain is improved. It is critical to have adequate anesthesia before attempting a closed reduction as pain and muscle spasm can prevent successful reduction of the hip joint.

Fractures of the Proximal Femur (Hip)

Hip fractures in general occur in an elderly population but can also be the result of high-speed motor vehicle accidents or falls. Hip fractures can be divided into three main categories based on the location of the fracture. These include intracapsular, intertrochanteric, and subtrochanteric fractures of the hip. The importance of the separate locations of hip fractures is mainly due to the blood supply to the hip. Intracapsular fractures of the hip that are displaced have likely disrupted the blood supply to the hip, and if not reduced and pinned, will ultimately go on to avascular necrosis (AVN). Intertrochanteric and subtrochanteric hip fractures usually do not have the blood supply disrupted and can be expected to heal even if left in traction.

Evaluation

Patients will usually have significant pain with any motion of the hip, and the extremity is usually shortened and externally rotated. They usually cannot bear weight. Occasionally, patients may have a valgus impacted or nondisplaced hip fracture, which can be difficult to detect on suboptimal X-rays (Figure 51.4). They may still be able to bear weight, although with a limp and some discomfort.

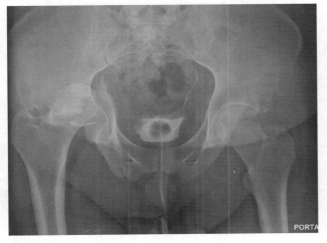

FIGURE 51.3 An acetabulum fracture with hip dislocation. Image by Paul T. Appleton, J. Kent Ellington, and John T. Kwon.

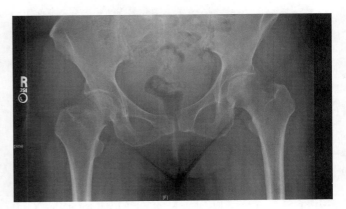

FIGURE 51.4 A valgus impacted femoral neck fracture. These are usually stable and have a low incidence of AVN. Image by Paul T. Appleton, J. Kent Ellington, and John T. Kwon.

Diagnosis

X-rays of the hip are diagnostic and important in determining treatment options and urgency. A lateral X-ray of the affected hip is also critical for evaluating femoral neck fractures to determine if the fracture is displaced and needs a formal open reduction versus a partial hip replacement.

Treatment

Treatment is variable based on the location of the hip fracture and will be discussed in the sections that follow based on the type of hip fracture.

Intracapsular fractures involve the femoral neck and can be either nondisplaced or displaced, which is important for determining treatment methods. Intracapsular hip fractures that are displaced have usually disrupted the blood supply to the femoral head and there is a high incidence of avascular necrosis to the hip. Replacing the femoral head with prosthesis is the preferred treatment in elderly patients (Figure 51.5). In young patients it is worth trying to reduce the fracture urgently and pinning it with screws or wires (Figure 51.6A and Figure 51.6B). If no operative options are available, nondisplaced femoral neck fractures should be treated with protected weight bearing for 12 weeks. Patients should be instructed on touch weight bearing—no more than 20 pounds of pressure on the leg—or the equivalent of as if they were walking on an eggshell and trying not to crush it. If the fracture is displaced and no operative intervention is possible, traction can be applied to the affected extremity for 4–6 weeks to allow pain to subside and some initial healing to take place.

In regard to extra-capsular hip fractures, fractures that are intertrochanteric or subtrochanteric should be treated with internal fixation using either an intramedullary rod or hip screw if available (Figure 51.7A and Figure 51.7B). These should be

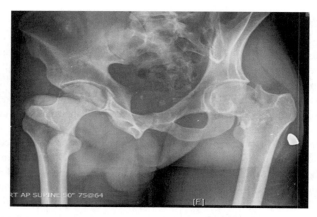

FIGURE 51.6A AP and view of a displaced femoral neck fracture in a younger patient from a gunshot. Image by Paul T. Appleton, J. Kent Ellington, and John T. Kwon.

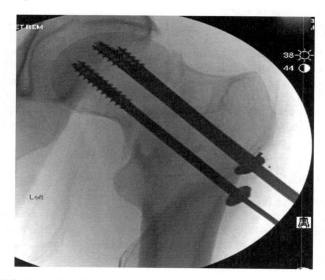

FIGURE 51.6B If possible, these should be reduced and treated with three cannulated screws (b). Image by Paul T. Appleton, J. Kent Ellington, and John T. Kwon.

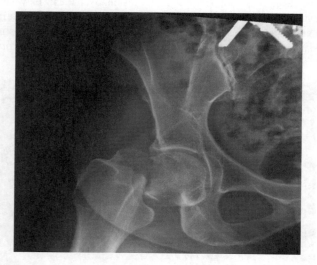

FIGURE 51.5 AP and lateral views of a displaced femoral neck fracture. Given the high risk of AVN, a hemiarthroplasty should be done for these injuries if resources are available. Image by Paul T. Appleton, J. Kent Ellington, and John T. Kwon.

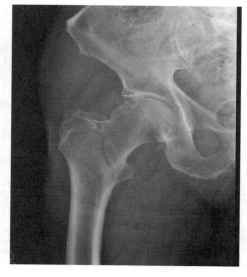

FIGURE 51.7A An intertrochanteric hip fracture. Image by Paul T. Appleton, J. Kent Ellington, and John T. Kwon.

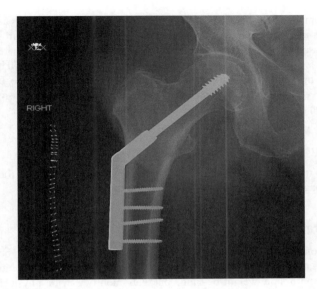

FIGURE 51.7B The intertrochanteric hip fracture treated with a sliding hip screw. Image by Paul T. Appleton, J. Kent Ellington, and John T. Kwon.

referred to tertiary facilities if resources are not available. If surgical intervention is not an option, traction should be applied for up to 8–12 weeks before mobilization has been started. If possible, weekly X-rays should be obtained to determine the position of the fracture as it is healing. Traction can be adjusted by adding or subtracting weight to improve the alignment. Be cognizant of complications for long-term traction, including deep venous thrombosis and pressure sores.

Femoral Shaft Fractures

Femoral shaft fractures are usually the result of high-energy trauma; however, they are becoming more common in low-energy accidents with the elderly population. If associated with a high-energy mechanism, one must be prudent in initial management of the patient, including fluid resuscitation, as a high volume of blood loss can occur with these injuries.

Evaluation

It is usually fairly obvious when a patient has a femur fracture as there is considerable pain and deformity given the magnitude of the injury. The affected limb will be shortened and malrotated, and there is often significant swelling in the thigh. A thorough neurovascular examination should be performed, keeping in mind that compartment syndrome can occur with this injury.

Diagnosis

If possible, X-rays should be obtained to confirm the diagnosis. It is important to try to include imaging of the ipsilateral hip as there is a high incidence of hip fractures associated with femoral shaft fractures. Patients should be splinted if possible with a long posterior splint extending from the hip joint and including the foot. Gentle traction can be pulled on the extremity as plaster hardens with the intent of decreasing some of the shortening.

Treatment

It is very difficult to treat femoral shaft fractures nonoperatively. Invariably, there is significant shortening and should the femur heal with this degree of shortening, permanent disability may result. If operating facilities are not present, traction can be utilized trying to hold the femur out to length while it heals to prevent a significant shortening deformity. Traction can be placed through a pin in the supracondylar region and just remain for 12 weeks, checking X-rays on a weekly interval and allowing the chance to adjust traction to help correct angulation. This is a very labor-intensive process, but if no other resources are available, this is a better option than casting. External fixators can also be placed to allow patients the opportunity to remain somewhat mobile rather than being confined to bed rest. There is also a much lower incidence of infection with external fixator placement than with open reduction internal fixation or placement of an intramedullary nail. Two to three pins should be place proximal to the fracture and two to three below the fracture and a bar placed between the pins, tightened after appropriate traction has been applied. One can use the contralateral leg to assess rotation and length while adjusting the external fixator. If available, internal fixation is the treatment of choice. If intra-operative fluoroscopy is not available, plating of the fracture is a good option assuming strict sterile techniques can be maintained, as an infection can be a devastating complication (Figure 51.8). The gold standard treatment for femur fractures remains intramedullary

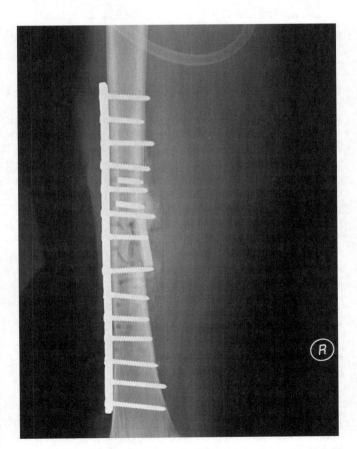

FIGURE 51.8 Plating of a femoral shaft fracture. Image by Paul T. Appleton, J. Kent Ellington, and John T. Kwon.

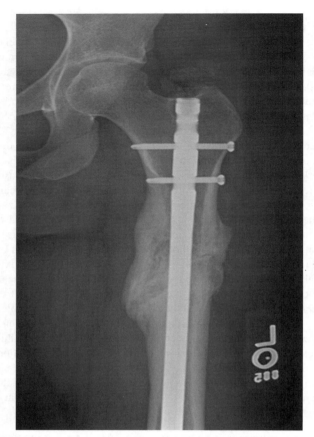

FIGURE 51.9 An intramedullary rod placed for treating a femoral shaft fracture. Image by Paul T. Appleton, J. Kent Ellington, and John T. Kwon.

fixation; however, significant resources must be available including the intramedullary devices and intra-operative fluoroscopy (Figure 51.9). Alternatively, if fluoroscopy is not available the SIGN nail is a viable option if the surgeon is familiar with the equipment and technique. Intramedullary implants can be placed in the femur after the fracture site is opened and the femoral canal hand reamed. This device allows locking of the nail to add stability to the construct without fluoroscopy. If a referral center is available, initial stabilization with a splint or skeletal traction followed by transfer is the preferred treatment algorithm.

Supracondylar Femur Fractures

Supracondylar femur fractures are fractures that occur in the femur just above or involving the knee joint. These fractures can be difficult to treat as any malreduction of the distal femoral joint surface can result in significant disabling arthritis and malalignment of the limb.

Evaluation

Like femoral shaft fractures, supracondylar femur fractures can be associated with high-energy mechanism. There is usually significant pain, swelling, and deformity of the limb. Fractures of the supracondylar area can be associated with similar deformity as femoral shaft fractures on examination. Again, a thorough neurovascular exam is important upon first encounter. In addition, there is less muscle and soft tissue covering the bone at this region, and it is important to look for open wounds caused by protruding bone. It is equally important to assess for injuries to the extensor mechanism (quadriceps tendon, patella, and patella tendon) around the knee.

Diagnosis

X-rays of the knee and femur are the mainstay to making the diagnosis of a supracondylar femur fracture (Figure 51.10).

Treatment

Nondisplaced fractures of the supracondylar femur can be treated in a cast or knee brace for 8–12 weeks. Patients should remain non–weight-bearing, but can mobilize with physical therapy once the pain has subsided. Patients should limit range of motion of the knee for the first month, but after initial healing has occurred, gentle range of motion of the knee may be commenced, although weight bearing should be limited for 3 months. Displaced fractures are more difficult to manage and, like femur fractures, one should consider local resources as operative treatment is advisable, if possible. If the fracture will be managed at a local facility and operative intervention is not an option, skeletal traction is the first treatment option. Traction pins should be placed in the tibia to avoid introducing a potential infectious source to the supracondylar area. Traction pins can be placed at the level of the tibial tubercle. Weekly X-rays of the distal femur should be obtained to assess alignment and allow adjustment of traction. While in traction, patients should not neglect the opportunity to do physical therapy in the form of quadriceps contraction as this will help maintain some muscle bulk/function once they are ready to commence ambulation. After 8 weeks, traction can be discontinued and patients can start range of motion of the knee. Weight bearing should be restricted for 12 weeks. If the resources are available, external fixation is also a viable option. This allows patients the opportunity to ambulate with crutches and not be restricted to bed rest as is the case with traction.

Because these fractures are so close to the joint, it is necessary to place a spanning external fixator across the knee with pins in the femur and pins in the tibia. External fixators should be left in place for 8–12 weeks followed by removal and placement in a knee brace. Full weight bearing can be started at 3 months, and range of motion of the knee should commence at 8 weeks. Definitive treatment of displaced supracondylar femur fractures involves external fixation if resources are available (Figure 51.11). Given the difficulty in managing these fractures nonoperatively, one should consider a referral to an appropriate facility if possible, especially in younger patients.

Patella Fractures

Fractures of the patella are usually the result of a direct blow or fall on the patella. Significant deforming forces are present

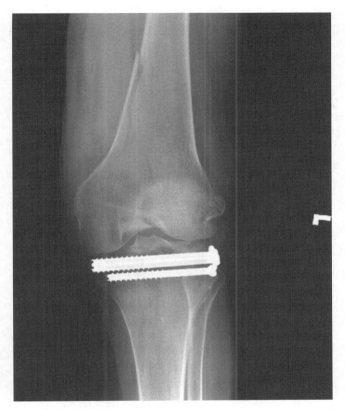

FIGURE 51.10 A supracondylar femur fracture. Image by Paul T. Appleton, J. Kent Ellington, and John T. Kwon.

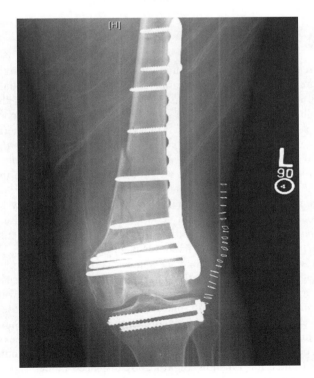

FIGURE 51.11 A supracondylar femur fracture treated with plates and screws. Image by Paul T. Appleton, J. Kent Ellington, and John T. Kwon.

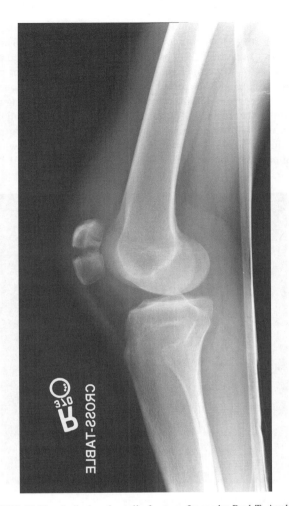

FIGURE 51.12 A displaced patella fracture. Image by Paul T. Appleton, J. Kent Ellington, and John T. Kwon.

around the patella, including the quadriceps (pulling proximally) and patella (pulling distally) tendons. The patella is critical in providing the link between these tendons and allowing active extension of the knee.

Evaluation

Patients are usually tender right over the patella, and there is often associated swelling and ecchymosis. Usually, they are unable to hold the knee extended. Often, there is a palpable step-off felt on the patella due to the displacement of the fracture.

Diagnosis

X-rays of the knee are diagnostic if available. Figure 51.12 shows a displaced patella fracture.

Treatment

Many patella fractures can be treated nonoperatively. If the fracture is nondisplaced or minimally displaced, a long leg cast that ends just short of the ankle is adequate to prevent knee flexion. The advantage to this injury as compared to many other lower extremity fractures is that patients can bear weight immediately with no consequence on fracture healing. The cast should be worn for 4–6 weeks and then patients can begin early mobilization with knee range of motion. Displaced patella fractures in young people should be treated operatively if possible. Simple tension band constructs with wires can be created to hold fractures in position during healing. Although helpful, these can be done without intra-operative fluoroscopy (Figure 51.13A and Figure 51.13B).

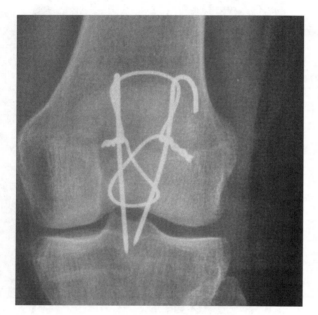

FIGURE 51.13A　A tension band construct using K-wires and simple wire can also be used to effectively treat patella fractures. Image by Paul T. Appleton, J. Kent Ellington, and John T. Kwon.

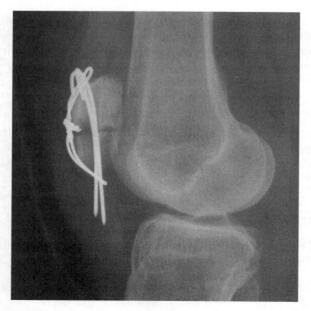

FIGURE 51.13B　A tension band construct using K-wires and simple wire can also be used to effectively treat patella fractures. Image by Paul T. Appleton, J. Kent Ellington, and John T. Kwon.

One should focus on maintaining quadriceps strengthening exercises early and allow range of motion at 4 weeks. Full weight bearing should be permitted.

Tibial Plateau Fractures

Fractures of the proximal tibia (plateau) can range from non-displaced/minimally displaced fractures of the joint surface to high-energy significantly displaced injuries. Some joint depression or displacement can be tolerated reasonably well; however, knee stability and associated ligamentous injuries are almost as important as the fracture.

Evaluation

Like supracondylar femur fractures, tibial plateau fractures can be associated with significant pain and deformity of the extremity, particularly in high-energy injuries. Compartment syndrome is not uncommon, and increased swelling and pain should be monitored closely. Open fractures can also occur frequently in higher energy tibial plateau fractures, and one must do a thorough examination of the skin and soft tissues in the setting of a plateau fracture.

Diagnosis

An X-ray of the knee is usually diagnostic. Subtle abnormalities should be looked for, including joint depression, which is most commonly on the lateral side of the knee joint.

Treatment

Treatment of non- or minimally displaced tibial plateau fractures can be a cast or knee immobilizer. Weight bearing should be restricted for 8–12 weeks depending on the severity of the injury. Stability of the knee should be assessed once pain control will allow examination. If there is depression on the lateral joint surface, even up to 2 cm can be tolerated as long as the knee is not unstable. Stability can be assessed by putting valgus stress on the knee (moving the foot laterally in relation to the knee). If there is not significant instability (more than 10 degrees as compared to the uninjured side), the fracture can likely be treated nonoperatively with good success. Displaced proximal tibia fractures—especially those that are higher energy—should be treated with operative fixation. Spanning external fixators, as described in the supracondylar femur section, can be effective (Figures 51.14 and 51.15). By pulling the limb out to appropriate length and alignment, good results can be achieved even with limited resources. Again, one must be cognizant of increased swelling and compartment syndrome that can develop in these injuries. External fixators should be left in place for 8–12 weeks, depending on severity of the injury, and weight bearing should be limited for 3 months. Significantly displaced injures should be referred to a facility capable of undertaking internal fixation if possible.

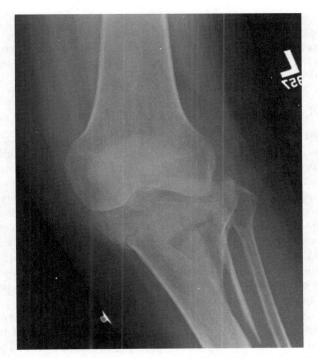

FIGURE 51.14 A tibial plateau fracture with some lateral joint line depression. Image by Paul T. Appleton, J. Kent Ellington, and John T. Kwon.

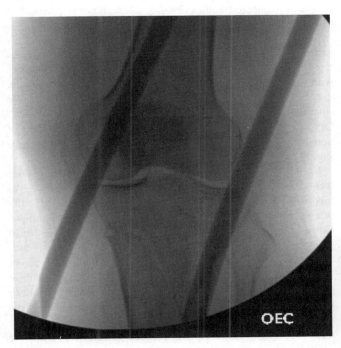

FIGURE 51.15 AP image following external fixator placement. Image by Paul T. Appleton, J. Kent Ellington, and John T. Kwon.

Tibia Shaft Fractures

Fractures of the tibia are often associated with high-energy mechanisms including road traffic crashes and falls from height. Because there is little soft tissue coverage over the tibia, these can often be open fractures where the bone comes through the skin.

In addition, compartment syndrome can be associated with these fractures, and it is prudent to be aware of this associated diagnosis.

Evaluation

On physical examination, there may be an obvious deformity in addition to soft tissue swelling. Compartment syndrome is not uncommon and typically presents as pain out of proportion to examination, swelling, and pain with passive motion of the toes or ankle. If compartment syndrome is present for long enough, patients may develop decreased sensation in the foot (particularly in the first web space on the top of the foot) where the deep peroneal nerve is often affected by swelling in the anterior muscle compartment of the tibia.

Diagnosis

X-rays of the tibia are diagnostic, but if not available, the pain and obvious deformity of the bone in its subcutaneous location are adequate. It is important to determine that the knee joint is not involved and that the fracture mainly involves the tibial shaft. Figure 51.16 shows a minimally displaced tibia shaft fracture.

Treatment

Open fractures should be treated with debridement and antibiotic prophylaxis if possible. Initial splinting may help with pain control. Many tibia fractures can be treated nonoperatively assuming one watches out for associated compartment syndrome. Tibia shaft fractures that do not involve the joint surface can be treated in a long leg cast for 6 weeks followed by a short leg cast for an additional 2–3 months. Weight bearing in the short leg cast can begin as pain permits. Casts can usually be discontinued at 3–4 months depending on healing (Figure 51.17). For inherently unstable fractures (significant angulation and inability to hold in a reasonable position) and those with compartment syndrome where casting would preclude close wound observation, external fixation is also an option. Two pins should be placed proximal and distal to the fracture and once alignment restored, the external fixator bars tightened. External fixators should remain in place for 2–3 months followed by a short leg–walking cast until

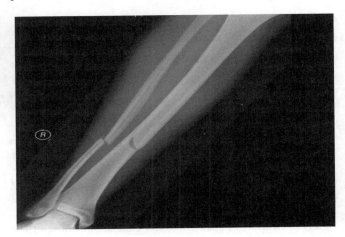

FIGURE 51.16 A minimally displaced tibia/fibula fracture. Image by Paul T. Appleton, J. Kent Ellington, and John T. Kwon.

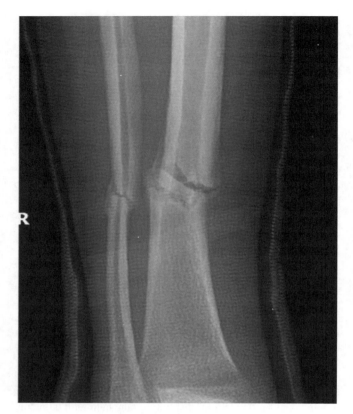

FIGURE 51.17 Healing of a tibia fracture in a cast after 3 months. Image by Paul T. Appleton, J. Kent Ellington, and John T. Kwon.

pain-free weight bearing is achieved. Plating of tibia fractures is discouraged as the poor soft-tissue coverage over this subcutaneous bone causes an unacceptably high complication rate. For unstable fractures where casting and/or external fixation is not an option, a referral to a tertiary care facility (if available) for intramedullary nailing should be considered. Similar to managing femur fractures, the SIGN nail is a viable option for fixing tibia shaft fractures assuming the surgeon is familiar with this technique. Most fractures of the tibia shaft can be treated successfully in remote hospitals where adequate cast material or external fixators are available.

Foot and Ankle Trauma

Lower extremity trauma, whether from high-energy mechanisms or from those seemingly more benign, can be a significant cause of impairment and disability. Often due to motor vehicle crashes, falls from height, or crush injuries, many foot and ankle injuries can be associated with more proximal skeletal injuries.

Aside from the injury itself, foot and ankle trauma causes significant disability due to affecting the use of the entire extremity via limiting weight bearing. This can affect a patient's ability to mobilize and causes management problems for the treating physician as the patient may need transportation for additional or definitive care.

There exists a wide spectrum of foot and ankle injuries, from those that may be limb- and life-threatening to those that result in little long-term disability. However, given the functional

requirements and daily demands placed on the lower extremity, injuries to the foot and ankle can severely impact a patient's ability to not only perform activities of daily living but also to make a living. This section is dedicated to the acute care of foot and ankle trauma to hopefully maximize your patients' outcomes.

Pilon Fractures

Pilon means "to ram or hammer" in French. Pilon fractures are an uncommon injury resulting in impaction injury to the articular surface of the distal tibia (plafond) (Figure 51.18). Pilon fractures can occur from either low- or high-energy mechanisms. Open fractures are more common in this fracture type due to the amount of energy transmitted to create the fracture and the thin soft-tissue envelope. The fibula is often intact. Associated injuries are common, with 30% of patients having ipsilateral injuries and 10% having bilateral injuries. Spine fractures can also occur and should be diligently evaluated. Compartment syndrome may develop after pilon fractures, and close monitoring is imperative. Lastly, neurovascular injuries can occur with these significant injuries.

A thorough evaluation of the skin for swelling, abrasions, and open fractures is necessary. Compartment syndrome must be ruled out and carefully monitored during the first 24 hours. The standard neurovascular exam is also performed. X-rays are performed of the ankle (anterior-posterior, mortise, lateral) and tibia (anterior-posterior, lateral). Often, a traction view of the ankle will help delineate fracture lines. A CT scan is very helpful, if available, to help guide preoperative surgical planning.

After examination and imaging, malaligned fracture patterns or fractures with shortening should be reduced and an external fixator should be applied. With highly comminuted fractures with significant soft-tissue injury, simple cast immobilization may be inadequate to stabilize the extremity—although all pilon fractures can be immobilized temporarily with splint placement. Open fractures should be urgently irrigated and debrided of nonviable tissue and bone. Antibiotics and tetanus prophylaxis should be administered upon presentation.

Unlike tibial shaft fractures, pilon fractures often require formal open reduction and internal fixation (ORIF) due to involvement of the distal tibial articular surface and difficulty in controlling for malalignment using nonoperative technique. However, given the high-energy mechanism leading to most pilon fractures, immediate ORIF is prohibitive as there is usually significant soft-tissue swelling. Due to a high incidence of wound healing problems with acute definitive fixation of most pilon fractures, spanning external fixation is recommended until swelling abates in 1–2 weeks' time (Figure 51.19). ORIF of the fibula can be performed simultaneously with external fixation as it restores length; however, skin incision placement needs to be carefully planned as not to interfere with future skin incisions. Any compromise in the soft-tissue envelope should preclude simultaneous fibula fixation. It is preferable to keep at least 8 cm between skin incisions to prevent vascular compromise to the skin bridge. Ultimately, patients should undergo ORIF in a staged fashion when soft-tissue swelling has resolved.

Fractures with minimal displacement can be closed reduced and placed into a well-padded splint with the ankle at a resting position. Although keeping the ankle at 90 degrees is often advocated to prevent Achilles contractures, in the trauma setting

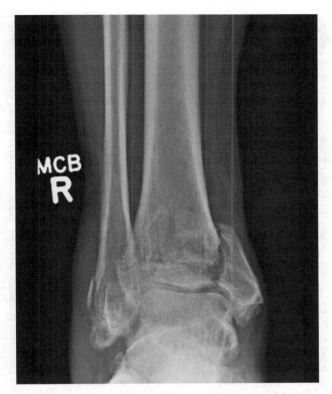

FIGURE 51.18 Pilon fracture showing intra-articular extension into the plafond. Image by Paul T. Appleton, J. Kent Ellington, and John T. Kwon.

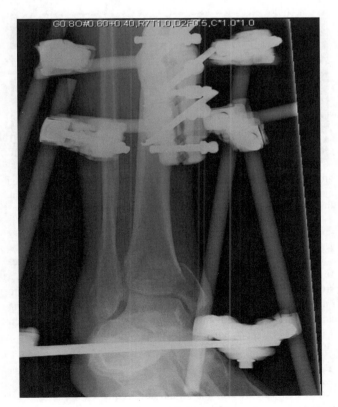

FIGURE 51.19 Placement of spanning external fixator for acute stabilization of a pilon fracture. Image by Paul T. Appleton, J. Kent Ellington, and John T. Kwon.

the ankle should be splinted in a position to best protect soft tissues and maintain vascularity as forcibly splinting the ankle at 90 degrees can cause increased fracture displacement, skin tenting, or neurovascular compromise. Regardless, strict elevation and non–weight bearing are imperative until ORIF is suitable. Patients should be checked every week, along with interval X-rays until ORIF is performed.

Infection and wound dehiscence are feared and serious complications may arise following pilon fractures. These can be reduced with thoughtful management of pilon fractures. ORIF is frequently delayed 2–3 weeks. Strict elevation and non–weight bearing is critical. Osseous and soft-tissue stabilization with either splinting or external fixation should be performed as soon as possible. Open fractures increase the incidence of soft-tissue compromise and infection. This can ultimately lead to amputation if severe.

Long-term complications are largely due to posttraumatic arthritis, pain, stiffness, and deformity. Not infrequently, these patients are converted to an ankle arthrodesis if pain is significant.

Ankle Fractures

The World Health Organization (WHO) declared the years 2000–2010 the bone and joint decade, largely due to the burden of musculoskeletal disease worldwide. A large percentage of this disease is from fractures and its sequelae. Ankle fractures are typically due to a rotatory deforming force applied to either a supinated or pronated foot, although a combined mechanism with associated axial load does occur. Ankle fractures are categorized into stable and unstable injuries. Stable injuries can be managed nonoperatively, whereas unstable injuries require ORIF.

Ankle fractures can occur from either low- or high-energy mechanisms. Careful examination of the foot and lower leg will help in an accurate diagnosis. A thorough evaluation of the skin for swelling, abrasions, and open fractures is necessary. The standard neurovascular exam is also performed. It is important to also palpate the proximal fibular for pain (this may suggest a Maisonneuve fracture). An open fracture should be irrigated and debrided of nonviable tissue and contamination urgently. Intravenous (IV) antibiotics and tetanus prophylaxis should be administered immediately. The standard three views of the ankle should be obtained non–weight bearing (AP view, mortis view, lateral view). If there is concern for a more proximal injury, proximal tibia/fibula X-rays are obtained. Associated injuries include cartilage abrasions, fractures, and osteochondritis dissecans (OCDs) to either the talus and/or tibial plafond and syndesmotic disruption.

After the examination and imaging, the patient should be placed into a well-padded splint. A closed reduction/manipulation may need to be performed and a three-point bend may need to be applied to maintain the reduction of an unstable ankle fracture and/or dislocation. Longitudinal traction is also necessary. Often the talus translates laterally and follows the fibula. Thus, a hand on the medial leg and a hand on the lateral ankle will assist in pushing the talus back under the tibia. Likewise, with a large associated posterior malleolus fracture, the talus translates posteriorly. The talus displaces posteriorly because of the loss of the bony support due to the posterior malleolus fracture. In this instance, the ankle may need to be plantarflexed approximately

30 degrees to keep the talus under the tibia. If the ankle is too unstable to be treated with splinting, a spanning external fixator may be required.

After reduction and splinting, ankle fractures should be seen within 5–7 days to evaluate for the need to change the splint to a cast and to monitor for displacement. Displacement in the splint is possible, and this could lead to tenting of the skin and full-thickness loss, especially medially. If severe, this can lead to a severe complication, which may lead to amputation if advanced soft-tissue coverage techniques are not available (free-flap tissue transfer).

Isolated Malleolar Fractures

Stable injuries are defined by a fracture of one side of the ankle. An isolated lateral malleolus fracture, isolated medial malleolus fracture, or isolated posterior malleolus can often be managed successfully with a non–weight-bearing cast for 6 weeks. Fibula fractures can be classified by the Danis-Weber classification based on the level of the fracture in relation to the syndesmosis. Weber A fractures are infra-syndesmotic, Weber B fractures are at the level of the syndesmosis, and Weber C fractures are supra-syndesmotic. All isolated lateral malleolus fractures below the level of the ankle joint (Weber A) can be managed with surgeon preference (brace, boot, cast) and weight bearing as tolerated.

However, there are times when isolated lateral malleolar fractures will require ORIF. Weber B ankle fractures are due to supination-external rotation forces. This is due to the fact that although only the lateral malleolus is fractured, an unstable injury results due to the deltoid ligament medially being torn, leading to a rotationally unstable injury pattern. These are called bimalleolar-equivalent injuries (Figure 51.20). This is commonly missed and can lead to displacement, arthritis, and deformity. Weekly X-rays are obtained to assess for displacement, which would require ORIF.

Weber C fractures are by definition unstable and typically require ORIF. These are fractures that occur above the ankle joint line and disrupt the syndesmosis, leading to instability.

Isolated medial malleolar fractures can at times be managed nonoperatively in a cast and non–weight bearing. If the fracture is nondisplaced or minimally displaced, it can be watched with interval X-rays to ensure that it does not displace. It is recommended to obtain X-rays every week for the first 2–3 weeks, then every 2–3 weeks until it has healed. There is a 10% rate of nonunion with nonoperative management of medial malleolus fracture, but the majority of those patients are asymptomatic.

Isolated posterior malleolar fractures are rare and can frequently be treated nonoperatively. If the fracture is less than 25% of the joint and is not displaced more than 2 mm, this can be treated in a non–weight-bearing cast for 6 weeks. ORIF may require anterior to posterior directed screws after the posterior malleolus is reduced, or may require a direct posterior approach between the peroneals and flexor hallucis longus and application of a buttress plate.

Bimalleolar and Trimalleolar Ankle Fractures

These types of ankle fractures always require surgery because they are unstable injury patterns. As little as 1 mm of displacement leads to an approximately 40% increase in talar contact

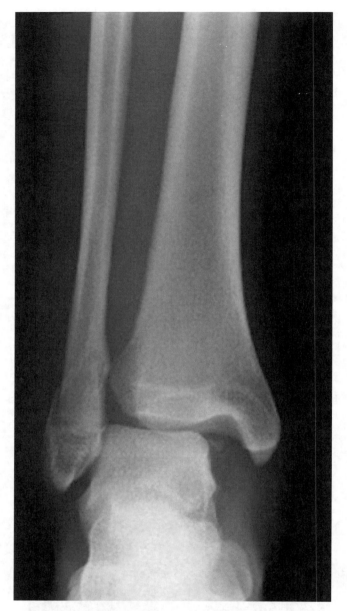

FIGURE 51.20 Bimalleolar equivalent ankle fracture with increased medial clear space indicating deltoid injury and unstable fracture pattern. Image by Paul T. Appleton, J. Kent Ellington, and John T. Kwon.

forces, leading to degenerative changes over time. Again, a careful examination and reduction and splinting are performed in a similar manner as above. Postreduction films are necessary to ensure proper alignment. Patients are kept non–weight bearing and ORIF is delayed until soft-tissues are appropriate, often within several days, but within 2 weeks if possible.

Ankle Dislocations

Ankle dislocations are uncommon and frequently are associated with at least one fracture of the ankle. These injury patterns, even in the low-energy setting, are frequently open and require urgent debridement and reduction. Often, the fractures can be repaired in the same setting, but repair should be delayed if the wound is grossly contaminated. If, after closed or open reduction with or without ORIF, the ankle is still unstable, an external fixator should also be applied. If it is purely an ankle dislocation (without fracture), the ankle should be reduced and casted when swelling has decreased. These injuries should be reduced quickly, as skin tenting and compromise is common. Patients should be made non–weight bearing. The cast should be removed in 4 weeks and motion allowed. At times, a closed reduction is not possible. This is due to anatomic blocks to reduction, which may necessitate an open reduction. Most commonly, the tibialis anterior tendon or posterior tibialis tendon can be entrapped and block reduction, but other structures around the ankle can also block reduction.

Talus Fractures

Talus fractures are uncommon and comprise approximately 0.85%–1% of all fractures (Figure 51.21). They can be from high-energy mechanisms or from lower energy twisting mechanisms. High-energy mechanisms often result in talar neck fractures with associated periarticular fracture-dislocations. These can be limb threatening as there is often associated neurovascular compromise to the foot, significant soft-tissue compromise, and a higher incidence of open fractures. As the talus and its articulations account for more than 90% of the motion of the foot and

ankle, these injuries can result in significant long-term disability if not treated appropriately.

The talus is mainly covered by articular cartilage and has a tenous blood supply. Fracture-dislocations can result in vascular compromise by disrupting the microcirculation or by causing intrinsic occlusion of the major vascular structures by bony displacement. AVN is a long-term potential complication.

Injury is often from a high-energy mechanism. Talus fractures are often associated with dislocations of the surrounding joints such as the tibiotalar, subtalar, and talonavicular joints. This can result in rotation of the talar body around an intact deltoid ligament, causing the body to rest between the posterior aspect of the medial malleolus and Achilles tendon. Or, a fracture-dislocation of the talar head/neck can cause dorsal displacement threatening the dorsalis pedis artery. Given the close proximity of the surrounding neurovascular bundles and thin soft-tissue envelope, these injuries must be managed in an expeditious manner.

A careful physical examination of the entire lower extremity, looking in particular for vascular compromise, is essential. One should immediately assess for open and skin-threatening injuries. The posterior tibial artery and dorsalis pedis artery should be assessed for palpable pulses, and distal perfusion should be assessed via capillary refill. The overall coloration of the foot should be assessed, as a blanched cold foot indicates severe vascular compromise. If any of the above are present and associated with a obvious deformity, an immediate reduction maneuver should be attempted prior to radiographic examination. Associated injuries to the ipsilateral and contralateral lower extremity should be examined as well as spinal pathology. X-rays of the ankle and foot should be obtained and ideally an AP, mortise, and lateral ankle series plus an AP and oblique view of the foot should be obtained. However, if resources are limited, the single lateral foot X-ray and mortise view of the ankle will be most instructive. CT scan is optimal and is instructive to better visualize smaller occult fractures, assess for comminution, and help with preoperative planning. However, this resource may not be readily available and is not often needed for the acute management of these injuries.

Talar neck fractures are classified per the Hawkins classification. Type I are nondisplaced, type II are displaced neck fractures with associated subtalar subluxation/dislocation, type III are associated with both subtalar and tibiotalar subluxation/dislocation, and type IV are type III injuries with an additional talonavicular subluxation/dislocation.

Type I fractures can be treated with simple splint immobilization and protected weight bearing. Type II–IV fractures require immediate reduction. If resources are available, conscious sedation using propofol or other anesthetic agents that allow for both analgesia and muscle relaxation is optimal. If unavailable, PO or IV pain medications should be administered with a combination of intra-articular analgesic agents (such as lidocaine) injected into the tibiotalar and subtalar regions. Reduction is obtained by a combination of maneuvers. Longitudinal distraction and plantar flexion of the forefoot is performed while simultaneously applying counter-traction and a varus/valgus moment on the heel to reduce the subtalar joint. If the tibiotalar joint is dislocated, the knee is bent to relax the Achilles tendon and the entire foot is distracted longitudinally to the long axis of the tibia. Once distraction is obtained, the foot is used as a lever and the talus

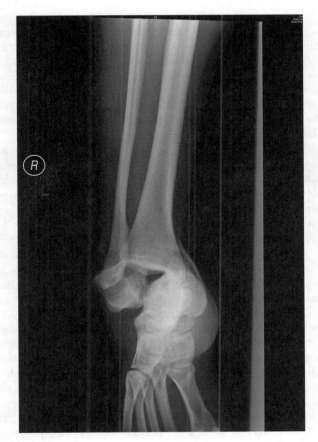

FIGURE 51.21 Talar neck fracture. Image by Paul T. Appleton, J. Kent Ellington, and John T. Kwon.

is forcibly pushed under the tibial plafond. Longitudinal distraction on the foot will often reduce a dislocated talonavicular joint. However, if the talonavicular joint remains unreduced, a repeat longitudinal force on the forefoot is applied, the heel is plantarflexed by grasping to calcaneal tuberosity, and a downward force is applied directly over the talar head.

Closed fracture-dislocations are associated with significant ligamentous and soft-tissue disruption but once reduced can be often maintained by splint/cast immobilization until transportation to definitive management is possible. If there is an open fracture-dislocation or severe trauma to the overlying soft tissues with residual gross instability, an external fixator in delta configuration can be applied. All patients should be non–weight bearing to the injured extremity with elevation to decrease further soft-tissue compromise.

Open talus fractures should be treated expeditiously. All open wounds should be immediately irrigated with sterile saline, any gross visible contamination manually removed from the wound, and a sterile dressing applied. The prompt administration of IV antibiotics and tetanus prophylaxis is essential.

Open talus fractures with an associated extruded talus are extreme cases. Management of these injuries follows the same principles for all open fractures but requires special considerations. Patients should be treated with immediate reduction, irrigation, and replacement of the extruded talus back into the wound with expeditious surgical management. Although there is a high rate of AVN, there can be a very low infection rate, and replacement of the extruded talus allows for more potential future reconstructive solutions.

Type II–IV fractures require surgical fixation although the rate of AVN increases with severity of injury.

Calcaneus Fractures

Calcaneus fractures account for approximately 2% of all fractures, and the calcaneus is the most frequently fractured tarsal bone (Figure 51.22). Most of these fractures occur secondary to high-energy injuries and cause considerable morbidity and socioeconomic burden as 90% occur in working individuals in their peak earning years. Ten percent of calcaneus fractures are open injuries, and there is an approximately 10% incidence of foot compartment syndrome. Many authors have recognized poor outcomes following this fracture and significant residual disability. Aside from open calcaneus fractures, most can and

should be treated in a staged fashion as significant trauma to the soft-tissue envelope often precludes immediate surgical fixation when required. In areas where resources are limited for definitive surgical fixation and the management of potential postsurgical complications, nonoperative treatment is a viable consideration. However, future disability can be significant and can take various forms such as the development of posttraumatic arthritis, impingement syndromes, reflex sympathetic dystrophy (RSD) and tarsal tunnel syndrome, chronic pain, and difficulties with shoe wear.

Calcaneus fractures are often intra-articular and involve the subtalar joint. While smaller fractures, such as those on the anterior process, can be a result of a twisting mechanism, most are due to high-energy axial load. Physical examination should look for skin threatening, neurovascular compromise, and associated injuries of the lower extremity. In addition, there is a 10%–15% association with spinal injuries due to mechanism, and a thorough spinal and neurologic examination should be performed. Non–weight-bearing X-rays of the ankle and foot should be obtained. In addition, a Harris heel view can give additional information regarding varus deformity, subtalar involvement, and heel shortening. Additional AP and lateral X-rays of the lumbosacral spine are indicated, if warranted, based on physical examination findings of tenderness, step-offs, or crepitus. If resources are limited and no other associated injuries are present, a single lateral X-ray of the foot gives the treating physician the most information regarding the nature of the fracture.

Closed reduction and restoration of normal anatomy of calcaneus fractures is difficult. Older techniques have been described which entail using vices and other mechanical means to establish medial and lateral compression of the tuberosity to reduce width and traction to restore length. These are usually ineffective at achieving long-term reduction and places risk to an already compromised soft tissue envelope. However, manual traction on the heel to attempt to correct the deformity can be attempted although compressive techniques are not recommended.

Simple splinting should be performed and the patient should be non–weight bearing with elevation of the affected extremity until definitive treatment can be obtained. A well-padded splint with multiple layers of cotton and ACE wraps help facilitate edema control and allow for comfortable mobilization of the injured patient. If surgical fixation is warranted, usually a period of 5–12 days is required to allow for the reduction of swelling. After 2–3 weeks, surgical fixation can be technically more difficult due to consolidation and malunion of the fracture and surgical reduction and fixation is only recommended if the appropriate resources, including a skilled surgeon, are available.

Open fractures should be treated expeditiously with immediate irrigation, decontamination, the administration of IV antibiotics and tetanus prophylaxis. Formal irrigation and debridement in the operating theatre is required. The open wound is often found medially and results from a sharp bony laceration from the displaced medial wall. Simultaneous surgical fixation through an attempted medial approach or more commonly used lateral approach is not advocated due to high complication rates. After irrigation and debridement the injured extremity can be simply immobilized in a splint. Early wound closure if possible has been shown to be advantageous.

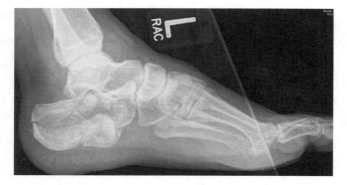

FIGURE 51.22 Intra-articular calcaneus fracture. Image by Paul T. Appleton, J. Kent Ellington, and John T. Kwon.

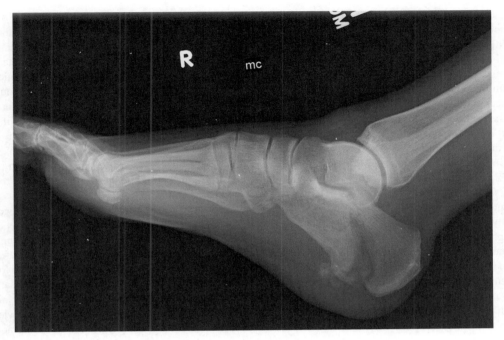

FIGURE 51.23   Calcaneal beak fracture. Image by Paul T. Appleton, J. Kent Ellington, and John T. Kwon.

Calcaneal beak fractures are those where the superior calcaneal tuberosity is displaced superiorly and deserve special consideration. (Figure 51.23) Fracture displacement often results in either an open injury posteriorly or significant skin tenting and threatening. These must be reduced as the risk of subsequent skin erosion and open fracture is high. Closed reduction is often unsuccessful as the Achilles tendon acts as a deforming force. Formal reduction is required and can be maintained either by formal open reduction internal fixation or by the percutanous placement of Kirshner wires. The extremity should be splinted in equinus so as to reduce the deforming force of the Achilles tendon.

Subtalar Dislocations

Subtalar dislocations are uncommon and are frequently mistaken for ankle dislocations. They are associated with other foot fractures and ankle fractures. Subtalar dislocations occur either medial or lateral and occur from inversion- or eversion-deforming forces, respectively. Lateral is less common (15%). If closed reduction is difficult, it is likely due to entrapment of the posterior tibialis tendon or flexor digitorum longus. Medial dislocations are more common and blocks to reduction are due to either the talonavicular joint capsule or extensor digitorum brevis. Closed reduction for either is accomplished with the knee flexed to relax the Achilles tendon along with longitudinal traction. After reduction, a non–weight-bearing cast is applied for 3 weeks, then early motion is started as stiffness is a common sequelae. The subtalar joint is inherently stable and typically does not require an external fixator.

Midfoot Fractures

Navicular fractures, cuboid fractures, and Lisfranc fracture-dislocations can be a source of considerable disability. Unless associated with other injuries, they are often closed injuries with less

risk for overall neurovascular compromise. However, they can be associated with significant soft-tissue injury, degloving, and skin threatening based on the mechanism. These injuries are often a result of a crushing mechanism, twisting injury, forced abduction/adduction, or axial loading longitudinally through the foot. There is a higher association with foot compartment syndrome with Lisfranc fracture-dislocations in particular.

Navicular fractures can occur through the body, tuberosity or avulsion type fractures of the surrounding capsular structures or of the posterior tibial tendon. Three views of the foot non–weight bearing are obtained. Careful physical examination is warranted. If a significant navicular body fracture with displacement occurs, the foot may be deformed in an adducted posture due to shortening of the medial column of the foot. If a navicular body fracture is associated with dorsal displacement, there can be significant threatening of the dorsal skin as well as intrinsic pressure on the closely related dorsalis pedis artery. While closed reduction rarely corrects the adducted position of the foot, it must be attempted in cases of dorsal skin threatening or neurovascular compromise. Longitudinal traction is applied to the forefoot to facilitate distraction through the midfoot. Dorsal pressure is then applied directly over the navicular body in a plantar direction. These injuries can be splinted and the patient made non–weight-bearing until definitive treatment can be obtained. A medially placed external fixation can be used to help maintain foot posture.

Cuboid fractures, also known as nutcracker fractures, are often a result of forced abduction of the foot. The cuboid is impacted between the 4th and 5th metatarsal bases and the anterior calcaneus. These injuries can range from simple anterior impaction of the cuboid to a highly comminuted cuboid body fracture. In distinction to navicular fractures, cuboid fractures often result in an abducted posture to the foot secondary to shorten of the lateral column. Three views of the foot non–weight bearing are obtained. Closed reduction and maintenance of column length is very difficult. External fixation is warranted if available to help maintain foot posture and can at times be used for definitive treatment. Otherwise these injuries can be splinted and the patient made non–weight bearing until definitive treatment can be obtained.

Lisfranc fracture-dislocations of the tarsometatarsal (TMT) joints are rare (accounting for <1% of fractures) but are significant injuries to the midfoot and are often a cause for significant morbidity due to the high association with the development of posttraumatic arthritis (Figure 51.24). The Lisfranc joints consist of the 1st through 5th TMT joints. Multiple ligamentous structures stabilize the midfoot with the plantar structures being stronger. The dorsal ligamentous and capsular structures are relatively weaker, and most dislocations occur dorsally due to this fact. Anatomically there is no intermetatarsal ligament between the 1st and 2nd proximal metatarsals. The Lisfranc ligament, a strong band connecting the medial cuneiform to the base of the 2nd metatarsal, helps stabilize this area.

Physical examination reveals a swollen and ecchymotic foot. Although gross vascular compromise is uncommon, the 1st intermetatarsal branch of the dorsalis pedis artery crosses the midfoot

in close proximity to the 2nd TMT and can be disrupted, leading to significant swelling and compartment syndrome. Depending on the direction of displacement (usually lateral), the foot can appear abducted and plantar flexed through the midfoot. Plantar midfoot ecchymosis is considered pathognomic for this type of injury. A careful neurovascular assessment should be performed. Given the higher association with compartment syndrome, signs and symptoms of compartment syndrome should be sought after. Aside from pain out of proportion, patients may complain of paresthesias or dysesthesias. The foot may be tense with associated fracture blisters. The classic sign of pain with passive motion is invariably present although has been shown to be less reliable with foot trauma.

Radiographic examination includes three views of the foot. Ideally, these are obtained weight bearing so as to accentuate any subtle displacement of the Lisfranc joints, although this can be difficult due to patient discomfort. The author's preference is to obtain three views of the contralateral uninjured foot for comparison. A small bony avulsion in the 1st/2nd intermetatarsal space, called the fleck sign, can reveal subtle Lisfranc ligament injury. If resources are limited, a weight-bearing AP and oblique view of the injured foot should allow for diagnosis. Several radiographic markers have been used to assess for subluxation or dislocation of the TMT joints. On the AP radiograph, the medial border of the 1st metatarsal should align with the medial border of the medial cuneiform. In addition, the medial border of the 2nd metatarsal should align with the medial border of the middle cuneiform. On the oblique X-ray, the medial border of the 3rd metatarsal should align with the medial border of the lateral cuneiform, and the medial border of the 4th metatarsal should align with the medial border of the cuboid. On the lateral X-ray the metatarsal bases should align with their corresponding cuneiforms without plantar or dorsal subluxation. One should keep in mind, however, the highly constrained nature of the midfoot structures, and any displacement, regardless of the view, should raise suspicion.

Immediate closed reduction of displaced injuries (>2 mm) is required. If available, conscious sedation is beneficial to facilitate reduction and to improve patient comfort. The most common direction of injury displacement is lateral and dorsal. With the hindfoot immobilized, the forefoot is grasped and longitudinal traction is applied. Using the forefoot as a lever, the metatarsals are reduced medially and plantarly.

The foot and ankle should be splinted and the patient should be made non–weight bearing. Any displacement visualized on plain radiographs is usually an indication for surgical fixation.

Forefoot Fractures

Fractures of the metatarsals and phalanges are common injuries, often resulting from "stubbing the foot," twisting injuries, or crush injuries. Although rarely limb threatening, open fractures of the toes can lead to infection, osteomyelitis, and progressive or systemic illness if untreated. Metatarsal fractures can also cause future disability in the form of malunion and metatarsalgia. Although the incidence of neurovascular injury is low, the treating physician should carefully monitor these patients for the development of later complications.

Physical examination is important to look in particular for open injuries or subtle punctures as many principles in the

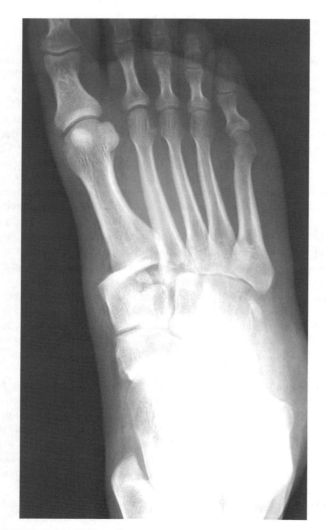

FIGURE 51.24 Lisfranc fracture-dislocation. Image by Paul T. Appleton, J. Kent Ellington, and John T. Kwon.

treatment of open fractures apply. If found they should be irrigated, with administration of i.v. antibiotics and tetanus prophylaxis. Although neurologic injury is often of little consequence acutely, neuropathy of the toes may present future difficulties with ulceration and infection. Vascular compromise of the toes from traumatic injury can similarly lead to future problems. If dry gangrene develops, this should be carefully monitored and the affected portions allowed to auto-amputate as a healthy base of granulation tissue develops under the ischemic area over time. If wet gangrene develops, surgical amputation is required. If the toe is ischemic from acute traumatic injury, expeditious amputation should be considered.

Plain radiographs are sufficient for metatarsal and toe fractures. Metatarsal fractures usually can be treated nonoperatively with simple immobilization and protected weight bearing. However, several exceptions apply, and if a skilled surgeon is available, then surgical fixation should be considered. Surgical indications for metatarsal fractures include: (1) fracture of the border metatarsals (1st and 5th), (2) multiple metatarsal fractures, (3) open fractures, and/or (4) metatarsal fractures with significant angulation, displacement, or shortening.

Toe fractures (phalangeal) can be usually treated nonoperatively with weight bearing in a stiff soled shoe. The involved toe can be "buddy taped" to the adjacent toes. This entails applying tape around the toes such that the adjacent toes act as a splint to ensure proper toe alignment. If the phalanx is high comminuted and displaced, an argument can be made for pin fixation, although this must be balanced by the availability of resources and the risk of infection.

Foot Compartment Syndrome

Severe trauma to the foot can lead to foot compartment syndrome. Foot compartment syndrome follows the same pathophysiology as compartment syndrome in other areas of the body and involves increased intracompartmental pressure leading to vascular and neurologic compromise and tissue necrosis. Management of foot compartment syndrome is controversial and varies considerably among practitioners.

Part of the controversy stems from foot compartment syndrome being a relatively new entity as described in the literature and the historic confusion regarding the foot compartments and their locations. For surgeons not familiar with the complex anatomy of the foot, assessing and releasing compartments can be technically difficult to perform safely and satisfactorily. In addition, surgical release not only puts the patient at risk for infection and wound healing complications, but in untrained hands also can lead to further neurovascular injury. Ultimately, the decision to surgically treat foot compartment syndrome relies on a careful risk-versus-benefit analysis.

Patients present after severe foot trauma with a swollen, tense, and ecchymotic foot. There may be associated degloving or open injuries which do not preclude the development of compartment syndrome. Patients often have severe pain and can complain of parasthesias or dysesthesias. Clinically, patients often have pain with passive toe movements, although this has been found to be of little value in diagnosis after foot trauma. Patients can have vascular compromise and ischemic toes.

The sequela of untreated foot compartment syndrome can be disabling, although rarely life- or limb-threatening, and include neurogenic claw toeing, metatarsalgia, neuritis, fibrosis, chronic pain and RSD.

Diagnosis is made clinically and confirmed via intracompartmental pressure testing, although the equipment required for this may not be readily available. The only treatment is surgical and involves multiple dorsal and medially based incisions to release all foot compartments. However, in settings where management of the potential complications of surgical release and appropriate resources are not available for the treatment of infection and wound dehiscence, ability to perform split-thickness skin grafting for closure, careful wound care, or availability of vacuum-assisted closure (VAC) therapy, we do not recommend surgical decompression.

Suggested Reading

Bucholz RW, Heckman JD, Court-Brown CM, et al. (eds.). *Rockwood and Green's Fractures in Adults*. 7th ed. Philadelphia: Lippincott Williams & Wilkins, 2010.

Browner BD, Green NE, Jupiter JB, et al. (eds.). *Skeletal Trauma: Basic Science, Management, and Reconstruction*. 4th ed. Philadelphia: WB Saunders, 1997.

COMMENTARY

Ankur B. Bamne, Korea

A vehicular accident is reported every 3 minutes and a death every 10 minutes on Indian roads.[1] Poor driving etiquette, lack of adequate safety in cheap modes of transport, and congested roads contribute to the higher incidence of motor vehicle accidents and subsequent trauma to the lower extremity in LMICs. It comes as no surprise that the Decade of Action for Road Safety (2011–2020) follows the Bone and Joint Decade (2001–2010) as declared by the WHO.

Even in major cities, LMICs lack Level 1 trauma centers. The first response teams are not in place to respond to motor vehicle accidents. Many trauma patients are transported to hospitals by untrained people. They are frequently taken to hospitals that lack the basic infrastructure to manage these multiply injured patients. Also, there is a significant delay in trauma patients reaching the hospital because of poor infrastructure. As a result, the morbidity and mortality rates for these accident victims are high.

Patients with a fracture and associated vascular injury frequently need amputation due to delay in getting medical attention within the window of limb salvage. Open injuries that might be considered for limb salvage in LMICs are commonly considered "nonsalvageable." Also, facilities for limb reimplantation following traumatic amputation are almost non-existing in most of the LMICs.

Many unique treatment modalities are used in LMICs which may be obsolete in high-income countries (HICs). Fixations of fractures of the shaft of femur with K-nail and Austin-Moore prosthesis (AMP) for hemi-arthroplasty are a frequent occurrence in India. Parts of external fixators such as connecting rod and clamps are sometime reused in other patients to decrease cost.

The burden of sequelae of infection is also profound in LMICs. Infected nonunions are a common occurrence as a result of poor operating conditions. These need even more advanced reconstruction techniques, but they are scarce in LMICs. Also, bone defects have to be managed with autograft in the absence of availability of allograft bone or bone graft substitutes.

Complications like compartment syndrome are underdiagnosed and undertreated, so they often lead to serious sequelae. Foot and ankle injuries are common because of the practice of working barefoot in the fields. These are again neglected, leading to serious consequences like infection, cellulitis, or necrotizing fasciitis, which can end up in amputation, especially in patients with diabetes mellitus. Many centers do not have facilities for advanced wound management like VAC, which makes treating soft-tissue defects a long and morbid process.

Thus, a huge gap exists in the management of trauma between LMICs and HICs. This has been described in various studies.[2,3] This needs to be addressed by increasing expenditures on healthcare and prioritizing the development of healthcare facilities.

Pelvic Fractures

Pelvic fractures are the result of high-energy trauma. They may be associated with injuries to the genitourinary tract and abdominal organs and result in significant morbidity and mortality. They are associated with significant blood loss, which is concealed. Limited resources in LMICs make managing these complex injuries difficult.

The pelvis may be conceptualized as a ring, with the sacrum posterior and the two innominate bones flanking on the sides. Stability is provided by the ligaments.

The mechanism of injury may vary from high-energy to low-energy. Physical examination may reveal swelling of the genitalia, bruising, and a positive pelvic compression test. An injury to the vaginal mucosa makes it an open fracture.

Frontal projection radiographs of the pelvis along with inlet and outlet views are the basic means of investigation. They are also the most important to ascertain the type and severity of injury. A CT scan may be helpful in preoperative planning.

Pelvic fractures are classified into three main types, APC, LC, and vertical shear. Each type has a typical mechanism of injury and characteristic radiographic patterns with varying grades of severity.

Early management of pelvic fractures includes compression of the pelvis either with a sheet or a pelvic binder. Stable injuries may be managed with restricted weight bearing on the affected side. External fixation may be used as a definitive or interim measure. Unstable injuries generally require internal fixation depending upon the type and severity of injury.

Fractures of the Acetabulum

Fractures of the acetabulum occur as a result of high-energy trauma. A common mechanism of injury is the dashboard type of injury, and it may be associated with posterior hip dislocation. On examination, hip movements may be painful. The lower extremity will have a flexion, adduction, and internal rotation attitude if associated with dislocation. A thorough neurovascular examination is mandatory. It is best to treat these injuries at a well-equipped tertiary trauma center and by surgeons well experienced in managing these injuries.

An AP radiograph of the pelvis along with Judet views are basic investigations for acetabular fractures. CT scans are extremely helpful in understanding the pattern of the fracture and planning the subsequent approach and fixation.

Stable, minimally displaced fractures may be treated conservatively. Associated hip dislocations need to be reduced on an emergency basis. Unstable injuries need internal fixation. The nature of the injury dictates the surgical approach.

Hip Dislocations

Hip dislocations may or may not be associated with acetabular fractures. Posterior dislocations are most common. The characteristic attitude of the limb may be an indicator of the direction of dislocation. Posterior dislocations will have a flexion, adduction, and internal rotation attitude whereas anterior dislocations will have an extension, abduction, and external rotation attitude. Shortening will be present in both the cases.

Closed reduction of the hip is done on an emergency basis under sedation. After reduction a check radiograph is important to confirm concentric reduction of the joint and to detect any fractures that may have been missed during the initial radiograph. Postreduction, restricted weight bearing is permitted.

Fractures of the Proximal Femur (Hip)

These fractures occur most commonly in the elderly as a result of osteoporosis; however, they also occur in the young as a result of high-energy trauma. They are broadly divided into intra-capsular, inter-trochanteric, and sub-trochanteric, as each of these types has specific management due to peculiar anatomy and vascular supply.

On examination, the extremity will be shortened and externally rotated and there will be tenderness around the hip region. Weight bearing is usually not possible. It is important to image the hip with both an AP and a lateral radiograph.

Intracapsular fractures generally disrupt blood supply to the femoral head and may lead to AVN of the femoral head. In young patients (less than 60 years old), urgent fixation of these fractures is done with canulated screws. In the elderly, a partial hip replacement (hemi-arthroplasty) may be considered to make them ambulate earlier. These fractures have a high rate on nonunion due to their intracapsular location and precarious blood supply.

Extracapsular hip fractures may be inter-trochanteric or sub-trochanteric. These are usually treated with internal fixation either with an intramedullary nail or a sliding hip screw. These have a good rate of union as compared to intracapsular fractures.

Femoral Shaft Fractures

Femoral shaft fractures usually occur as a result of high-energy trauma. They are usually associated with significant blood loss (almost 1000 ml). Hence, initial fluid resuscitation is important.

On examination, there will be swelling in the thigh region with gross shortening and deformity. There will be diffuse tenderness around the thigh. Careful inspection of the overlying skin should be done to rule out open fractures. A thorough neurovascular examination is important. Plain radiographs taken in two planes are usually diagnostic

Initial management includes volume replacement and splinting of the injured limb, preferably in a well-padded Thomas's splint. If operative facilities are not available, these fractures may be managed with traction. However, internal fixation with a locked intramedullary nail remains the gold standard for these fractures. Locked nails give rotational stability and prevent shortening. However, a standard operative room set up with intra-operative fluoroscopy is required.

Supracondylar Femur Fractures

Supracondylar femur fractures occur proximal to the knee joint. Proper management is important to prevent malalignment and subsequent secondary arthritis. These fractures are usually associated with high-velocity trauma. Clinical findings are similar to those seen with femur fractures. In addition, a hemarthrosis may be present in the knee joint. Thorough neurovascular examination is important because of proximity of the femoral artery and sciatic nerve to the femur in this region. Radiographs are usually diagnostic.

Nondisplaced stable fractures may be treated conservatively with a traction pin in the proximal tibia. Range of motion may be commenced after a month in traction. Weight bearing is restricted for 3 months. However, displaced or intra-articular fractures need operative fixation. This can usually be achieved with a plate or an intramedullary nail. Open fractures need debridement and external fixation with subsequent soft-tissue coverage.

Patella Fractures

The patella is the largest sesamoid bone in the body. It enhances the action of the quadriceps muscle. However, its superficial location in the anterior aspect of the knee makes it vulnerable to fractures by direct impact. Also, it may fracture due to sudden concentric contraction of the quadriceps.

Patients complain of pain over the knee joint. Active resisted knee extension may not be possible. However, it may be possible if the retinaculi are intact. A palpable step is often present over the patella. AP and lateral knee radiographs are adequate for the diagnosis.

Nondisplaced or minimally displaced patella fractures with intra-articular step-off of less than 2 mm can be treated conservatively in a cylinder cast (above-knee cast up to ankle) for 6 weeks. Displaced fractures need internal fixation. Tension band wiring works extremely well and is considered the gold standard for patella fractures. Early range of motion needs to be instituted to prevent stiffness.

Tibia Plateau Fractures

Tibia plateau fractures occur as a result of high-velocity injuries. They range from nondisplaced fractures to displaced fractures with joint surface depression. They may be associated with ligamentous injury around the knee. Open fractures are relatively common in this area. Compartment pressure needs to be monitored to detect evolving compartment syndrome.

AP and lateral radiographs are standard modalities for investigation. Oblique radiographs help to detect displacement. CT scan with 3 reconstruction is extremely helpful to delineate fracture anatomy and plan subsequent management.

Non- or minimally displaced fractures may be treated with a cast or knee immobilizer with restricted weight bearing. Displaced fractures need to be with internal fixation. Spanning external fixation may be used in case of open fractures or fractures with severe soft-tissue injury.

Tibia Shaft Fractures

Tibia fractures are the result of high-energy injuries. Because of little soft-tissue coverage on the medial aspect of tibia, open fractures are common in this location. Also they may be associated with a compartment syndrome.

History taking will reveal the mode of injury. On physical examination, swelling and deformity of the leg may be present. Range of motion of knee and ankle will not be possible due to pain. Also, pain out of proportion to injury is the first sign of compartment syndrome. X-rays are usually diagnostic.

Open fractures need debridement and external fixation. Nondisplaced fractures may be treated in a cast. Unstable fractures need internal fixation with an intramedullary nail, which allows early mobilization and weight bearing.

Pilon Fractures

Pilon fractures are the fractures of the distal articular surface of the tibia (plafond). These commonly occur due to high-energy trauma. Open fractures are also common in this area. Associated injuries include tibia plateau, pelvic, and spine fractures.

Initial management includes splinting and elevation. Immediate ORIF of these fractures is commonly prohibitive because of the soft-tissue swelling. One method to circumvent this problem is to apply a spanning external fixator and proceed with definitive internal fixation after swelling subsides in a week. Infection and wound dehiscence are serious complications following fixation of these fractures.

Ankle Fractures

Ankle fractures are relatively common and result from rotational force in varying positions of the foot. Ankle fractures may be stable or unstable. Stable fractures may be treated in a cast. Unstable fractures need ORIF after skin condition is permissive.

Ankle Dislocations

Ankle dislocations are relatively uncommon injuries. However, they are frequently open with a wound present medially. Emergent closed reduction is done to prevent soft-tissue complications. Associated fractures are managed with internal fixation.

Talus Fractures

Talus fractures are relatively uncommon. These may result from high- or low-energy mechanisms. These injuries may be limb-threatening. As the talus and its articulations account for more than 90% of the motion of the foot and ankle, these injuries can result in significant long-term disability if not treated appropriately. The talus has a precarious blood supply. AVN is a potential long-term complication. Also, soft-tissue injuries must be monitored carefully. Multiple views of the foot and CT scan are helpful in delineating the fracture anatomy. Closed reduction of these fractures should be performed immediately. Severe injuries need internal fixation. However, nonunion may develop in some of these patients.

Calcaneus Fractures

The calcaneus is the most frequently fractured tarsal bone. These fractures occur most commonly due to high-energy trauma and are associated with severe soft-tissue swelling. The spin should be screened to rule out fractures that are commonly associated with calcaneus fractures.

Immediate management includes splinting, elevation, and careful monitoring of the soft-tissue envelope. ORIF should be undertaken only when the soft-tissue condition is acceptable. A wrinkle sign has been described wherein the skin over the calcaneus wrinkles after the initial edema is settled. Open injuries need emergency debridement and stabilization.

Subtalar Dislocations

Medial dislocations of the subtalar joint are more common. Closed reduction is attempted and postreduction a cast is applied.

Midfoot Fractures

These injuries are a source of considerable disability. Lisfranc's fracture-dislocations are associated with a higher incidence of foot compartment syndrome. Different management strategies need to be employed depending upon the location of the injury.

Forefoot Fractures

These are relatively benign injuries; however, in the event of local infection or vascular compromise, they can become limb-threatening. Conservative management works well for most of these.

Foot Compartment Syndrome

Compartment syndrome results from swelling inside nonyielding compartments and compromises vascular supply. It is a commonly underdiagnosed and inadequately treated entity. Managing this condition needs advanced wound management measures postfasciotomy.

References

Chapter 1

1. World Health Organization. WHO Statistical Information System [Internet]. 2010. Available from: http://www.who.int/whosis/en/index.html.
2. Bickler S, Ozdegiz D, Gosselin R, et al. Key concepts for estimating burden of surgical conditions and unmet need for surgical care. *World Journal of Surgery*. 2010; 34(3): 374–80.
3. Global Initiative for Emergency and Essential Surgical Care [Internet]. World Health Organization. 2010. Available from:http://www.who.int/GIEESC.
4. Funk L, Weiser T, Berry W, et al. Global operating theater distribution and pulse oximetry supply: an estimation from reported data. *Lancet*. 2010; doi: 10.1016/S0140-6736(10)60392-3.
5. Murray CJ, Lopez AD. Global mortality, disability and the contribution of risk factors: Global Burden of Disease Study. *Lancet*. 1997; 349: 1436–42.
6. Jamison D. The Role of Surgery in Global Health. Presented at Harvard Symposium: Harvard Club, Boston, MA. November 5, 2010.
7. Debas HT, Gosselin R, McCord C, Thind A. *Surgery. In: Disease Control Priorities in Developing Countries*. 2nd ed. New York: Oxford University Press, 2006: 1,245–60.
8. Ozdegiz D, Hsia R, Weiser T, et al. Population Metric for Surgery: Effective Coverage of Surgical Services in Low-Income and Middle-Income Countries. *World Journal of Surgery*. 2008; doi: 10.1007/s00268-008-9799y.
9. Corlew DS. Estimation of the Impact of Surgical Disease Through Economic Modeling of Cleft Lip and Palate Care. *World Journal of Surgery*. 2010; 43(3): 391–6.
10. Ozdegiz D, Jamison D, Cherian M, McQueen K. The burden of surgical conditions and access to surgical care in low and middle income countries. *Bulletin of the World Health Organization*. August 2008; 86(8): 646–7.
11. Vos T. Improving the Quantitative Basis of the Surgical Burden in Low-Income Countries. *PLOS Medicine*. 2009; 6(9): e1000149.
12. Gosselin R, Gyamfi Y, Contini S. Challenges of Meeting Surgical Needs in the Developing World. *World Journal of Surgery*. 2011; 35: 258–261.
13. World Health Organization. Surgery at the District Hospital [Internet]. Accessed Jan 15 2011. Available from: http://www.who.int/surgery/publications/scdh_manual/en/index.html.
14. Kushner A, Cherian M, Noel L, et al. Addressing the millennium development goals from a surgical perspective: essential surgery and anesthesia in 8 low- and middle-income countries. *Archives of Surgery*. 2010; 145(2): 154–9.
15. McQueen K, Ozdegiz D, Riveillo R, et al. Essential surgery: integral to the right to health. *Health and Human Rights*. 2010; 12(1): 137–52.
16. Hodges SC, Mijumbi C, Okello M, et al. Anaesthesia services in developing countries: defining the problems. *Anaesthesia*. 2007; 62: 4–11.
17. Weiser TG, Regenbogen SE, Thompson KD, et al. An Estimation of the global volume of surgery: a modeling strategy based on available data. *Lancet*. 2008; 372(9633): 139–44.
18. World Health Organization. The World Health Report 2006—Working Together for Health [Internet]. 2006. Accessed Dec 12, 2010. Available from: http://www.who.int/whr/2006/en/.
19. Dubowitz G, Detlefs S, McQueen K. Global Anesthesia Workforce Crisis: A preliminary survey revealing shortages contributing to undesirable outcomes and unsafe practices. *World Journal of Surgery*. 2010; 34(3): 438–44.
20. United Nations UN. Millennium Declaration and Millennium Development Goals [Internet]. Accessed Jan 11, 2011. Available from: http://www.un.org/millenniumgoals/bkgds.html.
21. Pierce EC. The 34th Rovenstine Lecture: 40 years behind the mask: safety revisited. *Anesthesiology*. 1996; 84(4): 965–75.
22. World Health Organization. Safe Surgery Saves Lives [Internet]. Accessed Jan 15, 2011. Available from: http://www.who.int/patientsafety/safesurgery/en/.
23. Walker IA, Wilson IH. Anaesthesia in developing countries—a risk for patients. Lancet. 2008; 371: 968–69.
24. Ouro-Bangna Maman AF, Tomta K, Ahouangbevi S, Chobli M. Deaths associated with anaesthesia in Togo, West Africa. *Tropical Doctor*. 2005; 35: 220–22.
25. Hansen D, Gausi SC, Merikebu M Anaesthesia in Malawi: complications and deaths. *Tropical Doctor* 2000; 30: 146–149.
26. Buck N, Devlin HB, Lunn JN. The report of a confidential enquiry into perioperative deaths. London: Nuffield Provincial Hospitals Trust and the King's Fund, 1987.
27. Enohumah K, Imarenglaye C. Factors associated with anesthesia-related maternal mortality in a tertiary hospital in Nigeria. *Acta Anaesthesiologica Scandanavia*. 2006; 50: 206–10.
28. Rivello R, Ozdegiz D, Hsai RY, et al. The role of collaborative academic partnerships in surgical training, education and provision. *World Journal of Surgery*. 2010; 34(3): 459–65.

Chapter 2

1. Good Medical Practice In. London General Medical Council 2013.
2. Burdick EJ, Lederer W. *The Ugly American*. London: Gollancz, 1958.
3. Holt GR. Ethical conduct of humanitarian medical missions: II. Use of photographic images. *Archives of Facial Plastic Surgery*. 2012; 14: 295–6.
4. Politis GD, Schneider WJ, Van Beek AL, et al. Guidelines for pediatric perioperative care during short-term plastic reconstructive surgical projects in less developed nations. *Anesthesia and Analgesia*. 2011; 112: 183–90.

5. Schneider WJ, Politis GD, Gosain AK, et al. Volunteers in plastic surgery guidelines for providing surgical care for children in the less developed world. *Plastic and Reconstructive Surgery.* 2011; 127: 2477–86.

6. Schneider WJ, Migliori MR, Gosain AK, et al. Volunteers in plastic surgery guidelines for providing surgical care for children in the less developed world: part II. Ethical considerations. *Plastic and Reconstructive Surgery.* 2011; 128: 216e–22e.

7. Waisel DB. Let the patient drive the informed consent process: ignore legal requirements. *Anesthesia and Analgesia.* 2011; 113: 13–5.

8. Glickman SW, McHutchison JG, Peterson ED, et al. Ethical and scientific implications of the globalization of clinical research. *New England Journal of Medicine.* 2009; 360: 816–23.

9. Faden RR, Kass NE, Goodman SN, et al. An ethics framework for a learning health care system: a departure from traditional research ethics and clinical ethics. *Hastings Center Report.* 2013: S16–27.

10. Hunt MR, Schwartz L, Sinding C, Elit L. The ethics of engaged presence: a framework for health professionals in humanitarian assistance and development work. *Developing World Bioethics.* 2014; 14: 47–55.

11. Isaacson G, Drum ET, Cohen MS. Surgical missions to developing countries: Ethical conflicts. *Otolaryngology Head and Neck Surgery.* 2010; 143: 476–9.

Chapter 3

1. Tollefson TT, Larrabee WF,Jr. Global surgical initiatives to reduce the surgical burden of disease. *Journal of the American Medical Association.* 2012 Feb 15; 307(7): 667–668.

2. College of Surgeons in East Central and Southern Africa. College of Surgeons in East Central and Southern Africa. Available at: www.cosecsa.org/index.php/about-cosecsa/partners/. Accessed Oct 1 2013.

3. Galukande M, Ozgediz D, Elobu E, Kaggwa S. Pretraining experience and structure of surgical training at a sub-Saharan African university. *World Journal of Surgery.* 2013 Aug; 37(8): 1836–1840.

4. Derbew M, Beveridge M, Howard A, Byrne N. Building surgical research capacity in Africa: the Ptolemy Project. *PLOS Med.* 2006 Jul; 3(7):e305.

5. Nadler EP, Nwomeh BC, Frederick WA, Hassoun HT, Kingham TP, Krishnaswami S, et al. Academic needs in developing countries: a survey of the West African College of Surgeons. *Journal of Surgical Research.* 2010 May 1; 160(1): 14–17.

6. Petroze RT, Mody GN, Ntaganda E, Calland JF, Riviello R, Rwamasirabo E, et al. Collaboration in surgical capacity development: a report of the inaugural meeting of the Strengthening Rwanda Surgery initiative. *World Journal of Surgery.* 2013 Jul; 37(7): 1500–1505.

7. Frenk J, Chen L, Bhutta ZA, Cohen J, Crisp N, Evans T, et al. Health professionals for a new century: transforming education to strengthen health systems in an interdependent world. *Lancet.* 2010 Dec 4; 376(9756): 1923–1958.

8. Kinfu Y, Dal Poz MR, Mercer H, Evans DB. The health worker shortage in Africa: are enough physicians and nurses being trained? *Bulletin of the World Health Organization.* 2009 Mar; 87(3): 225–230.

9. Sheikh A, Naqvi SH, Sheikh K, Naqvi SH, Bandukda MY. Physician migration at its roots: a study on the factors contributing towards a career choice abroad among students at a medical school in Pakistan. *Global Health 2012.* Dec 15; 8: 43-8603–8-43.

10. Hagander LE, Hughes CD, Nash K, Ganjawalla K, Linden A, Martins Y, et al. Surgeon migration between developing countries and the United States: train, retain, and gain from brain drain. *World Journal of Surgery.* 2013 Jan; 37(1): 14–23.

11. Ozgediz D, Galukande M, Mabweijano J, Kijjambu S, Mijumbi C, Dubowitz G, et al. The neglect of the global surgical workforce: experience and evidence from Uganda. *World Journal of Surgery.* 2008 Jun; 32(6): 1208–1215.

12. Kruk ME, Pereira C, Vaz F, Bergstrom S, Galea S. Economic evaluation of surgically trained assistant medical officers in performing major obstetric surgery in Mozambique. *BJOG.* 2007 Oct; 114(10): 1253–1260.

13. Galukande M, Kaggwa S, Sekimpi P, Kakaire O, Katamba A, Munabi I, et al. Use of surgical task shifting to scale up essential surgical services: a feasibility analysis at facility level in Uganda. *BMC Health Services Research.* 2013 Aug 1; 13: 292-6963–13-292.

14. Kruk ME, Wladis A, Mbembati N, Ndao-Brumblay SK, Hsia RY, Galukande M, et al. Human resource and funding constraints for essential surgery in district hospitals in Africa: a retrospective cross-sectional survey. *PLOS Med.* 2010 Mar 9; 7(3):e1000242.

15. Sani R, Nameoua B, Yahaya A, Hassane I, Adamou R, Hsia RY, et al. The impact of launching surgery at the district level in Niger. *World Journal of Surgery.* 2009 Oct; 33(10): 2063–2068.

16. Chilopora G, Pereira C, Kamwendo F, Chimbiri A, Malunga E, Bergstrom S. Postoperative outcome of caesarean sections and other major emergency obstetric surgery by clinical officers and medical officers in Malawi. *Human Resources for Health.* 2007 Jun 14; 5: 17.

17. Cumbi A, Pereira C, Malalane R, Vaz F, McCord C, Bacci A, et al. Major surgery delegation to mid-level health practitioners in Mozambique: health professionals' perceptions. *Human Resources for Health.* 2007 Dec 6; 5: 27.

18. Ferrinho P, Sidat M, Goma F, Dussault G. Task-shifting: experiences and opinions of health workers in Mozambique and Zambia. *Human Resources for Health.* 2012 Sep 17; 10(1): 34-4491–10-34.

19. Lipnick M, Mijumbi C, Dubowitz G, Kaggwa S, Goetz L, Mabweijano J, et al. Surgery and anesthesia capacity-building in resource-poor settings: description of an ongoing academic partnership in Uganda. *World Journal of Surgery.* 2013 Mar; 37(3): 488–497.

20. Kimuli T, Meya D, Meya D, Tulsky J, Schecter W. Blood and body fluid exposures among surgeons in Mulago Hospital. *East and Central African Journal of Surgery.* 2011, Nov/Dec; 16(3).

21. Global Partners in Anesthesia and Surgery. Workforce Expansion. Available at: http://www.globalpas.org/projects/capacity-building/scholarships/. Accessed Oct 13 2013.

22. Magee WP, Raimondi HM, Beers M, Koech MC. Effectiveness of international surgical program model to build local sustainability. *Plastic Surgery International.* 2012; 2012: 185725.

23. Corlew S, Fan VY. A model for building capacity in international plastic surgery: ReSurge International. *Annals of Plastic Surgery.* 2011 Dec; 67(6): 568–570.

24. ReSurge International. ReSurge International: Training Doctors. Available at: http://resurge.org/impacting_the_world/training_doctors.cfm. Accessed Oct 5 2013.

25. Duke University. Duke Global Surgery. Available at: http:// surgery.duke.edu/about-departments/divisions-and-programs/ duke-global-surgery. Accessed Oct 5 2013.

26. Haglund MM, Kiryabwire J, Parker S, Zomorodi A, MacLeod D, Schroeder R, et al. Surgical capacity building in Uganda through twinning, technology, and training camps. *World Journal of Surgery.* 2011 Jun; 35(6): 1175–1182.

27. Global Surgery Initiative at UVA. Global Surgery Initiative at UVA: Teleconferences. Available at: http://virginiaglobalsurgery.wordpress.com/activities/international-teleconferences/. Accessed Oct 3 2013.

28. AMPATH. Donate to AMPATH. Available at: www.ampathkenya.org/donate. Accessed Oct 1 2013.

29. IVUmed. IVUmed's Annual Teach One, Reach Many Benefit. Available at: www.ivumed.org/current-news/benefit-2013/. Accessed Oct 1 2013.

30. Harvard Medical School. Paul Farmer Global Surgery Fellowship. Accessed Oct 6 2013.

31. Association for Academic Surgery. AAS/AASF Global Surgery Research Fellowship Award. Available at: http://www. aasurg.org/awards/fellowship_award_global.php.   Accessed Oct 6 2013.

32. Campbell A, Sherman R, Magee WP. The role of humanitarian missions in modern surgical training. *Plastic and Reconstructive Surgery.* 2010 Jul; 126(1): 295–302.

33. Aswani J, Baidoo K, Otiti J. Establishing a head and neck unit in a developing country. *Journal of Laryngology & Otology.* 2012 Jun; 126(6): 552–555.

34. Bill & Melinda Gates Foundation. Open LOI Global Health Grants. Available at: www.gatesfoundation.org/How-We-Work/ General-Information/Grant-Opportunities/Open-LOI-Global-Health-Grants/. Accessed Oct 1 2013.

35. Centers for Disease Control and Prevention. CDC Global Health Funding. Available at: www.cdc.gov/globalhealth/global healthfunding.htm. Accessed Oct 2 2013.

36. The Henry J. Kaiser Family Foundation. U.S. Funding for Global Health: The President's FY 2014 Budget Request. Available at: http://kff.org/global-health-policy/fact-sheet/u-s-funding-for-global-health-the-presidents-fy-2014-budget-request/. Accessed Oct 1 2013.

37. Ronald McDonald House Charities (RMHC). RMHC Global Grant Recipients 2011–2012. Available at: www.rmhc. org/RMHC_Grants_2012-2012.pdf?v = 1. Accessed Oct 5 2013.

38. World Health Organization. About the Department of Human Resources for Health. Available at: http://www.who.int/hrh/ about/en/. Accessed Oct 14 2013.

39. Republic of Rwanda. Human Resources for Health Program. 2013; Available at: http://hrhconsortium.moh.gov.rw/. Accessed Oct 24 2013.

40. Republic of Rwanda. Human Resources for Health: Program Overview. 2013; Available at: http://hrhconsortium. moh.gov.rw/about-hrh/program-overview. Accessed Oct 14 2013.

41. Brigham and Women's Hospital. BWH Global Health Hub: Clintons Visit HRH Program Faculty, Patients in Rwanda. 2013; Available at: http://bwhglobalhealthhub.org/?p=395. Accessed Oct 14 2013.

42. Rwandan Ministry of Health, Talks at Brigham and Women's Hospital, Boston, MA, USA and at the CUGH Consortium of Universities for Global Health March, 2013; 2013.

Chapter 4

1. Fisher QA, Politis GD, Tobias JD, et al. Pediatric anesthesia for voluntary services abroad. *Anesthesia and Analgesia.* 2002; 95(2): 336–50.

2. Magee WP, Vander Burg R, Hatcher KW. Cleft lip and palate as a cost-effective health care treatment in the developing world. *World Journal of Surgery.* 2010; 34: 420–7.

3. Politis GD, Schneider WJ, Van Beek AL, et al. Guidelines for pediatric perioperative care during short-term plastic reconstructive surgical projects in less developed nations. *Anesthesia and Analgesia.* 2011; 112(1): 183–90.

4. Schneider WJ, Politis GD, Gosain AK, et al. Volunteers in Plastic Surgery guidelines for providing surgical care for children in the less developed world. *Plastic and Reconstructive Surgery.* 2011; 127(6): 2477–86.

5. Leach LS, Myrtle RC, Weaver FA. Surgical teams: role perspectives and role dynamics in the operating room. *Health Services Management Research.* 2011; 24(2): 81–90.

6. D'Addessi A, Bongiovanni L, Volpe A, et al. Human factors in surgery: from Three Mile Island to the operating room. *Urologia Internationalis.* 2009; 83(3): 249–57.

7. Paige JT. Surgical team training: promoting high reliability with nontechnical skills. *Surgical Clinics of North America.* 2010; 90(3): 569–81.

Chapter 5

1. Hodges SC, Mijumbi C, Okello M., et al. Anaesthesia services in developing countries: defining the problems. *Anesthesia.* 2007; 62: 4–11.

2. Jochberger S, Ismailova F, Lederer W, et al. Anesthesia and its allied disciplines in the developing world: a nationwide survey of the Republic of Zambia. *Anesth Analg* 2008: 106(3): 942–948.

3. Zoumenou E, Gbenou S, Assouto P, et al. Pediatric anesthesia in developing countries: experience in the two main university hospitals of Benin in West Africa. *Pediatr Anesth* 2010; 20: 741–747.

4. Tobias JD. Administration of sevoflurane using other agent-specific vaporizers. *Am J Therapeutics* 1998; 5: 383–385.

5. Adriani J. *The Pharmacology of Anesthetic Drugs.* 4th ed. Springfield: Charles C Thomas; 1960.

6. Williams DG, Hatch DJ, Howard RF. Codeine phosphate in paediatric medicine. *B J Anaesth* 2001; 86: 413–421.

7. Gasche Y, Daali Y, Fathi M, et al. Codeine intoxication associated with ultrarapid CYP2D6 metabolism. *N Engl J Med* 2004; 351: 2827–2831.

8. Cox RG. Hypoxaemia and hypotension after intravenous codeine phosphate. *Can J Anaesth* 1994; 41: 1211–1213.

9. Shanahan EC, Marshall AG, Garrett CPO. Adverse reactions to intravenous codeine phosphate in children: A report of three cases. *Anesthesia* 1983; 38: 40–42.

10. Kahn LH, Alderfer RJ, Graham DJ. Seizures reported with tramadol. JAMA 1997; 278: 1661.

11. Johnson RE, Fudala PJ, Payne R. Buprenorphine: Considerations for pain management. *J Pain Symptom Manage* 2005; 29: 297–326.

12. Kussman BD, Sethna NF. Pethidine-associated seizure in a healthy adolescent receiving pethidine for postoperative pain control. HYPERLINK "http://www.ncbi.nlm.nih.gov/sites/entrez?cmd= search&term=%22Paediatr%20Anaesth%22%5bJour%5d%20 AND%201998%5bpdat%5d%20AND%208%5bvolume %5d%20AND%20349%5bpage%5d" \l "#" \o "Paediatric anaesthesia." *Paediatr Anaesth* 1998; 8: 349–52.

13. McNicol ED, Tzortzopoulou A, Cepeda MS, Francia MB, et al. Single-dose intravenous paracetamol or propacetamol for prevention or treatment of postoperative pain: a systematic review and meta-analysis. *B J Anaesth* 2001; 106(6): 764–765.

14. Duggan ST, Scott LJ. Intravenous paracetamol (acetaminophen). *Drugs* 2009; 69: 101–113.

15. Wininger SJ, Miller H, Minkowitz HS, et al. A randomized, double-blind, placebo-controlled, multicenter, repeat dose study of two intravenous acetaminophen dosing regimen for the treatment of pain after abdominal laparoscopic surgery. *Clin Ther* 2010; 32: 2348–2369.

16. Munro HM, Walton SR, Malviya S, Merkel S, et al. Low dose ketorolac improves analgesia and reduces morphine requirements following posterior spinal fusion in adolescents. *Can J Anesth* 2002; 49: 461–466.

17. Strom BL, Berlin JA, Kinman JL, Spitz PW, et al. Parenteral ketorolac and risk of gastrointestinal and operative site bleeding. *JAMA* 1996; 275: 376–382.

18. Christ G, Mundigler G, Merhaut C, et al. Adverse cardiovascular effects of ketamine infusion in patients with catecholamine-dependent heart failure. *Anaesth Intensive Care* 1997; 25: 255–259.

19. 17th WHO Essential Medicines List and the 3rd WHO Essential Medicines List for Children.

20. Diefenbach C, Kiinzer T, Buzellot CW, Theisohn M. Alcuronium: a pharmacodynamic and pharmacokinetic update. *Anesth Analg* 1995; 80: 373–7.

21. Gan TJ, Meyer T, Apfel CC, et al. Consensus guidelines for managing postoperative nausea and vomiting. *Anesth Analg* 2003; 97: 62–71.

22. Lee CH, Peng MJ, Wu CL. Dexamethasone to prevent postextubation airway obstruction in adults: a prospective randomized, double blind, placebo controlled study. *Crit Care* 2007; 11:R72.

23. Anene O, Meert KL, Uy H, Simpson P, et al. Dexamethasone for the prevention of airway obstruction: a prospective, randomized, double-blind, placebo-controlled trial. *Crit Care Med* 1996; 24: 1666–1669.

24. Habib AS, Gan TJ. Food and drug administration black box warning on the perioperative use of droperidol: a review of the cases. *Anesth Analg* 2003; 96: 1377–1379.

25. Hohnloser SH, Klingenheben T, Singh BN. Amiodarone-associated proarrhythmic effects: a review with special reference to torsade de pointes tachycardia. *Ann Intern Med* 1994; 121: 529–535.

26. Faber TS, Zehender M, Van de Loo A, Hohnloser S, et al. Torsades de pointes complicating drug treatment of low-malignant forms of arrhythmia: four case reports. *Clin Cardiol* 1994; 17: 197–202.

27. Prough DS, Roy R, Bumgarner J, Shannon G. Acute pulmonary edema in healthy teenagers following conservative doses of intravenous naloxone. *Anesthesiology* 1984; 60: 485–6.

28. Cuss FM, Colaco CB, Baron JH. Cardiac arrest after reversal of effects of opiates with naloxone. *Br Med J*. 1984; 288: 363–364.

Chapter 6

1. Buckenmaier C, Lee E, Shields C, Sampson J, Chiles J. Regional Anesthesia in Austere Environments. *Regional Anesthesia and Pain Medicine*. 2003; 28: 321–7.

2. Cote C, Lerman J, Anderson B (eds.). *A Practice of Anesthesia for Infants and Children*. 5th ed. Philadelphia: Saunders, 2013: 3.

3. Haynes AB, Weiser TG, Berry WR, Lipsitz SR, Breizat AH, Dellinger EP, Herbosa T, Joseph S, Kibatala PL, Lapitan MC, Merry AF, Moorthy K, Reznick RK, Taylor B, Gawande AA. A surgical safety checklist to reduce morbidity and mortality in a global population. *The New England Journal of Medicine*. 2009; 360: 491–9.

4. Brown D (ed.). *Regional Anesthesia and Analgesia*. 1st ed. Philadelphia: Saunders, 2005: 159–172.

5. Hadzic A (ed.). *Textbook of Regional Anesthesia and Acute Pain Management*. China: McGraw-Hill Co., 2007: 307–18.

6. Hadzic A (ed.). *Textbook of Regional Anesthesia and Acute Pain Management*. China: McGraw-Hill Co., 2007: 93–104.

7. Mariano E, Ilfeld B, Cheng G, Nicodemus H, Suresh S. Feasibility of ultrasound-guided peripheral nerve block catheters for pain control on pediatric medical missions in developing countries. *Pediatric Anesthesia*. 2008; 18: 598–601.

8. Oberndofer U, Weintraud M, Redl G. The use of ultrasound-guided regional anesthesia in a rural developing area in India for plastic and orthopedic operations. *Pediatric Anesthesia*. 2010; 20: 198–9.

9. Chin K, Perlas A, Chan V, Brull R. Needle Visualization in Ultrasound-Guided Regional anesthesia: Challenges and Solutions. *Regional Anesthesia and Pain Medicine*. 2008; 33: 532–44.

10. Hadzic A (ed.). *Textbook of Regional Anesthesia and Acute Pain Management*. China: McGraw-Hill Co., 2007: 753–67.

11. Cote C, Lerman J, Anderson B (eds.). *A Practice of Anesthesia for Infants and Children*. Philadelphia: Saunders, 2013: Table 41-2.

12. Weinberg G. Lipid Emulsion Infusion. *Anesthesiology*. 2013; 117: 180–7.

13. Lewis W (ed.). *Anatomy of the Human Body by Henry Gray*. 20th ed. Philadelphia: Lea & Febiger, 1918: Figure 807.

14. Lewis W (ed.). *Anatomy of the human body by Henry Gray*, 20th ed. Philadelphia: Lea & Febiger, 1918: Figure 797.

15. Hadzic, Admir. *Textbook of Regional Anesthesia and Acute Pain Management*. McGraw-Hill. 2007. Table 25-3.

16. Hadzic, Admir. *Textbook of Regional Anesthesia and Acute Pain Management*. McGraw-Hill. 2007. Table 35-1.

17. Hadzic, Admir. *Textbook of Regional Anesthesia and Acute Pain Management*. McGraw-Hill. 2007. Table 38-2.

Chapter 7

1. Hodges SC, Mijumbi C, Okelly M, McCormick BA Walker IA, Wilson IH. Anaesthesia services in developing countries: defining the problems. *Anaesthesia*. 2007; 62: 4–11.

2. World Health Organization. WHO Manual: Surgical Care at the District Hospital; 2003 [cited 2011 Oct 17]. Available from: HYPERLINK "http://www.who.int/surgery/publications/scdh_manual/en/" www.who.int/surgery/publications/scdh_manual/en/

3. Merson MH, Black RE, Mills AJ. International Public Health: Diseases, Programs, Systems, and Policies. 2nd Ed. Burlington (MA): Jones and Bartlett Publishers, Inc; 2006.

4. U.S. Census Bureau. Global Population Composition; 2002 [cited 2011 Oct 11]. Available from: www.census.gov/population/international/files/wp02/wp-02004.pdf

5. U.S. Census Bureau. International Data Base; 2011 [cited 2011 Oct 11]. Available from: http://www.census.gov/population/international/data/idb/country.php

6. UNICEF. *State of the World's Children Report*; 2011 [cited 2011 Oct 17]. Available from: HYPERLINK "http://www.unicef.org/sowc2011/pdfs/SOWC-2011-Statistical-tables_12082010.pdf" www.unicef.org/sowc2011/pdfs/SOWC-2011-Statistical-tables_12082010.pdf

7. Demographic and Health Surveys. STATcompiler; 2011 [cited 2011 Oct 17]. Available from: HYPERLINK "http://www.measuredhs.com/" www.measuredhs.com

8. The World Health Report. Geneva: World Health Organization; 2004 [cited 2011 Oct 17]. Available from: http://www.who.int/whr/2004/annex/topic/en/annex_3_en.pdf

9. The World Health Report. List of Member States by WHO regions and mortality stratum. Geneva: World Health Organization; 2004 [cited 2011 Nov 8]. Available from: http://www.who.int/whr/2004/annex/en/index.html

10. The World Health Report. Geneva: World Health Organization; 2004 [cited 2011 Nov 8]. Available from: http://www.who.int/whr/2004/annex/topic/en/annex_2_en.pdf

11. Bickler S, Ozgediz D, Gosselin R, Weiser T, Spiegel D, Hsia R, et al. Key concepts for estimating the burden of surgical conditions and the unmet need for surgical care. *World J of Surgery*. 2010; 34: 374–80.

12. Debas HT, Gosselin R, McCord C. Surgery. In: Disease Control Priorities in Developing Countries. 2nd ed. New York: Oxford University Press; 2006.

13. McQueen KAK. Anesthesia and the global burden of surgical disease. *International Anesth Clinics*. 2010; 48(2): 91–107.

14. Ozgediz D, Jamison D, Cherian M, McQueen K. The burden of surgical conditions and access to surgical care in low- and middle-income countries. *Bulletin of the World Health Organization*. 2008; 86(8): 646–7.

15. Dyer RA, Reed AR, James MF. Obstetric anaesthesia in low-resource settings. *Best Practice & Res Clin Obstet and Gyn*. 2010; 24: 401–12.

16. World Health Organization. Global Health Observatory Data Repository; 2011 [cited 2011 Oct 17]. Available from: http://www.who.int/gho/health_workforce/physicians_density/en/index.html

17. World Health Organization. Global Health Observatory Data Repository; 2011 [cited 2011 Oct 17]. Available from: http://apps.who.int/ghodata/?vid=92100

18. World Health Organization. Global Health Observatory Data Repository; 2001 [cited 2011 Oct 17]. Available from: http://gamapserver.who.int/gho/interactive_charts/health_workforce/PhysiciansDensity_Total/atlas.html

19. Ronsmans C, Holtz S, Stanton C. Socioeconomic differentials in caesarean rates in developing countries: a retrospective analysis. *Lancet*. 2006; 368: 1516–23.

20. Draulans N, Keikens C, Roels E, Peers K. Etiology of spinal cord injuries in sub-saharan Africa. Spinal Cord advance online publication October 11, 2011; 1–7. Available from: http://www.nature.com.ezproxy.welch.jhmi.edu/sc/journal/vaop/ncurrent/pdf/sc201193a.pdf

21. Mathers CD, Lopez AD, Murray CJL. The Burden of Disease and Mortality by Condition: Data, Methods and Results for 2001. In: Lopez AD, Mathers CD, Ezzati M, Jamison DT, Murray CJL, ed. *Global Burden of Disease and Risk Factors*. Washington, D.C. and New York: The World Bank and Oxford University Press; 2006 [cited 2011 Sept 8]. Available from: http://www.dcp2.org/pubs/GBD

22. Tait AR, Malviya S. Anesthesia for the child with an upper respiratory tract infection: still a dilemma? *Anesth Analg*. 2005; 100(1): 59–65.

23. Tait AR, Malviya S, Voepel-Lewis T, Munro HM, Seiwert M, Pandit UA. Risk factors for perioperative adverse respiratory events in children with upper respiratory tract infections. *Anesthesiology*. 2001; 95(2): 299–306.

24. Walker IA, Merry AF, Wilson IH, McHugh GA, O'Sullivan E, Thoms GM, et al. Global oximetry: and international anaesthesia quality improvement project. *Anaesthesia*. 2009; 64: 1051–60.

25. McCormick BA, Eltringham RJ. Anesthesia equipment for resource-poor environments. *Anaesthesia*. 2007; 62(Suppl. 1): 54–60.

26. World Federation of Societies of Anaesthesiologists. International standards for a safe practice of anaesthesia; 2008 [cited 2011 Sept 28]. Available from: HYPERLINK "http://www.anaesthesiologists.org/guidelines/" www.anaesthesiologists.org/guidelines/

Chapter 9

1. Nicholau, D. (2007). Postanesthesia Recovery. In R. Stoelting & R. Miller, *Basics of Anesthesia (Fifth Edition)*. (563–577). Philadelphia: Churchill Livingstone Elsevier.

2. World Health Organization. Surgical Safety Checklist. Available online at: http://www.who.int/patientsafety/safesurgery/ss_checklist/en/index.html. Accessed on June 22, 2011.

3. Mecca, RS. (2006). Postoperative Recovery. In P. Barash, B. Cullen & R. Stoelting, *Clinical Anesthesia (Fifth Edition)*. (1379–1403). Philadelphia: Lippincott Williams & Wilkins.

4. Lexicomp Online. Available online at: http://online.lexi.com/crlsql/servlet/crlonline. Accessed on June 22, 2011.

5. Tomlinson D, von Baeyer CL, Stinson JN, Sung L. A systematic review of faces scales for the self-report of pain intensity in children. Pediatrics. 2010 Nov; 126(5): e1168–98. Epub 2010 Oct 4.

6. Morgan, E.G., Mikhail, M., Murray, M. (2006). Local Anesthetics. In E.G. Morgan, M. Mikhail, & M. Murray, *Clinical Anesthesiology (Fourth Edition)*. (263–275). New York: Lange Medical Books/McGraw-Hill.

7. Doufas, AG. et al, *Best Practice & Research Clinical Anaesthesiology*; consequences of inadvertent perioperative hypothermia; Volume 17, Issue 4, December 2003: 535–549.

8. Alfonsi P, Postanesthetic shivering: Epidemiology, Pathophysiology and Approaches to prevention and management, Minerva Anesthesiol 2003: 69: 438–41.

9. Sasada, M, Smith, S. (2003). In M. Sasada & S. Smith, *Drugs in Anaesthesia & Intensive Care (Third Edition)*. Oxford: Oxford University Press.

10. Finfer, S, Bellomo, R. A comparison of albumin and saline for fluid resuscitation in the intensive care unit. *N Engl J Med.* 2004 May 27; 350(22): 2247–56.

11. Borgman, MA, Spinella, PC. The ratio of blood products transfused affects mortality in patients receiving massive transfusions at a combat support hospital. *J Trauma.* 2007 Oct; 63(4): 805–13.

Chapter 10

1. Hazinski MF, Nolan JP, Billi JE, et al. Part 1: Executive Summary: 2010 International Consensus on Cardiopulmonary Resuscitation and Emergency Cardiovascular Care Science with Treatment Recommendations. *Circulation.* 2010; 122: S250–75.

2. Sayre MR, Koster RW, Botha M, et al. Part 5: Adult Basic Life Support: 2010 International Consensus on Cardiopulmonary Resuscitation and Emergency Cardiovascular Care Science with Treatment Recommendations. *Circulation.* 2010; 122: S298–324.

3. Morrison LJ, Deakin CD, Morley PT, et al. Part 8: Adult Advanced Cardiovascular Life Support: 2010 International Consensus on Cardiopulmonary Resuscitation and Emergency Cardiovascular Care Science with Treatment Recommendations. *Circulation.* 2010; 122: S345–421.

4. Gaba DM, Fish KJ, Howard SK. *Crisis Management in Anesthesiology.* London: Churchill Livingstone, 1994.

5. Kleinman ME, de Caen AR, Chameides L, et al. Part 10: Pediatric Basic and Advanced Life Support: 2010 International Consensus on Cardiopulmonary Resuscitation and Emergency Cardiovascular Care Science with Treatment Recommendations. *Circulation.* 2010; 122: S466–515.

6. PALS Provider Manual ed. by Ralston, Hazinski, Zaritsy, Schexnayder and Kleinman. 2006. Published by the American Heart Association.

7. Little G, Niermeyer S, Singhal N, et al. Neonatal resuscitation: a global challenge. *Pediatrics.* 2010; 126: e1259–60.

8. Perlamn JM, Wyllie J, Kattwinkel J, et al. Part 11: Neonatal Resuscitation: 2010 International Consensus on Cardiopulmonary Resuscitation and Emergency Cardiovascular Care Science with Treatment Recommendations. *Circulation.* 2010; 122: S516–38.

Chapter 11

1. Keshavjee S, Farmer PE. Tuberculosis, Drug Resistance, and the History of Modern Medicine. *New England Journal of Medicine.* 2012; 367: 931–936.

2. Light RW, Macgregor MI, Luchsinger PC, Ball WC, Jr. Pleural effusions: the diagnostic separation of transudates and exudates. *Annals of Internal Medicine.* 1972; 77: 507–13.

3. White RE, Parker RK, Fitzwater JW, et al. Stents as sole therapy for oesophageal cancer: a prospective analysis of outcomes after placement. *Lancet.* 2009; 10: 240–6.

4. White RE, Mungatana C, Topazian M. Esophageal stent placement without fluoroscopy. *Gastrointestinal Endoscopy.* 2001; 53: 348–51.

5. Borgulya M, Ell C, Pohl J. Transnasal endoscopy for direct visual control of esophageal stent placement without fluoroscopy. *Endoscopy.* 2012; 44: 422–4.

6. Tanuah Y, Kendia K, Yangni Angate H, Aka D, Bakassa S, Yapobi Y, Kangah M, Coulibaly AO, Metras D. L'Aspergillome pulmonaire symptomatique: à propos de 71 cas opérés = Symptomatic pulmonary aspergilloma. 1994; 41(5): 315–318.

7. Tanuah Y, Kendia K, Yangni Angate H, Aka D, Bakassa S, Yapobi Y, Kangah M, Coulibaly AO, Metras D. Les Dilatations des bronches post-tuberculeuses: soixante seize cas opérés = Post-tuberculous bronchiectasis. *Médecined'Afriquenoire.* 1994; 41(6): 345–8.

8. Tanuah Y, Kendia F, Yangni-Angate H, Ehounoud H, Yapo P, Ouattara K, Kouassi K, Longechaud A, Brunet A, Coulibaly AO, Metras D. *Journal of the African Association of Thoracic and Cardio-Vascular Surgeons.* 2007; 2(1): 63–90.

9. Ciss G, Diarra O, Ba M, Ndiaye A, Kane O, Dieng PA, Sall Ka B, Ndiaye M. Pneumonectomie pour poumons détruits post- tuberculeux/Pneumonectomy for destroyed lung secondary to tuberculosis. *Journal of the African Association of Thoracic and Cardio-Vascular Surgeons.* 2007; 2(1): 63–90.

10. Ondo N'Dong F, Diallo OKF, Mbamendame S, et al. Pythorax: Aspects cliniques et thérapeutiques a Libreville. A propos de 24 cas./Empyema in Libreville, Gabon: 24 cases. *Journal of the African Association of Thoracic and Cardio-Vascular Surgeons.* 2007; 2(2): 124–8.

11. Diarra O, Ba M, Ndiaye A, et al. Pleuresies purulentes aux urgences chirurgicales: Etude retrospective de 34 cas au CHU de Dakar/Empyema at Dakar Teaching Hospital,senegal: 34cases. *Dakar Médical.* 2003; 48(2).

12. Kendja F, Ouede R, Ehounoud H, Demine B, Yapo Y, Tanuah Y, Yangni-Angate H. Traitement Chirurgical des Pachypleurites Secondraires Pythorax Chroniques: A propos de 141 cas. *Journal of the African Association of Thoracic and Cardio-Vascular Surgeons.* 2012; 7(1), 24–29.

13. Tanuah Y, Yangni-Angate H, Kangah M, et al. Aspects chirurgicaux des cancers broncho-pulmonaires en COTE D'IVOIRE/Surgical Management of lung carcinoma in Cote D'Ivoire. XVIIIe Annual congres of the West African College of Surgeons Monrovia, Liberia 24–31 January 1988.

14. Ondo N'Dong F, Diallo Owondo FK, Mbamendame S, et al. Cancers broncho-pulmonaires: prise en charge à Libreville à propos de 34 cas/Broncho-pulmonary cancers: Management in Libreville: 34 cases. *Bull Med Owendo.* 2009; 12(33).

Chapter 12

1. Raja AJ, Levin AV. Challenges of teaching surgery: ethical framework. *World Journal of Surgery.* 2003; 27: 948–51.

2. Silen W (ed.). *Cope's Early Diagnosis of the Acute Abdomen,* 22nd ed. Cary: Oxford University Press, 2010.

3. King M, Bewes P, Cairns J (eds.). *Primary Surgery: Non-Trauma, Volume 1.* Cary: Oxford University Press, 1990.

4. Choen RV, Aun F (eds.). *Tropical Surgery.* Switzerland: Karger AG, 1997.

Chapter 13

1. Higham J, Kang JY, Majeed A. Recent trends in admissions and mortality due to peptic ulcer in England. *Gut.* 2002; 50: 460–4.
2. Janik J, Chwirot P. Peptic ulcer disease before and after introduction of new drugs—a comparison from a surgeon's point of view. *Medical Science Monitor.* 2000; 6: 365–8.
3. Dore MP and Graham DY. Pathogenesis of duodenal ulcer disease: the rest of the story. *Baillieres Best Practice and Research Clinical Gastroenterology.* 2000; 14: 97–107.
4. Shapiro DS, Loiacono LA. Mean arterial pressure: therapeutic goals and pharmacologic support. In: Nichols D. Optimizing hemodynamic support in severe sepsis and septic shock. *Critical Care Clinics of North America.* 2010; 26(2): 289.
5. Chowdhury A, Dhali GK, Banerjee PK. Etiology of gastric outlet obstruction. *American Journal of Gastroenterology.* 1996; 91: 1679.
6. Matsui H, Shimokawa O, Hyodo I, et al. The pathophysiology of nonsteroidal anti-inflammatory drug induced mucosal injuries in stomach and small intestine. *Journal of Clinical Biochemistry and Nutrition.* 2011 March; 48(2): 107–11.
7. Chiba N. Ulcer disease and helicobacter pylori infection: etiology and treatment. In: McDonald J, Burroughs A, Feagan B, Fennerty B (eds.). *Evidence Based Gastroenterology and Hepatology.* 3rd ed. 2010: 102–38.
8. Branicki FJ, Coleman SY, Fok PJ, et al. Bleeding peptic ulcer: a prospective evaluation of risk factors for rebleeding and mortality. *World Journal of Surgery.* 1990; 14: 262.
9. Chen ZJ, Freeman ML. Management of upper gastrointestinal bleeding emergencies: evidence-based medicine and practical considerations. *World Journal of Emergency Medicine.* 2011; 2(1): 5–12.
10. King M, et al. *Primary Surgery, Vol. 1, Non-trauma.* Oxford Medical Publications, 1990: 172–3.
11. Barkun A, Bardou M, Marshall JK. Consensus recommendations for managing patients with nonvariceal upper gastrointestinal bleeding. Nonvariceal Upper GI Bleeding Consensus Conference Group. *Annals of Internal Medicine.* 2003, 139(10): 843–57.
12. Cappell MS, Friedel D. Initial management of acute upper gastrointestinal bleeding: from initial evaluation up to gastrointestinal endoscopy. *Medical Clinics of North America.* 2008; 92: 491–509.
13. Pacios E, Arias-Diaz J, Zuloaga J, et al. Albendazole for the treatment of Anisakiasis ileus. *Clinical Infectious Disease.* 2005; 41(12): 1825–6.
14. Krige JEJ, Kotze UK, Bornman PC, et al. Variceal Recurrence, rebleeding and survival after endoscopic injection sclerotherapy in 287 alcoholic cirrhotic patients with bleeding esophageal varices. *Annals of Surgery.* 2006; 244(5): 764–70.
15. Bendtsen F, Krag A, and Moller S. Treatment of acute variceal bleeding. *Digestive and Liver Disease.* 2008; 40(5): 328–36.
16. Riechle FA, Fahmy WF, Golsorkhi M. Prospective comparative clinical trial with distal splenorenal and mesocaval shunts. *American Journal of Surgery.* 1979; 1237: 13–21.
17. Grace ND, Conn HO, Resnick RH, et al. Distal splenorenal vs. portalsystemic shunts after hemorrhage from varices: a randomized controlled trial. *Hepatology.* 1988; 8: 1475–81.
18. Fischer JE (ed.). Portal hypertension and its treatment. In: *Fischer's Mastery of Surgery.* 5th ed. Philadelphia: Lippincott Williams & Wilkins, 2007.
19. Tavakkolizadeh A, Ashley SW. Operations for peptic ulcer. In: *Shackelford's Surgery of the Alimentary Tract.* 6th ed. Philadelphia: Saunders Elsevier, 2007.
20. Lam YH, Lau JY, Fung TM, et al. Endoscopic balloon dilation for benign gastric outlet obstruction with or without Helicobacter pylori infection. *Gastrointestinal Endoscopy.* 2004; 60(2): 229–33.
21. Gibson JB, Behrman SW, Fabian TC, et al. Gastric outlet obstruction resulting from peptic ulcer disease requiring surgical intervention is infrequently associated with Helicobacter Pylori. *Journal of the American College of Surgery.* 2000; 191(1): 32–3.
22. Behrman SW. Management of complicated peptic ulcer disease. *Archives of Surgery.* 2005; 140(2): 201–8.
23. Lipof T, Shapiro D, Kozol R. Surgical perspectives in peptic ulcer disease and gastritis. *World Journal of Gastroenterology.* 2006; 12(20): 2348–52.
24. Ly J, O'Grady G, Mittal A, et al. A systemic review of methods to palliate malignant gastric outlet obstruction. *Surgical Endoscopy.* 2010; 24: 290–7.
25. Kement M, Ozlem N, Colak E, et al. Synergistic effect of multiple predisposing factors on the development of bezoars. *World Journal of Gastroenterology.* 2012; 18(9): 960–4.
26. Chassin JL. Pyloroplasty, Heineke-Mikulicz. In: *Operative Strategy in General Surgery.* New York: Springer-Verlag, 1980.
27. Donahue PE. Foregut. In: *Acute Care Surgery: Principles & Practice.* New York: Springer, 2007.
28. Hoya Y, Mitsumori N, Yanaga K. The advantages and disadvantages of a Roux-en-Y reconstruction after a distal gastrectomy for gastric cancer. *Surgery Today.* 2009; 39(8): 647–51.
29. Kudsk KA, Croce MA, Fabian TC, et al. Enteral versus parenteral feeding. Effects on septic morbidity after blunt and penetrating abdominal trauma. *Annals of Surgery.* 1992; 215(5): 503–13.

Chapter 14

1. Stinton LM, Myers RP, Shaffer EA. Epidemiology of gallstones. *Gastroenterology Clinics of North America.* 2010; 39(2): 157–69, vii.
2. Morgenstern L. Carl Langenbuch and the first cholecystectomy. *Surgical Endoscopy.* 1992; 6(3): 113–4.
3. Gracie WA, Ransohoff DF. The natural history of silent gallstones: the innocent gallstone is not a myth. *New England Journal of Medicine.* 1982; 307(13): 798–800.
4. Shaffer EA. Epidemiology and risk factors for gallstone disease: has the paradigm changed in the 21st century? *Current Gastroenterology Reports.* 2005; 7(2): 132–40.
5. Adedeji A, Akande B, Olumide F. The changing pattern of cholelithiasis in Lagos. *Scandanavian Journal of Gastroenterology.* 1986; 124: 63–6.
6. Bekele Z, Tegegn K. Cholecystitis: the Ethiopian experience, a report of 712 operated cases from one of the referral hospitals. *Ethiopian Medical Journal.* 2002; 40(3): 209–16.

7. Rahman GA. Cholelithiasis and cholecystitis: changing prevalence in an African community. *Journal of the National Medical Association*. 2005; 97(11): 1534–8.

8. Thomson SR, Docrat HY, Haffejee AA, et al. Cholecystectomy in a predominantly African population before and after the advent of the laparoscopic technique. *Surgeon*. 2003; 1(2): 92–5.

9. Volzke H, Baumeister SE, Alte D, et al. Independent risk factors for gallstone formation in a region with high cholelithiasis prevalence. *Digestion*. 2005; 71(2): 97–105.

10. Azi MR, Wandwi WB. Cholelithiasis in Dar es Salaam, Tanzania. *Central African Journal of Medicine*. 1995; 41(10): 308–12.

11. Ostrow, B. Cholelithiasis, cholecystitis and cholecystectomy—their relevance for African surgeons. *Surgery in Africa—Monthly Review*. 2007; 16.

12. Hirota M, Takada T, Kawarada Y, et al. Diagnostic criteria and severity assessment of acute cholecystitis: Tokyo Guidelines. *Journal of Hepato-Biliary Pancreatic Surgery*. 2007; 14(1): 78–82.

13. Straub CM, Price RR, Matthews D, et al. Expanding laparoscopic cholecystectomy to rural mongolia. *World Journal of Surgery*. 2011; 35(4): 751–9.

14. Darko R, Archampong EQ. The microflora of bile in Ghanaians. *West African Journal of Medicine*. 1994; 13(2): 113–5.

15. Cameron JL. *Current Surgical Therapy*. 9th ed. Philadelphia: Mosby Elselvier, 2007.

16. Guttikonda S, Vaswani KK, Vitellas KM. Recurrent gallstone ileus: a case report. *Emergency Radiology*. 2002; 9(2): 110–12.

17. Sanai FM, Al-Karawi MA. Biliary ascariasis: report of a complicated case and literature review. *Saudi Journal of Gastroenterology*. 2007; 13(1): 25–32.

18. Lim JH, Kim SY, Park CM. Parasitic diseases of the biliary tract. *American Journal of Roentgenology*. 2007; 188(6): 1596–1603.

19. Javid G, Wani N, Gulzar GM, et al. Gallbladder ascariasis: presentation and management. *British Journal of Surgery*. 1999; 86(12): 1526–7.

20. World Health Organization. Soil-transmitted helminth (STH) infections are widely distributed in tropical and subtropical areas [Internet]. 2006. Accessed May 28 2011. Available from: http://www.who.int/intestinal_worms/epidemiology/map/en/index.html

21. Lazcano-Ponce EC, Miquel JF, Munoz N, et al. Epidemiology and molecular pathology of gallbladder cancer. *CA-A Cancer Journal for Clinicians*. 2001; 51(6): 349–64.

22. Randi G, Franceschi, S, La Vecchia C. Gallbladder cancer worldwide: geographical distribution and risk factors. *International Journal of Cancer*. 2006; 118(7): 1591–1602.

23. Surgical care at the district hospital. Geneva: World Health Organization, 2003.

24. Basu S, Giri PS, Roy D. Feasibility of same day discharge after mini-laparotomy cholecystectomy—a simulation study in a rural teaching hospital. *Canadian Journal of Rural Medicine*. 2006; 11(2): 93–8.

25. Thomas S, Singh J, Bishnoi PK, Kumar A. Feasibility of day-care open cholecystectomy: evaluation in an inpatient model. *ANZ Journal of Surgery*. 2001; 71(2): 93–7.

26. Mir IS, Mohsin M, Kirmani O, et al. Is intra-operative cholangiography necessary during laparoscopic cholecystectomy? A multicentre rural experience from a developing world country. *World Journal of Gastroenterology*. 2007; 13(33): 4493–7.

27. Gurusamy KS, SamrajK. Primary closure versus T-tube drainage after laparoscopic common bile duct stone exploration. *Cochrane Database of Systematic Reviews*. 2007a(1), CD005641.

28. Gurusamy KS, Samraj K. Primary closure versus T-tube drainage after open common bile duct exploration. *Cochrane Database of Systematic Reviews*. 2007b(1), CD005640.

29. Sergelen, O. Development of Laparoscopic Surgery in Mongolia [Internet]. 2006. Accessed March 13 2010. Available from: http://www.gfmer.ch/Medical_education_En/PGC_RH_2006/Reviews/pdf/Orgoi_laparoscopy_2006.pdf.

30. Strasberg SM, Hertl M, Soper NJ. An analysis of the problem of biliary injury during laparoscopic cholecystectomy. *Journal of the American College of Surgeons*. 1995; 180(1): 101–25.

31. de Santibanes E, Ardiles V, Pekolj J. Complex bile duct injuries: management. *The Official Journal of the Hepato-Pancreato-Biliary Association*. 2008; 10(1): 4–12.

32. Jupp J, Fine D, Johnson CD. The epidemiology and socio-economic impact of chronic pancreatitis. *Best Practice & Research Clinical Gastroenterology*. 2010; 24(3): 219–31.

33. Garg PK, Tandon RK. Survey on chronic pancreatitis in the Asia-Pacific region. *Journal of Gastroenterology and Hepatology*. 2004; 19(9): 998–1004.

34. Townsend CM, Beauchamp RD, Evers M, Mattox K. *Sabiston Textbook of Surgery*. 18th ed. Philadelphia: Elsevier, 2008.

35. Villatoro E, Mulla M, Larvin M. Antibiotic therapy for prophylaxis against infection of pancreatic necrosis in acute pancreatitis. *Cochrane Database of Systematic Reviews*. 2010(5), CD002941. doi:10.1002/14651858.CD002941.pub3.

36. Mulholland M, Lillemoe K, Doherty G, Maier R, Simeone D, Upchurch G. Greenfield's Surgery: Scientific Principles and Practice. Philadelphia: Lippincott, Williams and Wilkins, 2010.

37. Stamatakos M, Stefanaki C, Kontzoglou K, et al. Walled-off pancreatic necrosis. *World Journal of Gastroenterology*. 2010; 16(14): 1707–12.

38. Reid-Lombardo K, Khan S, Sclabas G. Hepatic Cysts and Liver Abscesses. *Surgical Clinics of North America*. 2010; 90(4).

39. Lin AC, Yeh DY, Hsu YH, et al. Diagnosis of pyogenic liver abscess by abdominal ultrasonography in the emergency department. *Emergency Medicine Journal*. 2009; 26(4): 273–75.

40. Wang CL, Guo XJ, Qiu SB, et al. Diagnosis of bacterial hepatic abscess by CT. *Hepatobiliary & Pancreatic Diseases International*. 2007; 6(3): 271–75.

41. Chavez-Tapia NC, Hernandez-Calleros J, Tellez-Avila FI, et al. Image-guided percutaneous procedure plus metronidazole versus metronidazole alone for uncomplicated amoebic liver abscess. *Cochrane Database of Systematic Reviews*. 2009(1), CD004886. doi: 10.1002/14651858.CD004886.pub2.

42. Mandell (ed.). *Mandell, Douglas, and Bennett's Principles and Practice of Infectious Diseases*. 7th ed. London: Churchill Livingstone, 2009.

43. Zhang W, McManus D. Concepts of immunology and diagnosis of hydatid disease. *Clinical Microbiology Review*. 2003; 16: 18–36.

44. Guidelines for treatment of cystic and alveolar echinococcosis in humans. *Bulletin of the World Health Organization*. 1996; 74: 231–42.

45. Schantz P, Kern P, Brunetti E, et al. *Tropical Infectious Diseases: Principles, Pathogens & Practice: Echinococcosis.* Philadelphia: Churchill Livingstone, 2006.

46. How to make normal saline [Internet]. 2004. Accessed June 3 2011. Available from: http://medicalcenter.osumc.edu/patiented/materials/pdfdocs/procedure/how-to/makenor.pdf.

Chapter 15

1. Sundaresan JB, DuttaTK, Badrinath S, et al. Study of hypersplenism and effect of splenectomy on patients with hypersplenism. *Journal, Indian Academy of Clinical Medicine.* 2005, 6(4): 291–6.

2. Bruce-Chwatt LJ. *Essential Malariology.* London: Heinemann Medical, 1980.

3. Malaria Rapid Diagnostic Test Performance: Results of the WHO product Testing of Malaria RDTS: Round 2 (2009), Geneva: World Health Organization, 2009.

4. World Health Organization. International travel and health: Situation as on 1 January 2011. Geneva, Switzerland: World Health Organization Press, 2011.

5. Schaefer KU, Khan B, Gachihi GS, et al. Splenomegaly in Baringo District, Kenya, an area endemic for visceral leishmaniasis and malaria. *Tropical and Geographic Medicine.* 1995; 47(3): 111–4.

6. De Cock KM, Lucas SB, Jupp RA, et al. Chronic splenomegaly in Nairobi, Kenya. I. Epidemiology, malarial antibody and immunoglobulin levels. *Transactions of the Royal Society of Tropical Medicine and Hygiene.* 1987; 81(1): 100–6.

7. Snow RW, Guerra CA, Mutheu JJ, et al. International funding for malaria control in relation to populations at risk of stable plasmodiumfalciparum transmission. *PLOS Medicine.* 2008; 5(7): e142.

8. Imananagha KK, Awotua-Efebo OE, Consul JI. Severe malaria in children: a proposal for clinical grading. *South African Journal of Child Health.* 2009; 3(10): 5–8.

9. World Malaria Report, Geneva, Switzerland: World Health Organization, 2009 Print.

10. *Guidelines for the Treatment of Malaria,* 2nd ed. Geneva: World Health Organization, 2010.

11. Osman MF, Elhkidir IM, Roger SO Jr., et al. Non-operative management of malarial splenic rupture: the Khartoum experience and an international review. *International Journal of Surgery.* 2012; 10(9): 410–4.

12. Manenti F, Porta E, Esposito R, et al. Treatment of hyperreactive malarial splenomegaly syndrome. *Lancet.* 1994; 343: 1441–2.

13. John AB, Ramlal A, Jackson H, et al. Prevention of pneumococcal infection in children with homozygous sickle cell disease. *British Medical Journal.* 1984; 288: 1567–70.

14. Gaston MH, Verter JI, Woods G, et al. Prophylaxis with oral penicillin in children with sickle cell anemia. *New England Journal of Medicine.* 1986; 314: 1593–9.

15. Ballet JJ, Jaureguiberry G, Deloron P, et al. Stimulation of T Lymphocyte-dependent differentiation of activated human B lymphocytes by Plasmodium falciparum supernatants. *Journal of Infectious Diseases.* 1987; 155: 1037–1040.

16. Stach JC, Ufrenoy E, Roffi J, et al. T-cell subsets and natural killer activity in Plasmodium falciparum-infected children. *Clinical Immunology and Immunopathology.* 1986, 38: 129–134.

17. Troye-Blomberg M, Romero P, Patarroyo ME, et al. Regulation of the immune response in Plasmodium falciparum malaria III. Proliferative response to antigen *in vitro* and subset composition of t cells from patients with acute infection of from immune donors. *Clinical and Experimental Immunology.* 1984; 58: 380–7.

18. Kremsner PG, Feldmeier H, Zotter GM, et al. Immunological alterations in uncomplicated Plasmodium falciparum malaria. Relationship between parisitaemia and indicators of macrophage activation. *Acta Tropica.* 1989; 46: 351–9.

19. Kremsner PG, Zotter GM, Felmeirer H, et al. Immune Response in Patients during and after Plasmodium falciparum Infection. *Journal of Infectious Diseases.* 1990; 161(5): 1025–8.

20. Boone KE, Watters DA. The incidence of malaria after splenectomy in Papua New Guinea. *BMJ.* 1995; 311: 1273.

21. Imbert P, Rapp C, Buffet PA. Pathological rupture of the spleen in malaria: Analysis of 55 cases (1958–2008). *Travel Medicine and Infectious Disease.* 2009; 7: 147–159.

22. Egwunyenga OA, Ajayi JA, Duhlinska-Popova DD. Malaria in pregnancy in Nigerians: seasonality and relationship to splenomegaly and anemia. *Indian Journal of Malariology.* 1997; 34(1): 17–24.

23. Stephenson LS, Latham MC, Kinoti SN, et al. Regression of splenomegaly and hepatomegaly in children treated for Schistosoma haematobium infection. *The American Journal of Tropical Medicine and Hygiene.* 1985; 34(1): 119–23.

24. Elliott DE. Schistosomiasis. Pathophysiology, diagnosis, and treatment. *Gastroenterology Clinics of North America.* 1996; 25: 599.

25. Cota GF, Pinto-Silva RA, Antunes CMF, et al. Ultrasound and clinical investigation of hepatosplenic schistosomiasis: evaluation of splenomegaly and liver fibrosis four years after mass chemotherapy with oxamniguine. *American Journal of Tropical Medicine and Hygiene.* 2006; 74(1): 103–7.

26. Sleigh AC, Mott KE, Hoff R, et al. Manson's Schistosomiasis in Brazil: 11-Year Evaluation of Successful Disease Control with Oxamniquine. *Lancet.* 1986; 327(8482): 635–7.

27. Kamel R, Dunn MA, Skelly RR, et al. Clinical and immunological results of segmental splenectomy in schistosomiasis. *British Journal of Surgery.* 1986; 73(7): 544–7.

28. Adam I, Elwasila E, Homeida M. Praziquantel for the treatment of schistosomiasis mansoni during pregnancy. *Annals of Tropical Medicine and Parasitology.* 2005; 99: 37.

29. Savioli L, Crompton DW, Neira M. Use of anthelminthic drugs during pregnancy. *American Journal of Obstetrics and Gynecology.* 2003; 188: 5.

30. Adam I, Elwasila E, Homeida M. Praziquantel for the treatment of schistosomiasis mansoni during pregnancy. *Transactions of the Royal Society of Tropical Medicine and Hygiene.* 2004; 98: 540.

31. Chulay JD, Bryceson AD. Quantitation of amastigotes of Leishmania donovani in smears of splenic aspirates with visceral leishmaniasis. *American Journal of Tropical Medicine and Hygiene.* 1983; 32(3): 475–9.

32. Troya J, Casquero A, Muñiz G, et al. The role of splenectomy in HIV-infected patients with relapsing visceral leishmaniasis. *Parasitology.* 2007; 134(5): 621–4.

33. Robays, J, Bilengue MM, Van der Stuyft P, et al. The effectiveness of active population screening and treatment for sleeping sickness control in the Democratic Republic of Congo. *Tropical Medicine and International Health.* 2004; 9: 542–50.

34. Verastegui M, Moro P, Guevara A, et al. Enzyme-linked immunoelectrotransfer blot test for eiagnosis of human hydatid disease. *Journal of Clinical Microbiology.* 1992: 1557–61.

35. Franquet T, Montes M, Lecuberri FJ, et al. Hydatid disease of the spleen: imaging findings in nine patients. *American Journal of Roentgenology.* 1990; 154: 525–528.

36. Dachman AH, Ross PR, Murari PJ, et al. Nonparasitic splenic cysts: A report of 52 cases with radiologic-pathologic correlation. *American Journal of Roentgenology.* 1986; 147: 537–42.

37. Davis A, Pawlowski ZS, Dixon H. Multicentre clinical trials of benzimidazole carmates in human echinococcus. *Bulletin of the World Health Organization.* 1986; 64: 383–8.

38. Skroubis G, Vagianos C, Polydorou A, et al. Significance of bile leaks complicating conservative surgery for liver hydatidosis. *World Journal of Surgery.* 2002; 26: 704–8.

39. Llenas-Garcia J, Fernandez-Ruiz M, Caurcel L, et al. Splenic abscess: a review of 22 cases in a single institution. *European Journal of Internal Medicine.* 2009; 20: 537–9.

40. Chiang IS, Lin TJ, Chiang IC, et al. Splenic abscesses: review of 29 cases. *The Kaohsiung Journal of Medical Sciences.* 2003; 19(10): 510–5.

41. Lee WS, Choi ST, Kim KK. Splenic abscess: a single institution study and review of the literature. *Yonsei Medical Journal.* 2011; 52(2): 288–92.

42. Zerem E, Bergsland J. Ultrasound guided percutaneous treatment for splenic abscesses: The significance in treatment of critically ill patients. *World Journal of Gastroenterology.* 2006; 12(45): 7341–45.

43. Nagem RG, Petroianu A. Subtotal splenectomy for splenic abscess. *Canadian Journal of Surgery.* 2009; 52(4): E91–2.

44. Reichel C, Theisen A, Rockstroh JK, et al. Splenic abscesses and abdominal tuberculosis in patients with AIDS. *Gastroenterology.* 1996; 34(8): 494–6

45. Bernabeu-Wittel M, Villanueva JL, Pachon J, et al. Etiology, clinical features and outcome of splenic microabscesses in HIV-infected patients with prolonged fever. *European Journal of Clinical Microbiology.* 1999; 18(5): 324–9.

46. Topal U, Savci G, Sadikoglu MY. Splenic involvement of tuberculosis: US and CT findings. *Gastrointestinal Radiology.* 1994; 4: 577–9.

47. Dixit R, Arya MK, Panjabi M, Gupta A, et al. Clinical profile of patients having splenic involvement in tuberculosis. *Indian Journal of Tuberculosis.* 2010; 57(1): 25–30.

48. Ng CY, Leong EC, Chng HC. Ten-year series of splenic abscesses in a general hospital in Singapore. *Annals of the Academy of Medicine, Singapore.* 2008; 37: 749–52.

49. ApisarnthanarakA. Computed tomography characteristics of hepatic and splenic abscesses associated with melioidosis: a 7-year study. *Journal of Medical Imaging and Radiation Oncology.* 2011; 55(2): 176–82.

50. Ool LL, Leong SS. Splenic Abscesses from 1987–1995. *American Journal of Surgery.* 1997; 174(1): 87–93.

51. Ikezawa K, Naito M, Yumiba T, et al. Splenectomy and antiviral treatment for thrombocytopenic patients with chronic hepatitis C virus infection. *Journal of Viral Hepatitis.* 2010; 17: 488–92.

52. Amin MA, El Gendy MM, Dawoud IE. Partial splenic embolication versus splenectomy for the management of hypersplenism in cirrhotic patients. *World Journal of Surgery.* 2009; 33: 1702–10.

53. 2004 Report on the Global AIDS Epidemic; 4th Global Report. Geneva, Switzerland: UNAIDS, 2004. Print.

54. Vallabhaneni S, Scott H, Carter J, et al. Atraumatic splenic rupture: an unusual manifestation of acute HIV infection. *AIDS Patient Care STDS.* 2011; 25(8): 461–4. Epub June 28 2011.

55. Solano T, Atkins B, Tambosis E, et al. Prevalance and clinical significance of splenomegaly in asymptomatic Human Immunodefieciency Virus Type I infected adults. *Clinical Infectious Diseases.* 2000; 30(6): 943.

56. Beral V, Peterman T, Berkelman R, et al. AIDS associated NHL. *Lancet.* 1991; 337 (8745): 805–9.

57. Kanavos P, Vandoros S, Garcia-Gonzalez P. Benefits of global partnerships to facilitate access to medicines in developing countries: a multi-country analysis of patients and patient outcomes in GIPAP. *Globalization and Health.* 2009; 5: 19.

Chapter 16

1. Kanumba ES, Mabula JB, Rambau P, et al. Modified Alvarado Scoring System as a diagnostic tool for acute appendicitis at Bugando Medical Centre, Mwanza, Tanzania. *BMC Surgery.* 2011; 17(11): 4.

2. Addiss DG, Shaffer N, Fowler BS, et al. The epidemiology of appendicitis and appendectomy in the United States. *American Journal of Epidemiology.* 1990; 132: 910.

3. Chavda SK, Hassan S, Magoha GA. Appendicitis at Kenyatta National Hospital, Nairobi. *East African Medical Journal.* 2005; 82(10): 526–30.

4. Mungadi IA, Jabo BA, Agwu NP. A review of appendicectomy in Sokoto, North-western Nigeria. *Nigerian Journal of Medicine.* 2004; 13(3): 240–3.

5. John SK, Joseph J, Shetty SR. Avoiding negative appendectomies in rural surgical practice: Is C-reactive protein estimation useful as a diagnostic tool? *National Medical Journal of India.* 2011; 24(3): 144–7.

6. Flum DR, Morris A, Koepsell T, et al. Has misdiagnosis of appendicitis decreased over time? A population-based analysis. *Journal of the American Medical Association.* 2001; 286(14): 1748–53.

7. Chianakwana GU, Ihegihu CC, Okafor P, et al. Adult surgical emergencies in a developing country: the experience of Nnamdi Azikiwe University Teaching Hospital, Nnewi, Anambra State, Nigeria. *World Journal of Surgery.* 2005; 29: 804–8.

8. Matthews JB, Hodin RA. Acute Abdomen and Appendix. In: *Greenfield's Surgery: Scientific Principles and Practice.* 5th ed. Lippincott Williams & Wilkins; 2010.

9. Birnbaum BA, Wilson SR. Appendicitis at the millennium. *Radiology.* 2000; 215: 337.

10. Arnbjornsson E, Bengmark S. Obstruction of the appendix lumen in relation to pathogenesis of acute appendicitis. *Acta Chirurgica Scandinavica.* 1983; 149: 789.

11. Jones BA, Demetriades D, Segal I, et al. The prevalence of appendiceal fecaliths in patients with and without appendicitis. A comparative study from Canada and South Africa. *Annals of Surgery.* 1985; 202: 80.

12. Lee SL, Walsh AJ, Ho HS. Computed tomography and ultra-sonography do not improve and may delay the diagnosis and treatment of acute appendicitis. *Archives of Surgery.* 2001; 136: 556.

13. Chung CH, Ng CP, Lai KK. Delays by patients, emergency physicians, and surgeons in the management of acute appendicitis: retrospective study. *Hong Kong Medical Journal.* 2000; 6: 254.

14. Golledge J, Toms AP, Franklin IJ, et al. Assessment of peritonism in appendicitis. *Annals of the Royal College of Surgeons of England.* 1996; 78: 11.

15. Andersson RE, Hugander AP, Ghazi SH, et al. Diagnostic value of disease history, clinical presentation, and inflammatory parameters of appendicitis. *World Journal of Surgery.* 1999; 23: 133.

16. Lane R, Grabham J. A useful sign for the diagnosis of peritoneal irritation in the right iliac fossa. *Annals of the Royal College of Surgeons of England.* 1997; 79: 128.

17. Izbicki JR, Knoefel WT, Wilker DK, et al. Accurate diagnosis of acute appendicitis: a retrospective and prospective analysis of 686 patients. *European Journal of Surgery.* 1992; 158: 227.

18. Berry J Jr, Malt RA. Appendicitis near its centenary. *Annals of Surgery.* 1984; 200: 567.

19. Silen, W. *Cope's Early Diagnosis of the Acute Abdomen.* 22nd ed. Oxford University Press, 2010: 86–104.

20. Carneiro F, Cifuentes E, Tellez-Rojo M, et al. The risk of Ascaris lumbricoides infection in children as an environmental health indicator to guide preventative activities in Caparaó and Alto Caparaó, Brazil. *Bulletin of the World Health Organization.* 2002; 80: 40–5.

21. Schulze SM, Chokshi RJ, Edavettal M, et al. Acute abdomen secondary to Ascaris lumbricoides infestation of the small bowel. *American Surgeon.* 2005; 71: 505–7.

22. Chandler ND, Parisi MT. Radiological case of the month. Yersinia enterocolitica masquerading as appendicitis. *Archives of Pediatrics & Adolescent Medicine.* 1994; 148(5): 527–8.

23. Rucinski J, Fabian T, Panagopoulos G. Gangrenous and perforated appendicitis: a meta-analytic study of 2532 patients indicates that the incision should be closed primarily. *Surgery.* 2000; 127: 136.

24. Grosfeld JL, Weinberger M, Clatworthy, Jr HW. Acute appendicitis in the first two years of life. *Journal of Pediatric Surgery.* 1973; 8(2): 285.

25. Rothrock SG, Pagane J. Acute appendicitis in children: emergency department diagnosis and management. *Annals of Emergency Medicine.* 2000; 36(1): 39.

26. Eryilmaz R, Sahin M, Alimoglu O, et al. The value of C-reactive protein and leucocyte count in preventing negative appendicectomies. *Ulus Travma Acil Cerrahi Derh.* 2001; 7(3): 142–5.

27. Alvarado A. A practical score for the early diagnosis of acute appendicitis. *Annals of Emergency Medicine.* 1986; 15(5): 557–64.

28. Rezak A, Abbas HM, Ajemian MS, et al. Decreased use of computed tomography with a modified clinical scoring system in diagnosis of pediatric acute appendicitis. *Archives of Surgery.* 2011; 146(1): 64–7.

29. Schneider C, Kharbanda A, Bachur R. Evaluating appendicitis scoring systems using a prospective pediatric cohort. *Annals of Emergency Medicine.* 2007; 49(6): 778–84.

30. Naaeder SB, Archampong EQ. Clinical spectrum of acute abdominal pain in Accra, Ghana. *West African Journal of Medicine.* 1999; 18(1): 13–6.

31. Ekenze SO, Anyanwu PA, Ezomike UO, et al. Profile of pediatric abdominal surgical emergencies in a developing country. *International Surgery.* 2010; 95(4): 319–24.

32. Wang LT, Prentiss KA, Simon JZ, et al. The use of white blood cell count and left shift in the diagnosis of appendicitis in children. *Pediatric Emergency Care.* 2007; 23(2): 69–76.

33. Macklin CP, Radcliffe GS, Merei JM, et al. A prospective evaluation of the modified Alvarado score for acute appendicitis in children. *Annals of the Royal College of Surgeons of England.* 1997; 79(3): 203.

34. Ho HS. ACS Surgery: Principles and Practice: *Appendectomy.* 6th ed. BC Decker, Inc; 2007.

35. Grunewald B, Keating J. Should the 'normal' appendix be removed at operation for appendicitis? *Journal of the Royal College of Surgeons of Edinburgh.* 1993; 38: 158.

36. Blair PM, Bugis PS, Turner LJ. Review of the pathologic diagnosis of 2,216 appendectomy specimens. *American Journal of Surgery.* 1993; 165: 618.

37. Truji M, Puri P, Reen DJ. Characterization of the local inflammatory response in appendicitis. *Journal of Pediatric Gastroenterology and Nutrition.* 1993; 16: 43.

38. Meier D. Opportunities and improvisations: a pediatric surgeon's suggestions for successful short-term surgical volunteer work in resource-poor areas. *World Journal of Surgery.* 2010; 34: 941–6.

Chapter 17

1. *Rutkow I. Demographic and socioeconomic aspects of hernia repair in the United States in 2003. Surgical Clinics of North America.* 2003; 83: 1045–51.

2. Jamison D, Breman J, Measham A, et al. (eds.). *Disease Control Priorities in Developing Countries.* 2nd ed. Washington DC: The World Bank and Oxford University Press, 2006.

3. Nordberg EM. Incidence and estimated need of caesarean section, inguinal hernia repair, and operation for strangulated hernia in rural Africa. *British Medical Journal (Clinical Research Edition).* 1984; 289(6437): 92–3.

4. Sanders DL, Porter CS, Mitchell KCD, et al. A prospective cohort study comparing the African and European hernia. *Hernia.* 2008; 12(5): 527–9.

5. Mbah N. Morbidity and mortality associated with inguinal hernia in northwest Nigeria. *West African Journal of Medicine.* 2007; 26: 288–92.

6. Gallegos NC, Dawson J, Jarvis M, Hobsley M. Risk of strangulation in groin henrias. *British Journal of Surgery.* 1991; 78(10): 1171–3.

7. Hair A, Paterson C, Wright D, et al. What effects does the duration of an inguinal hernia have on patient symptoms? *Journal of the American College of Surgeons.* 2001; 193(2): 125–9.

8. Dahlstrand U, Wollert S, Nordin P, et al. Emergency femoral hernia repair: a study based on a national register. *Annals of Surgery.* 2009; 249(4): 672–6.

9. Bay-Nielsen M, Kehlet H, Strand L, et al. Quality assessment of 26,304 herniorrhaphies in Denmark: a prospective nationwide study. *Lancet.* 2001; 358(9288): 1124–8.

10. Tongaonkar RR, Redy BV, Mehta VK, et al. Preliminary multicentric trial of cheap indigenous mosquito-net cloth for tension-free hernia repair. *Indian Journal of Surgery*. 2003; 65: 89–95.
11. Clarke MG, Oppong C, Simmermacher R, et al. The use of sterilized polyester mosquito net mesh for inguinal hernia repair in Ghana. *Hernia*. 2009; 13(2): 155–9.
12. Nordin P, Zetterstrom H, Gunnarsson U, et al. Local, regional, or general anaesthesia in groin hernia repair: multicentre randomized trial. *Lancet*. 2003; 362: 853–8.
13. Nordin P, Zetterstrom H, Carlssson P, et al. Cost-effectiveness analysis of local, regional and general anaesthesia for inguinal hernia repair using data from a randomized clinical trial. *British Journal of Surgery*. 2007; 94: 500–503.
14. Meier DE, OlaOlorun DA, Omodele RA, et al. Incidence of umbilical hernia in African children: redefinition of "normal" and reevaluation of indications for repair. *World Journal of Surgery*. 2001; 25(5): 645–8.
15. Lichtenstein IL, Shilman AG, Amid PK, et al. The tension free hernioplasty. *American Journal of Surgery*. 1989; 157: 188–93.
16. Beahrs OH, Beart RW (eds.). *Inguinal and Femoral Hernias. In: General Surgery*. Boston: Houghton Mifflin, 1980.
17. Shouldice EE. The Treatment of hernia. *Ontario Med Rev.* 1953; 20: 670.
18. Shillcut S, Clarke M, Kingsnorth A. Cost-effectiveness of groin hernia surgery in the western region of Ghana. *Archives of Surgery*. 2010; 145(10): 954–61.
19. Franneby U, Sandblom G, Nordin P, et al. Risk factors for long-term pain after hernia surgery. *Annals of Surgery*. 2006; 244(2): 212–9.

Chapter 18

1. *Albaran RG, Webber J, Steffes CP. CD4 cell counts as a prognostic factor of major abdominal surgery in patients infected with the human immunodeficiency virus. Archives of Surgery.* 1998; 133(6): 626–31.
2. Lord RV. Anorectal surgery in patients infected with human immunodeficiency virus: factors associated with delayed wound healing. *Annals of Surgery*. 1997; 226(1): 92–9.
3. Consten EC, Slors FJ, Noten HJ, et al. Anorectal surgery in human immunodeficiency virus-infected patients. Clinical outcome in relation to immune status. *Diseases of the Colon and Rectum*. 1995; 38(11): 1169–75.
4. Murray CJ, Lopez AD, Jamison DT. The global burden of disease in 1990: summary results, sensitivity analysis and future directions. *Bulletin of the World Health Organization*. 1994; 72(3): 495–509.
5. Demyttenaere SV, Nansamba C, Nganwa A, et al. Injury in Kampala, Uganda: 6 years later. *Canadian Journal of Surgery*. 2009; 52(5): E146–50.
6. Thanni LO. Epidemiology of injuries in Nigeria—a systematic review of mortality and etiology. *Prehospital and Disaster Medicine*. 2011; 26(4): 293–8.
7. Yunaev M, Ling A, Abbas S, et al. Abdominal tuberculosis: an easily forgotten diagnosis. *ANZ Journal of Surgery*. 2011; 81(7–8): 559–60.
8. Heller T, Goblirsch S, Wallrauch C, et al. Abdominal tuberculosis: sonographic diagnosis and treatment response in HIV-positive adults in rural South Africa. *International Journal of Infectious Diseases*. 2010; 14(Suppl 3): e108–12.
9. Jadvar H, Mindelzun RE, Olcott EW, et al. Still the great mimicker: abdominal tuberculosis. *American Journal of Roentgenology*. 1997; 168(6): 1455–60.
10. Radzi M, Rihan N, Vijayalakshmi N, et al. Diagnostic challenge of gastrointestinal tuberculosis: a report of 34 cases and an overview of the literature. *Southeast Asian Journal of Tropical Medicine and Public Health*. 2009; 40(3): 505–10.
11. Ozdogan M, Baykal A, Aran O. Amebic perforation of the colon: rare and frequently fatal complication. *World Journal of Surgery*. 2004; 28(9): 926–9.
12. Takahashi T, Gamboa-Dominguez A, Gomez-Mendez TJ, et al. Fulminant amebic colitis: analysis of 55 cases. *Diseases of the Colon and Rectum*. 1997; 40(11): 1362–7.
13. Primary Surgery Online. *Primary Surgery* [Internet]. 2008. Accessed March 1 2012. Available from: http://www.primary-surgery.org/start.html.
14. Raveenthiran V, Madiba TE, Atamanalp SS, et al. Volvulus of the sigmoid colon. *Colorectal Disease*. Jul 2010; 12(7 Online): e1–17.
15. Bogardus ST, Jr. What do we know about diverticular disease? A brief overview. *Journal of Clinical Gastroenterology*. 2006; 40(Suppl 3): S108–11.
16. Madiba TE, Mokoena T. Pattern of diverticular disease among Africans. *East African Medical Journal*. Oct 1994; 71(10): 644–6.
17. Bejar LM, Gili M, Infantes B, et al. Effects of changes in dietary habits on colorectal cancer incidence in twenty countries from four continents during the period 1971–2002. *Revista Espanola de Enfermedades Digestivas*. 2011; 103(10): 519–29.
18. Ginsberg GM, Lauer JA, Zelle S, et al. Cost effectiveness of strategies to combat breast, cervical, and colorectal cancer in sub-Saharan Africa and South East Asia: mathematical modelling study. *BMJ*. 2012; 344: e614.
19. Corman ML. *Colon and Rectal Surgery*. Philadelphia: Lippincott Williams & Wilkins, 2005.
20. Kirshtein B, Roy-Shapira A, Lantsberg L, et al. Use of the "Bogota bag" for temporary abdominal closure in patients with secondary peritonitis. *The American Surgeon*. 2007; 73(3): 249–52.

Chapter 19

1. Barleben A, Mills S. Anorectal anatomy and physiology. *Surgical Clinics of North America*. 2010; 90(1): 1–15.
2. Markell KW, Billingham RP. Pruritus ani: etiology and management. In: Steele, SR. *Surgical Clinics of North America*. 2010; 90(1): 130–132.
3. Cameron JL, Cameron AM (eds.). Management of Pruritus Ani. *In: Current Surgical Therapy*. 10th ed. Philadelphia: Elsevier, 2011: 243–5.
4. Finne CO, Fenyk JR. Dermatology and Pruritus Ani. In: *The ASCRS Textbook of Colon and Rectal Surgery*. 2nd ed. New York: Springer, 2011: 277–94.
5. Herzig DO, LU, KC. Anal Fissure. In: Steele, SR. *Anorectal Disease. Surgical Clinics of North America*. 2010; 90(1): 33–44.

6. JL and Cameron AM (eds.). Anal Fissure. In: *Current Surgical Therapy,* 10th ed. Philadelphia: Elsevier, 2011: 230–2.

7. Ricciardi R, Dykes SL, Madoff RD. Anal Fissure. In: *The ASCRS Textbook of Colon and Rectal Surgery.* 2nd ed. New York: Springer, 2011: 203–18.

8. JL and Cameron AM (eds.). Hemorrhoids. In: *Current Surgical Therapy.* 10th ed. Philadelphia: Elsevier, 2011: 223–9.

9. Sneider EB. Diagnosis and Management of Symptomatic Hemorrhoids. In: Steele, SR (ed.). *Surgical Clinics of North America.* 2010; 90(1): 17–32.

10. Singer M. Hemorrhoids. In: *The ASCRS Textbook of Colon and Rectal Surgery.* 2nd ed. New York: Springer; 2011: 75–202.

11. Vasilevsky CA. Anorectal Abscess and Fistula. In: *The ASCRS Textbook of Colon and Rectal Surgery.* 2nd ed. New York: Springer; 2011: 219–43.

12. Steele SR. Anorectal Abscess and Fistula-in-Ano: Evidence-Based Management. *Surgical Clinics of North America.* 2010; 90(1): 45–68.

13. Cameron JL, Cameron AM (eds.). Anorectal Abscess and Fistula. In: *Current Surgical Therapy,* 10th ed. Philadelphia: Elsevier, 2011: 233–240.

14. Steele SR (ed.). Evaluation and Management of Pilonidal Disease. *Surgical Clinics of North America.* 2010; 90(1): 113–24.

15. Papaconstantinou HT, Thomas JS. Pilonidal Disease and Hidradenitis Suppurativa. In: *The ASCRS Textbook of Colon and Rectal Surgery,* 2nd ed. New York: Springer, 2011: 261–76.

16. Cameron JL, Cameron AM (eds.). Pilonidal Disease. *Current Surgical Therapy.* 10th ed. Philadelphia: Elsevier, 2011: 261–7.

Chapter 20

1. Modlin IM, Kidd M, Lye KD. From the lumen to the laparoscope. *Archives of Surgery.* 2004; 139(10): 1110–26.

2. Harrell AG, Heniford BT. Minimally invasive abdominal surgery: lux et veritas past, present, and future. *American Journal of Surgery.* 2005; 190(2): 239–43.

3. Castadot RG, Magarick, RH, Sheppard L, Burkman RT. A review of ten years' experience with surgical equipment in international health programs. *International Journal of Obstetrics and Gynecology.* 1986; 24(1): 53–60.

4. Wiles WA, Wicks AC, Thomas GE. Peritoneoscopy in a developing country. *South African Medical Journal.* 1980; 57(5): 147–50.

5. Udwadia TE. Diagnostic laparoscopy. *Surgical Endoscopy.* 2004; 18(1): 6–10.

6. Gasim B, Fedail SS, Hakeem SE. Peritoneoscopy: experience in Sudan. *Tropical Gastroenterology.* 2002; 23(2): 57–60.

7. Missalek W, Mmuni K. Laparoscopy as a diagnostic method in internal medicine: experiences with 168 procedures at Kilimanjaro Christian Medical Centre, Moshi Tanzania. *Tropical Doctor.* 1991; 21(3): 113–6.

8. Ogbonna BC, Obekpa, PO, Momoh JT, Obafunwa JO, Nwana EJ. Laparoscopy in developing countries in the management of patients with an acute abdomen. *British Journal of Surgery.* 1992; 79(9): 964–6.

9. Purry NA. Peritoneoscopy in a developing country. *South African Medical Journal.* 1980; 57(14): 522.

10. Zanoni P, de Lalla F. Value of diagnostic laparoscopy in developing countries. *Tropical Doctor.* 1986; 16(4): 148–9.

11. Udwadia TE. Peritoneoscopy for surgeons. *Annals of the Royal College of Surgeons of England.* 1986; 68(3): 125–9.

12. Blum CA, Adams DB. Who did the first laparoscopic cholecystectomy? *J Minim Access Surg.* 2011 Jul-Sep; 7(3): 165–168.

13. NIH Consensus Statement, Gallstones and Laparoscopic Cholecystectomy. 1992: NIH.

14. Perez R C. Abordaje transvaginal de organos intrabdominales. Paper presented at the Cirugia 2010: XI Congreso Cubano de Cirugia.

15. Weiser TG, Regenbogen SE, Thompson KD, et al. An estimation of the global volume of surgery: a modelling strategy based on available data. *Lancet.* 2008; 372(9633): 139–44.

16. Baigrie RJ, Stupart D. Introduction of laparoscopic colorectal cancer surgery in developing nations. *British Journal of Surgery.* 2010; 97(5): 625–7.

17. Contini S, Taqdeer A, Gosselin RA. Should laparoscopic cholecystectomy be practiced in the developing World? The experience of the first training program in Afghanistan. *Annals of Surgery.* 2010; 251(3): 574.

18. Ozgediz DKS, Galukande M Dubowitz G, et al. Africa's neglected surgical workforce crisis. *Lancet.* 2008; 371: 627–8.

19. Doctors Pioneer Laparoscopic Surgery in Rivers State (Nigeria) [Internet]. 2009. Accessed Sept 8 2010. Available from: http://allafrica.com/stories/200901060261.html.

20. Me Cure Healthcare Limited. Medical Tourism [Internet]. 2010. Accessed March 14 2011. Available from: http://www.mecure.co.in/medical-tourism.html.

21. Science in Africa. Medical Tourism [Internet]. 2007. Accessed June 28 2010. Available from: http://www.scienceinafrica.co.za/2007/june/medicaltourism.html.

22. Orgoi S. Development of laparoscopic surgery in Mongolia [Internet]. 2006. Accessed March 9 2009. Available from: www.gfmer.ch/Medical_education_En/PGC_RH_2006/Reviews/pdf/Orgoi_laparoscopy_2006.pdf.

23. Akporiaye L. Trigen Survey: West African College of Surgeons. Port-Harcourt: Unpublished data. 2010.

24. Chadraabal U. Information of biliary track surgery in Mongolia. *Health Sciences University of Mongolia.* 2010.

25. The Business of Health in Africa: Partnering with the Private Sector to Improve People's Lives. 2008; Washington DC: International Finance Corporation, World Bank Group.

26. Udwadia TE, Udwadia RT, Menon K, et al. Laparoscopic surgery in the developing world. An overview of the Indian scene. *International Surgery.* 1995; 80(4): 371–5.

27. deVries C, Price RR. Global Sugery and Public Health: *A New Paradigm.* 1st ed. Sudbury Jones and Bartlett Learning, LLC, 2010.

28. Health Indicators 2006. (2007). Ulaanbataar National Center for Health Development.

29. Rahman GA. Cholelithiasis and cholecystitis: changing prevalence in an African community. *Journal of the National Medical Association.* 2005; 97(11): 1534–8.

30. Cadiere GB, Himpens J, Bruyns J. Laparoscopic surgery and the third world. *Surgical Endoscopy.* 1996; 10(10): 957–8.

31. Okrainec A, Smith L, Azzie G. Surgical simulation in Africa: the feasibility and impact of a 3-day fundamentals of laparoscopic surgery course. *Surgical Endoscopy.* 2009; 23(11): 2493–8.

32. Okrainec A, Henao O, Azzie G. Telesimulation: an effective method for teaching the fundamentals of laparoscopic surgery in resource-restricted countries. *Surgical Endoscopy.* 2010; 24(2): 417–22.

33. Straub CM, Price RR, Matthews D, et al. Expanding laparoscopic cholecystectomy to rural mongolia. *World Journal of Surgery.* 2011; 35(4): 751–9.

34. Asbun HJ, Berguer R, Altamirano R, et al. Successfully establishing laparoscopic surgery programs in developing countries. Clinical results and lessons learned. *Surgical Endoscopy.* 1996; 10(10): 1000–3.

35. Manning RG, Aziz AQ. Should laparoscopic cholecystectomy be practiced in the developing world?: the experience of the first training program in Afghanistan. *Annals of Surgery.* 2009; 249(5): 794–8.

36. World Health Organization. Declaration of alma-ata. (1978, 01 April 2006) [Internet]. 2006. Accessed March 4 2009. Available from: http://www.euro.who.int/AboutWHO/Policy/20010827_1.

37. Bullington M, Flick N, McLean G, et al. Sierra Leone Hospital Assessment: Adaptation of the WHO EESC Situational Analysis. 2010.

38. Spiegel DA, Choo S, Cherian M, et al. Quantifying surgical and anesthetic availability at primary health facilities in Mongolia. *World Journal of Surgery.* 2011; 35(2): 272–9.

39. Rodas E, Vicuna A, Merrell RC. Intermittent and mobile surgical services: logistics and outcomes. *World Journal of Surgery.* 2005; 29(10): 1335–9.

40. Mir IS, Mohsin M, Kirmani O, et al. Is intra-operative cholangiography necessary during laparoscopic cholecystectomy? A multicentre rural experience from a developing world country. *World Journal of Gastroenterology.* 2007; 13(33): 4493–7.

41. Misra M C, Kumar S. Total extraperitoneal (TEP) mesh repair of inguinal hernia in the developing world: comparison of low-cost indigenous balloon dissection versus direct telescopic dissection: a prospective randomized controlled study. *Surgical Endoscopy.* 2008; 22(9): 1947–58.

42. Shillcutt SD CM, Kingsnorth AN. Cost-effectiveness of groin hernia surgery in the Western Region of Ghana. Unpublished article submitted to *Archives of Surgery.* Plymouth Postgraduate Medical School, 2009.

43. Tongaonkar RR, Reddy BV, Mehta VK. Preliminary multicentric trial of cheap indigenous mosquito-net cloth for tension-free hernia repair. *Indian Journal of Surgery.* 2003; 65(1): 89–95.

44. JNC Limited. Turnkey Medical Equipment Services [Internet]. 2011. Accessed May 14 2011. Available from: http://www.jnciltd.com/

Chapter 21

1. Jemal A, Bray F, Center MM, et al. Global Cancer Statistics. *CA: A Cancer Journal for Clinicians.* 2011; 61: 69–90.

2. International Agency for Research on Cancer. Globocan [Internet]. 2008. Accessed March 31 2011. Available from: http://globocan.iarc.fr/.

3. Huo D, Ikpatt F, Khramtsov A, et al. Population differences in breast cancer: survey in indigenous African women reveals over-representation of triple-negative breast cancer. *Journal of Clinical Oncology.* 2009; 27: 4515–21.

4. Bird PA, Hill AG, Houssami N. Poor hormone receptor expression in East African breast cancer: evidence of a biologically different disease? *Annals of Surgical Oncology.* 2008; 15: 1983–8.

5. Stark A, Kleer CG, Martin I, et al. African ancestry and higher prevalence of triple-negative breast cancer: findings from an international study. *Cancer.* 2010; 116: 4926–32.

6. Ben Abdelkrim S, Trabelsi A, Missaoui N, et al. Distribution of molecular breast cancer subtypes among Tunisian women and correlation with histopathological parameters: a study of 194 patients. *Pathology Research and Practice.* 2010; 206: 772–5.

7. Thang VH, Tani E, Johansson H, et al. Difference in hormone receptor content in breast cancers from Vietnamese and Swedish women. *Acta Oncologica.* 2011; 50: 353–9.

8. Dey S, Soliman AS, Hablas A, et al. Urban-rural differences in breast cancer incidence by hormone receptor status across 6 years in Egypt. *Breast Cancer Research and Treatment.* 2010; 120: 149–60.

9. Jemal A, Center MM, DeSantis C, et al. Global patterns of cancer incidence and mortality rates and trends. *Cancer Epidemiology, Biomarkers & Prevention.* 2010; 19(8): 1893–907.

10. Kuzwar, Wayne. No Survival Benefit Found in LRT for Women Presenting With Metastatic Breast Cancer [Internet]. Dec 13 2013. Accessed Feb 25 2014. Available from: http://www.onclive.com/conference-coverage/sabcs-2013/No-Survival-Benefit-Found-in-LRT-for-Women-Presenting-With-Metastatic-Breast-Cancer#sthash.kF0BkxfC.dpuf.

11. Shulman LN, Willett W, Sievers A., and Knaul, FM. Breast cancer in developing countries: opportunities for improved survival. *Journal of Oncology.* 2010.

12. Sharma K, Costas A, Damuse R, Hamiltong-Pierre J, Pyda J, Ong CT... Meara JG. The Haiti breast cancer initiative: initial findings and analysis of barriers-to-care delaying patient presentation. *Journal of Oncology.* 2013.

Chapter 22

1. World Health Organization and UNICEF. Countdown to 2015 decade report (2000–2010): taking stock of maternal, newborn and child survival. Washington DC: 2010.

2. King M, Bewes PC, Cairns J, et al. (eds.). Primary Surgery—Volume I Non-Trauma. Oxford University Press, 1990.

3. World Health Organization. Integrated Management of Pregnancy and Childbirth. Managing complications in pregnancy and childbirth: a guide for midwives and doctors. Geneva: 2007.

4. Van DeVel de M, De Buck F. Anesthesia for non-obstetric surgery in the pregnant patient. *Minerva Anestesiology.* 2007; 73(4): 235–40.

5. Agdi M, Tulandi T. Surgical treatment of ectopic pregnancy. *Best Practice & Research Clinical Obstetrics and Gynaecology.* 2009; 23: 519–27.

6. Steigrad SJ. Epidemiology of gestational trophoblastic diseases. *Best Practice & Research in Clinical Obstetrics and Gynaecology.* 2003; 7(6): 837–47.

7. Early Amniotomy Shortens Delivery Time, But Doesn't Affect Outcomes. Paper presented at: Society for Maternal-Fetal Medicine (SMFM) 31st Annual Meeting: Abstract 6. Feb 10 2011.

8. World Health Organization WHO. Guidelines for the management of postpartum hemorrhage and retained placenta. Geneva. 2009.

9. *Hofmeyr GJ, Shweni PM. Symphysiotomy for feto-pelvic disproportion. Cochrane Database of Systematic Reviews.* 2010; Issue 10.

10. El-Hamamy E, B-Lynch C. A worldwide review of the uses of the uterine compression suture techniques as alternative to hysterectomy in the management of severe post-partum hemorrhage. *Journal of Obstetrics and Gynaecology.* 2005; 25(2): 143–9.

Chapter 23

1. Awori N, Bayley A, et al. *Primary Surgery: Non-Trauma 1.* New York: Oxford University Press, Inc., 1990.

2. Mann W (ed.). Culdocentesis. *UpToDate,* Waltham: 2011.

3. Mann W (ed.). Dilation and curettage. *UpToDate,* Waltham: 2011.

4. Jamison DT, Feachem RG, MAkgoba MW, et al. (eds.). Disease and Mortality in Sub-Saharan Africa. 2nd ed. Washington, DC: World Bank, 2006.

5 UNICEF. Goal: Improve Maternal Health. Accessed March 28, 2012. Available from: http://www.unicef.org/mdg/maternal.html.

6. Hogan MC, Foreman KJ, Naghavi M, et al. Maternal mortality for 181 countries, 1980–2008: a systematic analysis of progress towards Millennium Development Goal. *Lancet.* 2010; 375(9726): 1609–23.

7. Sharp H (ed.). Abdominal Myomectomy. *UpToDate,* Waltham: 2011.

8. Rock J, Jones HW. *TeLinde's Operative Gynecology.* 9th ed. Philadelphia: Lippincott Williams & Wilkins, 2003

9. Rock J, Jones HW. *TeLinde's Operative Gynecology.* 10th ed. Philadelphia: Lippincott Williams & Wilkins, 2008.

10. Zieman M (ed.). Surgical termination of pregnancy: First trimester. UpToDate, Waltham: 2011.

11. Barbieri R (ed.). Vaginal myomectomy for a prolapsed uterine leiomyoma. UpToDate, Waltham: 2011.

12. Falcone T, Zieman M (ed.). Surgical sterilization of women. UpToDate, Waltham: 2011.

13. Barbieri R (ed.). Spontaneous abortion: Management. UpToDate, Waltham: 2011.

14 Sharp H (ed.). Abdominal hysterectomy. *UpToDate,* Waltham: 2011.

15. Falcone T (ed.). Surgical treatment of ectopic pregnancy and prognosis for subsequent fertility. UpToDate, Waltham: 2011.

16. Sharp H (ed.). Oophorectomy and ovarian cystectomy. UpToDate, Waltham: 2011.

17. Cook J, Sankaran B, Wasunna A (eds.). *Surgery at the district hospital: obstetrics, gynaecology, orthopaedics, and traumatology.* World Health Organization. Geneva: World Health Organization: 1991.

Chapter 24

1. World Health Organization. Surgical Care at the District Hospital: Chapter 9. [Internet]. 2003. Available from: http://whqlibdoc.who.int/publications/2003/9241545755.pdf.

2. UNAIDS & WHO. WHO and UNAIDS announce recommendations from expert meeting on male circumcision for HIV prevention [Internet]. 2007. Available from: http://data.unaids.org/pub/PressRelease/2007/20070328_pr_mc_recommendations_en.pdf.

3. Bailey RC, Egesah O, Rosenberg S. Male circumcision for HIV prevention: a prospective study of complications in clinical and traditional settings in Bungoma, Kenya. Bulletin of the World Health Organization. 2008; 86(9): 657–736.

4. Schoen EJ. Ignoring evidence of circumcision benefits. *Pediatrics.* 2006; 118(1): 385–7.

5. Wein AJ, Kavoussi LR, Novick AC, et al. *Campbell-Walsh Urology.* 9th ed. Philadelphia: Saunders Elsevier, 2007.

6. World Health Organization. Report of an informal consultation on surgical approaches to the urogenital manifestations of lymphatic filariasis. Global Programme for the elimination of lymphatic filariasis. Accessed April 15–16, 2002. Available from: http://whqlibdoc.who.int/hq/2003/WHO_CDS_CPE_CEE_2003.38.pdf.

7. Baskin LS, Kogan BA, Duckett JW. *Handbook of Pediatric Urology.* Philadelphia: Lippincott-Raven Publishers, 1997.

8. Graham SD, Keane TE. *Glenn's Urologic Surgery.* 7th ed. Philadelphia: Lippincott Williams and Wilkins, 2010.

Chapter 25

1. Warf BC. Hydrocephalus in Uganda: predominance of infectious origin and primary management with endoscopic third ventriculostomy. Journal of Neurosurgery (Pediatrics 1). 2005; 102: 1–15.

2. Warf BC and the East African Neurosurgery Research Consortium. Pediatric hydrocephalus in East Africa: prevalence, causes, treatments, and strategies for the future. *World Neurosurgery.* 2010; 73(4): 296–300.

3. Warf BC. Comparison of one-year outcomes for the Chaabra™ and Codman Hakim Micro Precision™ shunt systems in Uganda: a prospective study in 195 children. *Journal of Neurosurgery (Pediatrics 4).* 2005; 102: 358–62.

Chapter 28

1. Long, JA. *Chalazion. Oculoplastic Surgery.* New York: Saunders Elsevier, 2009.

2. Hogewag M, Keunen JEE. Prevention of blindness in leprosy and the role of the vision 2020 programme. *Eye.* 2005; 19, 1099–1105.

3. Hersh PS, Zagelbaum BA, Cremers SL. *Ophthalmic Surgical Procedures.* 2nd ed. Thieme Publishing, 2009.

4. Montgomery MA, Bartram J. Short-sightedness in sight-saving: half a strategy will not eliminate blinding trachoma. *Bulletin of the World Health Organization.* 2010; 88: 82.

5. Burton MJ, Mabey DCW. The global burden of trachoma: a review. *PLOS Neglected Tropical Diseases.* 2009; 3(10): e460. doi:10/1371/journal.pntd.0000460.

6. World Health Organization. Prevention of blindness and visual impairment: Priority eye diseases, Trachoma. Available from: http://www.who.int/blindness/causes/priority/en/index2.html.

7. Reacher M, Foster A, Huber J. Manual: Trichiasis surgery for trachoma—The bilamellar tarsal rotation procedure. World Health Organization, 1998.

8. Krachmer JH, Mannis MJ, Holland EJ. *Cornea: Surgery of the Cornea and Conjunctiva—Volume 2.* 3rd ed. Mosby Elsevier, 2013.

9. World Health Organization. Visual impairment and blindness. Fact Sheet N0282, updated April 2011.

10. World Health Organization. Vision 2020. The right to sight. Global initiative for the elimination of avoidable blindness: Action plan 2006–2011. 2007.

Chapter 29

1. Malamed SF. *Handbook of Local Anesthesia.* 5th ed. Philadelphia: Elsevier, 2004.

2. Peterson LJ, Hupp JR, Ellis II E, et al. *Contemporary Oral and Maxillofacial Surgery.* 3rd ed. Philadelphia: Elsevier, 1998: 152, 153, 156, 179, 242–243.

Chapter 30

1. Lavy C, Sauven K, Mkandawire N, et al. State of surgery in tropical Africa: a review. *World Journal of Surgery.* 2011; 35(2): 262–71.

2. Gosselin RA, Gyamfi YA, Contini S. Challenges of meeting surgical needs in the developing world. *World Journal of Surgery.* 2011; 35(2): 258–61.

3. Taira BR, Kelly McQueen KA, Burkle FM, Jr. Burden of surgical disease: does the literature reflect the scope of the international crisis? *World Journal of Surgery.* 2009; 33(5): 893–8.

4. Zirkle LG, Jr. Injuries in developing countries—how can we help? The role of orthopaedic surgeons. *Clinical Orthopaedics and Related Research.* 2008; 466(10): 2443–50.

5. Spiegel DA, Gosselin RA, Coughlin RR, et al. The burden of musculoskeletal injury in low and middle-income countries: challenges and opportunities. *The Journal of Bone and Joint Surgery.* 2008; 90(4): 915–23.

6. Mock C, Cherian MN. The global burden of musculoskeletal injuries: challenges and solutions. *Clinical Orthopaedics and Related Research.* 2008; 466(10): 2306–16.

7. Atijosan O, Rischewski D, Simms V, Kuper H, Linganwa B, Nuhi A, et al. A national survey of musculoskeletal impairment in Rwanda: prevalence, causes and service implications. *PIOS One.* 2008; 3(7): e2851.

8. Lopez AD, Mathers CD, Ezzati M, et al. Measuring the Global Burden of Disease and Risk Factors, 1990–2001. In: Lopez AD, Mathers CD, Ezzati M, et al. (eds.). *Global Burden of Disease and Risk Factors.* Washington DC: World Bank, 2006.

9. Lopez AD, Begg S, Bos E. Demographic and Epidemiological Characteristics of Major Regions, 1990–2001. In: Lopez AD, Mathers CD, Ezzati M, et al. (eds.). *Global Burden of Disease and Risk Factors.* Washington DC: World Bank, 2006.

10. Mathers CD, Lopez AD, Murray CJL. The Burden of Disease and Mortality by Condition: Data, Methods, and Results for 2001. In: Lopez AD, Mathers CD, Ezzati M, Jamison DT, et al. (eds.). *Global Burden of Disease and Risk Factors.* Washington DC: World Bank, 2006.

11. Schein M. Seven sins of humanitarian medicine. *World Journal of Surgery.* 2010; 34(3): 471–2.

12. Butt MF, Dhar SA, Gani NU, Farooq M, Mir MR, Halwai MA, et al. Delayed fixation of displaced femoral neck fractures in younger adults. *Injury.* 2008; 39(2): 238–43.

13. Nadkarni B, Srivastav S, Mittal V, et al. Use of locking compression plates for long bone nonunions without removing existing intramedullary nail: review of literature and our experience. *The Journal of Trauma.* 2008; 65(2): 482–6.

14. Devnani AS. Simple approach to the management of aseptic non-union of the shaft of long bones. *Singapore Medical Journal.* 2001; 42(1): 20–5.

15. Crowley DJ, Kanakaris NK, Giannoudis PV. Femoral diaphyseal aseptic non-unions: is there an ideal method of treatment? *Injury.* 2007; 38 (Suppl 2): S55–63.

16. Cierny G, 3rd, Mader JT, Penninck JJ. A clinical staging system for adult osteomyelitis. *Clinical Orthopaedics and Related Research.* 2003; 414: 7–24.

17. Tetsworth K, Cierny G, 3rd. Osteomyelitis debridement techniques. *Clinical Orthopaedics and Related Research.* 1999; 360: 87–96.

18. Ismavel R, Samuel S, Boopalan PR, et al. A simple solution for wound coverage by skin stretching. *Journal of Orthopaedic Trauma.* 2011; 25(3): 127–32.

19. Craig DM, Sullivan PK, Herndon JH, et al. One-stage arm-preserving shoulder resection with latissimus dorsi flap for basal cell carcinoma. *Annals of Plastic Surgery.* 1988; 20(2): 158–62.

20. Stanbury SJ, Elfar J. The use of surgical loupes in microsurgery. *The Journal of Hand Surgery.* 2011; 36(1): 154–6.

21. Lubega N, Mkandawire NC, Sibande GC, et al. Joint replacement in Malawi: establishment of a National Joint Registry. *The Journal of Bone and Joint Surgery: British Volume.* 2009; 91(3): 341–3.

22. Stewart GD, Stewart PC, Nott ML, et al. Total joint replacement surgery in a rural centre. *The Australian Journal of Rural Health.* 2006; 14(6): 253–7.

23. Smith J, Okike K. Operation Walk Boston [Internet]. 2011. Accessed March 12 2013. Available from: http://operation-walkboston.blogspot.com/

24. King M, Bewes P, Cairns J et al. Background to surgery. In: *Primary Surgery, Vol 1.* Oxford: Oxford University Press, 1990.

25. Gosselin RA, et al. *World Journal of Surgery.* 2011 February; 35(2): 258–61.

26. *The Bangladesh Development Studies* Vol.28. No.1/2, March–June 2002.

Chapter 31

1. Bickler SW, Telfer ML, et al. Need for paediatric surgery care in an urban area of The Gambia. *Tropical Doctors*. 2003; 33(2): 91–4.

2. Ameh EA, Chirdan LB. Paediatric surgery in the rural setting: prospect and feasibility. *West African Journal of Medicine*. 2001; 20(1): 52–5.

3. Mhando S, Young B, Lakhoo K. The scope of emergency paediatric surgery in Tanzania. *Pediatric Surgery International*. 2008; 24(2): 219–22.

4. Bickler SW, Ameh EA. Surgical Care for Children. *A guide for primary referral hospitals*. MacMillan, Oxford, 2011.

5. Ameh EA, Bickler SW, Lakhoo K, Nowmeh BC, Poenaru D (Eds). *Paediatric surgery: a comprehensive text for Africa*. GlobalvHELP, Seattle, 2010.

6. Ouro-Bang'na Maman, AF, et al. Anesthesia for children in Sub-Saharan Africa—a description of settings, common presenting conditions, techniques and outcomes. *Paediatric Anaesthesia*. 2009; 19(1): 5–11.

7. Walker I, et al. Pediatric surgery in south-western Uganda: A cross-sectional survey. *Bulletin of the World Health Organization*. 2010. epub November 26, 2010.

8. Wall SN, et al, Reducing intrapartum-related neonatal deaths in low- and middle-income countries-what works? *Seminars in Perinatology*. 2010; 34(6): 395–407.

9. Hesse AA, Balint J. Nutritional Support. In: Poenaru DEA (ed.). *Pediatric Surgery in Africa*. 2010, Global HELP.

10. Nasir AA, Abdur-Rahman LO, Adeniran JO. Outcomes of surgical treatment of malrotation in children. *African Journal of Paediatric Surgery*. 2011; 8(1): 8–11.

11. Ameh EA, Chirdan LB. Neonatal intestinal obstruction in Zaria, Nigeria. *East African Medical Journal*. 2000; 77(9): 510–3.

12. Eckoldt-Wolte F, Hess AA, Krishnaswami S. Duodenal atresia and stenosis. In: *Pediatric Surgery in Africa*. 2010, Global HELP.

13. Rode H, Millar A. Jejuno-ileal atresia and stenosis. In: Puri P. *Newborn Surgery*. London: Arnold, 2003: 445–56.

14. Osifo DO, Evbuomwan I. Does exclusive breastfeeding confer protection against infantile hypertrophic pyloric stenosis? A 30-year experience in Benin City, Nigeria. *Journal of Tropical Pediatrics*. 2009; 55(2): 132–4.

15. To T, et al. Population demographic indicators associated with incidence of pyloric stenosis. *Archives of Pediatric and Adolescent Medicine*. 2005; 159(6): 520–5.

16. Nmadu PT. Alterations in serum electrolytes in congenital hypertrophic pyloric stenosis: a study in Nigerian children. *Annals of Tropical Pediatrics*. 1992; 12(2): 169–72.

17. Ekenze SO, et al. Profile of pediatric abdominal surgical emergencies in a developing country. *International Surgery*. 2010; 95(4): 319–24.

18. Ogundoyin OO, et al. Pattern and outcome of childhood intestinal obstruction at a tertiary hospital in Nigeria. *African Health Sciences*. 2009; 9(3): 170–3.

19. Abantanga FA, et al. Pneumatic reduction of intussusception in children at the Komfo Anokye Hospital, Kumasi, Ghana. *East African Medical Journal*. 2008; 85(11): 550–5.

20. Ekenze SO, Mgbor SO. Childhood intussusception: The implications of delayed presentation. *African Journal of Paediatric Surgery*. 2011; 8(1): 15–8.

21. St. Peter. Appendicitis. In: Holcomb G, Murphy J (eds.). *Ashcraft's Pediatric Surgery*. Philadelphia: Saunders, 2010.

22. Zhang HL, Bai YZ, Zhou X, et al. Nonoperative management of appendiceal phlegmon or abscess with an appendicolith in children. *Journal of Gastrointestinal Surgery*. 2013; 17(4): 766–70.

23. Campbell AM, Kuhn WP, Barker P. Vacuum-assisted closure of the open abdomen in a resource-limited setting. *South African Journal of Surgery*. 2010; 48(4): 114–5.

24. Lewing K, Gamis A. Lymphomas. In: Holcomb G, Murphy J (eds.). *Ashcraft's Pediatric Surgery*. Philadelphia: Saunders, 2010.

25. Hadley GP, Lakhoo K. Lymphomas. In: Poenaru DEA. *Pediatric Surgery in Africa*. 2010, Global HELP.

26. Moore SW, Schneider J, Schaaf HS. Diagnostic aspects of cervical lymphadenopathy in children in the developing world: a study of 1,877 surgical specimens. *Pediatric Surgery International*. 2003; 19(4): 240–4.

27. Moore S, Tsifularo N, Troebs R. Lymphadneopathy in African children. In: Poenaru DEA, et al. (eds.). *Pediatric Surgery in Africa*. 2011, Global HELP.

28. Moore, S.W., N. Tsifularo, and R. Troebs, Lymphadenopathy in African children. In: Poenaru DEA. *Pediatric Surgery in Africa*. 2010, Global HELP.

29. Hadley L, Lakhoo K. Lymphomas. In: Ameh E, et al. (eds.). *Pediatric Surgery in Sub-Saharan Africa*. 2011, Global HELP.

30. Mutalima N, et al. Impact of infection with human immunodeficiency virus-1 (HIV) on the risk of cancer among children in Malawi—preliminary findings. *Infectious Agents and Cancer*. 2011; 5: 5.

31. Margaron FC, Poenaru D, Northcutt A. Pediatric cancer spectrum in Kenya: a histopathologic review. *Pediatric Surgery International*. 2010; 26(8): 789–94.

32. Ekenze SO, et al. The burden of pediatric malignant solid tumors in a developing country. *Journal of Tropical Pediatrics*. 2010; 56(2): 111–4.

33. Wilde JC, et al. Challenges and outcome of Wilms' tumor management in a resource-constrained setting. *African Journal of Paediatric Surgery*. 2010; 7(3): 159–62.

34. Israels T, et al. Acute malnutrition is common in Malawian patients with a Wilms tumor: A role for peanut butter. *Pediatric Blood Cancer*. 2009; 53(7): 1221–6.

35. Davidson A, et al. Wilms tumor experience in a South African centre. *Pediatric Blood Cancer*. 2006; 46(4): 465–71.

36. Ekenze SO, Agugua-Obianyo NE, Odetunde OA. The challenge of nephroblastoma in a developing country. *Annals of Oncology*. 2006; 17(10): 1598–600.

37. Israels, R et al. SIOP PODC : clinical guidelines for the management of children with Wilms Tumor in a low-income setting. *Pediatr Blood Cancer*. 2013; 60(10): 5–11.

38. Rogers T, et al. Experience and outcomes of nephroblastoma in Johannesburg, 1998–2003. *European Journal of Pediatric Surgery*. 2007; 17(1): 41–4.

39. Pena A, Levitt M. Anorectal malformations. In: Holcomb G (ed.). Pediatric Surgery. Philadelphia: Saunders, 2010.

40. Poenaru D, et al. Caring for children with colorectal disease in the context of limited resources. *Seminars in Pediatric Surgery*. 2010; 19(2): 118–27.

41. Meier D. Opportunities and improvisations: a pediatric surgeon's suggestions for successful short-term surgical volunteer work in resource-poor areas. *World Journal of Surgery*. 2010; 34(5): 941–6.

42. Ekenze SO, Ngaikedi C, Obasi AA. Problems and outcome of Hirschsprung's disease presenting after 1 year of age in a developing country. *World Journal of Surgery.* 2011; 35(1): 22–6.

43. Abdur-Rahman LO, Cameron B. Hirschsprung's disease in Africa in the 21st century. *Surgery in Africa.* 2010.

44. Evbuomwon I, Lakhoo K. Congenital abdominal wall defects: exomphalos and gastroschisis. In: Poenaru DEA (ed.). *Pediatric Surgery in Africa.* 2011, Global HELP.

45. Sekabira J, Hadley GP. Gastroschisis: a third world perspective. *Pediatric Surgery International.* 2009; 25(4): 327–9.

46. Brandt ML. Pediatric hernias. *Surgical Clinics of North America.* 2008; 88(1): 27–43, vii–viii.

47. Hadley GP, Lakhoo K. HIV-AIDS and the pediatric surgeon. In: *Poenaru DEA. Pediatric Surgery in Africa.* 2010, Global HELP.

48. Sharma S, Gupta DK. Tuberculosis. In: *Poenaru DEA. Pediatric Surgery in Africa.* 2010, Global HELP.

49. Typhoid vaccines: WHO position paper. *Weekly Epidemiologic Record.* 2008; 83(6): p. 49–59.

50. Ameh EA. Typhoid ileal perforation in children: a scourge in developing countries. *Annals of Tropical Pediatrics.* 1999; 19(3): 267–72.

51. Clegg-Lamptey JN, Hodasi WM, Dakubo JC. Typhoid ileal perforation in Ghana: a five-year retrospective study. *Tropical Doctors.* 2007; 37(4): 231–3.

52. Ameh E, Abantanga F. Surgical complications of typhoid fever. In: Ameh EA, Bickler SW, Lakhoo K, Nowmeh BC, Poenaru D (Eds). *Paediatric surgery: a comprehensive text for Africa.* Global HELP, Seattle, 2010; 103–110.

53. Ekenze SO, kefuna AN. Typhoid intestinal perforation under 5 years of age. *Annals of Tropical Paediatrics.* 2008; 28(1) 53–8.

54. Chang YT, Lin JY, Huang YS. Typhoid colonic perforation in childhood: a ten-year experience. *World Journal of Surgery.* 2006; 30(2): 242–7.

55. Meier DE, Tarpley JL. Typhoid intestinal perforations in Nigerian children. *World Journal of Surgery.* 1998; 22(3): 319–23.

56. Abantanga FA, Wiafe-Addai BB. Postoperative complications after surgery for typhoid perforation in children in Ghana. *Pediatric Surgery International.* 1998; 14(1–2): 55–8.

57. Sawardekar KP. Changing spectrum of neonatal omphalitis. Pediatric Infectious Disease Journal. 2004; 23(1): 22–6.

58. Mullany, L.C., et al., Risk factors for umbilical cord infection among newborns of southern Nepal. *American Journal of Epidemiology.* 2007. 165(2): p. 203–11.

59. Amsalu S, Lulseged S. Tetanus in a children's hospital in Addis Ababa: review of 113 cases. *Ethiopian Medical Journal.* 2005; 43(4): 233–40.

60. Ameh EA, Nmadu PT. Major complications of omphalitis in neonates and infants. *Pediatric Surgery International.* 2002; 18(5–6): 413–6.

61. Ameh EA, et al. Fournier's gangrene in neonates and infants. *European Journal of Pediatric Surgery.* 2004; 14(6): 418–21.

62. Guvenc H, et al. Neonatal omphalitis is still common in eastern Turkey. *Scandinavian Journal of Infectious Diseases.* 1991; 23(5): 613–6.

63. Winani S, et al. Use of a clean delivery kit and factors associated with cord infection and puerperal sepsis in Mwanza, Tanzania. *Journal of Midwifery & Women's Health.* 2007; 52(1): 37–43.

64. Debe NM, Dahl M, Jonsbo F. [Omphalitis with fatal outcome in new-born baby boy]. *Ugeskr Laeger.* 2008; 170(3): 158.

65. Fraser N, Davies BW, Cusack J. Neonatal omphalitis: a review of its serious complications. *Acta Paediatrica.* 2006; 95(5): 519–22.

66. Moss RL, Musemeche CA, Kosloske AM. Necrotizing fasciitis in children: prompt recognition and aggressive therapy improve survival. *Journal of Pediatric Surgery.* 1996; 31(8): 1142–6.

67. Enwonwu CO, et al. Pathogenesis of cancrum oris (noma): confounding interactions of malnutrition with infection. *American Journal of Tropical Medicine and Hygiene.* 1999; 60(2): 223–32.

68. Ameh EA, et al. Necrotizing fasciitis of the scalp in a neonate. *Annals of Tropical Paediatrics.* 2001; 21(1): 91–3.

69. Mshelbwala PM, Sabiu L, Ameh EA. Necrotising fasciitis of the perineum complicating ischiorectal abscess in childhood. *Annals of Tropical Pediatrics.* 2003; 23(3): 227–8.

70. Lewis RT. Soft tissue infections. *World Journal of Surgery.* 1998; 22(2): 146–51.

71. Ogundiran TO, Akute OO, Oluwatosin OM. Necrotizing fasciitis. *Tropical Doctor.* 2004; 34(3): 175–8.

72. Derbew M, Ahmed E. The pattern of pediatric surgical conditions in Tikur Anbessa University Hospital, Addis Ababa, Ethiopia. *Ethiopian Medical Journal.* 2006; 44(4): 331–8.

Chapter 32

1. Parkin DM, Bray FI, Devesa SS. Cancer burden in the year 2000. The global picture. *European Journal of Cancer.* 2001; 37(Suppl 8): S4–66.

2. Pisani P, et al. Outcome of screening by clinical examination of the breast in a trial in the Philippines. *International Journal of Cancer.* 2006; 118(1): 149–54.

3. Calle EE, et al. Overweight, obesity, and mortality from cancer in a prospectively studied cohort of U.S. adults. *New England Journal of Medicine.* 2003; 348(17): 1625–38.

4. Sener SF, Grey N. The global burden of cancer. *Journal of Surgical Oncology.* 2005; 92(1): 1–3.

5. Adebamowo CA, Akarolo-Anthony S. Cancer in Africa: opportunities for collaborative research and training. *African Journal of Medicine and Medical Sciences.* 2009; 38(Suppl): 5–13.

6. Parkin DM. The global health burden of infection-associated cancers in the year 2002. *International Journal of Cancer.* 2006; 118(12): 3030–44.

7. Lee CL, Hsieh KS, et al. Trends in the incidence of hepatocellular carcinoma in boys and girls in Taiwan after large-scale hepatitis B vaccination. *Cancer Epidemiology, Biomarkers and Prevention.* 2003; 12(1): 57–9.

8. Harper DM, et al. Efficacy of a bivalent L1 virus-like particle vaccine in prevention of infection with human papillomavirus types 16 and 18 in young women: a randomised controlled trial. *Lancet.* 2004; 364(9447): 1757–65.

9. Mellstedt H. Cancer initiatives in developing countries. *Annals of Oncology*. 2006; 17 (Suppl) 8: viii24–viii31.

10. Farmer P, et al., Expansion of cancer care and control in countries of low and middle income: a call to action. *Lancet*. 2010; 376(9747): 1186–93.

Chapter 33

1. Smith PG, Pike MC, Taylor E, et al. The epidemiology of tropical myositis in the Mengo Districts of Uganda. *Transactions of the Royal Society of Tropical Medicine and Hygiene*. 1978; 72: 46–53.

2. Olson DP, Soares S, Kanade SV. Community-acquired MRSA pyomyositis: case report and review of the literature. *Journal of Tropical Medicine*. 2011; 970848.

3. Small LN, Ross JJ. Tropical and temperate pyomyositis. *Infectious Disease Clinics of North America*. 2005; 19: 981–9, x–xi.

4. Heckmann JG, Lang CJ, Haselbeck M, et al. Tropical pyomyositis. *European Journal of Neurology*. 2001; 8: 283–4.

5. Chauhan S, Jain S, Varma S, et al. Tropical pyomyositis (myositis tropicans): current perspective. *Postgraduate Medical Journal*. 2004; 80: 267–70.

6. Shepherd J, Stewart J. The surgery of sepsis. In: King M (ed.). *Primary Surgery*. Oxford: Oxford Medical Publishers, 1990: 52–64.

7. Dobson M, Fenton P, Fisher R, et al. Cellulitis and Abscess. In: Dobson M, Fisher R (eds.). *Surgical Care in the District Hospital*. Geneva: World Health Organization, 2003: 5-19–5-20.

8. Ojulong J, Mwambu TP, Joloba M, et al. Relative prevalence of methicilline resistant Staphylococcus aureus and its susceptibility pattern in Mulago Hospital, Kampala, Uganda. *Tanzanian Journal of Health Research*. 2009; 11: 149–53.

9. World Health Organization. Buruli Ulcer [Internet]. 2011. Accessed June 14 2011. Available from: http://www.who.int/buruli/en/.

10. Merritt RW, Walker ED, Small PL, et al. Ecology and transmission of Buruli ulcer disease: a systematic review. *PLOS Neglected Tropical Diseases*. 2010; 4: e911.

11. Walsh DS, Portaels F, Meyers WM. Buruli ulcer: Advances in understanding Mycobacterium ulcerans infection. *Clinics in Dermatology*. 2011; 29: 1–8.

12. Kibadi K, Boelaert M, Fraga AG, et al. Response to treatment in a prospective cohort of patients with large ulcerated lesions suspected to be Buruli Ulcer (Mycobacterium ulcerans disease). *PLOS Neglected Tropical Diseases*. 2010; 4: e736.

13. Herbinger KH, Beissner M, Huber K, et al. Efficiency of fine-needle aspiration compared with other sampling techniques for laboratory diagnosis of Buruli ulcer disease. *Journal of Clinical Microbiology*. 2010; 48: 3732–4.

14. Adu E, Ampadu E, Acheampong D. Surgical management of buruli ulcer disease: a four-year experience from four endemic districts in ghana. *Ghana Medical Journal*. 2011; 45: 4–9.

15. Wijers DJ. Bancroftian filariasis in Kenya I. Prevalence survey among adult males in the Coast Province. *Annals of Tropical Medicine and Parasitology*. 1977; 71: 313–31.

16. Taylor MJ, Hoerauf A, Bockarie M. Lymphatic filariasis and onchocerciasis. *Lancet*. 2010; 376: 1175–85.

17. Pfarr KM, Debrah AY, Specht S, et al. Filariasis and lymphoedema. *Parasite Immunology*. 2009; 31: 664–72.

18. Ahorlu CK, Dunyo SK, Asamoah G, et al. Consequences of hydrocele and the benefits of hydrocelectomy: a qualitative study in lymphatic filariasis endemic communities on the coast of Ghana. *Acta Tropica*. 2001; 80: 215–21.

19. Thomas G, Richards FO, Jr., Eigege A, et al. A pilot program of mass surgery weeks for treatment of hydrocele due to lymphatic filariasis in central Nigeria. *American Journal of Tropical Medicine and Hygiene*. 2009; 80: 447–51.

20. DeVries CR. The role of the urologist in the treatment and elimination of lymphatic filariasis worldwide. *BJU International*. 2002; 89(Suppl 1): 37–43.

21. Noroes J, Dreyer G. A mechanism for chronic filarial hydrocele with implications for its surgical repair. *PLOS Neglected Tropical Diseases*. 2010; 4: e695.

22. Shenoy RK. Management of disability in lymphatic filariasis—an update. *Journal of Communicable Diseases*. 2002; 34: 1–14.

23. Chen HC, Salgado CJ, Mardini S, et al. Humanitarian rescue medical action for patient with advanced lower extremity lymphedema. *Lymphology*. 2008; 41: 93–5.

24. UNAIDS. Epidemic Update [Internet]. 2010. Accessed June 14 2011. Available from: http://www.unaids.org/documents/20101123_GlobalReport_Chap2_em.pdf.

25. Pastorin J SA, Bascunana A, Giron JA, et al. International Conference on AIDS. Surgery in AIDS patients. *Journal of the International AIDS Society*. 1996 Jul 7–12; 1996: 301.

26. Becker K, Erckenbrecht JF. [Preoperative risk assessment and perioperative management of HIV-infected patients]. *Med Klin (Munich)*. 2001; 96: 26–31.

27. Dua RS, Wajed SA, Winslet MC. Impact of HIV and AIDS on surgical practice. *Annals of the Royal College of Surgeons of England*. 2007; 89: 354–8.

28. Carrillo EH, Carrillo LE, Byers PM, et al. Penetrating trauma and emergency surgery in patients with AIDS. *American Journal of Surgery*. 1995; 170: 341–4.

29. Schecter WP. Surgical care of the HIV-infected patient: a moral imperative. *Cambridge Quarterly of Healthcare Ethics*. 1992; 1: 223–8.

30. Cardo DM, Culver DH, Ciesielski CA, et al. A case-control study of HIV seroconversion in health care workers after percutaneous exposure. Centers for Disease Control and Prevention—Needlestick Surveillance Group. *New England Journal of Medicine*. 1997; 337: 1485–90.

31. Fry DE. Occupational risks of blood exposure in the operating room. *American Journal of Surgery*. 2007; 73: 637–46.

32. Whitby D, Howard MR, Tenant-Flowers M, et al. Detection of Kaposi sarcoma associated herpesvirus in peripheral blood of HIV-infected individuals and progression to Kaposi's sarcoma. *Lancet*. 1995; 346: 799–802.

33. Stewart S, Jablonowski H, Goebel FD, et al. Randomized comparative trial of pegylated liposomal doxorubicin versus bleomycin and vincristine in the treatment of AIDS-related Kaposi's sarcoma. International Pegylated Liposomal Doxorubicin Study Group. *Journal of Clinical Oncology*. 1998; 16: 683–91.

34. Dezube BJ. Management of AIDS-related Kaposi's sarcoma: advances in target discovery and treatment. *Expert Reviews on Anticancer Therapies*. 2002; 2: 193–200.

35. Simonart T. What is the role of surgery in the treatment of Kaposi's sarcoma? *Journal of the European Academy of Dermatology and Venereology*. 2007; 21: 573.

36. Allen PJ, Gillespie DL, Redfield RR, et al. Lower extremity lymphedema caused by acquired immune deficiency syndrome-related Kaposi's sarcoma: case report and review of the literature. *Journal of Vascular Surgery*. 1995; 22: 178–81.

37. Heim M, Wershavski M, Azizi E, et al. Rehabilitation considerations of prosthetic fittings for Kaposi's sarcoma amputees. *Disability and Rehabilitation*. 2000; 22: 734–6.

38. Kaposi Sarcoma, Abdominal Signs. 2011. Accessed June 14 2011. Available from: https://portal.surgicalcore.org/content/dx_kaposi_sarcoma_dx1.

39. Wheeler DW, Baigrie RJ. Palliative surgery for acute bowel obstruction caused by Kaposi's sarcoma in a patient with AIDS. *International Journal of Clinical Practice*. 2003; 57: 347–8.

40. Neville CR, Peddada AV, Smith D, et al. Massive gastrointestinal hemorrhage from AIDS-related Kaposi's sarcoma confined to the small bowel managed with radiation. *Medical and Pediatric Oncology*. 1996; 26: 135–8.

41. Ramdial PK, Sing Y, Hadley GP, et al. Paediatric intussusception caused by acquired immunodeficiency syndrome-associated Kaposi sarcoma. *Pediatric Surgery International*. 2010; 26: 783–7.

42. Wilson SE, Robinson G, Williams RA, et al. Acquired immune deficiency syndrome (AIDS). Indications for abdominal surgery, pathology, and outcome. *Annals of Surgery*. 1989; 210: 428–33; discussion 33–4.

43. Vukasin P. Anal condyloma and HIV-associated anal disease. *Surgical Clinics of North America*. 2002; 82: 1199–211, vi.

44. Schlecht HP, Fugelso DK, Murphy RK, et al. Frequency of occult high-grade squamous intraepithelial neoplasia and invasive cancer within anal condylomata in men who have sex with men. *Clinical Infectious Disease*. 2010; 51: 107–10.

45. Trombetta LJ, Place RJ. Giant condyloma acuminatum of the anorectum: trends in epidemiology and management: report of a case and review of the literature. *Diseases of the Colon and Rectum*. 2001; 44: 1878–86.

46. Lord RV. Anorectal surgery in patients infected with human immunodeficiency virus: factors associated with delayed wound healing. *Annals of Surgery*. 1997; 226: 92–9.

47. World Health Organization. Tuberculosis [Internet]. 2010. Accessed June 14 2011. Available from: http://www.who.int/mediacentre/factsheets/fs104/en/.

48. Freixinet J. Surgical indications for treatment of pulmonary tuberculosis. *World Journal of Surgery*. 1997; 21: 475–9.

49. Kundu S, Mitra S, Mukherjee S, et al. Adult thoracic empyema: A comparative analysis of tuberculous and nontuberculous etiology in 75 patients. *Lung India*. 2010; 27: 196–201.

50. Malhotra P, Aggarwal AN, Agarwal R, et al. Clinical characteristics and outcomes of empyema thoracis in 117 patients: a comparative analysis of tuberculous vs. non-tuberculous aetiologies. *Respiratory Medicine*. 2007; 101: 423–30.

52. Treat of tuberculosis: guidelines; 2010.

53. Akgul AG, Orki A, Orki T. Approach to empyema necessitatis. *World Journal of Surgery*. 2011; 35: 981–4.

54. Falzon D. Multidrug and extensively drug-resistant TB (M/XDR-TB): 2010 global report on surveillance and response. WHO Library Cataloguing-in-Publication Data 2010.

55. Farmer P, Bayona J, Becerra M, et al. The dilemma of MDR-TB in the global era. *International Journal of Tuberculosis and Lung Disease*. 1998; 2: 869–76.

56. Mitnick CD, Appleton SC, Shin SS. Epidemiology and treatment of multidrug resistant tuberculosis. *Seminars in Respiratory and Critical Care Medicine*. 2008; 29: 499–524 Epub 2008 Sep 22.

57. Pomerantz M, Brown J. The surgical management of tuberculosis. *Seminars in Thoracic and Cardiovascular Surgery*. 1995; 7: 108–11.

58. Kang MW, Kim HK, Choi YS, et al. Surgical treatment for multidrug-resistant and extensive drug-resistant tuberculosis. *Annals of Thoracic Surgery*. 2010; 89: 1597–602.

59. Kir A, Inci I, Torun T, et al. Adjuvant resectional surgery improves cure rates in multidrug-resistant tuberculosis. *Journal of Thoracic and Cardiovascular Surgery*. 2006; 131: 693–6.

60. Kir A, Tahaoglu K, Okur E, et al. Role of surgery in multidrug-resistant tuberculosis: results of 27 cases. *European Journal of Cardiothoracic Surgery*. 1997; 12: 531–4.

61. Pomerantz BJ, Cleveland JC, Jr., Olson HK, et al. Pulmonary resection for multi-drug resistant tuberculosis. *Journal of Thoracic and Cardiovascular Surgery*. 2001; 121: 448–53.

62. Shiraishi Y, Nakajima Y, Katsuragi N, et al. Resectional surgery combined with chemotherapy remains the treatment of choice for multidrug-resistant tuberculosis. *Journal of Thoracic and Cardiovascular Surgery*. 2004; 128: 523–8.

63. Yaldiz S, Gursoy S, Ucvet A, et al. Surgery offers high cure rates in multidrug-resistant tuberculosis. *Annals of Thoracic and Cardiovascular Surgery*. 2011; 17: 143–7.

64. Somocurcio JG, Sotomayor A, Shin S, et al. Surgery for patients with drug-resistant tuberculosis: report of 121 cases receiving community-based treatment in Lima, Peru. *Thorax*. 2007; 62: 416–21. Epub August 23, 2006.

65. Citak N, Sayar A, Metin M, et al. [Results of surgical treatment for pulmonary aspergilloma with 26 cases in six years: a single center experience]. *Tuberk Toraks*. 2011; 59: 62–9.

66. Awori N, Cairns J, Hankins G. Preventing Surgical Tetanus. In: King M, Bewes P (eds.). *Primary Surgery: Volume Two Trauma*. Oxford: Oxford Medical Publishers, 1990.

Chapter 34

1. Janis JE, Kwon RK, Attinger CE. The new reconstructive ladder: Modifications to the traditional model. *Plastic and Reconstructive Surgery*. 2011; 127(Suppl.): 205s–212s.

2. Semer NB. Local Flaps. In: *Practical Plastic Surgery for Nonsurgeons*. New York: Authors Choice Press, 2007: 111–20.

3. Gosman AA. Basics of Flaps. In: Janis JE (ed.). *Essentials of Plastic Surgery: A UT Southwestern Medical Center Handbook*. St Louis: Quality Medical Publishing, 2007: 20–38.

4. Thorne CT. Techniques and principles in plastic surgery. In: *Grabb and Smith's Plastic Surgery*. 6th ed. Philadelphia: Lippincott Williams and Wilkins, 2006.

5. Mathes S, Alpert B, Chang N. Use of the muscle flap in chronic osteomyelitis: experimental and clinical correlation. *Plastic and Reconstructive Surgery.* 1982; 69: 815.
6. Donelan MB. Principles of burn reconstruction. In: *Grabb and Smith's Plastic Surgery.* 6th ed. Philadelphia: Lippincott Williams and Wilkins, 2006.
7. Longacre J, Berry HK, Basom CR, et al. The effects of Z-plasty on hypertrophic scars. *Scandinavian Journal of Plastic and Reconstructive and Hand Surgery.* 1976; 10: 113.

Chapter 36

1. Wilhelmi BJ, Blackwell SJ, Miller JH, et al. Do not use epinephrine in digital blocks: myth or truth? *Plastic and Reconstructive Surgery.* 2001; 107: 393.
2. Singer AJ, Hollander JE, Subramanian S, et al. Pressure dynamics of various irrigation techniques commonly used in the emergency department. *Annals of Emergency Medicine.* 1994; 24: 36.
3. Stillman RM, Marino CA, Seligman SJ. Skin staples in potentially contaminated wounds. *Archives of Surgery.* 1984; 119: 821.
4. Conolly WB, Hunt TK, Zederfeldt B, et al. Clinical comparison of surgical wounds closed by suture and adhesive tapes. *American Journal of Surgery.* 1969; 117: 318.
5. Singer AJ, Quinn JV, Clark RE, et al: Closure of lacerations and incisions with octylcyanoacrylate: a multicenter randomized controlled trial. *Surgery.* 2002; 131: 270.
6. van der Eerden PA, Lohuis PJ, Hart AA, et al. Secondary intention healing after excision of nonmelanoma skin cancer of the head and neck: statistical evaluation of prognostic values of wound characteristics and final cosmetic results. *Plastic and Reconstructive Surgery.* 2008; 122(6): 1747–55.
7. Argenta LC, Morykwas MJ. Vacuum-assisted closure: a new method for wound control and treatment: clinical experience. *Annals of Plastic Surge*
8. Enoch S, Grey JE, Harding KG. *ABC of wound healing: nonsurgical and drug treatments. BMJ.* 2006; 332: 900.
9. Parrett BM, Matros E, Pribaz JJ, et al. Lower extremity trauma: trends in the management of soft-tissue reconstruction of open tibia-fibula fractures. *Plastic and Reconstructive Surgery.* 2006; 117(4): 1315–22.
10. Elliott KG, Johnstone AJ. Diagnosing acute compartment syndrome. *Journal of Bone and Joint Surgery.* 2003; 85: 625.
11. Malinoski DJ, Slater MS, Mullins RJ. Crush injury and rhabdomyolysis. *Critical Care Clinics.* 2004; 20(1): 171–92.
12. Talan DA, Citron DM, Abrahamian FM, et al. Bacteriologic analysis of infected dog and cat bites. Emergency Medicine Animal Bite Infection Study Group. *New England Journal of Medicine.* 1999; 340: 85.
13. Cruse PJ, Foord R. The epidemiology of wound infection. A 10-year prospective study of 62,939 wounds. *Surgical Clinics of North America.* 1980; 60(1): 27–40.
14. Bennett LL, Rosenblum RS, Perlov C, et al. An *in vivo* comparison of topical agents on wound repair. *Plastic and Reconstructive Surgery.* 2001; 108(3): 675–87.
15. Centers for Disease Control. Recommendations for Postexposure Interventions to Prevent Infection with Hepatitis B Virus, Hepatitis C Virus, or Human Immunodeficiency Virus, and Tetanus in Persons Wounded During Bombings and Other Mass-Casualty Events—United States, 2008 [Internet]. Available from: http://www.cdc.gov/mmwr/preview/mmwrhtml/rr5706a1.htm#top.
16. Centers for Disease Control. Rabies: Domestic Animals [Internet]. 2011. Available from: http://www.cdc.gov/rabies/exposure/animals/domestic.html.
17. Centers for Disease Control. Rabies: Medical Care [Internet]. 2011. Available from: http://www.cdc.gov/rabies/medical_care/index.html.
18. Baumann LS, Spencer J. The effects of topical vitamin E on the cosmetic appearance of scars. *Dermatologic Surgery.* 1999; 25: 311.
19. Levenson SM, Gruber CA, Rettura G, et al. Supplemental vitamin A prevents the acute radiation-induced defect in wound healing. *Annals of Surgery.* 1084; 200: 494.
20. Macdonald JM, Sims N, Mayrovitz HN. Lymphedema, lipedema, and the open wound: the role of compression therapy. *Surgical Clinics of North America.* 2003; 83: 639.
21. Desneves KJ, Todorovic BE, Cassar A, et al. Treatment with supplementary arginine, vitamin C and zinc in patients with pressure ulcers: a randomised controlled trial. *Clinical Nutrition.* 2005; 24: 979.
22. Hunt TK, Ehrlich HP, Garcia JA, et al. Effect of vitamin A on reversing the inhibitory effect of cortisone on healing of open wounds in animals and man. *Annals of Surgery.* 1969; 170: 633.

Chapter 37

1. Briggs SM, Schnitzer JJ. The World Trade center terrorist attack: Changing priorities for surgeons in disaster response. *Surgery.* 2001; 132(3): 506–12.
2. Briggs SM. Advanced Disaster Medical Response: *Manual for Providers.* Boston: Harvard Medical International, 2003.
3. Born C, Briggs SM, Ciraulo DL, et al. Disasters and mass casualties: II. Explosive, biologic, chemical, and nuclear agents. *Journal of the American Academy of Orthopedic Surgery.* 2007; 15(8): 461–73.
4. Briggs SM. Disaster Management Teams. *Current Opinion on Critical Care.* 2005; 11: 585–9.
5. Dewo P, Magetsari R, Busscher HJ et al. Treating natural disaster victims is dealing with shortages: an orthopaedics perspective. *Technology and Healthcare.* 2008; 16(4): 255–9.
6. Dhar SA, Bhat MI, Mustafa A, et al. Damage control orthopaedics' in patients with delayed referral to a tertiary care center: experience from a place where Composite Trauma Centers do not exist. *Journal of Trauma Management and Outcomes.* 2008; 29(2): 2.
7. Gill A, Lebel E, Blumberg N, et al. The orthopedic department activity within the IDF-MC field hospital in Haiti. Hebrew, English Abstract. *JIMM.* 2010; 7(2): 68–72.
8. Lin G, Yitzhak A, Batumsky M. Surgical strategies in an ongoing mass casualty disaster: Lessons learned from the experience of the Israeli IDF-MC field hospital in Haiti. Hebrew, English Abstract. *JIMM.* 2010; 7(2): 60.
9. Quintura, DA, Spectrum of pediatric injuries after a bomb blast. *Journal of Pediatric Surgery.* 1997; 32(2): 307–10.

10. Sagi R, Farfel A, Yitzhak A, et al. Challenges in operating pediatric division in a field hospital during disaster. Hebrew, English Abstract. *JIMM*. 2010; 7(2): 64–7.

11. Patel TH, Wenner KA, Price SA, et al. A U.S. Army Forward Surgical Team's experience in Operation Iraqi Freedom. *Journal of Trauma*. 2004; 57(2): 201–7.

12. Lin G, Lavon H, Gelfond R, et al. Hard times call for creative solutions: medical improvisations at the Israel Defense Forces Field Hospital in Haiti. *American Journal of Disaster Medicine*. 2010; 5(3): 188–92.

13. Spinella PC: Warm fresh whole blood transfusion for severe hemorrhage: US military and potential civilian applications. Critical Care Medicine. 2008; 36(Suppl): S340–5. 11. Spinella PC: Warm fresh whole blood transfusion for severe hemorrhage: US military and potential civilian applications. *Critical Care Medicine*. 2008; 36(Suppl): S340–5.

14. Bartal C, Zeller L, Miskin I, et al. Crush syndrome: saving more lives in disasters. Lessons learned from the early-response phase in Haiti. *Archives of Internal Medicine*. 2011; 171(7): 694–6.1.

15. Reis ND, Michaelson M. Crush injury to the lower limbs. Treatment of the local injury. *Journal of Bone and Joint Surgery*. 1986, 68(3): 414–418.

16. Nance ML. The Halifax disaster of 1917 and the birth of North American pediatric surgery. *Journal of Pediatric Surgery*. 2001; 36(3): 405–8.

17. Coleman CN, Weinstock D, Casagrande R, et al. Triage and treatment tools for use in a scarce resources-crisis standards of care setting after a nuclear detonation. *Disaster Medicine and Public Health Preparedness*. 2011; 5: 111–21.

18. Merin O, Ash N, Levy G et al, The Israeli field hospital in Haiti—ethical dilemmas in early disaster response. *New England Journal of Medicine*. 2010; 362(11): e38, Epub 2010.

Chapter 38

1. Jayaraman S, Sethi D. Advanced trauma life support training for ambulance crews. *Cochrane Database Syst Review*. 2010(1): CD003109.

2. American College of Surgeons Committee on Trauma. *Advanced Trauma Life Support for Doctors: Student Course Manual*. 2008: 1–24.

3. Ben-Galim P, Dreiangel N, Mattox KL, et al. Extrication collars can result in abnormal separation between vertebrae in the presence of a dissociative injury. *Journal of Trauma*. 2010; 69(2): 447–50.

4. Glasgow Coma Scale [image on the internet]. 2011. Accessed Jan 17 2011. Available from: http://www.google.com/imgres?imgurl = http://www.medicalscale1.com/wp-content/uploads/2010/11/glascow-coma-scale11.jpg.

Chapter 39

1. Paudel B, Shrestha B, Banskota A. Two faces of major lower limb amputations. *Kathmundu University Medical Journal*. 2005; 3(3): 212–6.

2. Litchfield MH. Agricultural work related injury and ill-health and the economic cost. *Environmental Science and Pollution Research*. 1999; 6(3): 175–82.

3. Gajewski D, Granville R. The United States Armed Forces Amputee Patient Care Program. *Journal of the American Academy of Orthopedic Surgery*. 2006; 14(10): S183–7.

4. Harding K. Major lower limb amputations in the Marshall Islands: incidence, prosthetic prescription, and prosthetic use after 6–18 months. `Pacific Health Dialogue*. 2005; 12(1): 59–66.

5. Ong BY, Arneja A, Ong EW. Effects of anesthesia on pain after lower-limb amputation. *Journal of Clinical Anesthesia*. 2006; 18(8): 600–4.

6. Petrisor B, et al. Fluid lavage in patients with open fracture wounds (FLOW): an international survey of 984 surgeons. *BMC Musculoskeletal Disorders*. 2008; 9: 7.

7. Gustilo RB, Anderson JT. Prevention of infection in the treatment of one thousand and twenty-five open fractures of long bones: retrospective and prospective analyses. *Journal of Bone and Joint Surgery, American volume*. 1976; 58(4): 453–8.

8. Gustilo RB, Mendoza RM, Williams DN. Problems in the management of type III (severe) open fractures: a new classification of type III open fractures. *Journal of Trauma*. 1984; 24(8): 742–6.

9. Feliciano DV, et al. Fasciotomy after trauma to the extremities. *American Journal of Surgery*. 1988; 156(6): 533–6.

10. Gregory RT, et al. The mangled extremity syndrome (M.E.S.): a severity grading system for multisystem injury of the extremity. *Journal of Trauma*. 1985; 25(12): 1147–50.

11. Bosse MJ, et al. A prospective evaluation of the clinical utility of the lower-extremity injury-severity scores. *Journal of Bone and Joint Surgery, American volume*. 2001; 83-A(1): 3–14.

12. Larrey D. *Memoires de Chirugie Militaire, Vol. 2*. Paris: Smith, 1812: 180–195.

13. Tintle S, et al. Traumatic and trauma-related amputations: part II: upper extremity and future directions. *Journal of Bone and Joint Surgery, American volume*. 2010; 92(18): 2934–2945.

14. Beaty C (ed.). *Campbell's Operative Orthopedics*. Philadelphia: Elsevier, 2007.

15. Ramachandran VS, Brang D, McGeoch PD. Size reduction using Mirror Visual Feedback (MVF) reduces phantom pain. *Neurocase*. 2009; 15(5): 357–60.

16. Forsberg JA, et al. Heterotopic ossification in high-energy wartime extremity injuries: prevalence and risk factors. *Journal of Bone and Joint Surgery, American volume*. 2009; 91(5): 1084–91.

Chapter 40

1. World Health Organization. A WHO Plan For Burn Prevention and Care [Internet]. 2008. Available from: http://whqlibdoc.who.int/publications/2008/9789241596299_eng.pdf.

2. Interplast. The Forgotten Global Health Crisis of Burns [Internet]. 2009. Available from: http://www.interplast.org/about/gfx/fs09_burns%20factsheet.pdf.

3. American Burn Association. Burn Incidence and Treatment in the United States: 2011 Fact Sheet [Internet]. 2011. Accessed 5/26/2011. Available from: http://www.ameriburn.org/resources_factsheet.php.

4. Norton D, Hyder A, Bishai D, Peden M. Unintentional Injuries. In: Jamison DT, World Bank, Disease Control Priorities Project (eds.). *Disease Control Priorities in Developing Countries*. 2nd ed. New York: Oxford University Press, 2006. Available from: http://www.worldbank.icebox.ingenta.com/content/wb/2302.

5. Mozingo D. Surgical Management. In: Carrougher G (ed.). *Burn Care and Therapy.* St. Louis: Mosby, 1998: 233–248.

6. van Hasselt E. *Burns Manual.* 2nd ed. Holland: Nederlandse Brandwonden Stitchting, 2008: 150.

7. Mlcak RP, Buffalo MC. Pre-hospital management, transportation, and emergency care. In: Herndon DN (ed.). *Total Burn Care.* 2nd ed. London: Saunders Elsevier, 2002: 67–77.

8. Warden GD. Fluid resuscitation and early management. In: Herndon DN (ed.). *Total Burn Care.* 3rd ed. London: Saunders Elsevier, 2007: 107–118.

9. Barrow RE, Herndon DN. History of treatment of burns. In: Herndon DN (ed.). *Total Burn Care.* 3rd ed. London: Saunders Elsevier, 2007: 1–8.

10. Saffle JR, Graves C. Nutritional support of the burned patient. In: Herndon DN (ed.). *Total Burn Care.* 3rd ed. London: Saunders Elsevier, 2007: 398–419.

11. Sanford-Smith J. *Eye Surgery in Hot Climates.* 3rd ed. Leicester: F.A. Thorpe Publishing Ltd., 2004.

12. Malaria No More. Learn About Malaria [Internet]. 2011. Accessed May 26 2011. Available from: http://www.malarianomore.org/malaria.

13. Atiyeh BS, Costagliola M, Hayek SN. Burn prevention mechanisms and outcomes: pitfalls, failures and successes. *Burns.* 2009; 35(2): 181–93.

Chapter 41

1. Younes RN, Gross JL, Aguiar S, Haddad FJ, Deheinzelin D. When to remove a chest tube? A randomized study with subsequent prospective consecutive validation. Journal of the American College of Surgeons 2002; 195: 658–62.

2. Bell RL, Ovadia P, Abdullah F, Spector S, Rabinovici R. Chest tube removal: end-inspiration or end-expiration? *The Journal of Trauma.* 2001; 50: 674–7.

3. Williams M, Carlin AM, Tyburski JG, Blocksom JM, Harvey EH, Steffes CP, Wilson RF. Predictors of mortality in patients with traumatic diaphragmatic rupture and associated thoracic and/or abdominal injuries. Am Surg. 2004 Feb; 70(2): 157–62.

4. Ondo N'Dong F, Ngo'o N'ze S, Mbourou JB, et al. Mortalité et Morbidité dans les Traumatismes et

5. Plaies Thoraciques à Libreville. Revue de 130 cas./Mortality and morbidity for thoracic trauma in Libreville,Gabon: 130 cases. Bulletin Médical d'Owendo. 1997; 6/18: 23–27.

6. Yapoby Y, Tanuah Y, Kangah M, et al. Les Traumatismes thoraciques (A propos de 46 cas)./Thoracic trauma: 46 cases in Cote d'Ivoire. Med Afr Noire. 992; 39(4): 278–82.

7. Yena S, Sanogoz Z, Sangare D, et al. Les traumatismes thoraciques à l'Hôpital du point "G", Mali/Thoracic trauma at "Point G hospital" in Bamako, Mali. Mali Medical. 2006; 21(1): 43–8.

Chapter 42

1. Hirschberg A MK. *Top Knife: The Art & Craft of Trauma Surgery.* London: TfM Publishing, 2005.

2. Souba WW, Fink M, Jurkovich G, et al. *ACS Surgery: Principles and Practice.* 6th ed. Ontario: Decker, B.C. Inc, 2007.

3. American College of Surgeons. *ATLS: Advanced Trauma Life Support for Doctors: Student Course Manual.* 9th ed. Chicago: American College of Surgeons, 2008.

4. Mulholl L, Doherty G, Maier R, Simeone D, Upchurch G (eds.). *Greenfield's Surgery: Scientific Principles and Practice.* 6th ed. Philadelphia: Lippincott Williams & Wilkins, 2010.

Chapter 43

1. Rosenstein D, McAninch JW. Urologic emergencies. *Medical Clinics of North America.* 2004; 88(2): 495–518.

2. Chandhoke PS, McAninch JW. Detection and significance of microscopic hematuria in patients with blunt renal trauma. *Journal of Urology.* 1998; 140(1): 16–8.

3. Miller KS, McAninch JW. Radiographic assessment of renal trauma: our 15-year experience. *Journal of Urology.* 1995; 154(2): 352–5.

4. Santucci RA, Wessells H, Bartsch G, et al. Evaluation and management of renal injuries: consensus statement of the renal trauma subcommittee. *BJU International.* 2004; 93(7): 937–54.

5. Bretan PN, Jr., McAninch JW, Federle MP, Jeffrey RB, Jr. Computerized tomographic staging of renal trauma: 85 consecutive cases. *Journal of Urology.* 1986; 136(3): 561–5.

6. Morey AF, McAninch JW, Tiller BK, et al. Single shot intra-operative excretory urography for the immediate evaluation of renal trauma. *Journal of Urology.* 1999; 161(4): 1088–92.

7. Voelzke BB, McAninch JW. The current management of renal injuries. *American Journal of Surgery.* 2008; 74(8): 667–78.

8. Carroll PR, Klosterman P, McAninch JW. Early vascular control for renal trauma: a critical review. *Journal of Urology.* 1989; 141(4): 826–9.

9. Presti JC, Jr., Carroll PR, McAninch JW. Ureteral and renal pelvic injuries from external trauma: diagnosis and management. *Journal of Urology.* 1989; 29(3): 370–4.

10. Selzman AA, Spirnak JP. Iatrogenic uretural injuries: a 20-year experience in treating 165 injuries. *Journal of Urology.* 1996; 155(3): 878–81.

11. Morey AF, Iverson AJ, Swan A, et al. Bladder rupture after blunt trauma: guidelines for diagnostic imaging. *Journal of Urology.* 2001; 51(4): 683–6.

12. Iverson AJ, Morey AF. Radiographic evaluation of suspected bladder rupture following blunt trauma: critical review. *World Journal of Surgery.* 2001; 25(12): 1588–91.

13. Gomez RG, Ceballos L, Cobern M, et al. Consensus statement on bladder injuries. *BJU International.* 2004; 94(1): 27–32.

14. Andrich DE, Mundy AR. The nature of urethral injury in cases of pelvic fracture urethral trauma. *Journal of Urology.* 2001; 165(5): 1492–5.

15. Mundy AR, Andrich DE. Urethral trauma. Part I: introduction, history, anatomy, pathology, assessment and emergency management. *BJU International.* 2011; 108(3): 310–27.

16. Mundy AR, Andrich DE. Urethral trauma. Part II: Types of injury and their management. *BJU International.* 2011; 108(5): 630–50.

17. Black PC, Miller EA, Porter JR, Weseells H. Urethral and bladder neck injury association with pelvic fracture in 25 female patients. *Journal of Urology.* 2006; 175(6): 2140–4.

18. Morey AF, Metro MJ, Carney KJ, et al. Consensus on genitourinary trauma: external genitalia. *BJU International.* 2004; 94(4): 507–15.

19. Wessells H, Long L. Penile and genital injuries. *Urologic Clinics of North America.* 2006; 33(1): 117–26, vii.

20. EO Olapade-Olaopa, SA Adebayo, OM Atalabi, AA Popoola, IA Ogunmodede and UF Enabulele. Rigid retrograde endoscopy under regional anaesthesia: a novel technique for the early realignment of traumatic posterior urethral disruption. *African Journal of Medicine and Medical Sciences.* 2002; 31, 277–280.

21. EO Olapade-Olaopa et al. On-site physicians at a major sporting event in Nigeria. *Prehospital and Disaster Medicine. 2006;* 21(1): 40–44.

Chapter 45

1. Mulligan R, Mahabir R. The prevalence of cervical spine injury, head injury, or both with isolated and multiple craniomaxillofacial fractures. *Plastic and Reconstructive Surgery.* 2010; 126(5): 1647–51.

2. Zorn J, Agag B, Agag R. Frontal sinus fracture. *Eplasty.* 2011; 11: ic5.

3. Miloro M, Ghali G, Larsen P, et al. *Peterson's Principles of Oral and Maxillofacial Surgery.* 2nd ed. Hamilton: BC Decker, Inc., 2004.

4. Sargent L. Nasoethmoid orbital fractures: diagnosis and treatment. *Plastic and Reconstructive Surgery.* 2007; 120(7): 16S–31S.

5. Mikrogianakis A, Valani R, Cheng A. *The Hospital for Sick Children: Manual of Pediatric Trauma.* Toronto: Lippincott Williams & Wilkins, 2008.

6. Zafar A, Penne R. Medial Wall Orbital Fracture [Internet]. eMedicine. 2010. Available from: http://emedicine.medscape.com/article/1219023.

7. Duane T, Schatz N, Caputo A. Pseudo-Duane's Retraction Syndrome. *Transactions of the American Ophthalmological Society.* 1976; 74.

8. Appling W, Patrinely J, Salzer T. Transconjunctival approach vs. subciliary skin-muscle flap approach or orbital fracture repair. *JAMA Otolaryngology—Head & Neck Surgery.* 1993; 119(9): 1000–7.

9. Baumann A, Ewers R. Transcaruncular approach for reconstruction of medial orbital wall fracture. *International Journal of Oral and Maxillofacial Surgery.* 2000; 29(4): 264–7.

10. Albright C, McFarland P. Management of midfacial fractures. *Oral Surgery, Oral Medicine, Oral Pathology.* 1972; 34(6): 858–79.

11. Danko I, Haug R. An experimental investigation of the safe distance for internal orbital dissection. *Journal of Oral and Maxillofacial Surgery.* 1998; 56(6): 749–52.

12. Galiano A, et al. Pediatric facial fractures: children are not just small adults. *RadioGraphics.* 2008; 28: 441–61.

13. Kim J, Huoh K. Maxillofacial (midface) fractures. *Neuroimaging Clinics of North America.* 2010; 20(4): 581–96.

14. Hull HF, Mann JM, Sands JC, et al. Toxic shock syndrome related to nasal packing. *Archives of Otolaryngology—Head and Neck Surgery.* 1983; 118: 791–4.

15. Jayawardena S, Eisdorfer J, Indulkar S, et al. Infective endocarditis of native valve after anterior nasal packing. *American Journal of Therapeutics.* 2006; 13(5): 460–2.

16. Allsop D, Kennett K. Skill and facial bone trauma. In: *Accidental Injury: Biomechanics and Prevention.* Berlin: Springer, 2002: 254–8.

17. Larrabee W, Makielski K, Henderson J. *Surgical Anatomy of the Face.* Philadelphia: Lippincott Williams & Wilkins, 2004.

18. Stanley R, Nowak G. Midfacial fractures: importance of angle of impact to horizontal craniofacial buttresses. *Otolaryngology—Head & Neck Surgery.* 1985; 93(2): 186–92.

19. Strauss H, Morgan M, Hamilton M. External fixation of facial fractures. *American Journal of Surgery.* 1979; 45(3): 144–50.

20. Montazam A, Anastassov G. Management of condylar fractures. *Atlas of the Oral and Maxillofacial Surgery Clinics of North America.* 2009; 17(1): 55–69.

21. American Academy of Pediatric Dentistry. Guideline on Management of Acute Dental Trauma [Internet]. 2010; 34(6). Available from: http://www.aapd.org/media/Policies_Guidelines/G_trauma.pdf.

22. Horswell B, Meara DJ. Pediatric Craniomaxillofacial Trauma. In: Miloro M, Ghali G, Larsen P, Waite P. *Peterson's Principles of Oral and Maxillofacial Surgery.* 3rd ed. Shelton: PMPH USA, 2012.

23. Wesson D, et al. *Pediatric Trauma: Pathophysiology, Diagnosis and Treatment.* New York: Taylor and Francis Group, 2006.

Chapter 46

1. Negrel AD, Thylefors B. The global impact of eye injuries. *Ophthalmic Epidemiology.* 1998; 5: 143–67.

2. Jackson H. Bilateral blindness due to trauma in Cambodia. *Eye.* 1996; 10: 517–20.

3. Brilliant LB, et al. Epidemiology of blindness in Nepal. *Bulletin of the World Health Organization.* 1985; 63: 375–85.

4. Thylefors B. Epidemiological patterns of ocular trauma. *Australia and New Zealand Journal of Ophthamology.* 1992; 20(2): 95–8.

5. Upadhyay M, et al. The Bhakptapur Eye Study: Ocular trauma and antibiotic prophylaxis for the prevention of corneal ulceration in Nepal. *British Journal of Ophthalmology.* 2001; 85(4): 388–92.

6. Ballal SG. Ocular trauma in an iron forging industry in the eastern province, Saudi Arabia. *Occupational Medicine.* 1997; 47(2): 77–80.

7. Whitcher JP, Srinivasan M, Upadhyay MP. Corneal blindness: a global perspective. *Bulletin of the World Health Organization.* 2001; 79: 214–21.

Chapter 47

1. Potter JK. Facial Soft Tissue Trauma. In: Janis Je (ed.). *Essentials of Plastic Surgery: A UT Southwestern Medical Center Handbook.* St. Louis: Quality Medical Publishing, 2007: 243–8.

2. King MH. Lesser face injuries. *Primary Surgery Vol. 2—Trauma.* Oxford University Press, 1986.

3. Semer NB. Facial Lacerations. In: Semer NB. *Practical Plastic Surgeons for Non-Surgeons.* Philadelphia: Hanley and Belfus, Inc, 2001: 145–59.

4. Mosser SW. Lip Reconstruction. In: Janis JE (ed.). *Essentials of Plastic Surgery: A UT Southwestern Medical Handbook.* St. Louis: Quality Medical Publishing, 2007: 324–36.
5. Epidemiological profile of scalping victim-patients treated at the Fundação Santa Casa de Misericórdia do ParaCaio B. Cunha; Raquel M.M. Sacramento; Bernardo P. Maia; Renan P. Marinho; Hilton L. Ferreira; Dov C. Goldenberg; Maria L. C. P. Menezes *Rev Bras Cir Plást.* 2012; 27(1): 3–8.
6. Stab wounds: Epidemiological profile of emergency room treatment. Robson C Zandomenighi, Douglas L Mouro, Eleine A P MartinsRev Rene. *Fortaleza.* 2011; 12(4): 669–77.
7. Magee WP, Burg RV, Hatcher KW. Cleft lip and palate as cost-effective health care treatment in the developing world. *World Journal of Surgery.* 2010; 34: 420–427.

Chapter 48

1. Go NK, DeVivo MJ, Richards JS. The epidemiology of spinal cord injury. In: Stover SL, DeLisa JA, Whiteneck GG, editors. *Spinal Cord Injury.* Gaithersburg: Aspen, 1995: 21–55.
2. Chiu WT, Lin HC, Lam C, et al. Review Paper: epidemiology of traumatic spinal cord injury: comparisons between developed and developing countries. *Asia-Pacific Journal of Public Health.* 2010; 22(1): 9–18.
3. Shrestha D, Garg M, Sing GK, et al. Cervical spine injuries in a teaching hospital of eastern region of Nepal: a clinic-epidemiological study. *Journal of Nepal Medical Association.* 2007; 46(167): 107–11.
4. Chacko V, Joseph B, Mohanty SP, et al. Management of spinal cord injury in a general hospital in rural India. *Paraplegia.* 1986; 24(5): 330–5.
5. Maharaj JC. Epidemiology of spinal cord injury in Fiji: 1985–1994. *Spinal Cord.* 1996; 34(9): 549–59.
6. Singh R, Sharma SC, Mittal R, et al. Traumatic spinal cord injuries in Haryana: An epidemiological study. *Indian Journal of Community Medicine.* 2003; 28(4): 184–6.
7. Reinhold M, Knop C, Beisse R, et al. Operative treatment of 733 patients with acute thoracolumbar spinal injuries: comprehensive results from the second, prospective, Internet-based multicenter study of the Spine Trauma Study Group of the German Association of Trauma Surgery. *European Spine Journal.* 2010; 10: 1657–76.
8. Solagberu BA, Ofoegbu CK, Abdur-Rahman LO, et al. Pre-hospital care in Nigeria: a country without emergency medical services. *Nigerian Journal of Clinical Practice.* 2009; 12(1): 29–33.
9. Harris MB, Sethi RK. The initial assessment and management of the multiple-trauma patient with an associated spine injury. *Spine.* 2006; 31(11): S9–S15.
10. Furlan JC, Fehlings MG. Cardiovascular complications after acute spinal cord injury: pathophysiology, diagnosis, and management. *Neurosurgical Focus.* 2008; 25(5): E13.
11. Hu R, Mustard CA, Burns C. Epidemiology of incident spinal fracture in a complete population. *Spine.* 1996; 21: 492–9.
12. Brown CV, Antevil JL, Sise MJ, et al. Spiral computed tomography for the diagnosis of cervical, thoracic, and lumbar spine fractures: Its time has come. *Journal of Trauma and Acute Care Surgery.* 2005; 58: 890–5.
13. Bachulis BL, Long WB, Hynes GD, et al. Clinical indications for cervical spine radiographs in the traumatized patient. *American Journal of Surgery.* 1987; 153: 473–8.
14. Radiographic assessment of the cervical spine in symptomatic trauma patients. *Neurosurgery.* 2002; 50: S36–S43.
15. MacDonald RL, Schwartz ML, Mirich D, et al. Diagnosis of cervical spine injury in motor vehicle crash victims: how many x-rays are enough? *Journal of Trauma and Acute Care Surgery.* 1990; 30: 392–7.
16. Sengupta DK. Neglected spinal injury. *Clinical Orthopaedics and Related Research.* 2005; 431: 93–103.
17. Rathore MF, Hanif S, Farooq F, et al. Traumatic spinal cord injuries at a tertiary care rehabilitation institute in Pakistan. *Journal of the Pakistan Medical Association.* 2008; 58(2): 53–7.
18. Rechtine GR, Bono PL, Cahill D, et al. Postoperative wound infection after instrumentation of thoracic and lumbar fractures. *Journal of Orthopedic Trauma.* 2001; 15: 566–9.
19. Rathore FA, Farooq F, Muzammil S, et al. Spinal cord injury management and rehabilitation: highlights and shortcomings from the 2005 earthquake in Pakistan. *Archives of Physical Medicine and Rehabilitation.* 2008; 89(3): 579–85.
20. Taugir SF, Mirza S, Gul S, et al. Complications in patients with spinal cord injuries sustained in an earthquake in Northern Pakistan. *Journal of Spinal Cord Medicine.* 2007; 30(4): 373–7.
21. Jain NB, Sullivan M, Kazis LE, et al. Factors associated with health-related quality of life in chronic spinal cord injury. *Archives of Physical Medicine and Rehabilitation.* 2006; 87(10): 1327–33.
22. Green BA, Eismont FJ, O'Heir JT. Spinal cord injury—a systems approach: prevention, emergency medical services, and emergency room management. *Critical Care Clinics.* 1987; 3(3): 471–93.

Chapter 51

1. Joshipura MK. Total trauma care: International perspective. *Hospital Today.* 1996; 11: 43–4.
2. Jain AK. Orthopedic services and training at a crossroads in developing countries Orthopedic services and training at a crossroads in developing countries. *Indian Journal of Orthopedics.* 2007 Jul–Sep; 41(3): 177–179.
3. Lavy CBD. Orthopedic training in developing countries. *Journal of Bone and Joint Surgery British Edition.* January 2005; 87-B(1): 10–11.

Appendix

Safety, Security, and Survival Considerations for Healthcare Providers in Remote, Hostile, and Disaster Areas

Mykel Hawke

Introduction

While highly skilled and essential to providing urgently needed care in low- and middle-income countries (LMICs) surgeons, anesthesiologists, and the entire healthcare workforce are generally unaware of and untrained for the potential survival and safety issues that are inherent in many LMICs and disaster settings. Elemental infrastructural shortcomings like a lack of food, water, or shelter; communication limitations; and even a hostile local environment can each pose essential dangers to the healthcare team. Each of these dangers, too, can cause an effort to fail before it has even begun.

Therefore, provided below is a primer for healthcare professionals in safety, security, and survival for LMICs. Although these points can be applied anywhere, they are often applicable to disaster-type settings in LMICs.

Safety

Travel to, Arrival in, and Movement through Country, Borders, and Danger Zones

Safety and security begins before you leave. It is generally a good idea to make sure all affairs are in order before you go, including wills, powers of attorney, care of all belongings, and responsibilities. As always, keep vaccines up to date and maintain good dental health as well; failure to do so can make you a burden to the visiting surgical team or make you operationally ineffective.

Ensure that you are fully insured for the endeavors you are undertaking. Most policies will not cover acts of war, force majeure, and so on. Read the fine print in your policy and make sure you are covered. The services of underwriters, for example Lloyd's of London, can also be considered, although this may be a costly option depending on the circumstances. Otherwise, understand what is not covered and either conform to those limits or make sure your reports comply within their parameters.

Always be sure you have any and all medical prescriptions on hand and in enough stock to see you through at least 30 days beyond your expected departure. Keep copies of the documents that support these as well. Be mindful that some countries have odd laws against would-be Good Samaritans: things such as condoms can be considered contraband.

Always make sure you have spares for things like glasses and prosthetics. Be sure that you have a way to store them so they are protected and secured from theft while you are working. Do not expect that you will have any privacy or personal space for security.

Once at the departure point, be mindful of those who would seek to harm or exploit you, especially in war relief efforts. It is important to have a good "link up" plan with many backups such as phone numbers, names, addresses, and maps before you leave your home. Many things can go wrong in mass casualty situations, and one must be ready to deal with all exigencies.

Travel with some emergency cash that is always on your person with your passport. Be ready to have property confiscated by authorities and be sure to be in compliance with all laws before you arrive. Be familiar with local scams; every country has its own unique set of scammers. Being prepared for these situations will be your best approach to negotiating through those who are seeking to exploit the confusion for their own gain.

How to Dress

What you wear will quickly say more about you than you may realize. It is generally a good idea to dress in an understated manner, so as to not flaunt wealth or invite robbery. Consider packing weight versus durability for deployments, and always consider cultural expectations. Many cultures like either bright clothes or very subdued colors. Try to go with clothes that are easy to wash, dry, repeat wear, and hide stains and blood while considering cultural norms. When all else fails, earth tones always work.

Avoid bringing jewelry or expensive watches. In fact, wear watches you don't mind losing, getting stolen, or even giving away. Maybe even bring a few for trade or gifts to special folks who volunteer to help. Sunglasses and hats are often helpful and healthful, but they can alienate the poor and suffering, be scary to those who see Americans as aggressors, and distinguish you as a target for those who are hostile to your attempts to help those with whom they disagree. Finally, footgear is the most important thing you wear as you will be on your feet all day, may have to travel by foot to render aid, or may have to escape by foot if crisis occurs. Pick the best you can for the environment and bring sandals to air feet and dry out footgear.

How to Pack

Try to travel with only one large bag and one small one, and be sure both have wheels, handles, and straps. Keeping a "go bag" containing everything you'd need to survive is a must: this small bag will become your lifeline should you have to evacuate for any reason. Keep it near you, stocked and ready to go. All the survival items listed below should be in it. The day you don't have an item is the day you will need it.

- Your big bag should have the main supplies you need to operate for the expected duration. When planning and packing, add one week for disasters or one month for wars, depending on circumstances.
- Your bags should be strong enough to protect your belongings and should able to be secured. After use, they must either be able to be stored without occupying too much space or be able to double as storage or as a table/platform once in base camp.
- Personal hygiene items should be minimal: soap, shampoo, razors, deodorant, and lotions. Consider time and water requirements, as well as being surrounded by folks who have nothing. Being clean is often enough. Mirrors are good and can double for survival signaling, rear security, brightening a small work space/quarters, and gifting on departure.
- Sleeping gear should always be considered: a bag, pillow, and hammock; poncho with some string/cordage/bungee; or a small tent and pad. Be tiny; be self-contained.
- All clothing should be based on environment, but consider a scarf or handkerchief as these make great emergency dressings, tourniquets, carry bags, slings, eye and face protection, washcloths, and do-rags, and have about a dozen other uses.
- Consider a small water kettle, cup boiler, or stove: multi-fuel types are best as they can burn a variety of liquid fuels that may be found locally, whereas propane may not be as readily available. You can make all water safe as soon as it hits a rolling boil to save fuel and stay healthy and hydrated. Water can also be used to make sweet drinks and salty broths. In general, plan on no electricity.
- Consider bringing a 1-week supply of minimal food as this can help you stay fed and operational and may help other healthcare providers should food become scarce during the first few days. You can always give it away to locals if you find food is not an issue on the ground. Consider a roll of toilet paper and wet wipes for the first few days as well.
- If a stove is not an option, consider water treatment tablets (one bottle is cheap and small).
- Always bring prescription medications, glasses, and contacts. Consider a small bottle of sunscreen and insect repellent when warranted; remember vector control will quickly become a serious problem in most postdisaster/war refugee camps.
- Bring a first-aid kit for personal use.
- Consider bringing a map of the region, compass, whistle, flashlight, and multi-tool knife for many uses, but primarily for emergencies like survival and escape.

Things to Avoid: What Not To Do

The main thing to avoid is to become a victim. Do not become a victim of crime, do not become another victim of circumstance by not being correctly prepared, and do not become a victim of violating local laws or customs.

In general, do not speak loudly or strongly about political, personal, or religious convictions. You are there to help, one human to another. Any opinions are best saved for friends you've made only after they have asked your opinions.

Base Operations

Communications

Communication is one of the easiest and most important things to remedy, and yet it is one of the most frequently forgotten aspects of logistics planning. Always make sure your mobile phone is set for international roaming. Set this up with your service provider *before* you leave the country. Most providers cannot or will not set up roaming from out of country for fear it is a criminal activity. Check for the best service providers and carriers in your target area before you go and consider getting a local plan. Do not plan on mail. Most countries have a limited postal capability and often of dubious integrity when it comes to packages, imports, taxes, fees, fines, and deliberate confiscation.

For any and all of your personal electronics, try to have your own backup power sources. If you cannot bring a personal handheld generator, try to bring solar rechargers that also have a hand crank.

Waste Disposal

Waste management will quickly become a huge issue and should be addressed right away. Not only will you need to urinate and defecate, so will every other healthcare provider, volunteer, patient, and homeless refugee. Latrines should be designated immediately and built to handle the volume of the situation, in a good location for the circumstances, and with respect to the local customs.

Morgue Operations

Morgues are an often-unconsidered reality for many healthcare providers, especially those responding to large-scale mass casualties such as genocides or earthquakes. A location for bodies must be designated, a way to identify or record them should be established, and some means to protect them from desecration should be instituted. This should be made very clear and transparent to indigenous populations, and their customs must be taken into account. Some cultures may forbid burial without markings or cremation, but burning may be the only way to control disease given certain hot climates. Also, there may need to be a way to handle limbs and medical waste, especially in situations when a large number of amputations are required (earthquakes, active conflict zones, etc.). Consider rats, cats, and dogs as potential pests at limb dumps and body holes. Extermination may be required for vector control, and local customs for killing these must be factored as well.

Camp Hygiene

Hygiene will be a vital aspect of any activity. There must be enough supplies to support basics like feeding and hydrating healthcare personnel, as well as taking care of medical needs such as sterilization and sharps disposal and control.

Waste will need to have designated collection areas and a removal plan. Trash can also become a black market item and, as such, special care needs to be taken when selecting where to store trash, who collects it, and what becomes of it. This could actually become a source of crime in a camp and a struggle for power. Individuals will need to be designated to police the camp and make sure trash is concentrated and collected, that washing areas are designated with water, and waste runoff areas planned and controlled. Cooking, showering, and other cleaning areas may have to be designated, managed, and controlled to ensure the camp is not only hygienic but also orderly. This will reduce friction that could quickly erupt into violence. Every bit of planning and management that can be done should be done.

Duties, Details, and Designs for Team, Group, or Camp

All medical personnel must be prepared to wear multiple hats and have additional duties. To maximize assets, take a survey to ascertain all skills sets found within the group and apply accordingly to the same to maximize all volunteer assets; always consider the motivation of volunteers in case of hidden agendas that can cause undue strife for the visiting surgical team. Try to task everyone not injured or ill with some extra duties. Keeping folks busy and feeling like they are still contributing something worthy will go a long way toward keeping peace and maintaining dignity for the victims.

Living Arrangements for Staff, Volunteers, and Other Personnel

Try not to have a major quality difference between the volunteers and the victims in terms of living arrangements. This disparity could cause violence to erupt. Try to respect cultural mores and not mix genders when not appropriate for the indigenous population. Likewise, volunteers should receive little to no extra benefits or privileges for their service.

Vehicles, Facilities, Power, Fuel, and Other Logistics

Vehicles are powerful tools. They must be safeguarded night and day. These can be commandeered and stolen at *any* time. Ensure a good driver is assigned to not only maintain the vehicle, but also to protect it within reason. The same holds true for any facilities, kitchens, food stores, medical supplies, fuel, generators, and so on. Everything must be secured and protected. Plan to keep all facilities so that they can be within sight of the core operations and staff to keep an added degree of security. Establish a policy for response should locals commandeer them.

Treatment Control

Long waiting lines can breed manipulation within the triage line. Try to monitor lines, or utilize trustworthy volunteers to observe and maintain fairness and balance. Double-check translators with other translators from time to time to make sure they are giving truest work.

Use of Local Assets and Development of Translators/Interpreters

This is a very delicate issue. Often the first native speakers encountered who can also speak English are used as interpreters. Great care must be used in screening them if there is a choice and time. These individuals will become major players and power brokers by default. They can say almost anything to a patient they don't like to offend the patient or harm the medic's reputation if they have any issue for any reason. As time permits, vet them and test them, change their duties and assignments, and always observe them with a mind toward ensuring honesty, integrity, and intentions.

Selecting and Training Indigenous Personnel for Support Operations

Initially, most operations will take whatever local assets and volunteers they can get. Staff should be mindful of the potential for clashes of cultural, political, financial, and religious differences between volunteers. Be ready to change personnel as needed; however, recognition of employee rights is even more essential than in other circumstances. *Always* handle sensitive matters privately, not in front of the public, but also *always* have witnesses in private, at least one from your team and one from the local population. This will maintain balance for rumor control should it come to that.

Planning and Protection

Often there will be no reliable power infrastructure in an initial disaster response setting. As such, it is best to project power needs and plan to bring the necessary power with you. Usually, generators, oils, fuel, parts, power cables, tools, manuals, and someone with skills to maintain them may be required, especially for large-scale power needs. Other forms of power may be more relevant in terms of lanterns, kerosene lamps, white gas stoves, or even flashlights and candles. Any needs should be considered, and there should be no expectation for local source supply procurement.

Whatever the power requirement may be, there will be a demand for power by others. Power will become a vital commodity that will warrant close management and understanding of needs beyond the medical program.

Weather Considerations

When a major weather catastrophe is not the reason for the medical deployment, then weather is often not considered by most medical planners. But a quick study of weather patterns at least one season behind and one head is always warranted in case spring is later or winter is ahead. A bit of preplanning could save the effort and avoid calamity and failure.

Culture

There is no limit to the amount of variables in this department, but a concerted effort must be made to understand whatever may be the norm for the people being treated. There are many things victims will overlook from their rescuers, but it takes only one simple, seemingly benign action to trigger a massive negative response, which in some cases may not be recoverable. Spend time on these variables and continue to inquire and disseminate as information is acquired. Most healthcare providers are sensitive to others by nature, but in the heat of stress and in the face of horrific calamity, we all have moments of frustration. Everyone on the team should be on alert for other team members when they experience these moments to make sure they get a temporary reprieve. It could mean the difference between a small loss of care and a huge loss of receptivity by the local populace.

Air, Sea, and Land Support Considerations

One main port will often be the obvious main route or port of entry in the immediate aftermath of a disaster response. However, there are often other routes that are well established and long used by locals. Do not forget to seek and explore these once on the ground.

Interactions and Relations with Other Entities and Agencies

Often, many volunteers, agencies, and other service entities are duplicating the same efforts. Try to utilize other assets when possible. Always offer some assistance or service in trade so as not to become a burden on another group. Share any information you have acquired and offer any extra contributions you can render. Be seen as a community contributor to ensure your visiting surgical team has the best chance of success. Seek to establish a command center for sharing information.

Security

Healthcare professionals frequently overlook security issues in LMICs, but they represent a crucial element to any dedicated medical effort. An understanding of some of the key points to maintaining a safe and secure environment will help ensure a successful experience. Local talent and imported specialists all require managing.

Kidnap and Ransom Situations

If the possibility of kidnapping exists, reconsider both the personal and programmatic risks and benefits of working in that context. Discuss the issue with the organization you are working with, and decide for yourself and your family whether its members are competent to deal with such issues. If they are not, do not go.

Hostage Threats and Situations

There is a trend in some regions for more hostile actions against medical personnel as a way of discouraging any outsiders from helping or as a method of frightening locals into avoiding acceptance of outside help. In almost all cases, a passive response will diffuse potentially violent situations.

Road Blocks (Legal and Illegal)

You will know if there are legal road blocks in your area of operation or, at least, how to identify what the official forces' uniforms and vehicles look like. If there are roadblocks, be prepared to stop and show papers. Be sure to disseminate the information among other aid workers, especially if improper measures are being implemented. Sometimes there may be illegal roadblocks by bandits or others. In these cases, difficult decisions must be made. Often these checkpoints are specifically set up for robberies, and in a lawless place, they may even attempt rape or murder. Attempting to stop early and drive another way may be advised, but there is a risk of instigating further aggression.

Attacks on Personnel, Facilities, Camp, Convoys, Minorities, or Other Groups

A part of any post-disaster operation is personnel management. Sometimes individuals or small groups will reach for violence out of frustration, desperation, or reaction. In these cases, aid workers should have at least some discussion and general plan for how to respond, whether it be evacuation, withdrawal, or cessation of operations until stability returns. In cases of direct acts of aggression toward medical personnel, a similar strategy needs to be considered and a tentative plan understood by all members of the team. Often, aggressive elements will be ill-defined and dispersed; guidance distributed beforehand can speed recovery time by reducing incorrect actions and possibly exacerbating the dilemma.

Whatever the course of action agreed upon for the aid workers, a similar plan should be embraced in response to attacks on minorities within the refugee camp. If you feel the need for security, at the first level, consider who can assist you and obtain assistance. Once the immediate threat has dissipated, it is essential to again consider the risks and benefits of your involvement within a changed context. Political and cultural implications in security selection should also be considered.

Conflicts within Camp, Clans, and Countries

Sometimes, conflicts will flare up between groups on any scale, and these exigencies must be given at least a cursory discussion in the planning phase, with a tentatively agreed-upon course of action accepted for each level. Often, many telltale signs of discontent and dissention are evident if the aid workers are attentive and ask questions about welfare, attitude, and morale. There is usually a group leader, and some form of negotiation and temporary appeasement through compromise can often diminish potentially disastrous scenarios.

Riots in Camp or in Close Proximity

In almost all cases, the difference between riot and other conflicts is that conflicts are between groups with leaders and hence some level of control. Riots by definition are mass chaos and violence. Usually, without force, the only option is to remain out of force's way in a secure area until the riot passes or is quelled by others.

Theft (Personal)

Theft is an unfortunate reality in most societies, especially where there is great loss and much suffering due to tragedy. Try to keep honest people honest either by not having valuables or by keeping them well secured and unknown to others. When theft happens, be prepared to let it go and try to solve it personally. You may inadvertently risk others being killed if a theft becomes public knowledge; some local leaders may seek a culprit, right or wrong, and may sentence him to death to save face for their community in front of the visiting medical workers.

Robberies (Supplies)

When robberies of supplies begin to take place, there is no choice but to address it head on. Increased security measures are warranted, and the group must decide how far they are willing to go to defend these supplies.

Personal Protection Measures (Passive and Active)

Always maintain situational awareness. Be sure to periodically change habits, routines, and routes to prevent plotting and planning by malfeasants. Keep things secure, including private and personal information that can be exploited. Have designated plans for return and meeting times. Have radios and communications plans for regular check-in times.

Group Protection Measures (Passive and Active Measures)

Passive measures may include designating travel buddies or teams, setting check-in and return times, and presetting destinations and routes with known and identifiable vehicles, outfits, and personnel. Active group measures may include traveling with security, the use of checkpoints, gate guards, and so on.

Camp Security

There will always be a need for security in any camp situation. While this goes against most medical notions of standard operations, security must be considered and implemented before it is needed. At the very minimum, establish security for the medical supplies and the medical personnel. Consider security of all aspects of the operation, from protecting patients, to protecting food and fuel, to protecting the laundry and rubbish.

Law, Government, Officials, and Politics

Finally, all official apparati must be considered. Sometimes these entities will be helpful and at other times they may be a hindrance or even hostile to outside aid. Respect must always be paid and administration adhered to; however, creative solutions may be required to render help when and where it is needed most.

Survival

Like safety and security, a basic understanding of and consideration for the necessary elements of survival are essential for success.

Individual, Small Team, Large Group, and Communal

The first requirement is to always have a plan. Plan for yourself, then your team, then the folks you are there to help. Consider the situation and determine how long you may need to survive and then factor logistics to realistically sustain that time frame. Being prepared makes you a better team member and provider. Preparedness allows you to be self-sufficient. A good rule of thumb is to always have a 24-hour supply of support on or near you. Keep a 3–7 day supply in your escape bag, workplace, and means of transport. Never leave base without all you need to survive or leave the country.

Water

Water is vital but weighs a lot, so while it is imperative to have some initial stock, the stores of water for mobile survival inherently must be small. For static survival, maximum storage is always recommended.

There are many methods of making water safe. Know them. Some include:

- Boiling
- Chemical treatment by bleach or iodine
- Ultraviolet (UV) light by the sun or UV wands
- Filtration by many methods

Food

Food is not as important, but generally a 3-day supply should be readily available and one should know how to procure some edibles from the area. This may take time, so always carry food supplement. Food becomes more important with illness, injury, bad weather, or high-duress scenarios.

Fire

It is always good to have a lighter or matches, but always have a backup such as a magnifying glass, magnesium bar, batteries, and chemicals. There are many ways to start a fire; know one alternative and carry a lighter. Fires can give warmth, provide light, signal, cook food, make water potable, keep insects away, and keep predators at bay. But they may not keep unwanted visitors away; use fires only by day and avoid smoke from green wood. Always have a tinder source, as fires can be tricky to start with just a lighter. Examples of good tinder include toilet paper, dressings, and tampons. Petroleum gauze from medical supplies is an ideal source.

Shelter

Shelter may be important in extreme temperatures or dangerous environments. Try to use your vehicles or a natural shelter, like a cave or tree, to save time and energy. Always carry a poncho, tarp, or even a trash bag. Your clothes are your first line of defense shelter.

Signals

Always carry a phone or radio, but when they fail, consider lights, sounds, whistles, air horns, and so on. A big part of signaling is a plan: know whom to signal, when and where. Know the emergency radio frequencies or numbers to dial and how to operate equipment. It may be prudent to develop an internal code for the aid workers in dangerous areas to let them know discreetly when to begin evasive maneuvers and where to link up. These load signals may be both in code words and a physical sign.

Navigation

It is critical to always know exactly where you are and where safe haven is in relation to you. Always have a plan on how to get there and know what it would take to drive, fly, boat, and walk. Know the terrain and have a compass. Consider the possibilities of having to walk out and bring others with you. Dress and pack accordingly, and live in this ready-to-go mobile and navigate mode.

Tools

This is an all-encompassing topic, but things such as a knife, flashlight, canteen, cup to boil water, spoon, and cordage are often overlooked and become extremely valuable resources in a survival mode. Give the tools in your kit a lot of thought based on your abilities and demands.

Medical

This one goes without saying for medical professionals, but have a standard medical kit that you and others can use. Consider the basics as well as the advanced medical needs. Often, band-aids and aspirin are the medical kit items used most frequently. Think off-label use, biggest bang for the buck, and wide application medications and supplies.

Barter

There are many extras that may—and should—be carried when space allows. They should be good all-rounders that double for personal survival, team utilization, and local trading and gifting. These may become items that "purchase" your survival in terms of a guide, translator, informant, or driver. Give thought to what is valued where you are going and maybe have some extras. Always think, plan, be ready, and be flexible. I give a special salute to all who study how to serve mankind and seek to alleviate suffering during times of tragedy.

Index

Note: Page references followed by *b*, *f*, or *t* indicate boxes, figures, or tables, respectively.